ENCYCLOPEDIA OF NURSING RESEARCH

ENCYCLOPEDIA OF NURSING RESEARCH

JOYCE J. FITZPATRICK, PHD

EDITOR-IN-CHIEF

 SPRINGER PUBLISHING COMPANY

Springer Publishing Company, Inc.
536 Broadway
New York, NY 10012-3955

Cover design by Janet Joachim
Acquisitions Editor: Sheri W. Sussman
Production Editors: T. Orrantia and Helen Song

97 98 99 00 01 / 5 4 3 2 1

Library of Congress Cataloging-in-Publication Data

The Encyclopedia of nursing research / Joyce J. Fitzpatrick, editor.
    p.   cm.
  Includes bibliographical references and index.
  ISBN 0-8261-1170-X (hardcover)
  1. Nursing—Research—Encyclopedias. I. Fitzpatrick,
Joyce J., 1944– .
  [DNLM: 1. Nursing Research encyclopedias. WY 13
E563 1998]
RT81.5.E53   1998
610.73'072—dc21
DNLM/DLC
for Library of Congress   98-15853
                               CIP

Printed in the United States of America

CONTENTS

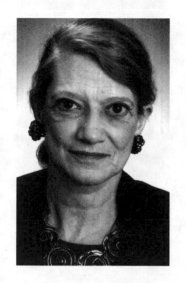

Joyce J. Fitzpatrick, PhD, RN, FAAN, is the Elizabeth Brooks Ford Professor of Nursing, Frances Payne Bolton School of Nursing at Case Western Reserve University in Cleveland, Ohio, where she was Dean from 1982 to 1997. Dr. Fitzpatrick is widely published in nursing literature, having received the American Journal of Nursing Book of the Year Award eight times. She is the Editor of the *Annual Review of Nursing Research* series, now in its sixteenth volume, and in 1997 she was appointed Editor of the National League for Nursing's journal *Nursing and Health Care Perspectives*. In November 1997, Dr. Fitzpatrick assumed the presidency of the American Academy of Nursing.

ADVISORY BOARD

Editor

Joyce J. Fitzpatrick, PhD, FAAN
Elizabeth Brooks Ford Professor
Frances Payne Bolton School of Nursing
Case Western Reserve University
Cleveland, Ohio

Faye G. Abdellah, EdD, ScD, FAAN
School of Nursing
Uniformed Services University of the Health
Sciences
Bethesda, Maryland

Joan Kessner Austin, DNS, FAAN
School of Nursing
Indiana University
Indianapolis, Indiana

Dorothy Brooten, PhD, FAAN
Frances Payne Bolton School of Nursing
Case Western Reserve University
Cleveland, Ohio

Marie J. Cowan, PhD, FAAN
School of Nursing
University of California-Los Angeles
Los Angeles, California

Suzanne Lee Feetham, PhD, FAAN
College of Nursing
University of Illinois at Chicago
Chicago, Illinois

Phyllis B. Giovannetti, ScD
Faculty of Nursing
University of Alberta
Edmonton, Alberta, Canada

Patricia A. Grady, PhD, FAAN
National Institute of Nursing Research
National Institute of Health
Bethesda, Maryland

Judith R. Graves, PhD, FAAN
Nursing Informatics Director
Virginia Henderson International
Nursing Library at Sigma Theta Tau,
International.
Indianapolis, Indiana

Laura L. Hayman, PhD, FAAN
Frances Payne Bolton School of Nursing
Case Western Reserve University
Cleveland, Ohio

Janet Heinrich, DrPH, FAAN
Director
American Academy of Nursing
Washington, DC

Ada Jacox, PhD, FAAN
College of Nursing
Wayne State University
Detroit, Michigan

Loretta Sweet Jemmott, PhD, FAAN
School of Nursing
University of Pennsylvania
Philadelphia, Pennsylvania

ix

PREFACE

This *Encyclopedia of Nursing Research* grew from a longstanding commitment of the publisher, Dr. Ursula Springer, and the Editor in presenting to the field of nursing, and to nurse scholars around the globe, a comprehensive, yet concise and authoritative guide to the study of nursing. Its conception followed 15 years of publication of the Annual Review of Nursing Research (ARNR), a series launched by Springer Publishing Company in 1983. Through these formative years of nursing science, I have had the privilege of serving as editor of the ARNR series, and most important, of witnessing the rapid growth of knowledge and expertise in nursing research.

Graduate students in nursing and nurse researchers will be the primary audience for this Encyclopedia. Yet, nurses in all phases of education, from basic to doctoral, from formal university and college-based programs to continuing education offerings, within all health systems will find this an important introduction to the key terms and topics of nursing research.

In this first edition, we considered it important to include a selective list of nursing research journals, national professional organizations, and key government agencies concerned with nursing research. Also, the reader will find the list of acronyms especially useful, as the jargon surrounding any professional field of study is sometimes staggering.

For all readers we have emphasized the interconnectedness of topics and terms. At the end of each entry there is a list of cross-referenced terms. And, of course, the alphabetical list of entries is provided to assist the reader in quickly finding the relevant term. While every effort was made to include the most comprehensive list of entries, based on both a literature review of key terms in journals and the ARNR series, and the expert advice of the Advisory Board members, we are cognizant of the fact that some terms may have been overlooked. We have already begun the work of the second edition. Thus, we encourage readers to advise the editor of new terms that should be added to the already extensive list.

This project has been one of the most rewarding endeavors of my professional career. It has been met with a great deal of professional interest, and, most important, an extra measure of enthusiasm, by students at all levels. The References section lists the most critical references on each topic. It is this attention to key references that may be of most use to graduate students who wish to pursue a topic in more depth.

It goes without saying that this publication would not have been possible without the experts in nursing research, those who authored the hundreds of entries. Each author, some of whom have authored multiple entries, deserves thanks for the written entries, and for the willingness to respond to strict guidelines and page and reference limitations. Distilling one's life work into a few hundred words is often the most difficult accomplishment.

This editor is indebted to the colleagues who served as member of the Advisory Board. I thank each of you for your willingness to plunge into yet another publishing project with me. I especially thank each of you for your insights and endless comments on possible entries and possible authors. I know that at times we might have seemed redundant in our requests for review of the various lists of entries. Please know that I appreciated each of your responses, and all of the efforts to identify topics and authors, especially in the startup phase of our endeavor.

As with any large continuing project such as this, there is a true team effort necessary for a quality project. First, my thanks to Dr. Ursula Springer, the publisher, for conceiving the project, and asking me to undertake the editing at a time when my commitments were at a peak. I am glad that I did not hesitate. To the Springer staff who facilitated the production at the many levels, I also owe a huge thank you. Most especially to Sheri Sussman from Springer who saw the project through its many stages.

As an editor, I have been fortunate to select editorial assistants, those who have been on the other end of the phone and E-mail to answer author questions and to shepherd the process throughout its production. First, a thanks to Rosalie Tyner who joined the project at its initiation and shortly thereafter returned to her first love of clinical nursing. But most especially, and consistently for the past year and a half, to Laree Schoolmeesters, a PhD student at Case Western Reserve University, Frances Payne Bolton School of Nursing, who lived and breathed *The Encyclopedia of Nursing Research* for many many months, days, and hours, who was introduced to the large world of nursing research publications through her day-to-day contact with authors. Laree has been a dream to work with, and is a large part of the timeliness of this publication.

Joyce J. Fitzpatrick

CONTRIBUTORS

Lauren S. Aaronson, PhD, RN, FAAN
*Associate Dean for Research and
  Professor
University of Kansas
School of Nursing
Kansas City, KS*

Faye G. Abdellah, EdD, ScD, FAAN
*Dean and Professor
Uniformed Services University of
  the Health Sciences
Bethesda, MD*

Ivo L. Abraham, PhD, RN, CS, FAAN
*Chief Executive Officer and Prin-
  cipal
Epsilon Group, LLC
Charlottesville, VA*

Dyanne D. Affonso, PhD, RN, FAAN
*Dean and Professor
Emory University
Nell Hodgson Woodruff School of
  Nursing
Atlanta, GA*

Jerilyn K. Allen, ScD, RN
*Associate Professor
The Johns Hopkins University
School of Nursing
Baltimore, MD*

Carole A. Anderson, PhD, RN, FAAN
*Dean and Professor
The Ohio State University
College of Nursing
Columbus, OH*

Gene Cranston Anderson, PhD, RN, FAAN
*Mellen Professor
Case Western Reserve University
Frances Payne Bolton School of
  Nursing
Cleveland, OH*

Patricia G. Archbold, PhD, RN, FAAN
*Professor
Oregon Health Sciences Univer-
  sity
School of Nursing
Portland, OR*

Carol A. Ashton, PhD, RN
*Director of Nursing Research
LDS, Cottonwood, and Alta View
  Hospitals
Salt Lake City, UT*

Regina C. Aune, PhD, RN
*Associate Professor; Lieutenant
  Colonel, USAF
Uniformed Services University of
  the Health Sciences
Bethesda, MD*

Joan Kessner Austin, DNS, RN, FAAN
*Professor
Indiana University School of
  Nursing
Indianapolis, IN*

Susan Auvil-Novak, PhD, RN
*Assistant Professor
Case Western Reserve University
School of Nursing
Cleveland, OH*

Kay C. Avant, PhD, RN, FAAN
*Associate Professor
University of Texas
School of Nursing
Austin, TX*

Judith A. Baigis, PhD, RN, FAAN
*Associate Dean for Research and
  Scholarship
Georgetown University
School of Nursing
Washington, DC*

Jane H. Barnsteiner, PhD, RN, FAAN
*Professor and Director
University of Pennsylvania
School of Nursing
Philadelphia, PA*

Cheryl Tatano Beck, DNSc, CNM, FAAN
*University of Connecticut
Storrs, CT*

Barbara E. Berger, PhD, RN
Clinical Assistant Professor and
    Clinical Scientist
University of Illinois at Chicago
    and University of Illinois at
    Chicago Medical Center
Chicago, IL

Nancy Bergstrom, PhD, RN,
    FAAN
Professor
University of Nebraska Medical
    Center
College of Nursing
Omaha, NE

Barbara Bishop MN, RN,
    FAAN
Editor
The American Journal of Mater-
    nal/Child Nursing
New York, NY

Suzanne Blancett, EdD, RN,
    FAAN
Editor-in-Chief
The Journal of Nursing Adminis-
    tration
Bradenton, FL

Carol E. Blixen, PhD, RN
Senior Nurse Researcher
Cleveland Clinic Foundation
Department of Nursing Education
    and Research
Cleveland, OH

Eleanor J. Bond, PhD, RN
Associate Professor
University of Washington
Department of Biobehavioral Nurs-
    ing and Health Systems
Seattle, WA

Joan L. Bottorff, PhD, RN
Associate Professor and NHRDP
    Health Researcher
University of British Columbia
School of Nursing
Vancouver, BC

Barbara J. Braden, PhD, RN,
    FAAN
Professor and Dean
Creighton University
Graduate School
Omaha, NE

Patricia Flatley Brennan, PhD,
    RN, FAAN
Professor
University of Wisconsin
School of Nursing
Madison, WI

Pamela J. Brink, PhD, RN,
    FAAN
Executive Editor
University of Alberta
Faculty of Nursing
Edmonton, Alberta

Dorothy Brooten, PhD, FAAN
Burry Professor and Dean
Case Western Reserve University
Frances Payne Bolton School of
    Nursing
Cleveland, OH

Emma J. Brown, PhD, RN
University of Pennsylvania
School of Nursing
Philadelphia, PA

Kathleen C. Buckwalter, PhD,
    RN, FAAN
Professor
University of Iowa
College of Nursing
Iowa City, IA

Helen Kogan Budzynski, RN,
    PhD, FAAN
Professor
University of Washington School
    of Nursing
Psychosocial and Community
    Health
Seattle, WA

Vern L. Bullough, PhD, RN,
    FAAN
Visiting Professor
University of Southern California
Department of Nursing
Northridge, CA

Cynthia F. Cameron, PhD, RN
Associate Professor and Associate
    Dean
The University of Manitoba
Faculty of Nursing
Winnipeg, Manitoba

Jacquelyn C. Campbell, PhD,
    RN, FAAN
Professor
Johns Hopkins University
School of Nursing
Baltimore, MD

Sara Campbell, MS, RN
Coordinator for Student Develop-
    ment and
Mennonite College of Nursing
Bloomington, IL

Victoria Champion, DNS, RN,
    FAAN
Associate Dean of Research
Indiana University
School of Nursing
Indianapolis, IN

Peggy L. Chinn, PhD, RN,
    FAAN
Editor
Advances in Nursing Science
University of Connecticut
Storrs, CT

Marlene Zichi Cohen, PhD, RN
Associate Professor
University of Maryland
School of Nursing
Baltimore, MD

Kathleen Byrne Colling, PhD,
    RN
University of Michigan
School of Nursing
Ann Arbor, MI

Inge B. Corless, PhD, RN,
    FAAN
Associate Professor and Director
Massachusetts General Hospital
Institute of Health Professions
Boston, MA

Cynthia L. Corritore, PhD
Assistant Professor
Creighton University
College of Business Administration
Omaha, NE

Marie J. Cowan, PhD, RN, FAAN
Professor and Dean
University of California, Los Angeles
School of Nursing
Los Angeles, CA

Diane Cronin-Stubbs, PhD, RN, FAAN
Professor
Rush University College of Nursing
Riverside, IL

Leah Curtin, ScD, RN, FAAN
Consultant
Cincinnati, OH

Jennifer P. D'Auria, PhD, RN
Assistant Professor
University of North Carolina
School of Nursing
Chapel Hill, NC

Barbara Daly, PhD, RN, FAAN
Associate Professor
Case Western Reserve University
School of Nursing
Cleveland, OH

Sabina DeGeest, PhD, RN
Assistant Professor
Katholieke Universitieit Leuven
Leuven, Belgium

Alice S. Demi, DNS, RN, FAAN
Professor
Georgia State University
School of Nursing
Atlanta, GA

Karen E. Dennis, PhD, RN, FAAN
Associate Professor
University of Maryland
School of Nursing
Baltimore, MD

Elizabeth C. Devine, PhD, FAAN
Professor
University of Wisconsin
School of Nursing
Milwaukee, WI

Nancy Diekelmann, PhD, RN, FAAN
Helen Denne Shulte Professor
University of Wisconsin
School of Nursing
Madison, WI

Sue K. Donaldson, PhD, RN, FAAN
Dean and Professor
The Johns Hopkins University
School of Nursing
Baltimore, MD

Rosemary Donley, PhD, RN, FAAN
Executive Vice President
Catholic University of America
School of Nursing
Washington, DC

Molly C. Dougherty, PhD, RN, FAAN
Editor
School of Nursing
University of North Carolina
Chapel Hill, NC

Karen Hassey Dow, PhD, RN
Associate Professor
University of Central Florida
School of Nursing
Orlando, FL

Jacqueline Dunbar-Jacob, PhD, RN, FAAN
Professor
University of Pittsburgh
School of Nursing
Pittsburgh, PA

Marsha L. Ellett, DNS, RN
Assistant Professor
Indiana University
School of Nursing
Indianapolis, IN

Veronica F. Engle, PhD, RN, FAAN
Professor
University of Tennessee
College of Nursing
Memphis, TN

Janet Enslein, RN, MA
The University of Iowa
College of Nursing
Iowa City, IA

W. Scott Erdley, RN, MS
State University of New York
School of Nursing
Buffalo, NY

Lois K. Evans, DNSc, RN, FAAN
Associate Professor
University of Pennsylvania
School of Nursing
Philadelphia, PA

Sarah P. Farrell, PhD, RN, CS
Assistant Professor
University of Virginia
Charlottesville, VA

Jacqueline Fawcett, PhD, RN, FAAN
Professor
University of Pennsylvania
School of Nursing
Philadelphia, PA

Suzanne Lee Feetham, PhD, RN, FAAN
Professor, Harriet L. Werley Research Chair
University of Illinois at Chicago
College of Nursing
Chicago, IL

Harriet R. Feldman, PhD, RN, FAAN
Editor
Pace University
Lienhard School of Nursing
Pleasantville, NY

Mary L. Fisher, PhD, RN
Associate Professor
Indiana University
School of Nursing
Indianapolis, IN

Joyce J. Fitzpatrick, RN, PhD, FAAN
Elizabeth Brooks Ford Professor
Case Western Reserve University
Frances Payne Bolton School of Nursing
Cleveland, OH

Jacquelyn H. Flaskerud, PhD, RN, FAAN
Professor
University of California
School of Nursing
Los Angeles, CA

Juanita W. Fleming, PhD, RN, FAAN
Professor and Special Assistant to the President
University of Kentucky
Lexington, KY

Beverly C. Flynn, PhD, RN, FAAN
Professor and Director
Indiana University School of Nursing
Institute of Action Research and Community
Indianapolis, IN

Marquis D. Foreman, PhD, RN
Associate Professor
University of Illinois at Chicago
College of Nursing
Chicago, IL

Jeanne C. Fox, PhD, RN, FAAN
Director, SRMHRC
University of Virginia
SE Rural Research Center
Charlottesville, VA

Marilyn Frank-Stromborg, EdD, JD, RN, FAAN
Professor
Northern Illinois University
Dekalb, IL

Maureen Frey, PhD, RN
Director of Research and Advanced Practice
Children's Hospital of Michigan
School of Nursing
Detroit, MI

Sara T. Fry, PhD, RN, FAAN
Professor of Nursing Ethics
Boston College
School of Nursing
Chestnut Hill, MA

Teresa T. Fulmer, PhD, RN, FAAN
Professor
New York University
School of Nursing
New York, NY

John F. Garde, CRNA, MS, FAAN
Executive Director
American Association of Nurse Anesthetists
School of Nursing
Park Ridge, IL

Susan Gardner, MSN, RN
University of Iowa
College of Nursing
Iowa City, IA

Carol Gaskamp, MA, RN
Associate Professor
Kansas Newman College
Division of Nursing
Wichita, KS

Carole Gassert, PhD, RN
Officer
American Medical Informatics Association
Rockville, MD

Denise H. Geolot, PhD, RN, FAAN
Deputy Director
Division of Nursing
Rockville, MD

Carol P. Germain, EdD, FAAN
Associate Professor and Chairperson
University of Pennsylvania
School of Nursing
Philadelphia, PA

Phyllis B. Giovannetti, RN, ScD
Professor and Associate Dean (Graduate)
University of Alberta
Faculty of Nursing
Edmonton, Alberta

Greer Glazer, RNC, PhD, FAAN
Professor
Kent State University
School of Nursing
Solon, OH

Jody E. Glittenberg, PhD, RN, FAAN
Professor
University of Arizona
College of Nursing
Tucson, AZ

Marion Good, PhD, RN
Assistant Professor
Case Western Reserve University
Frances Payne Bolton School of Nursing
Cleveland, OH

Patricia A. Grady, PhD, RN, FAAN
Director
National Institute of Health
National Institute of Nursing Research
Bethesda, MD

Judith Rae Graves, PhD, RN, FAAN
Director
Virginia Henderson Nursing Library
Sigma Theta Tau, Inc.
Indianapolis, IN

Margaret Grey, DrPH, RN, FAAN
Associate Dean for Research and Doctoral Studies
Yale University
School of Nursing
New Haven, CT

Hurdis M. Griffith, PhD, RN, FAAN
Dean and Professor
Rutgers College of Nursing
Newark, NJ

Deborah Gross, DNSc, RN, FAAN
Professor
Rush University
College of Nursing
Chicago, IL

Ira P. Gunn, CRNA, MLN
Consultant
El Paso, TX

Linda C. Haber, DNS, RN, CS
Clinical Specialist
Veterans Affairs
Northern Indiana Health Care System
Fort Wayne, IN

Edward J. Halloran, PhD, RN, FAAN
Associate Professor
University of North Carolina at Chapel Hill
Chapel Hill, NC

Charlene M. Hanson, EdD, RN, CS, FAAN
Professor
Georgia Southern University
Center for Rural Health & Research
Statesboro, GA

Gail A. Harkness, DrPH, RN, FAAN
Professor
University of Connecticut
School of Nursing
Storrs, CT

Roseanne Harrigan, EdD, CPNP, RN, FAAN
Dean and Professor
University of Hawaii
School of Nursing
Honolulu, HI

Emily J. Hauenstein, PhD, RN, CS
Associate Professor
University of Virginia
School of Nursing
Charlottesville, VA

Patricia Hayes, RN, MHSA
Co-Editor
Clinical Nursing Research
Edmonton, Alberta
Canada

Laura L. Hayman, PhD, RN, FAAN
Walter Professor
Case Western Reserve University
Frances Payne Bolton School of Nursing
Cleveland, OH

Janet Heinrich, DrPH, RN, FAAN
Executive Director
American Academy of Nursing
Washington, DC

Margaret Heitkemper, PhD, RN, FAAN
Professor
University of Washington
Department of Biobehavioral Nursing and Health
Seattle, WA

Marion M. Hemstrom, DNSc, RN
Assistant Professor
Case Western Reserve University
Frances Payne Bolton School of Nursing
Cleveland, OH

Beverly Henry, RN, PhD, FAAN
Editor
University of Illinois
College of Nursing
Chicago, IL

Suzanne Bakken Henry, DNSc, RN, FAAN
Associate Professor
University of California
School of Nursing and Graduate Group in Medical
San Francisco, CA

Nancy Olson Hester, PhD, RN, FAAN
Professor
University of Colorado
School of Nursing
Denver, CO

Martha N. Hill, PhD, RN, FAAN
Professor
Johns Hopkins University
School of Nursing
Baltimore, MD

Ada Sue Hinshaw, PhD, RN, FAAN
Dean and Professor
University of Michigan
School of Nursing
Ann Arbor, MI

Diane Holditch-Davis, RN, PhD, FAAN
Professor
University of North Carolina
School of Nursing
Chapel Hill, NC

Barbara J. Holtzclaw, PhD, RN, FAAN
Director of Research
University of Texas
Health Science Center
San Antonio, TX

William L. Holzemer, PhD, RN, FAAN
Professor and Chair
University of California
School of Nursing
San Francisco, CA

Lois M. Hoskins, RN, PhD, FAAN
Professor
The Catholic University of America
School of Nursing
Washington, DC

Sally A. Hutchinson, PhD, RN, FAAN
Professor
University of Florida
College of Nursing
Jacksonville, FL

Kathleen Huttlinger, PhD, RN
Professor
Samuel Merritt College of Nursing
Oakland, CA

Gail L. Ingersoll, EdD, RN, FAAN
Professor and Associate Dean of Research and
Vanderbilt University
School of Nursing
Nashville, TN

Pamela Magnussen Ironside, PhD, RN
Assistant Professor
Clarke College
Dubuque, Iowa

Sharol F. Jacobson, PhD, RN, FAAN
Professor and Director of Nursing Research
University of Oklahoma
Health Sciences College of Nursing
Oklahoma City, OK

Ada Jacox, PhD, RN, FAAN
Professor and Associate Dean for Research
Wayne State University
College of Nursing
Detroit, MI

Monica E. Jarrett, PhD, RN
Research Associate Professor
University of Washington
Department of Biobehavioral Nursing and Health
Seattle, WA

Loretta Sweet Jemmott, PhD, RN, FAAN
Associate Professor and Director
University of Pennsylvania
School of Nursing
Philadelphia, PA

John B. Jemmott, III, PhD
Professor
Princeton University
Department of Psychology
Princeton, NJ

Jean E. Johnson, PhD, RN, FAAN
Professor Emerita
University of Rochester
School of Nursing
Rochester, NY

Marion Johnson, PhD, RN
Associate Professor
University of Iowa
College of Nursing
Iowa City, IA

Dorothy A. Jones, EdD, RNC, FAAN
Associate Professor
Boston College
School of Nursing
Chestnut Hill, MA

Catherine F. Kane, PhD, RN, FAAN
Associate Professor
University of Virginia
School of Nursing
Charlottesville, VA

Gwen Brumbaugh Keeney, MS, RN
University of Illinois
College of Nursing
Chicago, IL

Maureen Keickeisen
Clinical Nurse Specialist
UCLA Medical Center
Department of Nursing
Los Angeles, CA

Lisa Kelley, RN, MA
University of Iowa
College of Nursing
Iowa City, IA

Mary E. Kerr, RN, PhD
Associate Professor
University of Pittsburgh
School of Nursing
Pittsburgh, PA

Shaké Ketefian, EdD, RN
Professor
University of Michigan
School of Nursing
Ann Arbor, MI

Hesook Suzie Kim, PhD, RN
Professor
University of Rhode Island
College of Nursing
Kingston, RI

Karin T. Kirchhoff, PhD, RN, FAAN
Professor
University of Utah
College of Nursing
Salt Lake City, UT

Katharine Y. Kolcaba, PhD, RN
Assistant Professor
University of Akron
College of Nursing
Akron, OH

Christine T. Kovner, PhD, RN, FAAN
Associate Professor
New York University
Division of Nursing
New York, NY

Heidi vonKoss Krowchuck, PhD, RN
Associate Professor
The University of North Carolina at Greensboro
School of Nursing
Greensboro, NC

Joan Kub, PhD, RN
Assistant Professor
Johns Hopkins University
School of Nursing
Baltimore, MD

Alice M. Kuramoto, PhD, RNC, FAAN
Professor
University of Wisconsin
School of Nursing
Milwaukee, WI

Hae-OK Lee, DNSc, RN
Assistant Professor
Case Western Reserve University
School of Nursing
Cleveland, OH

Elizabeth R. Lenz, PhD, RN, FAAN
Professor and Associate Dean
Columbia University
School of Nursing
New York, NY

Eugene Levine, PhD
Professor
Uniformed Services University of the Health Sciences
Bethesda, MD

Linda Lewandowski, PhD, RN
Assistant Professor
Johns Hopkins University
School of Nursing
Baltimore, MD

Ada M. Lindsey, RN, PhD, FAAN
Dean and Professor
University of Nebraska Medical Center
College of Nursing
Omaha, NE

Terri H. Lipman, PhD, CRNP
Assistant Professor/Clinical Nurse Specialist
University of Pennsylvania
Diabetes/Endocrinology
Philadelphia, PA

Juliene G. Lipson, RN, PhD
Assistant Professor/Clinical Nurse
University of California
Department of Community Health Systems
San Francisco, CA

Carol Loveland-Cherry, PhD, RN, FAAN
Associate Professor
The University of Michigan
School of Nursing
Ann Arbor, MI

Brenda L. Lyon, DNS, RN, FAAN
Associate Professor
Indiana University School of Nursing
Adult Health Nursing
Indianapolis, IN

Meridean Maas, PhD, RN, FAAN
Professor
University of Iowa
College of Nursing
Iowa City, IA

Susan L. MacLean, PhD, RN
Director
Research Science
Park Ridge, IL

Beverly Malone, PhD, RN
President
American Nurses Association
Washington, DC

Lucy N. Marion, PhD, RN, FAAN
Associate Professor
University of Illinois
College of Nursing
Chicago, IL

Karen S. Martin, RN, MSN, FAAN
Health Care Consultant
Martin Associates
Omaha, NE

Patricia A. Martin, PhD, RN
Director for Nursing Research
Wright State-Miami Valley College of Nursing and Health
Dayton, OH

Margaret Fisk Mastal, PhD, MSN
Clinical Coordinator
Kaiser Permanente
Springfield, VA

Linda J. Mayberry, PhD, RN
Adjunct Professor
Emory University
Nell Hodgson Woodruff School of Nursing
Atlanta, GA

Angela Barron McBride, PhD, RN, FAAN
Distinguished Professor and University Dean
Indiana University
School of Nursing
Indianapolis, IN

Maureen P. McCausland, DNSc, RN, FAAN
Associate Dean for Nursing & Chief Nursing
University of Pennsylvania
School of Nursing
Philadelphia, PA

Joanne Comi McCloskey, PhD, RN, FAAN
Distinguished Professor
University of Iowa
College of Nursing
Iowa City, IA

Kathleen A. McCormick, PhD, RN, FAAN
Agency for Health Care Policy and Research
Rockville, MD

Charlotte McDaniel, PhD, RN
Director and Clinical Professor
The University of Pittsburgh Medical Center
Pittsburgh, PA

Patricia McDonald, PhD, RN
Assistant Professor
Case Western Reserve University
School of Nursing
Cleveland, OH

Graham McDougall, PhD, RN
Associate Professor
Case Western Reserve University
School of Nursing
Cleveland, OH

Beverly J. McElmurry, EdD, FAAN
Professor and Associate Dean
University of Illinois at Chicago
College of Nursing
Chicago, IL

Mary Lynn McHugh, PhD, RN
Associate Professor
Wichita State University
School of Nursing
Wichita, KS

Mary J. McNamee, PhD, RN
Assistant Dean and Assistant Professor
University of Nebraska Medical Center
College of Nursing
Omaha, NE

Barbara Medoff-Cooper, PhD, RN, FAAN
Associate Professor
University of Pennsylvania
School of Nursing
Philadelphia, PA

Paula M. Meek, PhD, RN
Assistant Professor
University of Arizona
College of Nursing
Tucson, AZ

Janet C. Meininger, PhD, RN
Professor
The University of Texas at Houston
School of Nursing
Houston, TX

Afaf Ibrahim Meleis, PhD, RN, FAAN
Professor
University of California
Department of Community Health Systems
San Francisco, CA

Bonnie L. Metzger, PhD, RN, FAAN
Associate Professor
University of Michigan
School of Nursing
Ann Arbor, MI

Mathy Mezey, EdD, RN, FAAN
Professor
New York University
Division of Nursing
New York, NY

Margaret Shandor Miles, PhD, RN, FAAN
Professor
University of North Carolina
School of Nursing
Chapel Hill, NC

D. Kathleen Milholland, PhD, RN
Research Associate Professor
University of South Florida
Tampa, FL

Nancy Milio, PhD, RN, FAAN
Professor
University of North Carolina
School of Nursing
Chapel Hill, NC

Nancy Houston Miller, RN, BSN
Associate Director
Stanford University School of Medicine
Division of Cardiovascular Medicine
Palo Alto, CA

Susan M. Miovech, PhD, RNC
Clinical Instructor
University of Pennsylvania
School of Nursing
Philadelphia, PA

Pamela H. Mitchell, PhD, RN, FAAN
Professor
School of Nursing
University of Washington
Seattle, WA

Ethel L. Mitty, EdD, RN
Adjunct Assistant Professor
Associate Research Scientist
New York University
Division of Nursing
New York, NY

Doris M. Modly, PhD, RN, FAAN
Professor
Case Western Reserve University
School of Nursing
Cleveland, OH

Rita Black Monsen, DSN, MPH, RN
Professor and Chairperson
Henderson State University
Department of Nursing
Arkadelphia, AR

Ida M. Moore, DNSc, RN, FAAN
Associate Professor
The University of Arizona
College of Nursing
Tucson, AZ

Mary Lou Moore, PhD, RNC
Research Assistant Professor
Bowman Gray School of Medicine of Wake Forest University
Winston-Salem, NC

Shirley M. Moore, PhD, RN
Associate Professor
Case Western Reserve University
Frances Payne Bolton School of Nursing
Cleveland, OH

Patricia Moritz, PhD, RN, FAAN
Associate Professor
University of Colorado Health Sciences Center
School of Nursing
Denver, CO

Diana Lynn Morris, PhD, RN, FAAN
Case Western Reserve University
School of Nursing
Cleveland, OH

Evelyn Moses
Chief, Nursing Data and Analysis Staff
Division of Nursing
Rockville, MD

Barbara Munro, PhD, RN, FAAN
Dean and Professor
Boston College
School of Nursing
Chestnut Hill, MA

Carol M. Musil, PhD, RN
Assistant Professor
Case Western Reserve University
Frances Payne Bolton School of Nursing
Cleveland, OH

Mary Duffin Naylor, PhD, RN, FAAN
Associate Dean
University of Pennsylvania
School of Nursing
Philadelphia, PA

Leslie H. Nicoll, PhD, MBA
Editor-in-Chief
Muskie Institute of Public Affairs
University of Southern Maine
Portland, ME

Kathleen M. Nokes, PhD, RN, FAAN
Professor
CUNY, Hunter College
Hunter-Bellevue
New York, NY

Jane S. Norbeck, RN, DNSc, FAAN
Dean and Professor
University of California
School of Nursing
San Francisco, CA

Kathleen A. O'Connell, PhD, RN, FAAN
Professor
University of Kansas Medical Center
School of Nursing
Kansas City, KS

Ann L. O'Sullivan, PhD, CPNP, FAAN
Professor
University of Virginia
School of Nursing
Charlottesville, VA

Lisa Onega, PhD, RN
Assistant Professor
Oregon Health Sciences University
School of Nursing
Portland, OR

Judy G. Ozbolt, PhD, RN, FAAN
Professor
Vanderbilt University
School of Nursing
Nashville, TN

John R. Phillips, PhD, RN
Professor
New York University
School of Education
New York, NY

Linda R. Phillips, PhD, RN, FAAN
Professor
University of Arizona
College of Nursing
Tucson, AZ

Sally Phillips, PhD, RN
Director, Nursing Doctorate Program
University of Colorado
Health Sciences Center
Denver, CO

Bonita Ann Pilon, DSN, RN
Associate Professor for the Practice Nursing
Vanderbilt University
School of Nursing
Nashville, TN

Denise F. Polit, PhD
President
Humanalysis, Inc.
Saratoga Springs, NY

Sue Popkess-Vawter, PhD, RN
Professor
University of Kansas Medical Center
School of Nursing
Kansas City, KS

Diane Shea Pravikoff, PhD, RN
Director of Research/Professional Liaison
CINAHL Information Systems
Glendale, CA

Jana L. Pressler, PhD, RN
Assistant Professor
Pennsylvania State University
School of Nursing
University Park, PA

Linda C. Pugh, PhD, RNC
Director, Center for Nursing Research and
Pennsylvania State University
Center for Nursing Research
Hershey, PA

Joanne W. Rains, DNS, RN
Dean and Associate Professor
Indiana University East
Division of Nursing
Richmond, IN

Barbara Rakel, RN, MA
Advanced Practice Nurse
The University of Iowa
Hospitals and Clinics
Iowa City, IA

Gloria C. Ramsey, RN, BSN, JD
Project Director
New York University
Division of Nursing
New York, NY

Nancy E. Reame, PhD, MSN, FAAN
Professor
University of Michigan
Center for Nursing Research
Ann Arbor, MI

Richard W. Redman, PhD, RN, FAAN
Interim Associate Dean for Community
University of Michigan
School of Nursing
Ann Arbor, MI

Pamela G. Reed, PhD, RN, FAAN
Professor and Associate Dean for Academic
University of Arizona
College of Nursing
Tucson, AZ

Susan K. Riesch, DNSc, RN, FAAN
Professor and Associate Dean, Graduate Studies
University of Wisconsin, Madison
School of Nursing
Madison, WI

Mary Anne Rizzolo, EdD, RN, FAAN
Director
Interactive Technologies
Lippincott-Raven Publishers
New York, NY

Beverly L. Roberts, PhD, RN, FAAN
Associate Professor
Case Western Reserve University
Frances Payne Bolton School of Nursing
Cleveland, OH

Joyce Roberts, PhD, CNM, FAAN
Professor and Head
University of Illinois at Chicago
Department of Maternal–Child Nursing
Chicago, IL

Bonnie Rogers, DrPH, RN, FAAN
Associate Professor
University of North Carolina at Chapel Hill
School of Public Health
Chapel Hill, NC

Carol A. Romano, PhD, RN, FAAN
Director
National Institutes of Health Clinical Informatics Services
Bethesda, MD

Sheila Ryan, PhD, RN, FAAN
Dean and Professor
University of Rochester
School of Nursing
Rochester, NY

Virginia K. Saba, EdD, RN, FAAN
Clinical Associate Professor
Georgetown University
School of Nursing
Washington, DC

Marla E. Salmon, ScD, RN, FAAN
Professor
University of Pennsylvania
School of Nursing
Philadelphia, PA

Pamela J. Salsberry, PhD, RN
Associate Professor
The Ohio State University
College of Nursing
Columbus, OH

Loretta M. Schlachta, RN, MSHP
Clinical Director of Telemedicine
Strategic Monitored Services
New York, NY

Elizabeth A. Schlenk, PhD, RN
Assistant Professor
University of Pittsburgh
School of Nursing
Pittsburgh, PA

Madeline H. Schmitt, PhD, RN, FAAN
Professor
University of Rochester
School of Nursing
Rochester, NY

Susan M. Schneider, RN
Case Western Reserve University
Frances Payne Bolton School of Nursing
Richmond Heights, OH

Karen L. Schumaker, PhD, RN
Assistant Professor
University of California at San Francisco
School of Nursing
San Francisco, CA

Donald F. Schwarz, MD, MPH
Associate Professor of Pediatrics
University of Pennsylvania
School of Nursing and Medicine
Philadelphia, PA

Joan L. Shaver, PhD, RN, FAAN
Professor and Dean
University of Illinois at Chicago
College of Nursing
Chicago, IL

Nelma B. Shearer, MEd, MS
University of Arizona
College of Nursing
Tucson, AZ

Grayce M. Sills, PhD, RN, FAAN
Visiting Professor
Case Western Reserve University
Frances Payne Bolton School of Nursing
Cleveland, OH

Mary Cipriano Silva, PhD, RN, FAAN
Professor
George Mason University
College of Nursing and Health
Fairfax, VA

Carol E. Smith, RN, PhD
Professor
University of Kansas
School of Nursing
Kansas City, KS

Mariah Snyder, PhD, RN, FAAN
Professor
University of Minnesota
School of Nursing
Minneapolis, MN

Julie Sochalski, PhD, RN
Research Associate Professor
University of Pennsylvania
School of Nursing
Philadelphia, PA

Gwi-Ryung Son, RN, MN
Case Western Reserve University
School of Nursing
Cleveland, OH

Bernard Sorofman, PhD
Associate Professor
The University of Iowa
College of Pharmacy
Iowa City, IA

Susan M. Sparks, RN, PhD, FAAN
Senior Education Specialist
National Library of Medicine
Bethesda, MD

Janet Specht, PhD, RN
Research Scientist
University of Iowa
College of Nursing
Iowa City, IA

Theresa Standing, PhD, RN
Assistant Professor
Case Western Reserve University
Frances Payne Bolton School of Nursing
Cleveland, OH

Joanne Sabol Stevenson, PhD, RN, FAAN
Professor and Associate Dean
Rutgers University
College of Nursing
Newark, NJ

Barbara J. Stewart, PhD, RN
Professor
Oregon Health Sciences University
School of Nursing
Portland, OR

Kathleen S. Stone, PhD, RN, FAAN
Professor
The Ohio State University
College of Nursing
Columbus, OH

Ora L. Strickland, RN, PhD, FAAN
Professor
Emory University
Nell Hodgson School of Nursing
Atlanta, GA

Neville E. Strumpf, PhD, RN, FAAN
Associate Professor
University of Pennsylvania
School of Nursing
Philadelphia, PA

Eleanor J. Sullivan, PhD, RN, FAAN
Professor
University of Kansas
School of Nursing
St. Louis, MO

Susan Dale Tannenbaum, RN, BSN
Staff Nurse- Cardiac Unit
Johns Hopkins University
School of Nursing
Baltimore, MD

Anita J. Tarzian, MS, RN
Department of Acute Long-Term Care
University of Maryland
Baltimore, MD

Roma Lee Taunton, PhD, RN, FAAN
Professor
University of Kansas Medical Center
School of Nursing
Kansas City, KS

Ann Gill Taylor, RN, EdD, FAAN
Professor of Nursing
University of Virginia
Center for the Study of Complementary and Alternative Therapies
Charlottesville, VA

Debera Jane Thomas, DNS, RN, CS
Associate Professor
Florida Atlantic University
Boca Raton, Florida

Carol Lynn Thompson, PhD, RN
Associate Professor and Chair
University of Tennessee
College of Nursing
Memphis, TN

Mary E. Tiedeman, PhD, RN
Visiting Assistant Professor
Brigham Young University
College of Nursing
Provo, UT

Virginia P. Tilden, RN, DNSc, FAAN
Professor
Oregon Health Sciences University
School of Nursing
Portland, OR

Toni Tripp-Reimer, PhD, RN, FAAN
Professor and Associate Dean
University of Iowa
College of Nursing
Iowa City, IA

Barbara S. Turner, RN, DNSc, FAAN
Associate Dean
Duke University
School of Nursing
Durham, NC

Sharon Williams Utz, PhD, RN
Associate Professor and Chair
University of Virginia
School of Nursing
Charlottesville, VA

Barbara Valanis, DrPH, FAAN
Director of Nursing Research
Kaiser-Permanente
Center for Health Research
Portland, OR

Connie Vance, EdD, RN, FAAN
Dean and Professor
College of New Rochelle
New Rochelle, NY

Joyce A. Verran, PhD, RN,
FAAN
Professor
University of Arizona
College of Nursing
Tucson, AZ

Antonia M. Villarruel, PhD,
RN, FAAN
University of Pennsylvania
School of Nursing
Philadelphia, PA

Madeline Musante Wake, PhD,
RN, FAAN
Dean
Marquette University
College of Nursing
Milwaukee, WI

Patricia Hinton Walker, PhD,
FAAN
Dean and Professor
University of Colorado Health Sci-
ences Center
School of Nursing
Denver, CO

Lynn I. Wasserbauer, PhD, RN
Assistant Professor
University of Akron
College of Nursing
Akron, OH

Clarann Weinert, SC, PhD, RN,
FAAN
Associate Professor
Montana State University
College of Nursing
Bozeman, MT

Joan Stehle Werner, RN, DNS
Professor
University of Wisconsin-Eau
Claire
School of Nursing
Eau Claire, WI

Ann L. Whall, PhD, RN, FAAN
Professor
University of Michigan
School of Nursing
Ann Arbor, MI

Carolyn A. Williams, PhD, RN,
FAAN
Dean and Professor
University of Kentucky
Chandler Medical Center
Lexington, KY

Reg Williams, PhD, RN, FAAN
Associate Professor
University of Michigan
School of Nursing
Ann Arbor, MI

Holly Skodol Wilson, RN, PhD,
FAAN
Professor
University of California
School of Nursing
San Francisco, CA

Chris Winkleman
Case Western Reserve University
Frances Payne Bolton School of
Nursing
Cleveland, OH

Mary A. Woo, DNSc, RN
Assistant Professor
UCLA
School of Nursing
Los Angeles, CA

Marilynn J. Wood, RN, DrPH
Co-Editor
Clinical Nursing Research
Edmonton, Alberta
Canada

May L. Wykle, PhD, RN, FAAN
Professor and Associate Dean for
Community
Case Western Reserve University
Frances Payne Bolton School of
Nursing
Cleveland, OH

JoAnne M. Youngblut, PhD,
RN, FAAN
Associate Professor
Case Western Reserve University
Frances Payne Bolton School of
Nursing
Cleveland, OH

Renzo Zanotti, PhD
Professor
University of Padova
Padova, Italy

Jaclene A. Zauszniewski, PhD,
RN
Associate Professor
Case Western Reserve University
Frances Payne Bolton School of
Nursing
Cleveland, OH

LIST OF ENTRIES

ACRONYMS

A

AAAS American Association for the Advancement of Science

AACN American Association of Critical Care Nurses

AACN Association of American Colleges of Nursing

AAMSI American College of Medical Informatics

AAN American Academy of Nursing

AANA American Association of Nurse Anesthetists

AAP-CON American Academy of Pediatrics Committee on Nutrition

AAT Auscultated Acceleration Tests

ACC American College of Nurse Midwives Certification Council

ACE Angiotensin Converting Enzyme

ACMI American College of Medical Informatics

ACNM American College of Nurse-Midwives

ACNM DOA American College of Nurse Midwives Division of Accreditation

ACOG American College of Obstetricians and Gynecologists

AD Alzheimer's Disease

ADL Activities of Daily Living

ADN Associate Degree Nurses

ADRDA Alzheimer's Disease and Related Disorders Association

AFI Amniotic Fluid Index

AFRO Sub-Sahara Africa

AHCPR Agency for Health Care Policy and Research

AI Apolipoprotein

AI Artificial Intelligence

AIDS Acquired Immunodeficiency syndrome

AII High Density Lipoproteins Cholesterol Subclasses

AIII High Density Lipoproteins Cholesterol Subclasses

AJN *American Journal of Nursing*

AMA American Medical Association

AMIA American Medical Informatics Association

AMRO All countries of the Americas

ANA American Nurses Association

ANCOVA Analysis of Covariance

ANOVA Analysis of Variance

ANF American Nurse's Foundation

ANR *Applied Nursing Research*

APACHE Acute Physiology and Chronic Health Evaluation

APEX/PH Assessment Protocol for Excellence in Public Health

APIB Assessment of Preterm Infant's Behavior

APN Advanced Practice Nurse

APNA American Psychiatric Nurses Association

ARNR *Annual Review of Nursing Research*

ASQ Attributional Style Questionnaire

AWHONN Association of Women's Health Obstetrical and Neonatal Nurses

B

BBS Bulletin Board Services

BCRS Brief Rating Cognitive Scale

BDS Blessed Dementia Scale

BMI Body Mass Index

BPP Biophysical Profile

BSE Breast Self-Examination

BSN Bachelor of Science in Nursing

C

C/TCR Cultural/Transcultural Research

CA Conceptual Age

CABG Coronary Artery Bypass Grafting

CAI Computer Assisted Instruction

CAN Children's Action Network

CASQ Children's Attributional Style Question-
naire
CAT Computerized Axial Tomography
CAVE Content Analysis of Verbatim Explana-
tions
CBE Clinical Breast Examination
CCSE Cognitive Capacity Screening Examina-
tion
CD-ROM Compact Disk-Read Only Memory
CDC Center for Disease Control and Prevention
CDR Clinical Dementia Grading
CDS Computerized Decision Support
CE Continuing Education
CEO Chief Executive Officer
CES-D Center for Epidemiologic Studies Depres-
sion Scale
CFS Chronic Fatigue Syndrome
CHD Coronary Heart Disease
CHINS Community Health Information Net-
works
CHW Community Health Workers
CINAHL Cumulative Index of Nursing and Al-
lied Health Literature
CIS Clinical Information Systems
CIN *Computers in Nursing*
CLS Cognitive Levels Scale
CMG Case Mix Groups
CMV Cytomegalovirus
CNEP Community-based Nurse-Midwifery Edu-
cation Program
CNM Certified Nurse Midwife
CNO Community Nursing Organization
CNS Central Nervous System
CNS Clinical Nurse Specialist
COMMES Creighton Online Multiple Modular
Expert System
CONQUEST 1.0 Computerized Needs Oriented
Quality Measurement Evaluation System
CPR Computer-based Patient Record
CPRI Computer-based Patient Record Institute
CPT Current Procedural Terminology
CPU Central Processing Unit
CQI Continuous Quality Improvement
CRISP Computer Retrieval of Information on
Scientific Projects
CRNA Certified Registered Nurse Anesthetist
CST Contraction Stress Test
CT Computerized Tomography

CURN Conduct and Utilization in Nursing
CVD Cardiovascular Disease
CVI Content Validity Index

D
DASH Division of Adolescent and School
Health
DAT Dementia Assessment Inventory
DBP Diastolic Blood Pressure
DCCT Diabetes Control and Complications
Trail
DH Detrusor Hyperreflexia
DHEW Department of Health, Education, and
Welfare
DHHS Department of Health and Human Ser-
vices
DHIC Detrusor Hyperactivity Impaired Bladder
Contractility
DI Detrusor Instability
DM Diabetes Mellitus
DNA Deoxyribonucleic Acid
DNS Doctor of Nursing Science
DNSc Doctor of Nursing Science
DRG Diagnosis Related Group
DSD Detrusor Sphincter Dyssynergia
DSM-IV Diagnostic and Statistical Manual of
Mental Disorders Fourth Edition
DSN Doctor of Science in Nursing

E
EASQ Expanded Attributional Style Question-
naire
ECOSOC Economic and Social Branch of the
United Nations
EdD Educational Doctorate
EEG Electroencephalograph
EFM Electronic Fetal Monitoring
EKG Electrocardiogram
ELSI Ethical Legal and Social Implications
Branch of the National Human Genome Re-
search Institute
EMG Electromyogram
EMRO Countries of the Eastern Mediterranean
ENA Emergency Nurses Association
EOG Electrooculogram
EPSDT Early and Periodic Screening, Diagno-
sis, and Treatment
E.T. NET Educational Technology Network

ETS Endotracheal Suctioning
EURO Europe and the countries of the newly independent states of the former Soviet Union

F
FACT-G DOW
FDA Food and Drug Administration
FHP Functional Health Patterns
FHPAST Functional Health Patterns Assessment Screening tool
FICSIT Frailty and Injuries Cooperative Studies of Intervention Techniques
FIO2 Fraction of Inspired Oxygen
FIRST First Independent Research Support and Transition
FNP Family Nurse Practitioner
FNS Frontier Nursing Service
FROMAJE Function, Reason, Orientation, Memory, Arithmetic, Judgment, & Emotional Status
FSH Follicle Stimulating Hormone
FTE Full Time Employee
FY Fiscal Year

G
GDS Global Deterioration Scale
GI Gastro Intestinal
GnRH Gonadotropin Releasing Hormone
GNP Gross National Product
GPSS common computer languages
GPSS/H General Purpose Simulation Systems
GRASP Grace-Reynolds Application and Study of PETO

H
5-HIAA 5-hydroxyindoleacetic acid
HBV Hepatitis B Virus
HCFA Health Care Financing Administration
HCPAC Health Care Professional Advisory Committee
HCPCS [HCFA] Common Procedure Coding System
HCV Hepatitis C Virus
HDL High Density Lipoproteins
HDLC High Density Lipoproteins Cholesterol
HELP Healthy Evaluation Through Logical Processing
HFA Health for All

HHA Home Health Agency
HHAs Home Health Agencies
HHCC Home Health Care Classification
HIS Hospital Information Systems
HIV Human Immunodeficiency Virus
HL/7 Health Level Seven
HMG-CoA Class of lipid lowering drug
HMO Health Maintenance Organization
HPA Hypothalamic-Pituitary-Adrenal
HSA Health Services Administration
HSD Honestly Significant Difference
HSRS Hospital Stress Rating Scale
5-HT brain concentration of serotonin
HTN Hypertension

I
IADL Instrumental Activities of Daily Living
IASP International Association for Pain
IAV Interactive Video
ICD International Classification of Diseases
ICF Intermediate Care Facility
ICIDH International Classification of Impairments Disabilities and Handicaps
ICN International Council of Nurses
ICNP International Classification of Nursing Practice
ICU Intensive Care Unit
ID Inner Diameter
IDDM Insulin Dependent Diabetes Mellitus
IL-1 Interleukin 1
IL-6 Interleukin 6
INRUS Institute for Nursing Research in the Uniformed Services
IOM Institute of Medicine
IPA Independent Practice Associations
IQ Intelligence Quotient
IRB Institutional Review Board
ISH Isolated Systolic Hypertension
IU International Units
IVD Interactive Video

J
JCAHO Joint Commission on Accreditation of Healthcare Organizations
JONA *Journal of Nursing Administration*

K
KABC Kaufman Assessment Battery for Children

KAP Knowledge-Attitude-Practice
kg kilogram
KMC Kangaroo Mother Care

L
LAN Local Area Networks
LBW Low Birth Weight
LDLC Low density Lipoprotein Cholesterol
LH Leutinizing Hormone
LOS Length of Stay
LP-AI High Density Lipoproteins Cholesterol
   Subclasses
Lp{a} Lipoprotein (a)
LSD Least Significant Difference
LUNAR Learning and Using New Approaches
   to Research

M
M-f Masculinity-Femininity
MAIN Midwest Alliance in Nursing
MANOVA Multivariate Analysis of Variance
MARNA Mid-Atlantic Regional Nurse's Associ-
   ation
MCH Maternal Child Health
MD Medical Doctor
MDD Major Depressive Disorder
MeSH Medical Subject Headings
MHSR Mental Health Services Research
MI Myocardial Infarction
MIS Management Information Systems
MMSE Mini-Mental Status Examination
MNRS Midwest Nursing Research Society
MOS Medical Outcomes Study
MR Mental Retarded
MRB Manual Resuscitator Bag
MRI Magnetic Resonance Imaging
MS Master of Science
MSE Mental Status Examination
MSN Master of Science in Nursing
MTMM Multitrait Multimethod Matrix

N
N-M Nurse Midwives
NA Native American
NA Nurse Anesthetists
NAACOG Nurses Association of the American
   College of Obstetricians and Gynecologists
NANDA North American Nursing Diagnosis As-
   sociation

NCCS National Coalition for Cancer Survivor-
   ship
NCEP National Cholesterol Education Program
NCI National Cancer Institute
NCNR National Center for Nursing Research
NCSBN National Council of State Boards of
   Nursing
ND Doctor of Nursing
NEBHE New England Board of Higher Educa-
   tion
NEMC New England Medical Center
NF Nursing Facility
NHANES II National Health and Nutrition Ex-
   amination Surveys
NHANES III National Health and Nutrition Ex-
   amination Surveys
NHANES National Health and Nutrition Exami-
   nation Survey
NHIS National Health Interview Survey
NHLBI National Heart Lung and Blood Institute
NHRS National Health Record Survey
NIA National Institute on Aging
NIAAA National Institute on Alcohol Abuse and
   Alcoholism
NIC Nursing Interventions Classification
NICU Neonatal Intensive Care Unit
NIDA National Institute on Drug Abuse
NIDDM Non Insulin Dependent Diabetes Mel-
   litus
NIH National Institute for Health
NIH National Institutes of Health
NIMH National Institute for Mental Health
NINCDS National Institute of Neurological and
   Communative Disorders and Stroke
NINR National Institute for Nursing Research
NIS Nursing Information System
NLM National Library of Medicine
NLN National League for Nursing Research
NMDS Nursing Minimum Data Set
NOC Nursing Outcomes Measures
NONPF National Organization of Nurse Prac-
   titioner Faculty
NP Nurse Practitioner
NPO Nothing By Mouth
NRCS Nursing Research Classification System
NSAIDS Nonsteroidal Anti-Inflammatory Drugs
NSC National Safety Council
NSS Nursing Stress Scale

NST Non Stress Tests
NWHW Neighborhood Women's Health Watch

O
OAM Office of Alternative Medicine
OBSSR Office of Behavioral and Social Sciences Research
OD Outer Diameter
OD/ID Outer Diameter Inner Diameter ratio
OJKSN Online Journal of Knowledge Synthesis for Nursing
OSHA Occupational Safety and Health Administration

P
PA Physician Assistant
PACS Picture Archiving Communication Systems
PAR Participatory Action Research
PATCH Planned Approach to Community Health
PC Personal Computer
PCA Patient-Controlled Analgesia
PCP Phencyclidine
PCP Pneumocystis Carnii Pneumonia
PCU Pallative Care Unit
PEEP Positive End Expiratory Pressure
PET Positron Emission Tomography
PETO trade name product for GRASP
PHC Primary Health Care
PHS Public Health Services
PhD Doctor of Philosophy
PICU Pediatric Intensive Care Unit
PINI Patient Intensity for Nursing Index
PKU Phenylketonuria
PLST Progressively Lowered Stress Threshold
PMPM Prepayment for Services on a per Member per Month
PMS Premenstrual Syndrome
POTS Plain Old Telephone Services
PPO Preferred Provider Organization
PPVT-R Peabody Picture Vocabulary Test Revised
PSDA Patient Self Determination Act
PSS:NICU Parental stressor Scale Neonatal Intensive Care Unit
PUFA Polyunsaturated Fatty Acids

Q
QOL Quality of Life
QUALPACS Quality Patient Care Scale

R
r Pearson product-moment correlation coefficient
r² coefficient of Determination
R Multiple correlation
R² Measurement of amount of variance accounted for in the dependent variable
RARIN Retrieval and Application of Research in Nursing
RCT Randomized Clinical Trial
RDA Recommended Daily Allowances
RE Restraint Education
REB Regional Education Board
REC Restraint Education-with-Consultation (or Control)
REM Rapid Eye Movement
RN Registered Nurse

S
SBM Society of Behavioral Medicine
SCAMC Symposium on Computer Applications in Medical Care
SCU Special Care Units
SEARO Countries of South East Asia
SEM Structural Equation Modeling
SERPN Society for Education and Research and Psychiatric Mental Health Nursing
SIG Special Interest Group
SIMSCRIPT common computer languages
SLAM common computer languages
SMI Serious Mental Illness
SNOMED Systematized Nomenclature of Medicine
SPMSQ Short Portable Mental Status Questionnaire
SRCD Society for Research Child Development
SRE Schedule of Recent Experiences
SRRS Social Readjustment Rating Scale
STD Sexually Transmitted Disease
STT Sigma Theta Tau
STTI Sigma Theta Tau International
Sv02 mixed Venous Oxygen Saturation
SWAN Survey of Women Across the Nation
SWS Slow Wave Sleep

T
TB Tuberculosis
TC Total blood Cholesterol
TENS Transcutaneous Electrical Nerve Stimulation

TG Triglycerides
TIA Transient Ischemic Attacks
TISS Therapeutic Intervention Scoring System
TMIS Technicron Medical Information Systems
TNF Tumor Necrosis Factor
TPN Total Parenteral Nutrition
TPS Transaction Processing Systems
TQM Total Quality Management
TSNR Triservice Nursing Research Group

U
U.K. United Kingdom
U.S. United States
UAP Unlicensed Assistive Personelle
UCSF University of California San Francisco
UMLS Unified Medical Language System
UN United Nations
UNICEF United Nations Infants and Children Education Fund
UNLS Unified Nursing Language System
UPI Uteroplacental Insufficiency
USPHS United States Public Health Services

USUHS Uniformed Services University of Health Sciences
V
VAS Vibroacoustic Stimulation
VNA Visiting Nurses Association

W
WAN Wide Area Networks
WCHEN Western Interstate Commission for Higher Education in Nursing
WHO World Health Organization
WIC   special supplemental nutrition program for Women, Infants, and Children
WICHE Western Interstate Commission for Higher Education
WICHEN Western Council on Higher Education for Nursing
WJNR *Western Journal of Nursing Research*
WPRO Countries of the Pacific Rim
WSD Wholly Significant Difference
WWW World Wide Web

A

ACCESS TO HEALTH CARE

Well into the 1980s the discussion of access to health care centered on geographic, financial, and programmatic access to a wide array of basic outpatient and inpatient preventive and curative services targeted to a variety of disadvantaged populations. The emphasis was on need-based planning that would result in universal access for all Americans within a foreseeable future. By the mid 1990s the concept had undergone a remarkable change, resulting from ideological, political, demographic, technological, and policy trends. Access was redefined as the opportunity to buy private health insurance in a mushrooming privatized, profit-seeking market. The language of service systems, need, and underserved people was replaced by industry, financial risk, and paying customers, a lexicon adopted by the health professions, including nursing. Undoubtedly, the new context- and concept-laden language will increasingly affect nursing research. Depending on the path chosen, the profession's scholarship may or may not promote the public's health interests or universal access to care.

The new health care environment has several measurable dimensions that form the context for examining questions of access. These dimensions include the proliferation of managed care organizations, movement of Medicare and Medicaid into managed care systems, welfare reform, the decentralization of federal responsibility and deregulation, deficit reduction by all levels of government, the steady decline of health insurance coverage by employers, and growing gaps in health and income (Krieger, 1994). In total, these pose a quandary of increased need for access to health services and looming barriers to access for underserved, low-income groups and regions, pushing the prospects of universal access into an unforeseeable future.

This picture has major implications for research on access. Attention and resources might be directed toward the emerging industry systems and services, perspectives, and client issues. Alternatively, nursing research, while taking full account of the new contextual realities, might retain a focus on need-based access, extending it beyond small-scale client programs to total populations that are outside the interests of managed care organizations. Research designs could identify system barriers and organizational and policy implications for movement toward universal access.

A computerized search on access to health care services in the nursing and medical literature did not reveal major studies. Research was primarily on access to local, program-specific projects, evaluating patients' or caregivers' perceptions of service delivery in clinics and homes and often centered on diagnostic categories. Many studies sought to uncover barriers to care by selected populations, such as rural, African American, and Asian, mirroring the priorities of the overall financing and organization of U.S. health care. Where efforts were made to examine the practices of organizations—for example, hospitals or ambulatory sites—data came from personnel, ranging from nurse Chief Executive Officers (CEOs) and managers to unit staff.

Thus, perceptions rather than organization-level variables were used. Perceptions cannot be changed for the long term without policy-based changes in the organization or public policy bodies. Further, the limits of the personal health care system for health promotion and primary prevention of long-term illness due to chronic disease, damage from very low weight births, and accidents were rarely recognized.

The nature of the studies was such that they could not render policy-guiding directions, nor were attempts made to do so. That is, there were virtually no systemwide, organization- or policy-level studies examining variables such as Medicaid reform impacts or the financing or organization of delivery systems in managed care organizations, health centers, or health departments. Nor were there community-wide or national random sample studies. Virtually all studies were based on individual-level data, rather than organization- or policy-level data.

Notable exceptions were the organization-level, policy-directed studies led by Wood and Estes (1990) on the impact to services delivery following federal policy on diagnostic-related groups (DRGs) as a basis for public insurance payment and other cost-containment policies. These studies, which depicted shifts in the priorities, programs, staffing, and referral systems of hospitals and the spin-off effects on community-based health service organizations, showed subsequent impact on the access of eligible groups to care. This multistate, multiorganizational set of studies examined environmental variables (e.g., federal and state financing) and other policies, as well as resource-specific, organization-level variables such as staffing changes. In-depth interviews with leading organization incumbents could then be understood within these constraints, which shaped organizational programs, practices, and access priorities. As a result, policy implications could be drawn to guide resource commitments and allocation.

A crucial dimension of the emerging systems involves telemedicine, telecare, and telehealth, which provide services at a distance in rural and urban areas (Expert Panel, 1996). These electronic networks and related technologies, using computers, telecommunications, the Internet, electronic kiosks, voice mail, CD-ROMs, and videotape, extend current uses for medical consultations, x-ray readings, and electronic monitoring. They can utilize nurse practitioners in schools, public housing sites, senior centers, clinics, home care, health information, and community group communication. Research on the advantages and deficits of these uses is very limited.

For a decade, research and development in the nursing profession on information technology has been in informatics and the formation of data bases for institutional use, rather than consumer-oriented information. Rarely has attention been given to whether nurse units use electronic networks to promote community-based primary prevention and link community services to school, child care, senior, and other local service sites. Nor has there been any delineation of barriers (costs, training, support) to nurses and sites, clients, and community organizations. An empirical foundation for exploring and understanding these kinds of access issues is essential if nursing is not to become an appendage to the electronic network that is enveloping public health and medical care.

To address the growing need for health services access by disadvantaged groups, including an increasing share of blue-collar families, need-based access must be understood in the new marketing environment. To alter policy and organizational constraints, research must go beyond individual indicators (demographic or socioeconomic characteristics) or perceptions of patients or organizational incumbents. Research questions should focus on indicators of the organizations, systems, and policies that shape the patterns of behavior of managers, practitioners, and patients and the access profile of populations (welfare, Medicare and Medicaid beneficiaries, working poor families, and women). In addition to organization- and policy-level data, community variables on the living conditions and epidemiology of total populations provide insight on the distribution of health problems in a community. Managed care organizations, health departments, and other systems should use these community variables if accurate access assessments of their service arrangements are to address community-wide needs (Centers for Disease Control, 1996).

As suggested, organization variables include fiscal size and financing sources, resource allocations to services and personnel, and organizational linkages and service contracts, as well as perceptions of stakeholders. Additionally, the more immediate determinants of access to health plan selection include available choices, favorable premium costs and benefits coverage, and hours and sites of services. Needed indicators of access are those that reveal affordability, cultural acceptability, and geographic 24-hour access to useful information for primary and secondary preventive, acute, and chronic care. Finally, other aspects that shape access and availability of health-supporting services include managed care organization subcontracts with safety nets and providers for specific "carve-out" (family support and child care), enabling services (transportation, translation), and collaboration with local health departments (Milio, in press).

NANCY MILIO

See also
MANAGED CARE
RURAL HEALTH
TELEHEALTH
VULNERABLE POPULATIONS

ACTION SCIENCE

Action science is an approach to generating knowledge for practice by engaging practitioners in that process through reflection on their own behavioral worlds of practice (Argyris, Putnam, & Smith, 1985; Schön, 1983). Schön (1983) contrasts action science as advanced by these authors with the traditional, positivistic science, which he calls technical rationality. Technical rationality for professional practice is concerned with "knowing that," whereas action science is oriented to "knowing how" in practice. Although knowing how in practice contributes to the creation of knowledge that is not available from traditional research, what practitioners actually design in their practice may be limiting, routinized, and self-sealing. Hence, action science addresses generation of knowledge through reflection that fulfills the functions of discovery and change. Action science is primarily oriented to studying individual practitioners in their practice and generation of knowledge from individuals' practice; however, it can be applied to organizational behaviors and organizational intervention.

Putnam (1992) suggests that action science is based on three philosophical premises: (a) human practice involves meaning making, intentionality in action, and normativity from the perspective of human agency; (b) human practice goes on in an interdependent milieu of behavioral norms and institutional politics; and (c) the epistemology of practice calls for the engagement of practitioners in generating knowledge. Action science thus is a method and philosophy for improving practice and generating knowledge. Argyris (1987) suggests further that action science is an interventionist approach in which three prerequisites must be established for the research to ensue: (a) a creation of normative models of rare universes that are free of defensive routines, (b) a theory of intervention that can move practitioners and organizations from the present to a new desirable universe, and (c) a theory of instruction that can be used to teach new skills and create new culture.

Action science holds that actions in professional practice are based on practitioners' theories of action. Theories of action are learned and organized as repertoires of concepts, schemata, and propositions and are the basis on which practitioners' behavioral worlds are created in specific situations of practice. Argyris, Putnam, and Smith (1985) identify espoused theories and theories-in-use as two types of theories of action. Espoused theories of action are the rationale expressed by practitioners as guiding their actions in a situation of practice, whereas theories-in-use refers to theories that are actually used in practice. Theories-in-use are only inferable from the actions themselves, and practitioners usually are not aware of or not able to articulate their theories-in-use except through careful reflection and self-dialogue.

Argyris and Schön (1974) and Argyris, Putnam, and Smith (1985) identified Model I theories-in-use as a type that seals practitioners from learning and produces routinization and ineffectiveness in practice. Model II theories-in-use are proposed within action science as an intervention for Model I theories-in-use. Model II theories-in-use encompass principles of valid information, free and informed choice in action, and internal commitment. Reflection and learning are the two key processes necessary for the transformation from Model I theories-in-use to Model II theories-in-use. Action science, then, aims to engage both practitioners and researchers in this process of transformation through the creation of a normative model of rare universe and application of theories of intervention and instruction.

Knowledge of practitioners' theories-in use and espoused theories provides a descriptive understanding about the patterns of inconsistencies between theories-in-use and espoused theories revealed in actual practice. Through action science, practitioners engaged in Model II theories-in-use produce practice knowledge that informs their approach to practice without routinization or the self-sealing mode. In addition, action science generates knowledge regarding the process involved in self-awareness and the learning of new theories-in-use through reflective practice and practice design.

Research process in action science calls for the cooperative participation of practitioner and researcher through the phases of description, discovery of theories-in-use, and intervention. Transcriptions of actual practice by the researcher or narratives of actual practice by the practitioner are analyzed together in order to describe and inform reflectively the nature of practice and theories-in-use. Putnam (1996) suggests the use of the ladder of inference as a tool to discover practitioners' modes of thinking and action as revealed in transcripts or narratives. The research process is not oriented to the analysis of action transcripts or narratives by a researcher independent of the practitioner. It involves a postpractice face-to-face discussion (interview) between the researcher and the practitioner. Such sessions are used to get at the reconstructed reasoning of practitioners regarding critical moments of the practice and to provide opportunities for reflection on the thinking and doing that were involved in the practice. Through such sessions, the researcher also acts as an interventionist by engaging the practitioner to move toward new learning.

Nursing practice is a human-to-human service that occurs in the context of health care. Nurses practice within on-line conditions that are complex not only with respect to clients' problems but also in terms of organizational elements of the health care environment. Nursing practice is not based simply on linear translations of relevant theoretical knowledge that governs the situation of practice but has to be derived and designed from the nurse's knowledge of and responses to the competing and complex demands of the situation (Kim, 1994). In addition, as the action scientists suggest, nursing practice in general, as well as particular nursing actions, may be entrenched with routinization or frozen within Model I theories-in-use.

On the other hand, a great deal of nursing as practiced may be exemplary and creatively designed and enacted. The general aim of action science for nursing is then to improve nursing practice by freeing nurses from self-sealing practices and engaging them in the process of learning and participatory research (Kim, 1994).

HESOOK SUZIE KIM

See also
APPLIED RESEARCH
CLINICAL NURSING RESEARCH
EPISTEMOLOGY

ACTIVITIES OF DAILY LIVING

Measures of physical functional status such as activities of daily living (ADLs) and instrumental activities of daily (IADLs) have evolved over the past 40 years as important indicators of health status and disability. Disability refers to how an impairment or organic pathological change limits activities and functioning. As a measure of disability, ADLs refer to the basic tasks of everyday life, such as eating, bathing, dressing, toileting, and transferring. IADLs encompass the performance of a range of life activities more complex than those included in most ADL scales. They include activities necessary for independent function in the community, such as meal preparation, shopping, doing housework, traveling, and financial management.

Assessment of ADLs originated in clinical practice in rehabilitation as one way to measure performance, first for disability determination and later as an integral part of clinical management. These measures have been widely applied in clinical settings and population-based studies to define functional status and care needs, to guide health policy for aging and chronically ill populations, to evaluate treatment effectiveness, and to monitor the effects of disease on patients' day-to-day activities.

Nurse researchers have described the impact of illness on patients' physical functioning and tested interventions to improve ADLs and IADLs in populations with cardiac disease, AIDS, Alzheimer's disease, cancer, and numerous other conditions. In nursing research these measures of physical functioning are frequently evaluated as one dimension of functional status, quality of life, or broader measures of health status that also incorporate mental and social function.

Many different methods have been developed to rate individual ADLs or IADLs. Standard tests of an individual's performance conducted by a trained observer and questioning the individual about current level of functioning are two general approaches. Three standard forms of rating include (1) the degree of difficulty in performing certain activities, that is, how hard it is to perform an activity; (2) the degree of assistance or dependency, for instance, whether or not a person uses or needs assistance to perform an activity; and (3) whether or not an activity is performed (Jette, 1994). Another distinction in the measurement of ADLs and IADLs is whether the items on the scale ask what a person can do (person's physical capacity) or what a person does do (actual performance). An index asking what a patient can do may exaggerate the healthiness of the respondent by as much as 15% to 20% (McDowell & Newell, 1996). Most recent ADL indices utilize the performance approach for ADL items, using wording to assess the health reasons that a person did not do an activity. The choice of which rating scale to use depends on the researcher's conceptual definition of physical functioning and objectives of the research and can have a profound impact on the estimates of disability within and across studies.

Katz's Index of Activities of Daily Living was the first scale published in the 1950s. It was developed to study the effects of treatment on the elderly and chronically ill and has been widely used. As with all ADL scales, it is appropriate only when measuring severe levels of disability. Other well-known instruments of ADL indices include the PULSES, Barthel, Kenny, and the Medical Outcomes Study. IADL scales are commonly used with less severely handicapped populations; they have been more thoroughly tested for validity and reliability and may be more sensitive to minor changes in a patient's condition. IADL scales are often combined with ADL scales in one instrument to broaden the definition of disability. McDowell and Newell (1996) and Frank-Stromborg and Olsen (1997) have published descriptions of ADL and IADL scales along with their conceptual basis and psychometric properties.

As the proportion of our elderly population with chronic diseases increases, knowledge is needed about how to keep these individuals functionally independent and satisfied with their quality of life. Nurse researchers are in key positions to broaden and strengthen this line of research. Instruments must be refined or new ones developed, with sensitivity to the small but clinically meaningful changes observed as outcomes of nursing interventions. Most ADL and IADL scales were developed to rate a patient's condition at a single point in time. To determine change over time or after some therapeutic intervention, investigators frequently compare the difference noted in two or more repeated values of the single-state ratings. The sensitivity of existing instruments to small but clinically important changes has been largely untested.

Another direction for future nursing research is to determine what factors predict physical functioning and satisfaction with physical functional status in different populations. Research using measures of ADLs and IADLs has often overlooked the personal perspectives of patients and what changes in the particular disabilities are most important to them. A better understanding of predictive factors and personal preferences could lead to more effective planning and evaluation of therapeutic interventions. Future use of physiological indicators such as ADLs and IADLs may also include monitoring quality of care. Nurse researchers should be positioned to conduct these investigations and to assist clinicians to utilize research findings to improve quality of care.

JERILYN K. ALLEN

See also
COGNITIVE INTERVENTIONS
FUNCTIONAL HEALTH
OREM'S SELF-CARE DEFICIT
   THEORY OF NURSING
SELF-EFFICACY

ADHERENCE/COMPLIANCE

Adherence refers to the degree to which behavior corresponds to a recommended therapeutic regimen

(Haynes, Taylor, & Sackett, 1979). Numerous terms have been used to describe this behavior, including compliance, therapeutic alliance, and patient cooperation. Although the literature is filled with discussions of the acceptability of these terms and the differences between them, most investigators view the terms as synonymous and independent of the decision to engage in a particular therapeutic regimen. The most complete literature can be obtained from structured databases with the term *compliance*.

Adherence to health care regimens has been discussed in the literature since the days of Plato. However, little systematic attention was given to this phenomenon until the 1970s, when there was a proliferation of research. One of the first reviews of the literature was published in *Nursing Research* (Marston, 1970). Since that time there has been a profusion of research from a variety of disciplines. The majority of the research has focused on patient adherence, although there is a smaller body of literature on the adherence of research staff to clinical protocols and a growing body of literature on provider adherence to treatment guidelines.

One of the issues that continues to arise in discussions of patient adherence is patient autonomy. Is nonadherence a patient right or responsibility? This argument presumes that the patient is aware of his or her own behavior and has consciously decided not to follow a treatment regimen. The literature suggests that fewer than 20% of patients with medication regimens consciously decide not to engage in a treatment program. Those patients who have decided to follow the regimen but do not carry it out are unaware of episodic lapses in behavior or have difficulty integrating the health care regimen into their lives. The most common reasons given by patients for lapses in adherence are forgetting and being too busy. This group comprises on average 40% to 60% or more of patients in a treatment regimen.

The problem of nonadherence is costly in terms of dollars and lives. The National Pharmacy Council estimates that nonadherence to pharmacological therapies costs approximately $100 billion annually (Grahl, 1994). Although the cost of nonadherence to nonpharmacological therapies has not been estimated, the contribution to morbidity and mortality is high. Failures to quit smoking, to lose and maintain weight, to exercise regularly, to engage in safe sex practices, to avoid excess alcohol, and to use seat belts contribute significantly to declines in functional ability as well as to early mortality. Further data suggest that nonadherence to pharmacological as well as nonpharmacological therapies contributes to excess hospitalizations and complication rates (Dunbar-Jacob & Schlenk, 1996).

Poor adherence, then, is a significant problem of direct relevance to nursing. Nurse practitioners may prescribe or recommend therapies. Home health and community nurses provide education and assistance in carrying out health care advice. Hospital, clinic, and office nurses provide education regarding treatment plans. There is a need for intervention studies that will guide practice as nurses prepare and support patients in the conduct of treatment regimens.

Research on adherence is primarily focused on descriptive studies. In a review of the research conducted within nursing over the past 24 years (1972–1996), only 21 distinct adherence intervention studies were identified. The majority of the studies addressed adult patients (16 of 21). The studies focused on medication (5) or visit adherence (5), with less attention given to general regimen adherence (4), cancer screening (3), exercise (2), and immunization (1). The majority of the studies used either an educational intervention or ''nurse follow-up or visit.'' Two studies addressed modification of behaviors contributing to adherence, and four studies were theoretically driven. Three studies used the health belief model and one Orem's self-care theory. Only one study examined intervention effectiveness over time. Thus, the state of the research on adherence in nursing is rudimentary. The research on adherence is limited by the lack of attention to intervention studies, the narrow focus of the interventions, and the limited amount of theoretically driven research. This latter point may be related to the small number of theoretical frameworks addressed in the intervention research on adherence.

Future research on adherence should address strategies by which nurses can improve adherence to treatment regimens with attention directed toward various age groups, clinical populations, and regimen behaviors. The research would benefit from theoretical approaches to the problems of patient adherence and to the design of intervention strategies. Effective strategies delivered by nurses have considerable promise of a favorable impact on health outcomes and costs (Dunbar-Jacob & Schlenk, 1996).

This paper was supported in part by the National Institute of Nursing Research grant (5 P30 NR03924) and the National Heart, Lung, and Blood Institute grant (1 UO1HL48992).

JACQUELINE DUNBAR-JACOB

See also
ATTITUDES
ATTRIBUTION THEORY
RISK FACTORS
SELF-EFFICACY

ADMINISTRATION RESEARCH

Henry and colleagues (Henry, Moody, Pendergast et al., 1987) defined administration research as "concerned with establishing costs of nursing care, examining the relationships between nursing services and quality patient care, and with viewing problems of nursing service delivery within the broader context of policy analysis and delivery of health services" (p. 311). Since the 1970s, more emphasis has been placed on the importance of clinical (practice) research, resulting in many advances in nursing science. For example, there is an expansive knowledge in the prevention and treatment of skin breakdown; clinical management of acute and chronic pain; symptom management in areas of breathlessness, fatigue, and anxiety; preoperative preparatory teaching; social support in rural areas; and suctioning. However, there has not been equivalent emphasis on nursing administration research.

Early nursing administration research focused on factors influencing job satisfaction, recruitment, retention, turnover, motivation, and the characteristics of nurses. Later research focused on the category of nursing services, patient classification systems, incentives for nurses, decision-making models, change theory implementation, professional practice model structures, and most recently, effects of care delivery models and leadership characteristics of nurse executives.

Nursing administration research should be reprioritized and should become a required component of future research efforts. The health care environment is changing rapidly, and the focus on outcomes-based research has escalated in response to the need for cost-efficient and cost-effective delivery of services. It is as important to study the effects that contextual and organizational factors have on the delivery of nursing care as it is to study the effect of specific interventions. For example, Kraus and colleagues (Kraus, Dryer, Wagner, & Zimmerman, 1986) studied treatment and outcomes in 5,030 patients in intensive care units at 13 tertiary care hospitals. The differences in patient outcomes were attributed to the level of interaction and coordination of care between nurses and physicians, not to any specific intervention. Had this study's methodology not included variables related to communication patterns, a full understanding of the importance of the relationship between individual (patient) outcome and an organizational variable (communication patterns) would not have been discovered.

The study of how the structure and process of care affects outcomes of nursing is essential to understanding why certain interventions may differ across patient populations and clinical environments. Variables such as differences in role expectation and performance, workload, different care delivery models, governance structures, innovation readiness, levels of work satisfaction, size, and geographical location are examples of important variables that have been found to affect patient outcomes.

A balance between clinical research on patient outcomes and nursing care and understanding the context or environment in which that care occurs must take place if nursing is to determine what interventions are most effective and actually affect the health status of patients and families, communities, and organizations. Nursing administration research provides the methodologies to conduct the type of multidimensional work required to identify what factors affect the relevant variables and relationships that account for patient care differences.

CAROL A. ASHTON

ADOLESCENCE

Adolescence is a developmental stage distinct from childhood and adulthood. At what age the label *adolescence* is appropriate depends on the data source. The *Guide to Clinical Preventive Services* (U.S. Preventive Services, 1996a) uses ages 11 to 24 years. The most meaningful approach to this stage is to separate adolescence into three periods: (a) early adolescence, ages 10 to 14; (b) middle adolescence, ages 15 to 19; and (c) late adolescence, ages 20 to 24. During this transitional period adolescents reach physical and sexual maturity, develop more sophisticated reasoning ability, and make important educational and occupational decisions that will shape their adult careers.

Although the actual number of adolescents is increasing, this group represents a smaller proportion of the U.S. population; that is, the population represented by adolescents decreased from 14% in 1990 to 13.9% in 1993. In addition, the adolescent population now comprises 52% between the ages 10 and 14, compared to 48% between the ages 15 and 19. According to Day (1996) "baby boomers" are having children later in life, non-White populations are experiencing high fertility rates, and a large number of immigrants are in their 20s. Also, the percentage of adolescents within the White population (12.8%) is lower than that within the Hispanic (17.5%) or Black populations (17.1%). As a result of lower birth and immigration rates, the non-Hispanic White population under age 19 will be less than half of the U.S. population under age 19 by the year 2030. By 2000 the adolescent population between the ages of 10 and 19 will consist of 66% Whites not of Hispanic origin, 15% Blacks, 14% Hispanics, 4.5% Asians and Pacific Islanders, and 1% American Indians, Eskimos, and Aleuts; therefore, it is crucial for nurses to have cultural competence (Ozer, Brindis, Millstein, Knopf, & Irwin, 1997).

Most adolescent mortality and morbidity results from behavior and lifestyle and therefore is preventable (Elster & Kuznets, 1994). Many behavior patterns developed during adolescence continue into adulthood, and most of the leading health problems of adults are those associated with behaviors initiated early in life (e.g., smoking). In the past 10 years major advances have been made in understanding the health beliefs of adults and how these beliefs influence health-related behaviors. As our focus has turned to the early origins of health beliefs and behaviors, adolescence has increasingly become a focus of investigations. Researchers are making some progress in understanding how parental health attitudes and behaviors, social norms, peer pressures, and mass media affect teenagers' health-related beliefs and lifestyles. There is still much to learn regarding cognitive aspects (attitude, beliefs, perceptions), emotional aspects (feelings, concerns, moods, personality), social effects (norms, culture, environment, socioeconomic status), and biobehavioral (neurohormonal, psychoneuroimmunological) influences on the health practices of adolescents.

According to a survey by Thurber, Berry, and Cameron (1991), nurses were involved with adolescents regarding both health education and health appraisals. Nurse practitioners in primary care settings spend a significant amount of their time (25% to 48%) in the provision of health care to adolescents from diverse ethnic backgrounds. Before working with adolescents, nurses must understand how the egocentrism of this period influences behavior. Elkind (1984) described the "imaginary audience" as one consequence of adolescent egocentrism, that is, the assumption that everyone around them is watching them and is concerned about their appearance and behavior. Hence, they are very self-conscious and often go to extreme lengths to avoid what they are convinced will be mortifying experiences. Another consequence of the adolescent egocentrism and self-centeredness is the "personal fable," which is a set of beliefs in the uniqueness of one's feelings and of one's immortality. Others often describe this belief as "It won't happen to me"—the story we tell ourselves, whether having sex without protection, driving fast, smoking, or drinking, that other people may experience the negative consequences but not us.

Millstein, Petersen, and Nightingale (1993) offered an excellent overview of research on ways to promote health of adolescents. Two important concepts related to adolescent lifestyles are (a) how adolescents organize their lives and pattern their behavior in ways that put them at lower or higher risk for serious health problems and (b) how these patterns develop, persist, or cease at different times during the life span. Research topics include mental health, sexuality, diet and physical activity, oral health, substance abuse, violence, and safety.

The National Institute of Nursing Research Priority Expert Panel on Health Promotion (1993) recommended the following priorities for nursing research to yield significant understanding for improving the health of adolescents.

1. Examine the interactive effects of behavioral and biological processes, including the timing of developmental and social transitions on health behaviors.
2. Investigate family, school, and community strategies for adopting and maintaining health-promoting behaviors among teenagers in rural and urban settings. Special attention should be given to highly vulnerable youth who are economically disadvantaged, homeless, school dropouts, members of social or ethnic minority groups, immigrants, homosexuals, the alienated, chronically ill, or disabled.
3. Develop and test culturally appropriate, innovative health promotion interventions that incorporate both educational and contextual components in outreach settings, and focus on the collaboration of nurses with other health professionals.

Most of the health problems of adolescents have their origins in environmental or behavioral factors. Reducing adolescent morbidity and mortality requires strategies that involve multiple approaches delivered through multiple settings, including schools, the mass media, communities, families, and health care settings. In addition, legislation that prevents adolescents' access to cigarettes, alcohol, and guns can promote health. Regardless of the approach, it is essential that all nurses understand how to provide culturally competent health care for adolescents (Davis & Voegtle, 1994).

ANN L. O'SULLIVAN

See also
**PARENT-ADOLESCENT
RELATIONSHIPS/COMMUNICATION
REDUCING HIV RISK ASSOCIATED
SEXUAL BEHAVIORS AMONG
ADOLESCENTS
VIOLENCE AS A NURSING AREA
OF INQUIRY**

ADULT HEALTH

Human adulthood refers to the stages or phases of the life cycle after childhood and adolescence. It is the longest period of the life course. Physical, intellectual, educational, occupational, social, economic, spiritual, and health-related changes characterize the multiple stages of adulthood. The changes that take place in adulthood are of importance to nursing for two reasons. One is that adults, especially older adults, comprise the largest population served by nurses. The second is that adults are the parents or guardians of infants, children, and adolescents. Hence, adults are the direct or indirect targets of all of nursing care and patient or family education and counseling.

Ideally, nursing care and client education about self-care would be crafted to produce the maximum positive benefit for clients. Rarely are nursing actions designed to fit within the specific life stage, developmental stage, or personal contextual reality of adult clients.

History and Definitions of Terms

Adulthood. The study of adult development is a 20th-century phenomenon, ostensibly because people did not live long enough to merit inquiry in previous centuries. One notable exception was a treatise by Queletet published in 1842, entitled *A*

Treatise on Man and the Development of His Faculties. G. Stanley Hall and E. L. Thorndike were two early 20th-century scholars of the adult years. In mid-century, Erik Erikson (1959) published a set of life stages that expressed the middle-class norms of the 1940s and 1950s. Fortunately, he lived long enough to revise them and add additional stages as people lived ever longer. From 1960 through 1980, Bernice Neugarten (1968) and other investigators at the University of Chicago generated much of the work that serves as the foundation of extant theory on adult development.

The life-span perspective of adult development and aging is oriented to the scientific study of adult life stages and critical situations that most closely fits within the nursing goal to maximize quality of life for as much of the life span as possible. The life-span perspective focuses on change, continuity, and discontinuity over the life course. Each stage of adulthood has normative patterns, and as one stage folds into the next, personal changes occur and integration of these changes is necessitated. This process may produce anxiety, anger, frustration, and physiological stress responses during the transition while the conflicts between the old and the new self are resolved and the changes are integrated into the self system. These stress responses frequently present to health care providers in the form of accidents, chemical abuse, violence, or acute or chronic illness. The conditions are rarely perceived or treated within the developmental context. Rather, adults are decontextualized by health care professionals, who treat the immediate symptoms or condition while ignoring the adult context in which it occurs (Stevenson, 1993). Furthermore, health researchers, including nurse investigators, do not study health or care phenomena within the context of the adult life course.

Health. One conception of health with wide appeal in the medical community is attributable to Dubos (1965), who defined health as a state of equilibrium, adaptation, and harmony. Dunn (1980) went beyond mere equilibrium and devised the new concept of higher level wellness. Dunn's concept of higher level wellness embodied the idea of actualizing and maximizing human potential through the pursuit of three subgoals: making progress toward a higher level of functioning, having an open-ended expanding goal to seek a fuller potential, and progressing toward a more integrated and mature human existence through the entire life course. Pender (1996) attempted to incorporate both Dunn's actualizing focus and Dubos's concept of health as maintaining stability through adaptation to the environment. According to Pender, "health is the actualization of inherent and acquired human potential through goal-directed behavior, competent self-care, and satisfying relationships with others while adjustments are made as needed to maintain structural integrity and harmony with relevant environments" (p. 22). Recently, a group of WHO representatives redefined health as a "resource" for everyday life, not an outcome or end product to be obtained at some definable point in time. According to the WHO Ottawa Charter (Kaplun, 1992), good health is viewed as a resource that goes hand in hand with social, economic, and personal development, and it is a critically important resource for attaining and maintaining a high-level quality of life for the entire life course.

State of Knowledge on Adult Health

The prevailing theories about physical normality and the adult stages have changed since the 1960s. The prolongation of physical well-being has become a norm as humans are living ever longer, even in third world countries. Although the stages of adulthood differ by theorist, the middle stages have been expanded to accommodate the acceleration of longevity. Young adulthood lasts from about 18 to about 29; the core or traditional middle years encompass the years from 30 to 50 (50 was the average life span in 1900); the new middle years cover the years from about 51 to either 65 or 70, depending on the theorist. Young old age covers the period from either 65 or 70 to 75; middle old age extends to 85, and old-old age, or the frail age, is 85 and beyond. The latter three ages are relatively new designations and are evolving. It is quite likely that during the first three decades of the 21st century, as the baby boomers move into the higher age brackets, the old-old age designation will move upward and begin at age 90 or higher.

Different aspects of development are dominant in different stages of adulthood. The biological self reaches its peak in the middle 20s, and then a very gradual decline in physiological efficiency in organ systems occurs during the next seven or eight decades. The rate of change is mediated by genetics, lifestyle, and environment, but everyone experiences the decline. There is a rise in cognitive abilities in young adulthood that does not peak for most until middle age, and these abilities then decline at an even slower rate than the physical parameters. Emotional and spiritual development is postulated to continue well into old age and to peak near death for the cognitively and emotionally healthy. Any of these norms may be altered for individuals by genetics, mental or physical illness, catastrophic emotional events, or other significant situations. In the ideal world, health professionals would be cognizant of the developmental stage of each adult client and formulate care to match the needs and context of that stage (Stevenson, 1993). This ideal assumes that the necessary knowledge base exists, but it does not.

Critical Foci for Future Research

Although much has been learned, there is great difficulty in trying to separate the impact of lifestyle from what is ultimately possible for adult health under ideal conditions. This is true not only for the biological possibilities but also for the socioemotional realm and for the development of intellect, creativity, and wisdom. Much of the extant research is plagued by the inability of researchers to disentangle the overlay of familial and cultural expectations, cohort-specific life experiences, the environment, and idiosyncratic tendencies. What is generally considered normal for men or women during the major stages of adult life is open to criticism as being tied to specific historical periods (e.g., studies done in the 1950s or the 1980s), to expectations within an age cohort (e.g., those whose childhood spanned the Depression years or the Vietnam War), to gender differences that were influenced by prevailing values and expectations (e.g., pre–women's liberation or sexual liberation), or to physical adult health status in light of varying mores about smoking, fat intake, and exercise.

Cultural, cohort, and gender-expectation biases could be overcome to some extent with cross-cul-

tural or cross-sequential designs (Schaie, Campbell, Meredith, & Rawlings, 1989). These were first described by Schaie in 1964 and subsequently used by him and his colleagues in several studies, some of which are ongoing.

Nurse researchers are challenged to do more of their adult health research contextually tied to the specific adult ages and stages of the subjects (Stevenson, 1993). Most nursing research either erroneously lumps three or more distinct adult stages into one group (e.g., 25 to 60) or makes antitheoretical age categories (e.g., 25 to 45, 45 to 65, and 65 and above). Developmental and situational confounders abound in data categorized and analyzed in this way. Findings would be more valid and reliable, even about purely physiological phenomena, if scientifically based adult life stages were used as the grouping categories in research on adult health.

JOANNE SABOL STEVENSON

See also
CULTURAL/TRANSCULTURAL FOCUS
HUMAN BECOMING THEORY:
  PARSE'S THEORY OF NURSING
QUALITY OF LIFE
WELLNESS

ADVANCED PRACTICE NURSES

Definition

Conceptually, advanced practice nursing is described as the application of an expanded range of practical, theoretical, and research-based therapeutics to phenomena experienced by patients within a specialized clinical area of the larger discipline of nursing (Hamric, Spross, & Hanson, 1996). The history and evolution of advanced practice nursing is a tapestry of patient care provided by expert nurses who have expanded the boundaries and scope of the practice of nursing.

Advanced practice nurses (APNs) need basic core competencies to fulfill the advanced practice nursing role. These competencies include skills in expert clinical practice, consultation, teaching and coaching, research, leadership, collaboration, change agency, and ethical decision making (Hamric et al., 1996). APNs offer high levels of autonomous decision making in the assessment, diagnosis, and management of patients. Conceptually, the practice is nursing-based, with emphasis on health promotion, disease prevention, and education of patients and families. Advanced practice nurses must have a graduate degree in nursing in a chosen specialty and are differentiated by the ability to carry out direct, expert clinical practice. Although advanced practice nursing is an evolving field, currently the role of the APN is limited to nurse practitioners, clinical nurse specialists, certified nurse midwives, and certified registered nurse anesthetists, who provide direct clinical care for patients (American Nurses Association, 1993).

One of the hallmarks of advanced practice nursing is the commitment to collaboration with other disciplines. Advanced practice nurses work within the designated scope of practice and collaborate with or refer to other professional colleagues those patients and problems that fall beyond the expertise of APNs.

Research

Advanced practice nursing and the practice roles, issues, and evaluation of the four groups of APNs (nurse practitioners, certified nurse midwives, certified registered nurse anesthetists, and clinical nurse specialists) serve as a rich and comprehensive base for nursing research. Patient-centered outcomes research that explores outcomes of patients served by APNs is central to the health care system that is unfolding in the United States. The overused Office of Technology Assessment study of 1986, which evidenced the safety and satisfaction of using APNs to improve access to health care, can no longer be cited as the only research support for the education and practice of APNs. Health policy–based nursing research that explores workforce demographics, cost, reimbursement, and privileging, as well as the credentialing and regulation of APNs, is an undisputed data need. Nursing research focused in the realm of managed care and interdisci-

plinary, collaborative approaches to care is a highly sought after commodity. Research into the education and evaluation of APNs is critical to health policy forecasting and workforce planning.

Advanced practice nurse researchers who engage in clinical practice are the key to most of the research topics outlined above. Clinically based research networks that allow for multiple data generation on patient outcome are the single most important research agenda for the decade. Advanced nursing practice research, as a part of nursing as a whole, offers researchers the ability to explore new and expanding areas that support the use of expert nurses as competent, sought-after providers of primary and specialty care for the American people.

CHARLENE M. HANSON

See also
**CLINICAL NURSE SPECIALIST
EDUCATION: NURSE RESEARCHERS
    AND ADVANCED PRACTICE NURSES
NURSE ANESTHETISTS AND RESEARCH
NURSE-MIDWIFERY**

ALCOHOLISM

The DSM-IV diagnostic category of alcohol dependence is commonly called alcoholism. Alcohol dependence is a disease characterized by abnormal alcohol-seeking behavior that leads to impaired control over drinking (National Institute on Alcohol Abuse and Alcoholism [NIAAA], 1993). A diagnosis of alcohol abuse refers to a pattern of use that results in detrimental effects on health or social life that may eventually lead to alcohol dependence.

Alcohol dependence (alcoholism) is a primary, chronic disease with genetic, psychosocial, and environmental factors that influence its development and manifestations. Alcoholism results after prolonged, continuous, or periodic use of alcohol. Alcoholism is noted when control over drinking is impaired, when preoccupation with alcohol occurs, and when use continues despite adverse consequences. The disease often is progressive and fatal. Distortions in thinking, most notably denial, result (Sullivan, 1995).

Alcohol is a depressant drug and is the most commonly used and abused substance of addiction. It is widely available, can be legally acquired by persons over 21 (in most states), and is relatively inexpensive.

Prolonged use of alcohol results in numerous physiological and psychological effects. Alcohol is metabolized by the liver; women may metabolize alcohol less efficiently than men. Liver damage often occurs as a result of prolonged use. Alcohol-induced cardiovascular injury, immune system impairment, and neurological disorders also can occur. Alcohol withdrawal syndrome is usually mild and self-limiting but in about 5% of cases can result in delirium tremens, which can be potentially fatal.

In contrast with other health problems, there is no definitive physical finding or laboratory test for alcoholism. Tests for liver function reveal end-stage organ damage; they do not detect the primary disorder.

Alcohol use has occurred throughout recorded history. Alcoholism has often been considered a moral failing caused by the availability of alcohol. The temperance movement and Prohibition were attempts to control alcoholism. The establishment of Alcoholics Anonymous in the early 1930s and the acceptance of alcoholism as a medical condition in the mid-1950s were more therapeutic efforts to address alcoholism.

Reflecting absence of societal interest and the health care community's lack of understanding, research and clinical reports about alcoholism have been sparse in the nursing literature and in nursing science. Prior to 1989, studies of alcohol abuse or alcoholism were often descriptive, addressed nurses' attitudes toward clients with alcohol problems, or studied nurses who were recovering from alcoholism (Naegle, 1995). Nurse researchers who have contributed to the early literature on alcoholism include Haack, Hughes, Naegle, and Sullivan, among others.

In fact, information about alcoholism has been scant in nursing curricula. Thus, nursing students and presumably future clinicians and scientists were not aware of the extent of alcoholism as a health problem, and few studies of this serious illness were pursued. Nurses, however, care for clients with alcoholism regularly. It has been estimated that 30%

of hospitalized patients have disorders secondary to alcohol abuse, such as trauma, falls, cirrhosis, pancreatitis, or cardiovascular disease (NIAAA, 1993). Further, 15% to 20% of clients seen in primary care settings are estimated to have alcohol disorders (Fleming & Barry, 1992).

Recent initiatives by the federal government have attempted to ameliorate the lack of content and expertise in nursing education. Beginning in 1989, the National Institute on Alcohol Abuse and Alcoholism (NIAAA), the National Institute on Drug Abuse (NIDA), and the Office of Substance Abuse Prevention (now the Center for Substance Abuse Prevention) established initiatives to improve substance abuse education in schools of nursing through model curriculum projects and faculty development programs. Three curriculum models are now available, and more than 60 faculty fellows from 13 schools of nursing have been prepared through the federal faculty development grants; some have now received funding for alcohol research from NIAAA. Reports of this work, however, are in progress and not yet available in the literature. However, empirically based studies examining clinical interventions are beginning to appear in the literature (Mudd, Boyd, Brower, Young, & Blow, 1994; Wing & Thompson, 1995).

The potential for improved access to information about alcoholism exists through the curriculum models and the expertise of faculty, some of whom will continue alcohol research efforts and will encourage alcohol research among their students. It must be noted, however, that most schools of nursing do not have faculty trained in these projects and must rely on individual initiative to develop or enhance alcohol-related content.

Alcohol remains the most widely used and abused drug in America. Nurses will continue to encounter the consequences of alcohol abuse and dependence among their clients. It is essential that nurses be cognizant of the dire results of excessive alcohol consumption and be participants in the efforts to rehabilitate alcoholic clients. Although past research has focused on such issues as alcohol abuse content in nursing education or nurses with alcohol problems—both important topics—nonetheless, future research must target intervention strategies to improve the care of clients with alcohol disorders.

The health of millions of clients with alcohol problems depends on it.

ELEANOR J. SULLIVAN

See also
ADOLESCENCE
COGNITIVE DISORDERS
DRUG ABUSE
VIOLENCE AS A NURSING AREA
    OF INQUIRY

ALZHEIMER'S DISEASE

Alzheimer's disease (AD) is the most common form of the dementias, a group of illnesses that affect the brain, eventually resulting in death. Alzheimer's disease is a progressive neurological disorder that proceeds in stages over months or years and gradually destroys reason, memory, judgment, language, and functional ability, according to the Agency for Health Care Policy and Research Practice Guidelines (Costa, Williams, Somerfield, et al., 1996). Although cognitive impairment is a major symptom, changes in mood and personality often occur. In the early stages of the illness, AD is sometimes confused with delirium (an acute reversible mental confusion) or psychiatric depression; both conditions occur in older adults. Depression may be an early part of AD, when the individual is aware of a decline from previous level of competence and is having multiple memory problems.

Alzheimer's disease is characterized by an accumulation of cortical neuritic plaques and neurofibrillary tangles in excess of those found in normal aged persons (Berg, 1994) and can be diagnosed accurately only by brain biopsy or autopsy. Thus, most cases are diagnosed as probable AD. Computerized tomography is sometime used to show changes in the size and shape of the brain, which may indicate probable AD but is not a definite measure. Because of insufficient knowledge about the illness, criteria for probable AD have been developed only recently. These criteria are found in the *Diagnostic and Statistical Manual of Mental Disorders* (DSM-IIIR).

Approximately 4 million people are diagnosed with dementia of the Alzheimer's type, formerly thought to be a presenile disease. Its prevalence increases as individuals reach old age. It is estimated that 20% of those 80 and over can be expected to develop AD (Dungee-Anderson & Beckett, 1992). The diagnosis of early AD is based on mental status exams and changes in behavior rather than by laboratory instruments. Alzheimer's disease continues to baffle the health professions although much light has been shed on the illness since it was discovered in 1920 by the German physician Alois Alzheimer. In early assessment of the illness, differentiation must be made between AD and delirium and between AD and depression so that proper counseling can be established. Medications that may cause symptoms of cognitive impairment also need assessment.

Quality-of-Life Issues

Quality-of-life issues have been raised for persons with AD because of the progressive decline that occurs in several stages. Reisberg (1984) has identified nine different stages of the disease process. Thus, early identification of AD is extremely critical for planning quality care. Once the diagnosis of probable AD has been established, the question arises as to what type of care is needed. The AD patient may require minimal care in the early stages, but the need for care escalates as the individual experiences increased cognitive impairment. As the disease progresses, the quality of life changes, independent self-functions decrease, and the individual becomes totally dependent on caregivers. Loss of control of body functions and the inability to carry out the activities of daily living require continuous attention from caregivers, who are often family members.

Unfortunately, the direct care of the AD patient affects the quality of life of the caregiver and of family members who are forced to provide informal caregiving services. The term ''sandwich generation'' has been used to describe the plight of middle-aged women who are sometimes caregivers to parents with AD at the same time that they are caregivers to their children. These caregivers often need help to determine how best to care for their relatives with AD and how not to neglect their own health. Studies have shown that there is increased morbidity and mortality among caregivers of persons with AD (George & Gwyther, 1986).

The care of persons with AD has a major impact on nursing practice. Special care needs of dementia patients require appropriate nursing interventions at different stages of decline and for individual variation in symptomatology. The task is often difficult when the major goal is to maintain as much quality of life as possible for the patient. There is no known cure for AD, and therefore it is a major challenge for health care professionals. The emotional component that accompanies the illness affects formal caregivers as well as persons with AD and their families. The degenerative nature of the disease, together with the cognitive and functional impairment, requires an increasing amount of caregiving time. Determining the distinctions between stages of dementia is necessary for planning nursing interventions. Nursing care for the AD patient begins with accurate assessment, diagnosis of the stages, expected outcomes, care planning and implementation, and evaluation of effective interventions.

Nursing practice with patients who have AD is a field that is ripe for nurse researchers. Nursing care is the single mode of treatment for the disease even though a few drugs for improving memory are on the market. There is a particular need to develop specific models of care for this complex illness. Watson's (1988) nursing model of human care is one example of a framework that provides a conceptual basis for provision of nursing care to AD patients and their families. The nursing activity is intentional and based on a knowledge of the changing needs of the person with AD. The nurse is a key part of the human transaction and is equally important in the relationship with the family caregiver. Watson's model is based on a humanistic view of the individual.

Because of the severe mental impairment and functional decline manifested by the disease, nursing research is sorely needed to deliver competent nursing care to the AD patient. Patients need help with bathing, feeding, toileting, dressing, mobility, and communications, and the caregiver needs social support as well as help to plan care and to utilize community services. One problem is the tendency of AD patients to develop behavior problems (Wykle & Morris, 1994). In research studies of caregivers, behavior problems are listed most often as major stress inducers for the caregiver. Acting out behavior is sometimes related to excitement, inability to remember faces, and strange environments. Behavior problems such as wandering or actions brought about by delusions, disorientation, and communication problems, vary in these individuals depending on the disease course.

Part of the nursing assessment should include a psychiatric evaluation simply because AD patients often have high levels of anxiety and depression. The nursing practice theory of progressively lower stimuli therapy (PLST), developed by Buckwalter (1989), is designed to provide a nonstimulating environment that will cause less catastrophic behavior reactions. Recently, there has been a trend toward designing special care units for AD patients who are placed in a nursing home or hospital. These special care settings take into consideration the individual needs of the client as well as the type of staffing pattern necessary to provide quality care and maintain a safe environment. There is also a trend toward using alternative methods of intervention, such as massage therapy and horticulture therapy. Nevertheless, there is still much that is unknown about AD, its manifestations, and effective nursing interventions. This disease that profoundly affects older adults and their quality of life is a high priority for nursing outcome research.

MAY L. WYKLE
GWI-RYUNG SON

See also
**ALZHEIMER'S DISEASE: SPECIAL
   CARE UNITS IN LONG-TERM CARE
CAREGIVER
COGNITIVE DISORDERS
NEUROBEHAVIORAL DISTURBANCES
   OF THE OLDER ADULT: DELERIUM
   AND DEMENTIA**

ALZHEIMER'S DISEASE: SPECIAL CARE UNITS IN LONG-TERM CARE

Following "transinstitutionalization" of persons with dementia from state mental hospitals to community nursing homes in the 1960s and 1970s,

Coons (1983), Danford (1982), and Lawton (1975) pioneered the study of the effects of the environment on behavior among the demented. Their work influenced investigations of rehabilitative interventions (e.g., reality orientation, pet and music therapies, and behavioral and psychotherapies) designed to improve care for institutionalized persons with dementia. One result was the suggestion by nurses and others that integrating demented and nondemented residents may violate the rights of both parties and jeopardize quality of life and safety.

Special care units (SCU) in nursing homes for persons with Alzheimer's disease (AD) and related dementing disorders emerged rapidly in the 1980s. AD is the most prevalent type of dementia; however, the disease cannot be definitively diagnosed prior to autopsy. More than one cause of dementia often afflicts an individual, and persons with all types present many of the same care problems. For these reasons, SCUs usually serve persons with dementias of all types. Currently about 15% of nursing homes in the United States have an SCU. The number of SCUs may continue to increase for two or three decades because of growth in the number of elderly, the public's perception that SCU care is superior to traditional nursing home care, and the likelihood that SCUs will be profitable. However, other options for care, such as assisted living facilities, offer a lower cost advantage and may curtail the growth of SCUs.

Five key features are recognized as characterizing an SCU: (1) admission of residents with dementia, (2) special staff specification, selection, and training, (3) activity programming tailored to residents with dementia, (4) family programming and involvement, and (5) a segregated and modified physical and social environment. Although there is substantial consensus that these five features distinguish SCUs, there is disagreement about the specific nature of special programming, staffing, and services.

Care of persons with dementia and their families in all settings is an important aspect of gerontological and geropsychiatric nursing research as well as a National Institute for Nursing Research (NINR) priority. Leading nurse researchers in the care of persons with dementia on SCUs are Buckwalter, Maas, Hall, Matthew, and Ryden. Other research-

ers, primarily supported by NINR and the National Institute of Aging (NIA), also study SCUs.

Studies of Special Care Units

Hall and Buckwalter's (1987) progressively lowered stress threshold (PLST) model provided the conceptual framework for the development of many SCUs and for research to evaluate their effects. Descriptive studies have documented the characteristics of nursing homes that offer SCUs. State and regional surveys provide detailed information about the programs and practices of SCUs in particular geographic areas, and national surveys contribute information about structures, programming, and staffing that are characteristic of nursing facilities and SCUs nationwide. Survey results are limited by methodological differences that restrict comparisons.

Most early evaluative studies conducted by nurse researchers and others were single group efforts that assessed selected characteristics of residents with AD, family members, and staff at intervals before and after SCU admission. These studies documented some positive outcomes, including decreased nighttime wakefulness, improved hygiene, and weight gain in residents. Only half of the studies found improvement in resident physical function and behavioral symptoms. Confidence in these studies is compromised by small sample size, lack of rigor in design, potential researcher bias, and unclear outcome measure definitions.

Other studies compared outcomes for residents with dementia on a SCU with those in another setting, measuring selected characteristics of residents, family members, and staff caregivers at intervals. Only two studies revealed significant benefits for residents on the SCUs, contrasted with comparison residents, noting less functional decline (Rovner, Lucas-Blaustein, Folstein, & Smith, 1990), fewer catastrophic reactions, and increased social interaction (Maas & Buckwalter, 1990). Results for family members also were mixed, with one study finding significant decreases in feelings of depression, anxiety, guilt, and grief compared to family members in the control group (Wells & Jorm, 1987). Only one study found statistically significant reductions in staff stress and burnout and a statistically significant increase in job satisfaction (Maas & Buckwalter, 1990).

In 1991 the NIA Special Care Units Initiative supported 10 studies for 5 years to systematically study the characteristics and effects of SCUs. Preliminary results indicated few benefits for residents and family members or differences in costs of care in SCUs versus other settings. Staff caregivers, however, continue to report that persons with AD are better cared for and that staff can provide care more easily on SCUs (Work Group on Research and Evaluation of SCUs, 1996). Some investigators suggest that current instruments used in SCU research are inadequate to measure these staff perceptions.

Another group of studies measured specific interventions or modifications of SCUs rather than the SCU strategy as a whole. Nursing studies of pet therapy, music therapy, bathing, dressing, eating assistance, wandering deterrent strategies, specific environmental modifications, and staff training are among the interventions that have been systematically tested with positive effects for demented residents. Interventions to assist family members with their caregiving roles on SCUs also are being tested (Maas, Swanson, Reed, & Specht, 1996).

Large national nursing home data bases are now used to describe characteristics of facilities and SCUs and to study the cost of care on SCUs versus care on traditional nursing home units. Results support the findings from other studies that the cost of care on SCUs is comparable to costs on other units.

Issues in SCU Research

SCU field research is fraught with methodological problems that make achieving and maintaining rigorous study designs difficult. Potential sources of bias are inherent in the selection of study sites; resident, family, and staff subjects; and outcome measures. Overall better care in nonprofit versus for-profit homes, irrespective of the SCU, may explain results. Newer SCUs may have less impaired residents, and turnover of staff is greater. Differences in SCU size, nature of the environment, type of programming, admission and discharge policies,

the nursing care delivery system, staff ratios and staff mix, and the type and amount of staff training are some additional variables that influence outcomes. Administrators, clinicians, and family members usually determine whether or not a resident is placed on an SCU and may disrupt randomization by transfer of residents or staff. Residents are seldom randomly assigned to treatment groups within facilities because of contamination issues. Family members are assigned to groups because of their relationships to residents and staff by administrative decision. Subject attrition is a huge problem. Most studies employ quasi-experimental designs with nonequivalent control groups at the outset or experiments become quasi-experiments due to subject attrition. The myriad of resident, family, and staff characteristics, such as comorbidity, type of dementia, health, or education, pose measurement challenges.

Although development of standardized resident, family, and staff outcome measures has progressed, measures that capture clinically meaningful change may not be available due to floor or ceiling effects or inadequate sensitivity and validity with ethnic minority populations.

Summary and Future Research Recommendations

To date, research by nurses and others has not clearly established the efficacy of SCUs for residents with dementia, family members, or staff caregivers. Efforts to systematically document the cost effectiveness of SCUs also have not yielded clear results. The few positive findings from studies are counter to the prevailing views of nursing home providers and consumers. Most staff members believe that SCUs benefit residents and families as well as staff, who find it easier to care for demented residents on SCUs. Future nursing research must focus on documenting what is special about SCU care; refining measures of the SCU environment and programming; developing more sensitive outcome measures for residents, families, and staff; conducting larger multisite studies; evaluating the SCU strategy with minority populations; and using existing national datasets to analyze cost effectiveness.

MERIDEAN L. MAAS
JANET P. SPECHT

See also
ALZHEIMER'S DISEASE
MIDDLE-RANGE THEORIES OF
   DEMENTIA CARE
NEUROBEHAVIORAL DISTURBANCES
   OF THE OLDER ADULT: DELERIUM
   AND DEMENTIA
PHYSICAL RESTRAINTS FOR THE
   ELDERLY

AMERICAN ACADEMY OF NURSING

The idea of a national academy of nurses was first noted in the 1946 Rich Report ("Comprehensive Program," 1945). The Rich Report had been commissioned 2 years earlier by six major nursing organizations and contained an extensive plan for a national academy of nurses. The vision of the national academy put forth in the Rich Report did not receive attention in the massive welter of changes that was taking place in the large associations of professional nursing at that time.

At the 1964 biennial convention business meeting of the American Nurses Association (ANA), the House of Delegates received a motion from the floor to study and report to the next convention the feasibility of and/or a plan for the establishment of the American Academy of Nursing (AAN). The motion carried unanimously. From 1964 to 1972, various committees studied the idea of an academy and explored issues of purpose, membership, and the relationship to ANA. In 1972 the ANA board agreed to initiate the AAN and in January 1973 met to evaluate nominations and select charter fellows. The board of directors of the ANA selected the 36 charter fellows in 1973. During the next 9 years the governing council of the AAN selected the fellows. In 1981 the body of fellows elected a membership committee that was responsible for the fellow selection process. For the following 10 years

that committee selected candidates for fellowship and presented them to the total membership for vote. Successful ratification of the candidates by the fellowship was followed by induction into fellow status that occurred at the annual meeting. Since 1993 the selection process has been given to an elected Fellows Selection Committee that is charged with the responsibility for all aspects of the process (McCarthy, 1985).

Criteria for selection to fellowship are (a) membership in a state nurses association that holds membership in ANA, (b) evidence of outstanding contributions to nursing and health care, and (c) evidence of potential to continue to contribute to nursing and to the academy. In 1997 there are 986 active fellows, 146 emeritus fellows, and 19 honorary fellows.

> The purpose of the Academy is delineated in the Bylaws. The Bylaws state: The purpose of the Academy shall be to provide visionary leadership to the nursing profession and the public in shaping future health care policy and practice that optimizes the well-being of the American people through synthesis of scientific and philosophical knowledge as the basis for effective health care policy and practice. (American Academy of Nursing, 1996, Article 2)

The work of the fellows of the academy has been reflected over the years in many books and reports that have addressed the major issues confronting the profession. One of the most notable of the works of the fellows is the acclaimed "magnet hospital" study (McClure, Poulin, Sovie, & Wandelt, 1983), identifying what made certain hospitals attractive places for nurses to work: First, administration is supportive of professional nursing practice; second, there is a teaching-learning environment; and third, the process is open to change, and nursing has significant input into that change. The findings of this study continue to inform administrators, and it has been asserted that this study was a benchmark in the work of the academy. The report demonstrated that nurses could, should, and did claim the right to study their own domain and control their own turf. And, the study exemplified reframing as a valuable strategy for studying issues of public policy, that is, asking what is right and how to build on those features rather than asking what is wrong, the more typical approach.

In 1991, in collaboration with Mosby–Year Book Company, the academy adopted *Nursing Outlook* as its official journal. The work of the AAN is often presented in *Nursing Outlook*. The AAN currently has 12 expert panels that publish reports of their work in *Nursing Outlook* as well as in monographs and other periodicals.

GRAYCE M. SILLS

See also
AMERICAN NURSES ASSOCIATION
AMERICAN NURSES ASSOCIATION
COUNCIL FOR NURSING RESEARCH

AMERICAN ASSOCIATION OF COLLEGES OF NURSING

The American Association of Colleges of Nursing (AACN) is a national voice for baccalaureate and higher-degree programs in nursing. AACN's educational, research, governmental advocacy, data collection, publications, and other programs work to establish quality standards for bachelor's- and graduate-degree nursing education, assist deans and directors to implement those standards, influence the nursing profession to improve health care, and promote public support of baccalaureate and graduate nursing education, research, and practice.

AACN was founded in 1969 and represents more than 500 schools of nursing nationwide that offer baccalaureate, graduate, and postgraduate programs.

AACN is a leader in securing sustained federal support for nursing education and research, in shaping legislative and regulatory policy affecting nursing school programming, and in ensuring continuing financial assistance for nursing students. In addition, AACN's national databank reports the most current statistics available on student enrollments and graduations, faculty salaries, institutional resources, and other trends and conditions in baccalaureate and graduate nursing education.

In 1986, AACN directed the national panel that defined the knowledge and skills needed by graduates of America's bachelor's-degree nursing educa-

tion programs. AACN publishes and disseminates these baccalaureate "essentials" to nursing schools and policy makers throughout the nation and revises its teaching components to stay current with changing conditions in nursing and in health care. AACN also publishes core standards for the education of advanced practice nurses and all other registered nurses who are prepared at the master's-degree level, as well as indicators of quality doctoral nursing programs.

AACN's publications include the *Journal of Professional Nursing* and *SYLLABUS* newsletter, as well as a variety of books and directories.

Carole A. Anderson

See also
DOCTORAL EDUCATION
HEALTH POLICY
NURSING EDUCATION

AMERICAN MEDICAL INFORMATICS ASSOCIATION

The American Medical Informatics Association (AMIA) is a nonprofit membership organization. AMIA was consolidated in late 1990 following discussions among the Boards of Directors of the American Association for Medical Systems and Informatics (AAMSI), the American College of Medical Informatics (ACMI), and the Symposium on Computer Applications in Medical Care (SCAMC).

As stated in its strategic plan and policy manual, AMIA "is the premier association in the United States dedicated to the development and application of medical informatics in the support of patient care, teaching, research, and health care administration." AMIA's mission is "to advance the public interest through charitable, scientific, literary, and educational activities."

AMIA serves as an authoritative body in the field of medical informatics and represents the United States in the informational arena of medical systems and informatics in international forums.

Included among our 3,700 members are the developers of clinical information systems, academically based health care professionals devoted to the applications of computers in clinical care, and users of health care information systems. Members include physicians, nurses, educators, computer and information scientists, biomedical engineers, medical librarians, and academic researchers.

The American College of Medical Informatics (ACMI) is a college of elected fellows who have made significant contributions in the field of medical informatics. Initially incorporated in 1984, the organization later dissolved its separate corporate status to merge with two other organizations when AMIA was formed. ACMI now exists as an elected college of fellows within AMIA, with its own by-laws and regulations that guide the organization, its activities, and its relationship with AMIA.

AMIA's Advisory Council comprises 28 organizations with a broad span of influence and importance in medicine and biomedical engineering. This group has acted as a forum to discuss broad issues and to give AMIA advice on how to proceed on public policy issues. It is an important part of AMIA's strategic planning process and serves as a sounding board for discussion of a range of topics.

Carole A. Gassert

See also
CLINICAL INFORMATION SYSTEMS
COMPUTER-BASED DOCUMENTATION
IN PATIENT CARE
NURSING INFORMATICS

AMERICAN NURSES ASSOCIATION

The American Nurses Association (ANA) was established 100 years ago, in 1897. Created to promote the professional and educational advancement of nurses, the ANA has given nurses the vehicle through which to present issues affecting nursing and the general welfare of the nurse. In its 100-year history, the ANA has fostered nursing research, promoted nursing practice legislation, encouraged development of advanced and continuing education programs, and stimulated the establishment and implementation of standards of nursing practice, nursing service, and nursing education.

Isabel Hampton Robb, the first president of the ANA, reflected on the first 25-year period, "We . . . close the first quarter of a century of our history with the knowledge that our chief weakness during these years has come from the rapid increase in numbers, from the want of a professional and educational standard and from the scattering of our forces from lack of organization" (ANA, 1976, p. 38).

The national organization realized the need for studies and focused efforts in three areas: (a) selection and preparation of students in schools of nursing, (b) distribution of nursing services, and (c) status and employment conditions of nurses. A study supported by the Rockefeller Foundation resulted in the publication of *Nursing and Nursing Education in the United States*, best known as the Winslow-Goldmark Report of 1923. Another major study was commissioned to investigate the supply and demand for nursing services, a job analysis of nursing and nurse teaching, and the grading of nursing schools; it resulted in the book *Nurses, Patients and Pocketbook*.

In 1951 the ANA established the American Nurses' Foundation (ANF) as a research, education, and charitable affiliate. The foundation raises funds and supports a small grants program. The ANF supports pilot studies on priority issues for the profession, creates education programs, and publishes needed resources. ANF projects have included: (a) the Community-Based Health Care Project, which developed nurse/consumer partnerships in addressing community needs; (b) the Every Child By Two campaign for early immunizations for children; and (c) school health projects implemented through the ANA state nurses associations.

The ANA established the Council for Nurse Researchers in 1971. This council provided leadership in identifying future needs for the development of a strong research base for the profession. The ANA led efforts to develop a standard classification scheme for nursing languages and identified data elements that should be included in national health care data bases. The ANA also completed early research on ethical issues affecting nursing practice and clinical decisions.

The ANA is an advocate for nursing research, encouraging the establishment of the Nursing Research Grants and Fellowship Program in the U.S. Public Health Service in 1955. The initial federal programs focused on the preparation of nurse researchers. The ANA was the primary organization to lobby for funding for nursing research and education throughout the early development of nursing research in schools of nursing. In 1983 the ANA initiated and encouraged legislation to create an institute for nursing research at the National Institutes of Health (NIH). This effort led to the establishment of the National Center for Nursing Research at NIH in 1985 and to the ultimate legislation in 1993 that recognized the center as the National Institute of Nursing Research (NINR).

Besides lobbying for nursing research at the federal level, the ANA also has worked to set the direction and priorities for research, working with other nursing organizations and several federal agencies throughout the years. For example, the ANA supported efforts to develop the "Nurse Staffing and Quality of Care in Health Care Organizations Research Agenda," a national effort supported by the Agency for Health Care Policy and Research, the NINR, and the Division of Nursing of the Health Service Research Awards. The ANA has supported the National Nursing Research Roundtable (NNRR) from its inception. It also has held research conferences on a regular basis and encouraged the dissemination of research findings within the nursing community and to the public.

Research efforts within the ANA continue to focus on the nursing profession—quality and staffing. In 1995 there was a special initiative to identify the linkages between nurse staffing, hospital organization variables, and outcomes of nursing care. The ANA began pilot studies of "Nursing's Report Card for Acute Care" and tested the feasibility of using large state hospital databases to acquire data on nursing's quality indicators in relation to nurse staffing. It is also in the process of establishing a national database of nursing quality indicators.

JANET HEINRICH

See also
AMERICAN ACADEMY OF NURSING
AMERICAN NURSES ASSOCIATION
COUNCIL FOR NURSING RESEARCH

NATIONAL INSTITUTE OF NURSING RESEARCH

AMERICAN NURSES ASSOCIATION COUNCIL FOR NURSING RESEARCH

Historically, the American Nurses Association (ANA) has recognized the importance of nursing science and nursing research to the discipline of nursing and the scientific development of the profession (ANA, 1992b). In the second half of the 20th century, a period of rapid growth in nursing science, there has been great need to aggressively showcase nursing research to the federal government and state legislatures as well as to other health disciplines. Simultaneously, there has been great need to educate nurses themselves about the importance of research in ensuring the credibility of the discipline. These have been two major components of the ANA's research mission.

The ANA's long-standing recognition of the essential role of research has been manifested in its organizational structure, which traditionally has included a standing research committee. In the years that predated the creation of a nursing institute at the National Institutes of Health, the ANA's research mission was enacted by two ANA organizational bodies: the ANA Cabinet on Nursing Research and the ANA Council for Nurse Researchers.

The ANA Cabinet on Nursing Research (1985) assumed primary responsibility for educating others, including nurses, about nursing research, and to this end it produced a number of formal position statements and published documents. Position statements addressed a range of research topics, for example, *Representation of Nurses on Institutional Research Review Committees* (1974), *Statement on Nursing Research Facilities Needs in Academic and Clinical Research Institutions* (1988), and *Responsible Use of Animals in Nursing Research* (1988).

Publications by the ANA Cabinet generally were aimed at informing nurses, other disciplines, legislators, and the general public about the importance of nursing research to the health of the American people. Examples of such publications include (a) *Directions for Nursing Research: Toward the*

Twenty-First Century (ANA Cabinet, 1985); (b) *Research in Nursing: Toward a Science of Nursing* (Clinton & McCormick, 1987); (c) *Education for Participation in Nursing Research* (ANA, 1989); and (d) *Developing Taxonomies for Nursing Research* (Germain & Dodd, 1993).

The other research body of the ANA, the Council of Nurse Researchers, assumed primary responsibility for representing the interests of nurse researchers. In this role it assumed leadership for sponsoring biannual national and international research conferences so that nurse researchers might achieve shared goals of showcasing their findings to nursing and the public, enhancing the training of future nurse scientists, and networking within the nursing scientific community. In achieving these goals, the ANA Council for Nurse Researchers collaborated with the regional nursing research societies. By 1990 the ANA had restructured its organization by sunsetting all of the cabinets. Thus, at that time the Council for Nurse Researchers became the single ANA research committee.

By the 1990s, societal needs and forces had shifted toward fiscal restraint and a mandate to focus on clinical practice effectiveness and outcomes. The ANA (1992c) put forward a major initiative, captured in its publication *Nursing's Agenda for Health Care Reform*, to influence the nation's organization of health care delivery toward effective, accessible, affordable, and humane health care for all. This document called for a focus on verifying the essential role of nursing in achieving these goals and for measuring the effectiveness of nursing practice.

In 1994, the ANA's council structure evolved again; the Council for Nurse Researchers became the Council for Nursing Research. As indicated by the name change, its mission changed from one of primarily representing nurse researchers to one of primarily advancing the ANA's research agenda on behalf of the discipline, that is, to focus on scientific processes directed toward the generation and testing of nursing knowledge. This is the central concern of the ANA Council for Nursing Research. To that end, the ANA Council for Nursing Research

1. collaborates with other nursing research organizations to plan the national nursing research agenda that supports improved health of all people and the evolution of nursing practice;
2. promotes private and public support for nursing research;
3. plans and coordinates the dissemination of nursing research findings and research database development;
4. promotes increased exploration of the health care needs of culturally diverse populations; and
5. serves as a resource regarding ethics, culture, nursing practice standards of care, and human rights as they relate to nursing research.

VIRGINIA P. TILDEN

See also
AMERICAN ACADEMY OF NURSING
AMERICAN NURSES ASSOCIATION

APPLIED RESEARCH

In an attempt to differentiate between various types of research, the scientific community uses a myriad of terms, which, however, tend to fall into a discrete classification. On the one end, terms such as *basic*, *fundamental*, and *theoretical* research are used to refer to research focused on discovering fundamental principles and processes governing physical and life phenomena. On the other end, we find such terms as *applied*, *clinical*, *practical*, and *product* research. These refer to the application of the findings of basic/fundamental/theoretical research to generate research aimed at answering focused and problem-specific questions. Though it is the subject of ongoing debate, we assume that there are fundamental principles and processes that are core to the discipline and its central tenets of health, patient, nurse, and environment. In addition, we assume that nursing draws on fundamental principles and processes discovered in other disciplines to generate new knowledge about nursing and patient care.

Under these assumptions, we can define applied research in nursing. The etymology of *applied* goes back to the Latin *ad-plicare*, meaning to put something (a law, a test, etc.) into practical operation.

Applied research in nursing, then, refers to research aimed at concrete and practical issues and questions of concern to the delivery of nursing care. The most evident type of applied research is intervention research—from exploratory investigations to rigorous clinical trials. This type of applied research is aimed at providing answers to questions about the effectiveness and efficacy of nursing interventions.

Yet nonintervention (or descriptive) research may be categorized as applied research as well if it meets the general criterion of being focused on concrete and practical issues and questions about nursing care. For instance, understanding the dynamics of clinical and subclinical noncompliance in transplant patients and their relationship to the occurrence of adverse posttransplant events helps nurses and other health professionals in developing interventions to enhance adherence to prescribed drug regimens (De Geest, Borgermans, et al., 1995). Developing risk profiles for institutionalization among various cohorts of community-dwelling elderly furthers our knowledge base for designing preventive strategies and models of care for patients, caregivers, and families (Abraham, Currie, Neese, Yi, Thompson-Heisterman, 1994; Steeman, Abraham, & Godderis, 1997).

In addition to effectiveness and efficacy, applied research in nursing also refers to cost calculations of nursing interventions. Managing the costs of care is a major issue in health care, and health care workers need evidence about the cost-effectiveness of the interventions used. For instance, implementation of a modified isolation protocol incorporating only those elements with proven effectiveness in the care of heart transplant recipients can be a source of considerable cost savings (De Geest, Kesteloot, Degryse, & Vanhaecke, 1995). Clinical and cost comparisons of preoperative skin preparation procedures in coronary artery bypass graft (CABG) patients provide additional data to support the necessary process of altering routine nursing practice to evidence-based nursing (De Geest et al., 1996).

Ivo L. Abraham
Sabina De Geest

See also
CLINICAL NURSING RESEARCH

**COST ANALYSIS OF NURSING CARE
EVIDENCE-BASED PRACTICE**

ARTIFICIAL INTELLIGENCE

The term *artificial intelligence* (AI) was first used in 1956 at a computer conference at Dartmouth College. Artificial intelligence has been variously defined as: the design and operation of computer systems capable of improved performance based on (a) experience (i.e., learning), (b) the computerization of activities that people believe involve thinking (such as problem solving and decision making), and (c) the development of computer systems that exhibit what people describe as intelligence, or the ability to reason and learn from experience. All three defined areas—machine learning, decision making, and reasoning—have produced distinct lines of research.

Typical areas of AI research include cognitive models of human learning, machine learning models, case-based learning models, and neural network research. The Navy Center for Applied Research in Artificial Intelligence conducts advanced research in several of these fields, especially those of machine learning, sensor-based control of autonomous activity, integration of varieties of reasoning to support complex decision making, and neural networks. Other major centers of AI development are located at Massachusetts Institute of Technology, the University of Georgia, and SRI International (produces commercial AI products).

Four capabilities have been identified for a computer to be able to produce an artificially intelligent product. First, it must be programmed with natural language processing to enable successful communication in a human language. Second, it must have a strategy for knowledge representation so that it can store its own knowledge base as well as the information input by the user. Third, it must have programming that provides it with one or more information-processing and problem-solving strategies. Fourth, it must have machine learning strategies programmed. The research areas in AI that hold the most promise for nursing applications are machine learning, expert systems, and knowledge engineering and representation. The fourth requirement needs further definition because how a machine learns mimics a human process that may not be known to all readers.

Machine Learning

Much work has been done on machine learning and reasoning in Defense Department laboratories. Machine learning requires the machine to evaluate its own performance and to change its decision-making strategies when performance success drops below predetermined acceptability levels. In general, this area of research focuses on pattern recognition and pattern reconstruction. Pattern recognition is a major source of human understanding, and making changes in mental problem-solving patterns is one definition of learning. Learning has been defined as adaptation to new circumstances by extrapolating the parameters of the problem and the deficiencies of the old problem-solving pattern to newly constructed patterns. The new patterns are tested until a more successful pattern is found. Thus, pattern recognition and elaboration is defined as the nature of learning.

When machines are programmed to recognize ineffectiveness of existing patterns and to construct and test changes in those patterns until a new pattern proves more successful, they are considered to exhibit machine learning. This area of research has produced significant new knowledge and applications in the defense industry. Of greater interest to nursing, it also led to new understandings about human reasoning and ways to improve human thinking, problem solving, and decision making. Woolery et al. (Woolery, Grzymala-Busse, Summers, & Budihardjo, 1991) examined the use of machine learning for development of expert systems in nursing.

The term *AI* has been used to refer to both expert systems and true artificially intelligent systems. The confusion stems from differences among users in the meaning of the term *intelligence*. The AI literature discusses two capacities of human intelligence: reasoning and learning from experience. All expert systems reason; that is, they apply one or more problem-solving strategies to specific information provided by a user and produce expert advice (or

a decision) as a product. When humans perform this process, they are using reason. Some AI researchers add the requirement for machine learning to the definition of AI. Computer systems that are sophisticated enough to analyze their own performance and change their processing strategies in response to ''experience'' are said to learn. The capacity to learn is what differentiates AI from expert decision-support systems that do not achieve the level of true intelligence. It is typical to find the terms *AI* and *expert system* used interchangeably. However, the term *AI* should be restricted to systems that both reason and learn from experience.

Expert Systems

In nursing the majority of publications that list AI as a search keyword address computerized nursing expert systems, which are usually clinical decision-support tools. The terms *expert systems* and *decision-support systems* are used interchangeably. Primarily, these are systems that help support decisions about nursing assessment or care planning. Much work also has been done on nurse staffing and scheduling systems, such as the MEDICUS or GRASP systems. These are management decision support systems that could also be considered expert systems for management. Decision-support systems may serve as an on-line reference without much reasoning ability. Poison control centers use such systems to determine the lethality and antidotes (if any) to a variety of substances considered to be poisonous to human beings.

Other types of expert systems accept data input from the user and provide a recommended course of action based on a preprogrammed problem-solving strategy. Still others guide the user in the selection of one or more problem-solving algorithms. The latter system may not offer action recommendations but merely serve to support a logical, systematic approach to the user's own problem-solving abilities.

Knowledge Engineering and Knowledge Representation

Another line of nursing scholarship in the field of AI involves knowledge engineering in nursing

(Chase, 1988). Knowledge engineering is a subfield of AI that seeks to understand the ways in which nursing experts conceptualize and define nursing problems and how they think about developing problem-solving strategies. Knowledge representation studies focus on a component of knowledge engineering. This field seeks methods of representing (programming and storing) information and human thinking processes in the computer. Knowledge is ultimately extracted from study of the ways that highly successful experts mentally depict external reality (knowledge representation) and from study of experts' problem-solving techniques, strategies, and approaches.

Importance for Nursing

Just as a hammer is a tool that expands the power of the human hand, the computer is a tool that can expand the power of the human mind. Artificial intelligence can greatly enhance the power of human cognition. The knowledge base of health science has increased exponentially over the past 20 years. The amount and complexity of information available for clinical situations can easily exceed the ability of an unaided nurse to use that information clinically. The human mind evolved to function under relatively simple survival conditions, not to integrate multiple, highly complex, technical sources of information nor to calculate interaction effects and probable outcomes of many variables. Unassisted, people cannot do that kind of work with an acceptable degree of consistency. Yet that level of information processing is exactly what modern science (and the U.S. legal system) demands of nurses. When the requirements of a task exceed human performance parameters, people must have tools that expand their capabilities. Artificial intelligence is one type of tool that can be developed to support and expand nurses' cognitive abilities so that they function in the sophisticated health care environment.

MARY L. McHUGH

See also
COMPUTERIZED DECISION SUPPORT SYSTEMS

NURSING INFORMATICS REPRESENTATION OF KNOWLEDGE FOR COMPUTATIONAL MODELING IN NURSING: THE *arcs*© PROGRAM VIRTUAL REALITY

ATTITUDES

Definition

An attitude can be defined as the person's evaluation (like or dislike) associated with an object. An attitude object can be anything that is discriminated by the person. Attitudes lie within the person and predispose them to respond. These responses are typically divided into three types: cognitive, affective, and behavioral (Eagly, 1992). Cognitive responses are beliefs or thoughts associated with the attitude object. Affective responses consist of emotions such as positive or negative feelings associated with the object. Behavioral responses are actions toward the attitude object that reflect favorable or unfavorable evaluations (Stroebe & Stroebe, 1995). Attitudes are thought to be acquired both directly through personal experience with an attitude object and indirectly through social learning (e.g., classical conditioning and modeling) from other persons (Baron & Byrne, 1994).

Attitudes and Behavior

The primary reason attitudes are relevant for nursing practice is their power to affect responses, especially behavioral responses related to health. This relationship between attitudes and behaviors has long been studied by social psychologists. Current research indicates that attitudes are related to behavior, but the relationship is not a simple one. Although attitudes had long been assumed to influence behavior, early research failed to support a strong causal relationship between them. It was the inability to predict behavior from attitudes that led to new approaches to understanding the relationship between attitudes and behavior. Social psychology has two different schools of thought about how attitudes affect behaviors, reflected in two models: expectancy-value and automatic processing.

Expectancy-Value Model

The rationale behind the expectancy-value model is that the process linking attitudes to behaviors is a reasoned one. According to this model (Fishbein & Ajzen, 1975), attitudes influence behavior through behavioral intentions or the intention to engage in the behavior. The direct antecedents of these behavioral intentions are (a) the attitude toward the behavior and (b) the subjective norm, which is the person's perception of the extent to which important others think that he or she should engage in the behavior. Ajzen (1988) revised this model by including additional concepts. The most popular revision is the theory of planned behavior; it proposes an additional predictor of behavioral intention, perceived behavioral control, which is the person's perception of how easy or difficult it will be to perform the behavior. Proponents of expectancy-value models point out that the degree of correspondence between the specificity of the attitude and the specificity of the behavior is important. If the correspondence between level of specificity of the attitude and the behavior are similar, attitudes are stronger predictors of behavior. For example, an attitude toward a specific object (taking hypertension medication) would be a better predictor of the behavior of taking hypertension medication than would a more global attitude toward maintaining a healthy lifestyle. The major criticism of these models is that they do not account for the role of well-established habits nor behavior that occurs with little or no thought or planning.

Attitude Accessibility Model

The attitude accessibility model, which was developed by Fazio and Williams (1986), proposed that attitudes are not carefully reasoned as proposed in the above model. In contrast, this model proposes that attitudes are automatically accessed in memory without conscious awareness and influence behavior directly (Baron & Byrne, 1994). An important component of this model is attitude accessibility, or the ease with which attitudes can be brought from memory. The more accessible the attitude, the greater the strength of the association in memory between the attitude object and its evaluation, the more readily the attitude is activated, and the stronger the attitude's influence on behavior. Therefore, anything that would lead to an attitude becoming more accessible would lead to behaviors that are consistent with the attitude. For example, when the attitude is derived from direct experience with the attitude object, attitude accessibility is more rapid, and the relationship between attitudes and behavior is stronger (Eagly, 1992).

Implications for Nursing

The attitude-behavior relationship is relevant for nursing practice because nurses commonly intervene to assist persons in changing health behaviors. The expectancy-value model of attitude has been used much more extensively as a framework to guide health behavior than has the attitude accessibility model (Stroebe & Stroebe, 1995). The expectancy-value model is better developed than the accessibility model, and the process by which attitudes influence behavior is more specified. The expectancy-value model provides a framework on which to build nursing interventions by providing an understanding about the beliefs and perceptions that shape attitudes and subjective norms. These beliefs and perceptions are appropriate targets of intervention by nurses, and bringing about changes in them can ultimately influence health behavior. With further development the attitude accessibility model will have implications for nursing practice through improving our understanding of circumstances when intentions to stop negative health behaviors (e.g., overeating) are not predictive of the behavior (Stroebe & Stroebe, 1995). Eagly (1992) suggests that research combining both models will lead to a more complete understanding of the attitude-behavior relationship.

JOAN K. AUSTIN

See also
ADHERENCE/COMPLIANCE

ATTRIBUTION THEORY
BEHAVIORAL RESEARCH
SOCIETY OF BEHAVIORAL MEDICINE

ATTRIBUTION THEORY

Definition and Assumptions

Nursing has traditionally maintained that nursing assessment should build on patients' perceptions of their situation, and the central concern of attribution theory is people's intuitive assignment of causality. Attributions are important because individuals respond not to events per se but to their cognitive representations of those events.

An attribution is the inference that individuals make about the causes of either their behavior or that of another person. Attribution theory assumes that people are constructive thinkers searching to explain important events confronting them, then acting on their imperfect knowledge of causal structure in ways they consider to be appropriate. This theoretical perspective makes three broad assumptions: (1) individuals regularly attempt to assign causes for important instances of their behavior and that of others; (2) there are patterns that can be uncovered in this assignment of causes; (3) the particular causes that individuals attribute for a given event have important consequences for their subsequent motivation, emotion, and behavior.

Clinically Relevant Causal Attributions

Most of the clinically relevant research to date describing causal attributions and the consequences of various attributional patterns has been based on the work of Seligman (Peterson, Maier, & Seligman, 1993), Weiner (1986), and their associates. Attributions have been most frequently categorized in terms of locus (internal/external), stability (fixed/variable), controllability (controllable/uncontrollable), and globality (global/specific). There is considerable evidence that some of these dimensions have differential consequences for affect, expectancy, and behavior. For example, people feel maximum pride in a success situation when they attribute their performance to internal causes; failure attributed to internal causes results in more shame than when attributed to external causes. Failure attributed to variable causes results in a higher expectancy for future success than attributions to fixed causes; success attributed to stable causes results in higher expectations for future success than do attributions to unstable causes. Individuals are held more accountable for their mistakes when a failure is due to controllable factors. Those who tend to explain negative life events with internal, stable, and global explanations (learned helplessness) are more prone to depression than those who make external, unstable, and specific explanations for such events.

Another related line of inquiry has noted that actors and observers are both guilty of the fundamental attribution error—attributing more causal force to dispositional explanations ("she is a bad mother") than to situational explanations ("she was ineffective because of constraints in that situation"), though actors are given to making more use of situational attributions than are observers. The actor-observer effect, as this difference has come to be termed, builds on the notion first proffered by Heider "that people invoke as causal those factors that engulf their perceptual field" (Robins, Mendelsohn, & Spranca, 1996, p. 375). Because the situation is front and center in the actor's perceptual field but the actor is more noticeable to the observer than the situation prompting the actor, it is no wonder that explanations are greatly affected by these differences in points of view.

Methodology

Explanatory style has been measured by various methods, for example, the Attributional Style Questionnaire (ASQ), which was later expanded to become the Expanded Attributional Style Questionnaire (EASQ) and then developed into a 48-item forced-choice version; the Content Analysis of Verbatim Explanations (CAVE); and the Children's Attributional Style Questionnaire (CASQ). In various studies using these methods, a pessimistic explanatory style has been linked to poorer physical and mental health (Buchanan & Seligman, 1995).

Though these measurement techniques assess explanations for positive events, the explanations for positive events have been less predictive than explanations for negative events, in part because of fewer theoretical underpinnings. The cycle linking pessimistic explanatory style to illness remains to be fully explored. It is hypothesized that uncontrollable events lead to increased endorphins, which in turn interfere with the functioning of the immune system, thus limiting the ability to fight off infection and making illness more likely to occur.

Implications for Nursing

Nurses have made extensive use of attribution theory in their study of phenomena of concern to nursing: emotional health during divorce, adjustment in patients with lung cancer, weight outcomes, reaction to birth of an infant with a defect, gender differences in thinking about parent-child interactions, causal thinking when patients suffer from various diseases (e.g., myocardial infarction, mood disorders, or arthritis) and caregivers (e.g., dealing with Alzheimer's disease or schizophrenia). Findings have frequently confirmed some of the principal tenets of attribution research, that is, males are more given to explaining failure in terms of external factors (McBride, 1985). Actor-observer differences have been scrutinized, and largely confirmed, in patient-staff perceptions of a psychiatric ward, in successful relationships between severely disabled adults and personal care attendants, in patient-staff perspectives on rehospitalization of the severely mentally ill, and in seclusion or restraint of psychiatric patients. Contrary to one of the assumptions of attribution theory, nurses have found that causal thinking is not always reported when a problem surfaces, nor does it always appear to be linked to adjustment (Jacobsen, Lowery, & McCauley, 1992).

Future Directions

Cognitive therapy aimed at improving explanatory style in at-risk individuals (e.g., those given to owning failure but not success or those not in environ-ments that encourage a sense of self-efficacy) is fast becoming a staple in the repertoire of nursing interventions. It is prospective, longitudinal tests of such clinical interventions that should most occupy nurse researchers in the future, particularly in linking explanatory style with both the onset of illness and its course over time. Many questions of relevance to health remain: Do specific explanatory styles affect specific health outcomes? If explanatory style is a relatively stable personality trait, then how realistic is it to assume that short-term cognitive therapy can have long-term consequences? To what extent does the explanatory style of an entire culture contribute to an individual's thinking? What are the mechanisms by which a pessimistic explanatory style influences health? Does a pessimistic explanatory style increase the number of negative life events one experiences? Can explanations of a patient's behavior be described by the nurse in such a way as to mobilize the family caregiver?

Theoretical Advantages

Attribution theory has proved to be a useful theory for nursing, meeting the following basic prerequisites:

1. There is a correspondence between the concerns of the theory and the concerns of nursing.
2. The theory has clearly stated assumptions, key concepts, and an internally consistent body of relational statements.
3. Because the theory is concerned with behavioral change, it suggests prevention and intervention possibilities.
4. The theory has proved capable of testing with various patient populations and clinical phenomena.

ANGELA BARRON MCBRIDE

See also
ATTITUDES
COPING
SELF-EFFICACY

B

BASIC RESEARCH

Basic research includes all forms of scholarly inquiry for the purpose of demonstrating the existence or elucidation of phenomena. Basic research is conducted without intent to address specific problems or real-world application of knowledge. The discipline of nursing is primarily applied rather than basic, although basic research is a part of the discipline (Donaldson & Crowley, 1978). As a discipline and a science, nursing is informed by knowledge from basic and applied research, and nursing disciplinary knowledge is integrated into the broader context of the whole of human knowledge.

The origins of nursing research trace back to Florence Nightingale (Woodham-Smith, 1951). Over time, the majority of the scholarly work is best categorized as applied rather than basic research in that nursing research has been conducted for the primary purpose of solving problems related to human health. Nursing seeks knowledge from the perspective of the human experience of health. Human perceptions and experiences of health are studied with the intent to generate knowledge to solve problems through nursing care and practice.

There is a cadre of nurses who were doctorally prepared in the basic sciences, both social and biological, as part of the U.S. Public Health Service Nurse Scientist Training Program from 1962 until the late 1970s. Nurses with PhDs in basic sciences were prepared to contribute as basic researchers, and then they adapted their knowledge and skills to conduct nursing research. Despite the growing number and popularity of doctoral programs in nursing, small numbers of nurses continue to pursue degrees in the basic sciences in the United States. This educational path is used more often in countries where doctoral programs in nursing are not available. Another link between the basic sciences and nursing has evolved as a result of doctoral students in nursing pursuing a graduate minor in a basic science or a postdoctoral fellowship in a basic science. These basic research programs for nurses with doctoral degrees in nursing are facilitated by nurses with doctoral degrees in basic research disciplines. Nurse researchers often engage in basic research to generate knowledge that may lead to new perspectives for applied research in nursing.

All clinical research in nursing is by definition applied research. Studies using animal subjects are often applied rather than basic research in nursing. Animal research is categorized as applied research if the work is designed to answer a clinical question, such as how does mammalian (e.g., rat) skeletal muscle adapt to non-weight-bearing conditions equivalent to bed rest (Kasper, Maxwell, & White, 1996)? In contrast, research involving human subjects or human cells and tissue might be basic research, particularly if the intent of the study is to elucidate an inherent mechanism.

Some nurse researchers contribute significantly as basic researchers and serve as liaisons who translate basic research for utilization in applied nursing research. The accompanying Table 1 is a representative but not inclusive list of contemporary doctorally prepared nurse researchers with an example of published work. The nurse researchers have conducted basic research while maintaining a primary identity in nursing. The doctoral degrees of the researchers listed are in both the basic sciences and nursing.

Sue K. Donaldson

See also
APPLIED RESEARCH
NURSING SLEEP SCIENCE

TABLE 1   Selected Basic Researchers in Nursing

Nurse Researcher	Basic Research Topic	Index Locator
Baxendale-Cox, L.	Model for apical Na channels of frog skin	(1990) *Journal of General Physiology, 95*, 647–678
Bond, E. F.	Insulin-induced membrane changes in K(+)-depleted rat muscle	(1993) *American Journal of Physiology, 265*(1, pt. 1), C257–C265
Cahill, C. A.	Carotid sinus baroreflex control of beta-endorphin release in dogs	(1989) *American Journal of Physiology, 256*(2, pt. 2), R408–R412
Cowan, M. J., & Kogan, H.	Interrelationship of autonomic nervous system and voluntary motor control	(1990) *Journal of Electrocardiology, 23*(Suppl.), 85–94
Donaldson, S. K.	GTPγS and skeletal muscle excitation-contraction couping in rabbit fibers	(1997) *American Journal of Physiology, 272 (Cell Physiology, 41)*, C572–C581
Drew, B.	Genes encoding surface glycoprotein of *Pneumocystis carinii*	(1993) *Journal of Biological Chemistry, 268*, 6034–6040
Engler, M. B.	Omega-3, omega-6, omega-9 fatty acids and vascular smooth muscle tone	(1992) *European Journal of Pharmacology, 215*, 325–328
Engler, M. M., & Engler, M. B.	Aortic relaxation in response to omega-3 fatty acids in rats	(1996) *Gerontology, 42*, 25–35
Heitkemper, M. M., & Bond, E. F.	Ovarian hormone status and gastric and gastrointestinal motility in rats	(1996) *Nursing Research, 45*, 218–224
Kasper, C.	Contractile protein isoforms and transitions in developing rat skeletal muscle	(1988) *American Journal of Physiology, 254 (Cell Physiology, 23)*, C605–C613
Kearney, M. L.	Hypoxemia and cardiovascular response to intracranial hypertension in fetal lambs	(1993) *American Journal of Physiology, 265*, H1557–H1563
Lee, K. A., Shaver, J. F., Giblin, E. C., & Wood, N. F.	Sleep patterns and menstrual cycle phase	(1990) *Sleep, 13*, 403–409
Lynaugh, J.	Nature of history	(1987) *Nursing Research, 36*(4), 69
McCarthy, D.	Insulin-like growth factor-I and immune response in rats	(1995) *JPEN: Journal of Parenteral and Enteral Nutrition, 19*, 444–452
Metzger, B. L., & Therrien, B.	Autonomic cardiovascular responsiveness in humans	(1989) *Nursing Research, 38*, 326–330 (1989) *Nursing Research, 38*, 139–143
Miaskowski, C.	Antinociceptive and motor effects of opioid agonists in rats	(1991) *Brain Research, 553*, 105–109
Page, G. G.	Sexual dimorphism in natural killer cell activity in rats	(1995) *Journal of Neuroimmunology, (63)*1, 69–77
Perry, P. A.	Smooth muscle adrenoreceptor sensitivity in rats	(1988) *Canadian Journal of Physiology and Pharmacology, 66*, 1095–1099
Plös, K.	Horizontal gene transfer in *E. coli* isolates	(1989) *Infection and Immunity, 57*, 1604–1611
Radke, K. J.	Aldosterone and renal potassium conservation in the rat	(1996) *American Journal of Physiology, 270*, E1003–E1008

TABLE 1   Selected Basic Researchers in Nursing *(Continued)*

Nurse Researcher	Basic Research Topic	Index Locator
Reame, N. E.	Follicle-stimulating hormone and pulsatile luteinizing hormone secretion	(1996) *Journal of Clinical Endocrinology and Metabolism, 81,* 1512–1518
Schwertz, D., & Piano, M.	Phosphoinositide metabolism and 5-HT1C receptor modulation in rat brain	(1993) *European Journal of Pharmacology, 247,* 81–88
Therrien, B.	Spatial disorientation following hippocampal damage in rats	(1993) *Nursing Research, 42,* 338–343
Tripp-Reimer, T.	Genetic demography of human communities	(1980) *Human Biology, 52,* 255–267
Woods, N. F., Lentz, M. J., & Kogan, H.	Arousal, stress response, menstrual cycle in humans	(1994) *Research in Nursing and Health, 17,* 99–110
Zeller, J. M.	Type II Fc receptor for human IgG	(1993) *Cellular Immunology, 149,* 144–154

BEHAVIORAL RESEARCH

An examination of behavioral research is best begun by examining what it is and differentiating it from related areas of research. Behavioral research within nursing generally refers to the study of health-related behaviors of persons. Studies may include the following areas: (a) health-promoting behaviors such as exercise, diet, immunization, and smoking cessation; (b) screening behaviors such as mammography, breast self-examination, and prostate examinations; and (c) therapeutic behaviors such as adherence to treatment regimen, blood glucose monitoring, participation in cardiac rehabilitation programs, and treatment-related appointment keeping. The research spans medical and psychiatric populations. It is directed toward an understanding of the nature of behavior and health relationships and to the modification of behaviors that affect health. It has been estimated that over half of premature deaths could be prevented if health behaviors were altered.

Behavioral research has its roots in learning theories that arose in the early part of the 20th century. Classical or respondent conditioning was followed by instrumental or operant conditioning and evolved into the cognitive-behavioral theories that dominate the field today. In classical conditioning an unconditioned stimulus is paired with a conditioned stimulus, resulting in the development of a conditioned response. Much of the research emphasizes conditioned physiological responses. An example is found in the study of anticipatory nausea and vomiting during chemotherapy. In this case, chemotherapy (unconditioned stimulus) may induce nausea and vomiting. After several exposures to chemotherapy in a particular setting (conditioned stimulus), the setting itself may induce nausea and vomiting (conditioned response) prior to and independent of the actual administration of the chemotherapy (unconditioned stimulus). Another example is reciprocal inhibition or desensitization in which anxiety is viewed similarly as a conditioned response to stimuli. An incompatible response (relaxation) is paired with progressively stronger levels of the conditioned stimulus in order to inhibit anxiety responses.

With instrumental or operant conditioning, behavior is seen as arising from environmental stimuli or random exploratory actions, which are then sustained by the occurrence of positive reinforcement following the behavior. Laws have been established that address the identification of reinforcers, the schedules of administration of reinforcers for initiation and maintenance of behavior, and strategies for the extinction of behavior. In this model, motivation is seen as a state of deprivation or satiation with regard to reinforcers. Numerous strategies have evolved from this work, including but not limited to contracting and tailoring, which have been used in studies of patient adherence; token economies, which have been used in studies on unit management with the mentally ill or mentally retarded; and contingency management, which has been used in the promotion of treatment behaviors such as exercise.

As the operant model has expanded over time, self-management has evolved as a special case of contingency management. With self-management the individual is responsible for establishing intermediate goals, monitoring progress toward those goals, and administering self-reinforcement for success. Self-management has been studied particularly for chronic, long-term regimens such as those for diabetes, asthma, and cardiovascular disease.

In both of these models there is an emphasis on behavior rather than motivation or personality or relationships, beyond that of the reinforcing behaviors of significant others. The history of the behavior is of less interest than the factors that currently sustain the behavior. An empirical model is used with an assessment of the frequency or intensity of the behavior over time, the stimulus conditions that precede the behavior, and the consequent or reinforcing events that follow the behavior. Intervention is then directed to the specific areas targeted by the initial assessment. Detailed assessment continues through the course of intervention and often through a period following intervention to assess maintenance or generalization.

Recently, the cognitive behavioral models have grown in prominence. In contrast to the classical or instrumental models, where observable behavior is of interest, the cognitive-behavioral models emphasize the role of thoughts in behavior. Thoughts may also be referred to as covert behaviors. A number of theories have emanated from this model; the most commonly addressed by nurse investigators are the self-efficacy theory (Lorig, Chastain, Ung, Shoor, & Holman, 1989), the theory of reasoned action (Jemmott & Jemmott, 1991), the theory of planned behavior (Jemmott, Jemmott, & Hacker, 1992), the health belief model (Janz & Becker, 1984), and the common sense model of illness (Baumann, Zimmerman, & Leventhal, 1989). A related integrative model is Pender's health promotion model, which incorporates elements from the preceding theories (Lusk, Ronis, & Hogan, 1997).

Each of the cognitive-behavioral models identifies a cognitive feature as a major motivational determinant of behavior. Self-efficacy theory postulates the role of perceived capability to engage in a behavior under various conditions. The theory of reasoned action postulates that intention to engage in a behavior is significant and is influenced by beliefs regarding behavioral outcomes and attitudes toward the behavior. The health belief model postulates that one's perceptions about the illness in terms of its threat (severity and susceptibility), as well as the perception of the benefits and barriers to engaging in the behavior, influence intentions and subsequently behavior. However, the common sense model of illness proposes that the individual's own model of the illness influences his or her illness or treatment-related behaviors.

Behavioral research can be distinguished from psychosocial research, which tends to emphasize adjustment and coping as well as predictor and moderator variables arising from the psychological state or the social environment of the person. Behavioral research, including cognitive-behavioral studies, emphasizes behavior. In the classical and instrumental models, observable behavior is stressed. In the cognitive-behavioral model, both observable and covert behaviors are stressed. Within nursing, much of the behavioral research has addressed participation in treatment, exercise, sexual behaviors, health promotion, breast self-examination and mammography utilization, childbirth and maternal behaviors, behavioral symptoms of dementia, self-management in chronic conditions, management of alcohol or drug dependency, and the role of biofeedback in such behaviors as pelvic floor muscle exercise in incontinence and heart rate variability. Unlike psychosocial studies, factors such as personality, coping strategies, and socioeconomic status are not primary interests; however, they may be of interest in determining reinforcers and stimulus conditions.

There is an additional body of behavioral research that tends to be interdisciplinary in nature and is of relevance to nursing. There are studies in the community to modify health behaviors in a population and studies within multicenter clinical trials that attempt to influence the health behavior or protocol-related behaviors of research participants.

Also there is a broad set of studies to identify the relationship between behavior and disease etiology, such as studies of the role of exercise on the maintenance of function in the older adult, mechanisms of addiction in smoking behavior, and the effect of neurotransmitters on eating behaviors.

Given the prevalence of lifestyle behaviors that adversely affect health and the management of illness, research to understand and modify those behaviors would benefit the individual as well as the population. There is a need for nursing research to expand into the interdisciplinary arenas, particularly in the examination of health behavior change in the community, studies within multicenter clinical trials, and the etiological relationship between behavior and health and illness. Further, many of the studies in nursing have been descriptive in nature or have focused on the development of assessment instruments. Although few of the studies have examined how to intervene with behaviors that contribute to the development or progression of illness, this research would be useful to better direct interventions with patients.

This paper was supported in part by a National Institute of Nursing Research grant (5 P30 NR03924) and a National Heart, Lung, and Blood Institute grant (1 UO1HL48992).

JACQUELINE DUNBAR-JACOB

See also
ADHERENCE/COMPLIANCE
PATIENT CONTRACTING
SELF-EFFICACY
SOCIETY OF BEHAVIORAL MEDICINE

BENCHMARKING IN HEALTH CARE

Benchmarking is a structured process used to discover, compare, and incorporate the best practices of high-performing organizations for the purpose of improving the benchmarking organization's performance. It was first used in the late 1970s by the Xerox Corporation and soon became popular in other industries. The introduction of benchmarking in industry was aligned with total quality management (TQM) and continuous quality improvement

(CQI). When used correctly, benchmarking offers the opportunity for exponential improvement rather than the incremental changes most frequent with traditional quality improvement methods. As health care became more industrialized, with enormous pressure to increase efficiency, quality, and customer satisfaction, health care organizations began to adopt benchmarking. As in other industries, benchmarking is often used in conjunction with TQM, CQI, other quality assurance programs, or competitive analysis in health care organizations. It has been used to improve business processes, management processes, and clinical processes in health care organizations.

Benchmarking is most effectively introduced in an organization with a preexisting culture of process orientation and analysis. It is a continuous, ongoing process that requires planning, analysis, and adoption of new processes. Processes to be benchmarked are identified during the planning phase, and because benchmarking costs can be significant, it is important that the organization identify key processes for improving performance. Performance data to be used as benchmarks must be identified and available for analysis and comparison with selected high performers. Selection of organizations to benchmark against is another major decision during the planning phase. The organization may choose internal benchmarking to compare performance of similar operations or divisions within the organization, within one operation or division over time, or with findings from research literature.

However, to reap the full benefit of benchmarking the organization must move to external benchmarking and comparisons with other organizations. External benchmarking can be conducted with like organizations in a geographical region, with similar organizations in a collaborative project, with recognized high performers in health care, or with high-performance industries outside health care. Identification and comparison with high performers is costly and time consuming and may be more efficiently handled by a consulting group or benchmarking clearinghouse that does benchmarking for health care organizations and has access to data from similar organizations recognized as high performers.

Analysis requires two discrete sets of data: (1) the benchmarks, or performance measures, to be used in comparing the benchmarking organization's performance against the selected high performers; and (2) a thorough description of the operational process being benchmarked in the organization using benchmarking and the comparison organizations. This operational description is often referred to as process mapping and is essential to identifying practices in the comparison organizations that enable them to be high performers. Identification of these "best" practices is a necessary prerequisite to the analysis, identification, and adoption of practices that can improve the benchmarking organization's performance. Implementation of operational processes identified through benchmarking, followed by reevaluation of the selected performance measures, is a cyclical process that is repeated until performance goals have been reached and maintained over time.

Although benchmarking has the potential to assist health care organizations to make quantum improvements in operational and delivery systems, it also has the potential to increase stress and cost and to be counterproductive if used inappropriately or improperly. Because benchmarking is in its infancy in health care, a number of pitfalls must be avoided. A common problem is comparing the benchmarks (performance measures) and not looking at the process to find out how the high-performing organization achieves performance and how it differs from the benchmarking organization's performance. Truly effective benchmarking requires in-depth, personal examination of the reasons for the high performer's success. It also requires that performance and productivity measures be consistent with the philosophy and objectives of the organization (Smeltzer, Leighty, & Williams-Brinkley, 1997). Problems also may arise from an inadequate study design, inadequate data analysis, and inadequate preparation of the organization for benchmarking.

Benchmarking studies have only recently been published in health care literature. Many of these studies are reported as case studies that provide information about the process being used, the organizational changes made, and the outcomes achieved through the benchmarking process. Examples of business and management processes studied include workers' compensation process, admissions process, scheduling systems, and operating room use. Studies of benchmarking with clinical processes (Bankert, Daughtridge, Meehan, & Colburn, 1996; Czarnecki, 1996) and patient populations (Clare, Sargent, Moxley, & Forthman, 1995; Lauver, 1996) are reported in the literature and often contain cost information as well as patient outcomes. Although consulting organizations have accumulated comparative data from the organizations they service, this information may surface in the literature slowly, if at all. To determine the usefulness of benchmarking for achieving improvements in health care organizations, more evaluative studies are needed to assess the effectiveness of benchmarking for improving the cost and quality of services provided by health care organizations.

MARION JOHNSON

See also
CLINICAL PATHWAYS
QUALITY MANAGEMENT
QUALITY OF CARE, MEASURING

BIBLIOGRAPHIC RETRIEVAL SYSTEMS

Classifying knowledge in books and other documents is in the domain of library and information sciences. Books and other documents are considered "physical objects" that can be classified in a number of ways; however, subject classification is considered the most significant characteristic. Whereas scientists in a field identify the knowledge of the field, bibliographic classifiers organize the knowledge produced by the scientists (Landgridge, 1992). The classification system is used to index the literature and thus serves a purpose of location and retrieval of the indexed documents. When the classification system is accompanied by an alphabetical list of terms with cross-references, it is called a thesaurus (Landgridge).

The major bibliographic classification schemes dealing with the nursing literature are implemented in computerized bibliographic database retrieval systems for nursing and medicine. Computerized bibliographic databases based on specialty-subject thesauri are available for many other reference disciplines of psychology, education, sociology, and so forth.

Access to bibliographic databases is either through a search service offered by the primary developer of the classification system or is licensed for use by bibliographic retrieval services that provide access to multiple bibliographic databases. Fees for such services vary considerably. Databases may be offered via direct on-line searching (Internet, WWW) or by CD-ROM. Searching the online computer systems requires a computer and perhaps hardware (modem) and software for dialing the on-line systems, the Internet, or a library with a CD-ROM version of the database.

A bibliographic retrieval system is a special type of information retrieval system. The information that is stored (and retrieved) is citation of documents represented in the system. Citations commonly include the article author, title, and the exact location of the article (the title of the journal in which it is published, journal volume and issue number, and pages). Other document types (books, videos, etc.), if incorporated in the system, have descriptors appropriate for that document type. Other data that help to locate a specific document—for example, accession number and author address—will be added to the database by the producer of the system. Abstracts are usually included.

Computerized bibliographic retrieval systems have three components: (a) the classification system for the field of knowledge (subject headings, thesaurus, controlled vocabulary); (b) a database of documents indexed with the controlled vocabulary of the classification system; and (c) the retrieval system search engine (software). The quality of retrieval is a function of all three elements. The controlled vocabulary must adequately represent the literature in the field. Terms from the controlled vocabulary must be accurately assigned to the documents in the field. The search software logic with which searches are done facilitates certain types of searches and hinders others, thereby affecting the quality of the retrieval.

Limits of Bibliographic Retrieval Systems for Nurse Researchers

Vocabulary Issues. Nursing has long been dissatisfied with bibliographic databases that index the nursing literature. In part, this is because the vocabulary used by major vocabulary systems has not satisfactorily reflected nursing terminology. Systems oriented toward nursing literature overcome some of this difficulty by classifying things of importance in nursing but not in medicine, such as nursing theoretical frameworks.

Another long-standing disappointment in the profession has been the inability to locate nursing research by variables studied. This is because variable names are so far out on the classification tree that they are usually not suitable for subject headings. This makes sense because variables usually represent the new nomenclature in a field. These new terms are frequently renamed or incorporated into another term or they may disappear altogether. Vocabularies need more stability than is characteristic of research variable names. Because variable names are not included in bibliographic classifications, articles are not indexed by the names of variables studied in the research.

The results section of research articles, where the variable names reside, is rarely used for assigning index terms (Horowitz & Fuller, 1982). The identification of variable names as keywords by researchers is of little use. Currently, there is no way to tell whether an author-identified term or a classifier-assigned subject heading is a research variable name or just another topic the article is "about." It is fair to say that "aboutness" indexing has a serious impact on retrievals of interest to researchers (Weinberg, 1987).

Document Representation in the Database. Research document representation in nursing-related databases is a problem for several reasons. First, if a controlled vocabulary is inadequate for any reason, indexers cannot assign terms to adequately represent documents. Second, research by nurses that is published outside the field may be in journals that are not indexed by the database developers in the domain. Third, bibliographic databases are limited to the published research literature. Frequently, the published literature fails to reflect adequately the knowledge being generated in a field. Cost of publishing and availability of reviewers limit the number of articles that can be published. Publication bias against small studies with nonsignificant findings and perhaps of parochial interest works against publication of clinical research in nursing. With more focus on statistical meta-analysis strategies, these studies might be combined and thus yield valuable new knowledge. The consequence of large amounts of fugitive research lies not just in the invisibility of knowledge to the discipline but results in a significant waste of resources to duplicate work that has already been done or to identify work that needs to be done.

The Search Strategy

The strategy or "logic" that the software uses to search the database determines how documents can be retrieved and how accurately the document set of interest can be retrieved. Although other search strategies are becoming available, the primary search strategy used by bibliographic retrieval systems in nursing and related fields is based on Boolean logic. The searcher must fully understand the logic used by the search system and how it is implemented in the database of interest.

Boolean logic is based in set theory, which is a way of combining sets of things—in this case, search terms in documents. The *operators*, called Boolean operators, dictate how the documents containing the terms will be combined. The operator *and* causes all the documents containing one term, x, and all documents containing another search term, y, to be combined into the set of documents that contain both x and y. This set of documents is called the search result.

The operator *or* results in a set of documents that have either the term x or y. It includes the set of documents that have both x and y. Other common operators are *not, adjacent, includes, excludes, begins with*. Generally, the more Boolean operators a system makes available, the more accurate the search that can be performed.

Accuracy is a generic term that refers to the concepts of sensitivity and specificity of the search result. In Boolean search systems of bibliographic databases, sensitivity and specificity are inversely related: the search either results in many documents that are not relevant but includes most that are relevant or it results in a few of the most relevant documents being found but fails to turn up others of relevance.

In addition to Boolean operators, common bibliographic database retrieval systems will have tags that identify other salient features of documents in the field; for example, the language the article is written in, document type, and whether the article is about humans or other animals. These characteristics can be used to further delimit a search.

Scientific Knowledge

Researchers are interested in scientific findings, not documents (Doyle, 1986; Weinberg, 1987). All that can be obtained from a bibliographic database search is a list of citations of documents or perhaps the full text of some documents that may or may not contain research findings. The accuracy of these searches can be extremely low, depending on the complexity of the search.

The scientific knowledge is the research result or findings; however, bibliographic classification is done to organize the scientific knowledge produced after it has been embodied in documents (Landgridge, 1992). When viewed this way, perhaps the results of research should not be part of a literature classification system because the results are the knowledge, not the document with the knowledge. Or perhaps this was and is the only legitimate method available to library and information scientists when approaching the literature of all disciplines.

Nonetheless, research knowledge can be indexed by its variables (Graves, 1997; Weiner, Stowe, Shirley, & Gilman, 1981) and linked to its source (the researchers); if published, the dissemination history of the study (bibliographic citations) can be provided. The Virginia Henderson International Nursing Library makes the nursing research that is in the *Registry of Nursing Research* accessible by directly indexing the studies by variable names as well as by researcher and by subject headings (see "The Virginia Henderson International Nursing Library").

JUDITH R. GRAVES

See also
**CUMULATIVE INDEX OF NURSING
  AND ALLIED HEALTH LITERATURE**

ELECTRONIC NETWORK
THE ONLINE JOURNAL
  OF KNOWLEDGE SYNTHESIS
  FOR NURSING

BIBLIOMETRICS

Definition

Bibliometrics is broadly defined as the application of mathematical and statistical methods to published scientific literature in a disciplinary field (Pritchard, 1969). Bibliometric research methods are based on a literary model of science. Using bibliometrics, information scientists assume that published research documents reflect new knowledge in a scientific field and that references in these reports represent relationships among scientists and their work.

Relevance to Nursing

Bibliometrics is a useful research methodology for describing and visually representing the communication structure of a scientific field. It has been used successfully to evaluate such things as emergence, change, and communication networks in specialty areas. Bibliometric methods have been helpful in identifying the foundational fields (i.e., other scientific fields) that have driven the genesis of a new scientific field. They also can be used to identify prominent scientists or documents that have influenced the intellectual development of a scientific field. Thus, bibliometric studies may provide insights into the historical and sociological evolution of nursing science as well as the design of information retrieval systems in nursing.

Research Methods

Research questions addressed by bibliometric studies generally fall into one of four categories: (a) characterization of a scholarly community, (b) evolution of a scholarly community, (c) evaluation of

scholarly contributions, and (d) diffusion of ideas from within and across disciplines (Borgman, 1990). Citation data are often used in bibliometric studies and are generally collected from bibliographies, abstracting and indexing services, citation indexes, and primary journals. Typically, the references of research journal articles are analyzed in bibliometric studies. Bibliographic attributes such as authors, citations, and textual content are used as variables in bibliometric research.

Citation analysis is the best-known bibliometric strategy. It is a set of strategies for studying relationships among cited and citing literature in a scientific field. Bibliographic coupling and co-citation analysis use citation analysis to demonstrate linkage of citation data. In bibliographic coupling, the focus is on the citing literature; that is, the number of references two articles have in common reflects the similarity of their subject matter. In co-citation analysis the focus is on the cited literature, that is, the number of times two documents are cited together in the reference lists of later publications. Sets of co-cited document pairs may be grouped together and mapped, using graphical display techniques such as cluster analysis and multidimensional scaling. The unit of analysis for co-citation analysis studies can also be journals (journal co-citation analysis) or authors (author co-citation analysis). Co-word analysis is another bibliometric strategy based on the analysis of co-occurrence of keywords used to index documents or articles. This method is useful for mapping content in a research field or for tracing the evolution of networks of problems in a disciplinary field.

Bibliometric strategies are practical and may be applied to citation data that are readily accessible on citation indexes and on-line electronic databases. No subjective judgments are made by the researcher about what literature best defines a scientific field or specialty area. It is the scholars themselves who publish in the scientific literature that determine the intellectual base of the specialty area. However, citation data can portray only what the scientific community in a field of study has recognized by way of publication. In addition, bibliometrics does not have a theory that integrates the methods and techniques used in the analysis of citations. Therefore, it is important that the investigator clearly delimit the specialty area to be investigated, be familiar with the field of interest, and interpret citation data in conjunction with other sources of information relevant to the area of interest.

Review of Research

There have been at least five bibliometric investigations of the nursing literature. Garfield (1985), an information scientist, conducted a journal citation study on core nursing journals indexed in the 1983 *Social Sciences Citation Index*, using citation data from 1981 to 1983. Four bibliometric studies have been conducted by nurse researchers. Messler (1974) conducted a citation analysis investigating the growth of maternity nursing knowledge as reflected in published nursing practice literature from 1909 to 1972. Wilford (1989) used citation analysis techniques to study citation patterns depicted in the references of a random sample of 310 nursing dissertations from 1947 to mid-1987. Johnson (1990) conducted a bibliometric analysis using the technique of keyword analysis to describe the evolution of the holistic paradigm in the field of nursing. D'Auria (1994) used citation analysis techniques, including author co-citation analysis, to demonstrate the feasibility of using author co-citation analysis for identifying emerging networks of researchers in the subfield of maternal and child health nursing from 1976 to 1990. Further bibliometric analyses of the research literature from the general field or subfields of nursing will provide a baseline for describing and interpreting citation data in the field of nursing.

Future Directions

At this point in the development of nursing science, it is critical that nurse scholars create ways to increase the visibility and retrieval of scientific information being generated in the field. Bibliometric methods can provide a way to track disciplinary influences and the identities of nurse scientists and scientists from other disciplines whose interests are shaping the generation of scientific information in nursing. The findings of bibliometric studies will provide nurse scholars with a guide for scholarship for doctoral students and researchers in the field of nursing that may differ from information that has been passed down as traditional wisdom. Thus, the findings of bibliometric studies will open up new avenues for debate and hypotheses generation in regard to the evolution of nursing science.

As the nursing research literature continues to grow, rigorous and systematic bibliometric research of citation data may contribute working models of the development of nursing science that could be used to evaluate scientific progress. By discovering trends in disciplinary and interdisciplinary linkages, nurse scholars can identify underdeveloped or neglected areas of research in nursing science. Evaluating the degree of scientific activity in research areas would help nurse scholars determine if research resources are allocated correctly as well as assist them in determining the need for new journals and books in the field of nursing. It will also provide an avenue by which nurse scholars may access scientific information and prevent the loss of information generated in the field of nursing.

JENNIFER P. D'AURIA

See also
  NURSING STUDIES INDEX
  SIGMA THETA TAU
      INTERNATIONAL NURSING
      RESEARCH CLASSIFICATION
      SYSTEM

BIOFEEDBACK TRAINING

Biofeedback is training in the use of information linked with training in sensitivity to the body state. Patients learn to achieve awareness of the contrast between the ill and the healthy mind/body state. Patients are taught mastery in self-regulation in order to maintain the healthy state. The kind of information that is cogent is that which can be used for patients to monitor themselves. The premier tool of patient training for self-management of health is offering patients the capacity to track body processes that indicate health and illness. Thus, feedback of physical/emotional signals (biofeedback) to patients is by far the most potent kind of information for self-management of health care.

Feedback of biological and psychological status is not new, but the complexity of indicators of health status now available to patients is vastly proliferated. A decade ago minimal knowledge was available about processes that led to illness and indicators by which to judge the maladaptation. Information is now available about how illness develops in the body. Now, any number of self-management skills can be instituted to interfere with the illness process. For example, a person may monitor bone density, thus tracing or preventing the osteoporosis process, or monitor electroencephalographic (EEG) patterns, thus preventing memory loss. Health professionals know more about the mechanisms of body processes—what produces, prevents, or reverses the disease process. The challenge is to program that knowledge and provide technical and counseling expertise so that patients acquire solid skills in self-management of mind and body.

Psychophysiology is the clinical science that provides the basis for understanding health and disease processes in biofeedback and other self-management skills. This topic initially highlights the central neurocognitive processes that join emotions and cognitive activity with physiological processes. Next, biofeedback will be reported in the context of a larger framework of self-management training, in which a programmatic approach is developed for self-regulation of specific symptom patterns depictive of neural disregulation. Were space available, the cogency of biofeedback for a cadre of chronic functional disorders could be outlined that would capture the pertinence and importance of biofeedback and self-management in future health care.

Psychophysiology—the Interface Between Mind and Body

Biofeedback/self-management interventions are relevant for any dysfunction in which cognitive-emotional and physiological processes produce neural arousal or activation. These neural processes, when dysfunctional, can be demonstrated in neuro-endocrine excesses or deficits, immune suppression, cerebral hypoperfusion, EEG hypostimulation or hyperstimulation, and reactions in numerous peripheral organ responses, such as the skin, the cardiovascular system, and neural pathways. Neural dysfunction also can be diffusely manifested as general symptoms of fatigue, cognitive impairment, confusion, chronic pain, and insomnia. It is now understood that neural dyscontrol lies at the heart of most chronic manifestations for which no specific etiological origin has been delineated (Benarroch, 1993). These disease conditions are called diseases of disregulation, a state during which the brain's integrative functions, providing neural control of management of body processes, have gone awry. The enlarging field of psychophysiology provides understandings about how the brain-body interface becomes disregulated.

In a regulated state the brain and body maintain a homeostatic balance, adapting brain activity with biochemical action; hormonal flow; neural, respiratory, and circulatory activity; and peripheral organ performance. Continuous adaptations will prevent long-term disregulation. The brain is the major organ needed for adaptation. Consider the dynamic efforts taking place: cognitive-emotional information flow and the generation of the more subtle cellular and chemical adaptive activity. A stress response or its counterpart, adaptation, is determined by this brain processing.

The homeostatic model traces an adaptive state, whereas the disregulated model is known as a stress response. It is suggested that under stress, the homeostatic pattern achieved by prior adaptation is overridden, producing a tenuous and dysfunctional pattern of psychophysiological stress reaction. Over a prolonged time, chronic disease develops. Thus, in most chronic major illnesses there can be traced a configuration of symptoms that are neurally mediated, overlaying and interacting with a pathophysiological process of the original disease (Steptoe, 1991; Wolf, 1981).

More and more disease conditions are viewed with recognition of this dynamic, interactive dyscontrol. Hypertension, irritable bowel syndrome, chronic fatigue, and fibromyalgia, among other disorders, are examples of disregulation. Even diabetes, arthritis, and a large number of collagen diseases, such as lupus erythematosis, and neuromuscular diseases such as multiple sclerosis are discovered to be outcomes of the autoimmune process triggered by immunological disregulation and its neural control. Certainly, psychiatric disorders can be viewed as disregulatory diseases. The study of biochemical and neurohormonal links to brain mechanisms that control the disease process has expanded, creating this whole new definition of diseases of disregulation.

This understanding of processes of the brain indicates that the brain contains the central adaptive resources for recovery from illnesses or from stress responses. Biofeedback training offers a window into the mechanisms of the dysfunctions through physiological information. The focus of self-management interventions considers the behavioral and emotional changes that will alter psychopathophysiological processes.

Self-Management and Biofeedback

At the heart of biofeedback/self-management training is the concept that the mind/body interface is a self-regulatory system. Self-regulation is an automatic feedback system that runs effectively until negative input disrupts the cycle. A negative sign or symptom forces the body to strive for a reregulated state, sometimes at the expense of an adaptive balance, producing pathological equilibrium. The stress response is an example. Henry (1992) noted that a challenge perceived as easy to manage will elicit an initial active coping response and accompanying release of norepinephrine. Difficulties in managing the task will first change the neuroendocrine parameters, then produce other efforts at adaptation.

In Henry's animal model, the path toward pathology began with threat. As anxiety arose, the norepinephrine/epinephrine ratio decreased; as distress grew, cortisol levels rose, and a passive mode of coping was observable. The ratio of catecholamines to corticoids decreased as frustration and uncertainty grew. Finally, the model of posttraumatic stress syndrome emerged, with repression and denial expressed in impaired attachment and increased irritability. The corticoids paradoxically returned to normal, but lasting emotional trauma

remained. Such pathological reregulation is abundant in our own patient populations. But the model also fits for the less traumatized conditions in which anxiety, anger, and depression are dominant features.

Personal control is the cornerstone in the goal orientation of biofeedback/self-management training. In a disregulated condition the threat of lack of control is great. In studies demonstrating a sense of loss of personal control, the predictability of adaptation on the part of the subjects is tenuous. Self-control reflects a degree of self-competence. Very early in their series of studies of somatic complaints Pennebaker, Burnam, Schaeffer, and Harper (1977) found that there is a relationship between perception of control and the incidence of physical complaints. The mechanism of symptomatology seems to be unrelated to physiological functioning but related to the subject's self-control and understanding and prediction of events (Pennebaker et al., 1977; Tetrick & LaRocco, 1987).

A signal that self-management training is a success can be seen by restoration of personal control. Indeed, an operational analysis of personal control suggests that one can measure such indicators as the following:

1. Behavioral control in ability to influence or modify events.
2. Cognitive control by processing of information so as to reduce the cost of adaptation.
3. Decision control through taking opportunities to choose from a number of courses of action.

Personal control is clearly a matter of central focus in self-management training.

Biofeedback is a basic element of our repertoire of health care offerings. We do not always label it as such, nor do we use it to its maximum. We feed back weight, temperature, and blood pressure measures to patients. How often do we think to use photos, mirrors, or audiovisual tapes to inform persons of their general appearance as a mark of health status, as could be done in eating disorders, depression, or anxiety states? The more formal field of biofeedback training, on the other hand, is oriented to the physiological and cognitive-affective processes that are integral to the disregulatory diseases being treated. It has relied on instrumentation of measures such as digital temperature, electromyograph readings, skin conductance, heart rate, and EEG activity as indicators of maladaptive responses. The field places heavy emphasis on training in consciousness as the means for making use of information in achieving self-regulation.

Much of the success in biofeedback treatment has to do with the conceptual approach to the training. The roots of biofeedback training emerged from operant conditioning theory, embracing a limited concept of physiological training without recognition of the neural, cognitive-affective components that are now critical to present-day theory. Biofeedback training is more than merely physiological training of neural pathways. Rather, it is a cognitive event, that of information processing of biological signals. Feedback enables the subject to become consciously aware of the interface between bodily status, environmental events, and internal cognitive information. It provides behavioral strategies to alter physiological activity.

Biofeedback Mechanisms

Biofeedback as an intervention modality is only as effective as the specificity of information that is offered to the patient in relation to the symptom disorder. The specificity of the information is dependent on understanding how symptoms might be generated. Because mechanisms of illness are not simple and linear, the feedback is also likely to be convoluted. Thus, much feedback cannot easily be explained to patients as it is derived from bioinstrumentation. It would be a mistake to oversimplify biological signals as if they represented the mechanisms. The clinician's skill lies in focusing on a changing signal as an approximate and representative indicator of bodily processes in a chain of disregulatory activities. The following two examples are sketched to demonstrate the difficulties of the use of biological signals to help patients to self-manage chronic symptoms.

Hypertension Self-regulation. Information about control of heart rate is one method of training patients to control high blood pressure. This therapeutic protocol incorporates respiratory and heart rate biofeedback based on the work of Grossman (1991), who noted that control of cardiovascular system integrity by the central nervous system could be observed through the respiratory sinus arrhythmia. The coupling of respiratory and heart rate action is key, because respiration is under voluntary control and can be used as the training device. The patient is trained to breathe deeply, using abdominal muscles, and can be shown the tracing of respiratory sinus arrhythmia on the computer screen. By training to fit the excursions of respiration and respiratory sinus arrhythmia together, heart rate changes and, subsequently, blood pressure can be shown to lower.

Being taught the link of the sympathetic nervous system with blood pressure and the link of emotions and relaxation responses with sympathetic arousal, the mind/body connection is being made to help patients learn to control bouts of hypertension. At home, self-regulation of self-monitored labile hypertension can reduce the average blood pressure markedly.

Attention Deficit Disorder/Cognitive Impairment. A striking feature of many disorders in which attention is restricted and the ability to organize, plan, and concentrate is deficient is that the EEG pattern shows an inability to marshal the proper brain frequencies to allow these functions (Linden, Habib, & Radojevic, 1996; Lubar, 1991). A common EEG pattern is an excess of theta frequency, the slowest wave pattern in the spectral array of all frequencies. This is found in attention deficit/hyperactivity. It is seen in persons with mild closed head injuries, in elderly who are losing memory, and in any number of chronic symptom patterns such as chronic heart disease and chronic fatigue syndrome. Patients can be taught to inhibit theta brain activity and increase another dominant frequency. In this case the training must be extended over a time span long enough to reorganize the brain wave pattern and create a habitual state. Self-training can augment the laboratory feedback, using mental tasks and other stimuli to trigger the desired frequency pattern at home.

Summary

Today, self-regulating actions will go far in preventing the progress of pathology, obviating the need for more drastic medication management or surgical intervention. The role of biofeedback in nursing practice can be extensive when the time comes that nursing action is not directed by large institutions. A greater amount of autonomy of practice will be mandatory in outpatient practices caring for patients with chronic diseases. Biofeedback is an augmentation to traditional treatment and need not be seen as a replacement treatment, thus positioning persons to choose either biofeedback or another traditional therapy.

HELEN KOGAN BUDZYNSKI

See also
BEHAVIORAL RESEARCH
COPING
STRESS

BREAST CANCER

Breast cancer is a major health problem in the United States, affecting approximately 181,600 women, or 30% of new cancer cases in women in 1997. Research in breast cancer is highly relevant to women's health research and has been a major interest of several nurse researchers over a period of time. Breast cancer research is targeted as a high research priority of the National Cancer Institute (NCI) and the National Institute of Nursing Research (NINR). For instance, NCI funding for breast cancer research increased to nearly $450 million in 1994. In addition, NINR has supported studies to improve women's knowledge of and behavior in breast cancer prevention and detection and funded research that will lead to effective nursing interventions.

A review of breast cancer studies conducted by nurses from the early 1970s to the 1990s demonstrated four focused areas of research: early detection through breast self-examination (BSE), management of symptoms during treatment, psychosocial response of patient and family, and issues in long-term cancer survivorship. The major theoretical frameworks used in nursing research in breast cancer include the health belief model, the Roy adaptation model, and Orem's self-care deficit theory.

Screening and Early Detection Research

Nurse researchers have made significant contributions to our knowledge of early detection through BSE practice and the factors influencing the patient's ability to perform BSE (Champion, 1991). Early studies emphasized BSE rather than mammography, presumably because teaching and education were prime areas for nursing intervention. Mammography use has increased exponentially in this country, and nurses now aim their research toward predictors of mammography usage. In addition, nurse researchers must expand their focus to the triad of breast cancer screening modalities: BSE, mammography, and clinical breast examination (CBE).

Nurse scientists have also targeted screening and early detection activities for high-risk groups such as African Americans (Nemcek, 1989), Hispanics (Longman, Saint-Germain, & Modiano, 1992), rural populations, and older women (Lierman, Kasprzyk, & Benoliel, 1991). Nurse researchers continue to develop intervention studies addressing the reduction of barriers to breast cancer screening, particularly among the underserved and elderly populations (Ansell, Lacey, Whitman, Chen, & Phillips, 1994).

Diagnosis and Symptom Management

The second major contribution by nurses in breast cancer research pertains to issues in diagnosis and symptom management. Nurse researchers have improved our understanding of anxiety, critical thinking, decision making, care-seeking behavior, and preferential choice in treatment for breast cancer (Lauver, 1992; Lierman, 1988). Another cluster of studies focused on symptom management during treatment; they include hair loss, nausea and vomiting, fatigue, and pain in advanced cancer.

Intervention Studies to Manage Symptoms

Three notable areas of intervention by several nurse researchers included exercise as a means to improve well-being and fatigue (Mock et al., 1997), the use of a coach or partner to enhance adaptation to breast cancer (Samarel & Fawcett, 1992) and attentional fatigue (Cimprich, 1992).

Early investigations by Winningham and colleagues (Winningham et al., 1989) evaluated the effects of aerobic interval training in improving the functional capacity of breast cancer patients on adjuvant chemotherapy. This led to an increase in the number of intervention studies examining the effectiveness of exercise. In the most recent analysis, Mock and colleagues (in press) used an experimental design to test the hypothesis that women who participated in a walking exercise program during radiation therapy treatment for breast cancer would demonstrate more adaptive responses, as evidenced by higher levels of physical functioning and lower levels of symptom intensity, than would women who did not participate. Women in the exercise group maintained an individualized, self-paced, home-based walking exercise program, and the comparison group received usual care. Results showed significant differences between the two groups on the outcome measures. The walking exercise group scored higher on physical functioning and lower on symptom intensity, particularly on measures of fatigue, anxiety, and difficulty sleeping. Implications were that a nurse-prescribed and monitored exercise activity was an effective, convenient, and low-cost self-care activity to help reduce symptoms of breast cancer treatment.

Psychosocial Response

The third major area of breast cancer studies focused on psychosocial response. Researchers have examined adjustment of patients, spouses, children, and family to the impact of breast cancer over time, concerns about quality of life, threat of cancer recurrence, issues in self-transcendence, and improvements in emotional and spiritual well-being. Northouse (1995) conducted several studies evaluating the impact of women's cancer on the family. In a review of the literature, the consensus from studies on the emotional impact of breast cancer on spouses is an increase in number of reported psychosomatic concerns, increased feelings of anx-

iety and depression, and high distress levels. The strongest predictor of adjustment was the level of concurrent stress in the marital relationship. Northouse also found few studies of the impact of breast cancer on children and directed attention to developing future studies in this regard.

Future Directions

Nursing research in breast cancer has improved our understanding of response to chronic illness tremendously. In the future, nurse researchers will continue to develop programs of research in breast cancer, work collaboratively with other disciplines, and use their expertise in setting national health policy and helping to direct a national research agenda.

KAREN HASSEY DOW

See also
BREAST CANCER SCREENING
CANCER CARE CHEMOTHERAPY
CANCER SURVIVORSHIP
RADIATION THERAPY

BREAST CANCER SCREENING

Breast cancer is a disease for which there is no foreseeable cure, and indications are that incidence will remain high. The American Cancer Society estimates that more than 180,000 women will be diagnosed with breast cancer in 1997, and almost 44,000 will die (Parker, Tong, Bolden, & Wingo, 1997). Although breast cancer remains a significant form of cancer mortality for women, in 1996 an overall decrease in mortality was reported. Because treatment is extremely effective with Stage I tumors, increases in mammography screening have influenced breast cancer mortality. When discovered early, breast cancer victims may anticipate a 95% chance for complete cure. Prospective mortality-based studies have demonstrated the effectiveness of mammography screening, particularly in women 50–70 years of age, and therefore most organizations recommend periodic screening beginning at age 50.

Recently, mammography recommendations have been expanded to include women 40 to 49. Two Swedish trials (Anderson, 1997; Bjurstam, Bjorneld, & Duffy, 1997) and a meta-analysis (Smart, Hendrick, Rutledge, & Smith, 1995) have shown a mortality-based advantage for women in their 40s. Consequently, both the American Cancer Society and the National Cancer Institute now recommend screening beginning at age 40. Obviously, breast cancer screening by mammography does not magically become effective at age 40 or 50 or 60, and one mistake that fueled controversy was comparing one decade to another. Comparing women aged 40 to 49 with women 50 and over creates artificial boundaries that cause much confusion. Now that the American Cancer Society and National Cancer Institute are in agreement, energy may be focused on other issues.

The effectiveness of clinical breast examination is not as clear as that of mammography, although it is currently recommended. Some studies demonstrating a mortality decrease for mammography have included clinical breast examination, but the independent effect of the latter has not been studied. In addition, the efficacy of breast self-examination (BSE) has been documented, although not in randomized, prospective mortality-based trials. To date, retrospective studies have found that BSE may detect an earlier stage of disease or smaller tumor size. Gastrin and colleagues (Gastrin et al., 1994) reported a significantly lower mortality for a sample population of 28,785 women enrolled in a BSE program, compared to what was expected with the general Finnish population. Preliminary results of a randomized study for BSE have indicated no benefit, although definitive conclusions cannot be made (Thomas, Gao, Self, et al., 1997).

Despite its apparent effectiveness, breast cancer screening is not used to its fullest advantage. According to the National Cancer Institute's *Cancer Facts* for 1996, one-time screening rates may approach 70% to 74%, but rates were lower for minorities and women over 65. The rates for consistent mammography screening at recommended intervals are not good. Rates for mammography in 1996 ranged from 40% to 51% for women aged 50–64 and from 30% to 42% for women 65 and over. Rates for clinical breast examination were some-what higher, ranging between 60% and 75%. Recent data indicate that women may report BSE practice as frequently as seven to eight times a year but have low proficiency scores. In one study, mean proficiency scores were a little over half of what an optimal examination score would be (Champion, 1995).

Relevance to Nursing

It is obvious that breast cancer screening has the potential to reduce mortality and morbidity from this dreaded disease. Breast cancer screening rates, although increasing, are not optimal. Most problematic is the fact that women do not follow current recommendations for screening. Minority rates for follow-up are dismal, and access to care is a real issue. This health-promoting detection activity is of primary importance to nurses in all areas of practice. Nurses are in an optimal position to increase all three screening methods (mammography, clinical breast examination, and BSE). Interventions to promote mammography and teach BSE can be carried out during general health promotion or while women are being seen for other reasons. Clinical breast examination is a skill that should be learned by all nurse practitioners and conducted yearly on all women aged 20 and over.

Theoretical Variables Related to Breast Cancer Screening

Several important theoretical variables have been tested for relationships to breast cancer screening—in particular, mammography and BSE. The theory that has generated the most research is the *health belief model*. The *health belief model* was initially conceptualized in the early 1950s to predict preventive behaviors such as influenza inoculations (Rosenstock, 1966). As originally formulated, the *health belief model* included the variable of perceived threat to health, which included the concepts of risk of contracting the disease (perceived susceptibility) and personal cost should the disease be contracted (perceived seriousness). In addition, benefits and barriers to taking preventive action were predicted to influence the health behavior. In 1988, the concept of self-efficacy, or perceived confidence in carrying out a preventive behavior, was added to the health belief model.

Other theories that have been used to predict breast cancer screening have included Fishbein and Ajzen's (1975) theory of reasoned action, which postulates that two major concepts are related to breast cancer screening: (a) beliefs and evaluations of these beliefs and (b) social influence. Social influence is also composed of two components: beliefs of significant others and the influence of significant others on the individual. Most recently, the transtheoretical model has been tested with mammography use and found to predict behavior (Prochaska et al., 1994). This model defines the outcome in terms of stages of preparedness to engage in a health-promoting activity. In addition to the factors involved in these models, descriptive research suggests that breast cancer screening is influenced by knowledge, previous health habits, particular demographic characteristics, and health care systems. For example, physician recommendation has proved to be highly predictive of mammography use in many studies.

Studies of Breast Cancer Screening

A number of studies spanning over a decade have used various models to predict mammography screening. In general, attitudinal variables such as perceived susceptibility, perceived benefits to screening, and perceived barriers to screening have been predictive of mammography. Rakowski and co-workers (Rakowski et al., 1992) found that perceived pros (benefits) and cons (barriers) varied across stages of mammography. The most consistent predictors of mammography use have been physician recommendation and barriers. The latter have included perceived lack of need, fear of results, fear of radiation, cost, pain, time, and inconvenience. Recently, the transtheoretical model has been used for predicting mammography by postulating that women move through a series of stages from precontemplation, or not thinking about mammography, to maintenance of mammography over time.

Descriptive studies to predict BSE have spanned the past two decades. Again, the variables of perceived susceptibility, benefits, and barriers have been significantly related to BSE. A less significant prediction of BSE compliance has been physician recommendation. Instead, women who were taught personally and returned a demonstration have been found to comply at higher rates. A major problem with BSE research has been the measurement of outcomes. In many earlier studies women were asked how many times they examined their breasts, and this was used as the operational measure of compliance. Later, self-report proficiency scales were widely used. Research has shown that there is often little correlation between reported frequency and proficiency, indicating that even if women practice BSE, they may not be doing it proficiently enough to detect lumps.

Actual measurement of BSE proficiency also has been problematic. The best studies have used trained observers to watch women either complete BSE or identify silicon lumps embedded in models. Subjective norms, as identified in the theory of reasoned action, have been predictive in some studies. In summary, most research has identified low to moderate correlations between attitudinal variables and BSE. Perceived confidence for completing self-examination has been one of the strongest predictors.

Interventions for Breast Cancer Screening

Intervention research for both mammography and BSE has systematically built on the descriptive studies of earlier decades. Interventions have ranged from multistrategy community interventions to individual patient-oriented interventions. Many of the individually focused interventions targeted perceptions of risk, benefits, and barriers. Multistrategy interventions often targeted physician recommendation, which had been found to be an important predictor of mammography screening. Various ways of delivering messages have been tried, including the media, telephone delivery, tailored letters or postcards, and in-person counseling. Access has been identified as a problem, as shown by the fact that persons in health maintenance organizations (HMOs) consistently have higher rates of mammography screening than do patients in private medical practice. Access-enhancing interventions have included the use of mobile vans, which provide easier access for women with transportation problems. Costs of mammography for indigent women continue to be a problem, although agencies such as the American Cancer Society and Little Red Door have helped to defray these costs. Social network interventions have been effective with minority groups. Peer leaders can sometimes be important links for low-income, African American, or Hispanic women. In summary, most interventions, but especially those based on sound theory, have been successful in increasing mammography.

Interventions addressing BSE often focus on teaching women the correct skills for practice. Many of the interventions use educational strategies, with or without counseling, related to the theoretical constructs of perceived susceptibility, benefits, and barriers. Many studies have used reminder systems or self-prompts to increase practice. Interventions have ranged from handing out pamphlets to one-to-one teaching sessions with return demonstrations. Studies using models to identify lumps have been the most vigorous. Studies that include personal demonstrations, guided feedback, and both cognitive and personal instruction evidence the greatest increase in proficiency.

Implications for Practice

Descriptive and intervention studies based on similar theories of breast cancer screening have extended over the past two decades. The major differ-

ence in relation to promoting mammography is the addition of physician recommendation. Physician recommendation is important both because medical advice is related to mammography and because an order may be necessary to obtain a mammogram. For BSE, personal teaching has been found to be a most important predictor. We now know enough about breast cancer screening to make certain recommendations for nursing practice. For both BSE and mammography, clinicians must take into account the individual's perceptions about her susceptibility to breast cancer. If this perceived susceptibility is unrealistically low, efforts must be made to paint a more accurate picture. Perceived benefits and barriers to both mammography and BSE also should be addressed and individualized strategies developed. For BSE teaching, the set of skills needed to complete this exam and observation of proficiency will be important. A major future direction related to mammography will be to increase interval compliance.

Breast cancer screening research has broad implications for increasing other health behaviors, such as colorectal or prostate screening. Preventive behaviors such as the use of skin protection and adherence to low-fat diets can also be targeted for intervention trials. Finally, nurses must actively encourage public policy decisions that increase screening access for all people.

VICTORIA CHAMPION

See also
BREAST CANCER
WOMEN'S HEALTH RESEARCH

C

CANCER CARE: CHEMOTHERAPY

Definition and Overview of Chemotherapy

Chemotherapy is defined by the 1997 *Taber's Cyclopedic Medical Dictionary* (Thomas, 1997, p. 363) as "the application of chemical reagents that have a specific and toxic effect on the disease-causing microorganism." Chemotherapy is primarily associated with the treatment of cancer but can be used with other diseases. Historically, the overall goal of this treatment approach has been maximum cell kill with tolerable toxicity. The balance between these two approaches can result in life-threatening side effects.

The effects of chemotherapy are systemic and thus invaluable in the treatment of cancer, a disease characterized by micrometastatic spread. The purpose of chemotherapy can be cure, control, or palliation. Many cancers are cured by the administration of chemotherapy. Recent advances have resulted in extended disease-free intervals and prolonged survival in cancers that previously had poor prognoses. There are more than 50 chemotherapeutic agents in use, with new drugs being developed yearly. Despite the addition of new drugs to the armamentarium of agents that can be used to combat cancer, drug resistance remains a formidable problem.

Drug resistance can be temporary or permanent. Permanent, or phenotypic, drug resistance is genetically based and hypothesized to be the major factor in chemotherapy drug failure. Recent research indicates the existence of multidrug, or pleiotropic drug resistance. The strategies that have been developed to combat multidrug resistance include "(1) increasing intracellular drug concentration using high doses of drugs; (2) alternating noncross-resistant chemotherapy regimens; (3) use of monoclonal an-tibodies or conjugates to target P-glycoprotein; and (4) use of drugs to inhibit the function of P-glycoprotein" (Knobf & Durivage, 1993, p. 279).

Historical Perspectives. The first chemotherapeutic agents were hormones, estrogen and androgen, which were used in the 1940s in the treatment of breast and prostate cancer. Modern-day chemotherapy began with an accidental discovery during World War II of the toxic effects of poison gases, specifically exposure to mustard gas (nitrogen mustard). A derivative of this agent was used subsequently to treat patients with Hodgkin's disease; although not permanent, there was documented tumor regression. Nitrogen mustard is one of the oldest class of antineoplastic agents, titled alkylating agents. The next discovery, by Dr. Sydney Farber in the late 1940s, was that folic acid antagonists could be used successfully against acute leukemia in children. Folic acid antagonists constitute the plant alkaloids class of antineoplastic agents. In the 1950s, the chemotherapeutic classes of antitumor antibiotics and antimetabolites were introduced into the treatment of cancer.

Rationale for Use. Because cancer cells move through the five phases of the cell cycle as do normal cells, chemotherapeutic agents are classified according to the point in the cell cycle at which the agent's effect is exerted on the cancer cells. Chemotherapeutic agents affect both normal and malignant cells by altering cellular activity during one or more phases of the cell cycle. The two major classes of agents that have been established on the basis of their activity during the cell cycle are called cycle phase-specific and cell cycle phase-nonspecific. Cell cycle-specific drugs are those that are lethal only if the cell is dividing. Cell cycle-nonspecific are effective only against resting cells. There are some chemotherapeutic agents that are cell cycle-specific, phase-nonspecific. These are drugs that act on both resting and cycling cells.

Because chemotherapy drugs affect both cancer and normal cells, the cancer patient experiences many side effects during treatment. These include (a) nausea and vomiting, (b) diarrhea, (c) stomatitis, (d) fatigue, (e) anorexia, (f) bone marrow suppression, (g) organ toxicity (cardiac, neurological, hepatic), and (h) cystitis. Nursing research has focused on describing and designing interventions to lessen the side effects of the chemotherapy and on effective educational interventions to promote self-care.

Drug Development. Chemotherapeutic drugs enter the mainstream of clinical treatment through clinical trials. Implementation of clinical trials for new chemotherapy drugs is carried out by a multidisciplinary research team, including nurses serving in research and clinical roles. Clinical trials are the principal method for obtaining reliable evaluation of treatment effects and for examining the efficacy of new therapeutic drugs. There are four phases of clinical trials. Phase I studies the maximum tolerated dose for the delivery schedule of a specific chemotherapy drug. The purpose of Phase II studies is to determine the antitumor toxicity of the drug in a variety of cancers. Phase III studies define the role of a drug in a cancer treatment regimen, comparing the new drug with conventional treatments. Phase IV studies integrate a new agent into a proven treatment plan. At this point, the drug is known to be effective, but it is not authorized for widespread clinical use.

Initially, the primary role of the nurse in clinical trials was that of a data collector (data manager). The role of the nurse evolved to that of a research or protocol nurse, answering patient and family questions about the research study, providing education related to the study, accruing patients for the study, and observing patients' responses and toxicities. These research or protocol nurses were among the first nurses to participate as collaborators in cancer research. With the growth of oncology nursing master's and doctoral programs, the nursing role related to clinical trials has grown to be that of research collaborator and co-investigator. In this role the nurse is able to incorporate nursing issues into medical protocols. "Currently, oncology nurses enhance the care of patients with cancer through collaborative and independent nursing research that facilitates biomedical research outcomes, impacts severity of disease and treatment-related outcomes, and improves the patient's ability to live with a chronic illness such as cancer" (Jenkins, 1996, p. 4).

Evolving Role of Nursing in Chemotherapy

In 1991 and 1995 the Research Committee of the Oncology Nursing Society conducted a survey of the membership to determine the top nursing research priorities. In 1991 the top research priorities related to the administration of chemotherapy were quality of life, symptom management, outcome measures for interventions, and pain control; in 1995 they were pain control, quality of life, neutropenia, and patient education. In the past decade cancer nursing research has focused on documenting and describing the phenomenon of chemotherapy side effects. The focus has shifted to designing intervention studies that will provide direction for clinical decision making.

Nursing Research

Administration Issues. Considerable chemotherapy nursing research in the 1980s focused on the hazards to health professionals of administering chemotherapeutic drugs, a concern that developed after Falck's study (Falck et al., 1979) reported increased mutagenicity in the urine of chemotherapy nurses. Research studies during this period tended to assess the uptake of specific cytotoxic drugs in the urine of nurses handling these drugs or to look at the mutagenic changes that had occurred in their urine. Johnson and Gross (1982) were unable to find methotrexate in the blood and urine of nurses who administered this drug. The other focus of nursing research was to investigate compliance with Occupational Safety and Health Administration guidelines for the safe handling of cytotoxic drugs. Valanis and Shortridge (1987) investigated this area and documented inconsistent adherence to these guidelines. Although there was increased use of protective equipment among nurses, most nurses did not wear face protection when handling cytotoxic drugs except when cleaning up a spill.

Side Effect Issues. The side effects from the administration of chemotherapy affect all body systems and occur initially, throughout administration, and years later. The chemotherapy side effects that nursing research has focused on are nausea and vomiting, stomatitis, pain, and fatigue. Cotanch and Strum (1987) randomly assigned 60 patients who were beginning inpatient chemotherapy infusions to three groups: (a) experimental, (b) placebo, and (c) control. The patients who were taught progressive muscle relaxation had less frequency and duration of vomiting, less general anxiety, less physiological arousal, and greater caloric intake 48 hours following the drug infusion than those patients not taught progressive muscle relaxation.

Quality-of-Life Issues. Quality of life (QOL) became a critical outcome measure when the National Cancer Institute initiated a policy to include it as an outcome measure in all clinical trials. Cancer nursing has played a prominent role in encouraging clinical interest in QOL research. Nursing research in this area has been describing the phenomenon, developing instruments to measure it, and testing interventions to promote QOL. Many of the QOL nursing studies have investigated patient responses to treatment with cytotoxic drugs. Sarna (1989) described the effects of the initial cycle of chemotherapy on QOL and functional status in adults over 65 years of age with lung cancer.

Summary

The role of the nurse in relation to chemotherapy has changed dramatically over the past several decades. Initially, the research role of the nurse was that of a data collector assisting physicians involved in clinical trials. The research role of the nurse then evolved to conducting research independently of clinical trials and focusing on the hazards of administering cytotoxic drugs to patients and investigating the impact of nursing interventions on the side effects of the drugs. Nurses are now vital, equal participants and conduct their own studies within clinical trials. Quality-of-life nursing studies are

frequently the vehicle with which nursing joins with physicians in seeking to improve the care of cancer patients.

MARILYN FRANK-STROMBORG

See also
CANCER SURVIVORSHIP
COMFORT
GRIEF
PAIN MANAGEMENT
QUALITY OF LIFE

CANCER IN CHILDREN

The annual incidence of cancer in the United States is 14 cases per 100,000 children younger than 15 years of age and 20 cases per 100,000 adolescents between the ages of 15 and 18 years. There are approximately 11,000 new cases of pediatric cancers each year in the United States. There is evidence that the incidence of cancer is increasing among children more than in young and middle-aged adults. In fact, between 1974 and 1991 there has been a 1% average yearly increase in the incidence of all malignant neoplasms in children 14 years of age or younger. The increased rate has been greater in young children and for tumors of the central nervous system, rhabdomyosarcoma, retinoblastoma, and neuroblastoma (Gurney et al., 1996; Lukens, 1994).

The observed increase in pediatric tumors, especially among young children, has resulted in an increased interest in the potential contribution of environmental exposures in interaction with genetic factors. To date, little is known about environmental agents associated with an increased risk of childhood cancer; however, epidemiological studies of pre- and postnatal environmental exposures have only recently been initiated. Ruccione and colleagues (Ruccione, Waskerwitz, Buckley, Perin, & Hammond, 1994) queried 500 parents about their concerns about potential causes of their child's cancer. Environmental exposures were the most common concern; examples of environmental concerns reported by parents included air, water, and food quality, occupational exposures, and school exposures. The second most common category of concerns was health-related exposures such as medications, trauma, marijuana use, and extended family history of cancer.

Contributions of Nursing Research to the Care of Children with Cancer

Five-year disease-free survival from childhood cancer has increased from less than 10% in 1950 to 81% in 1993. Despite this dramatic improvement in survival from a previously fatal disease, cancer remains the leading cause of death from disease in children and adolescents. Nursing research in the 1970s focused primarily on the emotional responses of children with a terminal illness and on the impact of the child's illness and death on the family. Waechter's (1987) classic study, "Death Anxiety in Children with Fatal Illness," found that children with a terminal illness experienced feelings of isolation, loneliness, and anxiety about dying. As a result of these findings, the importance of open and honest communication with ill children about their illness and concerns was recognized.

Nurse researchers documented that the healthy siblings of the child with cancer also experience significant emotional distress. Kramer (1987) identified emotional realignment, separation, and the ill child's therapeutic regimen as sources of stress experienced by healthy siblings. Siblings often feel guilty that they are somehow responsible for the illness. Siblings identify anger and resentment toward the special attention and needs of the ill child, isolation, and vulnerability as to the fact that they may also become sick. Parents of children with cancer are faced with the challenge of caring for a child with a life-threatening illness. Research findings are controversial about the magnitude of the stress experienced by parents and the types of coping strategies they use. In general, there is evidence that parents experience significantly more life-change events, such as marital conflict and financial strain. Parents worry more about the health and future of the ill child and are more likely to be overprotective.

As survival from childhood cancer increased and greater numbers of children achieved long-term disease-free remission, nursing investigations shifted from a focus on terminal illness to living with a chronic life-threatening illness. The adverse effects of the illness and treatment on social competence, school and peer relationships have been documented by nurse investigators. Hockenberry-Eaton and colleagues (Hockenberry-Eaton, Kemp, & DiIorio, 1994) investigated predictors of stress experienced during treatment for childhood cancer. Findings from this multivariate study of 44 children receiving cancer treatment documented an increased physiological response to cancer stressors (epinephrine and norepinephrine) and the importance of family characteristics and social support in buffering the child's anxiety.

Quality of life for children and adolescents with cancer is a recent interest in nursing research. Quality-of-life research focuses on the social, physical, and emotional functioning of the child and adolescent and when appropriate, the family members (Bradlyn et al., 1996). Nursing studies have investigated disease- and treatment-related pain and the side effects of treatment such as nausea and vomiting. Hope and resilience are two factors that have been linked to positive quality-of-life outcomes for adolescents with cancer. Hinds's (1988) grounded-theory study of adolescent hopefulness in illness and health found that adolescents with cancer included "others" as well as "self" in their definition of hopefulness.

Nursing research on the late effects of childhood cancer has increased over the past 10 years. Late effects refer to the persistent adverse effects of cancer treatment on nonmalignant cells and tissues and the persistent psychological and economic consequences of surviving a serious life-threatening illness (Moore, 1995). Nursing studies have documented the adverse effects of central nervous system (CNS) treatment on cognitive, academic, and psychosocial functioning. Children who receive whole brain radiation, especially at an early age, are at high risk for these problems. *Survivors of Childhood Cancer: Assessment and Management* is an excellent summary of the late effects associated with cancer therapy. This book was co-authored by nurse investigators and advanced practice clinicians (Schwartz, Hobbie, Constine, & Ruccione, 1994).

Nursing Research in Childhood Cancer: Limitations and Future Directions

Nursing research in pediatric oncology has been hampered by the limited number of investigators. Furthermore, sample sizes are often constrained by the number of children with a specific diagnosis at a treatment center. The majority of studies have been descriptive in design. A final limitation has been the paucity of instruments that are appropriate for use with children with cancer and family members. For example, many instruments that have been used to investigate psychosocial questions were developed and evaluated on noncancer samples. Therefore, items may not be relevant to the cancer illness experience. Instruments to measure quality of life for children and adolescents with cancer are now being developed and tested.

Nursing research has gained increased recognition and support as an important component of the pediatric cooperative groups. The cooperative group mechanism is an excellent strategy for developing multisite studies that are essential for the sample size requirements of multivariate studies. As noted above, the majority of nursing studies have been descriptive and correlational. There are very few quasi-experimental studies that test the efficacy of interventions that target clinical problems. An important next step in pediatric oncology nursing research is to design intervention studies that target significant behavioral and biological sequelae of the cancer treatment and illness experience.

Conclusions

There has been great progress in the treatment of childhood cancer. In fact, it is estimated that, by the year 2010, 1 in 250 individuals between the ages of 15 and 45 years will be a survivor of childhood cancer (Bleyer, 1990). This dramatic improvement in survival results from a greater understanding of the biological basis of the disease and the use of aggressive multimodal therapy. The psychosocial consequences of living with a chronic life-threatening disease and the adverse effects of cancer treatment on quality-of-life outcomes will become increasingly important. Pediatric oncology nurses are in an ideal situation to investigate these problems and to test interventions for improving outcomes for children with cancer.

IDA M. (KI) MOORE

See also
CHRONIC CONDITIONS IN CHILDHOOD
FAMILY CARE
GENETICS IN NURSING RESEARCH
PAIN IN CHILDREN
PSYCHOSOCIAL EFFECTS OF CHILD CRITICAL ILLNESS AND HOSPITALIZATION

CANCER SURVIVORSHIP

Ten million cancer survivors are living in the United States today. The growing numbers are a result of improved cancer treatment, symptom management, and supportive care. A cancer survivor is defined as an individual who is living with, through, and beyond a diagnosis of cancer. Cancer survivors include individuals living through cancer treatment, those who are cancer-free, and those having intermittent recurrence or persistent or advanced disease. This definition differs from the traditional view of a cancer survivor as one who has lived at least 5 years after cancer diagnosis.

Cancer survivors have stressed the increased importance of and attention to quality-of-life (QOL) issues and have been instrumental in the growing debate in the larger political and health arenas on policy about cancer survivorship. The cancer survivorship philosophy reflects the personal experiences and wisdom of individuals who have ''been there.'' The philosophy is based on the emergence of a more informed and assertive health care consumer having an optimistic expectation of survival.

The National Coalition for Cancer Survivorship (NCCS), which addresses concerns of cancer survivors, has grown from a grassroots organization to one having regional and national prominence. Major health policy issues on survivorship have continued to develop since the First National Congress on Cancer Survivorship in 1995 to the establishment of the Office of Cancer Survivorship at the National Cancer Institute in 1996. The purpose of the office is to explore critical research issues and consequences of cancer treatment through an interdisciplinary approach.

Studies of cancer survivors have focused primarily on the pediatric cancer survivor, but much research needs to be done with adult survivors. The concerns of cancer survivors can best be viewed through a QOL framework, which is a personal sense of well-being that encompasses a multidimensional perspective of physiological, psychological, social, and spiritual well-being. Changes in one area or domain of QOL can influence changes in other QOL domains.

Nurse researchers have contributed to our knowledge of the QOL concerns of cancer survivors. They have participated in clinical trials evaluating late physiological effects and have investigated high-incidence concerns of cancer survivors (Ferrell & Hassey Dow, 1997). Ferrell, Hassey Dow, Leigh, Ly, and Gulasekaram (1995) described the QOL in a study of long-term cancer survivors. They used a mailed survey of three instruments—a demographic tool, the QOL–Cancer Survivors tool, and the FACT-G—sent to 1,000 members of NCCS. The QOL instruments were designed to elicit concerns of cancer survivors in four areas, or domains: physical, psychological, social, and spiritual well-being. They received 687 returned surveys (57%). The mean age of the sample was 49.6 years; 81% were female, 72% college-educated, 63% married, 66% working full- or part-time. Results indicated that fatigue, aches and pains, and fertility were problematic physical late effects. Psychological concerns included the recall of distress at initial diagnosis and fear of recurrent, metastatic, or second cancers. Fear of future tests, anxiety, and depression were also problematic, as were family distress, sexuality, and financial burdens. In addition, hopefulness and purposefulness were positive outcomes of surviving cancer.

Nurse scientists continue to investigate late physical effects of pain, fatigue, dyspnea, functional changes (immobility, incontinence, and lymphedema), sexuality and intimacy issues, and cognitive impairments (Blesch et al., 1991) among cancer survivors. Physiological late effects where more research is needed include the development of secondary cancers, recurrent cancer, and late organ effects on the cardiovascular, pulmonary, reproductive, and endocrine systems.

Psychosocial late effects identified in descriptive studies of cancer survivors include the fear of recurrence, fear of testing procedures and medical surveillance, emotional distress, depression, uncertainty over the future, loneliness, and isolation (Mahon, 1991; Northouse, 1981). Uncertainty over the future and fear of recurrence have been identified as major areas targeted for interventions, although support groups have traditionally addressed some of these psychosocial issues.

Living with cancer may necessitate a change over time in the meaning of work and actual work practices. Nursing research in this area has identified work-related dilemmas such as overcoming bias in the workplace, disclosure, reentry concerns, breach of confidentiality, and lack of resources in the workplace (Berry & Catanzaro, 1992). Berry and Catanzaro described nursing interventions to help survivors return to the workplace. They divided the interventions into two categories: personal factors and environmental factors. Personal factors included collaborating with other health disciplines, addressing knowledge deficits about side effects and discrimination issues, and discussing the meaning of work. Environmental factors included the facilitation of reintegration of treatment with life activities and encouraging the worker to establish regular communication.

Spiritual distress characterized by loneliness, despair, grief, loss, and uncertainty has been identified in cancer survivors by nurse researchers (Kahn & Steeves, 1993). Positive life changes include risk taking, improved decision making, hope, and transcendence. These descriptive studies lay the groundwork for the development of interventions aimed at reducing such burdens. Interventions to help cancer survivors in the search for meaning are future areas of research (Ersek, Ferrell, Hassey Dow, & Melancon, 1997).

Future Areas of Research

Services needed by cancer survivors include access to long-term follow-up, development of guidelines and standards for long-term follow-up, expanded models of psychosocial and rehabilitative support, and education and health maintenance of cancer survivors. Nurse researchers have collaborated with advocacy and survivorship groups to describe the long-term needs of cancer survivors and have developed valid and reliable instruments to measure quality of life in this population (Hassey Dow, Ferrell, Leigh, & Melancon, in press). With the growing population of cancer survivors, survivorship research is a fruitful area for continued investigation in the future.

KAREN HASSEY DOW

See also
   COPING
   GRIEF
   QUALITY OF LIFE
   SOCIAL SUPPORT

CAPITATION

Definition

Capitation is a form of payment for health services and is usually associated with managed care, which is rapidly replacing fee-for-service payments as a method of compensation. Kongsvedt (1995) defines capitation specifically as "prepayment for services on a per member per month (PMPM) basis" (p. 76). This means that providers or provider organizations would receive the same amount of dollars every month (PMPM rate) for each enrolled member regardless of how expensive the services were or whether the member actually received services. Capitation payments are usually calculated on the capitation equivalent of average fee-for-service revenues of the provider or provider organization (based on actual or existing data for the population of interest) and vary according to the age and gender of the enrolled members. In some cases, the capitation rate is also based on risk, or expected high utilization of service based on risk, or specific conditions such as use of illegal drugs, selected chronic illnesses, and so forth.

Historical Perspective

Although health care reform as a legislative agenda is no longer relevant, market-driven reform is rapidly changing the structure and terminology of health care delivery to managed care. Managed care has grown out of the need to control escalating health care costs and is rapidly becoming accepted as the way health care will be delivered in the future. However, managed health care organizations are not new. They grew out of the private sector when prepaid plans were implemented in health maintenance organizations (HMOs). In this model (implemented in the 1970s) providers first shared the risk of financing health care for an enrolled population. Providers, primarily physicians, were offered the choice of collecting a fee for service from the patient or having the HMO pay the physician directly out of a prepaid per capita payment (capitation) for health services. Any excess revenue generated above expenses could be shared by providers, and enrollees (members) were also able to save health insurance premiums by reducing unnecessary hospital admissions and length of stays. Currently, there are many forms of managed care organizations besides HMOs, but the challenge for all these provider organizations is to remove inefficiencies and reduce costs from the current fee-for-service systems and through capitation to improve the quality and coordination of care across the continuum.

Implications for Nursing Practice and Research

In many cases, one capitated payment is in place that covers care across the continuum. In other situations, a blended capitation rate such as $x PMPM may exist for primary care services, with an additional capitated pool of $xx for referral services, and $xxx for inpatient or institutional care. Capitation affects nurses in all care settings across the continuum, from the staff nurse in acute care to the home health nurse to the primary care nurse practitioner. Awareness of the value of prevention, health promotion, and coordination of care in order to reduce unplanned visits and unexpected admissions is key to success in a capitated, managed care system. New nursing roles of case management and primary care provider in community-based settings offer opportunities created by managed care and challenges to manage care within specific limited resources.

Uses in Research

Research related to capitation in the context of managed care is health systems or health services research or evaluation research. Holzemer and Reilly (1994) used the term *variations research* as an important strategy designed to improve the quality of care while controlling costs. They proposed an outcomes model (based on the work of Donabedian) that allowed for measurement of variability related to client or population (age, gender, risk, etc.), variability of providers (such as advanced practice nurses vs. physicians), variability of interventions or processes of care, and variability in outcomes of care (which may include quality indicators, costs, cost savings, and patient/provider satisfaction).

Research related to capitation may involve assessment of risk for population-based care and determining the appropriate capitation based on variability within different populations. Community health assessment performed by community health nurses may be used for these types of assessments. Research related to capitation may involve study of the different uses and types of providers or processes of care needed to achieve required outcomes at a particular price (capitation rate PMPM). Finally, the research may focus on the cost savings of a particular intervention, for example, transitional models of care between hospital and home or the use of case management models to reduce inappropriate utilization of care.

Issues

The unit of analysis in research related to capitation is of paramount importance. Nurse researchers may study the client and client characteristics, the provider or provider system, specific interventions, or outcomes. Outcomes research is of great interest to managed care companies that are implementing capitation models. These companies desire quality outcomes (functional and clinically relevant changes) in the client and client satisfaction with the care, and they want them in a cost-effective manner. Variations research is an attempt to control confounding variables such as risk, severity of illness, and client characteristics that influence outcomes of care. Risk adjustment of outcomes is complex but must be addressed in variations research. Use of information systems to obtain data related to costs and other outcomes from organizational databases must be addressed. The issue of decisions related to data substitution and use of proxies to handle missing data is a relevant issue for health systems researchers who study the impact or effectiveness of capitation in the context of managed care.

Finally, an important issue is educating practicing nurses, current nurse researchers, and future students in the risk, cost, and quality issues related to capitation in managed care. The rapid increase in managed care organizations and systems has introduced new terms and concepts into medical and nursing language.

PATRICIA HINTON WALKER

See also
**HEALTH CARE REFORM
   AND NURSING RESEARCH
HEALTH MAINTENANCE
   ORGANIZATIONS
HEALTH SYSTEMS DELIVERY
MANAGED CARE
TRANSITIONAL CARE**

CARDIOVASCULAR NURSING

Cardiovascular nursing is defined as the nursing care of individuals who have a known or predicted alteration in cardiovascular physiological function. Cardiovascular nursing research has focused on the development of knowledge related to both acute events (myocardial infarction, cardiac surgery) and chronic aspects of cardiovascular disease (hypertension, heart failure, cardiomyopathy, prevention of cardiovascular disease), and it encompasses individuals, families, and communities. To a large extent, the focus of research in cardiovascular nursing has followed advances and changes in medical care—intensive care hemodynamic monitoring, cardiac arrhythmia monitoring and treatment, coronary artery revascularization, cardiac rehabilitation, implantable devices (pacemakers and defibrillators), and cardiac transplantation. As technical advances were made in cardiac care, nursing research focused on parallel nursing issues regarding patient comfort and safety, cardiovascular responses to treatment, symptom monitoring, preparatory preoperative and postoperative teaching, medication and medical regimen compliance, discharge teaching for home recovery, and risk factor reduction.

Historically, research in cardiovascular nursing has been an important part of the development of nursing science and has included interdisciplinary research, experimental studies, and studies addressing biopsychosocial outcomes. In a review of the 12 years of research presented by the Council on Cardiovascular Nursing at the scientific sessions of the American Heart Association during 1972 through 1983 (Kinney, 1985), the focus of cardiovascular nursing research was on hemodynamic problems encountered in nursing practice, patient and family responses to cardiac events, patient assessment, and patient teaching and compliance. The theories guiding cardiovascular research have been as varied as the research topics and include theories of coping, self-efficacy, self-regulation, physiological mechanisms, psychology, and education. The Council of Cardiovascular Nursing of the American Heart Association has played a central role in supporting research in cardiovascular nursing. The American Heart Association has had sessions devoted to the report of cardiovascular nursing research at its annual scientific sessions; published a research journal, *Cardiovascular Nursing*; and provided funding for cardiovascular nursing research since the early 1970s. Another journal of historical importance to the dissemination of research in cardiovascular nursing is *Heart & Lung*, an interdisciplinary specialty research journal addressing research in pulmonary and cardiovascular health since 1972.

Intervention research has been a major focus of cardiovascular nursing. In a review of cardiovascular nursing research, Foster and colleagues (Foster, Kloner, & Stengrevics, 1984) found that most tested nursing interventions fell within the category of patient and family teaching, followed by rehabilitation progress, coping and stress-reducing interventions, and patient reorientation for postcardiotomy delirium. The most widely researched areas were myocardial infarction, cardiovascular procedures, and coronary precautions. More recently, intervention research has focused on assisting individuals with heart failure, hypertension, and sudden cardiac death, and on coronary artery disease risk factor reduction. However, the costs and efficiency of cardiovascular nursing interventions have been little studied, and with the exception of the work of Gortner and Gillis, replication and extension studies have been few.

Cardiovascular nursing has a group of nurses with sustained programs of research, such as Cowan's (1990) investigations of the usefulness of electrocardiography to determine myocardial infarction size and sudden cardiac arrest, Dracup's research on cardiac care unit monitoring, and Gortner and Gillis's studies of the effectiveness of a supportive education program to enhance home recovery outcomes following acute cardiac events. Also, the influence of spouses and other family members in providing social support for patients following cardiac events has been documented in programs of research by Artinian, Gillis, and Yates. A growing body of knowledge about risk factor prevention has been ongoing in the research efforts of Sivarajan, Hill, Allen, and Hayman. Recently, Grady, Jalowiec, and White-Williams have conducted a series of studies addressing the needs of cardiac transplantation patients, and Dunbar has reported care issues of patients with implantable devices.

Instrument development in cardiovascular nursing research has been limited. Ferrans and Powers' Quality of Life Index (Cardiac Version) has been found to be a psychometrically sound instrument to measure quality of life in several types of cardiac patients. Also, the Self-Efficacy Expectation Scale by Jenkins has gained wide use in determining patients' self-efficacy expectations about cardiac recovery behaviors, and Miller's Health Intention and Health Behavior Scales have shown considerable usefulness in measuring compliance with medical regimens after cardiac events.

Analysis of cardiovascular nursing studies indicates that few women and elders have been included; studies have consisted primarily of White, college-educated individuals living in or near urban areas. Additionally, few economic issues have been addressed, such as the cost-effectiveness of nursing interventions and nurse utilization. Although considerable knowledge has been built about how to enhance recovery following acute cardiac events, an important area of cardiovascular nursing that still needs development is the prevention of coronary risk factors, including smoking, obesity, hypertension, inactivity, and hyperlipidemia. Of particular interest are the social and psychological variables influencing long-term behavior change for cardiovascular health and risk reduction. There also has been a recent initiative in cardiovascular nursing to better understand the gender and cultural differences in symptomatology associated with the diagnosis and treatment of acute cardiac events. An additional area for knowledge development is the biobehavioral mechanisms associated with cardiovascular nursing problems, interventions, and outcomes. Because technology in cardiovascular care has made great advances, there has been an increased interest in quality of life issues for individuals with myocardial infarction, cardiac surgery, heart failure, implantable devices, and transplantation (Cowan, 1990).

An important area for knowledge development in pediatric cardiovascular nursing is risk factor reduction in children and the long-term developmental and psychosocial outcomes for children with invasive cardiovascular procedures. Another important future direction is increased understanding of the genetic predisposition to cardiovascular disease and the use of gene therapy. One of the challenges facing cardiovascular nursing in the next decade will be to balance the research initiatives in two important areas: cardiovascular disease prevention and health promotion and the development of appropriate nursing interventions to promote patient comfort, safety, and optimal outcomes associated with the application of technology.

SHIRLEY M. MOORE

See also
DEPRESSION AND CARDIAC DISEASE

HEMODYNAMIC MONITORING
HYPERTENSION
RISK FACTORS
SMOKING/TOBACCO AS
 CARDIOVASCULAR RISK FACTORS

CARDIOVASCULAR RISK FACTORS: CHOLESTEROL

Background and Definition

Coronary heart disease (CHD) due to atherosclerosis is a leading cause of morbidity and premature mortality in both men and women in the United States, the industrialized world, and many developing countries. The atherosclerotic process begins early in life and is influenced over time by the interaction of genetic and environmental factors. Substantial data generated from epidemiological and clinical studies implicate hypercholesterolemia, elevated serum total blood cholesterol (TC), as an independent risk factor for atherosclerotic CHD. The relationship between TC and CHD is continuous and graded; epidemiological evidence supports a direct relationship between the level of TC and the rate of CHD. Because most cholesterol in serum is contained in atherogenic low-density lipoproteins (LDL-C), the concentration of TC in most individuals is highly correlated with LDL-C.

The National Cholesterol Education Program (NCEP, 1988) defined hypercholesterolemia as TC levels ≥ 240 mg/dl (6.21 mmol/L) for individuals 20 years of age and older. Although the second report of the expert panel issued by NCEP (1993) reaffirmed the definition of hypercholesterolemia, the recommendations for treatment decisions were modified, with increased emphasis on CHD risk status as a guide to the type and intensity of cholesterol lowering. For U.S. children and adolescents, NCEP (1991) defined a serum TC level of <170 mg/dl (4.4 mmol/L) as acceptable and ≥ 200 mg/dl (5.17 mmol/L) as abnormally elevated. LDL-C levels were targeted as the basis for treatment decisions; LDL-C levels ≤ 110 mg/dl are considered acceptable.

Prevalence in the United States

In 1985 the National Heart, Lung, and Blood Institute (NHLBI) launched NCEP with the ultimate goal of reducing the prevalence of elevated blood cholesterol levels and thus reducing CHD morbidity and mortality in the United States. The potential impact of the NCEP guidelines was evaluated by using data collected as part of the National Health and Nutrition Examination Surveys (NHANES II) (Sempos et al., 1989) and NHANES III (Johnson, Rifkind, et al., 1993) and the NCEP (1993) guidelines and recommendations. From the data collection period in NHANES II (1976–1980) to the period in NHANES III (1988–1991), the proportion of adults with hypercholesterolemia (TC ≥ 240 mg/dl) decreased from 26% to 20%. Concomitantly, the proportion with desirable levels (TC < 200 mg/dl [5.17 mmol/L]) increased 44% to 49% (Sempos et al., 1993). Decreases in the age-adjusted percentage with hypercholesterolemia were similar for Blacks and Whites, although there appeared to be a larger shift for Whites toward desirable levels.

It is estimated, on the basis of 1990 population data, that approximately 52 million Americans 20 years of age and older would be candidates for dietary therapy, and approximately 12.7 million might be candidates for cholesterol-lowering drugs (Sempos et al., 1993). Although prevalence rates for hypercholesterolemia as defined by TC levels ≥ 240 mg/dl have decreased to 20% and are consistent with the goals articulated in *Healthy People 2000* (U.S. Department of Health and Human Services, 1990), substantial numbers of Americans continue to be at risk for CHD because of adverse lipid profiles. Nurses could be instrumental in creative approaches to case finding, assessment, and management across health care settings.

Detection and Evaluation

Measurement Considerations. NCEP (1993) recommendations specify that TC should be measured at least once every 5 years in all adults 20 years of age and over. High-density lipoprotein cholesterol (HDL-C) levels help to determine risk status and should be measured simultaneously if accurate re-

sults are available. Because TC levels are influenced by acute illness, trauma, pregnancy, change in dietary intake, and acute myocardial infarction, routine (initial) testing to determine baseline levels are not recommended when these conditions exist. The results of the initial TC measurement will determine if lipoprotein analysis (particularly LDL-C estimation) is appropriate. Because the LDL-C value is normally estimated from measurements that include triglyceride (TG), blood samples should be collected from individuals who have fasted for 9 to 12 hours. Measurement considerations apply to specimens collected from children and adolescents; however, the specifics of risk assessment and follow-up vary. For both groups, NCEP (1991, 1993) emphasizes the importance of basing treatment decisions on the average of two fasting LDL-C measurements.

Other Lipid and Lipoprotein Risk Factors. Epidemiological studies have demonstrated that low levels of HDL-C, independent of LDL-C, are a significant risk factor for CHD. Available evidence indicates that for every 1 mg/dl decrease in HDL-C, the risk for CHD increases by 2%–3%. HDL-C levels are inversely correlated with CHD rates over a broad range of HDL-C levels; higher HDL-C levels appear to be cardioprotective. Thus, current NCEP recommendations suggest HDL-C measurements as part of the initial CHD risk assessment of adults and classify HDL-C <35 mg/dl as a major risk factor for CHD and levels ≥ 60 mg/dl as a negative risk factor.

Although serum triglycerides (TGs) are not considered an independent risk factor for CHD, TGs are correlated with CHD rates in most prospective and case-control studies. Further, elevated TGs are often associated with reduced HDL-C levels. These associations have been observed in population-based and clinical studies of adults and children. Because no large-scale clinical trials have addressed the question of whether reducing TG levels in hypertriglyceridemic individuals will decrease the risk for CHD, the utility of treatment of TG levels remains questionable.

Several additional components of the lipoprotein system are under intense evaluation for their utility in predicting risk for CHD across the life span. Some of the important components include apolipoproteins B and AI; HDL-C subclasses LP-AI, AII, and AIII; small, dense LDL-C particles; and lipoprotein (a) (Lp[a]). Currently, no definitive clinical trial data are available to recommend routine use in clinical practice, and accurate and reliable measurements are not widely available (NCEP, 1993). Lipid specialists may choose to measure these components, however, in individuals at risk for familial or genetic dyslipidemias.

Associated Factors. Hypercholesterolemia frequently coexists with other CHD risk factors that must be considered in both primary and secondary prevention efforts. Nonmodifiable risk factors include family history of CHD, male sex, and age; modifiable factors include cigarette smoking, hypertension, obesity, physical inactivity, and diabetes mellitus. Although not considered an independent risk factor for CHD, dietary intake, particularly excess consumption of saturated fats and cholesterol, is an important exogenous determinant of serum TC and CHD risk. Additionally, selected psychosocial factors, including the hostility component of the type A behavior pattern and acute psychological stressors, have been associated with CHD. Social and environmental factors that contribute to the isolation of individuals (economic insecurity, lower educational level, absence of family and/or social support) also have been associated with CHD in observational studies. Because CHD is polygenic and multifactorial, assessment and management will be optimally accomplished by a multidisciplinary team approach. With expertise in the physiological and behavioral aspects of CHD, nurses are particularly well suited for leadership roles in clinical practice and research to enhance the art and science of CHD prevention and management.

Treatment

NCEP (1993) and the recommendations of the 27th Bethesda Conference (Fuster & Pearson, 1996) emphasize the importance of matching the type and intensity of risk factor management with the hazard for CHD events. These recommendations, applied to the management of hypercholesterolemia in adults, target LDL-C levels as the basis for clinical decisions; however, emphasis also is placed on the total CHD risk profile. The ultimate goal of treatment on the individual (patient) level is the reduction of premature morbidity and mortality by the most efficient, effective, and least intrusive methods. The cornerstone of treatment is dietary modification, with emphasis on reducing the intake of saturated fat and cholesterol and correcting any imbalance between caloric intake and energy expenditure. In addition to NCEP, numerous agencies, including the American Heart Association and the National Academy of Sciences, advocate dietary change as part of the individual and population approach to reducing the risk of CHD and other chronic diseases.

Considerable variation in response to dietary modification has been observed in both males and females across the life span. Variations in serum TC reductions (ranging from 3% to 14%) are attributable to individual differences in biological mechanisms, baseline TC levels, nutrient composition of baseline diets, and adherence over time to the prescribed dietary regimen. Essential to successful dietary intervention in both adults and children are the attitudes, knowledge, and skills of the health care provider in motivating and sustaining behavioral change. Although the expertise of a registered dietitian is important in developing the dietary intervention, nurses can be instrumental in promoting self-care and facilitating adherence over time. Nurses can assume leadership roles to design individualized, developmentally and culturally appropriate interventions that incorporate the patient's concerns, economic and social supports, and patterns of health-related lifestyle behaviors known to influence the lipid profile and risk factors for CHD.

For adults (and children over 2 years) with hypercholesterolemia, diet modification is presented in two steps. The Step I Diet has recommended the following intakes as a percentage of a total caloric intake: ≤ 30% fat (saturated fats, 8%–10%; polyunsaturated fats, up to 10%; monounsaturated fats, up to 15%); carbohydrates, 55%; protein, approximately 15%. Cholesterol intake should be no more than 300 mg/day. The Step II Diet is similar except for further reductions in saturated fat (< 7% of total calories) and cholesterol (< 200 mg/day). The type and intensity of treatment is determined by the initiation and goal LDL-C level as well as the presence of additional risk factors (see Table 1). If the goals of treatment are not achieved after 3 months on a Step I Diet, progression to a Step II Diet is recommended.

Pharmacological interventions will normally be considered for primary prevention of CHD in adults (without evidence of disease) if dietary modification and other lifestyle changes (weight control, increased physical activity) fail to reduce LDL-C to goal levels within a 6-month period. For these individuals, several factors will influence the type and timing of drug therapy: baseline LDL-C levels, age, gender, and menopausal status. Drug therapy should be considered for older individuals (men 45 years and older, women 55 years and older) whose LDL-C levels exceed 190 mg/dl. Although some

TABLE 1   Treatment Decisions Based on LDL-Cholesterol

Dietary Therapy		
	Initiation level	LDL goal
Without CHD and with fewer than 2 risk factors	≥160 mg/dL	<160 mg/dL
Without CHD and with 2 or more risk factors	≥130 mg/dL	<130 mg/dL
With CHD	>100 mg/dL	≤100 mg/dL
Drug Treatment		
	Consideration level	LDL goal
Without CHD and with fewer than 2 risk factors	≥190 mg/dL[a]	<160 mg/dL
Without CHD and with 2 or more risk factors	≥160 mg/dL	<130 mg/dL
With CHD	≥130 mg/dL[b]	≤100 mg/dL

[a]In men under 35 years old and premenopausal women with LDL-cholesterol levels 190–219 mg/dL, drug therapy should be delayed except in high-risk patients like those with diabetes.
[b]In CHD patients with LDL-cholesterol levels 100–129 mg/dL, the physician should exercise clinical judgment in deciding whether to initiate drug treatment.

Source: Executive Summary, National Cholesterol Education Program: Second Report of the Expert Panel on Detection, Evaluation, and Treatment of Evaluation, and Treatment of High Blood Cholesterol in Adults (1993), 14.

controversy exists regarding the initiation of drug therapy for young adults without evidence of CHD, the severity of LDL-C elevation is universally considered in the decision. Drug therapy for levels exceeding 220 mg/dl is appropriate in those with a family history of premature CHD or genetic dyslipidemias; however, it may be delayed for individuals with levels in the range of 190–220 mg/dl if no other risk factors are present. In those with evidence of CHD, where the clinical objective is secondary prevention, cholesterol-lowering drugs may be initiated prior to 6 months.

Because the decision to initiate drug treatment commits most individuals to long-term therapy, NCEP recommends comprehensive, careful assessment of the risks and benefits and maximal efforts devoted to lifestyle modification. In primary and secondary prevention efforts, pharmacological intervention normally begins with a single cholesterol-lowering agent and may proceed to combination therapy after a minimum of 3 months. The four classes of lipid-lowering drugs in current use include bile acid binding resins, niacin, HMG-CoA reductase inhibitors, and fibrates. In addition to baseline LDL-C levels, the presence of other lipid abnormalities (i.e., low HDL-C, high TG) or CHD risk factors, side effects, general health status, and cost issues are considered in the selection of the specific drug protocol. Combination drug therapy is more costly, requires more frequent monitoring and supervision by the health care provider, and exposes the patient to more risks. Thus, the decision to proceed with more aggressive combination drug therapy should be made with active involvement and counseling on benefits and risks for the patient.

For children (2 years of age and older) and adolescents with hypercholesterolemia, dietary modification is also recommended as the first mode of treatment. NCEP (1991) recommended adoption of the Step I Diet early in childhood as the population approach to reducing TC levels and risk for CHD. As in adults, progression to the Step II Diet normally occurs if LDL-C goals are not realized after a minimum of 3 months. Drug therapy for children with hypercholesterolemia is normally reserved for those 10 years of age or older who fail to respond after 6 to 12 months of aggressive dietary intervention as indicated by LDL-C levels of 190 mg/dl and for those nonresponders with LDL-C levels of 160 mg/dl and a positive family history of premature CHD or two or more other CHD risk factors. Currently, only the bile acid binding resins have proven efficacy, relative freedom from side effects, and apparent safety when used in children and adolescents (NCEP, 1991).

Niacin has been used without serious short-term effects in children with familial or genetic hyperlipidemias; however, the long-term safety of other lipid-lowering agents has not been established. In the absence of definitive, prospective data generated from clinical trials, pharmacological treatment of hypercholesterolemic children should be highly selective, as indicated by NCEP, with careful, continuous monitoring of growth and developmental processes as well as other indicators of health status.

Nursing Research and Practice

Programs of nursing and multidisciplinary research focus on CHD across the life span; results to date have contributed to the existing body of knowledge in this area of inquiry and have influenced clinical practice. As part of a multidisciplinary program of research on cardiovascular health promotion and risk reduction in childhood and adolescence, Hayman and colleagues (Hayman et al., 1995; Hayman et al., 1988) examined the genetic and environmental determinants of risk for CHD during the school-age years, adolescence, and the transition between these developmental phases. Collective results indicated the importance of a developmental, family-based profile approach with emphasis on preventive interventions beginning early in life. Consistent with NCEP recommendations for prevention and management of hypercholesterolemia in children and adolescents, the results targeted the environmental determinants of risk and emphasized the adoption of heart-healthy lifestyles early in life. Similarly, in a school-based intervention study of CHD risk factors, Harrell and colleagues (Harrell et al., 1996) demonstrated the importance of physical activity in reducing TC levels in children and the efficacy of an integrated approach to cardiovascular health executed in the school environment.

Nurse investigators and clinicians have participated in the development, implementation, and evaluation of models of care delivery focused on hypercholesterolemia as part of multiple risk factor management (DeBusk et al., 1994). Specifically, this multidisciplinary case management system demonstrated the effectiveness of nursing interventions in reducing LDL-C (and other risk factors) as part of secondary prevention of CHD in adults. These results emphasize the role of nurses and nursing in CHD prevention as well as the need for additional research on innovative models of care delivery that consider both cost and quality as outcomes.

Gaps in Knowledge and Practice

During the past two decades considerable data have accumulated regarding the distribution and determinants of cholesterol levels in both males and females across the life span. Although dietary intake and other health-related lifestyle behaviors are acknowledged as essential components of primary and secondary prevention of CHD, nonadherence to therapeutic regimens is a continuing challenge for both health care providers and consumers across settings. Although creative strategies designed enhance adherence have been developed, few have been tested in clinical trials for comparative efficacy (Burke, Dunbar-Jacob, & Hill, 1997). In addition, minimal research attention has been devoted to the development and maintenance of these behaviors in children and adolescents and in vulnerable populations at highest risk for long-term noncompliance. For both primary and secondary prevention of CHD, research is needed to inform and evaluate multidisciplinary models of care delivery designed to increase access, adherence, and health outcomes.

LAURA L. HAYMAN

See also
  DIABETES MELLITUS
  NUTRITION
  OBESITY AS A CARDIOVASCULAR
    RISK FACTOR
  PSYCHOSOCIAL INTERVENTIONS
    DECREASE MORTALITY AFTER
    CORONARY ARTERY DISEASE

SMOKING/TOBACCO AS CARDIOVASCULAR RISK FACTOR

CAREGIVER

The term *caregiver* is defined as the individual who assists ill persons, helps with a patient's physical care, typically lives with the patient, and does not receive monetary compensation for the help. A more descriptive definition of a caregiver is a person who not only performs common caregiver responsibilities of providing physical, social, spiritual, nursing, and technical care but also advocates for the ill person within health care systems and society as a whole.

The caregiver role is often expected and prepared for in relationship to elders, but rarely is there preparation for caregiving to one's child (ventilator-dependent children) or one's spouse (technological dependency on lifelong hemodialysis or total parenteral nutrition). The caregiver's relationship with the patient, the caregiver's age and developmental stage, the patient's illness severity, the suddenness and amount of the change in the patient's need for caregiving have been predictive of caregiver burnout in various illness populations such as cancer care with home chemotherapy, cardiac rehabilitation, muscle deterioration, and disease victims (Biegel, Sales, & Schulz, 1991).

Defining the role and tasks taken on by a caregiver gives a much better description of the daily lives and potential problems these individuals experience. The typical role of the caregiver includes direct patient care, familial and societal responsibilities, and financial management of the home and medical care. Complex decisions must be made about finances, as well as deciding daily about the patient's status. Direct patient care is much more than physical care. It also necessitates learning large amounts of information about illness, symptoms, medications, and technological treatments and about how to relate to health care professionals (Smith, 1995). Caregivers also must be prepared for and able to respond to emergencies. Familial or household responsibilities include continuing the caregiver's life tasks, whether as breadwinner, housekeeper, or both. Caregivers also have many indirect activities related to direct care, such as establishing a care schedule, maintaining the inventory of supplies, and negotiating with third-party payers.

The indirect familial caregiver tasks include designating others to assist with patient care and other familial tasks, communication and exchanging information, and maintaining decision making among appropriate persons. Societal expectations of caregivers are assuming financial costs, planning for long-term care, and advocating for the patient's best interest. Society also expects caregivers to be knowledgeable about health services and reimbursement mechanisms (i.e., being their own case managers) to ensure effective yet efficient care. Caregivers also have numerous expectations for themselves and from others around them to perform various psychosocial tasks such as coping with changes in role, grieving the loss of health and personality of their loved one, releasing tension, resolving uncertainty or guilt, and providing positive regard for those with whom they interact.

Because the caregiver definition is laden with tasks and expectations, it is no wonder that the major area of research has been caregiver burden, measured as both subjective and objective strain. The majority of burden studies have been descriptive and correlational and have resulted in identification of multiple factors associated with caregiver burden. Major factors recognized as being significant for burden are the characteristics of the care needed by the patient, which are often measured as illness demands. Numerous demographic, life developmental stage, and social support variables have been studied in relation to caregiver burden (Braithwaite, 1992). Findings vary from study to study, but individual variables, such as gender, psychosocial adjustment, other life stressors, and the meaning of the caregiving experience to the individual, are influential yet not universally predictive of caregiver burden (Biegel, Sales, & Schulz, 1991).

Historically, research on the topic of caregivers has come from the literature on aging in which burden and supportive interventions have been studied. Interventions tested include teaching mastery of caregiving tasks, social interventions such as support groups or telephone contacts, and direct clinical services such as counseling and respite care.

Outcomes of many of these intervention studies indicated that, in the short term, the interventions may reduce caregiver stress in a limited way, but the burden returns when the interventions stop. Research with midlife caregivers reveals the need for interventions on resource management (Smith, 1994b) and motivation to help (Smith, 1994a). Further research is needed to test more interventions and match the timing of the intervention with the developmental life stage of the caregiver.

Research should continue on the culturally related aspects of caregiving strategies used in various ethnic groups (Picot, 1995). Another contemporary focus in caregiving research should be the caregiving family, as research has clearly indicated that multiple members of families are involved in providing direct and indirect care both to the patient and in support of the primary caregiver (Smith, 1996). In addition to the caregiving family, the caregiving neighborhood or parish should be a focus of study. In some countries giving care is a way of life that extends to friends, neighbors, and society. In the Netherlands the term *mantlezork* is used to define caregiving. This term is translated as the ''care cloak,'' protecting not only the patient but also the caregiver. In this country, Share the Care, a program designed for the care of people with cancer, is an example of *mantlezork* (Capossela & Warnock, 1995).

CAROL E. SMITH

See also
COPING
ELDER ABUSE
FAMILY CAREGIVING
   TO FRAIL ELDERS
GRIEF
SOCIAL SUPPORT

CARING

There has been heightened interest in the concept of caring over the past 20 years. Many noted nurse theorists/philosophers and authors have written about the central role caring plays in our nursing ethic. Philosophy, theory, research, and practice models have emerged. Definitions of caring generally comprise five major conceptualizations (Watson, in press): caring as (a) a human trait, (b) a moral imperative, (c) an affect, (d) an interpersonal interaction, and (e) a clinical intervention. Research and theories of caring have come from many other fields, including feminist studies, sociology, education, philosophy, religious studies, ministry, ethics, arts, and humanities. Larson and Ferketich (1993) state, ''Caring is defined as intentional actions that convey physical care and emotional concern and promote a sense of safeness and security in another'' (p. 690). Swanson (in press) further defines caring as ''a nurturing way of relating to a valued other toward whom one feels a personal sense of commitment and responsibility.''

Several noted authors have conducted extensive reviews of the literature and specifically the research literature addressing caring (Sherwood, 1997; Swanson, in press; Watson, in press). Most of the authors in this field concur that the state of the science at this time is based on a very respectable amount of single, independent studies that identify and describe. The vast majority of the literature is qualitative in nature, describing caring as a concept, behavior, attitude, environment, or process. However, some focused attention has been given to instrument development and testing to measure this multidimensional phenomenon (Center for Human Caring, 1997), with most attempting to describe caring behaviors, attitudes, or skills of nurses or student nurses.

Sherwood (1997) conducted a meta-analysis of 16 qualitative caring research studies in nursing. She described four patterns in the description of nurses' caring from the patient's perspective: interaction, knowledge, intentional response, and therapeutic outcomes. Those patterns, with explanatory themes, defined caring within the content, context, process, and outcomes related to therapeutic or healing outcomes. Two types of caring knowledge content and skills were found: person and technical-physical. Sherwood recommends that this review provides the structure to define therapeutics of caring operationally, providing a foundation and direction for future research.

Swanson (in press) conducted a literary meta-analysis of published nursing research on the concept of caring and to propose a framework. This quantitative analysis encompasses the review of over 130 caring research articles on empirical outcomes from 1980 to 1996. Her findings were congruent with Sherwood's data. The data collection was from a variety of sources: patient charts, observations of practice, and surveys or interviews of patients, families, nurses, students, teachers, and other health care professionals. The relationships investigated included nurse-colleagues, nurse-patient/family, student-teacher, student-student, student-patients, health care provider–patient/family, and family caregiver–family member. Research findings were categorized into five hierarchical levels: capacity, commitment/concern, conditions, caring actions, and consequences. Level I comprises characteristics of persons with the *capacity* for caring, whether inherent or environmentally enhanced or diminished. Level II, *concerns/commitment*, focuses on beliefs and values that undergird caring actions. Level III describes *conditions*: patient-, nurse-, and organization-related circumstances that enhance or diminish the likelihood that caring will occur. Level IV describes *caring actions*, behaviors, or therapeutics. Level V focuses on *consequences of caring*, those intentional and unintentional outcomes of caring for provider and/or recipients of care.

The review of full texts, book chapters, and published theoretical and research articles over the past 16 years provides an inclusive repository of substantive knowledge developed toward the ongoing investigation of caring. Several criticisms have been levied about the state of the research to date. Some authors have raised the questions concerning the fact that, given the changes in health care today, with the relocation of patients to homes and community settings, a vast majority of the studies of nurses, patients, and students has taken place in acute care settings, with acutely ill clients. Future research should be conducted on community-based aspects of care and on recipients of care who are dealing with chronic or end-of-life issues. It is hypothesized that the responses and outcome findings will be vastly different in these populations. Questions about instrument development to date also have been raised. How can there be ontological congruence within instruments developed to mea-

sure a construct like caring with strategies such as forced choice, which violate basic tenets of a caring philosophy? Other authors express concern that our research is too individual, small, isolated, and focused and that it is time to move it forward.

The work of Sherwood (1997), Swanson (in press), and Watson (in press) all provide guidance for future directions for research. The assessment and understanding of caring through a merging of qualitative and quantitative, data-based nursing studies will play a major role in specifying the processes and interventions resulting in critical patient care outcomes. This work is consistent with public demands for health care reforms and can provide a foundation and direction for practitioners in the 21st century. Given the state of knowledge to date, it is time to move toward more sound empirical nursing science studies that can ground our practice and demonstrate measurably improved outcomes.

Swanson (in press) suggests that investigations be directed toward areas such as (a) development of measures that quantify caring capacity; (b) examination of the effects of nurturing and experience on caring capacity; (c) development of measures to quantify conditions that may be competing variables when investigating links between caring actions and their outcomes; (d) moving investigations from the individual as unit of analysis to the study of aggregates; (e) development of clinical trials for the refinement of protocols for caring-based therapeutics toward tested effectiveness in promoting healthy outcomes; and further (f) caring as a measurable commodity in the promotion of health and well-being. Strategies of investigation that aim at new conceptualizations and models that explain, predict, and prescribe may lead to instrument development that will further our knowledge of effective caring and healing therapeutic interventions toward a mid-range, evidenced-based model of caring praxis.

SALLY PHILLIPS

See also
ATTITUDES
COMFORT
EMPATHY
WATSON'S HUMAN CARE MODEL

CASE MANAGEMENT

Definition

There are multiple definitions of case management, and the specific definition frequently depends on the setting and model of case management that is used, the discipline that employs it, and the type of personnel used to accomplish the functions (Cohen & Cesta, 1997). Various case management models are used today as a method of improving health care delivery and controlling or reducing cost. Models include private case management, social case management, primary care case management, nursing case management, and insurance case management, known as the broker model (Conti, 1993). However, regardless of the model, core functions identified are integration of care across the continuum, coordination of services among providers, and direct delivery of services to meet patient needs, efficiently and effectively attending to cost and the use of resources (Cohen & Cesta, 1997; Weil & Karls, 1985).

Historical Perspective and Relevance

Case management as a concept and role function is not new. It had been used by mental health providers and social services for many years. The first federally funded demonstration project began in 1971 and was used to coordinate and provide comprehensive services for the individual (Merrill, 1985). Major emphasis in the past was on the recipient of care and the coordination of services to meet the needs of the patient or client (Weil & Karls, 1985). However, more recently, case management has become a dominant theme as a desired approach to care and cost savings in the context of market-driven health care reform.

The nurse case management model was first introduced in 1985 and is considered a relatively new outgrowth of primary nursing. This case management model "emphasizes early assessment and intervention, comprehensive care planning, and inclusive service system referrals" (Cohen & Cesta, 1997, p. 5). However, it is important to understand how nurse case management is similar to and different from other case management models. Social case management has most frequently been used for long-term management of elderly populations. The primary focus of this model is to maintain the independence of patients or clients using a multidisciplinary approach to care. Primary care case management is usually associated with the gatekeeper role and is based on the medical model of care, in which the patient's access to services is controlled by the physician. Medical/social case management focuses on long-term care of patients at risk for repeated hospitalizations. In this model, the case manager can be of a variety of disciplines, but the focus of care is control of resource utilization. Private case management models generally serve clients who prefer more personalized services and are outside publicly funded programs. The services offered in this model are usually tailored to individual and family needs. In the insurance case management or broker model, the case manager assesses the needs of the patient or client; matches appropriate health and community resources, with cost-effectiveness as the goal; and monitors client needs, provider services, and resources used (Conti, 1993).

Case management is a dominant theme in discussion related to the challenges of managing patients and resources in a cost-conscious health care delivery system. Managed care is another theme that dominates discussions related to providing quality care while controlling resources. Although managed care and case management are used to achieve effective management of care, it is important to differentiate between the two terms. Managed care can be described as a general system of care that has replaced fee-for-service systems of care for improved management of resources, costs, quality, and effectiveness of health services. Case management, on the other hand, is a process of care that may be used as one strategy to control costs and use of resources and services in a managed care system. In conclusion, nursing case management provides outcomes-oriented care with attention to appropriate length of stay, monitors use of patient care based on type of client, integrates and coordinates clinical services, fosters continuity of care in the context of interdisciplinary practice, and enhances patient and provider satisfaction (Ethridge &

Lamb, 1989; Henderson & Wallack, 1987; Zander, 1988).

Uses in Research

Research related to case management can be approached by evaluation research, experimental or quasi-experimental research, or qualitative research. However, because of the difficulties of matching or controlling for control and experimental groups, quasi-experimental research is frequently used. Research may focus on the processes of care (describing and differentiating case management models) or on the outcomes of care, which frequently include quality indicators, costs, or cost savings identified as decreased length of stay, decreased hospitalizations, or nonroutine visits to providers and emergency rooms. However, outcome studies must not dominate the research without attention to the structure and specific processes of care that may influence evaluation studies of case management.

Data collection may be facilitated through the use of patient questionnaires, self-report instruments used by nurses providing case management, and large data sets (from health care provider agencies or payers) used for secondary analysis.

Issues and considerations related to case management roles must be addressed, as this model of care is shaped by a changing health care environment. Two of the most significant issues related to the implementation of case management roles and research related to case management are educational preparation and ethical competence. Because the practice arena is changing rapidly, it has been difficult for educators to clearly define core competencies of the case manager and to be clear about the level of educational preparation. Also, the various models of case management require attention to the structure of care, whom the case manager works for, and the primary purpose of the case management role. These issues and questions will have an impact on research design and questions, depending on setting, type of case manager, and population managed by case managers.

Another critical issue related to case management that affects practice and research is that of ethics. Because many case managers face competing loyalties, the question of ensuring ethical competence becomes as important as clinical, intellectual, financial, and administrative competence. Cohen and Cesta (1997) identified six challenges to be addressed in practice and research as the role of case manager evolves: (a) fidelity to the unique needs of individual patients, (b) competing loyalties, (c) resolving role conflicts, (d) owning responsibilities to underserved populations, (e) identifying personal biases, and (f) balancing care for others with appropriate self-care.

PATRICIA HINTON WALKER

See also
HEALTH CARE REFORM
HEALTH SYSTEMS DELIVERY
MANAGED CARE
RESEARCH IN NURSING ETHICS
PRIMARY NURSING

CASE STUDY AS A METHOD OF RESEARCH

There are many references to case study in the literature, but there is little agreement about what a case study actually is. Case study is described by some as a research method (Yin, 1989), a data collection method, and a reporting method (Lincoln & Guba, 1985). Others argue that "case study is not a methodologic choice, but a choice of object to be studied . . . case study is defined by interest in individual cases, not by methods of inquiry" (Stake, 1994, p. 236).

Thirty years ago case study was a popular design for nursing research. Today it is used less frequently in nursing because of the development of more sophisticated methods of research. Disciplines such as nursing, medicine, psychology, sociology, anthropology, ethics, and history frequently use case study as a teaching method. Used as a research method, case study can be quantitative; but because of the narrative nature of the case study, it is often used as a qualitative method. Case studies can be as simple as a single, brief case or very complex, examining a large number of variables. It is also used for hypothesis testing and theory generation.

Characteristics

Generally, case study is defined as an intensive systematic study of an entity or entities with definable boundaries, conducted within the context of the situation and examining in-depth data about the background, environmental characteristics, culture, and interactions (Bromley, 1986). Used as a research method, case study can be exploratory, descriptive, interpretive, experimental, or explanatory (Yin, 1989). The level of analysis also varies from factual or interpretive to evaluative (Lincoln & Guba, 1985), with the unit of analysis a single person, family, community, or institution (Burns & Grove, 1997).

Case studies must be conducted within the context of the individual or group of individuals because beliefs and values are an integral element in defining and influencing the behavior and experience of people. To determine if the conclusions of a case study can be applied to other situations, the case-in-context must be delineated. Another characteristic of case studies is that they are present-oriented. Even though historical data about the entity being studied is included in the research, the study focus is on the present.

Purpose

One purpose of case study is to expand the understanding of phenomena about which little is known. The data then can be used to formulate hypotheses and plan larger studies. Other purposes of case study include theory testing, description, and explanation. For example, the intensive analysis involved in case study is appropriate to answer questions of explanation, such as why subjects think or behave in certain ways. The case study approach also can be used when a problem has been identified and a solution needs to be found. "Ideally, a case study attempts to integrate theory and practice by applying general concepts and knowledge to a particular situation in the real world" (Bromley, 1986, p. 42).

Research Process

The research process for case study design is similar to techniques used in other designs. First, the purpose and the research questions are developed. Questions of what, how, and why are appropriate for case study designs. A theoretical framework may be used to guide the case study. This helps identify assumptions that the researcher may have about the phenomenon at the beginning of the study.

At the outset of the study the unit of analysis must be clearly delineated. The unit of analysis can be an individual, family, organization, or event. Clearly identifying the unit of analysis has implications for data collection and the study protocol. The protocol should list how subjects will be recruited, what constitutes data (documents, letters, interviews, field observation, etc.), what resources will be needed, and a tentative time line for data collection. The protocol may need to be modified as the study progresses and problems emerge. The protocol also identifies a plan for data analysis and reporting the data.

There are two basic designs in case study research. The first is the single-case design, which is used when a case represents a typical, extreme, critical, unique, or revelatory case (Yin, 1989). Multiple-case designs draw inferences and interpretations from a group of cases. When the purpose of the study is theory generation, multiple-case design is appropriate. Multiple-case designs also are useful to add depth to explanatory and descriptive studies.

Data for case study can be quantitative or qualitative and often include both in the same study. To improve the rigor of the study, three principles of data collection are employed: (a) multiple sources of data are used; (b) a case study base is developed using field notes, audio- or videotapes, logs, documents, and narratives; and (c) an audit trail is evident whereby the reader can follow the researcher's process from question to conclusion (Lincoln & Guba, 1985).

Data analysis in case study is not well developed. Methods for analyzing qualitative data include content analysis, analytic induction, constant comparison, and phenomenological analysis. "Unlike statistical analysis, there are few fixed formulas [for data analysis] . . . much depends on an investigator's own style or rigorous thinking . . . and careful consideration of alternative interpretations'' (Yin, 1989, p. 105). Methods for analyzing quantitative data are similar to those in any quantitative study and would depend on the research questions.

Reporting

Case study reports are presented in a variety of ways, from formal written narratives to creative montages of photographs, videotape, and arts and craft work. Most case study reports in nursing, however, are formal written narratives. The written product of case study is often artistic in its composition. There are no rules or standardized ways to write a report, but most case studies include an explanation of the problem or issue and a detailed description of the context and processes surrounding the phenomenon under investigation. A discussion of the results is also included in the report, which can contain inferences about how these results fit with the existing literature and practice implications.

Rigor in Case Study

The standard measures of reliability and validity apply to case studies that are quantitative. The criteria used to evaluate qualitative case studies are what Lincoln and Guba (1985) call trustworthiness. When a study meets the criteria for credibility, transferability, dependability, and confirmability, it is considered to be trustworthy. Credibility of the interpretations is supported by techniques such as triangulation of data collection methods, negative case analysis, and checking the interpretation with the participants themselves. Transferability (or fittingness) is an indication of whether the findings or conclusions of the study fit in other contexts and fit with the existing literature. When another person is able to follow the researcher's audit trail or the process and procedures of the inquiry, then the study is considered to be dependable. Confirmability is achieved when the results, conclusions, and

recommendations are supported in the data and the audit trail is evident.

Conducting case studies requires a researcher who is flexible and comfortable with ambiguity. It is essential that the investigator be open to the idea that there is more than one ''truth.'' It is necessary for the researcher to be aware of his or her own assumptions, preconceived ideas and values, and of how these impact data collection and analysis.

Case studies are essential to nursing because they are an excellent way to study phenomena within the context in which they occur. Because nurses believe in the uniqueness of human beings, case study is a method to capture this uniqueness and afford a way to gain knowledge about human interaction and behavior as it is situated within time and culture.

DEBERA JANE THOMAS

See also
CONTENT ANALYSIS
NARRATIVE ANALYSIS
PHENOMENOLOGY
TRIANGULATION

CAUSAL MODELING

Causal modeling refers to a class of theoretical and methodological techniques for examining cause-and-effect relationships, generally with nonexperimental data. Path analysis, structural equation modeling, covariance structure modeling, and LISREL modeling have slightly different meanings but often are used interchangeably with the term causal modeling (Youngblut, 1994a). Path analysis usually refers to a model that contains observed variables rather than latent (unobserved) variables and is analyzed with multiple regression procedures. The other three terms generally refer to models with latent variables with multiple empirical indicators that are analyzed with iterative programs such as LISREL or EQS. A common misconception is that these models can be used to establish causality with nonexperimental data; however, statistical techniques cannot overcome restrictions imposed by the study's design. Nonexperimental data provide weak evidence of causality regardless of the analysis techniques applied.

Components

A causal model is composed of latent concepts and the hypothesized relationships among those concepts. The researcher constructs this model a priori based on theoretical or research evidence for the direction and sign of the proposed effects (Bollen, 1989). Although the model can be based on the observed correlations in the sample, this practice is not recommended. Empirically derived models capitalize on sample variations and often contain paths that are not theoretically defensible; findings from empirically constructed models should not be interpreted without replication in another sample.

Most causal models contain two or more stages; they have independent variables, one or more mediating variables, and the final outcome variables. Because the mediating variables act as both independent and dependent variables, the terms *exogenous* and *endogenous* are used to describe the latent variables. Exogenous variables are those whose causes are not represented in the model; the causes of the endogenous variables are represented in the model.

Causal models contain two different structures. The measurement model includes the latent variables, their empirical indicators (observed variables), and associated error variances. The measurement model is based on the factor analysis model. A respondent's position on the latent variables is considered to cause the observed responses on the empirical indicators, so arrows point from the latent variable to the empirical indicator. The part of the indicator that cannot be explained by the latent variable is the error variance generally due to measurement.

The structural model specifies the relationships among the latent concepts and is based on the regression model. Each of the endogenous variables has an associated explained variance, similar to R^2 in multiple regression. The paths between latent variables represent hypotheses about the relationship between the variables. The multistage nature of causal models allows the researcher to divide the total effects of one latent variable on another into direct and indirect effects. Direct effects represent one latent variable's influence on another that is not transmitted through a third latent variable. Indirect effects are the effects of one latent variable that are transmitted through one or more mediating latent variables. Each latent variable can have many indirect effects but only one direct effect on another latent variable.

Analysis Issues

Causal models can be either recursive or nonrecursive. Recursive models have arrows that point in the same direction; there are no feedback loops or reciprocal causation paths. Nonrecursive models contain one or more feedback loops or reciprocal causation paths. Feedback loops can exist between latent concepts or error terms.

An important issue for nonrecursive models is identification status. Identification status refers to the amount of information (variances and covariances) available, compared to the number of parameters that are to be estimated. If the amount of information equals the number of parameters to be estimated, the model is "just identified." If the amount of information exceeds the number of parameters to be estimated, the model is "overidentified." In both cases, a unique solution for the parameters can be found. With the use of standard conventions, recursive models are almost always overidentified. When the amount of information is less than the number of parameters to be estimated, the model is "underidentified" or "unidentified," and a unique solution is not possible. Nonrecursive models are underidentified unless instrumental latent variables (a latent variable for each path that has a direct effect on one of the two latent variables in the reciprocal causation relationship but only an indirect effect on the other latent variable) can be specified.

Causal models can be analyzed with standard multiple regression procedures or structural equation analysis programs, such as LISREL or EQS (see "Structural Equation Modeling"). Multiple regression is appropriate when each concept is measured with only one empirical indicator. Path coefficients (standardized regression coefficients, or βs) are estimated by regressing each endogenous variable on the variables that are hypothesized to have a direct effect on it. Fit of the model is calculated by comparing total possible explained variance for the just identified model with the total explained variance of the proposed overidentified model (Pedhazur, 1982). Data requirements for path analysis are the same as those for multiple regression: (a) interval or near-interval data for the dependent measure; (b) interval, near-interval, or dummy-, effect-, or orthogonally coded categorical data for the independent measures; and (c) 5 to 10 cases per independent variable. Assumptions of multiple regression must be met.

In summary, causal modeling techniques provide a way to more fully represent the complexities of the phenomenon, to test theoretical models specifying causal flow, and to separate the effects of one variable on another into direct and indirect effects. Although causal modeling cannot be used to establish causality, it provides information on the strength and direction of the hypothesized effects. Thus, causal modeling enables investigators to explore the process by which one variable might affect another and to identify possible points for intervention.

JoAnne M. Youngblut

See also
FACTOR ANALYSIS
STATISTICAL TECHNIQUES
STRUCTURAL EQUATION MODELING

CEREBROVASCULAR DISORDERS

The term *cerebrovascular status* was first attached to nursing research regarding patients with critical neurological conditions in 1984 by L. Claire Parsons at the University of Virginia (Parsons & Wilson, 1984). It appropriately captures the underlying dynamics and craniocerebral mechanisms that threaten neuronal integrity in patients with a variety of acute intracranial disorders.

Cerebrovascular status broadly encompasses the relationships among the components of the intra-cranial system: blood, brain, and cerebrospinal fluid. In such conditions as acute head injury and hemorrhagic stroke, trauma to brain tissues sets in motion a cascade of events that may create local ischemia as well as compensatory vasodilation of large areas of the brain to maintain adequate overall cerebral perfusion. If intracranial pressure begins to rise due to the increase in blood volume or if brain hemorrhage acts as a mass, cerebrospinal fluid may be moved into the spinal sac to attempt to keep cerebrospinal fluid and tissue pressure from rising. Ordinarily, changes in systemic blood pressure do not change local cerebral perfusion pressure because of a phenomenon called autoregulation. However, in the injured brain, autoregulation may fail and allow cerebral perfusion pressure to rise and fall with systemic blood pressure. Conversely, in acute conditions such as ischemic stroke, major arterial vessels of the brain may receive too little blood, creating ischemia distal to that artery and setting in motion the same injury cascade as with direct brain trauma.

Clinical nursing research with people who have either acute or chronic effects of cerebrovascular disorders has involved (a) protection from effects of secondary insults such as hypoxia, reduced perfusion pressure, and environmental triggers to these events and (b) restoration and rehabilitation following the primary effects of brain injury and stroke. Reviews of nursing research regarding patients with neurological disorders have shown that essentially no nursing research was done until the mid-1960s and that the body of literature has grown only since the 1980s (DiIorio, 1990). The majority of this research focused on critically ill patients with acute cerebrovascular problems. A smaller body of research has involved issues related to restoration and rehabilitation of people with chronic effects of cerebrovascular damage. That body of research also has grown since the 1980s but not nearly to the extent of the acute care– and trauma-focused research.

Despite the growing number of research studies in the area, relatively few nurse investigators have sustained programs of research in either acute or chronic areas of cerebrovascular problems. The only sustained programs in cerebrovascular responses of patients with increased intracranial pressure (ICP) to nursing interventions have been the groups of Dr. Pamela Mitchell, University of Washington; Drs. Ellen Rudy and Mary Kerr, University of Pittsburgh; and Dr. Claire Parsons and Lee Crosby, University of Arizona (see, e.g., Crosby & Parsons, 1992; Kerr, Rudy, Brucia, & Stone, 1993; Mitchell, Kirkness, Burr, March, & Newell, in press). Margo Hugo (1992) of South Africa is the only investigator who has published a series of studies in the area of nursing interventions and ICP outside the United States.

In contrast, long-term care programs in restoration and rehabilitation of people with cerebrovascular problems have been mostly in Scandinavia, in the work of Elisabeth Hamrin and Astrid Norberg with patients recovering from stroke and those with neurodegenerative diseases. Deborah Webb of Baylor built a program of systems of care to enhance recovery of stroke patients. Dr. Margaret Kelly-Hayes is a nurse investigator who has been active in the longitudinal Framingham study regarding epidemiology of stroke.

The largest body of studies has examined the effects of various bedside nursing care activities on ICP and cerebral perfusion pressure, indirect indices of the adequacy of perfusion to brain tissues. Extension, flexion, and rotation of the neck is the only activity that uniformly increased ICP and often decreased cerebral perfusion pressure. Other activities studied, such as being suctioned, being repositioned, having the head of the bed elevated, and being subjected to painful procedures and assessments showed highly individualized patient responses. Current research is attempting to identify better predictors regarding which patients are apt to respond adversely to these common nursing care activities. These patients are said to have the nursing diagnosis of decreased adaptive capacity, intracranial. They may be identified by abnormal intracranial waveform (elevated P_2 waveform), increased amplitude of waveforms, or large and sustained increase in intracranial pressure to stimuli. Level of ICP does not appear to be a good predictor (Mitchell, Kirkness, Burr, et al., in press).

The studies regarding recovery and rehabilitation from acute stroke are sufficiently scattered in focus to preclude a summary of findings. Studies continue in Scandinavia and the United States to determine the effect of interdisciplinary stroke care teams on functional outcomes and costs (Webb, Fayad, Wilbur, Thomas, & Brass, 1995). Thus far the evidence is mixed, with the positive effects on functional outcomes often confounded by bias in selection of experimental and control groups. The issues of specific therapy versus natural recovery in ameliorating such impacts as altered communication, mobility, and the like are still unresolved despite decades of research in a variety of disciplines.

The advent of thrombolytic therapy to reverse stroke in progress has reenergized public and professional interest in stroke prevention and early treatment. One hopes to see an active nursing research agenda in such areas as community interventions for stroke prevention as well as interventions designed to reduce secondary brain injury in both cerebrovascular trauma and completed stroke.

PAMELA H. MITCHELL

See also
COGNITIVE DISORDERS
CRITICAL CARE NURSING
HEMODYNAMIC MONITORING

CHILDBIRTH EDUCATION

Childbirth education, defined as specific preparation focusing on labor, birth, and early parenting, is widely accepted in the United States today. A majority of childbirth educators are nurses, and nurses are major contributors to research in childbirth education.

The underlying philosophy of childbirth educators includes the concept of birth as normal, natural, and healthy and the right of a woman to make informed choices. The research interests of nurses and childbirth educators have included identification of appropriate content, effective teaching strategies, and research on those practices that enhance the ability of a woman to give birth in a way that is both physically and emotionally safe and satisfying.

Although much of the content of childbirth education classes is derived from clinical practice, nurses have examined the teaching preferences of childbirth educators, learning interests of both men and women attending childbirth education classes, and the learning needs of adolescents. Studies have indicated that women attending childbirth education classes use fewer medications, have increased confidence in their ability to cope, and have a greater sense of control during labor.

A number of studies have focused on individual components of childbirth preparation, including relaxation, breathing, position, pushing style, and support. Relaxation is the most consistently advocated technique for reducing muscle tension and pain in childbirth. During the past three decades, relaxation has been investigated and used by a broad spectrum of health providers to promote comfort and to improve physiological and psychological health status. Stevens and Heide (1977) used three levels of relaxation (none, basic, feedback) and two levels of focusing (none vs. attention focusing). In a carefully controlled administration and evaluation of pain (cold-pressor pain) on six successive occasions, it was demonstrated that the techniques of attention focusing and relaxation decreased pain experience and increased pain endurance. The combination of focusing plus relaxation with feedback was the most successful combination over the full 4-minute exposure period. An additional finding from this study was that practice with the techniques improved the subjects' tolerance, whereas tolerance decreased in the control group. Although Stevens and Heide were not studying women in labor, their findings were consistent with principles of childbirth education.

Humenick and Marchbanks (1981) specifically linked mastery of neuromuscular dissociation, a relaxation practice technique in which some muscle groups are relaxed while others remain tense, and a specific birth outcome, to the amount of medication used during labor. The results of this study of 31 women indicated that women who were able to use more advanced neuromuscular dissociation techniques used less medication. The importance of feedback concerning relaxation was found to be important in both of these studies (Humenick & Marchbanks, 1981; Stevens & Heide, 1977). Breathing techniques are commonly viewed as a strategy to aid relaxation. In Koehn's (1992) study of 57 postpartum women, breathing techniques were perceived as the most effective strategy for coping with labor and birth.

Position and positional change in the first stage of labor promote comfort and facilitate labor. Tryon (1966) noted that position was one of the three most frequently used measures to promote comfort in labor, the other two being back massage and breathing techniques. Potential first-stage positions include an upright position (walking and standing), supine and lateral positions in bed, and sitting. Squatting, a useful position for second stage, was found to impede descent of the presenting part in the first stage. In the second stage, potential positions include lithotomy, standing, sitting, hands and knees, dorsal or lateral recumbent, and squatting.

More important than any single position for comfort is the opportunity for position change. Rossi and Lindell (1986) observed that when 50 women were given both freedom and support to choose position and breathing style for second stage, they chose nine different positions and three variations of breathing techniques; no adverse outcomes occurred in any instance. In addition to comfort and efficacy, position may be of value in rotating the fetus from a posterior to an anterior position (Andrews & Andrews, 1983). In a study of women who were more than 38 weeks pregnant but who were not in labor, four positions were found to facilitate rotation, all of which involved the women on her hands and knees, in contrast to a sitting position.

The concept of support has been a traditional part of childbirth preparation. Support from husbands and even from strangers has been found to reduce medication use, decrease the length of labor, and contribute to a more positive view of labor. Koehn (1992) reported that mothers found labor companion support to be the most effective coping strategy.

Research on practices that enhance the ability of women to give birth safely include those relating to routine practices, such as eating or drinking during labor, and studies of the disadvantages as well as the advantages of interventions such as amniotomy, medications, episiotomy, and cesarean birth. Although these procedures are not performed by nurses, it is the nurse as childbirth educator who provides information for women to make decisions. The practice of keeping women NPO during labor and the corollary practice of IV administration dates to an era when most women received general anesthesia at the time of birth. This practice has been questioned, particularly by those studies that show fasting does not necessarily result in an empty stomach. Amniotomy is often suggested as a means of shortening labor with no harmful side effects, but studies have shown limited or no effect on the length of labor and an effect on fetal heart rate variability.

Much medication research has centered on epidural anesthesia, the primary mode for pain relief during both first and second stages of labor. The use of epidurals has been found to increase oxytocin augmentation, instrumental delivery (forceps), and cesarean birth and to have clinical sequelae in both mothers and infants. Studies differ in the drug and the dose administered by the epidural route, making comparisons between some studies difficult.

Studies of the effect of episiotomy, once a routine part of most hospital births in the United States but not in other countries, have shown that episiotomies do not decrease or prevent perineal lacerations (including deep tears), pelvic floor muscle relaxation, or fetal brain damage and do not heal better than a vaginal tear. Nurse researchers and others have shown that perineal tears can be reduced by perineal massage and possibly by position at birth. Side effects of episiotomy include pain, dyspareunia, and anal incontinence.

The cesarean birthrate in the United States has risen from 5% in 1970 to more than 20% in the 1990s. Nursing studies by Andrews and Andrews (1983) and Mendez-Bauer and Wadell (1983), and studies from other disciplines have shown that basic nursing intervention taught in childbirth education classes, such as positioning and ambulation, can lower the rate of cesarean birth.

Future research must address the value and safety of common interventions and must be widely disseminated to health care providers. Although trials cannot randomly assign some women and partners to childbirth classes and others (who wished to go) to nonattendance, specific topics and techniques taught in classes (e.g., type of relaxation technique) can and should be tested in a randomized fashion. Such testing will reinforce the value of some strategies and identify strategies with limited usefulness.

MARY LOU MOORE

See also
  NURSE-MIDWIFERY
  PREGNANCY
  PRENATAL CARE: COMMUNITY APPROACH
  PREVENTION OF PRETERM AND LOW BIRTHWEIGHT BIRTHS
  RELAXATION TECHNIQUES

CHILD FAILURE TO THRIVE

Classification of Failure to Thrive

Failure to thrive is a term used to describe a deceleration in the growth pattern of an infant or child. Typically, the deceleration is a growth deficit whereby the rate of the child's weight gain is below the third to fifth percentile for age, based on standardized growth charts. A deceleration in a child's growth pattern can occur for any number of physiological reasons; but when a child's lack of weight gain is attributed to psychosocial factors rather than to organic or disease-related factors, the term *nonorganic failure to thrive* (NOFTT) is used.

Traditionally, the failure to thrive syndrome has been classified into three categories: organic, nonorganic, and mixed. Although the term NOFTT frequently is used in contemporary literature, most experts agree that the classification is not so clear because all cases of failure to thrive have an organic etiology (i.e., undernutrition).

Nonorganic failure to thrive is a common problem of infancy and early childhood, and researchers have documented a dramatic increase in its incidence since the late 1970s. It accounts for 3% to 5% of the annual admissions to pediatric hospitals and about 10% of growth failure seen in outpatient pediatrics. Infants with NOFTT typically present not only with growth failure but also with developmental and cognitive delays and signs of emotional and physical deprivation, such as social unresponsiveness, a lack of interactive behaviors, rumination, anorexia, and poor hygiene.

Historical Perspective

Infant nutrition has long been the focus of pediatric research. Holt (1897) was one of the first to describe marasmus, a significant infant nutrition problem and a condition similar to the failure to thrive syndrome described in contemporary literature. It was in 1915 that the term *failure to thrive* was first used in the pediatric literature to describe rapid weight loss, listlessness, and subsequent death in institutionalized infants. In the early 1900s, the mortality rate for institutionalized infants was near 100%, and few realized the importance of environmental stimulation and social contact for infant growth and development. It was during this time that the first foster home care program for institutionalized marasmic infants was developed. The home care program involved the identification and training of families, by nurses, to care for the ill infants, and it included a significant amount of nursing intervention to monitor the progress of the infants. Unfortunately, this early work was not recognized by the pediatric community, despite a 60% drop in the mortality rate of marasmic infants cared for in the foster homes.

It was not until 1945 that the concept of failure to thrive captured the attention of the psychiatric and pediatric communities. In a classic paper, Spitz (1945) described depression, growth failure, and malnutrition in 61 foundling home infants. He used the term *hospitalism* to describe the syndrome that he observed, and he proposed that a lack of emotional stimulation and the absence of a mother figure were the main contributors to infant growth failure. Spitz postulated that with adequate love, affection, and stimulation, the infants would grow. Researchers demonstrated weight gain in infants with hospitalism when stimulation and affection were provided. Thus, these findings provided a foundation for a failure to thrive theoretical framework based on maternal deprivation in institutionalized infants.

In the mid-1950s a number of case reports were published in the psychiatric literature that documented depression, malnutrition, and growth failure in infants living in intact families. These case studies were the first to report feeding and interactional difficulties between the mothers and their infants. Feeding episodes for the mothers were anxiety-provoking, which led the mothers to decrease both the frequency of infant feedings as well as their contact with the infants. Ethnologists and child development experts began studying institutionalized and noninstitutionalized infants to further define the concepts of maternal deprivation and failure to thrive. On the basis of several studies, researchers concluded that decreased maternal contact led directly to failure to thrive in the infants. From these works the maternal deprivation framework for failure to thrive was established, and the mother's role in the infant's well-being became a central focus. Support for this framework grew as data accumulated documenting the association between maternal neglect and failure to thrive in infants.

Current Perspective

The maternal deprivation framework predominated in the literature until the late 1970s, when a transactional framework was developed to explain the psychosocial correlates of NOFTT. The transactional framework proposed that an infant's growth and development were contingent on the quality of parental care, the nature of parent and infant interactions, and the ecological conditions impinging on the family. Furthermore, the transactional model recognized that the quality of the parent-infant interaction reflected infant characteristics as well as parent characteristics. Historically, the emotional deprivation component of NOFTT has been investigated more than the nutritional deprivation component. Although experts in NOFTT would agree that malnutrition is the primary biological insult, systematic studies investigating this element are lacking.

Nutritional deprivation again became the focus of NOFTT research in the early 1970s, when some researchers disputed the hypothesis that maternal deprivation was its principal cause. More recent evidence suggests that the environmental deprivation may occur before the undernutrition. Although the primary cause of NOFTT may never be fully understood, it is apparent that nutritional deficits are dependent on the environmental context in which they occur.

The transactional model of pediatric medicine is similar to the ecological model developed by pediatric nurses and used to explain NOFTT (Barnard & Eyres, 1979; Lobo, Barnard, & Coombs, 1992). The ecological model focused on the three major interaction components of the parent-child relationship: those of the child, the parent, and the environment. These interactions are synchronous and reciprocal. Barnard and her colleagues (Barnard et al., 1989) emphasized the importance of the parent's and child's physical and emotional characteristics, as well as the supportive or nonsupportive nature of the environment in understanding the interactions. Researchers have examined parent-child interactions by means of direct, structured observations during feeding and other situations and found that NOFTT infants were less vocal and interactive with their parents and that the parents of these infants were less able to determine their infants' needs, compared to NOFTT infants and their parents. From this it is evident that interference with the reciprocal process of the parent-child relationship disturbs the opportunity to attain optimal growth and development. Because growth problems, such as NOFTT in infancy, place a child at significant risk for developmental delays as a toddler, it is important to recognize the interactional problems between parents and their infants so that interventions aimed at improving interactions can begin early in the parent-child relationship.

HEIDI VONKOSS KROWCHUK

See also
**MOTHER-INFANT/TODDLER
RELATIONSHIPS
NUTRITION IN INFANCY AND
CHILDHOOD**

**PARENTING RESEARCH IN NURSING
SOCIETY FOR RESEARCH
IN CHILD DEVELOPMENT**

CHILD LEAD EXPOSURE EFFECTS

Childhood lead poisoning is recognized as the most important preventable pediatric environmental health problem in the United States. Lead poisoning is defined as exposure to environmental lead that results in whole blood lead concentrations ≥ 10 µg/dl (micrograms/deciliter). Most researchers would agree that all children are exposed to environmental lead. Exposure begins in the prenatal period when physiological stress mobilizes lead from its storage in maternal bone into the blood, whereby it easily crosses the placenta and is deposited in fetal tissue. Depending on the level of lead present in the environment, the exposure continues as infants and children develop. Absorption of lead is dependent on age and nutritional status; young children and those who have diets high in fats are most susceptible. Once ingested, lead is distributed in the blood and eventually is deposited in bone and teeth.

Whole blood lead levels greater than 10 µg/dl put children at risk for developing a variety of health problems (e.g., developmental delays, mental retardation, altered hemoglobin synthesis, nephropathy, encephalopathy, and even death). As a direct result of primary and secondary efforts at prevention of lead toxicity, blood lead levels among U.S. children have been significantly reduced within the past 20 years. The major sources of environmental lead exposure have been greatly decreased through the elimination of lead in gasoline, the banning of lead-based paint for residential use, and the elimination of lead solder from food and beverage cans. Despite the success of these efforts, lead poisoning continues to occur in about 9% of children 5 years of age and younger.

Historical Perspective

Childhood lead poisoning was first described in the late 1800s by Gibson and his colleagues (Gibson, Love, Hardie, Bancroft, & Turner, 1892), who encountered a case of peripheral paralysis in a young child and described the similarities of the case to that of chronic lead poisoning in adults. Gibson speculated that the source of the lead poisoning was paint, and he described the long-lasting effects of the exposure. Unfortunately, most of Gibson's observations were ignored, as the prevailing view of the time was that once a child survived lead poisoning, there were no lasting effects. In the mid-1940s, researchers studied lead-poisoned children and found that most of the children had long-term sequelae such as learning and behavior disorders and other cognitive deficits. These researchers postulated that lead poisoning produced long-term neurological deficits in children, even in the absence of central nervous system symptoms. This change in thought provoked researchers to conduct epidemiological investigations of the problem of lead poisoning, but it was not until the early 1970s that cross-sectional and longitudinal studies of low-level lead exposure were conducted.

These early studies of lead exposure involved simple comparisons of a lead-exposed group and a comparison group on intelligence test measures; significant differences usually were found. As knowledge accumulated and research strategies became more sophisticated, researchers began to assess the influence of covariates, such as parental intelligence, socioeconomic status, and parental education level (Gatsonis & Needleman, 1992). Though conflicting results were common, lead exposure and neurobehavioral deficits remained significantly associated.

Relevance to Nursing Research

Although few nurse researchers have investigated the effects of low-level lead exposure on the neurobehavioral development of children, low-level lead exposure certainly falls within the realm of the phenomena of concern to the discipline. The phenomenon is unquestionably of clinical significance; until all lead is removed from the environment, clinicians will be faced with both screening children for lead exposure and treating the effects of this preventable public health problem. The deleterious effects of lead exposure have been known for 100

years; however, progress in prevention has been slow. Some of the reasons for this are related to society's indifference to problems of poor and vulnerable populations. Until recently, lead exposure was thought to be a problem only for poor inner-city minority populations, and parenting practices were thought to contribute to the problem. Also, many considered the elimination of lead in gasoline and paint sufficient to eradicate the problem of lead poisoning. In 1992 the Centers for Disease Control (CDC) issued comprehensive guidelines for preventing and treating the problem of childhood lead exposure. These guidelines were issued after the CDC had accumulated large amounts of scientific evidence from animal and human studies that supported the hypothesis that the deleterious effects of lead exposure occur at levels previously thought to be harmless.

Review of Studies

The earliest studies of lead poisoning were conducted on children who had blood lead levels ≥60 μg/dl and were symptomatic. During the 1970s, researchers focused on children who had lead levels in the 40–50-μg/dl range but were asymptomatic. Conclusions about the effects of lead exposure were difficult to make from these studies because of their methodological shortcomings, such as small sample sizes, lack of control over extraneous variables, and lack of precise outcome measures. In 1979, researchers conducted a major investigation of large numbers of asymptomatic children and used shed deciduous teeth rather than blood lead to measure lead exposure (Needleman et al., 1979). These researchers controlled for major confounding variables and concluded that lead level was associated with lower IQ, decreased attention span, and poor speech and language skills in the children studied. Long-term follow-up of the children led the researchers to conclude that the effects of low-level lead exposure (equivalent to whole blood lead ≤25 μg/dl) persisted throughout young adulthood. Reading disabilities and failure to complete high school were behaviors exhibited by children who had elevated lead dentine levels at age 7.

Scientists criticized the work done by Needleman and his colleagues (1979) because the study lacked baseline data about early cognitive abilities of the subjects. For instance, it was proposed that the affected children may have had neurological deficits at birth that would induce certain behaviors (increased mouthing) that predisposed them to lead exposure. To address this issue, subsequent studies were designed to follow large numbers of subjects from birth through early school age; major outcomes (e.g., IQ level, motor development, cognitive development) were measured, and large numbers of covariates were controlled. Numerous investigators using comparable designs reported similar findings; thus, a solid consensus among investigators began to emerge that lead was toxic at extremely low concentrations. Research with lead-exposed primates strengthened the consensus, and the toxic level of lead was redefined by the CDC as whole blood lead ≤10 µg/dl.

Future Directions

Researchers continue to study the effects of low-level lead exposure on the development of children. Although these efforts are worthwhile, future efforts could focus on identifying mediators of lead exposure effects, investigating the effects of lowering blood lead levels (chelation) on the neurobehavioral outcomes of children, and investigating the effects of providing educational materials about reducing environmental lead exposure to families of low-level-exposed children. Any efforts that address primary prevention of the problem would help to protect thousands of children against the long-lasting effects of lead exposure.

HEIDI VONKOSS KROWCHUK

See also
  FAMILY HEALTH
  NUTRITION IN INFANCY
    AND CHILDHOOD
  UNINTENTIONAL INJURY OF INFANTS
  VULNERABLE POPULATIONS

CHRONIC CONDITIONS IN CHILDHOOD

Definition

There is no one accepted definition of a childhood chronic condition; however, a recent research con-

sortium on chronic illness in childhood recommended that it be defined on two levels: duration of the condition and impact on the child's functioning (Perrin et al., 1993). In a definition based on duration, a chronic condition is one that has lasted or is expected to last more than 3 months (Perrin et al.). This definition would include recurring acute conditions (e.g., repeated ear infections) as well as those that are expected from the onset to be long-term (e.g., diabetes). In a definition based on impact on the child, a chronic condition would be one that limits the child's functioning or leads to the child's receiving additional medical attention beyond that expected for a child the same age.

Prevalence

Prevalence estimates for childhood chronic conditions, or the number of children with chronic conditions at any given point in time, vary according to the definition used. Estimates of prevalence range from less than 5% to more than 30% (Newacheck & Taylor, 1992); they tend to be higher when the definition is based on duration and lower when the definition is based on impact on the child's functioning. For example, results from the 1988 National Center for Health Statistics report, which used the definition of an impairment or disease lasting more than 3 months, indicated that almost 20 million children (31%) had one or more chronic conditions. Of these, approximately 13.3 million children had one condition, 4.1 million had two conditions, and 1.8 million had three or more conditions (Newacheck & Taylor). The most frequently reported conditions in this study were respiratory allergies, repeated ear infections, and asthma. In contrast, estimates from the Survey of Income and Program Participation (1995) for 1991–1992, which used a definition based on impact on the child's functioning, indicated that 3.8 million children 17 years or younger (7.9%) had a chronic condition. In this study the estimated prevalence increased with age (e.g., 2.2% for 0 to 3 years to 9.3% for 15 to 17 years) and was higher in boys than in girls across all age groups. Conditions most frequently reported in this survey were learning disability, speech problems, mental retardation, asthma, and mental or emotional problems.

Research

A large amount of research has been carried out to investigate children with chronic conditions and their families. Most of the research has been guided by stress theory and has focused on child and family adaptation (Austin, 1991). This research has established that, compared to their general population peers, children with chronic conditions are at risk for psychosocial adaptation and academic achievement problems. Moreover, the families of these children are at increased risk for adjustment problems (Thompson & Gustafson, 1996).

Two major approaches are used in research on children with chronic conditions and their families: noncategorical and categorical. The major assumption behind the noncategorical approach is that there are many commonalities in the experience of families of children with chronic conditions. These researchers generally study samples in which many different chronic conditions are represented. An example of nursing research using this approach is work by Knafl and Deatrick (1990) in their study of family management style. In contrast, researchers using the categorical approach generally study samples that are homogeneous in regard to chronic condition. An example of nursing research using the categorical approach is the research on family factors related to behavior problems in children with epilepsy (Austin, Risinger, & Beckett, 1992). Even though there has been much discussion about which approach is better to use, the current thinking is that the purpose of the research should determine the approach used. For example, the categorical approach is better when disease-specific variables are important, and the noncategorical approach is better when social and psychological variables are of interest (Stein, 1996). In nursing, both approaches can provide important information that will improve nursing care of children with chronic conditions and their families.

JOAN K. AUSTIN

See also
CANCER IN CHILDREN
FAMILY THEORY AND RESEARCH
PAIN IN CHILDREN
PARENTAL RESPONSE TO NEONATAL
  INTENSIVE CARE UNIT

PSYCHOSOCIAL EFFECTS OF CHILD
  CRITICAL ILLNESS AND
  HOSPITALIZATION

CHRONIC GASTROINTESTINAL SYMPTOMS

Chronic gastrointestinal (GI) symptoms, including abdominal pain, bloating, constipation, dyspepsia, and diarrhea, affect approximately 8% to 22% of the U.S. population (Drossman et al., 1993; Longstreth & Wolde-Tsadik, 1993). Of those individuals who seek health care services for their symptoms, the majority are women of menstruating age (Drossman & Thompson, 1992). In many cases, the symptoms cannot be ascribed to a specific pathological or organic cause. The diagnosis of irritable bowel syndrome is applied to those individuals who experience abdominal pain and alterations in bowel function with no measurable pathology (Rome criteria). An outline of GI symptoms that characterize irritable bowel disease was developed by an international committee of experts who meet in Rome and has come to be known as the Rome criteria (Drossman et al., 1990). These criteria include (a) abdominal pain relieved by a bowel movement or associated with changes in stool consistency and (b) fewer or more frequent stools, harder or looser stools, straining, urgency, feeling of incomplete evacuation or passage of mucus, and bloating or feeling of abdominal distention (Talley, Phillips, Melton, Wiltgen, & Zinsmeister, 1989).

There are several etiological theories of irritable bowel syndrome. They include GI motility disorder, increased pain sensitivity, dietary factors such as intolerances (e.g., lactose) and low dietary fiber intake, autonomic nervous system imbalance, and psychiatric causes. The heterogeneity and chronicity of the problem, as well as the lack of a specific marker of irritable bowel syndrome, makes management particularly challenging. Nurses are frequently involved in the management of patients who experience GI problems, and thus empirical evidence is needed to determine etiological factors and mechanisms as well as interventions to alleviate symptom experiences and distress.

Research related to irritable bowel syndrome has been primarily conducted by medical researchers, in particular, gastroenterologists and psychiatrists and some basic scientists who have described GI motility patterns in symptomatic individuals. Researchers interested in symptoms and lifestyle factors have relied primarily on retrospective measures of symptom experiences as well as psychological state data. These studies have utilized patients recruited from tertiary care clinics who may represent one end of the continuum of patients with irritable bowel syndrome. In addition, although women predominate in studies of patients with irritable bowel syndrome, little or no attention is paid to menstrual cycle phase or menopausal status. Finally, there is limited study of ethnic variability in symptom experiences or health care seeking.

Recent nursing research utilizing both retrospective and prospective (daily diary) measures has focused on the relationships between chronic GI symptoms and the menstrual cycle (Heitkemper, Levy, Jarrett, & Bond, 1995), self-report of psychological distress (Jarrett et al., in press), self-report of stress (Levy, Jarrett, Cain, & Heitkemper, 1997) and physiological indicators of arousal (Heitkemper et al., 1996). In several of these studies, symptomatic women who sought health care for symptoms were compared with asymptomatic women as well as women with similar symptom levels who did not seek health care and thus did not have a formal diagnosis. These studies provided descriptive information about the fact that for some women GI symptoms are (a) closely linked with menstrual cycle phase (i.e., more symptoms in the late luteal phase compared to the follicular phase), (b) associated with higher self-report levels of psychological distress and stress, and (c) related to higher levels of urinary catecholamine and cortisol excretion.

Additional descriptive information collected in studies of both menstruating and midlife women indicate that dietary fiber is lower than the recommended daily intake in all groups of women. Preliminary data also suggest what has been found in the medical literature, that more women with irritable bowel syndrome report a history of or current experience with physical or sexual abuse, compared to nonsymptomatic women; however, additional work is needed.

Interventions for irritable bowel syndrome have included strategies to modify diet, produce relaxation, and pharmacologically manipulate motility or pain sensitivity. Intervention trials are plagued by the use of a heterogeneous sample, often including both diarrhea-prone and constipation-prone patients, the lack of a "gold standard" on which to measure improvement, reliance on retrospective symptom reporting for both sample selection and outcome measures, and a significant placebo effect in drug trials (Heitkemper et al., 1995). Well-designed clinical trials research examining multifaceted nonpharmacological therapies are needed to explore the benefits of dietary modification, relaxation techniques, education or reassurance on symptom experiences, health care seeking, and quality of life. It is unlikely that one therapy or therapeutic package will be beneficial for all patients. Therefore, studies must carefully describe symptoms as well as the biobehavioral characteristics of the samples prior to intervention. In this way, characteristics likely to be predictive of intervention success can be identified.

There are multiple opportunities for additional research in the area of chronic GI symptoms. More work is needed to understand the physiological basis, including motility and pain sensitivity, which may account for symptom occurrence. The interrelationships among other symptoms (e.g., insomnia, dysmenorrhea, and urinary incontinence) and irritable bowel syndrome should be clarified. Psychological factors such as psychiatric diagnoses, psychological distress, posttraumatic stress syndrome, and daily measures of stress must be further explored for their relationship to GI symptoms and bowel function. The natural course of functional GI symptoms is also poorly understood. For example, it is not certain whether children who experience chronic abdominal pain and constipation are more likely to manifest irritable bowel syndrome as adults. Finally, the outcomes of GI symptoms in terms of health care utilization, lost productivity, and impaired functional ability should be described in diverse samples of individuals.

MARGARET HEITKEMPER
MONICA E. JARRETT

See also
HYPERALIMENTATION
MENSTRUAL CYCLE

NUTRITION
STRESS
URINARY INCONTINENCE

CHRONIC ILLNESS

Chronic illness is a term used to denote clinical problems, particularly diseases of duration usually longer than 3 months that have frequent recurrences and that lack a cure (Clarke, 1994). Lubkin (1995), in a review of definitions of chronic illness, provided a definition that has a fit with nursing practice: "Chronic illness is the irreversible presence, accumulation, or latency of disease states or impairments that involve the total human environment for supportive care and self-care, maintenance of function, and prevention of further disability" (pp. 7–8). Nursing's focus on such chronic conditions as urinary incontinence constitutes an adjunct to these definitions and must be taken into consideration for completeness of chronic illness from nursing's perspective.

It is clear from these definitions that those who are chronically ill usually require long periods of care and observation to manage symptoms and the underlying pathology. A paradox of these conditions is that available therapies and strategies for control do not provide cure but are frequently vital for long-term survival. However, many patients have found adherence to some therapies and strategies difficult and stop using them, regardless of the potential danger of exacerbation of their illness. The complexity of factors involved in adherence to therapies probably is a multifactorial problem, involving physiological, behavioral, social, cultural, and economic factors that continue to require investigation.

Chronic illnesses can be placed in several groupings. For example, some chronic illnesses are life-threatening when there are treatments but no cures, and they require major life adjustments to maintain health, such as insulin-dependent diabetes mellitus (IDDM). Some are of uncertain origin and clinical pathway, may or may not be life-threatening, and there is no clear treatment, such as lupus and multiple sclerosis. Others have difficult clinical patterns and symptoms, usually affect functional ability but are not life-threatening, and treatment is symptomatic (e.g., osteoarthritis). Finally, some are not illnesses at all but chronic conditions that require clinical management; they occur frequently, have high health care costs, and are amenable to control (e.g., urinary incontinence).

Chronic illnesses also can be viewed from the perspectives of research foci. Considerable clinical nursing research has been carried out on aspects of chronic illness from the perspectives of prevention, adaptation, self-management, compliance and adherence, quality of life, function, symptom recognition and control/management, family involvement, cultural influences, and strategies for improved outcomes, such as patient education (Funk, Tornquist, Champagne, & Wiese, 1993; Gallo, Breitmayer, & Knafl, 1992; Lorig, Stewart, Ritter, et al., 1996; Roberson, 1992; University of California–San Francisco (UCSF) Symptom Management Faculty Group, 1992). Much of this work has been smaller-scale, limited-sample studies, but some represents strong programs of research (see Lorig, 1996).

There are a multiplicity of theoretical frameworks that can be used in chronic illness research. These come from a variety of nursing perspectives and are based in physiological, behavioral, social, cultural, and systems concepts. Corbin and Strauss (1991) proposed a chronic illness nursing management model based on a trajectory framework that several studies have used. Development and use of such models continue to be needed in nursing research.

Health care of chronically ill populations in the past has principally been managed from a disease-focused perspective, emphasizing acute care and control of exacerbations, and today it is managed from a more holistic, life-course, self-care, and community-based perspective. Chronicity of health problems leads people to seek nursing care for a variety of reasons; symptom control/management, assistance with coping, family adjustment, and educational needs are examples. One of the most important goals of care for those who have or are at risk for chronic illnesses is postponing the time of onset of chronic illness, symptoms, and associated disability and extending productive life. Self management and care are important goals of nursing practice and have been for some time (Connelly, 1987).

Chronic illness is an ongoing concern for health care providers and policymakers for a number of reasons; one is that increasing life expectancy presents the possibility of an associated increase in chronicity and disability, with an associated increase in health care costs. In the past, nursing research focused on chronic illness and chronicity as an important phenomenon in itself. Today nursing research is focusing increasingly on (a) specific conditions, such as cognitive impairment; (b) symptoms, such as pain; (c) adherence to specific disease treatments, such as blood glucose control for IDDM; and (d) intervention strategies, such as community-focused health care models. This change seems to be in response to new sources of research funding and other factors that are less clear. These new opportunities for research funding are important; however, developing conceptual coherence of the diverse aspects of chronicity is vital for increasing the scientific clarity of chronic illness research.

To strengthen chronic illness research, a cadre of nurse investigators continues to be needed, as there are a few nursing research centers but not many nurse scientists who are involved in this area. Examples of such centers are those at the University of Pittsburgh (chronic conditions), University of Michigan (cognitive impairment), University of California–San Francisco (symptom management), University of Pennsylvania (serious illness), and Stanford University (patient education). There are opportunities for substantial inquiry to be carried out in all aspects of chronic illness, particularly in the areas of primary and secondary prevention, assessment, symptom management, effectiveness of therapies and interventions, nursing-related outcomes, and costs.

It is also timely for nursing methodologies to include combined qualitative and quantitative designs, increased numbers of clinical trials, and inclusion of cost-effectiveness questions where feasible. Another aspect of scientific inquiry that it is timely for nursing research to continue to embrace is replication and substantiation. A hallmark of a scientific breakthrough is that a unique, cutting-edge finding can be replicated. It is this replication that leads to substantiation in which a clear scientific basis is developed for acceptance of the original results.

PATRICIA MORITZ

See also
  ADHERENCE/COMPLIANCE
  DIABETES MELLITUS
  HYPERTENSION
  OSTEOARTHRITIS
  URINARY INCONTINENCE

CHRONIC MENTAL ILLNESS

Chronic mental illness is more recently referred to as serious and persistent mental illness (SMI), in deference to the victims of psychiatric disorder and to reflect more accurately the intensity and course of various disease processes. SMI is considered to be a psychiatric condition that persists over time, with a variety of clinical courses and with varying intensity of disability. It presents diagnostic and treatment challenges to clinicians that are beginning to be addressed more directly in the empirical nursing literature. Stress diathesis models of causation and course, pharmacological and other biochemical models of intervention, and psychosocial models of course and intervention are all subsumed within a biopsychosocial framework. Selected empirical studies of SMI are presented chronologically.

Review of Major Studies

Slavinsky and Krauss (1982) compared a nursing social support intervention to a medication management intervention over 2 years in a sample of 47 persons with SMI. Contrary to the hypothesis, the medication group improved in socialization and satisfaction with care, indicating that psychiatric nurses should develop more complex treatment models combining low-stimulation, low-threat atmospheres with a social support emphasis to encourage gradual assimilation into the community rather than attachment to the treatment environment.

Harding and colleagues (Harding, Brooks, Ashikaga, Strauss, & Breier, 1987) interviewed 82 persons with SMI 20–25 years after their discharge into a rehabilitation project from the Vermont State Hospital. Over one-half of the sample had achieved considerable improvement or recovery. Previous longitudinal studies of shorter duration had found little or no change in function at follow-up. Subsequently, Harding and colleagues (DeSisto, Harding, McCormick, Ashikaga, & Brooks, 1987) completed a follow-up study with persons from a Maine state psychiatric facility with no psychiatric rehabilitation discharge program. Findings showed better function for the Vermont group at follow-up.

Hamera and colleagues (Hamera, Peterson, Handley, Plumlee, & Frank-Ragan, 1991; Hamera, Peterson, Young, & Schaumloffel, 1992) examined the process of self-regulation and symptom monitoring in persons with SMI, using the Self-Regulation Interview for Schizophrenia. Target symptoms indicative of the relapse prodrome were identified in a community-living sample of persons with schizophrenia. The majority of subjects' target symptoms were anxiety-related, occurred weekly or more often, and always occurred with decompensation. Though occurring less frequently, psychotic and depressive markers were rated significantly more troublesome than anxiety-based indicators. Subjects reported taking three or more actions to regulate the symptom. The most frequent action was to add new activities or focus on existing ones. A 1-year follow-up of 28 original subjects found that half of the subjects reported using the same indicator or an indicator from the same category.

The data provided support for a symptom self-regulation model. Subjects easily identified indicators of illness that were disturbing and represented the need for action when they were present. Baker's (1995) qualitative study of the ability of persons with schizophrenia to detect early signs lends support to the model of Hamera et al. Baker's interviews indicate that the level of disturbance caused by prodromal symptoms motivate individuals to take action to relieve the distress. The study further explicates the developmental process of individuals with schizophrenia becoming aware of the need to monitor their distress and take action when needed.

Fetter and Lowery (1992) applied attributional models to perspectives on psychiatric rehospitalization by 120 patients and 162 inpatient staff. Findings suggested that patients tended to give internal attributions for the illness relating to their readmission, believing that the cause was not under their control. Staff also were likely to ascribe internal attributions for the readmission but were more likely to see the cause as lack of patient effort, which is considered to be controllable by the patient. These important differences in attribution suggest implications for preventing rehospitalization and for nursing staff education.

The general psychiatric literature documents unexpected high morbidity and mortality rates in psychiatric populations, compared to populations with primarily medical diagnoses. An investigation of 25 persons with SMI recently discharged to the community (Murphy, Gass-Sternas, & Knight, 1995) documents the health risks and health promotion activities of this population. In semistructured interviews, subjects reported high tobacco use, low levels of physical exercise, poor oral health, high-risk sexual behavior, and limited medical and dental care. Health promotion activities included adequate sleep and limited use of alcohol and drugs. The subjects reported a strong interest in participating in health promotion programs. This study suggests that a focus on adequate mental and dental care and the development of health promotion programs for persons with SMI could have a positive impact on the physical and mental health of this population.

In a study of community mental health service delivery (Francis, Merwin, & Fox, 1995), personal characteristics and use of community services were evaluated as predictors of use of inpatient care by 446 clients of this community mental health service. Findings indicated that inpatient hospitalization was predicted by use of community service. Clients who received assistance in obtaining outpatient medical services were less likely to be hospitalized, and those receiving legal and housing assistance were more likely to be hospitalized. These findings suggest that lack of adequate housing and appropriately supervised living settings may be related to inappropriate use of inpatient care as a substitute for community residential placement. This study highlights the need to increase efforts to support nontraditional assistive services to psychiatric clients.

In a retrospective descriptive interview study of 43 persons with SMI in a variety of inpatient and outpatient settings, Chavetz (1996) examined individual life histories to determine the processes, conditions, and events that subjects considered influential in their clinical outcomes. The complex and rich descriptive nature of this qualitative study precludes a full explication here; however, the interviews suggest some general conclusions. The clients perceived the management of their psychiatric illness as a partial result of individual learning and personal decision making. They reported that medication played a pivotal role in illness management, and they acknowledged psychosocial factors such as acceptance of diagnoses, negotiation of treatment, obtaining environmental supports, and relationship development as important in coping with and managing the challenges of the illness.

Further, personal choices seem to involve trade-offs between support and protection; thus, these individuals may accept restricted lives in exchange for clinical stability. Though such restrictions may reflect a real resource deficit, they emphasize how these individuals have relinquished goals and aspirations over time to protect against personal vulnerability and avoid challenging situations. This study characterizes the complex nature of the disabilities associated with severe mental disorder and associated deficits in social and vocational resources, which must be addressed in the development of community nursing intervention programs.

In a similar vein, Perese (1997) investigated the effect of unmet needs of persons with SMI on their quality of life, emergency room usage, and rehospitalization events. In semistructured interviews with 73 persons with SMI and some family members, unmet needs were most frequently cited as lack of friends, social and vocational roles, group affiliations, and self-identity. Poor perceived quality of life was statistically associated with stigma, poor self-identity, and lack of employment. Rehospitalization and emergency room use were related to unmet needs for safety, money, and employment. As with other studies reported here, these findings suggest the need for the development of innovative and meaningful human services that address the complex nature of SMI and its sequelae, including physical, cognitive, interpersonal, resource, and vocational deficits.

Summary and Implications for Future Research

The studies reported here are atypical of the general base of nursing literature regarding SMI in that the samples are large, the methodology is quantitative, and the questions address the illness, its consequences to the individual, and implications for treatment development. The need for substantive nursing research is crucial and includes further investigation of (a) causal attributes and processes, (b) course and outcome, (c) clinical indicators of morbidity and mortality, and (d) symptom regulation and management. There remains a critical demand for empirical investigations to determine those interventions that specifically enhance symptom management, daily coping, adaptation, general health status, and quality of life.

CATHERINE F. KANE

See also

CHRONOBIOLOGY, CHRONOPHARMACOLOGY, AND CHRONOTHERAPY

Chronobiology

Temporal or time-related variance of biological systems has been evident for several thousand years. The Chinese have been aware for over 5,000 years that the effect of a drug is dependent on the time of administration. In Western civilization, the 18th-century botanist Linnaeus believed that a knowledgeable man could tell time without a watch while walking through a forest, noting only what flowers were open or closed. Several centuries later, knowledge of biological variation in living systems was incorporated into Western science.

Shortly after World War II, scientists from all over the world came together to explore the mechanisms of biological rhythms and methods for rhythm identification and quantification. This meeting resulted in a large empirical base in support of a biological time structure and supplied the theoretical underpinnings for the development of chronobiology (Auvil-Novak, 1997). Clinical applications of chronobiological principles are increasing our knowledge of health and disease and leading to increased effectiveness in disease prevention, diagnostic procedures, and therapeutic outcomes (Woods, Felver, & Hoeksel, 1996).

Traditionally, medical therapy has been based on the concept of homeostasis as developed by Walter Cannon. Homeostasis refers to a set of regulatory mechanisms that maintain the body's internal environment in a state of temporal equilibrium. Changes in biological functions are counteracted to balance and maintain a steady state. Cannon's work derived from the concept of *milieu interieur*, as advocated by the French scientist Claude Bernard. Bernard's work attempted to describe the internal consistency of the individual's environment and did not preclude the existence of temporal variation or rhythmicity in biological systems (Auvil-Novak, 1997).

Advances in technology and instrumentation over the past few decades allowed scientists and clinical practitioners to detect and record subtle rhythmic changes in the physiological parameters of individuals (Dunbar & Farr, 1996). The quantitative study of these rhythmic changes demonstrated that biophysical and biochemical processes vary with respect to time in a periodic, regular, and predictable manner (Farr, Keene, Samson, & Michael, 1984). Chronobiology is defined as the study of these rhythmic variations. Periods of rhythmic variation in organisms may extend from milliseconds to several years in duration. As a general classification, rhythms less than 20 hours in length

are designated as "ultradian," 20 to 28 hours in length as "circadian," and greater than 28 hours as "infradian." Rhythms of about a week are referred to as "circaseptan," about a month as "circamensual," and about a year as "circannual."

The majority of biological rhythms are endogenous in nature and evidence suggests that they are genetically predetermined. These periodic variations in physiological function may lead to time-dependent differences in response and adaptation to stimuli and therapeutic interventions. Further, rhythms may be adjusted in their timing by environmental factors that act as synchronizers, entraining agents, or "zeitgebers." Examples of synchronizers include light-dark cycles, meal timing, and other social stimuli. After a change in the timing of the synchronizer, the rhythm period usually adapts, albeit slowly, to the new synchronizer phase. However, the period of adaptation for each physiological rhythm is highly variable. The organism as a whole has a variety of rhythms, with different phases operating in synchrony. Disruptions in synchronizer exposure may alter the typical phase relationships of the different physiological parameters leading to either a "free running" state with a fixed period and no relation to clock time or a level of "internal desynchronization" that may occur as periodic metabolic functions adjust at different rates to the new synchronizer schedule.

Chronopharmacology

Chronopharmacology is the study of time-dependent variations in pharmacology, including the influence of biological rhythms on the kinetics and pharmacodynamics of medications. The administration of pharmacological agents may be timed so that the optimal tolerance or optimal effect of an agent may be enhanced. Chronopharmacology also encompasses the study of how treatment with pharmacological agents may alter individual biological time structure itself. With respect to human biological time structure and rhythmic aspects of the disease process, the timing of medication is critical to the safety and efficacy of pharmacotherapy. There are several aspects of chronopharmacology that have been well defined. These include (a) chronopharmacokinetics, or the rhythmic variations in the absorption, distribution, and elimination of an administered drug; (b) chronesthesy, or the rhythmic changes in biological susceptibility, including changes in quantity or quality of receptor, cell permeability, and metabolic processes within the cell; and (c) chronergy, or rhythmic changes in the desired therapeutic response as well as in the severity of toxicity of a drug. Clinical evidence to support circadian administration of various pharmacological agents is rapidly mounting (Auvil-Novak, Novak, & El Sanadi, 1996).

Chronotherapy

Clinicians do not routinely address environmental issues with respect to synchronizer input and biological time structure. Intensive care units and surgical wards introduce many environmental factors that may increase patients' susceptibility to acute and chronic responses to illness. Excessive noise, disturbing sounds, hospital routines, and clinician rounds may result in sleep deprivation and abnormal sleep patterns. Altered meal timing, absence of usual sleep-wake routines, lack of windows, and associated deprivation of light-dark cycles are examples of zeitgebers that may be altered by illness, the surgical process, and hospitalization of the individual (Novak & Auvil-Novak, 1996). Familiarity with an organism's time structure and changes in the different rhythms in states of health and disease have led to differential time-related treatments that may be more efficacious than monochronic treatment regimens. Chronotherapy, or treatment that is based on knowledge of biological time structure, is receiving increasing recognition in Western society. Chronotherapy can be defined as the use of treatment timed according to the stages in the sensitivity–resistance cycles of target (or nontarget) tissues and organs to enhance the desired effect or reduce the undesirable effects. The goal of chronotherapy is the optimization of treatment by tailoring drug administration or treatment modalities to the individual's biological time structure to enhance their efficacy and reduce toxicity (Auvil-Novak, 1997).

SUSAN E. AUVIL-NOVAK

See also
CRITICAL CARE NURSING
NURSING SLEEP SCIENCE
PAIN MANAGEMENT

CLINICAL DECISION MAKING

Clinical decision making is the process nurses use to gather patient information, evaluate the information, and make a judgment that results in the provision of patient care (White, Nativio, Kobert, & Enberg, 1992). Clinical decision-making ability is defined as the ability by which a clinician identifies, prioritizes, establishes plans, and evaluates data. From this process a judgment is identified (Grossman, Campbell, & Riley, 1996). Decision making is central to professional nursing and has vital links to patient care outcomes (Catolico, Navas, Sommer, & Collins, 1996).

Clinical decision making is a difficult topic to research in that it is hard to measure objectively. Various methods have been used to investigate decision making, depending on what is being examined. Studies have investigated the process, types, and quality of clinical decision making. Catolico and colleagues (1996) studied decision making of practicing staff nurses. It was demonstrated that nurses with better communication skills had a greater frequency of actual decision-making practices. Some researchers have looked at approaches such as informatics or algorithms to aid decision making. Akers (1991) showed that nurses who used algorithms to aid their decision making utilized more thorough patient assessment and a more informed nursing response, which resulted in better patient management. Another critical issue is the educational level of the nurses who are formulating decisions. Studies have explored the decision-making process of student nurses, staff nurses, and nurse practitioners. A group of nursing students were given didactic and interactive teaching sessions on clinical decision making. Those students' decision making was in accordance with the decision making of experts significantly more often than that of the student nurses who did not receive the decision-making content (Shamian, 1991).

When investigating the decision-making process, researchers have utilized simulations, together with interviews about the thought processes individuals use to reach decisions. The quality of decision making is defined as having the ability to make frequently required decisions (Catolico et al., 1996). That aspect of decision making has been studied by using computer-assisted simulations requiring nurses to make decisions in controlled clinical situations. To investigate clinical decision making by nurse practitioners, the nurses care for patients via computer and interactive videos.

Various factors have been shown to affect clinical decision making, such as the experience and the knowledge base of the nurse. Those with case-related experiences are more likely to choose appropriate interventions. A study of nurse practitioners by White and colleagues (1992) concluded that case content expertise is crucial for clinical decision making from the aspect of understanding the significance of the data acquired and in making the correct decision. Nurses' decision making is also affected by the sociodemographics of the patient. Sociodemographics such as age, sex, race, religion, and socioeconomic status can bias decision making. For example, chest pain in female patients may be of less concern because of the perception that heart disease and myocardial infarction are much less common in women. Advanced-practice nurses in specialty practices tend to generate fewer hypotheses in their clinical decision making. Those nurses must be cognizant that formulating a diagnosis early in the data-gathering phase precludes the possibility of considering all options (Lipman & Deatrick, 1997).

Decision making is critical to nursing practice. Gathering, organizing, and prioritizing data are major components of the process. Continued research in this area can foster the development of decision-making skills in novice nurses and cultivate high clinical decision-making ability in expert nurses.

TERRI H. LIPMAN

See also
**CLINICAL JUDGMENT
COMPUTER-AIDED INSTRUCTION
EDUCATION: NURSE RESEARCHERS
    AND ADVANCED PRACTICE NURSES
GENDER RESEARCH
NURSING ASSESSMENT**

CLINICAL INFORMATION SYSTEMS

There is confusion and no standard agreement on the definition of a clinical information system (CIS). Commonly found in the literature are descriptions of a hospital information system (HIS), which refers to both system architecture and software to support functions such as order entry, admission/discharge/transfers, billing, finance, accounting, maintaining personnel records, generating reports, and scheduled maintenance. A CIS is usually described as a system that contains clinical data about patients, such as laboratory data, medications given, patient observations, and x-ray and other imaging data. Most commercial systems are HISs but are moving rapidly toward becoming CISs. Therefore, a CIS will be defined as an automated, integrated system that contains system architecture (hardware and software) to support both clinical and administrative functions in a clinical environment. Ideally, a CIS should support a longitudinal database containing all relevant clinical information used to provide health care to individual patients at any point of system access and across the life span. A CIS should also contain sophisticated communication and decision support to facilitate decision making by any health care provider involved in the diagnosis, treatment, and evaluation of patient outcomes.

The development of the CIS has paralleled the rapid advances in computer technology. Since the early 1940s remarkable progress has been made, from Turing's work on formalizing a mathematical algorithm to "giant brain" mainframe computers such as the UNIVAC 1, from the individual printed unit to the central processing unit (CPU) on a chip to powerful personal computers (PCs) and including integrated local networks (LANs), wide area networks (WANs), and workstations functioning in almost any setting. The application of computer technology in health care also began in the late 1940s and 1950s, with initial work done by Technicron Medical Information Systems (TMIS)/ Lockheed at the El Camino Hospital in Sunnyvale, California. Warner's work in the late 1950s and 1960s at the LDS Hospital in Salt Lake City, Utah, led to the development of health evaluation through logical processing (HELP), a system that supports and guides decision making and analysis of physiological data. Barnett and associates at the Massachusetts General Hospital in Boston and Wrederhold at Stanford were also involved in early development of hospital information systems and clinical information systems.

Continued use of computer technology and a CIS is imperative in a rapidly changing health care environment. Two major challenges to developing future systems are (a) building systems on set standards for system infrastructure that provides connectivity and data sharing and (b) establishing uniform environments for the structure and processing of communication.

Clinical information system development will be critical to nursing research and practice but is currently problematic in three important areas: (a) lack of a standard nursing language (e.g., taxonomies) to facilitate communication and to establish common usable clinical databases, (b) the complexity of nursing decision making that makes decision support more difficult, and (c) the need to balance specificity of decision making about clinical care and to individualize interventions based on patient and family needs. The lack of taxonomies impedes the identification of key indicators or logical sequences and pathways that are required for nurse decision making. Thus, work such as the nursing minimum data set (NMDS), the *Nursing Intervention Classification* (NIC), and the nursing management data sets will be crucial to CIS development. Nursing research is difficult at best in the current environment because clinical records are disorganized, not standardized, and often incomplete. Reducing variation in how nurses communicate patient problems, interventions, and outcomes will facilitate the ability to test nursing interventions effectively. This is especially important with the increasing emphasis on outcomes-based practice and cost efficiency.

Research-based practice standards must be developed to serve as a decision-making guide for clinicians yet also provide flexibility when patient needs require adjustment. A CIS should accommodate ready access to the standards so that new clinicians can access a standard on-line. Ideally, the CIS will provide alert mechanisms and suggestions based on presenting information recorded in the clinical record. If nursing can develop usable and understandable taxonomies and research-based practice standards are in place, the state of our science will improve.

Future CIS development will be based on a tremendous need for connectivity so that any clinician can access patient information needed to provide clinical care. Interface and communications are and will continue to be costly endeavors yet are essential to moving toward an automated longitudinal data repository, a concept embraced by the National Library of Medicine. The future of CISs is not just ready, accurate, and convenient access to patient information but on-line access to research and clinical databases, interactive expert referrals, access to the latest treatment summaries, digital textbooks and journals in full text, transmission of imaging results, reporting systems linked to electronic mailboxes so that results and information are communicated to health care providers, and expansive networks linking peripheral sites to hospitals, clinics, and patient homes. The CIS should also be easy to learn and use, require minimal redundancy in data entry, and conform to predetermined data standards such as Health Level 7 (HL/7) so that all system components are able to communicate with each other.

Increasing access and communication creates threats to the security and confidentiality of sensitive personal information. Another issue is how user identification can be determined so that system use and access is appropriate. Each clinician may be assigned a unique log-on, or voice recognition may be used to identify the access points and level of security permitted.

Nursing will have a key role in continued CIS development. System infrastructure must be constructed to ensure that appropriate decision support is available and that the security and confidentiality of patient and provider data are maintained. Nursing research could become a part of everyday clinical practice and better focused on evaluating outcomes and responses to specific interventions. Administrative functions such as staffing and scheduling will be correlated with actual patient requirements and streamlined, and automated patient records can reduce unnecessary paperwork and facilitate communication across all relevant disciplines. Nurses will have to embrace the use of computer technology as one method that can assist in improving sound clinical practice. To maximize continued CIS development, nurses must be actively involved in defining nursing information needs with colleagues in information technology and those defining data set standards. Examples of active involvement include (a) the American Nurses Association Steering Committee on Databases to Support Nursing Practice, and (b) the International Council of Nursing's initiative for an International Classification for Nursing Practice.

CAROL A. ASHTON

See also
**COMPUTERIZED DECISION SUPPORT
    SYSTEMS
NURSING INFORMATION SYSTEMS
NURSING INTERVENTIONS
    CLASSIFICATION
NURSING MINIMUM DATA SET
OMAHA SYSTEM**

CLINICAL JUDGMENT

The research on clinical judgment is vast, covering more than 30 years. A comprehensive review of the research literature reveals several different descriptors that have shared meaning with judgment: decision making, problem solving, and clinical inference. Although several definitions for clinical judgment and decision making exist in the literature, the definition of clinical judgment guiding this work is derived from the American Association of Colleges of Nursing (1986): "Clinical judgment is the process of translating knowledge and observation into a plan of nursing action and the implementation of that plan for the benefit of the patient/ client" (p. 8). This body of knowledge can be characterized by an analysis of the purposes of the studies, populations studied, and research methods and designs used. Additionally, a brief discussion of future needs is addressed to researchers interested in further developing this knowledge area.

The body of knowledge related to clinical judgment is of significance not only to nursing education but, more important, to the discipline and practice of nursing. In recent history nursing has operated in structured environments with a strong interdisciplinary health care team readily available in the delivery of comprehensive care. Even acute care environments are changing, involving nurses in the delivery of acute care to clients with rapidly changing status and with increasingly ambiguous and complex data. In addition, the changing health care arena presents a myriad of opportunities for nurses to move out into more unstructured, autonomous environments, where clinical judgments are made independently, in isolation. In some instances rapid, complex judgments on client status are required, together with plans for intervention. Therefore, research in this area provides a foundation for understanding the structure and process of clinical judgment and some insights into the education of new health professionals and the retraining of practicing health professionals for jobs in more ambiguous, independent settings (home health, hospice, telephone triage, telemedicine, etc.) that require complex, accurate clinical judgment competencies.

Most of the research in the field of clinical judgment has been for the expressed purpose of identifying the structure and processes used in arriving at a clinical judgment. Numerous authors, since the early writing of Hammond (1964) and Kelly (1964) on clinical inference, have employed a variety of similar research strategies to delineate this process, and there is great congruity in the findings. Many researchers have described steps or procedures employed in arriving at judgments consistent with human problem-solving theory, first described by Newel and Simon (1972). A vast body of findings suggests that context and complexity of patient/ client situations have a strong influence on judgments. Additionally, authors have found that knowledge of the client and/or relationship with the client influences judgment. Although there is strong congruence in research findings of nursing clinical judgment with the strategies described in the cognitive processing and information processing literature, the process is found to be much less linear than believed in the past. A great deal of the research, although continually refining and describing the structure and process, attempts to compare and contrast the judgment of various groups of nurses, trying to discern some understanding of other influences contributing to the practitioner's performance and ability other than the complexity and context of the client encounter.

There is enormous congruity in the types of participants in the studies. Nursing students have been studied most frequently. These studies have ranged from comparing students of varying educational levels (diploma, associate degree, baccalaureate, upper division RN, graduate nurse practitioners) to comparing returning RNs with experience to generic students and new graduates to experienced nonstudent practicing nurses. A small sample of studies has focused on nurses in certain areas of practice (hospice, home care, primary care, critical care) and on nurse practitioners. More recent studies have been stimulated by the work of Benner (1984) in examining the practices of novice and expert nurses. These studies have tried to explicate the influences of education and experience on clinical judgment.

The study methodologies and designs have most commonly been qualitative, descriptive studies. Simulated patient encounters have been a popular vehicle for data generation, including direct, on-site, "over the shoulder" participant observation; video vignettes designed by individual researchers; vignettes marketed for teaching and evaluating competencies in clinical judgment; patient exemplars written by researchers in collaboration with clinical experts; written patient scenarios and case studies; critical incidents; and more recently, computer-generated simulated patient encounters. Examination of patient documentation records and logs and audio phone recordings has been less commonly used. Many of these studies have employed the "think aloud" strategy, first described by Newell and Simon (1972), to encourage stimulated recall as a strategy to examine the processes used in performing clinical judgments. Content analysis of verbal protocols is a common descriptive data analysis strategy. Grounded theory and the use of constant comparative analysis is the most frequently cited research methodology, but others cited more recently have included hermeneutics, phenomenology, and naturalistic inquiry. A relatively small number of studies have used quantitative designs.

A review of the recommendations forwarded by the authors conveys great congruence as well. Consistently, authors describe the need for educational reform that incorporates a more holistic approach to teaching clinical decision making, such as allowing students more opportunity for dialogue or to "think aloud" about patient encounters, examining case studies or exemplars of patient scenarios, and working more directly in the clinical area with experts and clinically competent faculty. Authors urge that more effective teaching strategies be developed and evaluated that stimulate critical thinking and have consistently argued that our educational systems have not adequately evaluated the competencies of our students in the area of clinical judgment and critical thinking. Nearly all authors encourage more research to explicate an understanding of the complexity of clinical judgments. There is strong support for nurse educators to (a) improve teaching strategies and curriculum delivery models to strengthen clinical judgment competencies and (b) conduct research that evaluates the effectiveness of these innovations.

The future holds a wealth of opportunities for research in this area. As nurses move out into more independent roles, clinicians with strong, efficient skills in clinical judgment will be highly sought out in the new health care system. Individuals prepared to function independently and to competently determine the need for collaboration will be ready for the needs of clients in the 21st century. Research on clinical judgment structure and processes, diagnostic skill accuracy, and acquisition of the competence and confidence to perform complex independent clinical judgments with clients will be essential. Nursing education is presented with vast opportunities to address new curriculum structures and delivery models. Research on innovative teaching strategies and their effect on strengthening the competency of clinicians in this area will be invaluable as schools of nursing move forward in a new paradigm characterized by distance education, video teleconferencing, telemedicine, Web-based courses, and regional, national, and international educational initiatives. Identification of educational strategies that teach, reinforce, and evaluate clinical judgment competency is needed immediately.

SALLY PHILLIPS

See also
CLINICAL DECISION MAKING
CLINICAL PATHWAYS
COMPUTER-AIDED INSTRUCTION
NURSING PROCESS

CLINICAL NURSE SPECIALIST

The functional roles of nurses, such as private-duty nurses, were part of the early specialization in nursing, but the emergence of today's contemporary, credentialed clinical nurse specialist (CNS) has followed a 40-year path of debate and controversy. The development of CNS as an advanced degree preceded and was causal in the unfolding of nursing as an applied science. A parallel development of the nurse practitioner movement often placed these two advanced preparations in opposition, as nursing leaders in the 1960s and 1970s wrestled with shaping the future of the profession. The controversy continues today in a tightening fiscal environment. A review of the growth of the movement will aid our understanding of why the controversy remains and perhaps give direction for finding solutions.

Following World War II many social changes emerged. The GI Bill was introduced, permitting people unable to afford higher education to obtain university degrees, particularly in nursing. Science exploded, especially in the area of health and nursing. Nurses returning from military service were also eligible for advanced education under the GI Bill.

During this same period the nursing role in hospitals had become stratified, with large numbers of nurses' aides and practical nurses providing direct patient care. Registered nurses were removed from the direct care role and placed in supervisory roles. The public complained about fragmented care. Obtaining advanced clinical preparation allowed the clinical specialist to return to the patient and give expert, direct care (Hamric & Spross, 1989). The impetus was for a changing role for nursing, and federal funding became the means to meet this end.

The National Mental Health Act, passed in 1946, provided federal funds for research and training of core disciplines, and psychiatric nursing was designated as a core discipline. In 1954, Peplau, at Rutgers University, developed a master's degree program focused on development of the first advanced practitioner—the psychiatric nurse. Other specialties were soon to follow. In 1963 the Professional Nurse Traineeship Program provided the financial support to develop graduate program content in advanced clinical nursing. By 1984 there were 129 accredited programs throughout the United States for preparing clinical nurse specialists. A national system of certifying these specialists was put into place, though certification was not mandatory (Hamric & Spross, 1989). This advanced preparation gave nurses new options in their careers, such as in the six subroles of the CNS: researcher, consultant, advanced clinician, educator, leader/manager, and collaborator. However, with the growth of the PhD in nursing in the 1970s and 1980s, the subrole of researcher remained more focused on discovering the gaps as well as utilizing research findings in clinical settings. The PhD was the expected degree for a nurse researcher.

From the beginning the CNS role was not without its critics. Research showed that expert patient care made a difference in recovery and in patient satisfaction, but there were early arguments about the cost-effectiveness of the CNS role. The CNS expert had problems in making this important role visible and accountable. Part of the criticism grew from the expansion of specialization in medicine as fewer physicians practiced primary care. By the mid-1960s there was a critical shortage of these physicians, and the public complained about lack of access to primary care. So two new "middle-level" health practitioners emerged: the physician's assistant (PA) and the nurse practitioner (NP). In 1965 the first PA program began at Duke University, and in that same year the NP program, under the direction of Loretta Ford, began at the University of Colorado as a continuing education program (Hamric & Spross, 1989).

The debate about the place of the NP role in the nursing profession became very hot—fueled by nurse leaders such as Martha Rogers, who perceived the role as subservient to the physician. She and many other nurse educators believed that NPs had left the profession, for nursing was seen as caring for the psychosocial needs of the patient and medicine dealt with curing the disease. This perception was held for almost 20 years by many nurse educator leaders. This perception kept NP education largely within the confines of continuing education programs. As the economic environment of the health care system began to change in the late 1980s, CNS positions in the hospitals began to be eliminated. With cost containment of managed care, a less expensive practitioner was sought, and the CNS was not that practitioner. Instead, the value of an NP zoomed, and positions could not be filled because of the shortage. Hence, the enrollment of graduate students in NP programs throughout the United States increased while those for CNS programs slumped. The NP found broad opportunities in the field of primary care that physicians had abandoned. The NP advanced preparation took over most graduate programs (McFadden & Miller, 1994).

This change has not been easy, as leaders attempt to shape the future through various advanced credentialing and regulation. At the time of this writing the debate continues. There are those who advocate a second license for advanced nursing practice, and this title would include CNS, NPs, nurse anesthetists, and nurse midwives. A significant problem, identified by the National Council of State Boards of Nursing, is the current variety and lack of consistency in state regulation and professional certification of advanced nursing practice (Minarik, 1992). Research is needed on this problem related to public health safety, quality of care, interstate mobility, access, scope of practice, and titling. This topic is being debated in multiple nursing forums. And, as that debate continues, a new type of CNS seems to be emerging, combining the clinical advanced knowledge with case and systems management. The role of the CNS is part of emerging new roles of advanced nursing practice in an unfolding managed care health care system (Higgins, Ponet, James, Fay, & Madden, 1994).

JODY E. GLITTENBERG

See also
ADVANCED PRACTICE NURSES
NURSE ANESTHETISTS AND RESEARCH
NURSE-MIDWIFERY
NURSE RESEARCHER IN THE
  CLINICAL SETTING
PRIMARY NURSING

CLINICAL NURSING RESEARCH

Clinical nursing research is both broadly and narrowly defined. Broadly, it denotes any research of relevance to nursing practice that is focused on care recipients, their problems and needs. This broad definition stems from the 1960s, when a major change occurred in nursing science. Prior to the 1960s the research of nurses had focused on nurses and the profession of nursing. Major questions of interest related to nursing education and the way in which nurses practiced within care delivery structures (i.e., hospitals). The reasons for these foci are many, but for the most part they stem from the dearth of nurses with advanced degrees at that time and the fact that nurses with advanced degrees were educated in other disciplines (e.g., education).

In the late 1950s and 1960s a major shift occurred, driven by three factors. First, leaders in nursing successfully lobbied for the institution of the nurse scientist program through the federal government, which provided financial support for nurses to be educated in the sciences (e.g., physiology, biology, anthropology, psychology). Second, nurse theorists such as Faye Abdellah, Virginia Henderson, Imogene King, Ida Orlando, Hildegard Peplau, and Martha Rogers began to formulate conceptual models to direct nursing practice, and attention was focused on designing research that more or less was guided by those models (or at least the substantive areas circumscribed by the models). Third, as more nurses attained advanced degrees, doctoral education with a major in nursing finally became a reality, and the focus of nursing research shifted more firmly away from nurses and nursing education to the practice of clinical nursing. The broad definition of clinical nursing research, then, was originally formulated to differentiate between the research conducted by nurses prior to the 1960s, which focused on nurses, to the major shift in focus on practice.

Strongly influenced by the establishment of the Center for Nursing Research (at present the Institute of Nursing Research) in the National Institutes of Health (NIH), clinical nursing research has recently taken on a narrower definition, modeled after the definition of clinical trials (large-scale experiments designed to test the efficacy of treatment on human subjects) used at NIH. This narrow definition limits clinical nursing research to only those studies that focus on testing the effects of nursing interventions on clinical or "nurse sensitive" outcomes.

In addition to an evolution in definition, clinical nursing research also has changed in form and complexity over time. Early clinical nursing research was characterized by a focus on circumscribed areas of inquiry using experimental and quasi-experimental methodologies. Investigators were few and tended to work in isolation. Prompted by metatheorists such as Dickoff, James, and Wiedenbach (1968) and methodologists such as Abdellah and Levine (1965) and Mabel Wandelt (1970), nurse scientists were advised to derive questions directly from problems encountered in their clinical practice and to strive to develop and test interventions to solve these problems. Often an investigator conducted single studies on different problems rather than series of studies focused on different aspects of the same problem. As a result, study results tended to be context-bound and limited in generalizability to other settings, samples, or problems. The relationship between theory development and research was discussed abstractly but not explicitly operationalized, and a philosophy of knowledge building, rather than problem solving, had not yet developed.

The next stage in the evolution occurred with the realization that little was known about many of the phenomena of concern to nurses. This heralded a period during which emphasis shifted away from experimental methods to exploratory/descriptive methods, such as grounded theory. Guided by the metaparadigm of nursing (person, nursing, health, environment), nurse scientists began focusing on discovering and naming the concepts of relevance for study in nursing, on delineating the structure of these concepts, and on hypothesizing about the relationships of these concepts in theoretical systems.

More recently, clinical nursing research has become clearly defined as a cumulative, evolutionary process. Investigators are still advised to derive questions from clinical problems, but the focus is on knowledge generation, specifically the generation and testing of middle-range theory (a theory that explains a class of human responses), for example, self-help responses, symptom experience and management, and family responses to caregiving. Because knowledge is viewed as cumulative, investigators usually study various aspects of one particular concept or response; studies build on one another, and each study adds a new dimension of understanding about the concept of interest. This approach to clinical nursing research requires investigators to use multiple methodologies in their programs of research, including (a) inductive techniques to discover knowledge from data; (b) deductive techniques to test hypotheses that are either induced or deduced; and (c) instrumentation to increase the sensitivity, reliability, and validity of the measurement system designed for the concept.

The methodologies being used include qualitative methods such as ethnomethodology, grounded theory, and phenomenology and quantitative methods ranging from traditional experimental methods and designs to less traditional methods, such as path analysis and latent variable modeling. Because human responses change over time based on contextual factors or treatments (independent variables) applied by the nurse investigator and because understanding the nature of change often is at the crux of the theory building, skills in measuring change also may be required. This has resulted in the need for many investigators to incorporate techniques such as time series analysis and individual regression into their research.

Understanding the human responses of concern to nurses can also require an understanding of cellular mechanisms that are best studied in animal models and a coupling of biological techniques such as radioimmunoassay and electron microscopy, with psychosocial techniques such as neurocognitive assessment or self-report of psychological states. In addition, measurement of different units of analysis (e.g., individual, family, organization) may be required, along with strategies for understanding the effect of care contexts (e.g., social, physical, organizational environments) on the human response of concern. Needless to say, single investigators rarely have all the skills needed to advance the understanding of a particular concept. As a consequence, single investigators are becoming more and more a thing of the past as teams of scientists, including nurses and individuals from other disciplines, collaborate in the knowledge-building endeavor.

Nursing is concerned with human responses and is based on the assumption that humans are holistic and embedded in history and various environments. Clinical nursing research is about generating a body of knowledge on which nurses can base practice. It is about assuring the efficacy and safety of nursing actions, substantiating the effect of nursing actions on patient outcomes, and conserving resources (costs, time, and effort) while effecting the best possible results. It is about identifying strategies for improving the health of the population and promoting humanization within a health care environment that has a natural tendency to be mechanistic, compartmentalized, and focused on short-term rather than long-term gain. It is about client advocacy, client protection, and client empowerment. The challenge of clinical nursing research is to develop an understanding of human response through theory generation and testing while developing measurement systems and using research methods that capture the holism of the client and the holistic nature of the health care experience.

LINDA R. PHILLIPS

See also
CLINICAL TRIALS
DOCTORAL EDUCATION
MIDDLE-RANGE THEORY
NATIONAL INSTITUTE
   OF NURSING RESEARCH
NURSE RESEARCHER IN THE
   CLINICAL SETTING

CLINICAL PATHWAYS

Clinical pathways are multidisciplinary care management plans that organize, sequence, and guide the patient care tasks and interventions for an epi-sode of care. These tools are known by a variety of names, including CareMaps® (registered trademark of The Center for Case Management, Inc.), care paths, multidisciplinary action plans, and anticipated recovery paths. Pathways are created by expert clinicians from the various professions that routinely care for a specific type of patient, such as those with diabetes or those in heart failure. These clinicians meet to discuss the current trends in the care of these case types, historical data from their institutions related to length of stay and resource utilization, and health sciences research pertinent to the patient population. Agreement is reached on the best practices, and those practices are documented, organized, and sequenced along a time line to generate a pathway.

Clinical pathways are composed of four critical components: (a) tasks and interventions, (b) patient outcomes, (c) a time line, and (d) capacity to capture variance data. Tasks and interventions are usually grouped by category, such as medications, diet, teaching, tests, and consults. Within the medication category, for example, all pertinent medications for each period of time are listed. This list of medications may be very specific, such as "digoxin .25 mg qd," or the list may be more generic such as "IV antibiotics." Patient outcomes are the milestones that clinicians agree are important to patient recovery and movement toward discharge or transition to the next level of care. Each outcome is stated in measurable terms, such as, "afebrile" or "verbalizes signs and symptoms of infection prior to discharge."

Like interventions, outcomes are associated with a specific time period, and expected outcomes vary over time. The time line organizes and sequences care by unit of time. Some case types are best managed by day of stay in an acute care facility. In that instance all interventions and outcomes are listed and evaluated at least every 24 hours. Some case types are so complex that changes in the patient's condition occur more frequently. Time lines are adjusted; interventions and outcomes are monitored after just a few hours, such as for a coronary artery bypass graft (CABG) patient in the immediate postoperative period. Most CABG pathways include targeted interventions in the first 12-hour period designed to accomplish specific outcomes, such as early extubation. In other settings the most appropriate unit of time may be weeks (rehabilitation hospital) or minutes (emergency department). Variance occurs when patients do not meet their expected outcomes within the allotted time frame.

Some pathways also define a variance when interventions are changed, such as adding a new medication or deleting an expected lab test. Variances are tracked for each individual patient and trended for all patients whose care is guided by the clinical pathway. Periodically, the expert clinicians who wrote the pathway review the data to find ways to improve the quality of the care provided. For example, if the variance data for patients undergoing hip replacement surgery show that 35% have difficulty tolerating clear liquids on postop Day 1 because of persistent nausea or vomiting, the multidisciplinary team may consider a focused study on the types and amount of anesthetic agents used during surgery, or they may evaluate the types of antiemetic interventions these patients receive. Variance data create the foundation for continuous quality improvement of the clinical care and are therefore a powerful tool for clinicians.

History of Clinical Pathways

Clinical pathways were first used at the New England Medical Center (NEMC) in Boston in the mid-1980s. Called critical pathways, these documents outlined the important interventions for each case type. Outcomes were not included on the early pathways. These first appeared in 1990 in some institutions. Outcomes are routinely included on pathways today. Karen Zander and Kathleen Bower were nurse leaders employed at NEMC and led the initial efforts at documenting the critical elements and sequence of care. Their efforts continue in their numerous articles and books tracing the evolution of pathways in American health care.

Clinical pathways today are employed as care management tools across the entire continuum of care. Home health, rehabilitation, mental health, acute care, subacute and long-term care sites have developed these guidelines to assist providers in managing both the quality and cost of health care.

Research

Many program evaluation studies have been published in the nursing and health care literature describing the impact of pathway use on the length of stay and cost of care. These studies are almost always nonexperimental in nature, with no control group and no randomization. Given the nature of health care work, it is understandably difficult for agencies to maintain experimental control while simultaneously delivering patient care. Consequently, pathways have not been shown to be a causal factor in decreasing length of stay or cost. However, they have been associated with such results in the vast majority of reports. Other positive findings include an increase in satisfaction among patients who were placed on pathways. Staff satisfaction results have been mixed, sometimes positive and sometimes negative. Concern about additional paperwork for nurses is the most frequently cited negative finding.

Importance of Pathways to Nursing and Health Care

Clinical pathways have changed the way clinicians think about and organize patient care. Prior to pathways, each discipline developed its own plan of care, often without communicating that plan to any other discipline. The act of creating a pathway, even before it is ever used, creates an opportunity for all disciplines to share their ideas and expertise about the best plan of care for specific populations of patients. The process by which these ideas are synthesized can influence all health care team members as they support the achievement of patient outcomes.

It is important to note that clinical pathways were introduced to the U.S. health care system by nurses. In addition, the pioneering work done by nurses in the United States has been exported to the United Kingdom, Singapore, Canada, Spain, Australia, and South Africa, where clinical pathways are known to be in use. Continued growth of this methodology across cultures and borders is expected in the future.

BONITA ANN PILON

See also
  ADMINISTRATION RESEARCH
  CLINICAL DECISION MAKING
  COST ANALYSIS OF NURSING CARE
  NURSING PROCESS
  QUALITY OF CARE, MEASURING

CLINICAL TRIALS

Definition

A clinical trial is a prospective controlled experiment with patients. There are many types of clinical trials, ranging from studies to prevent, detect, diagnose, control, and treat health problems to studies of the psychological impact of a health problem and ways to improve people's health, comfort, functioning, and quality of life.

Classification

The universe of clinical trials is divided differently by different scientists. Clinical trials are often grouped into two major classifications, randomized and nonrandomized studies. A randomized trial is defined as an experiment in which therapies under investigation are allocated by a chance mechanism. Randomized clinical trials are comparative experiments that investigate two or more therapies. Nonrandomized clinical trials usually involve only one therapy, on which information is collected prospectively and the results compared to historical data. Comparing prospective data with historical control data introduces biases from many sources. These potential biases are usually of such magnitude that the results of nonrandomized studies are often ambiguous and not universally accepted unless the therapeutic effect is very large. These same biases are not present to the same degree in randomized trials. Recent development and use of mega-trials represents one variation.

The mega-trial is a large, simple, randomized trial analyzed on an "intent to treat" basis. In mega-trials randomization serves to achieve identical allocation groups (equal distribution of bias) where there is poor experimental control and large between-subject variation. Results of mega-trials cannot readily be generalized because their conclusions are observations, not causal hypotheses and therefore not testable. Mega-trials can be repeated but not replicated. Mega-trials dispense with the scientific aim of maximum experimental control to remove or minimize bias and instead use randomization to achieve equal distribution of bias between groups (Charlton, 1995).

In clinical drug trials, following approval by the Food and Drug Administration (FDA), three phases of clinical trials begin. Phase I studies generally establish whether a treatment is safe and at what dosages. Phase II studies assess the efficacy of treatments after their safety and feasibility has been established in Phase I. Phase III studies compare effectiveness of Phase II treatments against currently accepted treatments.

Some scientists divide clinical trials into three groups: (a) exploratory (initial trials investigating a novel idea), (b) confirmatory (designed to replicate results of exploratory trials), and (c) explanatory (designed to modify or better understand an established point). Other scientists divide the universe into two groups, such as pragmatic (practical benefits to the overall subject population treated) and explanatory (Viscoli, Bruzzi, & Glauser, 1995).

Trends and Issues

Issues surrounding clinical trials include biasing, expense of clinical trials, small sample sizes, and ethical issues. There are many biases that can compromise a clinical trial, such as observer bias, interviewer bias, use of nonvalidated instruments, uneven subject recruitment by physicians, and individual subject factors. Recent concerns have focused on bias in sample selection.

To date, the majority of clinical trials have included a limited segment of the U.S. population, that is, mainly middle-class, married, White males with little to no inclusion of women and minorities. This lack of diversity in trial samples has yielded results that are not always generalizable and effective. Research also has demonstrated bias due to subject factors. For example, subjects were more likely to participate in clinical trials on multiple sclerosis if they had a higher than median income and were disabled from work (Schwartz & Fox, 1995). Suggested approaches to reduce selection bias include (a) using a broad recruitment base to reduce patient and physician biasing factors and (b) facilitating subject transportation to the study site.

Clinical trials are expensive and resource-intensive. As a result, subject numbers are generally limited to the minimum number needed to demonstrate a significant effect not caused by chance. However, small clinical trials may not provide convincing evidence of intervention effects. Small clinical trials are valuable in (a) challenging conventional but untested therapeutic wisdom, (b) providing data on number of events rather than number of patients and thus may be sufficient to identify the best therapy, and (c) serving as a basis for overview and meta-analysis (Sackett & Cook, 1993).

To deal with the issue of small sample sizes, meta-analysis is increasingly being used. Meta-analysis (quantitative overview) is a systematic review that employs statistical methods to combine and summarize the results of several trials. Well-conducted meta-analyses are the best method of summarizing all available unbiased evidence on the relative effects of treatment (Richards, 1995). In a meta-analysis the individual studies are weighted according to the inverse of the variance; that is, more weight is given to studies with more events. Arrangement of the trials according to event rate in the controls, effect sizes, and quality of the trials or according to covariables of interest supplies unique information. If carried out prospectively, the technique provides information on the need for another trial, the number of subjects necessary to determine the validity of past trends and the type of subjects who might be benefited.

Well-conducted cumulative meta-analyses offer the caregiver and the health care consumer answers regarding effectiveness of an intervention at the earliest possible date (Ohlsson, 1994). However, critics of the technique note the difficulties of comparing studies with different designs, data collection methods, and form of study variables (Tucker, 1996). Proponents of meta-analysis recommend evaluating meta-analyses by using a scoring method

that lists 23 items in six major areas: study design, combinability, control of bias, statistical analysis, sensitivity analysis, and application of results (Sacks, Reitman, Pagano, & Kupelnick, 1996).

Ethical issues in clinical trials include issues of informed consent, withholding of treatment, and careful monitoring of clinical trial results. Additional issues of informed consent include assuring that subjects thoroughly understand potential risks and benefits of participation and any effects on their care should they decide to withdraw at any point in the study. Issues of withholding treatment include increasing subject risk or subject benefit if there is reasonable evidence of positive effects of the intervention or treatment. Careful monitoring of the effects of interventions or treatment is necessary to stop the trial if there is associated morbidity or mortality and extending the intervention or treatment to the control group in the event of significantly positive treatment effects.

Recommendations

Clinical trials remain the principal way to collect scientific data on the value of interventions and treatment. However, in designing and evaluating clinical trials, rigor of method, including careful evaluation of potential biasing factors, is essential. Meta-analysis provides a summary of all available, unbiased evidence on the relative effects of treatment. However, rigor of methods used to conduct the meta-analysis also must be evaluated.

DOROTHY BROOTEN

See also
META-ANALYSIS
QUANTITATIVE RESEARCH
  METHODOLOGY
RESEARCH IN NURSING ETHICS
RIGHTS OF HUMAN SUBJECTS
SCIENTIFIC INTEGRITY

COGNITIVE DISORDERS

Cognition has been defined as the activity of knowing: the acquisition, organization, and use of knowledge. All of our mental abilities—perceiving, remembering, and reasoning—are organized into a complex system with the overall function of cognition. Other descriptions refer to the mental processes of comprehension, memory, judgment, and reasoning, as opposed to emotional processes (McDougall, 1990). These definitions provide variability in terminology and represent the paradigms or theories that guide research. Therefore, cognition is defined as the supraordinate construct that includes all mental operations, such as attention span, concentration, and memory. The literature is vast in this area because work occurring simultaneously in gerontology, neuroscience, nursing, psychiatry, and rehabilitation does not always cross over or interrelate.

The theories of adult cognition, such as genetic-epistemological (represented by Piaget), information processing (represented by the computer), psychoanalytic (represented by Freudian analysis), postformal (represented by dialectics), and psychometric (represented by intelligence testing), denote different disciplines and methods of research that are not always appropriate for application to clinical research and practice (Rybash, Hoyer, & Roodin, 1986). There is substantial knowledge development on 14 nursing diagnoses formulated for cognition, based on the work of the North American Nursing Diagnosis Association. They include altered thought processes, sensory/perceptual alterations, potential for injury, self-care deficit, knowledge deficit, altered growth and development, altered sexuality patterns, altered parenting, altered role performance, impaired adjustment, self-esteem disturbance, social isolation, ineffective family coping, and altered family process.

The generic terms *confusion* and *disorientation* are global and insensitive for determining the specific cognitive processes diminished or compromised. A content analysis of cognitive impairment research was implemented, and the following 11 screening instruments were found to be of most use in clinical practice: the Dementia Assessment Inventory (DAT), Brief Cognitive Rating Scale (BCRS), Blessed Dementia Scale (BDS), Cognitive Capacity Screening Examination (CCSE), Cognitive Levels Scale (CLS), Function Reason Orientation Memory Arithmetic Judgment Emotion (FROMAJE), Global Deterioration Scale (GDS),

Mini-Mental State Exam (MMSE), Mental Status Examination (MSE), Clinical Dementia Rating (CDR), and the Short Portable Mental Status Questionnaire (SPMSQ) (McDougall, 1990).

Screening instruments are best suited to measure the presence, absence, and severity of impairment. Older adults in various settings should be routinely screened for cognitive function and mental status by clinicians and health care providers. Recommendations from research and practice are specific. Because cognitive impairment often goes undetected in nonpsychiatric settings, routine screening of older medical patients is recommended. Selection of a screening instrument must be discriminating and based on a clearly understood purpose, that is, cognitive function, mental status, or combinations of those categories.

Screening instruments were designed to measure the presence, absence, and severity of cognitive impairment. Typically, adults with less than an eighth-grade education may be incorrectly identified as cognitively impaired. Screening instruments were never designed to be the sole measure of cognitive function or mental status. Data from 1983 show that a reduction in length of stay by 1 day through accurate assessment of cognitive function would save between $1 and $2 billion each year (Levkoff, Besdine, & Wetle, 1986). The common types of cognitive disorders will be defined for heuristic purposes.

Cognitive impairment is a term describing a disturbance in cognitive functioning. Cognitive functioning is a broad construct that includes a number of categories: attention span, concentration, intelligence, judgment, learning ability, memory, orientation, perception, problem solving, psychomotor ability, reaction time, and social intactness. The assessment of cognitive functioning need not include all of these dimensions, but typical screening instruments such as the MMSE include many of them and give the clinician and researcher a gross indication of whether cognitive impairment is present. Assessment of cognitive function and a complete mental status examination are essential components in the diagnosis of delirium, dementia, and pseudodementia (McDougall, 1995).

Alzheimer's disease is a progressive disorder marked by dementia and the accumulation of cortical neuritic plaques and neurofibrillary tangles in excess of those found in normal aging. The only accurate method of diagnosing Alzheimer's disease is to perform a brain biopsy or autopsy (National Institute of Neurological and Communicative Disorders and Stroke [NINCDS]–Alzheimer's Disease and Related Disorders Association [ADRDA], 1985). Without either of these two methods, the diagnosis is "possible" Alzheimer's disease. Criteria for the clinical diagnosis of Alzheimer's disease were developed only in 1984 (McKhann, Drachman, Folstein, et al., 1984), and they are not fully operational because of insufficient knowledge about the disease. The criteria are compatible with the current *Diagnostic and Statistical Manual of Mental Disorders* and the *International Classification of Diseases*.

The criteria for the diagnosis of probable, possible, and definite Alzheimer's disease are presented by McKhann and colleagues (1984). Probable Alzheimer's disease can be clinically diagnosed if there is a typical insidious onset of dementia with progression and if there are no other systemic or brain diseases that could account for the progressive memory loss and other cognitive deficits. Excludable disorders include drug intoxication, manic-depressive disorder, multiinfarct dementia, and Parkinson's disease. Examples of other disorders that may cause dementia include thyroid disease, vitamin B_{12} deficiency, luetic brain disease and other chronic infections of the nervous system, subdural hematoma, occult hydrocephalus, Huntington's disease, Creutzfeldt-Jakob disease, and brain tumors. There are numerous other disorders causing or simulating dementia that have not been mentioned (see Office of Technology Assessment, 1987).

The diagnosis of dementia cannot be made if delirium is present. Although the official nomenclature for the syndrome is delirium, it has been given many other names: acute confusional state, acute brain syndrome, confusion, metabolic encephalopathy, and toxic psychosis. Delirium is a transient mental disorder with a relatively rapid onset, a course that typically fluctuates, and a brief duration. The essential features of delirium are (a) reduced ability to maintain attention to external stimuli and to appropriately shift attention to new external stimuli and (b) disorganized thinking, as manifested by rambling, irrelevant, or incoherent speech. There is sensory misperception, a disordered stream of thought, and difficulty in shifting, focusing, and sustaining attention to both external and internal stimuli. Irrelevant stimuli can easily distract the delirious individual. Also common are perceptual disturbances that result in misinterpretations, illusions, and hallucinations. In addition, disturbances of sleep-wakefulness and psychomotor activity are present. Nurse investigators have contributed to understanding the phenomena of concern to gerontology nurses caring for patients with cognitive disorders.

Sundown syndrome is a common behavioral problem manifested in patients with cognitive impairments and resembles delirium. Nurses often describe it as the agitation, restlessness, confusion, and wandering behavior of older adults when the sun goes down. Risk factors that have been identified for sundown syndrome in the elderly include physiological factors, such as dehydration, mental impairment, frequent night awakening for nursing care, dementia, and urine odor, and psychosocial factors, such as being in a room less than 1 month, recent admission to facility, and higher evening levels of confusion (Evans, 1987).

This term *confusion* is used by nursing to describe general affect and behaviors of patients; however, it is not specific and appears to have a great deal in common with delirium. The issue seems to be whether the terminology belongs to another discipline (Foreman, 1993). Assessment of behavior and discrimination of terms are important for planning appropriate nursing care of patients with cognitive disorders.

GRAHAM MCDOUGALL

See also
ALCOHOLISM
ALZHEIMER'S DISEASE
CHRONIC MENTAL ILLNESS
COGNITIVE INTERVENTIONS
MIDDLE-RANGE THEORIES
  OF DEMENTIA CARE

COGNITIVE INTERVENTIONS

Cognitive interventions are designed to change some aspect of cognitive function, such as attention, concentration, or memory. An intervention may be defined as a programmatic attempt at altering the course of life-span development. Interventions may be classified as concrete technologies involving such parameters as the goal: enrichment, prevention, or alleviation; the target behavior: cognition, social interactions, or attitudes; the setting: family, classroom, community, or hospital; and the mechanism: training-practice, psychotherapy, or health delivery (Baltes & Danish, 1980). These interventions may be applied to many patient or client populations such as the elderly in long-term care and young head-injured individuals in rehabilitation settings. (See Psychosocial Interventions.)

The body of research literature or data-based publications is stronger in the specialty of gerontology. The burgeoning elderly population of the United States, some 31.6 million people as estimated by the 1989 census, represents one of the biggest challenges facing the nation today in health care. Adults 55 years of age and older complain of memory problems frequently. General or specific incidents of forgetting are often used by older adults to interpret the effectiveness of their memory ability and awareness. The treatment for negative self-evaluation of memory in normal, healthy elderly persons takes two forms. The most frequent intervention is simply to tell the individual, "Don't worry, there is nothing wrong with you." This advice is rarely heeded, and the person continues to seek help or silently remains concerned.

The second approach is for the older adult to attend memory training programs. Memory training programs designed for older adults operate on two basic assumptions: (a) older adults with less than optimal performance will benefit from intense exposure to memory aids, and (b) participation in training will increase the use of these memory aids. The aim of memory training is to teach older adults to use internal memory strategies such as elaboration and rehearsal and external strategies such as calendars and lists to enhance their remembering.

A review of 39 published studies of memory training with older adults documented that the elderly may improve their memory performance on episodic memory tasks (Verhaeghen, Marcoen, & Goossens, 1992). The training was most effective when carried out in groups, when subjects were younger, when sessions were relatively short (less than 90 minutes), and when pretraining was provided in imagery or relaxation techniques. These conclusions are valid only for memory performance on classical episodic memory tasks; however, nothing can be inferred about the impact of memory training on everyday memory performance or on metamemory (memory awareness). More research is needed in this area, and older adults should be encouraged to continue learning. Specific examples of cognitive interventions designed to improve cognitive function are presented as prototypes.

Memory Interventions

In the community, Dellefield and McDougall (1996) designed a study to test the effects of a 2-week, four-session group intervention with healthy older adults to increase memory self-efficacy and memory performance. A total of 145 community-dwelling older adults with an average age of 71 years participated in the study, which was based on Bandura's self-efficacy theory. The intervention significantly increased both memory self-efficacy and memory performance in the treatment group. In addition, the treatment group's perception of control in memory-demanding situations was strengthened, and their perception of negative changes in memory over time was diminished. The control group experienced a significant decline in memory self-efficacy over time. Memory performance was not significantly related to memory self-efficacy. Those individuals with depression had significantly lower memory self-efficacy scores than did those without depression; however, there was no difference in memory performance between depressed and nondepressed subjects. From the posttest to the follow-up period, depressed subjects receiving the intervention showed a significant decrease in memory self-efficacy, whereas nondepressed subjects showed no change.

Interventions for Cognitive Impairment

The International Classification of Impairments, Disabilities, and Handicaps (ICIDH) uses the three conceptual levels of impairment, disability, and handicap to facilitate the collection and use of data (Brown, 1993b). Handicap is defined by the World Health Organization (WHO) as a disadvantage that limits or prevents fulfillment of a role that is normal and depends on age, gender, and social and cultural factors. Both the nature and extent of handicap are important to assess within the framework of the Americans With Disabilities Act and the WHO model of disablement. Although rehabilitation professionals have developed numerous objective measures of cognitive disability, they have not produced subjective measures of handicap. The framework of handicap is useful to guide these interventions.

An increasing proportion of the elderly in the Unites States will live or reside in nursing homes during their life span. The nation's nursing home population grew by 24.2% in the 10-year period from 1980 to 1990 as reported in a recent 1990 Census Bureau report. Of the 500,000 to 600,000 individuals who suffer from strokes annually, most are older adults, with 90% over age 55 and 80% over age 65. Many of these individuals will most likely spend time in nursing homes.

Rosswurm (1991) developed an attention-focusing program to stimulate perceptual and cognitive processing, improve functional performance, and increase participation in group activities in three skilled nursing facilities. The findings showed that there were significant improvements in perceptual processing of information and in the social interactions of the persons in the attention-focusing group. Abraham, Neundorfer, and Currie (1992) implemented a study to test the effects of three cognitive-behavioral group interventions on cognition and depression in nursing home residents. Based on Beck's model of cognitive therapy, the 24-week interventions failed to reduce depression, hopelessness, or increase life satisfaction scores in the residents; however, they improved overall cognitive function. In another study of nursing home residents with severe cognitive impairment and behavior disturbances, Goddaer and Abraham (1994) used relaxing music with a slow tempo and an unpredictable rhythm to reduce agitation. The music had a therapeutic effect on the negative behaviors and significantly reduced agitation as well as exhibition of physical and verbal agitated behaviors.

Nursing has developed a body of knowledge related to the design, implementation, and testing of psychosocial and psychoeducational interventions that is broader in perspective than cognitive interventions (see Psychosocial Interventions).

GRAHAM MCDOUGALL

See also
CEREBROVASCULAR ACCIDENTS
FUNCTIONAL HEALTH
GERONTOLOGIC CARE
MUSIC THERAPY
SELF-EFFICACY

COHORT DESIGN

A cohort design is a time-dimensional design to examine sequences, patterns of change or growth, or trends over time (Burns & Grove, 1993). A cohort is a group with common characteristics or experiences during a given time period (Woods & Catanzaro, 1988). Cohorts generally refer to age groups or to groups of respondents who follow each other through formal institutions such as universities or hospitals or informal institutions such as a family (Cook & Campbell, 1979). Populations also can be classified according to other time dimensions, such as time of diagnosis, time since exposure to a treatment, or time since initiating a behavior. A cohort might be graduates of nurse practitioner programs in the years 1995, 2000, 2005 or siblings in blended families. Cohort designs were originally used by epidemiologists and demographers but are increasingly used in studies conducted by nurses and other researchers in the behavioral and health sciences.

In the most restrictive sense a cohort design refers to a quasi-experimental design in which some cohorts are exposed to a treatment or event and others are not (Cook & Campbell, 1979; Brink & Wood, 1989). The purpose of a cohort design is to determine whether two or more groups differ on a specific outcome measure. Cohort designs are useful for drawing causal inferences in quasi-experimental studies because cohort groups are expected to differ only minimally on background characteristics. Recall that a quasi-experimental design lacks random assignment of subjects to groups. Although the groups in a cohort design may not be as comparable as randomly assigned groups, archival records or data on relevant variables can be used to compare cohorts that received a treatment with those that did not. Because simple comparisons between cohorts may suffer from a number of design problems, such as biased sample selection, intervening historical events that may influence the outcome variable, maturation of subjects, and testing effects, a strong cohort design can account for many of these threats to the internal validity of a study (Cook & Campbell, 1979).

There are two major types of cohort design: cohort design with treatment partitioning and the institutional cycles design. In a cohort design with treatment partitioning, respondents are partitioned by the extent of treatment (amount or length) received. In the institutional cycles design, one or more earlier cohorts are compared with the experimental cohort on the variable(s) of interest. The institutional cycles cohort design is strengthened if a nonequivalent nontreatment group is measured at the same time as the experimental group. A well-planned cohort design can control for the effects of age or experience when these might confound results in a pretest-posttest design or when no pretest measures of experimental subjects are available (Cook & Campbell, 1979). Cohort designs might utilize a combination of cross-sectional and longitudinal data.

The term *cohort studies* broadly refers to studies of one or more cohort groups to examine the temporal sequencing of events over time. Cohort studies may eventually lead to hypotheses about causality between variables and to experimental designs. Most cohort designs are prospective (e.g., the Nurses' Health Study, in which 100,000 nurses were enrolled in 1976 and have been followed since) although some are retrospective.

There are a number of types of cohort studies. The panel design, in which one or more cohorts are followed over time, is especially useful for describing phenomena. Trend studies are prospective designs used to examine trends over time. In trend studies, different subsamples are drawn from a larger cohort at specified time points to look at patterns, rates, or trends over time (Polit & Hungler, 1995). Panel designs with multiple cohorts are used to study change in the variable(s) of interest over time, to examine differences between cohort groups in variables, and to identify different patterns between groups. In a panel study with multiple cohorts, the groups can enter the study at different points in time, and the effects of aging can be differentiated from the effect of being a member of a particular cohort group (Woods & Catanzaro, 1988). A prospective study is a variation of a panel design in which a cohort free of an outcome but with one or more risk factors is followed longitudinally to determine who develops the health outcome. The prospective design is used to test hypotheses about risk factors for disease or other health outcomes. Some authors limit the term *cohort study* to designs in which exposed and nonexposed subjects are studied prospectively or retrospectively from a specific point.

A major problem with prospective studies of all types is subject attrition from death, refusal, or other forms of loss. The loss of subjects in a prospective study may lead to biased estimates about the phenomena of interest.

CAROL M. MUSIL

See also
EPIDEMIOLOGY
POPULATIONS AND AGGREGATES
QUASI-EXPERIMENTAL RESEARCH
TIME SERIES ANALYSIS

COLLABORATIVE RESEARCH

Definition and Relevance to Nursing

Collaborative research involves cooperation of individuals, agencies, and organizations in the planning, implementation, evaluation, and dissemination of research activities. Ideal collaboration brings the perspectives of nursing practice, research, and education to bear on complex issues of health and nursing. The research process, context, design, and needed resources for collaborative projects are not unique within the research arena. The unique feature involves the configuration of a research team whose members bring varying expertise, perspectives, and authority within an institution or agency.

Two prevailing trends support collaboration, namely, constrained resources and sociopolitical accountability. With diminishing resources to fund research and to deliver health care, partnerships can be an effective and efficient way to use human, fiscal, and material resources. Pooling resources of a variety of individuals, agencies, and disciplines can maximize the potential of all participants and contribute to a greater outcome.

Related to scarce resources is the call for increased accountability of research efforts. If finite resources are to be allocated, society and specific funding sources ask that the project demonstrate societal relevance and a connection to public concerns. Through partnerships with consumers, communities, or current practitioners, relevant and timely issues are more likely to emerge as inquiry topics.

Potential collaborators fall into several categories. Individuals can come to the project with expertise in the research process or in a substantive clinical area. Individuals can contribute the perspective of education, service, or research. Agencies or institutions can participate as collaborators, bringing specific human or material resources. Population groups can contribute the perspective and wisdom of a community. Nursing literature also advocates international collaborative efforts.

Advantages and Disadvantages

Collaborative research involves multiple advantages. One potential advantage is a strengthened process and improved outcome through the contribution from multiple individuals with varying expertise and perspectives. Investigator bias can be reduced with multiple inputs. Multisite partnerships give a potential of larger sample size over a shorter time frame and the benefits of built-in replication. Resources and potential funding sources can be increased through collaboration. The possibility of greater dissemination of findings increases with more participants. Collaboration with clinical agencies can help identify potential student clinical placement and supports a context for research that is compatible with the realities of nursing practice. Additionally, innovations in nursing practice or policy are more likely to be adopted if those involved in implementation participated in the inquiry process. Finally, collaborative interaction can enhance professional creativity, collegiality, and productivity.

Although benefits exist, collaborative research also presents distinct disadvantages. Most disadvantages are related to interpersonal issues and the complexities of pulling together different perspectives, priorities, and styles. Teamwork requires clear communication, trust, openness, administrative coordination, and distinct role delineation. Without those features, the integrity of the research and the professional productivity of the collaborators are at risk. Another disadvantage of collaboration is the possibility of multiple review boards and organizational protocols. Collaboration also may add to the time commitment.

Models of Collaborative Research

Five major types of collaborative research described in the nursing literature are the traditional model, health care setting model, unification model, consortium model (Chenitz, Sater, Davies, & Friesen, 1990), and participatory action research (Rains & Ray, 1995). Each model has advantages and disadvantages.

In the traditional model, individual researchers from the same or different institutions work together. In this model, researchers learn from the expertise of each other. The usual equal distribution of experience and expertise means that the research tasks can be divided. The project ideas can be critiqued by two or more researchers with training in the research process or in a substantive area. Detrimental characteristics of the traditional model relate to the necessity of decreased teaching load for researchers with an educational appointment and the need for resources of funding and research assistance. Examples of the traditional model abound.

In the health care model, research occurs within a clinical institution under the leadership of an employed nurse researcher. Collaborators include the clinical staff and the nurse researcher. The strongest merit of this model is the development of practice-relevant research; and because clinicians are involved, there is ownership, accepted innovation, and practice based on scientific research. In this model, subjects are easily accessible, and interdisciplinary collaboration is easily arranged. Disadvantages involve the potential for poor generalizability, investigator bias, role conflict, and scarce research funding. An example of this model can be found in the work of Reiley and colleagues (Reiley et al., 1996).

In the unification model, academic researchers from educational institutions and clinicians from health care agencies collaborate as equal partners. Benefits include combined resources from education and service, practice-relevant research, and enhanced collegiality. Disadvantages relate to the complexity of blending two institutions' perspectives and priorities, the challenges of meeting time and place, and the need to decrease teaching or work load for the researchers. Kolanowski and Whall (1996) provide an example of the unification model involving an academician and a clinician researcher.

The consortium model involves individuals from multiple health care agencies in a geographic region. This model provides the benefits of cost sharing, large subject pool, decreased data collection time, and the momentum and inspiration of a shared project. Because of the geographic distance between sites, communication and decision making present major challenges. Multiple agencies also introduce multiple protocols or review boards. Researchers in this model often report an ambiguity regarding their role in the project. As an example of this model, Segeren (1994) described the North American Consortium in Nursing and Allied Health, a partnership of four institutions for the purpose of collaborative research.

The participatory action research (PAR) model combines community participation, research, and action to solve pressing social problems. This mode of inquiry involves the community as an equal partner at every step of the process. Benefits include empowerment of local communities, development of lay leadership, and resolution of real-life situa-

tions. Disadvantages involve a long time commitment and difficulty in obtaining funding. The example of the PAR model provided by Rains and Ray (1995) involved community health promotion through the Healthy Cities process.

Guidelines for Collaborative Research

Collaborative efforts can be enhanced by the explicit discussion and written communication of guidelines. Thiele (1989) mentioned three significant issues that require attention: "questions of authorship, contribution and recognition of effort" (p. 150). Written agreement among collaborators should clarify role responsibilities for each participant, decision-making processes, tentative time schedules, spin-off projects, and subsequent use of data. Engebretson and Wardell (1997) listed the requisite personal attributes as "trustworthiness, competence, and flexibility" (p. 43) and the requisite relationship attributes as "acceptance, validation, and commitment" (p. 44) and often synergy and fun.

JOANNE W. RAINS

See also
CONSORTIAL RESEARCH
HISTORY OF NURSING RESEARCH
NATIONAL INSTITUTES OF HEALTH
WORLD HEALTH ORGANIZATION
  COLLABORATING CENTERS

COMFORT

Definition

Comfort has been conceptualized for nursing as a holistic outcome of patient care. It is defined as the experience of having the needs for relief, ease, or transcendence met in four contexts of experience. Relief, ease, and transcendence as three types of comfort were derived from a concept analysis of comfort by Kolcaba and Kolcaba (1991). The four contexts for experiencing comfort are physical, psychospiritual, environmental, and social; they were derived from the literature on holism (Kolcaba, 1991).

Comfort care is nursing care that is intended to enhance a patient's comfort beyond its known baseline. Comfort care consists of goal-directed, comforting activities (process) through which enhanced comfort (product) is achieved. The process is initiated by the nurse, often in conjunction with the patient and family, after an assessment of the comfort needs of the patient. Because the specified product or goal is enhanced comfort, a successful process is evaluated by comparing comfort levels before and after nursing interventions. The process is incomplete until the product of enhanced comfort is achieved (Dretske, 1988).

Theory of Comfort

Kolcaba (1994) provides a theoretical framework for practicing comfort care and for generating nursing research about comfort. Briefly, the theory states that interventions should be designed and implemented to address unmet comfort needs of patients and their families. Patients and families are recipients of nursing care, and they perceive the effectiveness of nursing interventions in the context of existing intervening variables. Intervening variables are factors that recipients bring to the situation, such as financial status, existing social support, previous experience with health care, and religious beliefs. If recipients of nursing care perceive that their comfort is enhanced through effective nursing interventions, those interventions qualify as comfort measures. Such comfort measures strengthen patients and their families during stressful health care situations, thereby facilitating health-seeking behaviors.

Schlotfeldt (1975) discussed health-seeking behaviors in terms of those that are internal (fertility, healing), external (self-care, functional status), or leading to a peaceful death. Consistent with holism, conscious and subconscious experience influence motivation for health-seeking behaviors. Because health-seeking behaviors are constructive, they are reciprocally and positively related to comfort. In the theory of comfort, comfort is the immediate

goal of nursing interventions, and health-seeking behaviors, specific to the research questions(s), are subsequent goals.

Relevance to Nursing

As a heuristic device, comfort care plans for individual patients or patient/family situations have been designed for students who are learning to apply comfort care to their patients (Kolcaba, 1995) and families (Kolcaba & Fisher, 1996). There are several advantages for teaching comfort care. First, it is theory-based nursing. Second, it is satisfying to patients because it is individualized and holistic. Third, it is satisfying to students because they become aware of and are given credit for all comfort measures that they implement for their patients. Fourth, it is appropriate for diverse settings. Fifth, it is easy to learn because students are familiar with the concept of comfort through their own experiences.

After a brief introduction to the theory, nurses are able to practice comfort care without the heuristic device of plans. When comfort care is used as a framework for organizing nursing care, that care is more efficient because many comfort measures can be implemented during one patient encounter. Nurses and patients find comfort care satisfying and productive because enhanced comfort is theoretically related to progress in physical therapy, collaboration with new health regimens, or faster healing.

Research

The content domain of comfort provides a diagram for designing interventions and problem-focused questionnaires. Holistic interventions, such as massage, music therapy, art therapy, guided imagery, therapeutic touch, and comfort care itself, can be targeted to several aspects in the grid at one time. Unmet needs of patients or families in specific health settings can be identified, and specific interventions can be designed to meet those needs. Unmet needs also can be translated into items on questionnaires to determine baseline comfort and postintervention comfort. Comfort questionnaires should have positive and negative items relevant to the research setting to represent each aspect of the domain. Although comfort is state-specific, a successful intervention theoretically should demonstrate increasing comfort over time. Therefore, at least three repeated measures of comfort should be collected in an intervention study where increased comfort is a desired goal.

The theory of comfort directs research in several ways. First, it guides nurses to test relationships between particular holistic interventions and comfort; an effective intervention is positively and significantly related to an increase in comfort over time. Second, it guides nurses to test relationships between comfort and health-seeking behaviors. If the relationship is positive, nurses have a pragmatic rationale for enhancing their patients' comfort. Third, it guides nurses to construct predictive models for interventions that enhance comfort and facilitate desired health-seeking behaviors.

Observational studies have been conducted to determine what kind of comforting actions are important for patients and what the term *comfort* actually means to patients. These studies were about the process of comfort care; they did not define the outcome of comfort.

Quantitative comfort studies are in their infancy, primarily because comfort has been operationalized only recently. But instruments developed from the content domain of comfort were sensitive to group differences in comfort during the immobility period following cardiac catheterization for different types of restraints and to differences in comfort between community dwellers and hospital patients. Several intervention studies in which comfort is the desired outcome are in progress: effectiveness of music therapy for persons having dressing changes for burns, effectiveness of comfort care for postsurgical incontinence, and effectiveness of guided imagery for women who choose conservative therapy for early breast cancer.

Future Directions

To demonstrate that comfort is an important mission for nursing, further research is needed to determine the relationship between enhanced comfort and health-seeking behaviors. Decreased length of stay for hospitalized patients, decreased readmissions, faster progress during rehabilitation, and increased functional status related to enhanced patient comfort would interest administrators, funding agencies, and policymakers. Further research also is needed to replicate experimental studies that have demonstrated the effectiveness of holistic interventions. When nurses wish to test such interventions, they should use an outcome consistent with a holistic paradigm; comfort is such an outcome.

KATHARINE KOLCABA

See also
MUSIC THERAPY
NONTRADITIONAL THERAPIES
NURSE-PATIENT INTERACTION
PAIN MANAGEMENT
SCHLOTFELDT'S HEALTH SEEKING NURSING MODEL

COMMUNITY EMPOWERMENT

Community empowerment is a social action process. It enables people to increase their understanding and control over personal, social economic, and political influences to improve their lives. In this respect, empowerment is both a process, an action, and an outcome, the goals that are attained as a result of the action. There is a shift in relationships and decision-making power among individuals, groups, and social institutions at the local level as people attempt to gain control over their destinies in a changing social and political environment. Community empowerment occurs in a social context and is an interactive process of change where both communities and individuals are transformed. Public health experts recognize that powerlessness is a broad risk factor for disease and health problems; and thus, empowerment is a strategy for health promotion (Israel, Checkoway, Shulz, & Zimmerman, 1994; Wallerstein & Bernstein, 1994).

Historic roots of community empowerment may be found in the literature related to community psychology, social psychology, community organizing, critical theories, feminist perspectives, primary health care, and health promotion. The literature indicates that there is an emphasis on social justice as people act in political and social arenas. The concept of community empowerment is proactive, rather than reactive, as individuals and organizations apply their talents and resources in collective efforts to meet their community's needs.

A Brazilian educator, Paulo Freire (1970), suggested a dialectical model of community participation and adult learning in promoting social justice and equity. Freire advocated for participatory education in which people become actors in history rather than objects or recipients of services. As actors, they become empowered as individuals to identify their problems and solutions, transforming themselves as well as changing oppressive circumstances.

Concepts and theories related to citizen participation, problem solving, sharing for power, community organizing, community development, conflict management, and feminist theory are essential to community empowerment. The case study methodology is commonly used in the study of community empowerment.

Research Examples

Two case studies highlight the role of community conflict in the process of community empowerment during a 7-year relationship between neighborhoods and a graduate program in community health nursing (Flick, Reese, Rogers, Fletcher, & Sonn, 1994). Conflicts external and internal to the community were facilitators and barriers to the application of Freire's approach to community organizing. The authors concluded that both conflict management theory and empowerment education theory must be integrated in working with diverse communities.

Another case study reported on the De Madres a Madres partnership of a Houston inner-city Hispanic community and the Texas Woman's University College of Nursing (McFarlane & Fehir, 1994). empowerment of indigenous women was studied using feminist theory and Freire's empowerment education theory. Two results emerged: (a) the enhancement of individual women's self-esteem as well as the collective community esteem and (b)

the promotion and support of a unique economy, volunteer-based programs to enhance community building distinctly different from the market economy.

A third case study identified five concepts that linked community empowerment and action research in Healthy Cities (Flynn, Ray, & Rider, 1994). The concepts were focused on community, citizen participation, information and problem solving, sharing of power (equity and social justice), and quality of life. Although the case studies provided evidence that these concepts were applicable to empowering communities through the Healthy Cities process, additional research was needed to determine if this set of concepts includes the critical elements of community empowerment.

Future Research

Concepts related to community empowerment require further research. Although research is providing beginning evidence of the relevance of many of the concepts, studies should be replicated in other communities. As data collection measures are developed, there is a need to move beyond the case study approach. Questions for nursing research include the following: How does empowerment work? How do nurses, who occupy higher positions of power than the people with whom they frequently work, empower the community, or does the community empower itself? What resources do nurses bring to empowering the community? How is information used to empower the community? Are individual empowerment and community empowerment related? What are the conflicts that arise when there is a shift in power relationships? How are conflicts resolved? How are communities held accountable for their actions in the empowerment process? What are the facilitators and barriers to empowering the community through media advocacy strategies? Also, because empowerment may not be a fixed state, what facilities sustain community participation when resources are fixed or declining?

The challenges in research related to community empowerment are similar to those of community health research. Interdisciplinary skills are needed, particularly those of health educators who have established the conceptual background and beginning research on community empowerment. Nurses, too, are beginning to add to the body of knowledge in this area of scholarship and can take the lead in promoting interdisciplinary research collaboration. A particular challenge is funding of these research efforts. Funding may be more likely if community empowerment research is incorporated as part of larger community studies linked to the national health objectives.

The concept of community empowerment as a social action process results in a shift in power relationships in the community. Community empowerment should be studied in conjunction with other concepts and community processes, such as individual empowerment, conflict management, how information is used to achieve knowledge and action, and other social, economic and political considerations. The outcomes of empowerment, including social justice, have an impact on community health indicators and quality of life.

BEVERLY C. FLYNN

See also
COMMUNITY HEALTH
FEMINIST RESEARCH METHODOLOGY
**URBAN HEALTH RESEARCH: NURSING
    RESEARCH IN URBAN
    NEIGHBORHOODS**
VULNERABLE POPULATIONS

COMMUNITY HEALTH

Community health is influenced by environmental, biomedical, organizational, and behavioral factors and encompasses a broad definition of health. For example, good jobs, education, safe neighborhoods, access to health and social services, and recreation and leisure activities all promote community health. Community health is a process of health promotion and disease prevention in which community leaders identify community problems and assets, create consensus on goals, take action, and reach goals. Key aspects of this process are community develop-

ment and multisectoral interventions, including health policy and community participation. Ongoing community-wide efforts assess and monitor progress in achieving explicitly stated community goals, for example, those adapted from *Healthy People 2000* (U.S. Department of Health and Human Services [USDHHS], 1990).

Because the health of people is affected by broad contextual factors, nurses, particularly community health nurses, must collaborate with other disciplines in developing a knowledge base for community health. Useful theories and models that can be applied to the study of community health include cultural change theories, social change theories, critical theories, community development, diffusion of innovation, ecological models, community participation, community power, and community decision making.

Research Examples

Community health research can be classified in different ways. For example, categorical programs include large-scale interdisciplinary studies such as the Minnesota Heart Health Program, the Pawtucket Heart Health Program, and the Stanford Five-City Project. Noncategorical programs include Healthy Cities and action research. Epidemiological research includes community needs, assets assessments, and risk factors for disease. Finally, there are evaluations of community health interventions.

Increasingly, nurses are conducting community health research and involving other disciplines and the community in the process. A study of the immunization levels of Mexican American and White non-Hispanic infants enrolled in Arizona's Medicaid managed care demonstration project is an example of a categorical program. Although non-Hispanic infants received more immunizations by age 1 year than did Mexican American infants, it was found that when explanatory variables were controlled through multiple regression analysis, ethnicity was no longer a significant predictor of immunization levels. Significant predictors of higher immunization levels included fewer siblings, maternal education, and older mothers. It was concluded that health insurance and enrollment in managed care were not sufficient to ensure adequate immunizations (Moore, Fenlon, & Hepworth, 1996).

Participatory action research was conducted by a Healthy City in rural Indiana. Community leaders of a Healthy City accept a broad definition of health and promote broad community participation from all sectors of the community in decision making for health. In this study, public health nursing faculty were asked to work with community leaders to assess the community's needs and assets. Following an analysis of existing census and health data indicating high death rates for heart disease and cancer, compared to state and national statistics, community leaders and faculty developed a health survey that focused on lifestyle behaviors related to heart disease and cancer. The results were compared to *Healthy People 2000* (USDHHS, 1990) goals on selected behaviors, indicating sedentary lifestyles, cigarette smoking, and inadequate dietary choices. Community leaders identified smoking as a "winnable issue" for focus on community action and change. Community leaders used the data to support the development and passage of a city ordinance to create nonsmoking environments in all city buildings. They also used multiple strategies with various collaborators to reduce adolescent access to tobacco. The authors concluded that participatory action research contributes to community empowerment through community health action (Rains & Ray, 1995).

McMaster University and the University of Toronto conducted a systematic overview of the effectiveness of public health nursing interventions. Evidence about the effects of community health and development projects within the scope of public health nursing were reviewed. Twenty-four articles, representing 17 different projects, were judged on selected quality criteria relevant for the report. The positive outcomes of these projects included community leadership and problem solving, the creation of community social and environmental programs or services, the establishment of planning structures, and the impact on legislation (Ploeg et al., 1995).

Future Research

Opportunities for nursing research in community health are enormous. The growth of managed care is placing increased demands on state and local public health systems to assure the continuation of vital programs. Research in managed care and its impact on community health is needed to assure accountability of essential services. The extent to which underserved populations receive care within cost-containment strategies should be studied. The development of community coalitions for health throughout the country requires further study. Most major health programs—for example, Assessment Protocol for Excellence in Public Health (APEX/ PH), Planned Approach to Community Health (PATCH), Healthy Cities and Communities, and HIV/AIDS Community Planning—involve the development of community coalitions as part of the community health process.

Research is needed to explain under what conditions coalitions succeed in promoting community health programs and policies. How effective are these programs and policies in changing key community health indicators of success? Nursing interventions, such as nurse-managed clinics or community nursing centers, need further research. What are the critical factors that sustain successful nurse-managed services at the local level? To what extent are these services being integrated into the networks of provider services? Dissemination of research findings is also important. For example, what are the characteristics of successful nurse-managed services that can be applied elsewhere and in what types of communities?

Likewise, the challenges are enormous. Nurses can take the lead in interdisciplinary research collaboration. The skills for community health research require the expertise of many disciplines in addition to nursing, including epidemiology, health economics, medicine, dentistry, health policy, statistics, and urban planning. The challenge is to share the expertise of each discipline as well as share the credit and rewards of collaboration. Although the time is ripe for funding such research efforts, such funding is highly competitive in the current health care arena.

The concept of community health incorporates a broad definition of health, one that recognizes the multiple community factors that support and impinge on health. Scientific inquiry that includes both qualitative and quantitative research approaches is needed to further build the body of knowledge relevant to the theory and practice of community health.

BEVERLY C. FLYNN

See also
   COMMUNITY EMPOWERMENT
   EPIDEMIOLOGY
   HEALTH POLICY
   NURSING CENTERS
   MANAGED CARE

COMMUNITY HEALTH INFORMATION NETWORKS

Community health information networks (CHINs) are virtually uncharted waters for nursing research. CHINs, extensions of the electronic medical record, link providers, payers, and consumers electronically across a geographic area to informational databases. Originally, communication infrastructures accessed via computer were developed for the sharing of clinical and financial data by physicians, health care agencies, and payers. Such electronic linkages exist in the public sector in federal, state, and local government systems (e.g., Health Care Financing Administration, Centers for Disease Control); in the private sector, including ambulatory, managed care, and home health systems; and in international systems (e.g., Denmark and Sweden models). Recently, in some CHINs information about insurance benefits and health or wellness issues are being made available to consumers as well. Opportunities for nursing research exist around issues of nursing language in databases, the monitoring and reporting of the financial value of professional nursing, and the design and evaluation of electronic consumer information programs.

Language and Finance Issues

Nursing can be proud of its ongoing, research-based development of nursing languages that are available for inclusion in CHIN databases. Extensive research has been a part of developing language systems for nursing diagnoses, nursing interventions, and nursing outcomes. The American Nurses Association (ANA) has established specific criteria and standards for language development. Four nomenclatures have been recognized by the ANA (1995a) as having met all criteria: (a) nursing diagnoses as developed by the North American Nursing Diagnosis Association (NANDA); (b) the *Nursing Intervention Classification* (NIC); (c) the *Omaha System*; and (d) the *Home Health Classification System* (American Nurses Association, 1995a). The NANDA system classifies only nursing diagnoses, NIC solely classifies nursing interventions, and the last two nomenclatures contain data elements that address nursing diagnoses, interventions, and outcomes for community health nursing.

The discrete data elements in these four nursing nomenclatures, coupled with their specific coding schema, support their incorporation into electronic databases. However, incorporation is neither a universal nor a congruent occurrence. Rather, inclusion is erratic; it generally ensues as an institutional or network-specific process, and frequently, recognized nursing nomenclatures are incorporated selectively or not at all. Further, these languages are not scientifically mapped to each other, although the electronic *Uniform Medical Language System* (UMLS) at the National Library of Medicine, which includes these nomenclatures in its data base, has made some progress in this area. In short, barriers exist to the uniform inclusion of nursing nomenclatures in CHIN databases—sporadic, selective use of the different languages and lack of congruent linkages among them. Ongoing research in language development should continue, but additional research is needed to identify and overcome the barriers to incorporating recognized nursing languages into CHIN databases.

Due to the inconsistent incorporation of nursing languages into databases, financial information about the performance and outcomes of nursing work is ambiguous and incomplete. The costs and benefits of professional nursing to consumers and to health care organizations should be specified by (a) geographic locale (e.g., Northeast, Southwest, urban, rural); (b) setting (e.g., inpatient, outpatient, school, work site); (c) agency (e.g., hospital, nursing home, health maintenance organization, visiting nurse association); and (d) different consumer population types (e.g., the elderly, the well, perinatal women, those with diabetes, asthma, etc.). If nursing data elements are not present in CHIN databases, financial data cannot be determined, and the work of nurses will remain unspecified, essentially invisible. The value of nursing will remain unknown to nursing's constituents: employers, payers, other health professionals, and consumers.

Design and Evaluation of Health Information

Another realm for nursing's contribution is the design and evaluation of health information programs delivered electronically. As agencies develop and make such entities available to consumers via their CHINs, research is warranted to determine optimal formats of presentation and the impact of these programs on intended outcomes. For example, when a CHIN proposes to offer patients on-line access for preoperative preparation, information, and instructions, many questions surface. What is the best design or format for presenting the information and instructions? What are the benefits as related to telephone contacts or personal encounters? Does the individual patient have realistic expectations about what will happen to them during and after surgery? Have they followed the instructions and prepared adequately? Do members perceive such programs as adding value to their insurance plan and their health status? Is this a cost-effective way to deliver preoperative instructions? Does such a delivery mode meet legal criteria for documentation or must it be used in conjunction with other educational modes? Evaluation research can contribute valuable answers, forming a strong base for making future decisions about similar technological applications across CHINs. Nurses have historically conducted research about the value of education to consumers, which can be applied to the new technology.

Community health information networks are proliferating. Nurses must ensure that labels indicating the work and outcomes of nursing are stan-

dardized and included in network databases. Predicated on their inclusion is the subsequent specification of attendant financial information that will define the costs and benefits of nurses to their employers, professional associates, payers, legislators, and consumers. Finally, as CHIN developers and users devise novel ways to provide consumers access to health information, nurses can lend their scientific expertise when designing and evaluating the worth of such programs. Research is essential to establish valid, reliable information about professional nursing's value in the cost effective improvement of consumer health states.

MARGARET FISK MASTAL

See also
**HOME HEALTH CARE
 CLASSIFICATION (HHCC) SYSTEM
NANDA
NURSING INTERVENTIONS
 CLASSIFICATION (NIC)
NURSING OUTCOMES
 CLASSIFICATION (NOC)
UNIFIED LANGUAGE SYSTEMS**

COMMUNITY MENTAL HEALTH

Antecedents of the Community Mental Health Movement

The ebb and flow of social policy in the United States is marked by gradual shifts in public perception and evaluation of the problems that beset the society in any given era. Thus, the convergence of major societal trends gave rise to the Community Mental Health Centers Act of 1963; the first of these trends had arisen from the earlier passage of the National Mental Health Act (Public Law 79-489) in July 1946. This act created the National Institute of Mental Health (NIMH) and appropriated significant federal monies to support innovations in training, research, and practice in the field of mental health. The act designated four core mental health disciplines: psychiatry, psychology, social work, and psychiatric nursing (Bloom,1984).

Funds from this act allowed financial support for students and faculty at the undergraduate and graduate levels in psychiatric nursing.

This federal infusion of dollars into the states required that each state would have a central planning authority charged with the responsibility for planning and evaluating community-based mental health services, the first time in U.S. history that the federal government had assumed responsibility for what had for more than a century been the exclusive duty of the states. This latter fact is most often attributed to the efforts of Dorthea Lynde Dix, who sought to have the abysmal community-based mental health care of the 1840s (i.e., asylums, jails, almshouses) replaced by a system of state psychiatric hospitals.

In the decade after the passage of the Mental Health Act there was growth in the number of state mental hospitals as well as in the number of admissions. Subsequently, Congress enacted the Mental Health Study Act to examine the human and economic problems of mental illness, and the Joint Commission on Mental Illness and Health was established. At the end of a 5-year period the commission presented its report to President John F. Kennedy. Three months later the president transmitted a message to Congress in which he outlined a "bold, new approach." This message framed the substance of what was to develop as the Community Mental Health Centers Act of 1963. The act provided for federal money to be matched with local dollars for construction of community-based mental health centers. Planning grants were given to each state to inventory mental health needs and resources. The country was divided into some 1,500 catchment areas, with the idea that eventually each catchment area would have its own center. The act mandated five essential services: inpatient care, partial hospitalization, emergency services, consultation, and education. Later, five additional services were added to the mandate: precare and aftercare, diagnostic services, rehabilitation, training, and research and evaluation.

In the years since 1963, Congress has extended and amended the act several times. In 1977, President Jimmy Carter and his wife, Rosalynn Carter, brought to the White House a long-standing concern for the care and treatment of persons with mental disabilities and mental illness. President Carter's first act was to establish a President's Commission on Mental Health, with Mrs. Carter serving as honorary chair. The report of this 1977 commission contained more than 100 recommendations. The major recommendations were to provide universal access to treatment at reasonable cost to all who needed it and to work toward high quality of services. Specific recommendations focused on working with the community to lessen the stigma associated with mental illness by (a) developing community supports, (b) providing for careful protection of basic rights, (c) focusing on prevention, and (d) expanding the research base to increase the available knowledge. Thus, in 1980, when the Community Mental Health Centers Act was scheduled to expire, Congress began to work on the new legislation, Public Law 96-398, the Mental Health Systems Act.

However, the mood of the country had changed. President Carter was not reelected in 1980 and was succeeded by Ronald Reagan. The Reagan administration had promised less federal government intrusion into the affairs of state governments; thus, the proposal for block grants was accepted, and the previous 20 years of categorical grant experience were negated. In 1981 the budgetary provisions for the Mental Health Systems Act were repealed, and the system of block grants was established. There are, however, legacies from this era of community mental health.

Treatment Approaches in Community Mental Health

Prior to the 1960s, long-term therapies were normative. Short-term therapy, crisis interpretation, and mental health consultation are now standard practice in the field (Bloom, 1984; Lancaster, 1980). Each modality has made a major contribution to the therapeutic armamentarium of mental health practitioners. Equally important, if not more so, intellectual work of the community mental health era yielded a set of concepts that continue to prove useful to the ongoing study of body and mind relationships. The conceptual notions of early childhood interventions, genetic risks, the importance of healthy pregnancy to future well-being, and other concepts led to an approach that examines risk factors and the incidence of mental illness. This era also sowed the seeds for the beginning work on the relationship between stress and illness. This was reflected in the emphasis on community-based mental health education as a strategy for prevention (Beisser & Rose, 1972).

An integral feature of all aspects of the community-based approach was an emphasis on citizen participation at all levels—national, state, and local. This forged an interesting alliance of lay people with professionals. However, the continued vocal and sometimes adversarial participation of consumers and their families in the planning, delivery, and evaluation of mental health services is a major strength in the struggle to achieve parity for mental health care with all other health care.

In the latter part of the 1990s, the community-based mental health delivery systems are faced with the additional challenge of managed care. How well the states can respond to these emerging mandates is yet to be seen. Some states have begun to shape new systems from older community-based systems, with evaluations yet to be completed (Inglehart, Hiebert-White, & Zuercher, 1995). What is clear is that the institutional responses to the problems of mental health and mental illness are and continue to be shaped by prevailing belief systems. The decade of the 1990s has been called the "decade of the brain." It is to be expected, then, that the focus for research, treatment, and training will continue to shift away from some of the core values that have shaped community mental health programs.

GRAYCE M. SILLS

See also
MENTAL HEALTH IN PUBLIC SECTOR PRIMARY CARE
MENTAL HEALTH SERVICES RESEARCH
PSYCHOSOCIAL INTERVENTIONS
STRESS

COMPUTER-AIDED INSTRUCTION

Students and practitioners of nursing have an urgent need for expanded comprehension in a broad range of subjects. However, the explosion of knowledge and resources in nursing and other areas has overwhelmed the ability of traditional educational methods to allow rapid assimilation and dissemination of health sciences data. Since the 1960s, educators have examined the use of computers to enhance human learning (i.e., computer-aided instruction, also known as CAI). Computer-aided instruction can provide features to enhance dynamic and interactive education that are not available or easily accessible in traditional learning modalities.

Traditional learning modalities include reading textbooks and journals and attending lectures or formal classes. Although printed materials have the advantages of simplicity, convenience, and portability, they are constricted in their capacity to present information by size and weight limitations as well as their lack of ability to convey sound and movement. Moreover, even in printed materials with self-test modules, this form of learning is relatively passive and cannot meet many learners' needs for active participation. Lectures or classes have the advantages of simplicity and familiarity and may provide opportunities for learner-instructor interaction. However, this form of education requires that specific times be set aside for attending the lecture or class and for travel to and from the site. Additionally, lectures and classes cannot be adjusted to the varying levels of knowledge and interests of the participants. The limitations of traditional teaching methods for information, sound and movement capabilities, interactivity, time constraints, and customization of material can be addressed by well-designed CAI programs (Jaffe & Lynch, 1995).

Application of CAI in Nursing Education/Inservice

Nursing presents unique challenges to educators and administrators. Basic nursing education requires the acquisition of skills that may needs frequent review by students, and continuing education for licensed nurses often has to be available 24 hours a day, 7 days a week, to meet the need of all nursing shifts. Staffing of a skills lab or presentation of material by instructors for prolonged periods is limited by the economic and personnel constraints of the organization. Many investigators have demonstrated that the flexibility of CAI— being available around the clock, presenting material multiple times, and responding to individual learning needs—can increase nursing student and staff performance to a greater extent than traditional instructional methods can (Jelovsek & Adebonojo, 1993; Napholz & McCanse, 1994; Sittig et al., 1995). An additional advantage of CAI is that scoring is impartial, and users are less likely to have concerns about the judgment or subjectivity of a computer (Umlauf, 1990).

A wide variety of CAI programs are available to nurses and other health professionals. Topics of these CAI programs include cardiac dysrhythmias, heart sounds, funduscopic examination, dermatological disorders, advanced cardiac life support, drug calculations, specialty patient management case studies (such as internal medicine, critical care, oncology), anatomy, physiology, patient interviews, 12-lead electrocardiogram interpretation, and intravenous line insertion. These CAI programs are available for purchase from major health sciences publishers, and a few can be obtained free of charge from some major biomedical companies.

Application of CAI in Patient Education

In addition to basic and continuing nursing education and inservice, CAI can be a powerful adjunct to patient education, useful for both in-hospital and outpatient education. It provides a personalized, institution-independent, interactive learning environment that can be repeated as often as desired by the patient. Thus, CAI can reinforce patient education in an individualized, nonthreatening manner. Currently, there are multiple CAI programs available through major biomedical companies (pharmaceutical, equipment, and publishers) for patient education. CAI programs currently available for patient education are on such varied topics as hyperlipidemia, diabetes, stroke, breast self-examination, and HIV.

Effective CAI Teaching Strategies

Computer-aided instruction is not merely simple access to vast amounts of information (such as clini-

cal databases, MEDLINE, patient records) but is rather an interactive, classroom-independent, personalized learning activity. Integration of multimedia (i.e., text, sound, animation, and video) often is found in the latest CAI programs. A well-designed CAI program can rival the best of traditional classroom or lecture experience, but a poorly conceived or designed CAI program can give the user a poorer learning experience and far more frustration than conventional educational methods.

Much of effective CAI design is similar to that of superior traditional teaching, that is, identification of goal-oriented learning appropriate to the medium. However, additional considerations for effective CAI design include an intuitive program interface, technical support for faculty and students, and continuous reevaluation and improvement of the program and CAI approach (Dodge, 1997). Other considerations to remember when designing a CAI program or deciding whether or not to use one include the integration of multimedia, interactivity, and equipment requirements for the program.

Although CAI can offer an amazing range of versatility for presentation of information, the integration of multimedia components must be applied in an appropriate manner. Multimedia should be employed to enhance the learning experience without overwhelming or distracting the user. Interaction between the user and the program should allow not only for assessment of knowledge but also should provide opportunities for acknowledging correct or incorrect responses and be able to easily find and review materials to enhance understanding.

A serious drawback in the application and utilization of CAI is equipment requirements. CAI hardware needs for computer type, amount of memory, processing speed, hard drive space, printer, input device (keyboard, mouse, graphics pad, data glove), sound card, and CD-ROM device are not standardized and can vary widely between programs. Thus, it is important to remember that no matter how wonderful the CAI, it will be completely useless if the equipment required by the program is not available to the user.

Current and Future CAI Technology

Original CAI systems consisted of a computer and software, but rapid advances in technology have added interactive laser disks, CD-ROM, and the Internet to the rich selection of CAI opportunities. Software, interactive laser disks, and CD-ROM CAI programs are available on a wide variety of topics. They have advantages in terms of portability and user access, as long as equipment requirements for the CAI are met. However, these forms of CAI are platform-dependent (i.e., computer- and operating system–specific) and expensive, and the provided information cannot be altered. The time necessary to distribute materials for both these forms of CAI and printed textbooks or journals can delay dissemination of information. However, the disadvantages of the other forms of CAI are bypassed by the latest form of CAI, the Internet.

The Internet is a worldwide network of computers that allows access to a variety of information sites and services. Use of the Internet is growing at an exponential rate. Advantages of the Internet for CAI applications include platform independence, relatively low cost, immediate updating of information, and rapid, worldwide dissemination of information. In some cases, rapid language translation (e.g., between German, Japanese, Swedish, and English) of material is available at some sites. The sophistication and distribution of nursing and health sciences CAI sites on the Internet is astounding. These sites range from interpretation of hemodynamic waveforms to pediatric electrocardiography. There is an even greater proliferation of patient information sites for such things as heart failure, AIDS, breast cancer, alcoholism, diabetes, and sports medicine.

Despite the excitement and extraordinary promise of Internet-based CAI, potential users must exercise caution. The very nature of the Internet, where almost anyone can set up a site and place his or her own version or interpretation of facts on it without expert review, demands that users be particularly careful in utilizing information obtained in this manner. Information learned via Internet CAI should be validated with accepted traditional sources, and nurses should frequently review information on Internet sites before recommending them to their patients.

The rapid evolution and expansion of nursing knowledge demands a more efficient and personalized form of learning than is currently available through journal subscriptions (now so numerous and diverse that most clinicians cannot keep up with their reading) and occasional professional meetings. Computer-assisted instruction offers a personalized, interactive, classroom-independent, learning opportunity. These exciting teaching features, coupled with CAI's ability to organize hierarchies of information, can provide nurses with the skills for both basic and increasingly expert clinical conceptualizations. Although CAI probably will never completely supplant a truly inspired human teacher, it can enhance and enlarge the learning process for both nurses and their patients.

MARY A. WOO

See also
COMPUTER SIMULATION
ELECTRONIC NETWORK
NURSING EDUCATION
PATIENT EDUCATION
RESEARCH ON INTERACTIVE VIDEO

COMPUTER-BASED DOCUMENTATION OF PATIENT CARE

One of the most valuable aspects of automating information management and processing is that, properly done, the process of designing an information system calls into question the nature of the work and the use of information in performing the work. By increasing the quality, quantity, availability, and feasible uses of information, a well-designed information system actually transforms the work itself. Consideration of computer-based documentation of patient care thus raises questions about the nature of patient care and the purposes of documentation, as well as the ways in which computer technology can transform and improve the processes of care.

Patient care has long been depicted as a linear, stepwise process consisting of assessment, diagnosis, determination of therapeutic goals, selection and implementation of interventions, and evaluation of the results of interventions. Sometimes a feedback loop is shown so that evaluation actually occurs during a reiteration of the process; when the patient is reassessed, current diagnoses are compared with previous diagnoses and goals, and goals and interventions are continued or modified (Goodwin & Edwards, 1975). This view of patient care provides some useful insights into the process, but it is greatly simplified. In reality, a caregiver who is deliberately working through the process may perform several steps simultaneously. For example, while implementing the intervention of tracheal suctioning, the nurse is simultaneously assessing not only the patient's reaction to the treatment but the patient's (a) overall respiratory function, (b) skin condition, (c) cognitive and emotional status, and (d) ability to participate in care. This simultaneous, nonlinear quality of patient care poses challenges to information systems intended to support care.

Moreover, patient care is not just the care of one provider for one patient. Increasingly, patient care is understood as a multidisciplinary process in which the contributions of all caregivers interact and are modified by the interactions. Supporting patient care requires, then, that systems provide each caregiver with the information needed for professional practice within the requirements and constraints of that caregiver's discipline, with consideration for the care provided by other disciplines. It follows that information generated and entered by one discipline may have to be presented in a different, sometimes summarized form for use by other disciplines. And the care provided by all disciplines must be managed and ordered so that care activities complement rather than conflict with one another and occur in the sequence and at times most likely to benefit the patient.

The care of each patient is thus both sequential and simultaneous, discipline-specific and multidisciplinary. To add to the complexity, each caregiver is usually responsible for multiple patients. From the caregiver's perspective, patient care means, in addition to the considerations in caring for each patient, balancing the needs and priorities of all the patients for whom the caregiver is responsible and blending with the contributions and exigencies of all the other caregivers. To support patient care effectively, computer systems must take into account the full range of complexity confronting the caregiver.

If patient care is complex, documentation must reflect that complexity while fulfilling its several purposes. First, in the care of the individual patient, documentation provides a stable and ongoing record of what has been observed, inferred, and performed on the patient's behalf. This record enables all those caring for the patient to communicate with one another and, on the basis of information received and reviewed, to make better decisions. Computer systems that support recording, communicating, and retrieving information (sometimes in different forms) thus aid documentation.

The ability to organize and present in meaningful ways information gleaned from multiple sources is a valuable feature. Second, documentation of the care of an individual patient provides a record for retrospective review. Can something be learned from this case study to improve care in the future? Were there instances of negligence, malfeasance, or on the other hand, exemplary practice? Are the contributions of each discipline well represented in the documentation system, and is it possible to view the whole of multidisciplinary care at selected points in time to assess the interactions of patient events and interventions? Legal and regulatory bodies require that records of patient care be available for scrutiny.

A less traditional function of documentation, one that could scarcely be realized without electronic databases, is to provide data that can be aggregated across patients and analyzed statistically to evaluate the quality and effectiveness of patient care, to perform cost-effectiveness studies, and to conduct clinical research using the data of everyday practice. To support this function, computer systems must not only capture information related to patient care but also abstract key elements into aggregate databases amenable to statistical analysis. This use of documentation has great potential for improving patient care, but it also raises issues of privacy and confidentiality of patient care information. Debates that weigh the right to control the use of personal information against the right to receive high-quality care based on evolving knowledge are ongoing and not easily resolved (Institute of Medicine, 1997b). Certainly, the potential to use patient care information in research databases augments the already important issues of validity and reliability of information in the patient record.

With this understanding of the complexities of patient care and the functions of documentation, how can we judge applications of computer-based documentation of patient care? Those that were developed early in the history of health informatics often are discipline-specific: physician order-entry systems, nursing care planning and documentation systems, and the like. Although each discipline may view information entered by and for another discipline, these older systems do not support multidisciplinary practice. Nevertheless, they do facilitate recording and communication and save a little time (Blackmon et al., 1982; Pabst, Scherubel, & Minnick, 1996).

More recently developed systems structure multidisciplinary planning and documentation around "clinical pathways," time-sensitive sequences of care to be provided and expected patient responses. Although these systems support a multidisciplinary approach to the overall care plan, they vary in their ability to support variations from the clinical pathway and unanticipated diagnoses, goals, and interventions. Increasingly, both commercially available systems and privately developed ones include programs for abstracting selected data elements electronically and storing these data in repositories for subsequent analysis. The degree to which this can be done is limited in part by lack of data standards, especially, but not only, in clinical vocabularies (American Medical Informatics Association, 1994; Evans, Cimino, Hersh, Huff, & Bell, 1994; Henry & Mead, 1997).

Computer-based documentation of patient care is evolving toward the complex functions needed to support the realities of practice, but much remains to be done. Recommendations for the development of computer-based patient records are available in the Institute of Medicine's report *The Computer-based Patient Record* (1997a). An excellent description of desired features of future systems is contained in *Next-Generation Nursing Information Systems: Essential Characteristics for Professional Practice*, by Zielstorff, Hudgings, and Grobe (1993). As computer-based documentation of patient care evolves, the enhanced availability of discipline-specific and cross-discipline knowledge and information will increasingly transform both the direct effects and the interaction effects of each caregiver's contributions to patient care.

JUDY G. OZBOLT

See also
**CLINICAL INFORMATION SYSTEMS
CURRENT PROCEDURAL
    TERMINOLOGY-CODED SERVICES
NURSING INFORMATICS**

COMPUTER SIMULATION

Computer simulation is a general term for a model of a dynamic system, problem, or process. A model airplane is a physical simulation of an object. Computer simulation is a model of an abstract series of events (e.g., a clinical case study) or a process (e.g., nurse staffing). In nursing, computer simulation is used to describe two different types of applications. The first and most common type of simulation is actually a computerized case study, most often available on CD-ROM media. The researcher develops a model case that exhibits all the characteristics of a typical clinical situation. Actors are filmed performing the case, and the film is digitalized and written onto a CD-ROM disk. The second type is a computer simulation model of a process; it takes the form of a computer program in a simulation language such as GPSS/H (General Purpose Simulation System/H).

Case Study Simulations

In educational and clinical research settings, simulation usually refers to vignettes that are filmed and used for educational research, testing, or instructional purposes. Patient case studies are usually the topic of the simulation. However, many different topics may be suitable for teaching, testing, or educational research simulations. For example, Roberts, While, and Fitzpatrick (1996) examined clinical problem solving by using videotaped simulations in their research methodology. Yensen and Woolery (1995) proposed a "virtual" nursing college based on the use of multimedia teaching aids, including simulations of clinical problems. The National Council of State Boards of Nursing has been involved in the research and testing of computerized clinical simulations for possible use in nursing licensure exams (Krawczak & Bersky, 1995). Computer simulations may be digitalized and written onto CD-ROM, tape media, or diskettes for the computer.

In educational settings the learner is presented with the simulated clinical case study (Stewart, 1995). Usually, the student views a part of the case—for example, a simulated assessment. The student then enters nursing diagnoses, suggestions for further assessments, or other queries. The program evaluates the student's performance and may offer further educational material.

There are several benefits to this type of application. First, the student is able to practice nursing skills under conditions that protect patients from the possible errors of a neophyte. Second, students are able to progress at their own speed. Thus, ideal learning conditions can be provided to each student without inconveniencing or hindering the learning of any other student. Third, these applications can be cost-efficient by conserving the time and energy of teachers. Fourth, simulations can provide a more appropriate learning experience than clinical practicums. In a simulation the exact type of clinical problem needed to support lectures can be provided at the precise time the student needs that experience. Any instructor can identify with the frustration of trying to make patient assignments that fit the student's learning needs in the course curriculum. Fifth, simulations are often fun for the learner. Enjoyable learning experiences are more likely to result in acquisition and retention of knowledge than are tedious experiences.

There are some cautions about simulations as learning tools. First, development of a simulation can be difficult. Not every teacher has the flair and skill necessary to construct simulations. Second, development costs may be high. Commercial simulations are usually developed by a vendor (or a developer contracted by the vendor) and marketed nationally or internationally. Simulations ought to be reviewed by one or more experts, and the reviewers' time and efforts must be compensated. This process is time-consuming and may be too expensive for individual teachers. The expense of development may limit the topics suitable for educational simulations.

A third concern about simulations is their life cycle. A simulation can quickly become outdated by new scientific, diagnostic, or treatment discoveries. For example, a simulation addressing the care of a patient with a particular type of central venous catheter will become obsolete overnight if that product is recalled or replaced with a newer model. Orally presented classroom lectures can be updated in an hour or two so that the material taught matches clinical practice. Updating a simulation can take weeks or months. It also can be an expensive task for the vendor and for the educational institution.

Process Model Simulations

The term *simulation* also is used to describe computer models of dynamic processes. Process model simulations have been used extensively in engineering. Nursing applications, although not as common as those in engineering, are found in the literature. For example, McHugh (1989) used simulation modeling to examine the effectiveness of various nurse staffing decisions in hospitals. Process model simulation also has been used to support nursing management decisions (Blake, Carter, O'Brien-Pallas, & McGillis-Hall, 1995; McHugh, 1988).

Process model simulations defined. Process model simulations are actually computer programs. They model dynamic processes by instructing the computer to perform the mathematical calculations or other instructions needed to model a process. The program also collects data and creates a report and may create a data output file so that the results of the simulation can be saved, manipulated, and analyzed. Process model simulations are used when the process cannot be modeled efficiently by a simpler method, such as paper-and-pencil diagrams of the process or linear programming. Specifically, simulation is required when the process involves multiple variables that interact among each other, particularly when more than two of the variables function randomly.

Types of process model simulations. There are two types of process model simulations: discrete event and continuous simulation. Discrete event simulation is by far the most commonly used type of simulation in nursing applications. It is used when the state of the system being modeled changes only at discrete time points—for example, nursing staff changes at shift time changes or perhaps at other scheduled times when shifts overlap. In a continuous simulation one or more aspects of the modeled process change continuously over time; for example, models of wound healing would require continuous simulations. Different computer languages are required for the two types of simulations. Computer languages commonly used for process model simulation include GPSS, SIMSCRIPT, and SLAM.

Utility of process model simulations. Computer simulations of work processes have long been used in industry to support management decision making. Schriber's (1991) GPSS language text provides many examples of using simulation to determine such things as the optimal number of bank tellers to have on duty at various times of the day, the best way to schedule tugboats in a busy harbor, scheduling machines for optimal work flow in a manufacturing operation, and so forth. Health care managers have a powerful tool for improving the effectiveness of certain types of decisions. For example, computer simulation models can test the cost-effectiveness of various unit and bed allocation decisions for hospitals. Such a simulation can answer questions such as "How many patients will we have to send to another hospital if we have 12 beds in our emergency department versus 10 beds, and what will be the differential staffing costs of 10 versus 12 beds?"

Computer simulation offers nursing a new research methodology. Simulation modeling has long been accepted as a research methodology in engineering and business but has been used less often in nursing. Some kinds of nursing problems are not amenable to simulation. Research problems in which there are variables that are critical to the situation but cannot be specified in a simulation (e.g., psychodynamic processes) are not appropriate subjects for simulation research. However, process model simulations offer some advantages for studying problems that can be simulated. First and foremost, they allow study of multiple, random, and interacting variables. No unaided human brain can perform that kind of feat. Thus, simulation allows controlled study of subjects that it may not be possible to study in any other fashion.

Importance for Nursing

Simulation models can be effective, economical, and educational decision-support and research

tools. The education of nurses is an expensive task, and educational institutions and departments—like all other work environments in the United States in the 1990s—are being asked to do more with less. Simulations may help educators, managers, and researchers to fulfill that mandate. Educational simulations can offer the best education to a large number of students more conveniently and at less cost than traditional classroom teaching.

In research, simulation can offer great advantages. Simulation studies may cost much less than traditional research, with its expensive sampling and data collection strategies. Simulation involves no risk to human subjects. In permits absolute control over the research environment, thus allowing near-perfect experimental control over extraneous variables, which previously was available only in bench laboratory settings—a research environment that is not available for many nursing management studies. Finally, simulation can use time as a variable. Many years of simulated time can be processed in seconds in a computer simulation. Thus, simulation research can permit study of variables over very long periods of "time" yet produce the results in seconds.

Nurses are becoming more expert at using computers in education, administration, and research. As more and more nurses gain computer expertise, the importance of computer simulation to enhance quality, efficiency, and frugality also will rise. Computer simulations will become a part of the nursing profession of the future in education, clinical practice, administration, and research.

MARY L. McHUGH

See also
COMPUTER-AIDED INSTRUCTION
ELECTRONIC NETWORKS
NURSING EDUCATION
RESEARCH ON INTERACTIVE VIDEO
TELEPRESENCE

COMPUTERIZED DECISION SUPPORT SYSTEMS

The informatics literature variously defines computerized decision support (CDS) systems. This term may be used to describe any system that uses raw data to provide information that might help clinicians make decisions; but in the strictest sense, a CDS system is expected to transform raw data into information by combining different kinds of information, recognizing patterns, and presenting the new information to clinicians in a way that influences the immediate decision making. Computerized decision support systems vary in terms of complexity and scope, ranging from provision of integrated reports to use of inferencing methods to determine complex associations between pieces of information. Computerized decision support systems can be categorized according to their level of complexity. This categorization refers not only to the complexity of the output of the system but also to the complexity of the input data and the level of the decision making the system supports.

The lowest level is called transaction processing systems (TPS). These systems are the most common; they monitor and record day-to-day routine activities. An example would be a bedside system that a clinician uses to record patient assessment data. Decision making that is supported by a TPS relates to supervision and control of routine activities and has the goal of improving efficiency. The next level in complexity is management information systems (MIS). As input these systems use the data collected by TPS as well as external data from outside the current setting. For example, when making patient care decisions, an MIS would include data from the patient at hand as well as data from other patients with similar conditions. The goal of the MIS is to provide information that promotes effective decision making. The third category of CDS systems is decision support systems. These systems use internal and external data. Although their goal is the same as the MIS—that is, to facilitate effective decision making—they deal with problems that are relatively unstructured. For example, such a system might be used to predict how a new patient care treatment might affect the average duration of patient stay in an institutional setting.

Within the different levels of CDS systems, the scope of the system can also vary. Some CDS systems assist with a narrow range of decisions related to one nursing diagnosis or procedure. Others assist with a broad range of decisions. The Creighton

Online Multiple Modular Expert System (COMMES) is an example of an early system designed to provide consultation and nursing care plans for an extensive number of nursing and medical diagnoses (Cuddigan, Logan, Evans, & Hoesing, 1988).

Nursing research in the area of informatics has a history of perhaps 25 years, most of which has been heavily invested in the basic work necessary for the building of CDS. This basic work includes the development and identification of classification systems, taxonomies, vocabularies, essential data elements, and types of information used in nursing research and nursing decision making (Benner, 1984; Werley, Devine, Zorn, Ryan, & Westra, 1991). Although nurse informaticists have also developed circumscribed CDS by using these building blocks, research related to the accuracy of the decisions and the efficacy of these systems in improving outcomes is fairly limited. One study was located that tested the accuracy of a CDS system using assessment data with a forward-chaining inference engine to identify nursing diagnoses and interventions appropriate to the patient (Hendrickson & Paganelli, 1994). A few studies have moved beyond these basic issues to test the effectiveness of specific CDS in producing nursing decisions that result in better outcomes of care (Cuddigan et al., 1988; Petrucci et al., 1992).

In 1993 the National Institute of Nursing Research (NINR) constituted an expert panel on nursing informatics. This group examined the state of the science in nursing informatics and declared it to be in its infancy. The panel was charged with setting research priorities for nursing informatics as part of the National Nursing Research Agenda. In carrying out this mandate, the panel identified seven foci for research, and within each focus these experts assessed the state of the science and identified and prioritized more specific research need (NINR, 1993). The foci were (a) using data, information, and knowledge to deliver and manage patient care; (b) defining and describing data and information for patient care; (c) acquiring and delivering knowledge from and for patient care; (d) investigating new technologies to create tools for patient care; (e) integrating systems for better patient care; (f) integrating systems for better patient care; and (g) evaluating the effects of nursing information systems.

Health care delivery today is so complex that it is currently straining the resources of our country, and multifaceted clinical decisions are being made in an environment of rapidly escalating intensity. When CDS systems are developed to produce specific patient care protocols that have been validated through rigorous methodologies, these systems have the potential to decrease harmful variation in care, improve clinical decision making, optimize outcomes of care, and cut health care costs.

BARBARA BRADEN
CINDY CORRITORE

See also
CLINICAL PATHWAYS
COMPUTER-BASED DOCUMENTATION
    OF PATIENT CARE
INTERNATIONAL CLASSIFICATION
    FOR NURSING PRACTICE
NURSING INFORMATICS

CONCEPT ANALYSIS

Definition

Concept analysis is a strategy used for examining concepts for their semantic structure. Although there are several methods for conducting concept analysis, all of the methods have the purpose of determining the defining attributes or characteristics of the concept under study. Some uses of a concept analysis are refining and clarifying concepts in theory, practice, and research and arriving at precise theoretical and operational definitions for research or for instrument development. Concept analysis has been used in other disciplines, particularly philosophy and linguistics, for many years. However, the techniques have only recently been "discovered" by nurses interested in semantics and language development in the discipline.

Place in the Structure of Nursing Research

Concept analysis is a useful tool for nurses conducting research. Because the outcome of a concept analysis is a set of defining characteristics that tell the researcher "what counts" as the concept, it allows the researcher to (a) formulate a clear, precise theoretical and/or operational definition to be used in the study; (b) choose measurement instruments that accurately reflect the defining characteristics of the concept to be measured; (c) determine if a new instrument is needed (if no extant measure adequately reflects the defining characteristics); and (d) to accurately identify the concept when it arises in clinical practice or in qualitative research data.

Relevance to Nursing

Concept analyses were relatively rare in nursing research until the early 1980s but have increased dramatically in number over the past two decades. Concept analysis is particularly relevant to a young science such as nursing. The process, regardless of method, requires rigorous thinking about the language used to describe the phenomena of concern to the discipline. Doing a concept analysis causes the researcher to be much more aware of and sensitive to the use of language in research. A conscious awareness of the language chosen to represent phenomena is necessary if nursing scientists are to develop a comprehensible body of knowledge for the discipline.

It is also necessary for thoughtful practitioners to be aware of the language of the discipline. How nurses think about and describe the problems and solutions relevant to their practice is of paramount importance in helping the consumer of nursing care and the policymakers who influence the practice milieu to understand what nursing is and what nurses do. If nurses do not have a central core of well-defined concepts to describe their practice, then confusion and ambiguity will persist, and the development of nursing science will suffer.

Researchers and Methods

It is beyond the scope of this work to outline the various methods of concept analysis. However, there are some excellent sources of information on methods of concept analysis in nursing. Some of these are Walker and Avant's (1995) *Strategies for Theory Construction in Nursing* (3rd edition), Chinn and Kramer's (1995) *Theory and Nursing: A Systematic Approach* (4th edition), and Rodgers and Knafl's (1993) *Concept Development in Nursing: Foundations, Techniques, and Applications.* The major journals that publish concept analyses are *Advances in Nursing Science, Scholarly Inquiry for Nursing Practice,* and *Image: The Journal of Nursing Scholarship.* The major research journals also publish concept analyses on occasion, when the analysis is linked directly to the research report.

Future Directions

Concept analysis has become a useful adjunct to nursing research. The outcome of a concept analysis significantly facilitates communication between researchers and practitioners alike. By specifying the defining characteristics of a concept, the researcher or practitioner makes it clear what counts as the concept so that anyone else reading about it or discussing it understands what is meant. Being clear about meaning allows better communication between scientists and practitioners about the usefulness and appropriateness of nursing language.

There is considerable discussion in the literature about which method of analysis is the most useful. Regardless of the method used, however, concept analyses can contribute significant insights into the phenomena of concern to nurses.

KAY C. AVANT

See also
INSTRUMENTATION
PHENOMENOLOGY

CONSORTIAL RESEARCH

Consortial research is a form of collaborative research that can be used to increase the quantity and quality of nursing research within clinical settings (Mays et al., 1992). It involves cooperative efforts among researchers at several institutions. The sites have formal, well-defined administrative and working relationships that spell out agreed-upon roles and responsibilities.

Consortial studies are done for a number of reasons: (a) to achieve the required sample size when studying a low-prevalence disease; (b) to increase the ethnic diversity or other characteristics of a sample, thus increasing generalizability of results; (c) to shorten the timeline for conducting the study by simultaneously recruiting subjects at multiple sites; (d) to provide mentoring to more junior researchers and staff nurses; (e) to share resources, tasks, and costs when external funding is not available; and (f) to increase opportunities for replication and dissemination.

Consortial studies may be conceived by one or a few investigators, who draft the initial proposal then recruit colleagues at other sites to participate in the study. These other investigators may be involved in helping to refine the proposal before it is submitted for funding. When the purpose of the consortium is more focused on mentoring junior colleagues or is a way to share resources and costs, it is more likely that development of the proposal will be a group endeavor from the start. In the latter case, the choice of topic may be generated by an advisory or steering committee. Whichever approach is taken, the pool of ideas generated by expertise from several institutions creates synergy that leads to more creative and productive research.

To conduct these multisite studies, one site usually serves a coordinating function for the study. Most often in externally funded studies, the coordinating center is responsible for identifying or developing questionnaires or other data collection forms, for data collection and processing procedures, and for receiving and centrally analyzing the study data. The oversight role of the coordinating center includes development and implementation of a quality control plan to assure standardization of sample identification, recruitment, and data collection procedures. Scientific issues for the conduct of the study are usually managed by a steering committee, often composed of the principal investigator from each participating site and a few key individuals at the coordinating center. Standing or ad hoc subcommittees of the steering committee are often formed to propose standards and oversee the work on specific aspects of the study. For example, the subcommittees bring proposals for publications and presentations, participant safety and endpoints, or clinical aspects before the steering committee for approval. The degree to which the steering committee is involved in development of protocols, questionnaires, and so forth, as opposed to approving those developed by the coordinating center, varies by study and the reason the consortium was created.

In a consortium formed primarily for the purpose of sharing resources, mentoring junior researchers, replicating a previous study, or disseminating results, the steering committee may be composed of representatives appointed by each participating institution. In such cases the steering committee often serves the purpose of setting priorities for the activities of the consortium. Funding of studies conducted by a consortium may take several forms. When external funding is involved, the two most common types are (a) providing one large grant to a coordinating center, which then subcontracts with each clinical site, and (b) providing individual grants to each participating institution with a separate grant to the coordinating center. The first approach gives the coordinating center budgetary leverage when a site is not performing up to par. This is an advantage for involving a new site or increasing the number of subjects enrolled at existing sites by redistributing funds from the nonperforming site. The second approach requires that each site meet the commitments for the good of the overall study. A third model, used when external funding is not available, shares the cost of the research among participating institutions within the consortium.

In medical treatment research and public health prevention research, consortial arrangements have been a preferred structure for large randomized trials that must recruit substantial populations in a relatively short time, provide intervention, and have sufficient follow-up time to generate adequate statistical power to compare the effects of treatment on the study outcomes. Nursing has generally had less experience with this approach, although consortia of schools of nursing with several practice settings have been formed to facilitate the conduct of collaborative clinical nursing research (Rizzuto & Mitchell, 1988a, 1988b, 1990; Schutzen-

ofer & Potter, 1989; Zalar, Welches, & Walker, 1985).

It may be expected that consortial research will increase as nursing researchers do more experimental research. Another factor that may promote consortial research in nursing is the changing health care system. As health care systems increase the number of contractual arrangements in attempts to provide cost-effective, integrated care across the continuum of patient needs, consortial research is likely to become more common.

BARBARA VALANIS

See also
COLLABORATIVE RESEARCH
FUNDING
HEALTH CARE REFORM
    AND NURSING RESEARCH
MENTORING IN NURSING RESEARCH

CONTENT ANALYSIS

Content analysis is a data analysis technique that is commonly used in qualitative research and focuses on structuring particular topics or domains of interest from unstructured data. It is a time-consuming process that involves organizing, identifying, coding, and making categories from patterns of data that are reflective of the topics (Patton, 1990). The topics or domains of interest are descriptive names chosen by the researcher and are sometimes also referred to as category labels (Morse & Field, 1995). Historically, early content analysis focused on linguistic and observational data. However, in addition to information derived from interviews and casual or structured observations, researchers may analyze written text from special documents, archival records, field logs, and diaries or may develop schemes to analyze visual data from pictures or videotapes.

Content analysis begins with reading the text or written transcription of an interview, notes from an observation, or some other mode of data collection. The investigator reads the completed text and determines the main ideas or topics of the transcription or observation. The investigator then rereads the text and numbers and assigns a code to each segment or group of lines from the transcription. Sometimes this may also be called labeling. Segments may consist of a single word or line, multiple words or lines, one or more paragraphs, or a pictorial schema and may vary according to the chosen topic or topics. The codes developed by the investigator reflect some commonality, such as an action or behavior, an event, thought, concept, and so forth. Line segments or groups of lines are separated and are grouped into categories, and the categories are grouped according to the topics that were identified by the investigator.

Topics or domains of interest may be chosen prior to a study, as with a focused study, or after the first interview. A focused qualitative study centers on one particular area of interest or intent, such as metaphorical analysis or feminist research. Another kind of focused study might center on a particular phenomenon like leadership style, body adornment among adolescent girls, or a demonstration of how caring activities are performed, to name a few.

The researcher may also choose to develop topics after a first interview or observation. Sometimes the topics seem to arise naturally from the data, whereas at other times the researcher must decide on and develop the topics from the information given. Developing a topic may be similar to making an index for a book or file labels (Patton, 1990). The researcher reads through the transcript of the interview or observation and begins to sort and organize the interview data according to likenesses and similarities. The researcher usually gets a sense of the main topics that pervade the text soon after the transcribing process is complete and after the first reading. This organization of the data may be done by hand or by using one of the many computer software packages that are available to assist organization of qualitative data.

Morse and Field (1995) suggest using between 10 and 15 main topics per study. They caution against making topics too specialized as only very small amounts of data will be able to fit into each. On the other hand, too many topics can cause confusion, and the researcher may have difficulty in remembering what categories go into each topic as the study progresses and more data are collected. With each subsequent interview or observation, the topics may be combined or subdivided into multiple categories as the need arises. As repetitive patterns arise, relationships between the categories and then between topics may be seen. Often the relationships may occur at the same time or be concurrent with each other. For example, in a study of adolescent face care, the topics "blemish care" and "facial scrubbing" are related and occur at the same time. In the same study, the topic "facial preparation" occurs or is antecedent to the topics of "blemish care" and "facial scrubbing," whereas the topical area "making up the face" may occur as a consequence of one of the earlier categories that was formed (Huttlinger, 1985; Morse & Field). Some researchers choose to quantify part of the analysis by counting frequency and sequencing of particular words, phrases, or topics.

The major reliability and validity issues of content analysis involve the subjective nature of the researcher-determined topics or category labels. What should be included within each topic should be clearly defined and should be clearly different from the others so that the results are mutually exclusive. The easiest way to determine reliability in a study that uses content analysis is to have two or more readers, other than the researcher, agree that the topics are appropriate for a particular study and that data can easily be organized under each. This is typically carried out by having the researcher randomly choosing a part of the study and having the readers look over the text and the topics independent of each other. A consensus of the readers would indicate the study's reliability.

Validity in content analysis can be achieved by determining the extent that the topics represent what they are intended to represent. If the topics are based on a conceptual framework or a particular focus, they must be justified, described, and explained in terms of being representative of that conceptual framework or focus. Therefore, topics that are developed to reflect a conceptual framework or focus must be consistent with the original definitions described by that framework. However, because content analysis is often used in exploratory and descriptive research, a conceptual orientation may not be used (see Exploratory Research).

KATHLEEN HUTTLINGER

See also
DESCRIPTIVE RESEARCH

GROUNDED THEORY
NARRATIVE ANALYSIS
QUALITATIVE RESEARCH
RESEARCH INTERVIEWS
   (QUALITATIVE)

CONTINUING EDUCATION

The ultimate goal of continuing education (CE) and staff development in nursing is to enhance professional growth and to improve nursing care. There have been conflicting results in studies of whether CE has an impact on patient outcomes. It is assumed that the answer is positive; therefore, continuing professional education remains an important means of maintaining and updating nursing knowledge and skills.

Definition

The definition of CE in nursing can be defined in the broadest sense as all educational activities beyond the basic nursing program. The purpose of CE is to build on the educational and experiential bases for the enhancement of practice, education, administration, research, or theory development, to the end of maintaining and improving the health of the public (American Nurses' Association, 1990).

Review of Major Studies

Historically, there were few research studies in continuing nursing education prior to the 1960s. The studies conducted in the 1960s focused on describing the nurse personnel resources and the nurses' perceptions of their learning needs. The topics in the literature during the 1970s were the following: needs assessment, the characteristics of the nurse learners, the planning process, instructional methods, motivation factors for participation in CE, program evaluations, and learner evaluations.

The early 1980s was an era when mandatory CE for relicensure was gaining momentum across the nation in all health professions. Comparison studies were conducted with registered nurses in states that had mandatory requirements and nurses in states

that did not. Research findings revealed that mandates were useful for a minority of unmotivated nurses to participate in CE. In the 1990s, research included change in learner behavior (attitude and knowledge change of nurses caring for AIDS patients), development of CE models based on the adult education conceptual framework, evaluation of effective teaching strategies (critical thinking, distance learning, concept maps), and cost analysis studies.

The majority of studies in CE and staff development explored knowledge and attitudinal change in the behavior of the nurse learner rather than improved patient care. However, professional associations, health care agencies, and individual nurses expect benefits from nurses' participation in continuing nursing education. These assumed benefits include improved quality of care, competence, personal benefits, and social benefits, such as shorter hospital stays for patients. Dr. del Bueno was one of the early researchers who found that there were other factors than CE that made a difference or change in practice and that CE alone does not make a difference.

Few researchers have examined the interaction of the many factors affecting changes in practice. Is a CE program viewed successful only to the extent that a recommended practice or behavior is implemented? Peden, Rose, and Smith (1992) used the Cervero and Rottet model, which recognized the CE program as only one component of behavior change. The individual, nature of change, and the social system are additional factors that influence behavior change.

Henry (1989) provided a detailed overview of 73 studies that were conducted on the evaluation of in-service education, orientation, and CE. These evaluation studies focused on the measurement of learner outcomes (60%) and learner behavior change (42%). Very few studies focused on patient impact (1%) and cost-effectiveness (10%). Turner (1991) stated that it is not clear from the literature whether continuing nursing education provides what is expected. In a mailed survey to 244 registered nurses, Turner found no significant relationships identified between the costs and benefits of continuing nursing education.

Research findings indicated that continuing nursing education programs increase knowledge and change attitudes. Some studies assumed that if there was a knowledge and attitude change, there would also be improvement in patient care, which has not always been measured or documented.

Waddell's (1991) meta-analysis research provided a thorough review of existing studies and confirmed the positive effects of CE on nursing practice. This was the first major meta-analysis research conducted in the field of continuing nursing education to determine the extent to which continuing nursing education had a positive effect on nursing practice. The meta-analysis on 34 studies supported the hypothesis that CE positively affects nursing practice. However, 35% of the studies failed to report any reliability and validity information on the instruments used to measure change. Audit and observation were the two basic kinds of measurements used for recording change in practice. Waddell recommended a cost-effective, valid, and reliable instrument for measuring nursing practice.

There are some major issues when measuring the impact of CE on nursing practice. There may be a lack of tools to measure changes in knowledge, skills, values, and attitudes. Studies focused on concrete uses of knowledge that are direct and observable often exclude conceptual changes in thinking, judging, and evaluating. Few studies examined how nurses use the knowledge they gain from CE. Sherwood (1996) used a qualitative inquiry to provide new dimensions to existing knowledge about how nurses use information from CE in practice. Sherwood developed a categorical model from which further study can determine linkages of a process-oriented model. Change indicators were the infrastructure linking the implementation in professional practice.

Methodology

Most of the studies utilized nonexperimental designs followed by quasi-experimental designs, and few used experimental designs. A majority of the research in continuing nursing education has been of a descriptive, exploratory design. Controlled experimental studies in continuing nursing education have been difficult to conduct because of the many variables of a social system, human behavior, and other extraneous factors. Qualitative research methodology has been infrequently used in conducting continuing nursing education studies.

Many needs-assessment instruments and methods require further refinement and testing to establish the validity and reliability of the instruments and the process. The complexity of the needs-assessment process is related to several factors: the difficulty in defining the term *need*, the diverse characteristics and unique learning needs of adult learners, and the use of numerous and varied methods to subjectively and objectively identify needs and establish priorities. The needs-assessment issue raises questions concerning the projective technique of identifying needs, the extent to which individuals are aware of their needs, and possibly the extent to which individuals may or may not wish to take responsibility for learning new materials.

Peer review and performance review by the nurse's supervisor are more objective measures of verifying improvements in patient care than attendance records and improvement in knowledge and attitude posttests following a CE program. Motivation to change is an individual choice, and there is no guarantee that nurses who attend CE programs will be motivated to make changes in their nursing practice. Very few studies have included as a variable the individual's desire to change.

Future Directions

In the future, nurse researchers will have to replicate currently existing studies, develop reliable and valid instruments for measuring patient outcomes and learner behavior change, and test evaluation models in continuing nursing education. There is also a need for more collaborative research projects with university professors, staff development educators, and other health professionals in the field. Much emphasis has been placed on the direct impact of improved quality of patient care as a result of continuing nursing education. Maybe there is not a direct link between continuing professional education and improved patient care but only a direct relationship to change in the behavior of the professional nurse.

ALICE M. KURAMOTO

COPING

Coping in nursing research is most often defined by using the definition and theoretical framework of psychologists Lazarus and Folkman (1984). They define coping as "constantly changing cognitive and behavioral efforts to manage specific external and/or internal demands that are appraised as taxing or exceeding the resources of the person" (p. 141). In these and other theorists' works, coping is conceptualized as part of a dynamic process consisting of a stressor, appraisal, resources, coping, and outcomes.

Hundreds of studies have been conducted by nurse researchers on stressors requiring coping. Most examine coping with illness or disease and medical treatment in catastrophic situations. Studies examining coping in chronic illness are prominent. Jalowiec (1993), in a 10-year review of nursing research on coping, found that the most frequent illness or treatment situations studied were cancer, heart disease, and major surgery. The majority of this research focused on coping by adult patients, followed in frequency by parents of ill children, spouses of patients, and family caregivers. Recently, more research has been conducted in the areas of child and adolescent coping (Garvin & Ryan-Wenger, 1997).

Lazarus and Folkman (1984) conceptualize stress as a person-environment transaction of two concomitant appraisals: appraisal of the significance of a stressor for the well-being of the person (primary appraisal) and appraising what might be done about the stressor (secondary appraisal). They also distinguish between two types of coping, problem-focused and emotion-focused. Nurse researchers investigate problem-focused coping as behavioral efforts at "doing something to relieve the problem" (p. 44); emotion-focused coping is defined as "coping that is directed at regulating emotional response to the problem" (p. 150).

Coping is usually studied in nursing research in response to one or more stressors, which can be defined as an "internal or external event, condition, situation, and/or cue" that has the potential to bring about or actually activates significant physical, psychological, social, or spiritual reactions (Werner, 1993, p. 20). Stressors studied in nursing research can be categorized as normative (expected) and catastrophic (unpredictable, infrequent). They are further differentiated as having or not having to do with health, illness, or treatment for these conditions (Werner, 1993).

Resources for coping studied in nursing research can be categorized as social resources such as social support, psychological resources such as hardiness and self-efficacy, spiritual resources, and others, such as finances and education. The resource most studied is social support. In an extensive review, Artinian (1993) found that 81% of the nursing research studies on coping resources examined social support. Similar results were reported in the review of Underwood and Ruiz-Bueno (1997). Results have been mixed as to whether social support acts as a buffer between stressors and health outcomes (buffering hypothesis) or if it has a direct effect on health outcomes (main effects hypothesis). This trend points to the need to study specific functions of resources in specific situations and in specific phases of illness or treatment.

On the basis of their reviews, Artinian (1993) and Underwood and Ruiz-Bueno (1997) reached several other conclusions. First, the context (e.g., chronic vs. acute illness) determines social support needs. Second, perceived availability of support is sometimes more strongly related to coping effectiveness than is the actual support received. Third, social support has both positive and negative effects. Finally, there appears to be a negative association between social support used as a coping resource and the outcomes of depression and anxiety.

Within the subcategory of psychological resources, hardiness is most studied in nursing research on coping (Artinian, 1993; Underwood & Ruiz-Bueno, 1997). The relationship of hardiness to health outcomes is still unclear. Likewise, the effect of control (perception that life is under personal control or that health can be controlled) is to date unclear. Trends in results suggest less control relates to negative health outcomes such as depression and anxiety.

Coping can be differentiated as coping style or coping behaviors (strategies). Coping style suggests typical responses across situations, whereas coping behaviors refer to what people actually do when faced with a stressor. Nurse researchers study coping behaviors much more frequently than coping styles.

Coping behaviors have been found to differ according to illness phase and associated stressors and to other factors, such as resources. People in all types of health and illness situations use a mix of problem-focused and emotion-focused strategies (Garvin & Ryan-Wenger, 1997; Jalowiec, 1993). Theoretically, problem-focused strategies are specifically tailored to the situation, although more global emotion-focused strategies are used across situations (Lazarus & Folkman, 1984).

Jalowiec's (1993) 10-year review identified five major coping behaviors used by patients, family members, and caregivers in illness situations, as follows:

1. Optimism. Jalowiec suggests that the strategy of optimism's effectiveness lies in its impetus to take constructive action, to think of additional options, and/or to retain cognitive control of stressful situations.
2. Social support. Using positive social support generally results in favorable health outcomes. Social support may function through provision of aid or assistance, bolstering self-esteem, ventilation of feelings, provision of information or advice, presence of a confidante, advocacy, and/or assisting with responsibilities.
3. Use of spiritual resources. This may involve prayer and relying on a greater power.
4. Control. Trying to maintain control aimed at the situation or at one's own emotions is exercised by obtaining information or by engaging in action. Jalowiec hypothesizes that control coping works by altering stressor appraisal or by influencing choice of coping behaviors.
5. Acceptance of the situation. This is found most often in situations where there are few other options.

Other, less frequent coping strategies found through nursing research include coping by distraction, denial, information seeking, reprioritization, shifting responsibilities, lessening expectations, compromising, comparing oneself to others, careful planning, taking one day at a time, tuning in to one's own body, and self-talk (Garvin & Ryan-Wenger, 1997; Jalowiec, 1993).

Further generalizations across studies: (a) coping changes from acute to chronic stages (based on longitudinal results), (b) less desirable coping strategies are associated with negative health outcomes, and (c) coping strategies perceived by subjects as most effective are often not those they engage in most frequently (Jalowiec, 1993). Coping outcomes most frequently studied by nurse researchers include recovery after illness or surgery, physiological indices, knowledge, distress level, adjustment, and quality of life or life satisfaction (Jalowiec).

Jalowiec's (1993) extensive review also indicated that approximately two thirds of the designs to study coping were descriptive and correlational, and one fifth were qualitative. Over 90% were cross-sectional. Frequency of longitudinal designs has increased throughout the past decade (Garvin & Ryan-Wenger, 1997). Most studies employ self-report instruments as methods. Instruments most used are the Jalowiec Coping Scale, the Ways of Coping Checklist, and Billings and Moos's Coping Scale. Tools most often used to measure family coping include instruments by McCubbin, Damrosch, and Hymovich (Jalowiec, 1993). Use of interviews in qualitative studies is increasing. Numerous nurse researchers are engaged in research regarding coping.

In summary, coping is the topic of extensive efforts in nursing research. Nurses study coping behaviors more frequently than coping styles and often employ the theoretical definition of coping by Lazarus and Folkman (1984). Five major ways of coping by patients and family members include optimism, social support, spiritual resources, control, and acceptance. Nurse researchers studying coping have most often used self-report methods and cross-sectional descriptive and correlational designs, although the number of longitudinal studies has increased over the past decade.

JOAN STEHLE WERNER

See also
   SELF-EFFICACY
   SOCIAL SUPPORT
   STRESS

COST ANALYSIS OF NURSING CARE

Cost analysis of nursing care reflects a body of administrative studies that focus on the determination of nursing costs to deliver care to aggregates or individual clients in a variety of settings, employing a variety of practice models and analysis tools.

Evolution of the Concept

Much of the history of research in the cost analysis of nursing care has been in efforts to "cost out" nursing services for the purpose of measuring productivity, comparing costs of various nursing delivery models, charging individual patients for true nursing costs, and relating nursing costs to other cost models, most notably Diagnosis Related Group (DRG) categories. Many studies were conducted to explain nursing costs in relation to proprietary acuity systems. The need and motivation for these costing efforts have evolved with the economic underpinnings of the health care system, as have the methodologies and setting focus. For example, most studies in the 1980s were performed in acute care hospitals.

Today, cost analysis of nursing care focuses on justifying the cost-effectiveness of professional practice models, evaluating redesign efforts, and monitoring and controlling nursing costs within an ever tightening, cost-conscious health care environment. Within the context of rising capitation penetration, cost analysis is essential to accurate capitation bidding and financial viability of the parent organization. As "best practices" benchmarking pushes the envelope of competitive bidding, demonstrating cost-effective nursing practice becomes essential to securing managed care contracts. Studies that look at nursing costs for episodes of illness across the continuum of care are needed. The concept of cost also must expand to include human as well as fiscal costs for amount and quality of care provided.

Relevance to Nursing

Cost analysis research is a type of nursing administrative research that concentrates on evaluating financial aspects of the delivery of nursing care. More recently, this type of research has been performed in a multidisciplinary fashion under the rubric of health services administration research.

Cost analysis studies always have been relevant to decision making by nursing administrators in selecting delivery models and justifying budgets, but such studies may become central to the survival of the entire profession in the future. As cross-trained, unlicensed assistive personnel (UAPs) proliferate, nurse administrators must struggle to prove the cost-effectiveness of professional nursing practice. Larger questions of appropriate skill mix cannot be determined solely on the basis of cost per hour of service, cost per case, or cost per DRG. New studies are needed that will combine traditional cost analysis with differential outcome analysis to secure a larger picture of the true cost-benefit ratio for specific nursing models.

Major Studies

The most notable characteristic of cost analysis studies is the variety of definitions, variables, and measurement tools used in the studies. Eckhart

(1993) performed a comprehensive review of 73 published studies focusing on costing-out nursing. These studies began in the early 1980s and extended through works published in 1990.

Because of the impact of DRGs, length of stay (LOS) was a consistent variable. Length of stay was found to correlate highly to nursing work performed whether measured by acuity indexes, nursing care hours, nursing costs, patient charges, or percentage ratio of nursing costs to hospital costs. These studies focused on inpatient settings, so little is known about cost analysis of nursing in the nonacute settings that are the emerging focus of health care. Not all DRG categories have been studied, and there has been little validity or reliability reported on the instruments used to measure related variables. Definitions critical to this area of study must be standardized. For example, decisions on whether direct and indirect costs include salary and benefits have been inconsistent. Which nursing staff are included in direct care calculations? What support services are included in indirect care calculation? What role should overhead and depreciation costs of nursing-related resources play?

Another major area of dispute is the lack of a standard measurement of acuity because of the proprietary nature of most acuity systems. One study (Phillips, Castorr, Prescott, & Soeken, 1992) compared Grace-Reynolds Application and Study of PETO (a tradename product for GRASP) and Medicus acuity systems to the Patient Intensity for Nursing Index (PINI). PINI significantly correlated with both systems ($p < .0001$), but the shared variability was only 44% and 49%, respectively. Shared variability between GRASP and Medicus was only 34, and it was concluded that the two acuity systems do not measure nursing resource use in the same way. Neither system was predictive of the PINI items "knowledge deficit, emotional status, severity of illness, or potential for injury." Such PINI items as hours of care, task or procedure complexity, and mobility were significant predictors of both Medicus and GRASP scores (Phillips et al., 1992). These findings seemed to indicate that task aspects of professional practice are measured by these systems, but interpersonal and observational aspects may not be fully appreciated. This work was confirmed by Cockerill, Pallas, Bolley, and Pink

(1993), whose study compared case costs for patients across six acuity systems. "When different workload measurement tools are applied to the same patients, clinical and statistical differences are witnessed in estimated hours of care" (p. 348). These variances in costs were up to 30%. It is impossible to distinguish between true differences in case costs and measurement error across institutions in these circumstances. Therefore, estimates of nursing costs based on acuity system will vary. More study is needed to normalize acuity systems before cross-institutional data will be meaningful.

Another fertile area for cost analysis is to evaluate cost differences among professional practice models. However, most of these studies use proprietary practice models that are difficult to duplicate in other settings. Additionally, some of these studies employ variables not traditionally associated with cost studies, such as self-management and shared governance models rather than or in addition to skill-mix delivery system models. New variables are identified in these studies that do influence nursing costs, such as nursing turnover, ratio of productive to nonproductive hours, and nursing satisfaction. Russo and Landcaster (1995) evaluated unlicensed assistive personnel models relative to cost-effectiveness, quality patient outcomes, and customer satisfaction. More complex issues emerge for this type of analysis. Relative productivity across discipline levels, recruitment, training, turnover, and impact on quality must be added to the equation.

Future Directions

Given the advent of capitation, cost analysis of nursing services will have to take new directions. As critical pathways (benchmark performance tools) evolve as care guides, the costs of pathway changes for nursing delivery, patient outcomes, and case costs must be calculated. What are the most efficient and effective pathways toward resolution of a given health problem? What practice setting is appropriate for patients at each step of the pathway? For example, when is it safe to transfer a fresh open-heart surgery patient from critical care to a stepdown environment? (Earliest transfer to a least costly delivery mode saves money.) These calculations may be critical for institutions to secure managed care contracts in a cost-competitive environment. Determining what activities can be safely eliminated from a pathway without negatively affecting care outcomes will have cost and resource savings as we move to "best demonstrated practices." Determining the costs and benefits for parallel nursing treatment options could similarly affect the state of nursing science.

Finally, we must move toward a cost-benefit analysis model that incorporates the outcomes of practice. This aspect has been especially elusive, given the "generic" and group nature of nursing practice. With multiple nursing providers each having its impact on a patient's care, how do we separate the relative contributions of each person or each subspecialty of nursing practice that a patient may experience in the course of care from contributions of other disciplines?

MARY L. FISHER

See also
BENCHMARKING IN HEALTH CARE
CAPITATION
HEALTH SYSTEMS DELIVERY
NURSING PRACTICE MODELS
NURSING WORKLOAD
    MEASUREMENT SYSTEMS

CRITICAL CARE NURSING

History

In the history of nursing the development of the specialty of critical care is fairly recent, paralleling the growth and development of intensive care units (ICUs) in the 1960s and 1970s. The first ICUs were areas in the hospital designated for the care of patients recovering from anesthesia who required close monitoring during a period of physiological instability. Recognition of the efficiency and effectiveness gained from segregating any patients who required intensive nursing care for a short period of time was spurred by experiences in managing

groups of critically ill patients, such as those injured in the Boston Coconut Grove fire of 1942 and victims of the polio epidemics of the 1950s. The development of the mechanical ventilator and advances in coronary care led to recognition of the need for specialized skills and knowledge bases among nurses caring for these patients.

The first specialty organization was formed by nurses in coronary care. As electrocardiographic monitoring became a routine tool in the care of many patients and critical care broadened to include the care of patients other than postanesthesia and those with cardiac disease, the American Association of Critical-Care Nurses (AACN), originally named the American Association of Cardiovascular Nurses, was formed in 1969 (Lynbaugh & Fairman, 1992). This was rapidly followed by the development of continuing education programs, formal recommendations for critical care curricular content in undergraduate programs, and a certification program. By 1992, AACN membership had grown to over 75,000 nurses (Rudy & Grenvik, 1992). The organization has had a major role in encouraging research through its own small grants program, through joint funding initiatives with corporations, and through its two research-oriented journals, *Heart and Lung* and *American Journal of Critical Care*.

Research Trends

From the outset, critical care has been a research-intensive discipline, both in medicine and in nursing. The initial narrow focus on maintaining physiological stability of the cardiopulmonary system undoubtedly contributed to the early commitment to research-based practice. Phenomena of interest can be described as falling into five broad areas: (a) the critical care environment, (b) critical care nurses, (c) monitoring techniques, (d) interventions, and (e) outcomes of critical care.

Environment. Interest in studying the environment of critical care began with observation of postcardiotomy delirium in open heart surgery patients in the 1960s. Efforts to describe this phenomenon and identify causative factors soon broadened to include all forms of delirium and disorientation, grouped under the heading "ICU psychosis." This syndrome is a transient psychotic state characterized by confusion, visual and auditory hallucinations, and sometimes paranoid ideation. It is thought to be related to a variety of physiological, psychological, and environmental factors.

Most research in this area has been descriptive and correlational in nature. Although the reported incidence of ICU psychosis has decreased over the years, there have been no controlled studies that have confirmed or precisely explained the interaction among dependent and independent environmental variables. Characteristics of the ICU environment that have been consistently implicated in studies and have been the target of changes in environment and care routines include sleep deprivation, social isolation, and multiple sources of unusual sensory stimulation, such as lighting and noise (Noble, 1982).

Critical Care Nurses. During the first decade of critical care development, there was considerable interest in studying the practitioners of this new specialty. In general, research projects were aimed at describing characteristics of nurses who chose this area of practice, comparing them with non-ICU nurses. In addition to looking for demographic differences, there was particular interest in the effects of working in the ICU environment on stress levels and the effects of stress, such as burnout and rapid turnover. Although there was some initial evidence that ICU nurses might be subject to increasing levels of situational stress, results over time became more equivocal, and interest in this line of inquiry has lessened.

Monitoring Techniques. Physiological monitoring has been the hallmark of critical care since its inception. Until the recent emphasis on reducing the cost of expensive services, the most common reason for ICU admission was either for frequent and close physical assessment by nurses or for monitoring of some physiological parameter that required specialized technology not available on the general hospital ward, such as electrocardiography or intracranial pressure monitoring. It is understandable, then, that studies of monitoring techniques have been so prevalent. In a review of critical care practice research conducted in the decade 1979 to 1988 (VanCott, Tittle, Moody, & Wilson, 1991),

the most common content areas were the effect of patient position on hemodynamic parameters (11%), cardiac output measurement (6%), and coagulation studies (5%).

Intervention. Interventional studies have become more frequent in the recent past. The majority of these studies have focused either on psychosocial interventions, such as teaching, communication techniques, or family support, or on specific nursing procedures, such as suctioning or chest tube drainage procedures. Like much of nursing research, most of the intervention studies have been limited by small sample sizes. In the review mentioned above, the average sample size was 41 (VanCott et al., 1991). In addition, these studies have typically used investigator-designed instruments, making comparisons across studies difficult, although the use of standardized acuity rating systems, such as APACHE or TISS, to describe study populations and control for acuity have become more common.

One very promising approach to the problem of small sample sizes is the AACN research program of large, multisite studies coordinated by an AACN research team. These investigations, termed "Thunder Projects," have enabled researchers to conduct large, tightly controlled studies of nursing problems specific to critical care. For example, the most recently completed project was a comparison of the effectiveness of heparinized versus nonheparinized flush solutions for maintaining patency of arterial catheters. This study, which supported the practice of heparinizing flush solutions, had a sample of 5,024 subjects (AACN, 1993). The current Thunder Project is examining comfort measures used with common critical care procedures.

Outcome Research. As is occurring in other disciplines, there has been a recent trend toward emphasizing outcomes research in critical care focused particularly on use of quality management tools such as critical pathways; new systems of care, such as case management; and alternative environments of care, such as special care units and observation units. It has been estimated that critical care accounts for 15% to 20% of total hospital costs (Berenson, 1984; Rudy & Grenvik, 1992). There is no question that the high cost of critical care in the context of a national commitment to reducing health care spending will continue to make testing of more cost-effective approaches to care a research priority.

Future Research Directions

Critical care research is expected to continue to concentrate in the areas of monitoring techniques, specific procedural interventions, and outcomes research. AACN's research priorities for the 1990s include ventilator weaning procedures, hemodynamic monitoring techniques, measurement of tissue oxygenation, and nutritional support modalities (Lindquist et al., 1993). Because the organization is so influential in supporting and directing research, their priorities probably accurately predict the major trends in research in this specialty.

In addition to the need for more multisite studies in order to generate adequate sample sizes, there continues to be a need for the development of valid and reliable instruments that can measure outcomes, other than physiological parameters, that are sensitive to nursing interventions. In addition, many of the previously reported intervention studies should be replicated and tested with varying populations.

BARBARA DALY

See also
CARDIOVASCULAR NURSING
ENDOTRACHEAL SUCTIONING
HEMODYNAMIC MONITORING
NURSING OCCUPATIONAL INJURY
  AND STRESS
PHYSIOLOGICAL MONITORING

CULTURAL/TRANSCULTURAL FOCUS

A cultural/transcultural focus is the study of the human-made environment shared by a group seeking meaning for its existence. Nurse investigators pursue this focus for current and potential problems relevant to nursing and health care. The scientific basis for culturally aware, appropriate, sensitive, competent, or congruent nursing care is growing

but is still deficient. The impact of available cultural research on patient care has been limited, as the topic receives only cursory emphasis in most curricula or practice settings, and relatively few educators and clinicians are cultural experts. In light of population projections that racial and ethnic minorities will be the majority in the United States by 2030 and abundant evidence that their health needs are not being met, more and better nursing research on culture is urgently needed.

Several perspectives on cultural/transcultural research (C/TCR) exist. To some, the terms are essentially synonymous and questions of disciplinary origin are unimportant. From an anthropological perspective, research on one culture is intracultural or a case study, research that contrasts cultures is cross-cultural, and research that looks for concepts that transcend cultures is transcultural. Leininger (1995) regards *cross-cultural* as a term from anthropology that insufficiently captures nursing concerns. She considers *transcultural* a better reflection of a formal, worldwide area of study and practice about culture and caring within nursing.

C/TCR is found in a great variety of nursing and nonnursing research and clinical journals. The *Annual Review of Nursing Research* has published critical reviews of cross-cultural nursing and of research on Native American and Hispanic health. Searchers are cautioned that (a) the names of racial or ethnic groups are often used only as descriptive labels, and findings do not advance true cultural knowledge; (b) race, culture, and ethnicity lack consensual definitions and are often used interchangeably; (c) acceptable names for groups change over time, place, or population (e.g., Negro, Black, Afro-American, African American); (d) data bases on special populations are often nonexistent or inadequate; and (e) findings ascribed to culture are often not distinguished from the effects of socioeconomic status, history, or political structures.

Frequently used frameworks include Leininger's (1995) culture care theory, self-care, health belief models, stress and coping, feminist theory, self-efficacy, and transitions. Critical evaluations of the appropriateness of these existing frameworks, particularly self-care and health belief models, for non-White or non-Western cultures are needed and are emerging. With the rise of the constructivist paradigm, research using illness representations, explanatory models, and theory-generating approaches is increasing. A concern about some work in the grounded theory and phenomenological traditions is naïveté about the barriers to frank cross-cultural communication, regardless of efforts to assess the quality of the data. Frequently used strategies for data collection include focus groups, ethnography and miniethnography, participant observation, personal and telephone interviews, and questionnaires.

The overwhelming majority of C/TCR has been intracultural, descriptive, small scale, and nonprogrammatic. The typical methodology is an interview or questionnaire study on health beliefs and practices or scores on a concept (like social support or self-efficacy) of one designated group. Single studies conducted by one nurse using small convenience samples are the norm. Multidisciplinary C/TCR has been rare outside of larger funded studies.

Examples of programmatic C/TCR include studies of health concepts and service utilization among Hispanic immigrants (also longitudinal), diabetes among Hispanics, AIDS-related testing and counseling for Latina and Asian women, and health needs of Middle Eastern women. Immigrants and refugees have received considerable programmatic attention. Studied groups include Greek, Polish, and illegal Irish immigrants; Cuban and Haitian immigrants, Afghan refugees and immigrants; and Cambodian and Thai women. Several comprehensive reviews of research issues with refugees have been published.

Community-based interventions are a relatively recent, much needed C/TCR focus. Outstanding efforts include a community and nursing collaboration to promote prenatal and postnatal care for Hawaiian, Filipino, and Japanese women, a rural community intervention for self-care of arthritis, a self-care intervention for Hispanic arthritics, and a program to empower Hispanic women to meet community health needs (McFarlane & Fehir, 1994).

Interest in measurement issues in C/TCR is burgeoning. Frequently measured concepts include acculturation (in Hispanics), depression, locus of control, self-care, self-efficacy, self-esteem, stress, and coping. Positive features include the exploration of the existence and interpretation of constructs in another culture (such as the nature of social support among Navajo women), the development of culturally appropriate instruments with community assistance, interpretation of instruments in light of cultural knowledge (such as studies of the HOME scale and the NCAST Teaching scale with American Indians), and emphasis on rigorous translation and cultural equivalence of instruments. The Health Promoting Lifestyle Profile is undergoing extensive study with Spanish-speaking samples and with persons of lower socioeconomic status.

A literature on methodology also has emerged. Becker and colleagues (Becker et al., 1992) have provided recommendations for health behavior research in diverse populations. Nurses have described research access to and acceptance by African Americans and Native Americans. Several investigators have agreed that therapists and clients or researchers and participants need not be matched on ethnicity or gender. Meleis (1996) has proposed that C/TCR be planned and evaluated using the criteria of contextuality, relevance, communication styles, awareness of identity and power differentials, disclosure, reciprocation, empowerment, and time.

Needs in C/TCR include more emphasis on cross-cultural and transcultural research than on intracultural research, more multidisciplinary and programmatic research, and progression from descriptive to intervention studies. Interventions should be designed with community involvement to assess the felt needs of communities and enable them to meet their own health needs. Studies of cultures not defined by race or ethnicity, such as rural and occupational cultures, are needed. Studies of cultural perspectives on ethics are urgently needed, as Western and biomedical ethics are certainly not a cultural universal. Folk and alternative healing practices and their possible combination with biomedical approaches should be studied systematically and sensitively; federal funding for such studies is now available. Studies of cultural adaptations of care in the home setting and the development of brief, rapid strategies for cultural assessment are necessary to ensure that culture is considered in the era of managed care, case management, and ever briefer inpatient stays. Finally, more interdisciplinary and collaborative research on culture is needed.

There are at least two major barriers to the advancement of C/TCR in nursing. First, the short funding cycle of most grantors is ill-suited to the demands of C/TCR, particularly if community partnerships and interventions are desired. Second, the full potential of C/TCR findings will not be realized until nursing students are better educated about the influence of culture on nursing care and health outcomes. A recent monograph by the American Academy of Nursing (1995) provides an excellent summary of the status of cultural knowledge in American nursing and guidelines for its desired future.

SHAROL F. JACOBSON

See also
**HEALTH OF AFRICAN AMERICANS
IMMIGRANT WOMEN
LEININGER'S TRANSCULTURAL
    NURSING MODEL
MINORITY POPULATIONS: ASIAN
    AMERICANS
MINORITY POPULATIONS: HISPANIC
NATIVE AMERICAN HEALTH**

CUMULATIVE INDEX TO NURSING AND ALLIED HEALTH LITERATURE

In the late 1940s, although *Index Medicus* existed for the biomedical literature, there was no index to the few nursing journals published at the time. Individual librarians took it upon themselves at their particular hospital or school of nursing to index the journals they received for their own population, a tremendous "duplication of effort and expenditure" as well as "waste on a national scale" (Grandbois, 1964, p. 676). One such librarian in Los Angeles, Ella Crandall, used 3 × 5 index cards to meet the needs of nurses on the staff of White Memorial Hospital and later, Los Angeles County Hospital. This index, which began as an internal project, was published as *The Cumulative Index to Nursing Literature* in 1961, a cumulation of indexing covering the period 1956 to 1960. Seventeen journals were included in this publication—from the *American Journal of Nursing* and *Nursing Re-*

search to the *American Association of Industrial Nurses Journal*. The "red books," as this publication became known, were well received in the nursing community (Raisig, 1964) and became a familiar part of nursing education throughout the United States.

Over the next three decades and more the *Index* grew and changed, reflecting the changes taking place in the profession itself. As would be expected, many indexing terms are similar or identical to those used in the indexing of biomedical journals. There are some important differences, and many terms added to the thesaurus demonstrate the development and growth of the nursing profession, both as a practice and as a science. The thesaurus is composed of a hierarchical tree structure that is used to index the most specific focus of the material. Broad categories include "Anatomy," "Diseases," and "Health Care," among others. An example of this hierarchy would be

Social Control
  Human Rights
    Patient Rights
      Treatment Refusal

An article specifically concerning a patient who was unwilling to accept care would be indexed with the most specific term—"Treatment Refusal." A more general article might be indexed using the "Patient Rights" term. Increased emphasis on nursing research, specialty and advanced practice, and managed care has resulted in indexing terms such as phenomenology, survival analysis, family nurse practitioners, case management, and nursing intensity. Research terms describing design, methodology, analysis, and data collection have been added, as have the names of nursing specialties, organizations, and classification systems.

Aside from the terms used, the materials indexed are different from those in indexes of the biomedical and other literature. Books and book chapters, pamphlets and pamphlet chapters, dissertations, audiovisuals, and consumer health and patient education materials are just a few of the other types of materials indexed. Because of the difficulty in obtaining these materials they are often defined as elusive or fugitive literature.

Other changes have taken place over these years. Recognizing that the boundaries of nursing intersect with many other health care disciplines, "Allied Health" was added to the *Index* title in 1977, resulting in *The Cumulative Index to Nursing and Allied Health Literature* (CINAHL®). There are 17 such disciplines covered, including physical therapy, occupational therapy, and communicative disorders. In 1983 the CINAHL® electronic database became part of several on-line services and was released as a CD-ROM in 1989. Individual access via the Internet is available as well.

Recent years have seen the development of CINAHL-created documents as part of the database. These include research instrument descriptions, clinical innovations, accreditation materials, and legal case descriptions. The database can no longer be viewed as only a bibliographical database, although that continues to be its primary function.

Throughout the nearly 40 years of its existence, the primary goal of the organization has been to connect nursing—and later allied health—professionals with materials written about and for them. The basic premise underlying the existence of the *Index* is that effective and knowledgeable practice depends on access to materials describing or studying that practice. These materials may be present in a variety of formats and from a variety of sources. Whereas indexing began with fewer than 10 journals, the current journal list includes more than 1,000 titles. Content other than that listed above includes practice guidelines, practice acts, standards of practice, critical pathways, and even full text of some journal articles. This is far too much material for any individual to subscribe to or otherwise acquire randomly, making an index essential (Pravikoff, 1993). "Increased emphasis on professionalization of nursing and clinical competence" (p. 33), changes in health care delivery, and ever increasing time pressures make any tool that assists in gathering information critical to practice. Searching this material on a regular basis should be a professional obligation of members of all health care disciplines for the duration of their careers.

DIANE SHEA PRAVIKOFF

See also
BIBLIOGRAPHIC RETRIEVAL SYSTEMS

BIBLIOMETRICS
NURSING STUDIES INDEX
THE ONLINE JOURNAL
   OF KNOWLEDGE SYNTHESIS
   FOR NURSING
SIGMA THETA TAU
   INTERNATIONAL NURSING
   RESEARCH CLASSIFICATION
   SYSTEM

CURRENT PROCEDURAL TERMINOLOGY-CODED SERVICES

Current procedural terminology (CPT) codes are listed in *Physicians' Current Procedural Terminology*, a manual published annually by the American Medical Association (AMA). All services or procedures that are reimbursed within the health care system are listed among the approximately 7,000 codes in the CPT manual. The codes are used universally by public (Medicare and Medicaid) and private (commercial insurance) payers as the coding system for payment purposes. They also are used by policymakers reforming the payment system and health care providers involved in system restructuring and reorganization. Within health maintenance, managed care, or other types of capitated organizations, CPT codes are used to monitor, track, categorize, and evaluate services.

Rightly or wrongly, payment denotes value in most organizations. Until they are included in the reimbursement system, nurses will never be fully valued as contributors in the business of health care or seen as mainstream providers by policymakers, insurers, or owners and managers of health care systems. Therefore, there has been an attempt by nurse researchers, policymakers, and professional associations to explore the degree to which nurses perform CPT-coded services and to examine the interrelatedness of CPT-coded services and nursing services.

Information on performance of CPT-coded services is useful when nurses want to argue successfully that they should be included as providers in the reimbursement system. If nurses can begin by demonstrating that they are providing services and procedures that are currently being reimbursed, most commonly to physicians and health care organizations, they can more easily argue for nurse reimbursement. Also, they can more easily join policymakers who make decisions on reimbursement.

One of the first surveys of registered nurses (RNs) providing CPT-coded services or procedures was published in the *American Journal of Nursing* (*AJN*) (Griffith, Thomas, & Griffith, 1991). A total of 4,869 RNs returned the questionnaire and in addition voluntarily contacted the principal investigator through 150 phone calls or letters. Clearly, the topic struck a nerve among nurses. The average number of coded services performed by the respondents was 27, with a range of 0 to 60. Considering the large number of codes in the CPT manual, this number appears small. But the average number of codes used by the individual physician and the number accounting for the majority of costs is also relatively small. Only 107 codes comprised 56.9% of all Medicare procedures at the time of the survey (Health Care Financing Administration and Bureau of Data Management and Strategy, 1990).

Associate degree nurses (ADN) and baccalaureate-prepared nurses (BSN) performed significantly more coded services than did master's-prepared (MS) and diploma-prepared nurses. Diplomates and ADNs received significantly more MD supervision than did those with either MS or BSN degrees. Overall, the nurses reported very little MD supervision when performing the coded services. Registered nurses who had practiced fewer than 10 years performed significantly more coded services than did those practicing more than 10 years.

To build on the *AJN* survey data that described activities of generalist nurses, random sample surveys were conducted to estimate the degree to which nurses in nine nursing specialty associations were performing CPT-coded procedures and how frequently they performed them (Griffith & Robinson, 1993). The respondents included 74 school nurses, 67 enterostomal nurses, 53 family nurse practitioners (FNPs), 43 critical care nurses, 43 oncology nurses, 40 rehabilitation nurses, 39 orthopedic nurses, 34 nephrology nurses, and 25 nurse midwives. Expert panels in each specialty were used to identify codes used in the development of specialty-specific questionnaires. The number of CPT codes on the questionnaires ranged from 233 for FNPs to 58 for school nurses. The mean number of coded services performed by individual respondents ranged from 79 (FNPs) to 18 (school nurses). Individual respondents performed 0–162 codes. Supervision by physicians was infrequent. Charges to Medicare in 1988 for the coded services included in the survey were $22,793,427.34 (aggregate allowable charges).

Following these research efforts, the American Nurses Association (ANA) has joined other organizations working under the auspices of the AMA CPT editorial panel, which proposes, revises, and approves CPT codes for the manual. Since 1993 nursing has been represented on the Health Care Professional Advisory Committee (HCPAC). In collaboration with specialty nursing organizations, ANA has surveyed, proposed, and revised codes for urinary biofeedback, psychiatric services, home visits, evaluation and management services, and nursing facility visits. The focus is on providing codes that can be utilized by nurses in all clinical and advanced practice roles (K. J. Bradley, personal communication, September 5, 1997).

In 1994, the ANA, along with Nursing Organization Liaison Forum, conducted a survey of nurses and found that most were unaware of how revenue was generated in their practice setting. Advanced practice nurses represented 46.1% of the sample ($N = 104$); another 22.1% were nurse administrators or managers; multiple specialties were represented. Respondents were asked to identify coding used in their practices based on 600 CPT and 200 HCPCS (Health Care Financing Administration [HCFA] Common Procedure Coding System) codes identified by an expert panel as common to nursing practice. Respondents indicated that 99% of such codes pertained to their practice. Evaluation and management services (office visits) were the most common (Sullivan-Marx & Mullinix, 1998).

HURDIS M. GRIFFITH

See also
COMPUTER-BASED DOCUMENTATION OF PATIENT CARE
HEALTH CARE FINANCING ADMINISTRATION
MANAGED CARE

D

DATA ANALYSIS

Data analysis is a systematic method of examining data gathered for any research investigation to support conclusions or interpretations about the data. Although applicable to both qualitative and quantitative research data analysis is more often associated with quantitative research. Quantitative data analysis involves the application of logic and reasoning through the use of statistics, an applied branch of mathematics, to numeric data. Qualitative data analysis involves the application of logic and reasoning, a branch of philosophy, to nonnumeric data. Both require careful execution and are intended to give meaning to data by organizing disparate pieces of information into understandable and useful aggregates, statements, or hypotheses.

Statistical data analysis is based in probability theory and involves using a number of specific statistical tests, or measures of association between two or more variables. Each of these tests or statistics (e.g., t, F, β, χ^2, ϕ, η, etc.) has a known distribution that allows the calculation of probability levels for different values of the statistic under different assumptions—that is, the test (or null) hypothesis and the sample size, or degrees of freedom.

Specific tests are selected because they provide the most meaningful representation of the data in response to the research questions or hypotheses posed. The selection of specific tests, however, is restricted to those for which the available data meet certain required assumptions of the tests. For example, some tests are appropriate for (and assume) nominal data, others assume ordinal data, and still others assume an interval level of measurement. Although each test has its own set of mathematical assumptions about the data, all statistical tests assume random sampling.

Several statistical computer programs (e.g., SPSS, SAS, LISREL, EQS) can aid the investigator with the tedious and complex mathematical opera-tions necessary to calculate these test statistics and their sampling distributions. These programs, however, serve only to expedite calculations and ensure accuracy. Because the investigator must understand the computer programs to use them appropriately, there is a hidden danger in the ease with which one may execute such programs. For valid data analysis, the investigator must fully understand the underlying statistical procedures and the implied assumptions of these tests in order to apply them appropriately.

The logic of null hypothesis statistical data analysis is one of *modus tollens*, denying the antecedent by denying the consequent. That is, if the null hypothesis is correct, our findings cannot occur; but our findings did occur, so the null hypothesis must be false. However, Cohen (1994) and others have convincingly argued that, by making this reasoning probabilistic for null hypothesis statistical testing, we invalidate the original syllogism. Moreover, for decades scientists from different disciplines have questioned the usefulness and triviality of null hypothesis statistical testing (see Labovitz, 1970; Le-Fort, 1993; Loftus, 1993; Rozeboom, 1960; Walker, 1986, for examples from sociology, psychology, public health, and nursing). Consequently, increased attention to the factors that contribute to findings of statistical significance is warranted; and power, effect sizes (for substantive significance), sample sizes, and confidence intervals are receiving increased attention in quantitative data analysis.

In contrast to quantitative data analysis, which requires that the investigator assign a numeric code to all data prior to beginning the analyses, qualitative data analysis consists of coding words, objects, or events into coherent or meaningful categories or themes as part of the actual data analyses. Also, because qualitative data analysis involves nonnumeric data, there are no statistical probabilistic tests to apply to their coding.

Historically, qualitative data coding has been done manually, but more recently computer programs (e.g., NUDIST) have been developed to aid the investigator in this laborious effort. However, as with the computer programs for quantitative analyses, those for qualitative data analysis are merely aids for the tedious and error-prone tasks of analysis. Using them still requires that the investigator make the relevant and substantive decisions and interpretations about codes, categories, and themes.

Quantitative data analysis allows for statistical probabilistic statements to support the investigator's interpretations and conclusions. Qualitative data analysis depends more exclusively on the strength and logic of the investigator's arguments. Nonetheless, both types of data analysis ultimately rest on the strength of the original study design and the ability of the investigator to appropriately and accurately execute the analytic method selected.

LAUREN S. AARONSON

See also
CAUSAL MODELING
CONTENT ANALYSIS
FACTOR ANALYSIS
NARRATIVE ANALYSIS
STRUCTURAL EQUATION MODELING

DATA COLLECTION METHODS

Nurse researchers use a wide variety of methods for collecting data (the pieces of information used to address a research problem), and these methods vary on a number of important dimensions. One dimension involves whether the data being collected are quantitative or qualitative. Until the 1980s, nurse researchers predominantly used methods of collecting quantitative data (information in numeric form) that could be analyzed by statistical techniques. The collection of quantitative information tends to involve highly structured methods in which exactly the same information is gathered from study participants in a comparable, prespecified way. Although quantitative data collection remains the most frequently used approach, nurse researchers have shown increasing interest in collecting qualitative data (information in narrative form). Researchers collecting qualitative data tend to have a more flexible, unstructured approach to collecting information, relying on ongoing insights during data collection to guide the course of further data gathering.

Another important dimension concerns the basic mode of data collection. The most frequently used modes of data collection by nurse researchers are self-reports, observations, and biophysiological measures. The accompanying table shows examples of specific data collection methods crossed on these two dimensions.

Self-reports involve the collection of data through direct questioning of people about their opinions, characteristics, and experiences. Self-reports can be gathered orally by having an interviewer ask study participants a series of questions—in writing by having participants complete a paper-and-pencil task or, less frequently, by having participants engage in some other activity, such as sorting cards. Structured, quantitative self-report data are usually collected by means of a formal, written document or instrument that specifies exactly what questions are to be asked. The instrument is called an interview schedule when the data are collected orally and a questionnaire when the data are collected in writing. Interviews can be conducted either in person or over the telephone. Interviews and questionnaires often incorporate one or more formal scales to measure certain clinical data (e.g., fatigue) or a psychological attribute (e.g., attitudes toward nursing homes). A scale typically yields a composite measure of responses to multiple questions and is designed to assign a numeric score to respondents to place them on a continuum with respect to the attribute being measured (e.g., depression). A less frequently used method of collecting structured self-report data is referred to as a Q-sort, which involves having the participant sort cards with words or phrases on them according to some continuum (e.g., most like me–least like me).

Self-report methods are also used by researchers who are primarily interested in qualitative data. When self-report data are gathered in an unstructured way, the researcher typically does not have a specific set of questions that must be asked in a specific order or worded in a given way. Instead, the researcher starts with some general questions and allows respondents to tell their stories in a natural, conversational fashion. Methods of collecting qualitative self-report data include completely unstructured interviews (conversational discussions on a topic), focused interviews (conversations guided by a broad topic guide), focus group interviews (discussions with small groups), life histories (narrative, chronological self-disclosures about an aspect of the respondent's life experiences), and critical incidents (discussions about an event or behavior that is critical to some outcome of interest). Although most unstructured self-reports are gathered orally, a researcher can also ask respondents to maintain a written diary of their thoughts on a given topic. Projective techniques, although not always considered a form of self-report, encompass a variety of data collection methods that rely on the participant's projection of psychological traits in response to vaguely structured stimuli (e.g., a Rorschach test). Projective techniques almost always solicit qualitative data, but the data can sometimes be quantified. Self-report methods are indispensable as a means of collecting data on human beings, but they are susceptible to errors of reporting, including a variety of response biases.

The second major mode of data collection is through observation. Observational methods are techniques for collecting data through the direct observation of people's behavior, communications, characteristics, and activities, either directly through the human senses or with the aid of observational equipment such as videotape cameras. Researchers who collect qualitative observational data do so with a minimum of researcher-imposed structure and interference with those being observed. People are observed, typically in social settings, engaging in naturalistic behavior; the researcher makes notes of his or her observations in narrative form. A special type of unstructured observation is referred to as participant observation: the researcher gains entry into the social group of interest and participates to varying degrees in its functioning while gathering the observational data.

Structured observational methods dictate what the observer should observe and how to record it. In this approach the observers often use checklists to record the appearance, frequency, or duration of preselected behaviors, events, or characteristics. Alternatively, the observer may use a rating scale to measure dimensions such as the intensity of observed behavior. Observational techniques are an important alternative to self-report techniques, but judgmental errors and other biases can pose a threat to the validity and accuracy of observational data.

Data for nursing studies may also be derived from biophysiological measures, which can be classified as either in vivo measurements (those performed within or on living organisms) or in vitro measurements (those performed outside the organism's body, such as blood tests). Biophysiological measures are quantitative indicators of clinically relevant attributes; they require specialized technical instruments and equipment. Qualitative clinical data—for example, descriptions of skin pallor—are gathered not through technical instruments but rather through observations or self-reports. Biophysiological measures have the advantage of being objective, accurate, and precise and are typically not subject to many biases.

Although most nursing research involves the collection of new data through self-report, observation, or biophysiological instrumentation, some research involves the analysis of preexisting data, such as are available through written documents. Clinical records, such as hospital records, nursing charts, and so forth, constitute rich and relatively inexpensive data sources. A variety of other types of documents (e.g., letters, newspaper articles) can be used as data sources for both qualitative researchers (e.g., those conducting historical research) and quantitative ones (e.g., researchers doing a quantified content analysis).

The collection of data is often the most time-consuming and costly activity in the research process. It is also a challenging task that requires creativity, the ability to adequately match the research question with the appropriate approach, and the ability to work within budgetary constraints.

DENISE F. POLIT

See also
CONTENT ANALYSIS
DATA MANAGEMENT
PARTICIPANT OBSERVATION
PHYSIOLOGICAL MONITORING

DATA MANAGEMENT

Data management is generally defined as the procedures taken to ensure the accuracy of data, from data entry through data transformations. Although often a tedious and time-consuming process, data management is absolutely essential for good science.

The first step is data entry. Although this may occur in a variety of ways, from being scanned in to being entered manually, the crucial point is that the accuracy of the data be assessed before any manipulations are performed or statistics produced. Frequency distributions and descriptive statistics are generated. Then each variable is inspected, as appropriate, for out-of-range values, outliers, equality of groups, skewness, and missing data. Decisions must be made about dealing with each of these. Incorrect values must be replaced with correct values or assigned to the missing values category. Outliers must be investigated and dealt with. If a categorical variable is supposed to have four categories but only three have adequate numbers of subjects, one must decide about eliminating the fourth category or combining it with one of the others. If continuous variables are skewed, data transformations may be attempted or nonparametric statistics employed.

Once each variable has been inspected and corrected where necessary, new variables may be created. This might include the development of total scores for a group of items, subscores, and so forth. Each of these new variables also must be checked for outliers, skewness, and out-of-range values. The creation of some new variables may involve the use of sophisticated techniques such as factor and reliability analyses.

Prior to each statistical test, the assumptions underlying the test must be checked. If violated, alternative approaches must be sought. Careful attention to data management must underlie data analysis. It ensures the validity of the data and the appropriateness of the analyses.

BARBARA MUNRO

See also
DATA ANALYSIS

DATA COLLECTION
VALIDITY

DATA STEWARDSHIP

Data and information are the symbolic representation of the phenomena with which nursing is concerned. Data are defined as discrete entities that are objective; information is defined as data that are structured and organized and that have meaning or interpretation. Information that has been synthesized so as to identify and formalize interrelationships is referred to as knowledge. When one term represents all three types of content, it is usually *information*. From this perspective, data are viewed as the raw material on which nursing knowledge and science are developed. Data stewardship refers to the responsibility to manage, administer, attend to, and take charge of the universe of relevant nursing data.

Nursing data issues revolve around several factors. The first relates to identification of the universe of relevant nursing data. Currently, there is no consensus regarding what data elements make up a minimum nursing data set nor what data elements are required to capture nursing diagnoses, interventions, and outcomes. Systems to label or name these elements also are inconsistently defined. Next, the complex nature of nursing phenomena poses measurement difficulties. Measurement is the process of assigning numbers to objects to represent the kind or amount of a character possessed by those objects. It includes qualitative means (assigning objects to categories that are mutually exclusive and exhaustive) and quantitative measures (assigning objects to categories that represent the amount of a characteristic possessed) (Waltz, Strickland, & Lenz, 1991).

Unlike other biological sciences, few nursing phenomena can be measured by using physical instruments with signal processing or monitoring. Measurement difficulties occur because nursing consists of a multiplicity of complex variables that occur in diverse settings. If one is able to identify what significant variables should be measured, then one is challenged with the difficulty of isolating those variables to measure them. Ambiguities and abstract notions must be reduced to set up concrete behavioral indicators if measurement is to be meaningful. Measuring nursing phenomena also requires the acknowledgment of the "fuzzy" and complex nature of nursing phenomena and the richness of the meaning contained in the context of the data. Finally, the value and use of data that are not coded or numeric, such as whole text data, must be studied to understand their benefits and boundaries for representing nursing phenomena. Content analysis of nursing data and their usefulness have to be further explored (National Center for Nursing Research, 1993).

Processing data implies the transfer of data in raw form to a structured, interpreted information form. Information has characteristics of accuracy, timeliness, utility, relevance, quality, and consistency. Data stewardship suggests that attention be paid to these characteristics. For example, accuracy is of concern at the level of judgment in collecting data as well as at the level of the data collected. Quality of data and information is related to the ability and willingness of clients to disclose information as well as to the nurse's ability to observe, collect, and record it. Reliability refers to random measurement errors such as ambiguities in data interpretation. These measurement errors that affect clinically generated data can occur at the point of care delivery, the time of documentation, and when data are retrieved or abstracted for studies (Hays, Norris, Martin, & Androwich, 1994).

With the advent of automated data processing and computerized information systems, decisions about data content, control, and cost need careful consideration. The content and design decisions concern format, standardized languages, level of detail, data entry and retrieval messages, and interfaces with nonclinical data systems. A primary concern of clinicians is the amount of time invested in harvesting data and recording it. Minimum time investment, with maximum clarity and comprehensiveness of data collected and recorded, is needed. Redundancy must be eliminated. Decisions related to content of data demand stewardship to ensure privacy, confidentiality, and security, especially when data are in electronic form. Requirements for legitimate access to data must be managed to facilitate the flow of clinical data while simultane-

ously restricting inappropriate access. There is a cost associated with the use and development of automated data bases; however, accuracy, reliability, and comprehensiveness of information should not be sacrificed because of cost.

Data stewardship poses challenges and responsibilities for nurses in building knowledge bases. Standardization of terms of data is critical, and coordination and synthesis of current efforts are needed. If nurses are to be stewards of their data, then further study should focus on the following areas: (a) the definition and description of the data and information required for patent care, (b) the use of data and knowledge to deliver and manage patient care, and (c) how one acquires and delivers knowledge from and for patient care (National Center for Nursing Research, 1993).

CAROL A. ROMANO

See also
DATA COLLECTION METHODS
DATA MANAGEMENT
NURSING MINIMUM DATA SET
RELIABILITY

DECISION MAKING ABOUT END-OF-LIFE CHOICES

The American Nurses Association (1992b) has issued four position statements on nursing's role in end-of-life decisions. These statements concerned the Patient Self-Determination Act (PSDA), comfort and pain relief for dying patients, nurses' involvement in decisions to forgo artificial nutrition and hydration, and do-not-resuscitate (DNR) orders. The Patient Self-Determination Act statement addressed the nurse's responsibility to facilitate informed decision making. The statement on forgoing artificial nutrition and hydration spoke to the ability of "competent adults" to evaluate and express their values and their right to have those preferences respected; this included the individual's preferences as expressed in an advance directive. Individuals who have "never been competent" included mentally disabled and mentally ill individuals. The DNR statement indicated that nurses' concerns with

DNR orders included lack of documentation regarding how a DNR decision was made. It addressed the rights of competent as well as incompetent patients (through their surrogates). However, none of these statements addressed the nurse's role, responsibility, and participation in determining a patient's capacity to make these decisions nor in assessing the patient's understanding of the decisions made. All four statements fail to distinguish between legal competency and clinical capacity.

Nursing research on nurses' actions with regard to assessment of decisional capacity and decision making about end-of-life choices is sparse. In a review of 182 charts, Palmateer and McCartney (1985) found that nurses used the term *disoriented* to describe mental status and rarely provided a behavioral description of "confusion." Their survey of nurses revealed that less than half of nurses interviewed knew about the early changes indicative of dementia. Brady (1987) reported that nurses documented that patients were confused when they exhibited disruptive or resistive behavior. Using a small convenience sample ($N = 70$) composed of undergraduate and graduate nursing students from a university-based school of nursing, psychiatric mental health nurses, and home health nurses, Weisensee and colleagues (Weisensee, Kjervik, & Anderson, 1994) found that nurses inadequately document nursing home residents' memory deficits or ability to follow simple directions and used short-term memory loss as a sign of incompetence. They report that a national survey of schools of nursing found that most nursing students receive some age-related content but that faculty preparedness in this area is extremely variable (Solon, Kilpatrick, & Hill, 1988).

Williams and Engle (1995) found that health care professionals, overall, predominantly used orientation and verbal function as indices of competence. In their interview survey, it appeared that nurses did not use decision-making ability or comprehension of a decision's consequences as criteria in their assessment. They suggest that nurses may be using the terms *alert* and *oriented* interchangeably. In general, these studies were limited by their small sample size and by the fact that standard definitions for key terms, such as *decisional capacity*, *confusion*, and *disorientation* were not established a priori.

There are several fruitful areas for nursing research. Consistent with nursing's role in encouraging and assisting patients to make decisions about end-of-life choices, it is vitally important to learn how nurses differentiate between competence and decision-specific capacity: what cues and patterns they look for and how this affects their conclusions, actions, and plans of care. *Competence*, a legal term, is presumed unless there is evidence that, overall, an individual is unable to manage personal or financial affairs, or both. *Capacity*, a clinical term, is based on the observation or test of specific abilities: (a) to make a choice, (b) to understand the situation and its implications, (c) to manipulate information rationally, and (d) to appreciate the nature of the situation (i.e., its consequences pursuant to giving or withholding consent).

A universal view of capacity as either fully present or absent is not supported medically or legally. For medical decision making, the specific competence needed to appreciate the nature, consequences, and alternatives of treatment options is known as decision-specific capacity. An individual may be capable of making some decisions but not others. Most older people retain sufficient cognitive capability to make some, but not necessarily all, decisions. Research has shown that physicians and psychiatrists know the legal standard for competence but apply it incorrectly, thereby undermining patient autonomy (Markson, Kern, Annas, & Glantz, 1994). Nothing is known about how well nurses approximate patients' mental status and decisional capacity in comparison to their professional colleagues.

Another area of research is nurses' understanding of the purposes of mental status assessment tests. Often used as a surrogate for decision-making capacity, tests such as the Mini-Mental Status Examination (MMSE) or Short Portable Mental Status Questionnaire (SPMSQ) were not designed or validated as tests of legal competence or decisional capacity (see Mezey, Stokes, & Rauckenhurst, 1995). Low scores do not automatically imply a complete absence of decisional capacity, nor do high scores confirm its presence. As found by others, Mezey, Teresi, Mitty, Ramsey, and Goldstein (1997) demonstrated that nursing home residents with mild Alzheimer's disease/dementia retain the ability to make a treatment choice. Even some residents with extremely low MMSE scores had sufficient decisional capacity to execute a health care proxy. These are residents who are frequently denied the exercise of their right to make this kind of health care decision on the basis of mental status assessment scores. Understanding, a key aspect of capacity, can be affected by language skills and nuance, sensory deficits, illness, depression, anxiety, medication, and education. Nursing research in this area might compare patients' ability to follow simple directions for self-care with their scores on standardized mental status assessment tests.

Capacity determination should rely on a composite picture of clinical data, not the least of which should be observations of an individual's functional ability. Such observations in a clinical or domiciliary setting would include a person's orientation, behavior, memory, ability to follow simple directions, ability to communicate and state wishes, and compliance with care regimens. Appropriate assessment of an individual's ability to make end-of-life choices should prevent two types of errors: (1) preventing competent individuals from making their own decisions and (2) failing to protect incompetent individuals from the harmful effects of a poor decision. An individual with limited verbal and social skills might be incorrectly assessed as incapacitated, whereas an individual with appropriate and acceptable verbal and social skills might be assessed as capable of reaching a health care decision when they are, in fact, incapable of doing so.

Research on the validity and reliability of nursing observations might remove barriers to patients' exercise of their right to make end-of-life decisions and prevent these kinds of errors. Physicians as well as the courts rely on nursing data, and thus it is urgent to investigate nurses' operative definitions of key mental status and cognitive, affective, and behavioral descriptors within and across settings and by level of professional education. Such research also could include faculty knowledge and understanding.

Basic descriptive research is needed on nurses' understanding of end-of-life decision making, for example: What is their knowledge about how advance directives (i.e., living will and durable power of attorney for health care) facilitate autonomous decision making? What is their understanding of the differences between withholding, withdrawing, and forgoing treatments or interventions? How do nurses assess whether or not a patient understands the particular decision(s) to be made or that have been made? Nurses are instrumental in helping proxy decision makers learn more about what individuals want and do not want at the end of their lives and understand the treatment options. Yet nothing is known about nurses' roles in proxy decisions nor about how nurses interpret, document, and communicate a patient's verbal instructions. Finally, additional research is needed about nurses' experiences with and communication of the patient's interest in assistance with dying.

ETHEL L. MITTY
MATHY D. MEZEY

See also
COGNITIVE DISORDERS
**DECISION MAKING: ADVANCE
  DIRECTIVES**
DEPRESSION AMONG OLDER ADULTS
NURSING ASSESSMENT

DECISION MAKING: ADVANCE DIRECTIVES

Historically, nurses have played a crucial role in helping people and promoting patient choice. Patients and families look to ''their'' nurses for information, advice, and support when facing difficult health care decisions. This relationship offers unique privileges and responsibilities. The Code of Ethics of the American Nurses Association (ANA) states that nurses must support patient autonomy and provide care according to the patient's wishes (ANA, 1985a). A survey of nurses conducted in 1994 by the ANA found that one of the most critical ethical issues facing nurses today is the end-of-life decision (ANA, 1997). Thus, advance directives are relevant to nurses. Advance directives, living wills, and the durable power of attorney for health care are mechanisms whereby individuals are able to exercise control over their bodies and direct the kind of care they want or do not want in the event that they lack decision-making capacity at the time a medical decision must be made. They affect nursing practice and have an impact on the ethical values of society at large.

A living will is a document that provides specific instructions to health care providers about the type of health care choices and treatment an individual would or would not want in order to prolong life. An individual may execute a living will to instruct health care professionals not to administer any "extraordinary treatment," "heroic treatment," "artificial treatment," or "life support" in the event of terminal illness. However, living wills also can be used to give instructions and/or directions about the kind of medical treatment an individual wants to have administered. Although most states recognize living wills, they are not recognized by statute in New York, Massachusetts, and Michigan.

A durable power of attorney for health care is a document that permits individuals to designate another person to make health care decisions for them should they lose decision-making capacity. The person appointed to make decisions is called a health care proxy, health care agent, attorney-in-fact, or surrogate.

Patient Self Determination Act

The Patient Self Determination Act (PSDA), a federal law effective December 1991, attempted to ensure that all patients are advised about their right to accept or refuse medical or surgical treatment and their right to execute an advance directive (Omnibus Budget Reconciliation Act of 1990, 1991). The intent of the act was to encourage early, full, and ongoing communication between health care professionals, patients, and families, when appropriate, about care at the end of life. All institutions that receive Medicare and Medicaid funding must advise patients about this right, document in the medical record whether the patient has an advance directive, implement advance directive policy, and provide staff and community education about advance directives. In addition, institutions are prohibited from refusing to provide care if an individual has not completed an advance directive.

Advance directives should become effective only when it is determined that the individual is incompetent and lacks decision-making capacity. As long as the patient retains decision-making capacity for the particular decision at hand, his or her decisions govern. When the patient is deemed to lack decision-making capacity, the surrogate decision maker is authorized to make all treatment decisions on behalf of the patient in accordance with the patient's stated wishes, whether rendered in writing or given verbally. However, in situations where the patient has never been competent and/or there is no clear and convincing evidence of what the person would have wanted, the surrogate decision maker will be called on to make decisions on the basis of what he or she believes is in the "best interest" of the patient.

Research to date on nurses' actions in facilitating patients' autonomous decision making and in implementing the PSDA is sparse. Mezey, Mitty, Rappaport, and Ramsey (1997) found that nurses are central to the implementation of the PSDA. Nurses disseminate advance directive materials, are responsible for asking whether the patient has an advance directive, and are involved in PSDA education to inform patients about their rights (Fleming & Scanlon, 1994; Wetle, Walker, & Blechner, 1994). A number of studies identified reasons that patients do or do not formulate advance directives (Berrio & Levesque, 1996; Cugliari, Miller, & Sobol, 1995; Mezey, Ramsey, Mitty, & Leitman, 1995). Reasons given by patient respondents for executing an advance directive are (a) wanting to make up their own mind, (b) feeling that it would help their families if they knew what was wanted, (c) having the peace of mind it would give, and (d) not wanting to be kept alive in a coma and with "tubes and wires." Reasons given by patients for not executing an advance directive were that (a) they needed more information, (b) their family would decide what to do, (c) their doctor would do what was right, (d) they never heard about advance directives, and (e) they want everything possible done.

Nursing research is needed on how nurses meet the letter and spirit of the PSDA to support patients' rights to make decisions about their health care. This research is necessary for informed ethical nursing practice. Important issues that should be explored include but are not limited to nurses' understanding about advance directives. What are the practical clinical implications for the use of living wills and durable powers of attorney for health care? What do these documents provide for and not provide for? How does this affect on the care of patients, particularly those who are terminally ill? What is the role of the nurse vis-á-vis the patient, family, and other members of the health care team? What is the role of the nurse in advance directive education for the surrogate decision makers?

Nurses play an important role in ongoing PSDA education, and part of the education should include the surrogate decision maker. This individual is thrust into the world of medical decision making and often is not provided with the information or is unable to comprehend—at that time—all that is necessary to make an informed choice. It is important to understand better how the nurse may further support surrogate decision makers. Further research is needed to determine how nurses might better assist patients, families, and surrogate decision makers to understand the medical and nursing treatments being proposed. It is imperative that individuals understand the language used and the treatments being proposed, to ensure that individuals are able to make informed decisions. Finally, further research is needed to determine the impact of race, culture, ethnicity, and religion on medical decision making of the patient, family, and nurse.

Today there are many more discussions about decision making and advance directives. Careful thinking, open communication, and further research are essential to foster a climate that is both supportive of and conducive to medical decision making. Nurses must continue to be part of this process, and nurse-based research, by and about nurses, will further that end.

GLORIA C. RAMSEY
MATHY MEZEY

See also

DELPHI TECHNIQUE

The Delphi technique is a research method used to identify key issues, to set priorities, and to improve decision making through aggregating the judgments of a group of individuals. The technique consists of using a series of mailed questionnaires to develop consensus among the participants without face-to-face participation. It provides the opportunity for broad participation and prevents any one member of the group from unduly influencing other members' responses. Feedback is given to panel members on the responses to each of the questionnaires. Thus, panel members communicate indirectly with each other in a limited, goal-directed manner.

The first questionnaire that is mailed asks participants to respond to a broad question. The responses to this questionnaire are then used to develop a more structured questionnaire. Each successive questionnaire is built on the previous one. The second questionnaire requests participants to review the items identified in the first questionnaire and to indicate their degree of agreement or disagreement with the items, to provide a rationale for their judgments, to add items that are missing, and to rank-order the items according to their perceived priority. On return of the second questionnaire the responses are reviewed, items are clarified or added, and the mean degree of agreement and the ranking of each item are computed. In the third questionnaire, participants are asked to review the mean ranking from the second questionnaire and again to indicate their degree of agreement or disagreement and give their rationale if they disagree with the ranking. Additional questionnaires are sent until the group reaches consensus. Many variations of this procedure have been used, the number of questionnaires used ranging from three to seven.

To be eligible to participate as a panelist in a Delphi study the respondent should (a) be personally concerned about the problem being studied, (b) have relevant information to share, (c) place a high priority on completing the Delphi questionnaire on schedule, and (d) believe that the information compiled will be of value to self and others (Delbecq, Van de Ven, & Gustafsen, 1975).

Several disadvantages of the Delphi technique limit its application. First, there must be adequate time for mailing the questionnaires, their return, and their analysis. Second, participants must have a high level of ability in written communication. And third, participants must be highly motivated to complete all the questionnaires.

The Delphi technique was first developed by the Rand Corporation as a forecasting tool in the 1960s, when investigators found that results of a Delphi survey produced better predictions than round-table discussions. The technique was later used to solicit opinions of experts on atomic warfare as a means of defense. It has since been applied in diverse fields, such as industry, social services, and nursing because of its usefulness and accuracy in predicting and in prioritizing.

The Delphi technique has been used in nursing studies to identify priorities for practice and research. The American Nurses Association Center for Nursing Research (1980) used the technique to identify national research priorities for the 1980s; Demi, Meredith, and Gray (1996) used it to identify priorities for urological nursing research; Lewandowski and Kositski (1983) and Lindquist and colleagues (Linquist et al., 1993) used it to identify research priorities for critical care nursing; and Lindemann (1981) surveyed members of the American Academy of Nursing to identify and prioritize issues important to nursing in the next decade. In a creative application of the method Demi and Miles (1987) attempted to achieve consensus on the parameters of normal grief by enlisting a panel of experts in the field of grief and mourning.

ALICE S. DEMI

See also
DATA COLLECTION METHODS

DEPRESSION AMONG OLDER ADULTS

The most common mental health disorder in late life is depression. It is often manifested as a recurrent illness or as a comorbid condition occurring with chronic health disease. Among older adults living in the community, 3% have a major depression and 10% to 14% have depressive symptoms.

Depression has a wide severity and morbidity range and is conceptualized as an abnormal mood state, a pattern of symptoms, or a clinical syndrome ranging from sadness to major depression.

As a mood state, depression is a universal human condition. In general, persons of all ages who experience a lowering of mood or transient feelings of sadness claim to be depressed. Clinically, the concept of depression is used to indicate a collection of symptoms, such as sadness, reduced ability to experience pleasure, pessimism, inhibition, retardation of action, and a variety of physical complaints. Symptoms of depression have been classified into types: physical, emotional, cognitive, and motivational (Beck, 1978).

Emotional symptoms of depression include sadness, dejection, anxiety, irritability, distress, disappointment, frustration, extreme negativity, overt hostility, intense anger, and inability to derive pleasure from previously satisfying activities. Cognitive symptoms include pessimism, negative self-evaluation, expectation of failure, self-blame, learned helplessness, disturbance in thought processes, inability to concentrate, and impaired decision making. The inability to complete even simple tasks, lack of initiative to perform daily activities, procrastination, avoidance of responsibility, and psychomotor retardation or agitation are referred to as motivational disturbances. Physical symptoms of depression are loss of appetite, sleep disturbances, loss of libido, and diffuse aches and pains. Psychosomatic complaints are more dominant in older individuals than in younger persons. Older persons also have a tendency to mask sad moods. Finally, interpersonal aspects of depression are likely to include withdrawal from social activities, increased dependency, acquiescence, dysfunctional communication patterns, and proneness to interpersonal tension and conflict.

Generally, a nursing diagnosis of a major depression is made if five of the following symptoms have been present for at least 2 weeks: changes in appetite, weight loss or gain, agitation, fatigue and loss of energy, feelings of hopelessness and guilt, and suicidal ideation. Be aware that cognitive impairment symptoms may be marked in the older person with depressive illness and may be mistaken for dementia. Differentiation between dementia and depression is a critical part of the nurses' assessment.

As a clinical syndrome, depression is usually qualified by an adjective to specify a particular type or form. Clinically, forms of depression include reactive, agitated, and psychotic. In addition, depression has been classified as endogenous (due to internal processes) or exogenous (due to external factors), terms that refer specifically to etiology. Moreover, depression is called primary when not preceded by any physical or psychiatric condition and secondary when preceded by another physical or psychiatric disorder. Finally, depression has been classified as acute (less than 2 years duration) or chronic (more than 2 years).

As a clinical entity, depression comprises attributes and characteristic signs and symptoms, including a definitive type of onset, course, duration, and outcome. The *Diagnostic and Statistical Manual of Mental Disorders* (DSM IV) (American Psychiatric Association, 1994) classifies clinical depression into major, minor, and dysthymic subtypes. Major depression refers to a clinical depression that meets specific diagnostic criteria as to duration, impairment of functioning, and presence of a cluster of physiological and psychological symptoms. Minor depression includes fewer depressive symptoms than does major depression. Dysthymia consists of fewer symptoms than are expressed in major depression but more than in minor depression, and it is more chronic.

Many theories of depression have been presented through the years. The earliest discussions of depression are in the psychoanalytic literature, where depression is viewed as mourning or melancholia (Freud, 1957). According to this perspective, loss, which may be conscious or unconscious, is central to both mourning and melancholia. Mourning is qualitatively different from melancholia in that the external world becomes impoverished and empty in mourning, and the internal world, including one's ego, feels the loss in melancholia. Psychoanalysts believe that the person experiences ambivalent feelings toward the lost object, which results from high dependency needs. Because the expression of dependency needs has the potential for destroying relationships with others, feelings of dependency, frustration, and hostility are repressed.

When the loss of the loved object occurs, negative feelings of anger and hostility are unleashed against oneself.

Peplau's interpersonal theory in nursing describes depression as a painful experience occurring as a way of managing anxiety when an individual's self-esteem is threatened. The energy of anxiety is displayed as anger turned inward toward the self, and the individual experiences feelings of overwhelming guilt, hopelessness, and suicidal ideation. Thus, depression can be a life-threatening illness and a serious concern for health care providers for older adults because of the potential for suicide.

Behavioral theories of depression emphasize social learning and environmental responses or stimuli that cause or maintain feelings of sadness. For learning theorists, the concept of reduction in reinforcement is central. Reinforcement is defined by the quality of one's interactions with the environment so that, when one is faced with a loss, behaviors previously reinforced by the lost object or person decrease. This theory is relative for elderly persons, who suffer a multitude of losses in their later years. Depression therefore is attributed to a reduction in activity due to a decrease in positive reinforcement that comes from significant others. Feelings of depression are elicited when a behavior receives little or no reinforcement. In addition, lower levels of behavioral activity result in a further reduction of positive reinforcement from the environment. Therefore, both activities and rewards decrease. Behavior theorists believe that changing a person's behavior directly through positive social interactions is the best way of reducing depressive symptoms.

The self-control model of depression is a behavioral perspective from which people are viewed as capable of exercising control over their behavior (Rehm, 1997): they do not merely react to external influences but exert control over the environment. This theory of depression includes cognitive aspects because depressed persons are believed to have deficits in self-monitoring (reflected in pessimism and hopelessness), self-evaluation (reflected in low self-esteem), and self-reinforcement (reflected in excessive self-punishment and negative self-statements).

Cognitive theories of depression postulate that depressive symptoms are experienced because of disturbances in thinking that lead to false beliefs and ideas. Cognitive and behavioral theories of depression are sometimes closely related, especially when thought processes are instrumental in self-reinforcing and self-evaluating activities. The original learned helplessness theory of depression postulated that the belief that one has no control over outcomes in one's life is the basis for depression (Seligman, 1975).

The attributional theory is similar to Beck's cognitive theory of depression, which proposes that depression is primarily a result of the tendency to view the self, the future, and the world in an unrealistically negative manner. This distorted, negative view of self, world, and future has been referred to as the "negative cognitive triad" (Beck, 1978). According to this theory, depressed persons regard themselves as unworthy, incapable, and undesirable; they expect failure, rejection, and dissatisfaction and perceive most experiences as confirming these negative expectations. The major symptoms of depression (affective, behavioral, somatic, and motivational) are viewed as direct consequences of this negative cognitive set.

Most recently, biochemical theories of depression have emerged and attained credibility. Electrolyte disturbances, including increases in intracellular sodium and decreases in intracellular potassium, have been reported to occur with depression. In addition, neurophysiological alterations have been identified through electrophysiological studies of evoked potential and electroencephalography, demonstrating increased right hemisphere activity and decreased left hemisphere activity in the brain of depressed persons. Hormonal or neuroendocrine factors also have been related to depression, including decreases in estrogen, hypothyroidism, and hyperadrenalism. Finally, the neurochemical changes in the neurotransmitters, especially in the biogenic amines that act as central nervous system and peripheral neurotransmitters, have been documented in cases of depression. The biogenic amines, including catecholamines (dopamine, norepinephrine, and epinephrine), serotonin, and acetylcholine, have been hypothesized to be causally related to depression.

Specific biochemical theories have been proposed. The catecholamine hypothesis states that some, if not all, depressions are associated with an absolute or relative deficiency of catecholamines, particularly norepinephrine, at functionally important receptor sites in the brain. A competing explanation for the etiology of depression lies in the serotonin hypothesis, which specifies that there is a deficiency in serotonin in persons with depression. Empirical evidence of deficits in either norepinephrine or serotonin or both has provided an important rationale for the usefulness of antidepressant medications that are specifically designed to increase the concentration of norepinephrine, serotonin, or both, in the brain.

However, the precise etiology of depression remains unknown; that is, no single theoretical explanation is sufficient from a holistic nursing perspective. In fact, there is mounting evidence that there is probably multiple causation, including genetic, biochemical, and psychosocial factors that contribute to one's vulnerability to depression. Evidence for this model of depression lies in the success of multimodal treatment approaches for depression that may include antidepressant medication, psychotherapy, diet therapy, light therapy, and electroconvulsive therapy.

Depression severely affects quality of life in older persons because of the nature of the symptoms, which can lead to total inability of the individual to care for self and to relate to others. There is a potential for persons with depression to negatively affect family members and others around them. Not surprisingly, only 2% to 4% of elders in the community seek mental health services. Most depressed elders are seen by general practitioners for psychosomatic complaints. Part of the symptomatology of depression is a focus on physical problems and requires the practitioners to carefully assess for depressive symptoms. Suicide is a factor in the depressed older adult. The suicidal rate for individuals aged 80 and over is twice that of the general population and is particularly high in older White males. Interestingly, most suicidal elders had recently visited a general practitioner prior to their suicidal act. Direct assessment of suicidal potential should be a routine part of any assessment of dementia in elders.

Although depression follows a finite course and will eventually dissipate unless the person commits suicide, the life of the individual can be particularly miserable. For some time there was reluctance on the part of psychiatric practitioners to treat depression aggressively in older adults. This attitude was partially based on Freud's notion that individuals could not benefit from psychotherapy after age 50. However, we have learned that older adults will respond favorably to antidepressant medications and the psychotherapies. Electroconvulsive therapy, once disregarded because of the crude method of application, is now seen more favorably as a mode of treatment for depressed older adults who do not respond to medications. Due to modern technology electroconvulsion therapy is believed to be a safe and effective treatment for depression in older adults when other therapies fail. Additional therapies that are found to be useful by nurses are life review, guided imagery, and family and group therapy.

Research in depression among older adults has been ignored in the past and is a neglected area, where much more nursing research is needed. It is critical that nurses assume a leadership role in disseminating information about the outcomes of a variety of treatments that can be used for depression in later life. There is a particular need to examine suicide in late life and to develop better assessment instruments for the purpose of detecting sources of suicide ideation in elders.

MAY L. WYKLE
JACLENE A. ZAUSZNIEWSKI

See also
ATTRIBUTIONAL THEORY
COGNITIVE DISORDERS
PEPLAU'S THEORETICAL MODEL
SUICIDE

DEPRESSION AND CARDIAC DISEASE

Studies using randomized experimental designs, large sample sizes, and advanced statistical analyses have documented a rate of approximately 15%–18% severe depression following a myocardial infarction (MI) (Ahern et al., 1990; Frasure-Smith, Lesperance, & Talajic, 1993). Depression is related to mortality, morbidity, and other psychosocial factors after an MI.

Relationship of Depression to Mortality

Severe depression is an independent predictor of mortality. Frasure-Smith et al. (1993) assessed 222 patients hospitalized post-MI, using the DSM-III-R psychiatric diagnosis of major depression (American Psychiatric Association, 1994). Sixteen percent of persons with an acute MI met the criteria for major depression. By 6 months, 17% of the 12 patients who later died were severely depressed.

In the Cardiac Arrhythmia Pilot Study of patients with significant ventricular arrhythmias (recorded 6–60 days after an MI), depression was a significant predictor of mortality or cardiac arrest within 1 year. The relationship of depression to mortality was significant even after controlling for history of prior MI, ejection fraction, beta-blocker or digitalis use, presence of transmural infarcts, and presence of runs of premature ventricular complexes on the 24-hour electrocardiogram at baseline (Ahern et al., 1990). The most frequent causes of death in severely depressed patients post-MI are reinfarction, arrthythmias, and congestive heart failure (Frasure-Smith et al., 1993). There has been a long-standing impression that symptoms of depression are common in patients with coronary artery disease.

Relationship of Other Psychosocial Factors to Depression

A history of major depression has been consistently reported as being established before the onset of acute MI in 44%–56% of the patients who are depressed post-MI (Freedland, Carney, Lustman, Rich, & Jaffe, 1992). Other studies have found that nearly 66% of patients with MI have some psychosocial distress, other than depression, primarily anxiety (Hackett, 1985). Although not completely studied, hypothetically, the psychosocial prognosis for severely depressed cardiac patients is poor, resulting in decreased quality of life, poorer social and physical functional status, perceived loss of energy, less likelihood to return to work, lack of initiative to perform optimal activities of daily living, and less likelihood of cardiovascular risk factor modification of health behaviors (Conn, Taylor, & Wiman, 1991). The mechanism by which depression causes mortality and poorer clinical outcomes in cardiac patients is unknown; however, it may alter motivation for healthy behavioral modification (i.e., smoking cessation, exercise) and adherence to medication (Carney, Freedland, Rich, & Jaffe, 1995).

Biological Indices Related to Depression and Cardiac Disease

Plasma norepinephrine concentrations are increased in patients with severe depression (de Villiers et al., 1987). The evidence of increased norepinephrine concentrations suggests a potential mechanism for the effects of depression on mortality and ventricular arrhythmias in cardiac patients as an altered autonomic nervous system, resulting in increased sympathetic activity (Carney et al., 1995).

Heart rate variability, an index of the autonomic nervous system balance, can further describe altered autonomic function and mortality in cardiac patients. Kleiger et al. (1987) reported that low heart rate variability increased the risk of death by a factor of 5.3 in 850 persons followed for 31 months after an MI. Lombardi et al. (1987) reported increased sympathetic and decreased parasympathetic activity, as measured by heart rate variability, immediately after an MI. The heart rate variability "normalized" in most people within 6 months after the MI.

Sudden cardiac arrest survivors have low heart rate variability, specifically suggestive of a loss of parasympathetic activity (Cowan, Kogan, Burr, Hendershot, & Buchanan, 1991). Not many studies have investigated heart rate variability in cardiac patients with severe depression.

Cortisol is increased in 40%–60% of depressed patients. The hypothalamic-pituitary-adrenal (HPA) axis, along with the noradrenergic system, are two of the most studied biological systems in relation to depression; both may coexist dysfunctionally in depressed patients (de Villiers et al., 1987). Arousal of the HPA axis, as manifested by increased cortisol secretion and resistance of plasma cortisol to suppression after dexamethasone administration, is common in major depressive disorders. Among depressed patients, norepinephrine measurements were significantly positively related to cortisol measurements in relation to dexamethasone administration (i.e., with the cortisol nonsuppressors).

Not many studies have reported on cortisol and norepinephrine levels in severely depressed cardiac patients. However, increased concentrations of cortisol have been found to occur within 72 hours of symptoms of acute MI. The magnitude of the cortisol response was positively correlated with infarct size as calculated by total creatinine kinase MB fraction enzyme release ($p < .0001$), and very high levels were predictive of mortality ($p < .05$) (Bain et al., 1992).

The serotonergic system has a role in the disturbed behaviors of depression, such as mood, sleep, sexual activity, and appetite (Meltzer, 1990). The brain concentration of serotonin (5-HT) is lowered in depressed subjects, and decreasing trytophan, the precursor of 5-HT, can induce severe depression in recovering depressed persons. Also, postmortem studies of suicide victims have indicated that brain 5-HT or its metabolite, 5-hydroxyindoleacetic acid (5-HIAA), is reduced. The most common measurement of serotonergic activity in depressed patients is the basal concentration of 5-HIAA in cerebrospinal fluid. Platelets have been used as a measurement of serotonergic mechanisms in severe depression because the processes of 5-HT uptake and binding sites in platelets are comparable to those in brain 5-HT sites (Meltzer, 1990). Plasma serotonin can potentially augment coronary vasospasm in coronary arteries with endothelial injury and/or augment intracoronary thrombosis contributing to an MI.

In summary, severe depression after acute MI is a predictor of mortality within 1 year. The most frequent causes of deaths are recurrent MIs, arrhythmias, and congestive heart failure. Severe depession is related to increased catecholamines, cortisol, and decreased serotonin.

MARIE J. COWAN

See also
DEPRESSION AMONG OLDER ADULTS

PSYCHOSOCIAL INTERVENTIONS
  DECREASE MORTALITY AFTER
  CORONARY ARTERY DISEASE
QUALITY OF LIFE
RISK FACTORS

DESCRIPTIVE RESEARCH

The *Oxford English Dictionary* defines research as "a search or investigation undertaken to discover facts and reach new conclusions by the critical study of a subject or by a course of scientific inquiry." *Descriptive* is defined as consisting of or concerned with a portrayal in words or detailed graphic account of observable things or qualities, without influence of one's feelings or values (Brown, 1993a). Descriptive research encompasses a broad range of research activity in nursing and has comprised the majority of nursing studies. Early research efforts were focused on descriptive epidemiological studies. Nightingale's pioneering work is a well-known example of this type of research. Well schooled in mathematics and statistics, Nightingale created elaborate charts demonstrating morbidity and mortality trends of soldiers during and after the Crimean War. Her detailed record keeping and graphic representation of these data convinced officials of the need to improve sanitary conditions for soldiers, which drastically reduced mortality rates (Cohen, 1984).

Historical Context

The progress in descriptive research activity in nursing has been influenced by several events and movements over the past several decades: advanced degree education in nursing, philosophical debate about the role of nursing and nursing research in the scientific community, establishment of centers for nursing research, and the formation of an agenda for knowledge development in nursing.

With the help of federal traineeship money, the earliest doctorally prepared nurses obtained degrees in basic science programs. The adoption and rejection of the logical positivist view of science helped clarify linkages between philosophy, theory, and method. At one extreme, nurse scientists and theorists argued that the future of nursing knowledge development lay in empirical studies that allowed for repeated observational statements under a variety of conditions. It was believed that one ultimate truth could be found after repeated objective observations, which would eventually lead to discovery of universal laws.

Critics of the logical empiricist approach argued that truth is influenced by history, context, and a chosen methodology and is constantly in a state of flux. What is humanly unobservable one day may be observable with the help of technological innovation another day. Ultimately, facts and knowledge are not static or theory-neutral (Poole & Jones, 1996). Although logical positivism is no longer espoused in nursing theory and science, its role was crucial in initiating dialogue about what nursing knowledge is and how research in nursing should be advanced. These dialogues have helped swing the pendulum from valuing experimental research as the gold standard in nursing to recognizing the important role of descriptive and exploratory research.

Knowledge Development in Nursing

Over the years, nursing leaders have struggled to establish which approach to knowledge development is appropriate and necessary for nursing. Dickoff, James, and Wiedenbach's (1968) four levels of theory for nursing included the most basic type, factor-isolating theory, as the product of descriptive studies, with higher level theories built on the necessary base of this first level of theory. Stevenson (1990) depicted a stepwise conceptualization of research in nursing, with exploratory research at the bottom and utilization in practice at the top. Descriptive research was thought to build on exploratory research findings and to provide a foundation of support for intervention studies, with the ultimate goal of utilizing research findings in practice. Reynolds, Timmerman, Anderson, and Stevenson (1992) encouraged nurse researchers to employ meta-analysis techniques to descriptive research. Meta-analysis is a useful statistical tool that synthesizes extant nursing research, but it has largely been applied only to experimental studies. Application of this technique to descriptive studies can help determine when a phenomenon is ready for testing with intervention studies.

Descriptive studies often are used when little research has been done in an area, to clarify and define new concepts or phenomena, to increase understanding of a phenomenon from another experiential perspective, or to obtain a fresh perspective on a well-researched topic. Also, the formulation and testing of measurement tools (e.g., to measure depression, anxiety, or quality of life) employ descriptive research techniques. The development and refinement of these tools will continue, with increasing emphasis on outcomes research as nurses are required to demonstrate how their interventions make a difference for their patients.

Types of Descriptive Research

Public and private funding of nursing research has allowed for an expansion of nursing knowledge based in research. Of the many studies funded by National Institute of Nursing Research, Sigma Theta Tau, and private foundations, descriptive research continues to command a large portion of research dollars. Descriptive research can employ quantitative or qualitative (including naturalistic) methodologies. Quantitative descriptive methodologies include surveys, measurement tools, chart or record reviews, physiological measurements, meta-analyses, and secondary data analyses. Qualitative descriptive methodologies include interviews, focus groups, content analyses, reviews of literature, observational studies, case studies, life histories, grounded theory studies, concept analyses, ethnographic studies, and phenomenological studies. Many qualitative methodologies employ exploratory as well as descriptive techniques.

Of 519 listings in CINAHL for 1996 under "descriptive research," the methodologies used included 252 surveys or measurement tools; 88 interviews, content analysis, or focus groups; 4 grounded theory studies; 19 observation studies; 4 ethnographies; 1 case study; 5 phenomenological inquiries; 2 secondary data analyses; 9 reviews of literature; 50 chart reviews; and 97 physiological

measurements (some studies used more than one methodology; 28 were not classified or were not research studies). Additional naturalistic and phenomenological studies were accessed separately under those index headings. Thus, a large portion of descriptive research involves the use of surveys or measurement tools, physiological measurements, and interviews. Other naturalistic or qualitative methodologies (e.g., ethnography, grounded theory, phenomenology) have become more available to nurse researchers in the recent past and continue to add to the descriptive research knowledge base in nursing.

Future Trends

Many nursing organizations and associations have delineated priorities for a nursing research agenda that include clarifying philosophical underpinnings of holism, research on care and caring, health promotion, disease prevention and wellness, development of knowledge about the family and social support networks, and research on minority groups and culturally different views of health and illness (Stevenson, 1988). Adding to nursing's knowledge base in these areas will require using descriptive research along with other research methodologies and incorporating the results of these studies into nursing practice and research endeavors.

ANITA J. TARZIAN
MARLENE ZICHI COHEN

See also
EXPLORATORY STUDIES
QUALITATIVE RESEARCH
QUANTITATIVE RESEARCH

DIABETES MELLITUS

Diabetes mellitus is one of the most common chronic illnesses in the United States, with an estimated 16 million individuals who have diagnosed or undiagnosed diabetes, the majority having noninsulin-dependent diabetes (NIDDM). The total direct and indirect costs of diabetes are approximately $92 billion per year. Diabetes is responsible for about 400,000 deaths annually and was the seventh leading cause of death by disease in 1995. Diabetes is a leading cause of cardiovascular disease, stroke, hypertension, blindness, kidney disease, nerve disease, amputations, dental disease, and complications of pregnancy. Furthermore, these complications disproportionately affect minority populations for as yet unknown reasons. Several of the objectives of *Healthy People 2000* (U.S. Department of Health and Human Services, 1990) reflect the need to correct the substantial morbidity and mortality from this disease by vigorous case finding and management.

The recently released findings of the Diabetes Control and Complications Trial (DCCT) demonstrate the importance of nursing care for reducing the mortality and morbidity associated with diabetes (DCCT Research Group, 1993). The DCCT compared intensive with conventional diabetes therapy to determine the effects on the development and progression of early vascular and neurological complications of insulin-dependent diabetes (IDDM). In a cohort without retinopathy, the risk for developing retinopathy decreased 76% with intensive therapy, and in a secondary prevention cohort, the progression of retinopathy was slowed by 54%. Microalbuminuria was reduced by 39%, albuminuria by 54%, and clinical neuropathy by 60%. Although intensive therapy was associated with severe hypoglycemia and clinically significant weight gain, there were no differences between those in the intensive treatment group and those in the conventional group in mean total scores on a quality of life measure. On the basis of these findings, the researchers and the American Diabetes Association recommend *intensive treatment* for the care of patients with IDDM. Because nurses often are responsible for follow-up care of intensively treated patients, these recommendations point to the need for ongoing nursing research in diabetes care.

The majority (90%) of individuals with the NIDDM are obese; therefore, increases in rates of obesity and sedentary lifestyle will contribute to an increase in rates of NIDDM, as will the aging of the population and increased availability of screening to more groups. Increased age is associated

with more obesity, and increased screening will find more latent cases. There has been a burgeoning of research in NIDDM, particularly in pharmacological treatment and exercise-diet interventions. Furthermore, because the relationship between poor glycemic control and diabetes complications appears to be the same for IDDM and NIDDM, the findings of the DCCT are being applied to management of NIDDM. The translation of these research findings to practice provides numerous opportunities for nursing research.

Traditionally, nursing has had a significant, key role in the multidisciplinary care and education of patients with diabetes. Management of diabetes requires that people with the disease significantly modify their lifestyle to adjust to a demanding treatment regimen. Long-term outcomes of avoiding or minimizing complications may be dependent on a complex series of interactions between biomedical and behavioral factors. Nursing research on the care of patients with diabetes has focused on four areas: descriptive studies dealing with *psychosocial adjustment* to diabetes; biobehavioral studies focusing on the relationship of various psychosocial parameters with metabolic control in diabetes; studies of the physiology of diabetes and its complications; and studies of diabetes care in the delivery of health care.

Studies of psychosocial adjustment to diabetes focus on either children and adolescents or adults. Dr. Margaret Grey's program of research examined the incidence of poorer adjustment in young children and the process of adjustment over time in children newly diagnosed with IDDM (Grey, Cameron, Lipman, & Thurber, 1995). Her work complements the work of other disciplines demonstrating that diabetes in childhood is associated with an increased risk of psychosocial difficulties. Similar work has been accomplished in adults, as summarized recently by Pollock (1993), who found in a number of studies that psychosocial functioning is associated with health-related hardiness and engagement in health promotion activities. Clearly, these problems are multifactoral and as such need a complex, multivariate approach.

Dr. Grey also has examined the impact of adjustment on *metabolic control* in children. Findings demonstrated that poorer psychosocial adjustment was associated with poorer metabolic control in both younger children and adolescents and that this relationship varied by the type of coping behaviors used by the children. Similar work has been accomplished by researchers in other fields studying adults with both type I and type II. Dr. Gail D'Eramo Melkus studied health care practices of African American women with NIDDM. The majority of studies examining these relationships used small samples obtained from one clinical site, examined simple bivariate relationships, and were not part of an overall theoretical approach to a program of research.

There are studies of the physiology of diabetes and its complications. Diabetes is a disease of relative or absolute lack of insulin secretion, which causes significant complications. Dr. Donna Hathaway at the University of Tennessee is the major nurse researcher whose program of research specifically deals with physiological aspects of diabetes care. She has been examining the relationship of quality of life to metabolic and physiological outcomes in patients with diabetes, and her work has focused on autonomic function and quality of life in adult kidney and pancreas-kidney transplant patients (Hathaway et al., 1993).

Finally, there are studies of diabetes care in health care delivery. Nurses have long been accepted as part of the diabetes care team, primarily as educators about diabetes. Dr. Sharon Brown conducted a number of meta-analyses of the diabetes education literature, concluding that patient teaching has positive outcomes in adults with diabetes. More recent work focused on the potential for interventions to affect knowledge as well as psychosocial adjustment and metabolic control (Brown & Hedges, 1994). Work on the impact of education on metabolic control in patients with NIDDM demonstrated that only minimal weight loss is necessary to improve metabolic control (D'Eramo-Melkus, Wylie-Rosett, & Hagan, 1992). Dr. Brown's most recent work on culturally sensitive management furthers the applicability of more general approaches to African American women with diabetes and the work of advanced practice nursing in caring for patients with diabetes. There have been few studies of the impact of other nursing interventions on patient outcomes specific to diabetes although there are several such studies currently in progress evaluating the impact of interventions such as coping skills training and culturally specific educational programs.

Some progress has been made in understanding these related and complex issues in the managements of patients with diabetes. A review of the chronic illness literature in pediatric nursing concluded that conceptually based interventions should be developed and appropriate outcomes measured. This conclusion is equally true of the literature on diabetes. The majority of the literature is descriptive and limited in scope to small clinical samples. Much research in diabetes is atheoretical, limiting the ability to develop theory and to apply findings across settings. There is much to be accomplished in studying diabetes care.

MARGARET GREY

See also
CHRONIC ILLNESS
CULTURAL/TRANSCULTURAL FOCUS
OBESITY AS A CARDIOVASCULAR
    RISK FACTOR
WEIGHT MANAGEMENT

DISASTER NURSING

Background

The dictionary defines disaster as ''a calamitous event, especially one occurring suddenly and causing great loss of life, damage, or hardship, as a flood, airplane crash, or business failure'' (*Webster's American Dictionary*, 1997). Disasters occur naturally, caused by forces of nature such as floods, hurricanes, and earthquakes, or they are nonnatural and man-made, such as war and the Oklahoma City bombing. Disasters are usually multistressor events that require a wide range of responses on the part of all emergency workers and health care providers. Disaster nursing comprises a part of the total response required to handle a disaster situation.

Disaster nursing requires individuals to respond to event, occupational, and emotional stressors

TABLE 1   Examples of Major Data Collection Methods for Nursing Research

General Method	Quantitative Approaches	Qualitative Approaches
Self-reports—oral	Structured in-person interview Structured telephone interview	Unstructured in-person interview Focused interview Focus group interview Life histories Critical incidents interview
Self-reports—written	Structured questionnaire Self-report scales (e.g., Likert, semantic differential, visual analog scale) Structured daily diary	Unstructured daily diary
Self-reports—other	Q-sort	Projective techniques
Observation	Observational checklists Observational scales	Participant observation Unstructured nonparticipant observation
Biophysiological	In vivo quantitative measures (e.g., blood pressure readings) In vitro quantitative measures (e.g., bacterial counts)	
Written documents	Clinical and other quantitative records Existing documents for quantified content analysis	Existing documents (e.g., letters, essays, newspaper articles)

while at the same time creating organization out of chaos, treating the injured, and determining the resources available. Often, nurses and other emergency personnel are at risk of personal injury themselves because of their efforts. Particularly in the case of natural disasters, they also may be victims (Stuhlmiller, 1994). Disasters are critical incidents that demand exceptional skills from the health care responders. Prior preparation for disaster situations is imperative. Successful management of a disaster event is predicated on the prior strategic planning for such events and the implementation of primary prevention by disaster workers—primarily, nurses and physicians (Bissell, Becker, & Burkle, 1996).

The immediate consequence of experiencing a disaster is psychological distress, which can include symptoms of dissociation, anxiety, and avoidance behavior, and experiencing reminders of the trauma. Research demonstrates that individuals who experience a major disaster will continue to experience many stressful changes, related to both the damage from the disaster and the intrapsychic

consequences of coping with the disaster in the following months (Koopman, Classen, & Spiegel, 1997). A disaster's effects reach beyond the immediate victims and include the victims' families and communities and the disaster workers.

Much of the initial research conducted with respect to disasters began with physicians' observations of war, the oldest nonnatural disaster. "Nostalgia" was a term used by Civil War physicians to describe soldiers' symptoms of generalized weakness, heart palpitations, and chest pain. Physicians studying the early wars of this century noted a clustering of trauma-related symptoms. In World War II they used such terms as "shell shock," "battle fatigue," and "war neuroses" to describe these symptoms. From these observations systematic research concerning disasters began (Fullerton & Ursano, 1997). The current body of knowledge regarding disasters and their effects is rooted in studies focusing on the emotional, psychological, and psychiatric implications, especially posttraumatic stress disorder, that surround a variety of modern-day disasters such as the Vietnam and Gulf wars; the Sioux City, Iowa, plane crash; Hurricanes Hugo and Andrew; and floods in the Midwest.

Nursing Care

Six percent to 7% of the U.S. population is affected annually by disasters. Disasters and trauma are costly events that affect the psychological and physical health and well-being of individuals (Fullerton & Ursano, 1997). Disaster nursing entails dealing with the immediate triage of victims, treatment of life-threatening trauma, and the care required in the weeks and months following such events. One of the tasks of nurses and other health care providers is to implement primary prevention by informing individuals about expected stressors, educating them about the importance of sleep and rest, and providing victims with the skills necessary to help them gain a sense of control over their situation (Ursano & Fullerton, 1997). People who are traumatized by a disaster may react in a variety of ways in their attempt to cope with the enormity of what has happened. Some may cry, others may become hysterical, still others are quiet, and some are almost catatonic, with a blank affect. Shock, denial, and disbelief, as well as acute symptoms of posttraumatic stress disorder, are commonplace in disasters. Some individuals may handle the immediate ordeal, then collapse later (Davis, 1996; Steefel, 1993).

Disaster nursing takes place wherever the disaster occurs, and this prehospital care requires considerable improvisation and flexibility. Research has demonstrated that both theoretical and practical experience, as well as prior planning for disaster scenarios, are critical to effective coordination and management of a disaster. Nurses who have had more emergency experience are better prepared to deal with sudden and unexpected events. They tend to approach such situations more systematically in assessing and comprehending what has happened, what needs to be done, and the extent of the injuries. Such nurses express confidence in knowing what to do and see themselves as capable of coping with the situation. Disasters can be described as "load and go" or "stay and play" (Suserud & Haljamae,

1997). Load-and-go situations require minimal interventions and rapid transport to trauma centers or hospitals in the immediate vicinity of the disaster. Stay-and-play disasters usually occur in areas removed from immediate access to trauma centers and hospitals. These kinds of disasters require triage, basic life support activities, retriage, and on-site treatment of the injured.

Although having nurses skilled in emergency lifesaving interventions in unusual and unexpected situations is an unstated requirement of disaster nursing, there are several risks to rescue workers themselves that must be considered. Rescue workers are exposed to event, occupational, and organizational stressors. The stressors unique to rescue workers, including nurses, are the perceptions surrounding role functioning, organizational conflicts, the impact of memories of previous rescues, and the greater exposure to death and mutilation (Stuhlmiller, 1994). Because of exposure to these stressors, nurses are vulnerable to psychological distress unless they are well prepared to function in a disaster situation, are debriefed within 24 hours of the experience, and understand that primary prevention is as important for them as for the victims of the disaster. Much further research must be conducted regarding the nurse's individual meanings of participation in disaster situations and the coping mechanisms and resources utilized by nurses that enable them to do their work (Stuhlmiller).

REGINA C. AUNE

See also
COPING
JOB STRESS
**NURSING OCCUPATIONAL INJURY
  AND STRESS**

DISCOURSE ANALYSIS

Discourse analysis is a method that has multiple meanings referring to a wide range of analytical procedures. Such methodological diversity has resulted not only from various philosophical traditions that treat discourse differently but also from conceptualization of discourse analysis by diverse disciplines that emphasize different aspects or meanings of discourse. Discourse is viewed as an appropriate subject matter for research by various disciplines, including linguistics, philosophy, anthropology, sociology, psychology, information science, literary criticism, journalism, and practice disciplines such as nursing and medicine.

Although the term *discourse* in relation to discourse analysis is defined and used differently in linguistics and in other disciplines, discourse refers to language-in-use as connected speech or written texts produced in social contexts, rather than in terms of single sentences considered in terms of grammar and syntax. Discourse analysis deals with texts of conversations and written texts produced among individuals, as well as those produced within larger social, historical environments such as journal articles or newspaper accounts, that are not directed to specific individuals as their audiences. Discourse as the object of analysis is usually obtained from natural occurrences rather than from constructions designed solely for the purpose of analysis as either exemplary or ideal cases. This orientation to natural texts as the focus of discourse analysis is a shift from the pioneering work of Harris (1952) in linguistics.

The term *discourse* in discourse analysis is commonly accepted as a mass noun with the above definition. However, the use of "a discourse" or "discourses" can often be found in discourse analysis with the poststructural, critical perspective, as in M. Foucault's work (1972). But the current literature abounds with both usages of the term (i.e., "discourse" and "a discourse"), not necessarily used consistently within one specific perspective.

Discourse analysis has its historic origin in the ancient Greek differentiation of grammar and rhetoric in language use (van Dijk, 1985). Although the study of rhetoric was differentiated from the study of grammar in linguistics throughout the centuries, it was not until the middle of the 20th century that a more formal approach to discourse analysis gained its appeal in linguistics. Hence, "pragmatics" in linguistics emphasizing discourse analysis has been separately developed, in contrast to the study of language proper that focuses on formal grammatical, syntactical, and morphological struc-

tures. Following this modern revisit in linguistics, many other disciplines have begun to take discourse as the proper subject of their scientific study. Although there are cross-disciplinary discussions of the methodology and application of various approaches of discourse analysis, there is no unified, integrated approach to discourse analysis. The literature across the disciplines suggests that there are at least three general perspectives within discourse analysis: (a) the linguistic perspective, (b) the conversation perspective, and (c) the ideology/critical perspective.

Linguistic Perspective

The linguistic perspective takes discourse as text produced by language use in either speech or writing. Thus, discourse text for this perspective can be from interpersonal conversations, written texts, or speech expositions such as testimonies. This perspective encompasses the formal pragmatics in linguistics, sociolinguistics in sociology, and ethnography of communication and ethnopoetics in anthropology. Hence, within this perspective there are several different methodological approaches to discourse analysis. Even within each orientation there are variations in the ways discourse texts are analyzed, depending on the frame within which various contextual features are brought into the analytic schema.

The formal pragmatics that had its beginning with Harris (1952) has been recast by speech act theory in the philosophical tradition of Searle (Searle, Kiefer, & Bierwisch, 1980) and Austin (1975) and also by poetics of the literary study. Discourse analysis from the formal pragmatics orientation addresses such aspects as speech competence with respect to discursive rules, text grammar, discourse comprehension, or discourse organization.

Sociolinguistics as a branch of sociology is a study of language use within the functional paradigm of sociology, which views social life in relation to larger social structures such as gender, status, social class, role, and ethnicity. Sociolinguists are concerned with ways in which people use different linguistic forms according to macrostructural and contextual differences.

Anthropological approaches in the linguistic perspective are ethnopoetics and ethnography of communication. Ethnopoetics is the study of oral discourse as speech art in the tradition of literary analysis and is concerned with the structures of verbal aesthetics. The focus is on the poetic patterning of discourse within different cultures. On the other hand, ethnography of communication, advanced by Hymes (1964), is concerned with general language use as practiced in specific sociocultural context. Ethnography of communication, done either from the cross-cultural, comparative orientation or from the single-culture orientation, is based on the assumption that discourse should be studied, positing it within the dynamics and patterns of discourse events in a given cultural context. In all these branches of the linguistic perspective, the emphasis is on the linguistic forms as used in social life.

Conversation Perspective

The conversation perspective takes discourse as conversational texts; it has been developed from the ethnomethodological tradition of Garfinkel in sociology. In this tradition, Sacks (1967) and others pioneered conversation analysis as a form of discourse analysis. Conversation analysis views discourse as a stream of sequentially organized discursive components that are designed jointly by participants of conversation applying a set of social and conversational rules. Conversation analysis studies rules that participants in conversation use to carry on and accomplish interaction, such as topic organization, turn taking, and use of response tokens. In recent years, however, conversation analysis has extended to include behavioral aspects of interaction (e.g., gesture, gaze, and laughter) as its analytical components. The use of transcripts and transcription symbols has been extensively developed in this perspective.

Ideological/Critical Perspective

Discourse analysis in the ideological/critical perspective differs from that in the other two perspectives in its emphasis on the nature of discourse as historically constructed and constrained idea and knowledge. Discourse in this perspective is not considered in terms of linguistic form or interactive patterning. Rather, discourse is not only what is said or written but also the discursive conditions that produce imagined forms of life in given local, historical, and sociocultural junctures and thus is embedded in and with power and ideology.

This perspective was represented by poststructuralists such as Foucault (1972) and Lyotard (1984), who viewed discourse analysis not simply as an analytical process but as a critique and intervention against marginalization and repression of other forms of knowledge and discursive possibilities. Foucault (1972) treats discourses in relation to rules tied to specific historical conditions of usage and as power relations. Hence, discourse analysis in this perspective is oriented to revealing sociohistorical functions and power relations embedded in statements of talks and texts as well as what Foucault called "systemic archives," of which statements form a part.

The foregoing discussion indicates that discourse analysis is not a unified approach to studying language use. Although three perspectives are identified for this method, there is a blurring of differences among the perspectives. The method, however, remains multidiscipline-oriented. In nursing, discourse analysis is being applied with all three perspectives. Discourse analysis with the linguistic perspective has been applied to study discourse comprehension in client-nurse interactions or discourse organization of nurses' notes and to analyze various discourses on such topics as abortion, individualized care, and professionalism in the nursing literature related to macrostructural or contextual factors.

On the other hand, discourse analysis with the conversation perspective has been applied to the study of turn taking and topic organization in client-nurse interactions and to examine the dynamics of home visiting. Within the ideological/critical perspective, discourse analysis has been applied to examine nursing documentation as a form of power relations, to analyze discourse of nursing diagnosis in the nursing literature, and to explicate the language of sexuality, menopause, and abortion as power relations and ideology. Written texts produced by clients and nurses and client-nurse conversations, as well as texts in the public domain, are the rich sources for applying discourse analysis to study the language-in-use from these perspectives.

HESOOK SUZIE KIM

See also
ETHNOGRAPHY
NURSE-PATIENT INTERACTION

DOCTORAL EDUCATION

Doctoral education in nursing includes two general types of programs offering three different types of degrees. One type of doctoral program offers the first (entry-level) professional degree in nursing. The second is an advanced degree (postbasic) program that leads to either the academic, research-oriented doctorate (the doctor of philosophy degree [PhD]) or the professional, also termed clinical or applied doctorate (the doctor of nursing science or doctor of science in nursing degree). Designed to be analogous to doctor of medicine programs, entry-level doctoral programs in nursing typically admit students who have earned baccalaureate or higher degrees in other disciplines and offer the doctor of nursing (ND) degree after approximately 4 years of full-time study. This type of doctoral program not only prepares students for entry into the practice of generalized nursing but also provides many of the bases for future leadership in the profession. It does not, however, provide advanced practice specialty preparation. The first entry-level doctoral program in nursing was established at Case Western Reserve University in 1979.

Currently, over 65 institutions offer advanced-degree doctoral programs in nursing, and more are being planned. Over three fourths of existing programs offer the academic doctorate, the purpose of which is to prepare graduates for a lifetime of scholarship and research. In recent years the trend has been toward offering the PhD degree, undoubtedly due in part to the universal recognition, acceptance, and prestige that this degree enjoys nationally and internationally. In fact, a number of institutions have recently shifted from offering the professional doctorate in nursing to offering the academic doctorate.

Curricula for programs leading to the academic doctorate typically contain a core of required courses addressing nursing theory, metatheory, and theory development strategies and various aspects of research methodology and statistics. Additionally, students usually are required to develop expertise in a specialized area of nursing knowledge and research by selecting courses in nursing and related disciplines (cognates), becoming involved in hands-on research-related experiences such as practical and research assistantships, and by conducting a major independent research project and writing the dissertation. Half or more of the credits focus on research methodology. On the average, full-time students complete doctoral study in 4 years: 2 years to complete the course work and an additional 2 years to complete the dissertation.

The professional doctorate (DNS, DNSc, DSN) is offered by programs that, at least theoretically, emphasize advanced clinical, administrative, or policy-related practice and leadership. These programs are focused on applied rather than basic research and on applying and testing new knowledge in practice. In actuality, when the curricula of the two types of advanced-degree doctoral programs have been compared, there were few differences; most reflected a research orientation that is typical of academic doctorates. Despite the current trend toward the PhD, the need exists for professional-degree doctoral programs that are different from those offering the academic doctorate. Skilled clinical leaders and administrative innovators are needed to improve practice, provide policy-making leadership, and guide the discipline through the monumental changes occurring in health care.

Curricula for such programs would include core courses in nursing theory, issues, research methodology, and statistics; courses and practicum experience designed to develop a high level of expertise in a specialized area of nursing practice; and a major research project and dissertation. The research project often is applied in nature, for example, a study designed to evaluate an innovative intervention or program. Graduates would be prepared to assume positions as clinical researchers, clinical administrators, clinical faculty (often with joint academic and clinical appointments), collaborative practitioners or designers of innovative roles, such as being responsible for measuring and improving outcomes in clinical settings.

Historically, doctoral nursing education began at Teachers College, Columbia University, and at New York University in the 1920s. After a 30-year hiatus during which no new programs were opened, interest in doctoral education was rekindled; and by the end of the 1970s, a total of 18 programs had been initiated. During the 1980s the number of programs more than doubled, and with the rapid increase in programs and enrollments came concern about maintaining high quality. The American Association of Colleges of Nursing took a leadership role in developing indicators of quality regarding student and faculty qualifications, curriculum content, administrative patterns, and support resources to assure that doctoral nursing programs would adhere to the same standards as those in established disciplines.

The 1990s has been an era of refining the discipline's ideas about the nature of scholarship and of doctoral education and fine-tuning of doctoral programs. Emphasis on defining, establishing, and maintaining quality has continued. In addition, considerable attention has been paid to the substantive foci of doctoral nursing programs, that is, the substance of what is being taught and learned and the specialty areas in which students are being prepared to develop knowledge or guide practice. The latter differ from program to program, with a particular school's strengths, particularly the expertise of its faculty, reflected in the specialties it offers at the doctoral level. There is movement away from a disproportionate focus on process to greater emphasis on the content that constitutes the input to and products of the scientific process.

During recent years there also has been increased attention to assuring that doctoral curricula include experiences that prepare graduates for the roles they will assume following graduation. For example, the requirement exists in some programs that students who aspire to academic positions take a teaching assistantship or a teaching practicum. There has also been a trend toward combining programs to allow more streamlining and efficiency, either between levels (e.g., combined master's and doctoral programs in nursing) or within a given level but between disciplines (e.g., combination of a doctoral nursing program with a master's program in another field, such as public health or business administration).

A number of patterns and trends that represent departures from earlier patterns can be said to characterize doctoral nursing education during the last quarter of the 1990s. The first has been a tendency for the total enrollment in and graduations from doctoral programs in the United States to remain relatively stable. A second trend, the continuing and growing tendency for doctoral students to enroll part-time, leads to concern that there will not be sufficient numbers of nurse scientists and educators to meet the discipline's future needs. A third trend is the increasing tendency for students to enter doctoral study from clinical, in addition to academic, backgrounds. Finally, an important trend has been the rapid growth in the numbers of doctoral nursing programs in institutions outside the United States. A concomitant interest has arisen in international collaboration to deliver high-quality doctoral education.

For individuals, the doctorate is the pinnacle of attainment in nursing education, and for institutions it is the pinnacle of academic attainment. The virtually universal acceptance of the doctorate as the terminal degree signifies nursing's status as a true academic discipline.

ELIZABETH R. LENZ

See also
AMERICAN ASSOCIATION OF COLLEGES OF NURSING EDUCATION: NURSE RESEARCHERS AND ADVANCED PRACTICE NURSES NURSING EDUCATION

DRUG ABUSE

Drug abuse is a subcategory of psychiatric illnesses known as substance-related disorders according to the DSM-IV (American Psychiatric Association [APA], 1994) and categorized by the specific drug used. Drugs of abuse include alcohol, amphetamines, caffeine, cannabis (marijuana), cocaine, hallucinogens, inhalants, nicotine, opioids, phencyclidine (PCP), sedatives, hypnotics, and anxiolytics (antianxiety agents). Abuse or addiction to several substances, including alcohol, is common.

According to the DSM-IV, there are two categories of substance-related disorders: abuse and dependence. Substance abuse is diagnosed when a pattern of hazardous or maladaptive use continues in spite of serious health, social, economic, or psychological consequences but symptoms do not meet the criteria for substance dependence. Substance dependence meets the criteria for substance abuse but is a more severe form of the disorder and is characterized by increasing dosages and frequency of dosages, tolerance, and the manifestation of withdrawal symptoms when the amount of substance is reduced or stopped.

Alcohol is the most widely used and abused drug in this country; its abuse and dependence are reported elsewhere in this text. Nursing research with other drugs of abuse and dependence are reported here.

Drugs of abuse also may be categorized as legal or illegal according to cultural and societal determinations. The use of some drugs is legal in America but illegal elsewhere (e.g., alcohol in Saudi Arabia) and vice versa (e.g., peyote in South America). Designating a drug as illegal makes its use criminal and results in devastating consequences to individual users, their families, communities, and even innocent bystanders.

Some categories of drugs that have medicinal uses (e.g., opioids, sedative-hypnotics) are controlled by the Drug Enforcement Agency, and their dispensation is restricted to licensed pharmacists, physicians, and registered nurses. Use of other drugs, such as heroin, is illegal regardless of how they are used. Furthermore, legal drugs may be used illicitly. For example, prescription drugs may be misused by their intended client or sold for misuse by others.

Nursing research has been slow to recognize the serious health and social problems of drug abuse and dependence. Although sparse, early studies primarily addressed alcohol problems; but when drug abuse was studied, the focus was on nurses' attitudes toward drug abusers, the incidence of drug addiction among nurses, or characteristics of nurses addicted to drugs. Studies addressing nursing care of the drug-abusing client were virtually nonexistent until recently, when some empirical intervention studies have appeared in the literature (Barton, 1991; Lindenberg, Gendrop, Nencioli, & Adames, 1994; Nyamathi, 1991; Zauszniewski, 1995).

Recognizing the need for information about alcohol and drug abuse and dependence, the federal government initiated two programs to meet that need. First, curriculum model grants were offered by the National Institute on Drug Abuse (NIDA), the National Institute on Alcohol Abuse and Alcoholism (NIAAA), and the Office of Substance Abuse Prevention (now known as the Center for Substance Abuse Prevention). Three model projects are complete and available for nursing schools. Second, the three agencies offered training grants for faculty selected from a variety of specialty clinical areas in schools of nursing to acquire expertise in substance abuse disorders. More than 60 faculty from 13 schools of nursing have been prepared through these grants, and some are now funded by NIDA or NIAAA to conduct research in drug abuse, although results of this work are not yet available in the literature.

Drug abuse and dependence are serious health and social problems in this country. Nurses have the potential to intervene with substance-abusing clients and improve outcomes, but research is needed to determine appropriate and effective nursing interventions. The health and well-being of clients, their families, and their communities depend on improved care in substance abuse nursing.

ELEANOR J. SULLIVAN

See also
ADOLESCENCE
ALCOHOLISM
HIV/AIDS: CARE AND TREATMENT
HOMELESS HEALTH
VIOLENCE AS A NURSING AREA
    OF INQUIRY

DYSPNEA

Definition

Dyspnea is the subjective sensation of difficult breathing. The origin of the word is the Greek *dys*, "abnormal or disordered," and *pnoia*, "breathing." Today it is a term used by clinicians to represent the subjective phenomena, with "shortness of breath" more often used to represent objective phenomena. The language used by patients regarding dyspnea has been factored into 19 descriptors (Simon et al., 1990), including such characteristics as "my breath does not go in all the way," "my breathing requires effort," "my chest feels tight," "I feel I am suffocating," "I feel that my breathing is rapid," and "I can't get enough air." Patients with a similar pathology are likely to use similar descriptors more often. For example, those with asthma tend to use the word *tight*. Healthy subjects also reliably report clusters of dyspnea descriptors.

Significance

Dyspnea is the most common reason for an emergency department visit by patients with asthma, chronic obstructive pulmonary disease (COPD), and heart failure. It also is associated with mortality and delayed weaning from mechanical ventilation. Some systems use dyspnea level as a criterion in determining disability. Millions of dollars are spent annually in symptom management and lost hours of work due to dyspnea.

The symptom of dyspnea may be acute, as in a tension pneumothorax; stimulus-related, as in exertional dyspnea; or chronic, as in emphysema. In acute states the symptom may be assistive in diagnosis. In episodic or chronic etiologies a common patient-initiated intervention is to decrease activity. Though the symptom severity may be reduced at first, the longer-range consequence may be deconditioning. Social interactions also may be reduced and depression increased. Quality of life is threatened as dyspnea frequency and intensity increase.

Mechanisms and Related Variables

Perceptual phenomena involve cerebral interpretation. The mechanisms and neural pathways that send messages to the brain for interpretation differ, however. Pain is a perceived phenomenon with specific pair receptors and a known neural pathway. Dyspnea lacks a common pathway but rather obtains messages from a number of peripheral and central receptors. Precise mechanisms for specific types of dyspnea continue to be investigated.

The brainstem is believed to be involved in some types of dyspnea, including but not limited to the chemoreceptor response to pH and CO_2. Oxygen level has very limited effect on dyspnea; many patients who are dyspneic have normal oxygenation levels, and those who are hypoxic generally have minimal improvement in dyspnea when normal oxygenation levels are reached. Oxygen cost has been moderately related to dyspnea but may have closer links to activity than to oxygen itself.

Ventilatory muscles, chest wall, lung, and airway receptors also have been identified as sources of information to make the interpretation of dyspnea. Stretch and irritation account for some stimuli. It has been proposed that a disproportional relationship between length and tension in the muscle spindle is also a stimulus. The theory has been expanded to involve a mismatch between outgoing motor signals to the respiratory muscles and incoming afferent signals.

Dyspnea is a multifactorial phenomenon. Carrier, Janson-Bjerklie, and Jacobs (1984) developed a model to organize the variables related to dyspnea. The variables were grouped into personal, health status, situational, patient-coping strategies and self-care behaviors, and therapeutic management strategies. Lung function values, work of breathing, fatigue, anxiety, and depression are often used covariates in dyspnea research.

Research

As with all subjective phenomena, the patient's report of the experience is considered valid. The similarity of dyspnea descriptors used by patients with similar pathologies supports the appropriateness of this assumption. The validity of many dyspnea measures today has been well established.

Reliability of dyspnea measures has been demonstrated by high correlations between the amount of resistive load added to the airway and the level of dyspnea intensity. Sensitivity was demonstrated when patients were able to discriminate between small changes in the resistive load added to the airway. Within-subject reliability regarding kinds of dyspnea remains to be examined.

Often the clinician is forced to rely on recall data regarding dyspnea. Because changing situational and personal variables can influence dyspnea over time, the question arises, how reliable is recall data? Meek and Lareau (1997) found that there was no statistical difference between actual and 2-week recall of average, greatest, and least dyspnea in males with severe COPD.

It has long been noted that patients with chronic dyspnea report lower levels of dyspnea than someone experiencing acutely the same level of physiological abnormality. It is proposed that developed coping strategies over the course of symptoms account for some of this difference. It is expected that we will better understand this difference as more is known about the mechanisms of dyspnea.

The cycle of dyspnea–inactivity–deconditioning–dyspnea also has been reported in numerous studies. Thompson (1990) showed that some patients could accurately predict how far they could walk before dyspnea would stop them, but some subjects underestimated their walking distance by as much as the distance of a football field during a 12-minute walk test. The fear of not being able to walk to the grocery or out to the mailbox because of predicted dyspnea can set up classic fear immobility. A major premise of pulmonary rehabilitation has been to break this inactivity cycle of dyspnea and to serve as a fear desensitization. Patients have reported reduced dyspnea and demonstrated greater walking distances and improved physical conditioning without direct improvements in pulmonary function after completing a pulmonary rehabilitation course.

A number of other effective coping strategies have been examined. Activity modification and energy conservation, symptom monitoring, relaxation techniques, education, and self-management of medication regimen have been effective. Positioning—sitting up, leaning forward, or resting their arms on their knees—decreases dyspnea for some. Abdominal breathing, paced breathing, or pursed-lip breathing are appropriate for some types of dyspnea.

Less nursing research has been conducted in the acute care setting. Gift, Moore, and Soeken (1992) examined the relationship of dyspnea, depression, and anxiety in asthma patients. Knebel, Janson-Bjerklie, Malley, Wilson, and Marini (1994) focused on dyspnea during weaning from mechanical ventilation. Thompson (1997) studied the pattern of dyspnea during tracheal suction of mechanically ventilated intensive care patients. The use of a fan blowing on the face of a patient with COPD has dramatic effects for some patients but not all—why? Many questions about dyspnea in the acute care population are yet to be examined. Within-subject comparison studies also are needed regarding dyspnea types and intensities and interventions for patients with acute exacerbations of chronic cardiopulmonary disease.

Future Directions

The search of mechanisms of dyspnea must continue in order to better understand this complex phenomenon. Much of the progress regarding dyspnea assessment and management can be attributed to the multidisciplinary community of scholars that meets annually and converses regularly. Such exchanges are vital to future advancement. Multidisciplinary as well as intradisciplinary efforts are encouraged in order to integrate the knowledge into practice decisions.

CAROL LYNN THOMPSON

See also
CHRONIC ILLNESS
COPING
ENDOTRACHEAL SUCTIONING
FATIGUE
QUALITY OF LIFE

E

EDUCATION: NURSE RESEARCHERS AND ADVANCED PRACTICE NURSES

Nurse Researchers

Nurse researchers at a minimum hold an earned doctorate. Many nurse leaders hold the view that nurses are needed with doctorates in nursing, education, and related disciplines. Doctorates include PhD, EdD, DNS, and ND degrees. The PhD and EdD are thought appropriate for the nurse researcher, and the DNS and ND are designed for clinicians who test nursing theories in a broader clinical context. The success of the nurse researcher is dependent on employer support for research, collaboration with peers, availability of library resources, computer services, and access to research populations.

Advanced Practice Nurses

Advanced practice nurses (APN) in care provider roles are nurse practitioners (NP), nurse anesthetists (NA), and nurse-midwives (N-M), for which master's level education is appropriate, although not all current practitioners hold master of science in nursing (MSN) degrees. There are at present more than 200 APN programs, most of which do offer the MSN degree. The curriculum, philosophy, and model for the MSN degree reflects other master's degree programs. In addition, nursing education must meet public health requirements as well as the students' need to acquire knowledge and education in order to work at a high level. Advanced practice nurses offer an economical complement or alternative to physician health care. As primary health care providers, they can provide high-quality care in a variety of settings, such as workplaces, schools, day-care centers, and others. Advanced practice nurses can provide from 60% to 80% of primary care that traditionally has been the purview of physicians. Nurse anesthetists provide anesthetic services and serve as sole providers for 49% of hospitals; nurse midwives provide full maternity care and can handle 90% of deliveries.

The curriculum model contains three components, with the main focus on the clinical role:

1. The core content must provide a foundation for the MSN specialties that may be pursued.
2. The content must provide for the students' direct patient and clinical services at an advanced level.
3. The specialty curricula include clinical and didactic content as prescribed by the specialty's official organizations.

Master's degree candidates are expected to acquire critical-thinking and decision-making skills. They must learn to assess accurately, plan, intervene, and evaluate health or sickness in clients and patients as well as communicate effectively and sensitively. All have prescriptive authority.

Specialty Organizations and Requirements for Credentials

Nurse Practitioner. The National Organization of Nurse Practitioner Faculty (NONPF) sets curricular guidelines requiring 500 hours of clinical practice in addition to classroom instruction under qualified, master's degree–credentialed, clinical nurse practitioners. However, most nurse educators have doctoral degrees.

Nurse Anesthetist. The Council on Accreditation of Nurse Anesthesia Educational Programs fixes requirements for the supervision of students by a credentialed faculty member, which should be in a 1:1 ratio initially and in the latter stage of the course a 1:2 ratio. The instructor must be a certified registered nurse anesthetist. Nurse anesthetists are prepared to work independently, as they may be the only providers of anesthesia care in some settings. The Council on Certification of Nurse Anesthetists requires that each student administer a minimum of 450 anesthetics and a minimum of 800 hours of anesthesia.

Nurse-Midwives. The American College of Nurse-Midwives (ACNM) is the professional association of certified nurse-midwives (CNMs). There are approximately 5,200 CNMs in the United States and its territories.

The Division of Accreditation (DOA) of the ACNM establishes the criteria for pre-accreditation and accreditation of education programs in nurse-midwifery. These criteria are the basis for the accreditation process, which is a joint activity involving both nurse-midwifery education programs and the DOA. The DOA of the ACNM is recognized by the U.S. Department of Education as an accrediting agency.

The graduate program provides all the essential components of the nurse-midwifery curriculum and is incorporated into a program of professional studies leading to an academic degree at the master's or doctoral level. Upon successful completion of the nurse-midwifery program, a graduate is eligible to sit for the national examination in order to become a CNM.

Core Curriculum

The core curriculum articulates the content that is the educational foundation of all graduate students regardless of specialty. Certain core courses are common to all APN programs. The general graduate core educational content includes research; policy, organization, and financing of health care; ethics; professional role development; theoretical foundations of nursing practice; human diversity and social issues; and health promotion and disease prevention. The core curriculum also includes advanced health and physical assessment, advanced physiology and pathophysiology, and advanced pharmacology.

Advanced practice nurses must be able to make sound clinical and management decisions based on astute diagnosis and assessments of their clients' or patients' problems. Advanced practice nurses may well provide the first contact or entry into health care as they work in many underserved areas without physician presence. The APN must have the skill to make physical and psychological assessments based on thorough history taking and observation of signs, symptoms, and pathophysiological changes in the client or patient.

In addition, the APN must have an understanding of normal physiology as well as a recognition of pathological mechanisms and appearances in order to make valid assessments followed by a management plan for the patient. The ability to understand and communicate with a client or patient is vital and basic. The understanding and use of pharmacological agents for the management of client health is necessary. Not only must the APN have a good understanding of the kinetics and dynamics of drugs, but it is critical to understand their effects at the cellular level and the consequent result of drug administration in the organism as a whole. In this area the APN should be cognizant of the various governmental and legal ramifications and requirements for drug administrations.

FAYE G. ABDELLAH

See also
ADVANCED PRACTICE NURSES
DOCTORAL EDUCATION
NURSE ANESTHETISTS AND RESARCH
NURSE-MIDWIFERY
PRIMARY NURSING

ELDER ABUSE

Elder mistreatment is a complex syndrome that can lead to morbid or even fatal outcomes for those afflicted. *Mistreatment* is the term used to describe outcomes from such actions as abuse, neglect, exploitation, and abandonment of the elderly, and it affects all socioeconomic, cultural, ethnic, and religious groups. It is estimated that between 700,000 and 1.2 million cases of elder mistreatment occur annually in this country (Pillemer & Finkelhor, 1988). The National Center on Elder Abuse 1991 survey, conducted by adult protective service agencies and state units on aging, documented an estimate of over 250,000 reports of elder mistreatment in that year (Tatara, 1993).

The term *elder mistreatment* has been defined by Hudson (1989) as "destructive behavior that is directed toward an older adult, occurs within the context of a relationship connoting trust and is of sufficient intensity and/or frequency to produce harmful physical, psychological, social and/or financial effects of unnecessary suffering, injury, pain, loss and/or violation of human rights and poorer quality of life for the older adult" (p. 16). In her seminal study, Hudson (1991) conducted a three-round Delphi survey with a national panel of 63 elder mistreatment experts to develop a taxonomy that now serves as the basis for research in the field and her ongoing program of nursing research (Hudson, 1991, 1994; Hudson & Carlson, 1994). Abuse is aggressive or invasive behavior, actions, or threats inflicted on an older adult and resulting in harmful effects for the older adult. Neglect is the failure of a responsible party to act so as to provide what is prudently deemed adequate and reasonable assistance that is warranted to ensure that the older adult's basic physical, psychological, social, and financial needs are met; the neglect results in harmful effects for the older adult (Hudson, 1989).

Physical abuse may include hitting, kicking, punching, and other physical contact. *Neglect* is the term used for inadequate care, which may be intentional or unintentional. Intentional neglect is the omission of appropriate care, which can readily lead to serious functional decline or death, for example, the intentional withholding of food or medicine. Unintentional neglect is a different situation. It occurs when an individual providing care to an elder person does not have the requisite knowledge and skills to provide such care appropriately. Finally, self-neglect, which is reportable in some states, occurs when an elder, either knowingly or unknowingly, lives in such a manner that his or her health is likely to deteriorate or already has done so.

Exploitation is fraudulent activity in connection with an older person's property or assets, and abandonment is defined as the deliberate and abrupt withdrawal of services in caring for an elderly person. Restriction as a form of elder mistreatment has recently been examined in an investigation of caregiver behaviors that have fewer social sanctions but may be equally deleterious to the older person (Fulmer & Gurland, 1996).

Nationally, the leading reason for mistreatment referral is neglect of elders, which accounts for over half of all cases that reach adult protective services hotlines or offices. Evidence suggests that only 1 in 14 elder mistreatment cases is reported to some public agency. Underreporting of elder mistreatment is a concern because elders may have disease symptoms or age-related changes that mask or mimic mistreatment symptoms, making assessment of mistreatment complex. Moreover, few clinicians have been trained in elder mistreatment assessment and intervention, which has also led to underreporting. Elder mistreatment is not new, but the term and the related literature have developed only in the past two decades. With an unprecedented number of individuals living beyond the age of 65 and even beyond the age of 85, clinicians and nurses must be sensitive to the possibility of elder mistreatment.

Theories for elder mistreatment causality have been posited. The dependency theory refers to the amount of care an elder person requires and is related to stressed caregiver research, which describes overwhelmed caregivers who lose their control or stop providing reasonable care. Conversely, there are data that reflect the caregiver's dependency on the elder (for shelter, money, etc.), which puts the elder at risk. Transgenerational violence theory refers to children who learn violent behavior as normal and then become violent and abusive as they grow older. This might be viewed from a learning theory perspective, although some have looked at it as a retribution act: an adult child may strike back at a parent or caregiver who was once abusive. The psychopathology of the abuser theory refers to any nonnormal caregiver, such as substance abusers (alcohol, drugs), psychiatrically impaired individuals, or mentally retarded caregivers. The number of mentally retarded elders over 65 years of age has grown substantially over the past decade, creating situations where mentally retarded or disabled offspring become caregivers for very elderly parents.

Elder mistreatment is a relatively new construct within the domain of family violence research. Early studies looked at the prevalence of elder mistreatment from a variety of perspectives: acute care, community nursing care, and the nursing home setting. Differences in operational definitions, methodological concerns, and the lack of national random samples have made it difficult to understand the conditions under which elder mistreatment is likely to occur. The National Committee for the Prevention of Elder Abuse has pointed out "that such basic questions as to the prevalence and incidence of abuse, risk factors and barriers to seeking and accepting help have not been answered" (Tatara, 1993, p. 37). Although reporting of elder abuse and neglect has been improved and there has been an increase in education and training, there is still a great need for empowerment of elders, preventive measures, and improved systems coordination.

Recent work by Hudson and Carlson (1994) provided a lexicon for elder mistreatment, operationalizing terms that can be used more effectively in practice. The outcome variables in elder mistreatment are challenging to name. Bruises have multiple causality in elders, who may be taking coumadin or have a history of frequent falling. Elders with cognitive impairment may report abuse appropriately, but no credence is given because of their deteriorated mental status. There is no Denver developmental screen for aging that enables the clinician to understand what an 80-year-old looks like and what conditions are likely to represent elder mistreatment. More researchers must be attracted to this field in order to conduct the studies that can begin to clarify the multiplicity of variables.

Signs and symptoms of elder mistreatment might include unexplained bruises, fractures, burns, poor hydration, reports of hitting or any other violent behavior against the elder, sexually transmitted disease in institutionalized elders, unexplained loss of money or goods, evidence of fearfulness around a caregiver, or the subjective report of abuse. It is especially difficult to evaluate the demented elder for mistreatment; a careful and thorough interdisciplinary team approach is required.

The American Medical Association's *Diagnostic and Treatment Guidelines on Elder Abuse and Neglect* (Aravanis et al., 1992) provides guidelines for the assessment of abuse and neglect of elders as well as flowcharts for assessing and intervening in elder mistreatment. Special attention is given to an elder's lack of decision-making capacity in an abusing situation. In such cases appropriate use of guardians should be reviewed. Elders may be inappropriately labeled confused when they choose to return to an abusing situation. For example, a mother may prefer to live with an abusing daughter rather than face the prospect of an unknown caregiver. Overzealous protection of a competent elder is a form of ageism that infantilizes the older individual and takes away his or her autonomy. Each state has elder mistreatment reporting laws or requirements, which professional nurses should become familiar with. A key practice implication in this field is the inclusion of a family violence question in the history and attention to any signs or symptoms in the physical exam that might appropriate follow-up in suspected cases.

TERRY FULMER

See also
  CAREGIVER
  COPING
  FALLS
  FAMILY CAREGIVING
    TO FRAIL ELDERS
  VIOLENCE AS A NURSING AREA
    OF INQUIRY

ELECTRONIC NETWORK

In general, a network is composed of a minimum of two connected points. For example, one person talking with another, face-to-face, can constitute a network. Telephone networks connect at least two people using transceivers, wire, switches, and computers. Television networks connect large numbers of people. An electronic network is considered to be the connection or linking of two or more computers to allow data and information exchange. Electronic computer networks may be as small as two computers or as large as the Internet, considered to be a network of networks.

The goal of networks is information exchange and may or may not be bidirectional. Person-to-person conversations, even if using some sort of intermediary like the telephone, are usually bidirectional. Television and some computer network applications may be unidirectional; however, bidirectional computer networks are the most common. Examples include local area networks (LAN), which may serve a department; larger networks called wide area networks (WAN); and the Internet. Intranets, which are the internal deployment of Internet technologies, are becoming more and more common.

Electronic networks are exciting tools for nursing and will be increasingly important in information acquisition and dispersion. Electronic networks, such as the Internet and the World Wide Web (WWW), not only provide a means of communicating but also facilitate collaborative research, promote education regardless of geographic limitations, and allow access and acquisition of needed resources. Electronic networks will continue to affect areas integral to nursing, such as a lifetime electronic health record, nursing research, increased interdisciplinary collaborative research, education without walls for patients and nurses, and nursing knowledge acquisition and information exchange.

Nursing and Electronic Networks

Although the essence of nursing has been a network, that is, the nurse-patient relationship, there is limited nursing research of electronic networks. Brennan, Moore, and Smyth (1991) and Ripich, Moore, and Brennan (1992) investigated the use of electronic networks to facilitate nursing support of home care clients and their caregivers. They concluded that a computer network is an excellent tool to facilitate support and information exchange among caregivers and between nurses and caregivers for patients with AIDS and Alzheimer's disease.

There are anecdotal reports and case studies to support nurses' use of electronic networks. Sparks (1993) has been instrumental in her advocacy and promotion of electronic networks and resource availability for nurses. In the early 1990s she championed the Educational Technology Network (E.T.-Net). E.T.Net promoted the exchange of information and ideas for nurses, nurse educators, and nursing students. It was the first international electronic network managed by a nurse. Barnsteiner's (1993) and Graves's (1993) work with nursing resource availability (Online Journal of Nursing Knowledge Synthesis and the Virginia Henderson STTI Electronic Library, respectively) and DuBois and Rizzolo (1994) in the *American Journal of Nursing's* AJN Network to promote continuing education for nurses are additional examples of nursing use of electronic networks.

As information technology increases in use and health care requires increased efficiency, nurses will rely more and more on information technology as one tool for providing the best possible patient care. Local electronic networks, such as clinical information systems, will include other larger networks so that nurses will have the best information resources to assist nursing care. Research concerning the effects of electronic networking on nurses and other health care professionals, as well as on patients and their families, is needed. Electronic networking should be examined as an independent variable through the inclusion of electronic networks in all stages of the research process. This research will promote the advancement of health and patient care by providing the scientific foundation for the appropriate application of electronic networking technologies.

W. Scott Erdley
Susan M. Sparks

See also
INTERNET
THE ONLINE JOURNAL OF KNOWL-
EDGE SYNTHESIS FOR NURSING
VIRGINIA HENDERSON INTERNA-
TIONAL NURSING LIBRARY
WORLD WIDE WEB

EMERGENCY NURSING RESEARCH

Over 80,000 emergency nurses provide emergency health care to 94 million individuals each year in the United States. These nurses practice in a wide variety of settings: community, military, federal, state, and local government emergency departments; prehospital settings; clinics and HMOs; and free-standing emergency centers. Emergency nurses provide care to a broad and diverse population, encompassing newborns to the elderly, primary care through critical care, prevention to resuscitation, frontier to large urban populations, and air and ground transport. Emergency nurses serve as the link between the community and the hospital when coordinating care for individuals returning to their homes; transferring to other facilities, such as nursing homes; or when admitted to the inpatient hospital. Like other nurses, emergency nurses also are clinicians, managers, educators, researchers, and leaders in government affairs and public health policy. Diversity is the word that describes the specialty of emergency nursing.

Research Agenda

The breadth of emergency nursing practice demands an equally diverse research agenda to provide emergency nurses with the knowledge to improve health care. As the professional organization for emergency nurses, the Emergency Nurses Association (ENA) provides direction, resources, and research and educational programs to develop a body of knowledge for emergency nursing and emergency health care.

To guide emergency nursing research, ENA and the ENA Foundation developed eight research initiatives that provide direction for an evolving research agenda. These initiatives include (a) mechanisms to assure effective, efficient, and quality emergency nursing care delivery systems; (b) effective and efficient outcomes of emergency nursing services and procedures; (c) factors affecting nursing practice; (d) influence of health care technologies, facilities, and equipment on emergency nursing practice; (e) factors affecting health care cost, productivity, and market forces to emergency services; (f) ways to enhance health promotion and injury prevention; (g) methods for handling complex ethical issues related to emergency nursing care; and (h) mechanisms to assure quality and cost-effective educational programs for emergency nursing.

The success of a research agenda is dependent on a strong research culture and a cadre of research scientists to conduct, disseminate, and utilize research in emergency nursing practice. Emergency nursing has a small but growing number of researchers. ENA member demographics document that emergency nurses have the education and experience to contribute to the research agenda. About 41% of the members have baccalaureate degrees; 14%, master's degrees; and 0.6%, doctoral degrees. A third of the members (31%) are currently advancing their education. Emergency nurses also have strong clinical expertise; 49% have practiced in emergency nursing for more than 10 years. Over half (59%) of the nurses spend at least 75% of their time providing direct patient care. Given the education and clinical expertise of emergency nurses, there is a great potential to increase the number of emergency nurse researchers.

In 1995 and 1996 the ENA Research Committee developed the LUNAR (Learning and Using New Approaches to Research) project to help emergency nurses develop research skills while participating in a national multisite study. Over 150 nurses attended a research training program, with 115 nurses in 89 emergency departments completing the research study. These nurses collected data on the characteristics of 12,422 patients seeking emergency care. A new multisite study, LUNAR II, will continue to develop the research culture and skills of emergency nurses.

Research Funding

In addition to developing a research culture and emergency nurse researchers, funding to support the agenda is needed. In 1991 the ENA Foundation was established to provide funding for peer-reviewed research, and by 1997, 29 studies had been funded. The majority of these studies were conducted in an emergency department, using a variety of research methodologies. The studies focused on family needs and behavior (4); patient satisfaction (2); prevention and education (3); domestic violence and violence in the emergency department (4); pain intervention (2); treatment modalities, interventions, or technology (6); and nurses' education, preparedness, decision making, or regulations affecting practice (8). All eight of the research initiatives were addressed by the studies—most frequently, emergency nursing care delivery systems (10), effective and efficient outcomes of care (7), factors affecting practice (6), and the influence of health care technologies (5). To a lesser extent, studies targeted initiatives for health care economics and management (1), health promotion and injury prevention (4), ethics (3), and educational programs (4).

ENA also supports a national research program. Each year a national data base survey is sent to all emergency departments to identify changes in demographics, services, utilization, and staffing. An ongoing survey of the demographic characteristics of emergency nurses also is maintained. A 2-year follow-up survey will determine changes in the knowledge, involvement, and needs of emergency nurses concerning public and professional motor vehicle injury–prevention programs. Other research includes the development and testing of a management data set, a survey on violence in the workplace, a study testing the effectiveness of trauma critical pathways, and a study examining practice outcomes of nurses with and without verifications in trauma nursing and pediatric emergency nursing.

Research Dissemination

Dissemination of completed research also is important for the continued development of research within emergency nursing. The ENA Research Committee conducted a literature search from 1989 through 1994 to identify the topics and initiatives that emergency nurses addressed in their published and presented research. The literature review showed that emergency nurse researchers primarily published their research in the *Journal of Emergency Nursing*. This journal and research abstracts from ENA conferences were the main sources of information used to identify the type of research conducted and disseminated by emergency nurses.

The information from the initial literature search and a recent review (1994–1996) indicated that emergency nurses used a variety of qualitative and quantitative methodologies and targeted a broad population of individuals and issues. Research on effective and efficient outcomes of emergency nursing care (48 studies) and factors affecting emergency nursing practice (43 studies) were disseminated most often. Also addressed were emergency nursing care delivery systems (29), health promotion and injury prevention (23), and health care technologies (23). Fewer emergency nurse researchers focused on educational programs for emergency nursing (6 studies), health care economics and management (5), and ethical issues (4).

Research by emergency nurses has increased steadily for the past 5 years and has the potential to increase rapidly with new research educational programs and grant funding. Past research addressed the needs of emergency nurses to provide care to a wide variety of patients in diverse settings. All eight of the ENA research initiatives were investigated by a variety of research methodologies. In the future an increased focus on ethics, health care economics, outcomes of care, health technology, and health promotion is expected because of the changes occurring in emergency health care.

SUSAN L. MACLEAN

See also
   ACCESS TO HEALTH CARE
   CLINICAL DECISION MAKING
   DISASTER NURSING
   VIOLENCE AS A NURSING AREA
       OF INQUIRY

EMPATHY

The concept of empathy in nursing has received considerable attention as a central "helping" component in the nurse-patient relationship. Although there is some evidence that empathy was prevalent in nursing interactions as early as the late 1800s (Sutherland, 1993), it was not until Carl Rogers's 1957 address to the American Nurse's Association on the essential characteristics of a therapeutic relationship that nurses began to examine seriously the concept of empathy and its application to nursing practice. Early nursing authors called for increased awareness of empathy and its therapeutic value.

Since that time there has been an uncritical and overwhelming acceptance of the importance of empathy in nursing. Nevertheless, after years of use and a growing body of literature related to empathy, conceptualization of the term remains incomplete, studies of nurses' empathetic ability appear contradictory, and evidence of the beneficial effects of empathy on health care outcomes is inconclusive (Bennett, 1995; Morse, Anderson, et al., 1992; Pike, 1990; Sutherland, 1993). Recently some authors have begun to question the usefulness and appropriateness of empathy in nursing practice (Pike; Morse, Anderson, et al., 1992).

Empathy has been described as a complex "bidirectional interpersonal" phenomenon, and as such it has eluded simple definition (Bennett, 1995, p. 37). A cursory review of the literature reveals a wide range of definitions, including descriptions of empathy as a trait, a state, an interpersonal process, a feeling, a sensitivity, an attitude, and an ability. In many cases authors struggle to offer clear definitions. There have been several attempts to clarify meaning and components of empathy and to determine areas of consensus. An analysis of the concept of empathy, based on a review of psychological and nursing literature, revealed four components of empathy: moral, emotive, cognitive, and behavioral (Morse, Anderson, et al., 1992). For example, emotional empathy is the arousal or responsive component resulting in empathic insight and followed by an emotional response. The empathetic response is felt by the caregiver on perception of the emotional distress within the other.

Although nurses have not focused on all components of empathy, Bennett (1995) indicates that there is consensus that empathy involves both cognition and affect in a multistage, cyclical process. However, models used in nursing to illustrate the process of empathetic communication have been simplistic. One exception to this is the model proposed by Morse, Bottorff, Anderson, O'Brien, and Solberg (1992). Attempts to differentiate empathy from related concepts, such as intuition and inference, is an important step toward conceptual clarity (Morse, Miles, Clark, & Doberneck, 1994). In summary, nurses' dependence on definitions from research on empathy in other fields such as counseling psychology has precluded description of how empathy may exist in nurse-patient interactions. A strong conceptualization would be particularly useful to nurses, but this remains a continuing challenge (Gagan, 1983; Morse et al., 1994).

Empathy has been a central concept in a large number of research investigations over the past two decades. Nurse researchers have attempted to measure levels of empathy, identify characteristics of empathetic nurses, describe factors that influence ability to empathize in nursing, describe functional levels of empathy as they are demonstrated in nursing, evaluate the effectiveness of educational programs on empathy, and document patient outcomes. Most studies focusing on empathy have been descriptive, using questionnaires or interviews. Evaluations of educational programs have been based on quasi-experimental designs.

Despite the amount of time and energy devoted to investigating empathy and its uses in nursing practice, our understanding of empathy has expanded very little. Several authors have concluded that knowledge development has been hampered by methodological problems, including the inadequacies of instruments used to measure empathy, use of small samples, cross-sectional designs, and inadequate analytical methods (Bennett, 1995; Morse, Anderson, et al., 1992). Progress also has been hampered by a lack of empathy research in nursing focused on the development or testing of theory about empathy and its uses in nursing as well as the lack of attention to other aspects of therapeutic rapport (genuineness, warmth, trust) so that the specific contribution of empathy is clearly delineated (Bennett, 1995). Others have noted the exclusive attention of researchers to measuring the observable, objective components of empathy (i.e., cognitive and behavioral) while ignoring the subjective, nonmeasurable components (i.e., moral and emotive) as an important obstacle to understanding empathy (Morse, Anderson, et al., 1992).

There are many questions that remain unanswered in relation to empathy. Readers may want to refer to the extensive list of key questions that Bennett (1995) has developed. Of fundamental importance will be delineation of how empathy is practiced in the various clinical settings, when and where empathy should be used, and the patient outcomes (positive and negative) that can result when nurses use empathy. If multidimensional conceptualizations of empathy are to be used as a basis for research, this will have direct implications for the selection of appropriate measures and designs to reflect this complexity. Finally, it is important that nurses remain open to the possibility that other concepts, yet to be identified and described, may represent significant components of the nurse-patient relationship better than concepts borrowed from other disciplines, such as empathy (Morse et al., 1994).

JOAN L. BOTTORFF

See also
ATTITUDES
NURSE-PATIENT INTERACTION
NURSE-PATIENT RELATIONSHIP
NURSING EDUCATION

ENDOTRACHEAL SUCTIONING

Definition

Endotracheal suctioning (ETS) is a common nursing intervention to remove mucus and debris from the tracheobronchial tree by the insertion of a suction catheter through the endotracheal tube and the application of vacuum during catheter withdrawal to aspirate tracheal secretions. Endotracheal suctioning is usually performed every 1–2 hours or as needed to maintain airway patency and arterial oxygenation. There are insufficient research data to identify the most significant clinical indicators of need for ETS. However, clinicians report the following clinical cues that indicate need: (a) color, (b) breath sounds, (c) respiratory rate and pattern, (d) coughing, (e) presence of secretions in the tubing, (f) saw-toothed flow-volume loops on the mechanical ventilator, and (g) blood oxygen levels.

The ETS procedure has a number of components, including hyperoxygenation (increased inspired oxygen), which can be delivered via either the ventilator or a manual resuscitation bag; hyperinflation (volume of inspired air above baseline tidal volume); open versus closed ETS through an adapter or in-line suction catheter to maintain mechanical ventilation; and postoxygenation. Associated variables include (a) saline instillation for the purpose of irrigation, (b) suction catheter size, (c) level of negative suction pressure, (d) depth of suction catheter insertion, (e) application of negative pressure either continuously or intermittently, (f) duration of negative pressure application, and (g) number of hyperoxygenation/hyperinflation suction sequences. Despite almost 70 years of research, controversy continues regarding the most efficacious ETS procedure. Although components of the ETS procedure have been well researched, the utilization of research findings has been variable in the clinical setting. The components of the ETS procedure have been developed to prevent the complications associated with the procedure.

Complications

The majority of research has been conducted to develop techniques to minimize the most common complication, hypoxemia. Hypoxemia, which is the lowering of blood oxygen levels, may result from the disconnection of the patient from the ventilator during the procedure and/or the removal of oxygen from the respiratory tract during the application of vacuum. Researchers have documented other side effects, which include (a) atelectasis, (b) bronchoconstriction and tracheal trauma, (c) alterations in arterial pressure (hypotension and hypertension), (d) increased intracranial pressure, (e) cardiac arrhythmias, (f) cardiac arrest, and (g) death. Atelectasis results from the insertion of a suction catheter with an outer diameter that is too large for the inner diameter of the endotracheal tube, causing catheter impaction and the removal of respiratory gases from distal alveoli with the application of vacuum. Bronchoconstriction and tracheal trauma result when the catheter stimulates the bronchial smooth muscle and inner lining of the trachea.

Hyperoxygenation/Hyperinflation

Hyperoxygenation/hyperinflation is a component of the ETS procedure used to prevent hypoxemia.

Hyperoxygenation is the administration of a fraction of inspired oxygen (FiO_2) greater than the patient's baseline FiO_2, either prior to (prehyperoxygenation) or following (posthyperoxygenation) suctioning. Hyperinflation is defined as the delivery of a breath of inspired air greater than the patient's baseline tidal volume. Research has shown that patients who receive no form of hyperoxygenation/hyperinflation with ETS show a significant decline in arterial blood oxygen. A critical evaluation of the research examining the effect of hyperoxygenation/hyperinflation on suction-induced hypoxemia shows variability in the techniques and the results. However, despite the conflicting findings, investigators have documented that 3–4 hyperoxygenation breaths at 100% oxygen and 135%–150% of tidal volume has been effective in preventing suction-induced hypoxemia (Stone & Turner, 1989). Researchers have recently documented that hyperinflation followed by ETS may cause a decrease or an increase in mean arterial pressure, and this may be due to the number of hyperoxygenation/hyperinflation suction sequences.

Ventilator versus Manual Resuscitation Bag

Hyperoxygenation/hyperinflation breaths can be delivered using either a manual resuscitation bag (MRB) or a ventilator. Investigators have reported inconsistently on the ability of different MRBs to deliver 100% oxygen. Research has shown that consistency is improved when the MRB has a reservoir of 1,000–2,000 cc attached to an oxygen source at a flow rate of 15 l/min or flush and adequate time is allowed for refill from the reservoir. Recent studies comparing the ventilator and the MRB, which have controlled important intervening variables, have concluded that hyperoxygenation/hyperinflation breaths delivered via the ventilator have resulted in elevated blood oxygen levels that are superior or equivalent to the MRB in preventing suction-induced hypoxemia. Investigators also have determined that the MRB produces a greater increase in airway pressure, arterial pressure, and heart rate compared to the ventilator. Hence, the ventilator is the preferred mode for delivering hyperoxygenation/hyperinflation breaths (Stone, 1990).

Open versus Closed ETS

Closed ETS through an adapter or in-line suction catheter permits uninterrupted ventilation, oxygenation, and positive end expiratory pressure during ETS. Without hyperoxygenation there is a greater decline in blood oxygen levels with open ETS than with closed ETS. With hyperoxygenation, via the ventilator or MRB, the decline in blood oxygen levels is equivalent or less with closed ETS.

Associated Variables

Although saline instillation prior to ETS is common clinical practice, there is inconclusive research to support any physiological benefit, and it may actually cause a decline in blood oxygen levels (Raymond, 1995). The relationship between the outer diameter (OD) of the suction catheter and inner diameter (ID) of the endotracheal tube can be a significant factor in the development of atelectasis during ETS. Researchers recommend an OD/ID ratio of 1:2. This can be achieved with a 14-mm French catheter and an endotracheal tube of 7, 8, or 9 mm. As the level of negative pressure or suction applied to the catheter influences the degree of tracheal trauma, negative airway pressure, secretion recovery, and hypoxemia, researchers recommend a suction pressure of 100–120 mmHg. The suction catheter should be advanced down the endotracheal tube without the application of vacuum until gentle resistance is met, reducing mechanical stimulation of the tracheal tissue, which may cause bradycardia, premature atrial contractions, and increased intracranial pressure (Kerr, Rudy, Brucia, & Stone, 1993). The catheter should be withdrawn a few centimeters prior to the application of vacuum to prevent catheter wedging, and the vacuum can be applied either continuously or intermittently with no significant difference in tracheal trauma while withdrawing the catheter in a rotating motion (Czarnik, Stone, Everhart, & Preusser, 1991). The duration of suction application should be no more than 10 seconds.

The number of hyperoxygenation or hyperinflation suction sequences or catheter passes should be limited to no more than two per episode, as research data indicate that there is a cumulative increase in arterial pressure, heart rate, and intercranial pressure with each pass (Stone, Bell, & Preusser, 1991). If additional suction passes are needed, 5–10 minutes should elapse to allow the patient's hemodynamic variables to return to baseline. The patient should be assessed for changes in blood pressure, heart rate, arrhythmias, and increased intracranial pressure, and the patient's ability to tolerate the procedure should be documented. The lungs should be auscultated to assess airway clearance, and the character of secretions (amount, color, and viscosity) should be recorded following ETS.

Future Research

Further research is needed to identify the important clinical indicators of the need for ETS, the effectiveness of saline instillation, methods to reduce the complications associated with ETS, and clinical trials to determine the most efficacious and cost-effective ETS procedure in different patient populations across the life span.

KATHLEEN S. STONE

See also
    CLINICAL NURSING RESEARCH
    CLINICAL TRIALS
    ENDOTRACHEAL SUCTIONING
        IN NEWBORNS
    HEMODYNAMIC MONITORING
    PHYSIOLOGICAL MONITORING

ENDOTRACHEAL SUCTIONING IN NEWBORNS

Background

Endotracheal suctioning (ETS) in newborns is the sterile procedure used to remove accumulated secretions and debris from the artificial airway of newborn infants. Newborns with respiratory compromise have an endotracheal tube inserted and are placed on mechanical ventilation to support their respiratory efforts. Because the endotracheal tube is placed through the glottis and resides in the trachea, the mucociliary elevator, which is responsible for moving secretions and debris from the trachea and bronchi to the pharynx, is halted. This results in secretions accumulating and pooling at the tip, around the sides, and within the lumen of the endotracheal tube. The pooled secretions inhibit ventilation and oxygenation, which can lead to tube occlusion and respiratory arrest. Currently, ETS is the only method used to removed the secretions and ensure patency of the endotracheal tube.

Endotracheal suctioning in the newborn routinely follows chest physiotherapy. It is also used for the following indications: (a) visible secretions in the endotracheal tube, (b) rhonchi on auscultation of the chest, (c) changes in breath sounds, (d) cyanosis, (e) oxygen desaturation, (f) agitation, (g) increased carbon dioxide tension, and (h) changes in end-tidal carbon dioxide waveforms. If it is suspected that the artificial airway may be compromised due to partial or complete occlusion, ETS is the first and immediate intervention initiated.

The Procedure

Endotracheal suctioning consists of inserting a sterile catheter through the endotracheal tube into the trachea and applying negative pressure to remove any accumulated secretions and debris within the lumen or at the tip of the endotracheal tube. The procedure may include the following interventions: (a) instillation of normal saline, (b) use of supplemental oxygen, (c) varying amounts of negative pressure, (d) different types of negative pressure applied (continuous or intermittent), and (e) different methods used to give supplemental breaths (the ventilator or a manual resuscitation bag).

Endotracheal suctioning is not a benign procedure. Associated complications include hypoxemia, atelectasis, bradycardia, tissue trauma, transient bacteremia, and increased intracranial pressure. The frequency with which ETS is performed varies with the needs of the infant; it may be required every hour or every 24 hours. The goal is to suction as often as the infant needs suctioning yet as infrequently as possible to minimize the complications associated with ETS. For detailed information on each step of the ETS procedure, readers should consult a textbook on care of the newborn infant.

Research on ETS in Newborns

The ETS procedure in the newborn was adapted from our knowledge base of ETS of adult patients. Research on ETS in infants began in the 1960s, when Brandstater and Muallem (1969) associated the degree of atelectasis with ETS. A summary of the major findings follows.

Supplemental oxygen should be increased prior to, during, and following ETS, with continual monitoring of the infant's oxygenation status to minimize suction-induced hypoxemia (Raval, Yeh, Mora, & Pildes, 1980). The introduction of pulse oximetry has enabled the nurse to monitor in real time the changes in oxygenation levels during the ETS procedure. As a result, supplemental oxygen can be adjusted during the procedure to maintain optimal status. Previous dependency on measures with significant lag times, such as arterial blood gases or transcutaneous oxygen monitors, did not allow for individualized supplemental oxygenation of the infant.

Additional breaths given during and after suctioning can minimize the degree of suction-induced atelectasis (Brandstater & Muallem, 1969). Research is needed on the most effective method for giving the breaths, by means of the ventilator or the manual resuscitation bag. Each method has a cadre of advocates, but a highly controlled and rigorous study is needed to answer the question. Previous research on ETS in newborns was not helpful, as procedure was not presented in enough detail to determine if the manual resuscitation bag or the ventilator was used.

Tracheal tissue trauma results from ETS when the suction catheter rests on or touches the tracheal epithelium while negative pressure is applied. Limiting the depth of catheter insertion to not more than 1 cm past the endotracheal tube tip and limiting the negative pressure to 75 mmHg or less will help prevent tracheal epithelial trauma (Kleiber, 1986).

Increased intracranial pressure is problematic in this fragile population; both ETS and mechanical ventilation are known to cause increases in intracranial pressure. Limiting the depth of the catheter insertion, the negative pressure, and the length of time that negative pressure is applied will limit the increases in intracranial pressure during ETS (Stone & Turner, 1989). Not all questions concerning ETS have been answered; recent debates include (a) whether the use of normal saline with ETS is justified, (b) how to determine noninvasively the need for ETS, and (c) the efficacy of the ETS procedure.

Future Directions in ETS Research

Changes in technology have created new avenues for research in ETS. The use of high-frequency ventilation resulted in the need for new methods to clear the airway of infants, but at this time there is no research. Nitric oxide therapy has meant that the infant cannot be removed from the ventilator for suctioning. The use of in-line suction catheters with nitric oxide therapy allows mechanical ventilation and oxygenation to continue during ETS. Limited data on in-line suction catheters are available for the adult population, but infant and newborn data are lacking. The timing of ETS following intratracheal instillation of surfactant still needs investigation because of the widespread use of exogenous surfactant therapy. Anecdotal data from adults has identified pain, discomfort, and feelings of panic associated with the ETS. Newborns are not medicated prior to ETS, but future research may change this practice. Noninvasive alternatives are also sought for endotracheal suctioning, but at this time none appear on the horizon.

BARBARA S. TURNER

See also
ENDOTRACHEAL SUCTIONING
PAIN IN CHILDREN

EPIDEMIOLOGY

Epi (upon), *demos* (people), and *logos* (thought) are the Greek words from which *epidemiology* was derived. Epidemiology is the study of the distribution and determinants of states of health and illness in human populations. Although epidemiological concepts can be traced to ancient times, the science of epidemiology emerged in England in the mid-1800s, when cholera was killing thousands of people, particularly in London. Primarily due to the work of John Snow, a British physician, and William Farr, the registrar general for England and Wales, cholera was ultimately traced to contaminated water obtained from a frequently used pump in the middle of a Soho square. This was accomplished by use of the population count provided by Farr and the detailed records of cases and deaths by Snow (1855). As an early epidemiologist, Dr. Snow outlined the frequency and distribution of cholera, calculated rates, and found evidence of a cause or determinant of the outbreak. He logically organized data, recognized and analyzed a natural experiment, and did so prior to the era of bacteriology. Florence Nightingale, a contemporary of William Farr and John Snow, was influenced significantly by their work.

Since that time epidemiology has been traditionally associated with the study of infectious diseases, and measures of prevention and control have centered on altering the characteristics of the infectious agent, host, or environment. However, the scope of epidemiology now has been expanded to the study of the distribution and determinants of noninfectious conditions and variables that contribute to the maintenance of health. Also, epidemiological methodology is widely accepted in planning and evaluating health services.

Both the epidemiological process and the nursing process have evolved from the problem-solving process. Nurses use the epidemiological process to assess community (group) needs, identify factors that influence those needs, plan and implement prevention and control measures, and evaluate outcomes. Epidemiology is (a) a methodology that is used to study the distribution and determinants of states of health and (b) a body of knowledge that results from the study of specific health conditions. Nurses use the body of knowledge about specific conditions in making competent and successful clinical decisions. For example, nurses assess individuals according to risk factors that have been associated with various conditions, such as HIV infection, coronary artery disease, and cancer. Interventions that focus on reducing an individual's modifiable risk factors then can be implemented.

Descriptive Epidemiology

The rate is the primary measurement used to describe the occurrence of a health problem. A rate is defined as a measure of the quantity of a disease or state of health in a specific population within a given period of time. It is a proportion that includes a factor of time, where

$$\text{Rate} = \frac{\begin{array}{c}\text{Number of conditions or events}\\\text{occurring in a period of time}\end{array}}{\begin{array}{c}\text{Population at risk during}\\\text{the same period of time}\end{array}} \times \text{Base multiple of 10}$$

Rates are the best indicators of the risk, or probability, that a particular condition will occur. An incidence rate or occurrence rate measures the probability that people without a particular condition will develop that condition over a period of time. Mortality rates are incidence rates. Often, incidence rates for groups exposed to a potential risk factor are compared with the incidence rates for those not exposed. This comparison results in a relative risk ratio. A relative risk greater than 1.0 indicates that the risk is greater in the exposed group.

A prevalence rate measures the number of people in a given population who have a specific, existing condition at a given point in time. Most morbidity rates are prevalence rates. Specific rates are more detailed rates, calculated for population subgroups. They are used to define the distribution of the condition by person (age, sex, ethnicity, or other demographic or biographic characteristics), place, or time. Adjusted rates have been standardized, removing the effect of differences in the population. Rates are commonly adjusted for age, removing age as a factor in the interpretation of the rates.

Epidemiological Observational Studies

There are three types of observational epidemiologic studies: cross-sectional (survey), case-control (retrospective, or ex post facto), and cohort (longitudinal, or prospective) studies. Intervention epidemiological studies are experimental or quasi-experimental in design. Cross-sectional studies produce prevalence data, cover a range of topics and serve many purposes. The U.S. National Health Survey, administered by the National Center for Health Statistics (NHRS), Bureau of the Census, since 1956, consists of a series of ongoing surveys and provides the only nationwide source of data for the prevalence of acute and chronic illness, disabilities, functional problems, and health needs and the use of health care resources. The three general programs include the National Health Interview Survey (NHIS), the National Health and Nutrition Examination Survey (NHANES), and the National Health Record Survey (NHRS) (Chyba & Washington, 1990; Kovar, 1989).

Case-control studies compare patients who have a specific health condition with controls who do not have the condition. This design retrospectively examines both groups for possible exposure or causative factors. Case-control studies are often the first step in hypothesis testing and allow feasible investigation of rare conditions, chronic diseases, and the long-term effects of exposure that often occur as occupational hazards. The first evidence of the relationship between smoking and cancer was documented by a case-control study (Doll & Hill, 1950). This classic study obtained information on smoking history and other variables from a large sample of patients with lung cancer and from controls who did not have the disease. A significant association between smoking and lung cancer was demonstrated. Case-control studies are often performed when investigating an outbreak. Following the identification of an unusual syndrome in 1981, case-control studies identified the risk factors that were ultimately linked with HIV infection and AIDS (Peterman, Drotman, & Curran, 1985).

Cohort studies are prospective studies that follow a group of people forward to determine health outcomes. They are often conducted after a hypothesis has been preliminarily tested through a case-control study. The Framingham Heart Study is a classic example. Initially, a cohort of 6,507 men and women were selected, and they have been examined every 2 years since 1948. The information gained from this study has contributed significantly to the knowledge base of risk factors for coronary artery disease (Dawber, 1980). The Nurses Health Study, initiated in 1976, is another large, well-known cohort study. It has produced much information regarding women's health issues.

Epidemiological Intervention Studies

Preventive intervention studies use the experimental method and are based on primary prevention, seeking to reduce the risk of acquiring a specific health condition among a healthy group of people. For example, a community-wide, smoking-prevention, quasi-experimental study was conducted as a part of the Minnesota Heart Health Program (Perry, Kelder, Murray, & Klepp, 1992). Throughout the follow-up period, smoking rates were significantly lower in the intervention community than in the comparison community. Therapeutic intervention studies or clinical trials are focused on concepts of secondary prevention. These studies attempt to determine the ability of intervention to decrease or prevent recurrence of symptoms and to improve the outcomes for individuals with specific health conditions. One such trial examined the effects of early photocoagulation for persons who have developed diabetic retinopathy (Early Treatment Diabetic Retinopathy Study Research Group, 1991). Clinical trials of drug therapy for various conditions are other examples.

Epidemiology is the methodology of preventive medicine, the study of the distribution and determinants of states of health and illness in human populations. Calculation of incidence and prevalence rates are used to measure the occurrence of a state of health or illness in a population within a given time period. Descriptive epidemiology examines variation in the distribution patterns, using cross-sectional surveys, case-control studies, and prospective cohort studies. Analytic intervention studies attempt to identify the determinants of states of health and illness and identify a cause-and-effect relationship between an exposure and outcomes. Preventive intervention studies focus on primary prevention among healthy populations. Therapeutic intervention studies are focused on secondary prevention, attempting to determine the ability of an intervention to influence outcomes for individuals with specific health problems.

GAIL A. HARKNESS

See also
INFECTION CONTROL
POPULATIONS AND AGGREGATES
RISK FACTORS
SECONDARY DATA ANALYSIS

EPILEPSY

Definition

Epilepsy refers to a chronic condition characterized by recurrent *seizures*. A seizure is a temporary alteration in functioning caused by abnormal discharge of neurons in the central nervous system (Holmes, 1987). The exact nature of the seizure depends on the function of the brain cells that are affected by the abnormal discharge. Seizures are classified into two major types: *partial* and *generalized*. Partial seizures, which occur when the electrical discharge remains in a circumscribed area of the brain, can be broken down further into elementary or complex divisions. With elementary partial seizures, the person's consciousness is not impaired. With complex partial seizures, there is some impairment of consciousness. In some persons with partial seizures, the abnormal discharge spreads throughout the brain and is referred to as a partial seizure with secondary generalization.

Generalized seizures occur when the discharge affects both brain hemispheres and results in a loss of consciousness. The two most common types of generalized seizures are generalized tonic clonic (grand mal) and absence (petit mal). In generalized tonic clonic seizures, the person typically stiffens all over in the tonic phase, has jerking movements of the arms and legs in the clonic phase, and is incontinent of urine. Following the seizure the person is commonly sleepy. In absence seizures, there are a few seconds of loss of consciousness. The person generally stares blankly and sometimes rotates the eyes upward. An absence seizure begins and ends abruptly (Dreifuss, 1996).

Prevalence

Epilepsy affects over 2 million persons in the United States. The cumulative incidence to age 80 years is 1.3% to 3.1%. Incidence rates are highest among those under 20 years of age and over 60 years of age. The trend is for the frequency of epilepsy to be decreasing in children and to be increasing in the elderly. Rates are slightly higher for men than for women. The prevalence of active epilepsy, defined as having had a seizure in the past 5 years or taking daily antiepilepsy medication, is between 4.3 and 9.3 per 1,000. In approximately 70% of new cases of epilepsy there is no specific identified cause. In the remaining 30% the risk factors for epilepsy are severe head trauma, infection in the central nervous system, and stroke. In the United States the prevalence of epilepsy is lower in Whites than in non-Whites, although the reasons for these differences are not clear (Hauser & Hesdorffer, 1990).

Prognosis and Treatment

Remission of epilepsy, defined as 5 years without seizures, is more common among persons with generalized seizures, those with no neurological deficits, and those with a younger age of onset. Approximately 70% of persons with epilepsy can be expected to enter remission (Hauser & Hesdorffer, 1990).

The major treatment of epilepsy is *antiepilepsy medication*. Most epilepsy is well controlled with such treatment, but approximately 20% of persons continue to experience seizures despite treatment with antiepilepsy medications. When partial seizures originate from a well-defined focus in an area of the brain that could be excised without serious neurological deficits, surgery to remove the affected part of the brain is an option. Other treatments for epilepsy have been tried with limited success. The ketogenic diet, which consists of food high in fat and low in carbohydrates, has been used since the 1920s. Recently, there has been increased interest in the ketogenic diet as a treatment. Other alternative treatments used experimentally include acupuncture and biofeedback.

Quality of Life Issues

The impact of epilepsy on the quality of life can be quite diverse. Although most persons with epilepsy have few if any limitations, some have severe problems that prevent them from engaging in fully productive lives. The exact prevalence of problems is difficult to establish because most studies have been carried out on clinic samples, that is, persons with seizures that are more difficult to control. Problems most commonly found in children include anxiety, poor self-concept, social isolation, depression, behavior problems, and academic underachievement (Austin, 1996b). The most common problems found in adults with epilepsy are unemployment, depression, social isolation, and problems with adjustment. Unemployment may be twice as high in persons with epilepsy as in the general population (Hauser & Hesdorffer, 1990). Factors generally associated with quality of life problems are severe and frequent seizures, presence of other conditions or deficits, chronic condition, negative attitudes toward having epilepsy, and lack of a supportive family environment.

Nursing Practice and Research

Research to guide the nursing care of persons with epilepsy is limited. Many quality of life problems experienced by persons with epilepsy are related to a poor psychosocial adjustment to the condition. Nurses can play a key role in helping persons make a positive adjustment to epilepsy. Research is needed to understand the factors that lead to adjustment problems. Moreover, research that tests nursing interventions is needed to guide nursing care designed to prevent and reduce the development of adjustment problems. More nursing research is needed on teaching self-management to persons with epilepsy. Nurses should play a major role in

developing knowledge to provide a research base for nursing practice with persons with epilepsy.

JOAN K. AUSTIN

See also
BIOFEEDBACK TRAINING
CHRONIC ILLNESS
QUALITY OF LIFE

EPISTEMOLOGY

Epistemology is the study of the nature of knowledge and truth and is recognized as one of the two main branches of philosophy (the other being metaphysics or ontology). Epistemology investigates the origins, methods, types, and validity of knowledge. As such, these investigations are foundational to the development of a body of knowledge and thus foundational to any science. If one assumes that the primary aim of nursing research is to develop a body of knowledge that is a base for practice, then there is by necessity a direct relationship between epistemology and nursing research. One can hardly discover, find, or create knowledge without some idea of what one is looking for or when one has successfully discovered or found it.

Over the past 30 years nursing has considered epistemic questions and recognized their foundational nature. The focus of much of the work in academe during the 1960s and 1970s was nursing epistemology. For example, the discussion concerning the nature of science and theories was an attempt to explicate criteria of knowledge, and Barbara Carper's (1978) classic piece on the fundamental patterns of knowing addressed the types of knowledge central for nursing practice. The focus of much of the work in the 1980s and 1990s has been on the feminist, poststructuralist, and critical theory frameworks as foundation for the development of nursing knowledge (Omery, Kasper, & Page, 1995). These approaches recognize the social context and characteristics of the investigator as significant.

To begin any discussion of epistemology, one must recognize that the work in this area is in response to the skeptic. Justification of knowledge makes sense only against a backdrop of the possibility that this may not be the case. Such a justification becomes key to the development of nursing science and practice because of its required knowledge base. If the skeptic is right, and knowledge is not possible, then nursing science and practice are likewise not possible. Thus, this discussion is highly relevant and important to the development of nursing.

Much of what has been done in nursing is a reflection of the questions and issues raised within philosophical circles. To examine and review nursing's work to date these questions will be used: What are the origin(s) of knowledge? What are the proper methods to acquire knowledge? What are the types of knowledge? What are the criteria for knowledge?

What are the origins of knowledge? The debate in philosophical circles has concentrated on the role of reason versus the senses in the acquisition of knowledge. The rationalists (e.g., Descartes) rely on reason as the genuine source of knowledge, whereas the empiricists (e.g., Locke, Berkeley) rely mainly on experience. The nursing version of this question has centered on a debate about the inability of sense experience to provide knowledge of patient problems. For example, is it enough to view the objective signs and symptoms of pain, or do we need to know something about the patient's reflections on these sensations to know of that patient's pain? Whereas setting up the problem as dichotomous may be efficient for discussion purposes, most recognize that the extreme exclusive position (i.e., holding only empiricism or rationalism as the origin of knowledge) is not tenable.

What are the proper methods to acquire knowledge? Methods have followed the origins problem discussed above. Induction and hypothesis testing have been linked to empiricism, and deduction has been linked to rationalism. Nursing has transformed this problem into a somewhat different issue. The struggle over methods in nursing has been based in a qualitative-versus-quantitative methodological debate that in many cases missed the mark. This debate has focused on which method is appropriate for acquiring knowledge and has frequently been set up as an either/or choice. The deeper issue in this controversy, frequently not recognized, is the prior question of origins and whether knowledge is found in experience, one's reasoning, or perhaps a combination of both.

What are the types of knowledge? The main distinction made in philosophy in this century has been between knowledge gained through "acquaintance" compared with knowledge gained through "description." Knowledge gained through acquaintance is knowledge of the self through introspection or of the external world through the perception of some quality or person directly through sense data. Knowledge gained through description is knowledge gained of others without direct apprehension and includes historical and scientific knowledge. Within nursing the best example of work completed in this area is Carper's (1978) ways of knowing, conceptualized as ethics, empirics, aesthetics, and personal knowledge. Aesthetics and personal knowledge are examples of knowledge gained by acquaintance; empirical and ethical knowledge are examples of knowledge gained by description.

What are the criteria for knowledge? The criteria for knowledge have generally been tied to a discussion of justified, true belief, with two theoretical perspectives receiving attention: the coherence theory of truth and the correspondence theory of truth. However, any discussion of criteria of knowledge leads into metaphysical questions about what are the fundamental entities in the world. In nursing this discussion has taken many forms, including a debate regarding the nature of reality.

Nursing epistemology reflects the fundamental questions and distinctions that philosophers have struggled with for centuries—the origins, methods, types, and criteria of knowledge. The heart of the struggle in nursing is not only a debate about the nature of knowledge per se but also about the role of social forces in steering the questions. These debates are likely to continue as they move the discipline to new understandings about these foundational issues.

PAMELA J. SALSBERRY

See also
MIDDLE-RANGE THEORY
PHENOMENOLOGY
PHILOSOPHY OF NURSING
SCIENTIFIC DEVELOPMENT

ETHICS OF RESEARCH

The ethics of research—defined as what one morally ought to do in conducting, disseminating, and implementing the results from systematic investigation or scholarly inquiry—are determined by both traditional and changing social values. These values vary within and among cultures worldwide; therefore, all researchers must carefully avoid ethnocentrism and cultural imposition. However, within the preceding context, two points cannot be disputed: (a) all research has ethical dimensions, and (b) all research must be ethical.

Historical Perspectives

Blatant violations of human rights occurred during the 1930s to the early 1970s. They resulted in public outrages and eventually led to the establishment of the following major codes of conduct for ethical research: the Nuremberg Code, the Declaration of Helsinki, and the National Commission for the Protection of Human Subjects of Biomedical and Behavioral Research (also known as *The Belmont Report*).

The preceding events, as well as rapid advances in science and technology, led to several important policy documents and ethical guidelines for nursing research. The policy documents include the 1980 and 1995 American Nurses Association's (ANA, 1995b) *Nursing's Social Policy Statement*. The ethical guidelines for nursing research include the ANA's 1975 and 1985 *Human Rights Guidelines for Nurses in Clinical and Other Research* (ANA, 1985c), as well as the recent ANA-sponsored monograph, *Ethical Guidelines in the Conduct, Dissemination, and Implementation of Nursing Research* (Silva, 1995).

Ethics of the Conduct of Research

The conduct of research with humans imposes strong moral obligations on nurse researchers. Once the ethics of the research proposal have been approved by an institutional review board or its equivalent, subject (or participant) selection usually occurs. The decision of whom to include and exclude from a study places the following moral burdens related to the ethical principle of justice on the researcher: (a) how to weigh the ethical pros and cons of using vulnerable persons as subjects, (b) how to avoid consistently selecting subjects based solely or primarily on ease of accessibility or any personal attribute that is not essential to the study's objectives, and (c) how to avoid overuse or underuse of any group of subjects.

Once subjects are selected, they should be given sufficient and unbiased information about all important aspects of the study and their role in the study before agreeing to participate. In addition, subjects' comprehension of information about the study and the informed consent process should be ascertained initially and throughout the study as indicated. Subjects have the right to stop participation in a study at any time and without fear of retaliation. The preceding steps are based on the ethical principles of autonomy and respect for autonomy. If subjects are not autonomous, proxy consents must be obtained.

The ethical conduct of research also focuses on the ethical principle of nonmaleficence (do no harm). The researcher must understand that the possibility of harm or potential harm can occur to subjects at any time while conducting research. Therefore, the researcher must carefully weigh any benefits against therapeutic harms (i.e., harms that are necessary to produce a greater good in the conduct of the research). However, therapeutic harms always require moral justification, and under no circumstance should the subject be used solely for the advancement of science.

The ethical principle of nonmaleficence also applies to scientific misconduct. Scientific misconduct is viewed as an intended act of deception that deviates from a discipline's ethical norms. It typically takes the form of plagiarism, irresponsible authorship, data falsification, data fabrication, and questionable research practices. Nurse researchers should be familiar with their organization's policies and procedures about scientific misconduct. In addition, nurse researchers should be aware of the Office of Research Integrity, which focuses on federal regulations to deter scientific misconduct.

When an interdisciplinary team is involved in the conduct of research, the principal investigator should be clearly designated and should assume overall accountability for the study. He or she is responsible for the supervision of all team members, including research assistants. Each team member must not only assume accountability for a part of the research but also must understand how that research builds on that of other team members. Finally, all members of the interdisciplinary research team must come to a common understanding of what the ethics of research means for their study.

The conduct of research with animals also has ethical import because of past and current cruelty to them and because of the increased need for basic research in nursing. The guiding ethical principles for researchers are (a) to use animals for studies only when necessary and (b) to inflict the least amount of harm and suffering to the fewest number of animals while still attaining research objectives. In addition, only species of animals appropriate to the study should be used, and humane treatment should be accorded them. Such treatment includes, but is not limited to, good hygiene, sufficient space for species, nutritious food, clean water, and appropriate social environment. Finally, before studies with animals are conducted, researchers must obtain the approval of institutional animal care and use committees or their equivalent.

Ethics of the Dissemination of Research

Some scholars and ethicists would argue that significant research of high quality that is not disseminated presents an ethical issue because persons who could benefit from that research are denied that benefit. Furthermore, undisseminated research cannot be implemented into practice. The ethics of the dissemination of research also involves researchers and peer reviewers. Researchers as authors have an ethical obligation to clarify primary and coauthor credits as soon as possible during the preparation of a manuscript; to designate when the manuscript is part of a larger study; to submit a manuscript to only one editor at a time; to present accurate, unbiased, relevant, and appropriately documented information in the manuscript; to notify appropriate persons when scientific misconduct is detected in one's own or other studies; and to avoid the use of retracted or invalid study results.

Researchers as peer reviewers have an ethical obligation to be objective in their review of research manuscripts and timely in their return of them, to offer constructive critiques that demonstrate respect, to avoid any conflicts of interest, and to maintain anonymity of authors and confidentiality of content until the manuscript is published.

Ethics of the Implementation of Research into Practice

The research literature indicates that many practitioners of nursing lack the education needed to understand research or to use the findings in practice. This lack of knowledge and comprehension diminishes these nurses' autonomy and puts them at risk for potentially unsound ethical decision making about research utilization. Therefore, persons responsible for implementation of research into practice must assist practitioners of nursing to critique research for scientific and ethical merit and for clinical applicability. This critique includes the insight that studies typically are replicated before being implemented into practice. Furthermore, persons implementing research into practice must ensure that strong and ethical administrative support exists so that implementation can begin, continue, and terminate if necessary without causing harm to patients, staff, or the organization.

In summary, the most important aspect of research is that it be ethical. Although the ethics of research are complex, nurse researchers should respect these ethics and incorporate them into their studies or scholarly inquiries now and in the future.

MARY CIPRIANO SILVA

See also
DOCTORAL EDUCATION
INFORMED CONSENT
RESEARCH DISSEMINATION
RIGHTS OF HUMAN SUBJECTS

ETHNOGRAPHY

The term *ethnography* translates as ''the written description of the folk (people/nation).'' However, the term is currently used to refer to both a specific naturalistic research method and the written product of that method. As a research process ethnography is a comparative method for investigating human behavior and patterns of cognition through observations in the natural setting. As a written product, ethnography is a descriptive analysis of the beliefs, behaviors, norms, and patterns of a culture. The focus on culture and cultural processes is central to ethnography and is one of the ways in which ethnography differs from other naturalistic methods, such as grounded theory (the study of basic social processes) and phenomenology (the study of the individual's lived experience).

Ethnography was developed primarily by anthropologists as they sought to understand other cultures and traditions. Although ethnography remains the primary research method in anthropology, it is employed by several other disciplines, most notably sociology, psychology, education, and nursing. As the method was adopted outside anthropology, the focus of study shifted from small-scale or tribal societies to areas more closely linked with the discipline adopting the method. For example, the study of small urban social communities was undertaken by sociologists from the Chicago School, investigations of schools as microcosms of society were addressed by educators, and the health beliefs and lay systems of ethnic groups were targeted by nurse anthropologists.

In the discipline of nursing, ethnography was introduced into the literature primarily by nurse anthropologists beginning in the late 1960s. Two seminal articles appearing in *Nursing Research* by Elizabeth Byerly (1969/1990) and Antoinette Ragucci (1972/1990) laid the foundation for future nurse ethnographers. As doctoral education came to be sponsored through the nurse scientist program, several nurses chose anthropology as a focus of doctoral study. This first generation of nurse anthropologists who conducted ethnographies included pioneers such as Madeleine Leininger, Agnes Aamodt, Pamela Brink, Margarita Kay, Elizabeth Byerly, and Oliver Osborne. A second generation of nurse anthropologists included Juliene Lipson, Evelyn Barbee, JoAnn Glittenberg, Marjorie Muecke, Janice Morse, and Toni Tripp-Reimer. Later, as schools of nursing developed their own doctoral

programs, some nurse ethnographers (Mildred Roberson and Joyceen Boyle) began to be trained within schools of nursing.

Ethnographic Variation

There are several different traditions subsumed under the term *ethnography*. Each of these has emerged with its own particular historical context, and each addresses somewhat different elements of culture. However, each of these approaches may be used fruitfully in nursing research, given the appropriate research question. Although there are over a dozen distinct ethnographic traditions, examples of four will be provided to demonstrate the diversity of approaches within ethnography.

An early ethnographic approach developed by Boas around the turn of the century is termed historical particularism. The central tenets of this approach are that each culture has its own long and unique history and that all elements of a culture are worthy of documentation. A typical product of historical particularism is the creation of cultural lists or inventories. This approach has been used in nursing research to identify specific folk treatments used in ethnic groups and to generate items to be used later in the construction of structured instruments.

Functionalism is a second ethnographic tradition. Here, however, the task of ethnography is to describe the structural elements and their interrelated functioning in a culture. This approach historically has been the most widely used in nursing research. A prominent example is that of Leininger's sunrise model.

The goal of ethnoscience, a third ethnographic tradition, is to discover folk systems of classification to determine the ways people perceive and structure their thinking about their world and to identify the rules that guide decision making. The taxonomy known as the Nursing Interventions Classification (NIC) was derived by using the ethnoscience approach.

Symbolic ethnography is a fourth approach, which is rapidly growing in application in nursing research. Here, investigators view culture as a system of shared meanings and symbols. They further believe that cultural knowledge is embedded in "thick descriptions" provided by cultural members. Most nursing research that deals with informants' explanatory models use this ethnographic tradition.

Ethnographic Fieldwork

Fieldwork is the hallmark of ethnographic research. Fieldwork involves the investigator's immersion in the target community for long periods of time in order to gain understanding for contextualizing the ethnographic data. Stages of fieldwork include (a) field entry, (b) development of relationships, (c) data collection, (d) data manipulation, (e) data analysis, and (f) termination. Many of these stages, particularly (b)–(e), overlap in time.

In conducting fieldwork an investigator may employ several strategies for data collection, including participant observation, informal interviews, structured interviews, pictures and videotapes, census and other statistical data, historical documents, projective tests, and psychosocial surveys. The variety of research strategies that are appropriately employed is another way in which ethnography differs from most other naturalistic methods. Further, ethnographers may use quantitative data to augment qualitative data. However, the mainstay strategies of ethnography rest in participant observation and informant interviews. If the focus of the ethnography concerns the cognitive realm (attitudes, beliefs, schemata) of the members of the culture, then interviewing is the primary strategy. On the other hand, if the focus of the ethnography involves structural features or patterns of behavior, then observations are the primary strategy. The majority of ethnographies, however, use a combination of strategies.

Methods used for data manipulation include strategies for taking notes and making memos, coding strategies, and indexing systems. More recently, computerized software programs such as ETHNO-GRAPH and NUD*IST have been fruitfully employed to aid in the management of data. Methods used in data analysis include matrix, thematic, and domain analysis.

In summary, ethnography is a method designed to describe a culture. The ethnographer seeks to understand another way of life from the perspective of a person inside the culture (emic view). Participant observation and informant interviewing are the major strategies used during fieldwork. The specific ethnographic tradition used by the investigator determines the form of the ethnographic product.

TONI TRIPP-REIMER
JANET ENSLEIN
BARBARA RAKEL
LISA ONEGA
BERNARD SOROFMAN

See also
GROUNDED THEORY
PARTICIPANT OBSERVATION
PHENOMENOLOGY
QUALITATIVE RESEARCH
RESEARCH INTERVIEWS
 (QUALITATIVE)

EVALUATION

Evaluation is a method for measuring the effect of some purposeful action on a particular situation. It is often described as an assessment of worth. In evaluation, both anticipated and unanticipated outcomes are important and are included in the discussion of findings and the publication of results. The purpose of evaluation is to provide information for decision makers who usually have some stake in the outcome of the intervention.

Evaluation methods have been categorized along a continuum ranging from simple assessment, in which informal practices are used to look for indication of outcome, to evaluation research, in which research methods are used to allow for generalization to other comparable situations (Ingersoll, 1996a). In actuality, the use of informal practices for determining intervention outcome is never appropriate. Consequently, the term *evaluation* should suffice for all efforts in which a systematic process is used to determine the effect of some intervention on some anticipated outcome. The research component of the term is assumed. No matter what the purpose of the evaluation, the issue of rigor is always foremost, and the methods and measurement approaches used should involve the same level of attention given to any research method.

According to Rossi and Freeman (1985), evaluations serve one of three purposes: (1) to conceptualize and design interventions, (2) to monitor implementation of some intervention, or (3) to assess the utility of some action. In the first type of evaluation, studies focus on (a) the extent of the problem needing intervention, (b) who should be involved in or targeted for the intervention, (c) whether the intervention proposed will address the problem or the needs of individuals, and (d) whether the chance for successful outcome has been maximized.

In the second type of evaluation, studies focus on what is done; they generally are referred to as process evaluation studies. These studies also determine whether the intervention is reaching the targeted population and whether what is done is consistent with what was intended. Process evaluations are essential for determining cause and effect, although they are not sufficient by themselves for measuring impact. That is where evaluation researchers often get into trouble. They stop collecting data once they describe what was done; therefore, process evaluation methods have tended to be viewed with disfavor, which is unfortunate. Although they are insufficient by themselves, they are absolutely necessary for determining whether the intervention caused the outcome and if so, how—and if not, why not.

In the third type, studies determine both the degree to which an intervention has an impact and the benefit of the intervention in relation to the cost. The degree of impact is referred to as the intervention's effectiveness, and the degree of cost is referred to as its efficiency (Rossi & Freeman, 1985).

Recent writings on evaluation focus on the need for theory to guide the investigation and frame the results. Authors have identified theories that range from those targeted solely for the purposes of designing evaluations to those directed at the expected relationships between intervention and outcome. For example, behavioral theories often are used to develop interventions targeted at changing health behaviors; they also are used to select measures for determining impact. Evaluation theories, on the other hand, focus on the purpose of the study— whether it is for determining what goals or outcomes should be examined, how the treatment should be developed and delivered, or under what conditions certain events occur and what their consequences will be. Chen (1990) has defined these two types of evaluation theory as normative (the first type) and causative (the second). Normative theory is derived from prior knowledge, usual practice, or theory. Causative theory is empirically based and specifies causal relationships between intervention and outcome.

Measuring the true effect of the intervention often is difficult. Evaluation studies are subject to the same measurement and analysis problems associated with other designs. In addition, Ingersoll (1996) has summarized several others that are important to evaluation research. Among these is the need to measure the extent of the intervention introduced, which is frequently absent from reports of evaluation studies. This information assists in demonstrating cause-and-effect relationships and clarifies what magnitude of the intervention is required before an effect is seen. It also helps to prevent the potential for Type III, IV, and V evaluation errors, which affect statistical conclusion validity and generalizability validity.

Type III evaluation error is an error in probability and results in solving the wrong problem instead of the right problem. It usually occurs when the program is not implemented as planned and when insensitive measures are used to determine effect. Type IV error occurs when the evaluator provides information that is useless to stakeholders. Type V error involves confusing statistical significance with practical significance, which ultimately leads to Type IV error (Ingersoll, 1996).

Evaluation is key to measuring intervention magnitude and effect. To assure that evaluations are useful, however, steps must be taken to design them according to some meaningful conceptual framework; and close attention must be paid to maximizing the rigor of the methods, analysis, and rejection of alternative hypotheses. Approaches to quality control recommended for other nonexperimental, quasi-experimental, and experimental designs are appropriate. With attention to these aspects of the evaluation process, evaluations become an effective means for extending nursing science.

GAIL L. INGERSOLL

See also
BENCHMARKING IN HEALTH CARE
NURSING ASSESSMENT
NURSING PROCESS

EVIDENCE-BASED PRACTICE

The growing trend for the use of research findings to serve as the basis for treatment decision making represents an important departure from more traditional approaches to care such as tradition and intuition. The term *evidence-based practice* refers to the use of clinical research findings to assist health care providers in making clinical decisions about patient care. Research-based practice is designed to eliminate the freelance behavior of individual health care professionals and provide each patient with optimal care for their actual or anticipated problems.

Moving to evidence-based practice entails four distinct steps. The first step is formulating the question to be addressed. The second step is gathering the research and getting the evidence correctly synthesized. Step three is developing research-based practice protocols, and Step four is applying the protocols in practice. The first two steps are part of the research synthesis process, and the fourth step is a component of research utilization.

Formulating the Question

The first step in evidence-based practice, formulating the question, involves determining whether it is a researchable topic or if research has been done on the topic. The topic must be clearly and specifically defined (e.g., heparin vs. nonheparinized flush for intermittent intravenous devices). Also, the topic should be sufficiently narrow as to have a discrete body of research to review. This leads to the search for original and review articles to locate findings that may be useful for direct practice.

Synthesizing the Research

The volume of research and the sophistication of study designs has dramatically increased over the past 30 years. There are now over 400,000 titles indexed by the Library of Medicine each year. Using the techniques of integrative review, it is possible to organize and synthesize research on topics of interest, to identify patterns, trends, gaps, and future directions for interventions and research.

Carrying out a research synthesis entails locating and gathering information on a topic, organizing it, summarizing and interpreting it, determining the validity of it, and then determining the practice considerations. This may be a descriptive analysis or a meta-analysis of completed research. A synthesis should contain details about the studies that are reviewed, and it should provide information about the state of the science on the topic. Efforts must be made to identify the limitations and weaknesses of studies and to search for explanations of varying results across studies. Practice recommendations should cite the evidence on which they are based and state the strength of the evidence.

Protocol Development

It is possible to develop research-based practice standards and protocols for all situations for which there is adequate evidence to allow drawing of recommendations from evidence to real-life clinical situations. Research-based practice protocols are developed once the synthesis of the research is completed and the practice recommendations are gleaned. Protocols may be created by organizations, institutional committees, or individual practitioners. They may be created by government agencies such as the Agency for Health Care Policy and professional organizations such as the American Association of Critical-Care Nurses.

Formal systems and structures within individual health care settings ensure the development and implementation of research-based practice protocols. Existing structures such as standards, procedures, and quality improvement committees lend themselves to protocol development activities. The performance improvement structure can be employed for identification of problem areas as well as for encouraging the use of research-based solutions.

Protocol Application

There is an interplay between the evidence, the institution, the individual practitioner, and the patient with protocol application, and hence there will never be a "one recommendation fits all" situation. Critical appraisal is necessary in the application of research-based practice protocols. There is a need to continue to examine the research base and look to these findings to enhance patient care; however, the research evidence is not always a substitute for clinical judgment. One must always consider individual patient differences when applying research-based practice protocols.

Not every research-based practice will fit into every institution. Consideration of the level of care and the resource availability is essential. In the case of the individual practitioner, components of resistance to change also must be taken into account. Different principles and rationales used by practitioners account for individual variations in practice. These individual differences are what has spurred government bodies and individual institutions to become increasingly involved in setting policies. Evidence-based care is the application of clinical research findings in the right way, at the right place, at the right time. It requires a balance between the research evidence and the circumstances of application.

JANE H. BARNSTEINER

See also
CLINICAL NURSING RESEARCH
QUALITY OF CARE, MEASURING
RESEARCH UTILIZATION

EXPERIMENTAL RESEARCH

True experiments have the potential to provide the strongest evidence about the hypothesized causal relationship between independent and dependent variables. Experiments are characterized by manipulation, control, and randomization. The quality of experiments depends on the validity of their design (Cook & Campbell, 1979; Wasserbauer & Abraham, 1995a, 1995b).

Manipulation

Manipulation means the researcher actively initiates, implements, and terminates procedures. In most instances, manipulation is linked to the independent variable(s) under consideration. Essential to manipulation is that the researcher has complete control over the process. The researcher decides what is to be manipulated (e.g., selected nursing intervention protocols), to whom the manipulation applies (e.g., samples and subsamples of subjects), when the manipulation is to occur according to the specification of the research design, and how the manipulation is to be implemented.

Control

Manipulation implies and is impossible without researcher control over extraneous sources that might affect and lead to incorrect scientific conclusions. Control aims "to rule out threats to valid inference." It also adds precision, the "ability to detect true effects of smaller magnitude" (Cook & Campbell, 1979, p. 8). Unlike laboratory studies where total control is often possible, in clinical research control is a relative matter. The researcher has the responsibility for ensuring as much control over extraneous forces as possible.

Control also includes "the ability to determine which units receive a particular treatment at a particular time" (Cook & Campbell, 1979, p. 8). This refers to control over two *processes* that determine who gets what at what time. The first process is the researcher's use of random methods to assign subjects to treatments. This is the preferred method of exerting control over subjects and their treatment as, theoretically, it ensures that known and unknown extraneous forces inherent to subjects are dispersed equally across the different treatment options. This may not always be possible, in which case the second process comes into play—that of structuring the assignment process in such a way that major, known extraneous forces are controlled.

Commonly used design strategies include blocking, matching, and counterbalancing. In blocking the potentially confounding variable is incorporated into the study design as an independent variable. Subjects are then randomly assigned within each block. In matching, a weaker but very common method of control, the researcher identifies one or more extraneous (usually up to three) variables to be controlled. As soon as a subject is recruited for one of the treatment groups, the researcher then tries to find subjects for the other group(s) identical to the first subject on the specified matching variables. Counterbalancing occurs when the researcher is concerned that the order in which treatments are administered influences the results. When counterbalancing is used, all subjects receive all treatments; however, the order of administration of treatments is varied.

Randomization

Randomization entails two separate processes: (a) random selection of subjects from the population and (b) random assignment of subjects to treatment and control conditions. Random selection is the process of randomly drawing research subjects from the population about which the researcher wants to gain knowledge and to which the researcher hopes to generalize the findings of a study. Random assignment entails allocating sampling units (e.g., patients) to treatment and control conditions by using a decision method that is known to be random (e.g., coin toss, random drawing, use of random tables, computer-generated random sequences of options). Random selection is virtually nonexistent in intervention studies in nursing; moreover, a large proportion (55.3%) of nursing intervention studies do not even use random assignment methods (Abraham, Chalifoux, & Evers, 1992).

Validity of Designs

Cook and Campbell (1979) review four types of validity of research designs, potential threats to

each, and strategies to remedy these threats. Statistical conclusion validity addresses the extent to which, at the mathematical/statistical level, covariation is present between the independent and dependent variables (i.e., the extent to which a relationship exists between the independent and dependent variables). Internal validity refers to whether an observed relationship between variables is indeed causal or, in the absence of a relationship, that indeed there is no causal link. Construct validity of putative causes and effects refers to whether the causal relationship between two variables is indeed "the one" and tries to refute the possibility that a confounding variable may explain the presumed causal relationship. External validity refers to the generalizability of an observed causal relationship "across alternate measures of the cause and effect and across different types of persons, settings, and times" (Cook & Campbell, 1979, p. 37). Validity of any type is not a yes/no issue of whether or not it is present. Rather it is a matter of degree, determined by the extent to which the researcher has tried to cope with the various potential threats to each type of validity.

Ivo L. Abraham
Lynn I. Wasserbauer

See also
QUANTITATIVE RESEARCH
QUANTITATIVE RESEARCH
   METHODOLOGY
QUASI-EXPERIMENTAL RESEARCH

EXPLORATORY STUDIES

Exploratory studies are those that investigate little-known phenomena for which a library search fails to reveal any significant examples of prior research. These kinds of studies have been very useful in nursing research in finding out more about nursing-related problems that occur in all areas of clinical practice, administration, and academe. Typically, an exploratory study will use a small sample and will focus on one particular area of interest or on one or two variables. The following are the kinds of research questions that might indicate an exploratory study in nursing: What is it like being a pregnant teenager? What kinds of patients need home care? What health-promoting behaviors do cafeteria workers engage in? What is the lived experience of military widows?

Since the intent of exploratory research is to find out and explore unknown phenomena, it is considered Level I research (designed to elicit descriptions of a single topic or population) and is reflected in many of the early research studies in nursing. An examination of the kind of research designs that were used in nursing just 25 to 30 years ago reveals a predominance of exploratory studies and includes such examples as (a) staff nurse behaviors and patient care improvement (Gorham, 1962), (b) the self-concept of children with hemophilia and family stress (Garlinghouse & Sharp, 1968), and (c) women's beliefs about breast cancer and breast self-examination (Stillman, 1977).

Exploratory studies are still very useful. They can be found in nursing journals and are often thought of as an initial step in the description of a researchable problem. There are many reasons for an exploratory study. Such studies are particularly useful when the investigator seeks to gather baseline information on a particular variable, like loneliness, widowhood, anxiety, or culture. Other researchers may wish to investigate a process about which little is known, such as the types and meanings of caring behaviors among elderly nursing home residents or the meaning of loss of a nursing role. Exploratory research may focus on one concept that has not been described in any great detail in the literature, such as isolation or comfort, or researchers may initiate an exploratory study to determine the feasibility of or need for a more extensive study or to establish baseline information that could lay the groundwork for a future study.

Regardless of the intent of exploratory research, a flexible design that enables the researcher to investigate and examine all aspects of a phenomenon is encouraged. Flexibility in the design allows the researcher to explore all kinds of emerging ideas and to change direction, if needed, as data are collected and analyzed. Thus, exploratory research is not limited to one particular paradigm but may have either a quantitative or qualitative design. Studies that propose a hypothesis and seek to provide a measure of a phenomenon as a description employ a quantitative design. One example of an exploratory study that uses a quantitative design is described by Schaefer, Swavely, Rothenberger, Hess, and Williston (1996). In this study the researchers described the nature and frequency of sleep pattern disturbances in patients who were recovering from coronary artery bypass graft (CABG) surgery.

Qualitative or naturalistic designs generally explore phenomena in the natural setting in which they occur and are commonly carried out by using semistructured or open-ended interviewing techniques and by observation. There are multiple approaches associated with qualitative research, but they all focus on those aspects of human behavior that are difficult to measure in numerical terms. One example of an exploratory qualitative study that used a grounded theory approach is that by Fleury, Kimbrell, and Kruszewski (1995). In this study the investigators sought to describe the healing experiences of 13 women who recovered from an acute cardiac event. Verbal transcripts were analyzed to find out more about the important issues and concerns of women during the recovery process.

Any critique of exploratory research would include the facts that these studies are limited in scope and focus, are not generalizable to a larger population, and cannot be used as a basis for prediction. In spite of these limitations, however, exploratory studies are useful to uncover or discover information about little-known phenomena or single concepts, to explore the existence of relationships between and among variables, to find out more about human behavior in a naturalistic setting, to lay the groundwork for more systematic testing of hypotheses, and to determine the feasibility for a more in-depth study.

KATHLEEN HUTTLINGER

See also
DESCRIPTIVE RESEARCH
PHENOMENOLOGY
PILOT STUDY

F

FACTOR ANALYSIS

Factor analysis is a multivariate technique for determining the underlying structure and dimensionality of a set of variables. By analyzing intercorrelations among variables, factor analysis shows which variables cluster together to form unidimensional constructs. It is useful in elucidating the underlying meaning of concepts. However, it involves a higher degree of subjective interpretation than is common with most other statistical methods. In nursing research, factor analysis is commonly used for instrument development (Ferketich & Muller, 1990), theory development, and data reduction. Therefore, factor analysis is used for identifying the number, nature, and importance of factors, comparing factor solutions for different groups, estimating scores on factors, and testing theories (Nunnally & Bernstein, 1994).

There are two major types of factor analysis: exploratory and confirmatory. In exploratory factor analysis, the data are described and summarized by grouping together related variables. The variables may or may not be selected with a particular purpose in mind. Exploratory factor analysis is commonly used in the early stages of research, when it provides a method for consolidating variables and generating hypotheses about underlying processes that affect the clustering of the variables. Confirmatory factor analysis is used in later stages of research for theory testing related to latent processes or to examine hypothesized differences in latent processes among groups of subjects. In confirmatory factor analysis, the variables are carefully and specifically selected to reveal underlying processes or associations.

The raw data should be at or applicable to the interval level, such as the data obtained with Likert-type measures. Next, a number of assumptions relating to the sample, variables, and factors should be met. First, the sample size must be sufficiently large to avoid erroneous interpretations of random differences in the magnitude of correlation coefficients. As a rule of thumb, a minimum of five cases for each observed variable is recommended; however, Knapp and Brown (1995) reported that ratios as low as three subjects per variable may be acceptable. Others generally recommend that 100 to 200 is advisable (Nunnally & Bernstein, 1994).

Second, the variables should be normally distributed, with no substantial evidence of skewness or kurtosis. Third, scatterplots should indicate that the associations between pairs of variables should be linear. Fourth, outliers among cases should be identified and their influence reduced either by transformation or by arbitrarily replacing the outlying value with a less extreme score. Fifth, instances of multicollinearity and singularity of the variables should be deleted after examining to see if the determinant of the correlation matrix or eigenvalues associated with some factors approach zero. In addition, a squared multiple correlation equal to 1 indicates singularity; and if any of the squared multiple correlations are close to 1, multicollinearity exists. Sixth, outliers among variables, indicated by low squared multiple correlation with all other variables and low correlations with all important factors, suggest the need for cautious interpretation and possible elimination of the variables from the analysis. Seventh, there should be adequate factorability within the correlation matrix, which is indicated by several sizable correlations between pairs of variables that exceed .30. Finally, screening is important for identifying outlying cases among the factors. If such outliers can be identified by large Mahalanobis distances (estimated as chi square values) from the location of the case in the space defined by the factors to the centroid of all cases in the same space, factor analysis is not considered appropriate.

When planning for factor analysis, the first step is to identify a theoretical model that will guide the statistical model (Ferketich & Muller, 1990). The next step is to select the psychometric measurement model, either classic or neoclassic, that will reflect the nature of measurement error. The classic model assumes that all measurement error is random and that all variance is unique to individual variables and not shared with other variables or factors. The neoclassic model recognizes both random and systematic measurement error, which may reflect common variance that is attributable to unmeasured or latent factors. The selection of the classic or neoclassic model influences whether the researcher chooses principal-components analysis or common factor analysis (Ferketich & Muller, 1990).

Mathematically speaking, factor analysis generates factors that are linear combinations of variables. The first step in factor analysis is factor extraction, which involves the removal of as much variance as possible through the successive creation of linear combinations that are orthogonal (unrelated) to previously created combinations. The principal-components method of extraction is widely used for analyzing all the variance in the variables. However, other methods of factor extraction, which analyze common factor variance (i.e., variance that is shared with other variables), include the principal-factors method, the alpha method, and the maximum-likelihood method (Nunnally & Bernstein, 1994).

Various criteria have been used to determine how many factors account for a substantial amount of variance in the data set. One criterion is to accept only those factors with an eigenvalue equal to or greater than 1.0 (Guttman, 1954). An eigenvalue is a standardized index of the amount of the variance extracted by each factor. Another approach is to use a scree test to identify sharp discontinuities in the eigenvalues for successive factors (Cattell, 1966).

Factor extraction results in a factor matrix that shows the relationship between the original variables and the factors by means of factor loadings. The factor loadings, when squared, equal the variance in the variable accounted for by the factor. For all of the extracted factors, the sum of the squared loadings for the variables represents the communality (shared variance) of the variables. The sum of a factor's squared loadings for all variables equals that factor's eigenvalue (Nunnally & Bernstein, 1994).

Because the initial factor matrix may be difficult to interpret, factor rotation is commonly used when more than one factor emerges. Factor rotation involves the movement of the reference axes within the factor space so that the variables align with a single factor (Nunnally & Bernstein, 1994). Orthogonal rotation keeps the reference axes at right angles and results in factors that are uncorrelated. Orthogonal rotation is usually performed through a method known as varimax, but other methods (quartimax and equimax) are also available. Oblique rotation allows the reference axes to rotate into acute or oblique angles, thereby resulting in correlated factors (Nunnally & Bernstein, 1994). When oblique rotation is used, there are two resulting matrices: a pattern matrix that reveals partial regression coefficients between variables and factors and a structure matrix that shows variable to factor correlations.

Factors are interpreted by examining the pattern and magnitude of the factor loadings in the rotated factor matrix (orthogonal rotation) or pattern matrix (oblique rotation). Ideally, there are one or more marker variables, variables with a very high loading on one and only one factor (Nunnally & Bernstein, 1994), that can help in the interpretation and naming of factors. Generally, factor loadings of .30 and higher are large enough to be meaningful (Nunnally & Bernstein, 1994). Once a factor is interpreted and labeled, researchers usually determine factor scores, which are scores on the abstract dimension defined by the factor.

Replication of factor solutions in subsequent analysis with different populations gives increased credibility to the findings. Comparisons between factor-analytic solutions can be made by visual inspection of the factor loadings or by using formal statistical procedures, such as the computation of Cattell's salient similarity index and the use of confirmatory factor analysis (Gorsuch, 1983).

JACLENE A. ZAUSZNIEWSKI

See also
MEASUREMENT AND SCALES
STATISTICAL TECHNIQUES

FALLS

A fall is an unintentional slip, trip, or drop from an upright position, resulting in the person landing on the floor. A near fall occurs when an environmental object or person prevents the person falling from landing on the floor. A fall may be associated with a fear of future falls; and subsequently, persons may restrict their activities or seek assistance, making them more dependent and less active. Injury, disability, and death are serious sequelae of falls, making this a critical issue to the person, the nurse, and society.

Risk Factors

Although the etiologies for a fall and near fall may be similar, persons at risk for each type may be different. Research has focused primarily on falls. Being female and over 65 years of age have been found to be risk factors for falls in all settings (community, long-term care facility, and hospital). However, these factors have very low sensitivity for identifying those at greatest risk. Thus, the number of risk factors has been used as an indicator of the degree of risk.

Most research on falls has not been guided by theory. However, the ecological model of functional health (Hogue, 1984) describes the interaction among environment, personal competence, and cognitive appraisal as contributing to falls. This model provides direction for identifying sets of factors that predict the probability of falls. Environmental risk factors include poor lighting, low contrast among important elements of the environment (e.g., poor contrast between edge of step and next step or between floor and wall), clutter and loose objects on the floor (e.g., children and rugs). Although not commonly categorized as environmental factors, other risk factors are medications, treatments for disease, and policies of health care facilities (e.g., use of restraints or ensuring exercise). These environmental factors may increase the risk of falls, but the personal competence determines whether an individual can recover from an unexpected disruption in posture.

The physical competencies associated with falls include poor balance, poor muscle strength, postural hypotension, impaired gait, and sensory losses (e.g., poor vision, impaired proprioception, and altered vibratory and vestibular information). Psychological competencies include cognitive impairment and depression. Cognitive appraisal, as an evaluative judgment of the environment and personal competencies, contributes to falls in this model but was rarely considered in past research on falls. However, cognitive appraisal is required for persons to determine their ability to move about safely and to identify hazards in the environment; it is integral to decisions about how and when to participate in activities. The accuracy of such judgments will affect whether activities are appropriately limited or adaptations are made in performing them.

Prevention and Intervention Programs

Most fall prevention programs in hospitals and nursing homes use risk factors to identify those persons at highest risk for a fall. Nearly all fall prevention programs include age, gender, and number of medications to identify those at risk. The most frequent interventions used in these programs focus on removing hazards from the environment, instructing the person to ask for help when ambulating or transferring, and ensuring that the person can easily call for help. In some nursing homes, motion monitors are placed on a wrist or ankle that send sound signals to alert the nursing staff when the person moves. However, these programs do not address the physical and psychological factors that place a person at risk for a fall.

Removing environmental hazards in the home has had limited success in reducing the rate of falls. In the community, investigators have assessed these hazards and developed individualized interventions to remove or minimize them. Investigators noted that many elderly adults were willing to make only a few changes and were more interested in interventions directed at physical risk factors. Moreover, Northridge, Nevitt, Kelsey, and Link (1995) demonstrated only a weak association between home hazards and falls, and the vigorous elderly adult was more likely to fall when more hazards were present than was the frail elderly adult.

Research of interventions targeted to specific physical risk factors is emerging. In a meta-analysis of exercise interventions in the program Frailty and Injuries: Cooperative Studies of Intervention Techniques (FICSIT), exercise reduced the rate of falls in elderly adults in nursing homes and in the community (Province et al., 1995). These results may be attributed to exercise-related increases in muscle strength and balance and improvements in gait.

Although exercise is a promising intervention to reduce falls, multidimensional interventions targeted to physical, psychological, and environmental factors associated with falls may be more effective. For example, Tinetti and associates (1994) demonstrated the effectiveness of an intervention that included assessment of risk factors for falls in elderly adults living in the community, and then they implemented an individualized treatment program targeted at each risk factor. This multidimensional program reduced the rate of falls and can be used as a model to develop similar interventions for evaluation in other settings.

Although research on falls started in the 1950s, more is needed to develop risk assessments that have adequate sensitivity and specificity and to develop more effective interventions targeted either to the specific populations at greatest risk for falls or to specific risk factors. This knowledge will provide direction for nursing assessment and intervention.

BEVERLY L. ROBERTS

See also
GERONTOLOGIC CARE
NEUROBEHAVIORAL DISTURBANCES
   OF THE OLDER ADULT: DELERIUM
   AND DEMENTIA
PHYSICAL RESTRAINTS
   FOR THE ELDERLY
PSYCHOSOCIAL INTERVENTIONS

FAMILY CARE

The definition of family care is influenced by how it is defined and examined in research of family members caring for other family members and how it is applied in policies related to family caregivers (Gilliss & Knafl, 1997). Family care is considered normative, that is, care provided within a family role, such as parental care of a child. Family care is also care beyond the expected family roles, such as that provided to other family members due to illness, disease, or disability. Research on family caregivers, also called informal caregivers, includes five primary areas: (a) parental care of normal infants and children, (b) care of children with chronic illness, (c) care of an ill spouse, (d) an adult child caring for a parent with physical and/or mental impairment, and (e) grandparents caring for grandchildren (Campbell & Patterson, 1995; Kristjanson & Ashcroft, 1994).

The parental care of infants and children is considered normative, care expected within the parental role. This research examines the mother-infant dyad, with more limited attention to the father-child dyad. Researchers have also examined parental expectations of the spouse in contributing to the care of the infant and child.

A second area is research examining the care of the child with a chronic illness or disability. This research includes low-birthweight infants, children with chronic illness, and children defined as medically fragile and requiring technological support for survival. Although this care places additional demands on the family members and family system, it is to some degree considered normative for the parent to care for the child. Nursing research includes the examination of factors affecting families' abilities to care for these children, the development of family management styles, and patterns of family responses (Feetham, 1993; Gilliss & Knafl, 1997). Nursing research is beginning to apply models of family strengths, assets, and resiliency rather than models of deficit and burden. Investigators have examined parental decision making related to the care of children with birth defects and other health problems. It has been identified that care decisions are based on what is considered the role of a good parent in protecting and doing the best for the infant or child (Campbell & Patterson, 1995; Gilliss & Knafl).

The definitions related to caregivers is a significant variable in research of spouse caregivers. Caregiving is not always distinguished from aid or assistance given as part of the normal exchange in family relationships. As a result of family structure and norms, care provided by family caregivers may be perceived and reported differently according to the family member's gender. For example, husbands report giving more care than wives, as caregivers report activities that are not ordinary for them or that are not part of their normal responsibilities. In contrast, a wife caring for an ill husband may not consider her normative activities, such as cleaning, as caring for the spouse within the context of the his illness (Walker, Pratt, & Eddy, 1995).

For practice and research it is recommended that care activities be differentiated between instrumental activities of daily living (IADL), such as laundry, shopping, and meal preparation, and activities of daily living (ADL), such as dressing, feeding, and toileting. In the National Health Interview Survey, men aged 75 and older reported needing help with IADL less frequently than women did, but men and women reported needing assistance with ADL equally. Another consideration is that ADL is an aspect of health care, whereas IADL involves primarily household tasks. It is also important to determine, when a care activity is performed, whether the care recipient is dependent on the assistance provided (Walker, Pratt, & Eddy, 1995).

An area of increasing research of family-informal caregivers is studies examining the responses of children caring for their aging and ill parents. Conceptually, researchers have used theories of stress and burden within the context of deficit models. In these studies the dependent variables are negative outcomes such as depression, fatigue, and other physical symptoms. Reviews of caregiving research note that many studies do not differentiate family roles and gender issues. Generational expectations are an important variable in research on adult children caring for their parents. For example, daughters may distinguish tasks they do in their own households from tasks they perform to assist their parents. Cleaning one's own house is a normative task, whereas cleaning a parent's home is caregiving. For a son caregiver, differentiating both gender and intergenerational caregiving tasks is important (Walker, Pratt, & Eddy, 1995).

A fifth area is grandparents caring for grandchildren. These studies tend to be descriptive and to identify the burdens experienced by men and women who assume the care of their grandchildren. As grandparents, rather than parents, these caregivers may not be eligible for societal sanctions and

resources, such as aid to dependent children. They may be elderly or in compromised health and may be grieving the loss of their own child or his or her inability to care for the children. Grandparents may also assume IADL for their children and ADL for their grandchildren when a grandchild is ill or disabled.

The samples used in research on family caregiving have tended to be purposive and convenience of families where a member assumes care. Quantitative and qualitative methodologies have been used, with some studies including interventions. A limited number of the family care studies apply family theoretical frameworks or conduct the studies within the context of the family. For example, using a theoretical framework of stress, some measures of family-related variables may be added, rather than framing the research within a family construct such as hardiness. Traditionally in studies of caregiving, data are collected from the caregiver and the care recipient; however, attention has not been given to these individuals as family members within family systems. In addition, a concept receiving limited attention in the context of family care is the health-promotion, disease-prevention roles of families (Feetham, 1993).

To inform policymakers, data are needed to document the incidence when family members are unwilling or unavailable for care. All areas of family care research can add significant knowledge to our understanding of families and of the interventions necessary to support families in caregiving (Feetham, 1993).

SUZANNE L. FEETHAM

See also
CAREGIVER
CHRONIC CONDITIONS IN CHILDHOOD
FAMILY HEALTH
PARENTING RESEARCH IN NURSING

FAMILY CAREGIVING TO FRAIL ELDERS

Family caregiving to frail elders is defined as the processes by which family members provide care, support, and assistance to elders who require help because of illness, memory problems, or frailty. For many years the family has provided the majority of long-term care to frail elders in community settings. Indeed, the health care system could not meet the needs of frail elders without the care provided by informal caregivers. In the past decade, changes in health and social policies have meant that the family is increasingly expected to assume a role in the acute care of elders in the home.

Because of their expertise in care processes, nurses are in a position to assist families in developing the knowledge and skill needed to provide care to frail older family members. Assisting families in this way has traditionally been the responsibility of home health nurses, but the increasing use of outpatient strategies to manage complex health problems in combination with early hospital discharge and use of skilled nursing facilities for acute care means that nurses in many settings have the potential to influence family caregiving.

Research on family caregiving to frail elders in the United States began in the late 1970s with the publication of a cross-national survey that debunked the myth that the American family abandons its elders to nursing home care (Shanas, 1979). Since that time, data from multiple national studies indicate that families provide over 80% of the personal and medically related care given to community-residing elders and that most caregivers are women, spouses, or adult children, retired and in poorer health than would be expected based on their age and gender. Primary caregivers often spend more effort in caregiving activities than a full-time job requires.

The first wave of research on caregiving focused on describing its negative effects on the caregiver, known variously as burden, strain, and stress. This work provided unequivocal evidence that caregiving for elders is difficult for the caregiver. It also led to an understanding of some of the factors that predict the negative responses to caregiving. Being female rather than male and being the spouse of the care receiver rather than a nonspouse are linked to higher levels of strain. High elder dependency is associated with higher levels of strain. Caregivers who provide more care report more strain. Higher levels of such variables as affection,

reciprocity, mutuality—all related to the quality of the relationship between the caregiver and care receiver—are associated with lower levels of strain. Likewise, higher levels of feelings of preparedness for caregiving are associated with lower levels of strain.

Less is known about positive responses to caregiving. Some studies indicate that caregivers experience satisfaction with and personal meaning from the caregiver role. Such rewards of caregiving are associated with lower levels of strain.

The quality of care provided by families needs further exploration. To date, most of the work in this area has focused on the recognition of poor-quality care and abuse—two important areas for nursing. Nursing interventions, however, are often focused on improving the quality of care provided by families; thus, we need a better understanding of good-quality family care.

The phenomenon of caregiving to persons with dementia has been explored more fully than caregiving to other special populations. Families find the secondary symptoms of dementia (e.g., wandering, agitation) particularly difficult. Increasingly, researchers are investigating caregiving in other special populations (e.g., cancer, Parkinson's disease). Recent studies have compared caregiving processes by race and ethnicity. This is an extremely complex area of research. For example, there is some evidence that caregiving processes are similar between Black and White families; measures used in these studies were developed in the dominant White culture and may not be appropriate for other groups. Concepts such as filial piety have been identified in studies of family care in Asian cultures. Evidence supports the existence of both similarities and differences in caregiving by culture and national origin.

Two excellent summaries of early caregiving research can be found in Horowitz (1985) and Givens and Givens (1991). The interested reader is referred to these sources for thoughtful analyses of the research on family caregiving in relation to nursing research and practice.

Although numerous theoretical perspectives have been brought to bear on family caregiving, two have had a major influence on knowledge development in nursing: theories of stress and coping and interactionist theories. Researchers who focus on family caregiving to elders with dementia and on the caregiver have tended to approach this area from the intraindividual perspective of stress and coping theory, whereas researchers interested in explicating caregiving processes and on improving care to the frail elder through work with the family have used the interpersonal interactionist perspective. Theoretical perspectives have influenced instrument development in caregiving. Measures of such concepts as caregiver stress and burden are used by researchers focused on stress and coping. Measures of such concepts as role strain and rewards are used by researchers focused on interactional caregiving processes.

Finally, more attention is now being given to interventions with caregivers or caregiving families; see Gallagher, Lovett, and Zeiss (1989), Collins, Givens, and Givens (1994), and Archbold and Stewart (1996) for a review of caregiving interventions. Nurses have been active in developing, administering, and evaluating psychoeducational interventions, expanded in-home care, transitional care models, and cognitive stimulation. Nurses are an important component of health services interventions for frail elders and their families (e.g., the channeling demonstrations, the social health maintenance organization). One conclusion from reviewing this work is that nurses have a key role in preparing and supporting families in caregiving activities and in identifying high-risk caregiving situations. Because of the increasing reliance on the family for care of frail elders, it is possible that too great a burden has been placed on the smallest social unit in society. It is critical that we turn our attention to understanding the costs to families of such changes in policy.

PATRICIA G. ARCHBOLD
BARBARA J. STEWART

See also

CAREGIVER
COPING
NEUROBEHAVIORAL DISTURBANCES
   OF THE OLDER ADULT: DELERIUM
   AND DEMENTIA
STRESS

FAMILY HEALTH

No universal definition of *family* has been adopted by the legal and social systems, family scientists, or the clinical disciplines that work with or study families. How the family is defined determines the factors that will be examined to evaluate the health of individual family members and the family unit. When examining health in the context of the family, the family can be defined as constituting the group of persons acting together to perform functions required for the survival, growth, safety, socialization, and health of family members. These functions include the care of ill and disabled members (Campbell & Patterson, 1995). Health and well-being are basic concepts to nursing science and practice. Research on health has focused primarily at the level of the individual and has demonstrated the interdependence between the health of the individual family members and the family (Campbell & Patterson, 1995; Feetham, 1997). Less is known of health from the family's perspective, as the interpretation of wellness and illness in relation to the family unit is a recent phenomenon.

Identification of healthy families has focused on family interaction patterns, family problem solving, and patterns of responses to changes in the family system. Factors influencing family health include (a) genetic forces; (b) physiological and psychological responses of individual family members; (c) cultural influences; and (d) the physical, social, economic, and political environments, including resources. Researchers have shown that health and risk factors cluster in families because members often have similar diets, activity patterns, and behaviors, such as smoking and alcohol abuse, as well as a common physical environment. These definitions and concepts of family health provide a framework for determining measurable outcomes of family health while also accounting for the diversity in family structure (Feetham, 1997).

The definition of family health is also consistent with a concept included across many definitions of health—that it is a dynamic state of being in which the developmental and behavioral potential of an individual is realized to the fullest extent possible (Broering, 1993; World Health Organization, 1976). Therefore, effective interventions with families incorporate an understanding of what health means to individual family members and to the family as a unit and how the environment influences their health actions. The family has been described as the primary social agent in the promotion of health and well-being (Campbell & Patterson, 1995; Carnegie Council on Adolescent Development, 1995); therefore, our knowledge of the family and its relationship to the health of its individual members is central to research related to health promotion and to families experiencing illness and disability (National Institute of Nursing Research, 1993; Pender, 1990).

SUZANNE L. FEETHAM

See also
**ADOLESCENCE
FAMILY CARE
FAMILY THEORY AND RESEARCH
GENETICS IN NURSING RESEARCH
PARENTING RESEARCH IN NURSING**

FAMILY THEORY AND RESEARCH

Family refers to any group whose members are related to one another through marriage, birth, or adoption. Burgess's (1926) description of a family as a unit of interacting personalities is still relevant to how families are viewed today. Because of the variety of family forms, theorists and researchers should provide their own definitions of family.

Significance for Nursing

Nursing has long been interested in families as the context for individual members and has focused more recently on the family as a whole. Families have been a component of studies of psychiatric illness, caregiving, violence, adaptation to chronic illness in both children and adults, and cardiac conditions and other acute illnesses. Family transitions, including grieving, transition to parenthood for adolescent mothers and married couples, and adaptation to divorce, remarriage, and stepfamilies, also have been studied. Nurses have published reports

in major family journals as well as in nursing research and specialty journals and the new *Journal of Family Nursing*.

Family Theory

Scholars from various disciplines have studied families, using diverse approaches. Theories presented here (except for stress theory) are based on descriptions provided by Klein and White (1996).

The central focus in exchange theory is on the individual and what motivates his or her actions. Individuals are viewed as rational and self-interested, seeking to maximize rewards and avoid costs. Individuals compare their own situation to others in the same circumstances and to others in different circumstances. In exchange theory the family is viewed as a collection of individuals. The family group is considered to be a source of rewards and costs for individual members. Exchange theory could be used by nurse researchers to investigate the processes of family negotiation and problem solving.

Like exchange theory, conflict theory assumes that individuals are motivated by self-interest. Individuals compete for scarce resources, which include knowledge, skills, techniques, and materials. Resources provide a potential base for the exercise of power. Conflict within the family is seen as the result of inequity of resources among individuals. Because conflict is both endemic and inevitable, a primary focus in the study of families is how they manage conflict. Haber and Austin (1992) used conflict theory to explore strategies and outcomes of marital decision making.

Concepts of symbolic interactionism include interaction patterns, meanings and definitions, symbols, sense of self, and role expectations. Socialization is the process by which individuals acquire the symbols, beliefs, and attitudes of their culture. Individuals construct a sense of self and meanings for events and things through interactions with other people and with the environment. Role involves each person's adjusting behavior to what he or she thinks the other person is going to do. Children and adults have particularly significant interactions in the context of the family. Likewise, roles that develop within the family are a crucial component of the individual's self-image. Killeen's (1993) transactional model of the self reflects factors important in symbolic interactionism.

The family as a whole is the focus of family systems theory. All parts of the system are interconnected, and therefore, changes in one part of the system influence all other parts of the system. Subsystems are smaller units of the system, such as individuals and dyads. Boundaries define who participates in the family and who participates in each subsystem. Boundaries exist between family members, between subsystems, and between the family system and the external environment. The degree of permeability of boundaries (open or closed) refers to the extent of impediments to the flow of information and energy. A homeostatic system dynamically maintains equilibrium by feedback and control. Woods, Haberman, and Packard (1993) utilized family systems theory in their study of family functioning when the mother is chronically ill.

The central concept in the ecological approach is adaptation. The child always develops in the context of family-type relationships, and that development is the outcome of the interaction of the person's genetic environment with the immediate family and eventually with components of the environment. The individual is embedded in four nested systems. The microsystem is the immediate setting in which the person fulfills his or her roles, such as family, school, or place of employment. The mesosystem refers to the interrelations between two or more settings in which the developing person actively participates. The exosystem consists of external settings that do not include the person as an active participant but instead include systems (such as the legal system) that affect the person's immediate settings. Macrosystem refers to culture. Bishop and Ingersoll (1989) used the ecological framework in their research on the effects of marital conflict and family structure on self-concepts of children.

Family development theory focuses on systematic changes experienced by families as they move through stages of their life course. Family stage is an interval of time in which the structure and interactions of role relationships in the family are noticeably distinct from other periods of time.

Shifts from one family stage to another are called transitions. Family development theory emphasizes the dimensions of time and change. Using family development theory, Mercer, Ferketich, DeJoseph, May, and Sollid (1988) investigated the effect of stress on family functioning during pregnancy.

The double ABCX model is an extension of Hill's (1958) original ABCX family stress model, in which A refers to the stressor event and related hardships, B refers to resources, and C to perception of A (McCubbin & Patterson, 1983). The crisis, X (the amount of disruptiveness or disorganization), emerges from the interaction of the event, resources, and perception of the event. The family's accumulation of life events and added stressors over time (Aa, pileup of demands) influences family adaptation both directly and indirectly through Bb (adaptive resources) and Cc, which is the perception of X, Aa, and Bb. Austin's (1996a) study of family adaptation to childhood epilepsy is based on a modification of the double ABCX model.

Research

Research on families typically is an effort to test theoretical propositions or to develop theory. Although family research reflects different theoretical orientations, a common concern is the most appropriate unit of analysis. Is the concept of interest a property of the individual, dyad, or the family as a whole? For example, can families as a whole or only individual members perceive? Another recurring issue in family research is how to construct family variables if discrepant reports are provided by different members of the same family. As family scholars address these problems, they can better explain the complexities of family life and ultimately provide guidance for intervention.

LINDA C. HABER

See also
FAMILY HEALTH
PARENT-ADOLESCENT
**   RELATIONSHIPS/COMMUNICATION**
PARENTING RESEARCH IN NURSING
PRESCHOOL CHILDREN
SOCIAL SUPPORT

FATIGUE

Fatigue is a universal symptom associated with most acute and chronic illnesses. It also is a common complaint among otherwise healthy persons and is cited as one of the most prevalent presenting symptoms in primary care practices. Defining fatigue, however, has challenged scientists for years. To date, no biological marker of fatigue has been identified. Because nursing is interested in symptoms and symptom management, fatigue is of major concern for nurse researchers and clinicians. Fatigue was named one of the top four symptoms for study by an expert panel on symptom management convened by the National Institute of Nursing Research.

The North American Nursing Diagnosis Association (NANDA, 1994) defines fatigue as "an overwhelming sustained sense of exhaustion and decreased capacity for physical and mental work" (p. 62). A number of nurse researchers have studied fatigue and have offered various proposals for categorizing it. Researchers at the Center for Biobehavioral Studies of Fatigue Management at the University of Kansas School of Nursing offer an alternative view of fatigue: "The awareness of a decreased capacity for physical and/or mental activity due to an imbalance in the availability, utilization, and/ or restoration of resources needed to perform an activity" (Aaronson et al., in press). This definition is not inconsistent with the NANDA definition. However, it adds a generic understanding of potential causes of fatigue, which may vary in different situations, to facilitate studying the mechanisms of fatigue in different clinical conditions. This addition also allows for a clearer conception of fatigue as a biobehavioral phenomenon.

Investigators who have focused on categorizing fatigue generally distinguish acute fatigue from chronic fatigue. Piper (1989) identifies acute fatigue as protective, linked to a single cause, of short duration, with a rapid onset, perceived as normal, generally occurring in basically healthy persons, with minimal impact on the person and usually relieved by rest. On the other hand, chronic fatigue is perceived as abnormal, has no known function or purpose, occurs in clinical populations, may have many causes, is not particularly related to exertion, persists over time, has an insidious onset, is not usually relieved by rest, and has a major impact on the person (see Potempa, 1993, for a review of chronic fatigue).

In the research and clinical literature, fatigue related to childbearing (see Milligan & Pugh, 1994, for a review) and fatigue related to cancer (see Irvine, Vincent, Bubela, Thompson, & Graydon, 1991; Smets, Garssen, Schuster-Uitterhoeve, & de Haes, 1993; Winningham et al., 1994, for reviews) have received the most attention. However, even these areas remain largely understudied and poorly understood. Although fatigue has been studied in a number of chronic illnesses, such as multiple sclerosis and rheumatoid arthritis, cancer-related fatigue is somewhat unique in that it is often associated with the treatment for cancer (both radiation and chemotherapy) that is most troublesome to the individual. In fact, fatigue associated with cancer treatment has been cited as a major reason for prematurely discontinuing treatment.

One of the more puzzling manifestations of fatigue is what is currently called chronic fatigue syndrome (CFS). Chronic fatigue syndrome is a diagnosis used for cases of severe and persistent fatigue for which no specific cause has been identified (see Fukuda et al., 1994, for the current full-case definition of CFS). Under varying names (e.g., neurasthenia, myalgic encephalomyelitis, postinfectious or postviral syndrome) a similar syndrome of unexplained, chronic, persistent fatigue has been documented in the literature since the late 19th century. Preliminary evidence from controlled studies and extensive clinical descriptions point to both a hypothalamic-pituitary-adrenal disorder (Demitrack et al., 1991) and an immune system disregulation (Bearn & Wessley, 1994) as likely central mechanisms operating in CFS.

Difficulty in studying, understanding, and treating fatigue is largely due to its ubiquitous nature and the unknown, multiple causes of fatigue. Moreover, untangling the relationship between fatigue and depression further confounds investigations of fatigue. Although fatigue is an identified symptom of depression as identified by the American Psychiatric Association, long-standing chronic fatigue, unrelated to an existing affective disorder, may precipitate depression. Further, although the hypothalamic-pituitary-adrenal axis is implicated in both CFS and depression, some evidence suggests a different pattern of neuroendocrine disturbance in CFS from that seen in depression (Ray, 1991).

A lack of consistent, valid, and reliable measures of fatigue also contributes to problems studying and understanding fatigue. Early work on fatigue in the workplace was conducted by industrial psychologists, hygienists, and the military. Consequently, these measures focused on healthy individuals and fatigue experienced at the time of measurement. More recent concern about the debilitating and distressing health effects of fatigue in clinical populations has led to the development of other measures, targeting fatigue in ill persons.

However, because there is no known biochemical test or marker for fatigue and because fatigue is first and foremost a subjective symptom, most measures of fatigue in healthy or ill populations rely on self-reports. Although a number of different self-report measures of fatigue can be found in the current literature, each taps a different aspect of fatigue or assesses fatigue in a specific clinical condition. When different measures of fatigue are used in different studies, it is difficult to know if discrepant findings result from substantive differences in fatigue or simply to the differences in the measures.

In sum, although there may be many causes of fatigue, each may ultimately be traced to a disruption in either the hypothalamic-pituitary-adrenal axis, the immune system, or both. If so, then continued investigations into CFS may lead to a better understanding of fatigue in other, clearly diagnosed clinical problems. Until work is done that suggests specific treatments for fatigue, nursing intervention studies that target ameliorating fatigue in different clinical populations must continue. Although rest generally alleviates acute fatigue, currently there are no known methods to eliminate the fatigue that plagues persons with various chronic illnesses or those whose fatigue is secondary to the treatments for their chronic illness. Using standardized measures, fatigue is a fertile area for nursing research.

LAUREN S. AARONSON

See also
CHRONIC ILLNESS

JOB STRESS
PREGNANCY
YOUNG WOMEN AND DEPRESSION

FEMINIST RESEARCH METHODOLOGY

Definition

Feminist research methodology refers to a perspective that espouses research on women, by women, and for women, with the use of rules for gathering evidence whereby feminist principles are applied to research. Feminist research methodology does not seek merely to be nonsexist, but to take person's lived experience as the methodological starting point for all knowledge-development efforts bearing on girls and women. This means refusing to rely solely on the loosely structured beliefs that pass for "givens" or "common sense" truths about the phenomenon under study.

By refusing to assume beforehand that any beliefs about women's experiences are necessarily true, the expectation is that the researcher is better prepared to *see clearly*, to be critical, and to complete a systematic investigation not only of their diseases but dis-eases. In women's health research it is difficult to rely on data from earlier studies of the menstrual cycle, exercise, or child rearing because of the many recent changes in the social context. For example, the notion that the "empty nest" is associated with depression in midlife women is a conceptualization that was embedded in a world where the majority of women did not work outside the family.

History

In the past three decades, women's health research as a subset of women's studies has become distinct and with it an emphasis both on conducting nonsexist research (e.g., eschewing traditional biases) and on asserting a new sensibility that positively values women's points of view and a holistic approach to health.

There has been much to critique in traditional research methods. Methods have not distinguished sex differences from gender-related differences (e.g., differences due to lack of opportunity rather than genetic ability) and have overemphasized gender differences when they account for relatively little variance. There has been a systematic preference for the so-called objective perspective of the (usually male) researcher over that of the female subject. The actor-observer effect, disclosed in tests of attribution theory, noted that actors make more use of situational attributions than do observers, so it is not surprising that male researchers have described some single mothers as "overprotective" when those mothers would have emphasized the demands placed on them by an absent father. Because women's behavior has traditionally been explained in terms of male-as-norm theoretical frameworks, female behavior has been pejoratively labeled, describing as dependent the woman whose husband is the breadwinner and not labeling in that way the man whose wife bakes the bread, cleans, and cares for their children. Indeed, research on women has been defined largely in terms of childbearing and child rearing.

Sometimes sample selection has been biased by using women employed in low-level positions and men employed in high-status professions to represent employed women and men. The possibility that the gender of the experimenter and choice of setting may have differential effects on women and men has been ignored; for example, young male interviewers in a "macho" cardiac rehabilitation setting may not be sensitive to how alien older women feel in such an environment. Inappropriate instruments have been used to evaluate women's behavior, for example, the Masculinity-Femininity (Mf) scale of the Minnesota Multiphasic Personality Inventory to operationalize femininity in women when the validity items for establishing femininity originally involved a criterion group of gay men. Because "main" effects have been sought over "interaction" effects, women have been excluded from research when they acted in unexpected ways (Denmark, Russo, Frieze, & Sechzer, 1988).

New Methodological Directions

Feminist research methodology has encouraged some new positive directions. Women have been encouraged to develop research careers. Federal guidelines now require women to be included as subjects in all studies related to their experience, and men are not to be excluded as subjects when the focus is on the traditional concerns of females. Context-stripping methods have been called into question because they ignore the extent to which social integration is associated with lower rates of disease and quality of life; grounded-theory methods have been encouraged because they permit the individual to discuss fully the lived experience (Keddy, Sims, & Stern, 1996). The emphasis is increasingly on doing research *with* women rather than *on* women.

Feminist Methodology in Nursing Research

Because one of its basic tenets is the person-environment fit, nursing has long been concerned about the importance of context in understanding health behavior. Nurses were among the first to question a preference for the so-called objective view of the researcher over the subjective view of the patient and to emphasize the lived experience (MacPherson, 1983; McBride & McBride, 1981). They took the lead in menstrual cycle research, which underscored the extent to which there is more to midlife women's health than menopause, and in the use of the diary/health journal as a way to analyze the complexity of women's reality (Woods, 1993). The establishment of the National Center for Nursing Research in 1986, along with the concurrent growth of doctoral nursing programs, meant that there were more women scientists to approach seriously women's health and caregiving (rather than cure-finding) research. Nursing also has extended the notion of a feminist research methodology to include the development of a feminist pedagogy in teaching (Gray, 1995).

Future Directions

Although nonsexist research methods have gained ground when judged in terms of the most egregious biases, and the concerns of women are no longer automatically given short shrift, the prevailing scientific model still reifies an empiricist, positivist, objective paradigm. Feminist researchers have challenged the very nature of science and how we search for knowledge, but reductionism remains dominant in the sciences. It remains true that context-stripping methods are easier to implement, particularly for the beginning researcher who does not have the skills to handle multifactorial designs.

Matters are complicated by the fact that some qualitative researchers discuss their approach with more enthusiasm for their methods than specificity about why their methods are appropriate to explore a particular phenomenon. Even feminists have tended to treat women as a monolithic group, thus ignoring the special concerns of minority women, who are even more affected by contextual matters (e.g., poverty, violence, and racism) than their White sisters. There remains a significant discrepancy between the methods espoused by feminist researchers and those actually utilized. Nevertheless, the future will increasingly demand that health researchers use biopsychosocial models to frame their programs of study and develop new ways of analyzing human experience within interlocking contexts.

Angela Barron McBride
Sara Campbell

See also
ATTRIBUTION THEORY
GENDER RESEARCH
GROUNDED THEORY
RESEARCH CAREERS
VULNERABLE POPULATIONS

FETAL MONITORING

Fetal assessment is part of the process of providing prenatal care. It involves early identification of real or potential problems and enables the achievement of the best possible obstetric outcomes. Fetal assessment involves low-tech and high-tech modalities such as fetal movement counting (kick counts), electronic fetal monitoring (EFM), nonstress tests (NST), vibroacoustic stimulation (VAS), auscultated acceleration tests (AAT), contraction stress tests (CST), amniotic fluid index (AFI), biophysical profiles (BPP), and Doppler velocimetry. The basis

for all of these testing modalities is evaluation of certain biophysical parameters related to the developmental and health-related patterns of fetal behavior in utero. Adequate uteroplacental function is necessary for these patterns of healthy behavior. Uteroplacental insufficiency (UPI) has been shown to be the cause of at least two thirds of antepartal fetal deaths (Gegor & Paine, 1992).

Electronic fetal monitoring will serve as the focal point for this discussion as it is the basic intervention used in fetal assessment. Electronic fetal monitoring as an electronic data gathering and data processing device was developed during the 1960s. By the end of the 1970s almost all major obstetrical units had at least one monitor, and 70% of all women in labor in the United States were monitored (Bassett, 1996). In addition to its use in monitoring fetal status during labor, modifications of EFM have been developed for antepartal fetal assessment to determine optimal fetal development and diagnose conditions of actual or potential fetal compromise (e.g., NST, CST, VAS, BPP).

Currently, controversies rage over the appropriate place of EFM in obstetric care. It was introduced into clinical practice on the basis of animal studies and became widely used, with no controlled assessment of its effectiveness in improving the outcome of delivery (Smith, Ruffin, & Green, 1993). It was supposed to provide more accurate fetal assessment with the accompanying prompt identification of fetal compromise. Early retrospective studies suggested that EFM was associated with fewer infants born with low Apgar scores, lower neonatal mortality rates, and better neurological outcomes. More recent, better controlled, prospective studies have failed to demonstrate improved fetal outcomes. What was discovered was that an increased incidence of invasive procedures and cesarean deliveries occurred among monitored women (Smith et al., 1993).

Larsen (1996) discussed the probable reasons that the use of EFM has not been the shining beacon of perinatal assessment it was purported to be. He states two reasons: obstetricians had unrealistic expectations, and the clinical use was more difficult than anticipated. Later studies have shown that intrapartal events do not play as important a role as earlier thought in the pathogenesis of brain damage in neonates. Asphyxia could not be consistently linked with specific heart rate patterns. Likewise, no statistical association between acidosis and developmental outcomes have been supported. These later problems are probably related to harm or changes that occur before labor ensues (Larsen).

The major problem is the risk of misinterpretation of the EFM tracing. Monitored women are subjected to unnecessary interventions if normal variations are mistaken for signs of asphyxia. Additionally, unsatisfactory technique gives a false perception of safety and increases the risk of erroneous decisions (Larsen, 1996). Current concerns are focused on the best ways to prevent or reduce inappropriate use of EFM and develop the best ways to assess and monitor fetal development and safety in labor.

The American College of Obstetricians and Gynecologists (ACOG) and the Association of Women's Health, Obstetrical, and Neonatal Nurses (AWHONN, formerly Nurses Association of the American College of Obstetricians and Gynecologists [NAACOG]) have developed standards and guidelines for practice concerning fetal assessment and the use of EFM (ACOG, 1989; NAACOG, 1991). These standards of practice determine the accepted conduct of antepartal and intrapartal care and provide the core of safe practice. It is the responsibility of all nursing and medical health care providers to be proficient in the use and interpretation of EFM and other intervention modalities employed in perinatal health care delivery. Other recommendations include using EFM as a diagnostic rather than a screening tool and not as a substitute for supportive health care personnel. Additionally, specific indications, such as oxytocin induction or augmentation of labor, an abnormal fetal heart rate by auscultation, twin gestation, hypertension or preeclampsia, dysfunctional labor, meconium staining, vaginal breech delivery, diabetes, or prematurity, should be present (Smith et al., 1993).

Further prospective studies should be conducted to try to determine the optimal balance of intermittent or continuous EFM and auscultation and the other modalities of fetal assessment and pregnancy management. Rigorous study protocols and close attention to the principles of scientific inquiry are needed so that study results will be reliable and valid. The major concerns of perinatal care should be optimal and cost-effective outcomes for mother and infant, without concern for protection of the caregiver from litigious actions.

SUSAN M. MIOVECH

See also
NICU PRETERM INFANT CARE
PREGNANCY
PREVENTION OF PRETERM AND LOW-BIRTHWEIGHT BIRTHS

FEVER/FEBRILE RESPONSE

Definitions

Fever is an abnormally high body temperature that occurs as a host response to pyrogens. A synonym for fever is pyrexia; hyperpyrexia refers to high fever. Body temperature elevation is only one of the complex of signs and symptoms of the febrile response. Febrile temperatures and associated rise in cytokines may have some beneficial effects in fighting infectious disease. Pyrogens cause the hypothalamus to readjust to a higher set point range (see Thermal Balance), but thermoregulatory function remains intact. This differentiates fever from hyperthermia, a potentially lethal condition in which neurologically damaging high temperatures result from dysfunctional thermoregulatory functions.

Febrile episodes are characterized by three phases, reflecting the rise and fall of circulating pyrogens. Initially, the chill phase occurs when thermostatic mechanisms are activated to raise body temperature to the newly elevated set point range. Vasoconstriction decreases skin perfusion, conserving heat but making the skin feel cold. Shivering generates heat and is stimulated by sensory inputs that detect discrepancies between existing temperatures and the new set point. The plateau phase follows when body temperature rises to the new set point level and warming responses cease. Finally, falling pyrogen levels lead to the defervescence phase, characterized by diaphoresis and vasodilation.

Relevance to Nursing

Although fever management of a palliative nature is well established in nursing care, methods of care have changed little over the past century. Early traditions reflected limited state of scientific knowledge and were empirically based. Elevated body temperature was thought to be the cause, rather than the result, of febrile illness. Intervention was therefore geared toward lowering body temperature. Current clinical practice lags behind recent discoveries that fever offers beneficial host responses. Cooling the body is counterproductive, is distressful to patients, and may cause compensatory overwarming. Recently, nurse researchers began testing nursing interventions based on thermoregulatory dynamics to (a) insulate thermosensitive areas of skin from cooling to reduce shivering, (b) facilitate heat loss from less thermosensitive regions without chilling, and (c) restore fluid volume and improve capillary blood flow to skin. Fear of neural damage resulting from protein denaturation during high fevers is justified at temperatures over 42°C.

However, true fevers are often self-limiting and remain well below this level. Body temperatures of about 39°C may have immunostimulant and antimicrobial effects. This makes comfort the primary reason for giving antipyretic drugs in low-grade fever. Shivering is more easily stimulated during fever, even with mild cooling. In extremely high fevers, aggressive cooling with conductive cooling blankets and ice packs causes vigorous febrile shivering. Shivering is physically exhausting and distressful to patients. Nurses are usually the consistent clinical observers of patients' body temperature, febrile patterns, physiological correlates, and sensory responses; thus, issues of measurement are of significance to nursing practice and research (see Thermal Balance).

Historical Perspective

Febrile symptoms are nonspecific responses to both infectious and host defense activities, so many symptoms and interventions are generalizable. Although research in fever management in other disci-plines tends to be concerned with controlling underlying infection with drugs, nursing research has focused on managing symptomatology of and responses to fever and fever therapy, regardless of etiology. Nurse researchers began, in the early 1970s, to examine methods of cooling the body during fever without stimulating shivering or causing temperature drift. Some were concerned about metabolic and cardiorespiratory effects of fever on vulnerable patients with cancer or HIV infection. The set point theory of temperature regulation was central to intervention studies, but mechanisms were not well understood until an endogenous pyrogen was postulated. Identification of endogenous pyrogens, cytokines, and other biological messengers continues and offers measurable biomarkers of fever as a host response.

Major Studies

Responsible nursing research on fever is well supported by scientific underpinnings in physiology, physics, biochemistry, and psychoneuroimmunology. Studies are often interdisciplinary and diverse in nature, varying from laboratory studies with humans and animals to clinical studies in hospitals and homes. Little research exists to clarify the ideal time or schedule for monitoring fever patterns even though circadian variations in temperature are well documented. Samples and colleagues (Samples, Van Cott, Long, King, & Kersenbrock, 1985) found that the 6 p.m. temperature of adult hospitalized medical-surgical patients effectively identified 30 of 38 patients who were febrile at any time during the day.

Such may not be the case when patients have abnormally expressed levels of cytokines, as in HIV disease. Taliaferro and Richmond (1996) found routine once-a-shift monitoring inadequate to capture fever episodes in 50 HIV-infected adults hospitalized for febrile illnesses. No temperature from a particular time of day predicted whether a fever had occurred during that 24-hour period. Only 15 febrile episodes were found with routine measurements, but 52 were detected with 2-hour monitoring.

Studies of febrile symptom management by Holtzclaw (1996) evolved from earlier intervention tests to suppress drug-induced, febrile shivering in patients with cancer. An intervention to insulate thermosensitive skin regions during the chill phase of fever was not only effective in reducing shivering (see Shivering), but it improved comfort. This preliminary work provided the basis for a comprehensive febrile symptom management protocol, currently being tested with febrile HIV-infected persons in the hospital and at home. Early findings document the effects of fever on hydration and cardiorespiratory effort (Holtzclaw, 1996). Insulative coverings are used as interventions to suppress chilling, and systematic oral fluid replacement is used to reduce the metabolic, cardiorespiratory, and fluid expenditures related to fever. Fatigue levels, thermal comfort, rate-pressure product, and febrile shivering are monitored in relation to the febrile episode. Dehydration is monitored by body weight, serum osmolality, and urine specific gravity in hospitalized patients, but a fever diary and home visits document changes in patients at home.

A growing awareness that cooling measures exert distressful and sometimes harmful effects has stimulated inquiry surrounding procedures commonly used to cool patients. There is evidence that a gradual, less drastic reduction in body temperature evokes fewer adverse responses during aggressive cooling treatments for fever. A comparison of cooling blanket temperatures (Caruso, Hadley, Shukla, Frame, & Khoury, 1992) demonstrated that warmer settings effectively lower body temperature as well as cooler levels, without stimulating distressful shivering. Morgan (1990) compared acetaminophen-treated subjects who were grouped into those receiving sponge baths, those on hypothermia cooling blankets, and those receiving only the antipyretic drug. No statistical differences were found in the degree of heat loss between the three groups, but the sponging required the greatest amount of nursing time. Shivering was prevalent in the group receiving the hypothermia treatment. Given the distress and time expenditure imposed by either of the traditional cooling techniques done by nurses, the use of the drug alone was preferable.

Future Directions

Today's nurse scientist is prepared to investigate many of the questions that remain unanswered in fever care. As investigators acquire skills and resources for these biological measurements, they can be used to quantify and qualify the effects of fever and fever intervention. Research is needed to demonstrate effects of elevated body temperature, cooling interventions, and measures to support natural temperature-stabilizing mechanisms. Fever may provide study variables, with body temperature, cytokines, and biochemical correlates as the outcome of interest. The febrile episode itself may be the context of other questions for study. The psychoneuroimmunological factors surrounding sleep, irritability, and tolerance of febrile symptoms remain untapped topics. Likewise, the metabolic toll of fever on nutritional variables and measures of energy expenditure also are important but relatively untouched areas of research for nursing.

BARBARA J. HOLTZCLAW

See also
FATIGUE
NUTRITION
SHIVERING
THERMAL BALANCE

FITZPATRICK'S RHYTHM MODEL

Fitzpatrick (1989) presented a rhythm model as the field of inquiry for nursing. Person, environment, health, and nursing are defined and related in her model. All of these elements have been linked with the idea of meaning as essential to life. Meaning is seen as the most crucial piece of human experience, necessary to enhance and maintain life. Fitzpatrick incorporated Rogers's (1983) postulated correlates of human development as a basis from which to differentiate, organize, and order life's reality.

Fitzpatrick (1989) recognized the importance of information systems as part of the field of inquiry within her rhythm model for nursing. By asserting that nursing knowledge is fundamentally inseparable from the strategies and structures that represent it and that nursing informatics comprises a new focus to manage the technologies involved in nursing, Fitzpatrick suggested that information systems be linked to nursing knowledge development.

Correlates of Human Development

Rogers's (1983) correlates of shorter, higher frequency waves that manifest shorter rhythms and approach a seemingly continuous pattern serve as Fitzpatrick's (1989) foci for hypothesizing the existence of rhythmic patterns. Rogers's position that the human life span approximates transformation with human development aimed toward transcendence has been incorporated within Fitzpatrick's descriptions of life perspective. The developmental correlate whereby time seems timeless represents a beginning of Fitzpatrick's theorizing regarding temporal patterns. Motion patterns have been derived from Rogers's proposal of motion seeming to be continuous with development. Consciousness patterns are aligned with Rogers's idea that one progresses from sleeping to waking and from there to a pattern that is beyond waking. The correlates of "visibility" becoming more ethereal in nature and "heaviness" approaching a more weightless phase serve as the basis for Fitzpatrick's perceptual patterns.

Definitions

Person and Environment. Fitzpatrick's (1989) definitions of person and environment are from her interpretations of Rogers's (1983) developmental correlates and explanations of person and environment. Envisioned as patterns within a pattern, or rhythms within a life rhythm, Fitzpatrick's rhythm patterns serve as the specifications for person and environment. Occurring within the context of rhythmical person/environment interaction, indices of holistic human functioning are identified by Fitzpatrick as temporal, motion, consciousness, and perceptual patterns. Fitzpatrick's writings are consistent with the Rogerian position regarding person and environment being open systems in continuous interaction.

Fitzpatrick (1989) has asserted that the four indices of human functioning are intricately related to health patterns throughout the life span, and these indices are rhythmic in nature. In a projection of Rogers's (1983) principle regarding the continuous interaction of persons and their environments, Fitz-

patrick postulated the dynamic concepts of congruency, consistency, and integrity as complementary with rhythmic patterns. The nonlinear character of patterns by Rogers has supported Fitzpatrick's incorporation of Rogers's specifications regarding four-dimensionality.

Health. Fitzpatrick (1989) stated that health is a basic human dimension undergoing continuous development. She offered heightened awareness of the meaningfulness of life as an example of a more fully developed phase of human health.

Nursing. The ontogenetic and phylogenetic interactions between person and health are regarded as the essence of nursing. Fitzpatrick (1989) attended not only to relationships within or between these interactions but also included latent relationships external to person and health. Nursing interventions were interpreted as facilitating the developmental process toward health. Fitzpatrick stated that nursing interventions can be focused on enhancing the developmental process toward health so that individuals might develop their human potential.

Relationships among Concepts

Because person and environment are integral with one another and have no real boundaries, environment is implied when the term *person* is used. The human element is treated as an open, holistic, rhythmic system that is described by temporal, motion, consciousness, and perceptual patterns. Fitzpatrick's (1989) conception of person is augmented by awareness of the meaningfulness of life or health. The meaningfulness of life is manifest through a series of life crisis experiences with potential for growth in one's meaning for living. Nursing's central concern is focused on person in relation to the dimension of meaning within health.

Major Studies, Researchers, and Methodology

Fitzpatrick's (1989) conceptualizations have been investigated by graduate students in nursing at the master's and doctoral level. Studies looking at temporality in combination with adult and elderly populations, temporality in association with psychiatric clients, and temporality in relation to terminally ill individuals provide a base for the existence of temporal patterns. However, from a holistic perspective of life span, use of the model is absent in nursing research focused on the infant, child, and adolescent notions of temporality.

Both younger and elderly groups have been addressed in investigating motion (Roberts & Fitzpatrick, 1983). Nevertheless, patterns of consciousness have been examined exclusively in older age groups (Floyd, 1982).

Different types of perceptual patterns, that is, perception of color and music, have been investigated. Because one's perception would seem to be dependent on a present pattern of consciousness, these studies seem to be related to patterns of consciousness.

Empirical support for the existence of nonlinear temporal patterns emerged from a number of research endeavors and helped to identify the need for generating questions about ways to measure the experience of time. The prevalence of temporal distinctions on the basis of differences in development were apparent in at least one study (Fitzpatrick & Donovan, 1978). A sense of timelessness was described as being characteristic of behaviors identified among the dying.

Pressler, Wells, and Hepworth (1993) are investigating methodological issues relevant to very preterm infant (< 30 weeks gestation) outcomes based on the idea of the existence of microrhythms within some larger rhythmic pattern. By applying time series techniques and fuzzy subsets to the analysis of longitudinal data collected in the neonatal intensive care unit (NICU) environment, this study is examining single-subject results for generalization across individuals. In general terms, the sequelae and risks associated with the NICU for very preterm neonates indicate that information processing deficits, attention deficit, and hyperactivity disorders are not uncommon during the preschool and school-age years. It is speculated that these problems might reflect these infants' inabilities to cope with stresses or care received while in the NICU environment.

Relationship to Other Theories

Borrowing from some of her own ideas about temporality, Fitzpatrick (1989) has hypothesized the field of inquiry for nursing knowledge development by outlining nursing inquiry of the past. She has traced major historical milestones of nursing research and identified important events leading up to present day research in nursing.

In cooperation with two colleagues, Fitzpatrick (Fitzpatrick, Wykle, & Morris, 1990) attempted to specify the field of inquiry for nursing in the area of geriatric mental health. Through the development of collaborative, interdisciplinary teaching, research, and practice relationships, Fitzpatrick et al. (1990) described how organizational theory could be used to support the development of a collaboration model for promoting the mental health of elderly persons across care settings. Intervention research with elderly populations was used to determine ways for improving the understanding, treatment, and rehabilitation of the mentally ill. The significance of Fitzpatrick's ideas lies in how rhythmic methodologies might be used to develop nursing knowledge and provide external validity to the model.

JANA L. PRESSLER

See also
ROGER'S SCIENCE OF UNITARY
 HUMAN BEINGS

FORMAL LANGUAGES

The National Center for Nursing Research (now the National Institute of Nursing) Priority Panel on Nursing Informatics (1993) defined nursing language as

> . . . the universe of written terms and their definition comprising nomenclature or thesauri that are used for purposes such as indexing, sorting, retrieving, and classifying varied nursing data in clinical records, in information systems (for care documentation and/or management), and in literature and research reports. . . . Determining the way

that nursing data are represented in automated systems is tantamount to defining a language for nursing. (p. 31)

This report also differentiated between clinical terms, which represent the language of practice, and definition terms, which represent the language of nursing knowledge comprising theory and research. The distinction between language that supports practice versus language that supports theory and research is blurring as the state of the science in this area moves toward nonambiguous, that is, definitional, concept representations that can be aggregated and abstracted into the existing standardized coding and classification systems (Henry & Mead, 1997). In addition, standardized coding and classifications systems are being designed for multiple purposes; for instance, the *Nursing Interventions Classification* (NIC) is used as an organizing framework for intervention literature in the *Cumulative Index of Nursing and Allied Literature* as well as for clinical and research purposes. The term *formal language* is used synonymously with standardized coding and classification systems in this section.

Standardized language for nursing has developed within the framework of the nursing minimum data set, comprising five data elements specific to nursing: (a) nursing diagnosis, (b) nursing interventions, (c) nursing outcomes, (d) intensity of care, and (e) unique RN provider number (Werley, Devine, & Zorn, 1988). The American Nurses Association's Steering Committee on Databases to Support Nursing Practice has recognized four systems as part of a unified nursing language system (McCormick et al., 1994). Standardized language systems demonstrated to have some utility for nursing care are summarized in Table 1.

North American Nursing Diagnosis Association (NANDA) Taxonomy 1

NANDA Taxonomy 1 is a classification of nursing diagnosis organized by human responses (NANDA, 1992). Related factors and defining characteristics are included for each diagnosis. Extensive work is underway to enhance and refine the taxonomy.

NANDA Taxonomy 1 is the most widely implemented formal nursing language in both paper-based and computer-based systems.

Nursing Interventions Classification

Nursing Interventions Classification is a categorization of both direct and indirect care activities performed by nurses (McCloskey & Bulechek, 1996). Each intervention consists of a label describing the concept, the definition of the concept, and a set of related activities or actions. The three-tiered taxonomy contains 6 domains (physiological-basic, physiological-complex, behavioral, safety, family, and health system), 27 classes, 433 interventions, and related nursing activities for each intervention. Davis (1995) operationalized the nursing activities from two published standardized care plans for patients with *Pneumocystis carinii* pneumonia with intervention terms from NIC. Carter and associates (Carter, Moorhead, McCloskey, & Bulechek, 1995) demonstrated the usefulness of NIC in implementing clinical practice guidelines for pain management and pressure ulcer management.

Home Health Care Classification

The *Home Health Care Classification* (HHCC) includes 20 home health care components, 147 nursing diagnoses (NANDA plus additional home care diagnoses), 166 nursing interventions modified by 4 types of nursing actions (assess, care, teach, and manage), and discharge status (improved, stabilized, or deteriorated) (Saba, 1992a). Recent studies by Parlocha (1995) and Holzemer and colleagues (Holzemer, Henry, Dawson, et al., 1997) have demonstrated the utility of the HHCC for categorizing nursing care activities for home care patients with a diagnosis of major depressive disorder and for hospitalized patients with HIV/AIDS, respectively.

Omaha System

The *Omaha System* (Martin & Scheet, 1992) consists of standardized schemata of nursing diagnoses, interventions, and ratings of outcomes for patient problems. The problem classification schema in-

TABLE 1   Examples of Standardized Coding and Classification Systems with Utility for Nursing

System	Problems	Interventions	Outcomes
NANDA Taxonomy 1*	x		
Current Procedural Terminology		x	
Nursing Interventions Classification*		x	
Nursing Outcomes Classification			x
Omaha System*	x	x	x
Home Health Care Classification*	x	x	x
SNOMED International	x	x	x
Patient Care Data Set	x	x	x

*Recognized by the American Nurses Association as part of a unified nursing language system.

cludes 40 client problems, 2 sets of modifiers, and clusters of signs and symptoms. The intervention schema is a taxonomy of 4 intervention categories and 62 targets or objects of nursing interventions. In the outcomes schema, patient progress in relationship to specific problems is rated on the dimensions of knowledge, behavior, and status. The *Omaha System* is the dominant formal language for clinical and research purposes in the community setting.

Nursing Outcomes Classification

The *Nursing Outcomes Classification* is a list of 190 nursing-sensitive outcomes with definitions, indicators, and measurement scales (Johnson & Maas, 1997). The outcomes are currently limited to the individual patient or family caregiver. Fourteen different measurement scales are associated with the 190 outcomes. For instance, bowel elimination and quality of life are rated on a 5-point scale ranging from extremely compromised to not compromised, whereas caregiver performance, direct care, and breastfeeding maintenance are rated from not adequate to totally adequate. There has been extensive testing and validation of the *Nursing Outcomes Classification* by the research team; however, the system has not been widely implemented or tested due to the recency of its publication.

Significant Works in Progress

Ozbolt (1996) and associates continue to refine an atomic-level set of standardized problem and activ-

ity terms for the acute care environment. Grobe (1996) and colleagues are utilizing natural language processing techniques to examine both the content and structure of nursing documentation as an extension of the work on the *Nursing Intervention Lexicon and Taxonomy*. At the international level, the International Council of Nursing is working on the creation of an international classification of nursing practice to accompany the existing World Health Organization classifications (Mortensen & Nielsen, 1996).

Health care classification systems such as the *International Classification of Diseases: Clinical Modification* and the *Physician's Current Procedural Terminology* (CPT) are widely available and utilized; however, no single nursing classification system or set of systems is as ubiquitous. Consequently, a few investigations have examined the feasibility of using standardized health care classifications not specifically designed for nursing in order to describe nursing diagnoses or patient problems (Henry, Holzemer, Reilly, & Campbell, 1994) and nursing interventions (Griffith & Robinson, 1992; Griffith & Robinson, 1993).

Current Procedural Terminology

The CPT comprises more than 7,000 codes designed to be used for reimbursement of health care services provided by physicians; as such, these terms are present in numerous state and federal databases. Two studies have examined the extent to which nurses perform CPT-coded services. The first study by Griffith and Robinson (1992) surveyed 100 randomly chosen members of the American Association of Critical Care Nurses. The mean number of CPT code activities performed by the nurses was 59, with a range of 15 to 78; 28 were performed by more than 70% of the respondents. In the second study, the investigators (Griffith & Robinson, 1993) sampled 100 randomly chosen nurses from each of nine nursing specialty organizations. Specialty-specific questionnaires were developed that reflected inclusion of codes judged by a specialty panel to be performed by members of the specialty. Study results showed that the mean number of CPT-coded functions ranged from 79 for family nurse practitioners to 18 for school nurses. The findings of these studies provided evidence that nurses perform many CPT-coded functions and that some functions are performed with great frequency (e.g., multiple times in a single day).

In contrast, Henry and colleagues (Henry, Holzemer, Randell, Hsieh, & Miller, 1997) compared the frequencies with which 21,366 nursing activity terms could be categorized using NIC and CPT codes. Nursing activity terms ($N = 21,366$) were collected from patient interviews, nurse interviews, intershift reports, and patient records and were categorized using NIC and CPT codes. There were significantly ($p < .0001$) greater numbers of nursing activity terms that could be categorized in the NIC system than in the CPT, thus providing evidence for the superiority of NIC in representing nursing activity data.

Systematized Nomenclature of Human and Veterinary Medicine (SNOMED)

SNOMED International is a compilation of nomenclatures organized into 11 modules: (a) topography; (b) morphology; (c) living organisms; (d) chemicals, drugs, and biological products; (e) function; (f) occupation; (g) diagnosis; (h) procedure; (i) physical agents, forces, and attributes; (j) social context; and (k) general (Coté, Rothwell, Palotay, & Beckett, 1993). A study by Henry and associates (1994) demonstrated that nurses use terms other than NANDA diagnoses (i.e., symptoms, signs,

medical diagnoses) to describe patient problems and that SNOMED terms, other than the NANDA diagnoses included in SNOMED (e.g., symptoms, medical diagnoses), were exact matches for terms used by nurses in their clinical documentation.

The body of evaluation literature related to standardized coding and classification systems suggests that although every language system described serves the purpose for which it was designed, no single system is adequate to serve all purposes (Chute, Cohn, Campbell, Oliver, & Campbell, 1996). Of particular note is the need for more atomic-level (less abstract) data representations. Ozbolt's *Patient Care Data Set*, the evolving axes of the *International Classification of Nursing Practice* (Nielsen & Mortensen, 1996), and the activities associated with the NIC interventions are all examples of atomic-level data. Other investigators note also the need for formal representations of these data to facilitate nonambiguous definitions and multiple uses of the language terms for computer-based systems (Henry & Mead, 1997).

SUZANNE BAKKEN HENRY

See also
**HOME HEALTH CARE CLASSIFICATION
NANDA
NURSING MINIMUM DATA SET
NURSING OUTCOMES CLASSIFICATION
SNOMED INTERNATIONAL**

FUNCTIONAL HEALTH

Functional health has been viewed as a requirement for independent living and is the ability to engage in daily activities related to personal care, socially defined roles, and recreational activities. Performance of these activities is integral to quality of life and to living independently and safely, particularly for elderly adults with adverse effects of aging and disease. Functional health is one dimension of health in the metaparadigm of nursing.

Although functional health represents well-being, most nomenclature used in research and clinical practice reflects its deficits. Researchers and clinicians have used different terms for deficits in functional health, including disability (Nagi, 1991), frailty (Lawton, 1991), functional limitation (Johnson & Wolinsky, 1993), and handicap (World Health Organization, 1980). Researchers and clinicians add to the confusion in nomenclature and theoretical definitions by using these terms to label other concepts.

The inconsistency in the nomenclature and theoretical definitions have limited the development of a theory of functional health. Several theories have been used to guide research on deficits in functional health. The World Health Organization (1980) model lacks conceptual clarity and theoretical consistency, and this makes operationalization and establishing relationships difficult. In the model by Johnson and Wolinsky (1993), functional limitations are sometimes confused with factors affecting these limitations, and perceived health is used as a proxy for functional limitations. In a proposed model of functional status, Leidy (1994) recommended nomenclature and definitions of this concept and others related to functional status that added to the conceptual confusion in this area.

Models of Functional Health

Three models, useful to guide research because they are theoretically clear and consistent, have been used in many research studies, and they add concepts and relationship that provide direction for future research. Hogue's (1984) model of functional health depicts the interplay between the environment and personal competencies (physical and psychological) and the influence on health. A strength of this model is the inclusion of cognitive appraisals of the environment and personal competencies as evaluative judgments that can be used in decisions about what activities to participate in and how. Cognitive appraisal is related to coping and adaptation, strategies to maintain the fit between the environment and personal competencies necessary to maintain functional health.

Nagi's (1991) model of disability is conceptually clear, logically consistent, and useful in interpreting current and past research. Disability (poor functional health) is the result of a sequence of temporal relationships. Pathology or lifestyle contributes to

impairments that are anatomic, physiological, and psychological, causing functional limitations at the level of the whole person (e.g., poor memory or inability to get up from a chair). Functional limitations then lead to disability, that is, the inability to perform daily tasks or roles independently. Unique in this model is the notion of thresholds where a certain amount of change must occur before change in a subsequent concept is observed. There is potential for nurses to use thresholds to identify persons at risk for functional limitation or disability. Although poorly developed in this model, the definition of the situation is conceptualized as affecting these relationships and is consistent with cognitive appraisal from Hogue's (1984) model.

An extension of Nagi's (1991) model of disability is the model of the disablement process (Verbrugge & Jette, 1994). This process describes the interplay between the extraindividual factors and intraindividual factors that is consistent with person-environment fit found in Hogue's (1984) model of functional health. Aspects of these two factors are more developed than in the models previously described.

Activities of Daily Living

Because functional health is the ability to engage in everyday activities, a plethora of research has focused on daily activities related to personal care (ADLs) and tasks related to providing food and shelter and caring for the home (IADLs). ADLs are hierarchically structured by the complexity of the motor skills required. IADLs are dependent on the same motor skills but are more dependent on cognitive capabilities (Johnson & Wolinsky, 1993). Johnson and Wolinsky also determined that ADLs and IADLs are highly related and may represent a continuum of the same construct.

The theoretical definitions of ADLs and IADLs are well established. First, empirical indicators were obtained by self-report. Many researchers noted that the accuracy of these responses could not be verified and could be adversely affected by cognitive impairment, social desirability, or minimization of dependency. Thus, observational indicators were developed to address the inadequacies of self-report. Although they may reflect what the person is able to do, observational measures may not reflect what a person actually does. Hence, both types of measures have limitations and provide different types of information.

A significant amount of research has focused on physical and psychological factors contributing to independence in ADLs and IADLs. Characteristics of gait, dynamic and static postural stability, and muscle strength were physical factors affecting these activities. Moreover, upper body function (e.g., muscle strength and range of motion of the arms used in reaching) has been related to ADLs, whereas lower body function (e.g., muscle strength of the legs used in ambulation and transfers) have been associated with IADLs (Lawrence & Jette, 1996). Relevant psychological factors included cognitive impairment and depression. Certain types of social support were factors contributing to dependency in daily activities; however, men and women used different types of social support in response to limitations in ADLs and IADLs (Roberts, Anthony, Matejczyk, & Moore, 1994). The role of the environment has not been well established except for the increase in dependency noted during hospitalization and long-term residence in a nursing home. Although there is beginning to be evidence that the relationship between actual abilities and perceptions of them is low, how these perceptions influence decisions people make about what activities to perform and how have not been well studied.

More nursing research is needed to identify thresholds in factors related to declines in functional health and to identify factors and processes by which people make decisions about performing daily activities. This knowledge could provide directions for assessment in populations at risk for poor functional health and might lead to more sensitive assessment strategies. A greater understanding of the interplay between environmental and personal factors affecting functional health may lead to multidimensional interventions that are more effective than single interventions targeted to one factor.

BEVERLY L. ROBERTS

See also
COGNITIVE DISORDERS

DEPRESSION AMONG OLDER ADULTS
FAMILY CARE
SOCIAL SUPPORT

FUNCTIONAL HEALTH PATTERNS

Definition

A functional health pattern (FHP) is a manifestation of an individual's behavior and responses across time. The typology of 11 functional health patterns identifies and defines each, as follows: (a) health perception–health management, (b) nutritional-metabolic, (c) elimination, (d) activity-exercise, (e) cognitive-perceptual, (f) sleep-rest, (g) self-perception–self-concept, (h) role relationship, (i) sexuality-reproductive, (j) coping–stress tolerance, and (k) value-belief (Gordon, 1982).

The organization of the FHP assessment framework provides a structure to examine a sequence of behaviors and responses within each pattern area. Subjective and objective data obtained during the assessment facilitates pattern construction for an individual, family, or community. Data from all of the functional health patterns' areas are assessed within the context of age and stage of development, culture and ethnic background, current health status, and environment.

A functional health pattern is both mutually exclusive and interactive, reflecting a holistic perspective. To determine a patient's responses and arrive at a clinical judgment all of the patterns' areas must be assessed. Often data obtained about one pattern area may be best understood in relation to information assessed in other patterns. A pattern may be described as functional, potentially dysfunctional, or dysfunctional. Behaviors (cues) obtained during an FHP assessment can be used to generate a tentative nursing hypothesis (e.g., nursing diagnosis). Each individual responds uniquely to the human experience. Judgments about this are described as probabilistic and noncausal.

Description

Historically, assessment tools were developed to assess different clinical populations, frequently duplicating medical information. The lack of a consistent nursing assessment framework resulted in inadequate data and limited information about nursing's contribution to care outcomes. The National League for Nursing prompted a shift away from nursing's task focus to one that was patient-centered. Forty schools of nursing participated in a survey that generated a classification list of the nursing's 21 problems (Abdellah, 1959). Later, in 1966, Henderson classified the 14 basic needs. This work identified human needs, articulated nursing functions, and helped direct nursing care toward patient responses. Gordon's (1982) typology of 11 FHPs provided a structure for organizing and documenting patient behavior over time.

The FHP framework offers nurses a consistent structure for identifying human responses and autonomous nursing interventions. This focus is consistent with the professional standards of nursing practice and *Nursing's Social Policy Statement* (American Nurses Association, 1995b). The FHP framework has been disseminated through textbooks and specialty publications as well as scholarly journals. It has been presented at numerous conferences and workshops; in hospitals, nursing homes, and ambulatory settings; nationally and internationally. In addition, academic nursing curricula have incorporated the FHP framework into courses across specialties.

Research

The FHP framework provides nurses with an opportunity to know the patient in a unique way. Through a series of semistructured interview questions each pattern is assessed as the individual life story unfolds. When additional information is required, nurse uses branching questions to elicit new perceptions. This qualitative approach to data collection leads to the isolation of data bits (or cues) that help formulate tentative diagnostic statements and reflect phenomena of concern to nursing.

Many clinical investigations have used the FHP framework as a structure for data collection. These studies describe patient responses to phenomena (e.g., eating disorders, sleep disturbances). Other investigations have used the FHP framework to validate cues associated with a particular nursing diagnosis. Nurses working in clinical specialties (e.g., ambulatory surgery, oncology, rehabilitation, and cardiovascular nursing) have used the FHP framework to identify patient responses throughout illness and recovery. Nurse administrators using data from FHP assessments report using findings to predict nurse and patient mix. Nursing educators have used FHP assessment data to evaluate clinical reasoning skills and diagnostic accuracy.

Currently, research is underway to clinically test an assessment screening tool using the 11 FHPs. The Functional Health Pattern Assessment Screening Tool (FHPAST) is a patient-completed instrument (Foster & Jones, 1997). The tool currently contains 58 items and organizes responses to each item on a 4-point Likert scale. Psychometric properties have been established with well adult populations. Initial data analysis reveals the emergence of four factors (general health status, health behaviors, health risks, and dysfunction) with alpha coefficients ranging from .74 to .90 for the factors and .89 for the total scale. The FHPAST assesses data across all pattern areas and is easily administered. The tool offers a quantitative measure of patient responses and identifies cues requiring further exploration.

Relevance to Nursing

The FHP framework provides nurses with a structure for organizing data that reflect responses and perceptions across individuals families and communities. The FHP (a) provides a framework to identify tentative nursing diagnoses, (b) helps link problem identification with interventions and nurse-sensitive outcomes, (c) creates a data base that can be computerized, (d) establishes a mechanism to document patient responses across populations and settings, and (e) identifies a way for nurse administrators to relate patient complexity with staffing patterns.

The FHP framework has been used to complement existing conceptual frameworks and expand nursing knowledge. "To combine these patterns with conceptual frameworks, the patterns are thought of as areas of self-care agency (Orem,

1980), adaptation (Roy, 1980), . . . or manifestations of the life pattern'' (Gordon, 1982, p. 108; Rogers, 1970). Other theories (e.g., Newman, 1997) focus on story telling as the vehicle for uncovering meaning and patterning of the whole. A complete FHP assessment uses story telling and organizes information within the health patterns to reflect behavior. Data from this assessment can also be used to isolate complex life themes, manifested by specific behaviors.

Future Directions

The functional pattern framework will continue to be used in academic and clinical sites throughout the United States and internationally. However, time constraints and decreased length of hospital stay may compromise its use and limit documentation of nursing assessment data. Research using the FHP framework will continue to refine phenomena amenable to nursing intervention. Movement toward the development of an International Classification of Nursing Language will promote the use of a consistent nursing assessment framework and increase validation of phenomena across countries. The testing and refinement of the FHPAST can help monitor patient responses over time and facilitate documentation and computerization of assessment data. The use of the FHP framework can expand nursing knowledge, isolate human experiences in illness and wellness, promote creative interventions, and help articulate nurse-sensitive outcomes.

DOROTHY A. JONES

See also
   INTERNATIONAL CLASSIFICATION
      FOR NURSING PRACTICE
   NURSING ASSESSMENT
   NURSING DIAGNOSES
   NURSING INTERVENTIONS
      CLASSIFICATION

FUNDING

Funding is the provision of money or other resources to carry out a research proposal, usually for a specific period of time. Resources may be money, time, or people to carry out the scientific work. Funding may be intramural (coming from an individual's place of employment, such as a university) or extramural (coming from a source that is external to the recipient or the recipient's place of employment, such as a federal or state agency or a private foundation). Extramural funding almost always is preceded by a scientific or technical review for merit by experts who are considered peers of intended applicants. At times there is also a second-level review made to determine the goodness of fit between the proposed project and the program that will fund it. Many research institutions also have instituted internal peer review of scientific merit for intramural funding.

In addition to scientific merit, proposals are usually reviewed for human subject safety, animal welfare if animal models are proposed, and the reasonableness of the scientific return for the overall cost of the research to be undertaken. This last focus is designed to provide opportunity for consideration of cutting-edge research in comparison to research that may be very well designed but may not provide new knowledge. It also provides opportunity for discussion of new, highly innovative research that may lead to future advances. Organizations that fund research are looking for scientifically superb proposals focused on cutting-edge health problems and issues where the expenditure is reasonable given the complexity of the study (for application strategies, see Reif-Lehrer, 1995; Ries & Leukefeld, 1995; Rush, Gullion, & Prien, 1996). This does not mean cheap, but it does mean that cost and scientific return are in balance (Torgerson, Ryan, & Ratcliffe, 1995).

Funding sources for nursing research are numerous and varied. Such support could be funding for the conduct of research or for research training and career development for nurse scientists interested in a mentored research experience. The National Institute of Nursing Research at the National Institutes of Health (NIH) is the principal federal source. It announces its research interest areas on the NIH homepage and through the literature (e.g., Cowan, Heinrich, Lucas, Sigmon, & Hinshaw, 1993; Grady, Harden, Moritz, & Amende, 1997). However, other NIH institutes and offices that fund clinical research with a specific focus, such as cancer, heart disease, or complementary therapies, are also important resources for nurse investigators. All the institutes at NIH accept and encourage investigator-initiated research. Therefore, it is advisable not to wait for publication of information about an exact topic; if the general topic is related to the institute's mission, contact them to discuss specific ideas. These and similar sources with specific interests should be pursued because their use enlarges the resources available for nursing research.

Information about research interests of the NIH and its institutes can be found through the NIH homepage at http://www.nih.gov. The Centers for Disease Control and Prevention are an important source for prevention and health promotion research and demonstration projects and can be contacted at http://www.cdc.gov. Also, the Agency for Health Care Policy and Research funds research on general health services, care delivery models, outcomes, and health care costs. Information about its research interests can be found at http://www.ahcpr.gov. Generally, federal agencies make their research interests known through their homepages or through contacts with staff listed on the homepages. Also, some agencies provide access to information about funded research. The NIH provides this through the Computer Retrieval of Information on Scientific Projects (CRISP) database, available through the NIH homepage under grants and contracts. Other nonpublic sources of funding are foundations, product and drug companies, and business corporations.

Foundations usually have highly targeted interest areas or specific populations of interest. For example, the W. T. Grant Foundation is interested in children; the Robert Woods Johnson Foundation is interested in end-of life care, home care, and economics of health care projects, among others. Many foundations have homepages; for example, Robert Woods Johnson's is http://www.rwjf.org. The *Foundation Directory* and various on-line programs available through libraries are good sources of information on national, regional, and local foundations. Product and drug companies frequently seek clinical investigators to assist with human testing, and nurse investigators have been active in this area. There are research grant programs available for small businesses to test products and to transfer technology into useable health products. The NIH, the Food and Drug Administration, and other federal agencies that fund clinical research are sources for these funds. Funding from entities that may have a vested interest in a particular outcome from the research they support requires special consideration that offices of university-sponsored programs usually can provide (Loos, Shortridge, Adaskin, & Rock, 1994).

PATRICIA MORITZ

See also
GRANTSMANSHIP
NATIONAL INSTITUTE
   OF NURSING RESEARCH
NATIONAL INSTITUTES OF HEALTH
RIGHTS OF HUMAN SUBJECTS

G

GENDER RESEARCH

Gender is an old term used in linguistic discourse to designate whether nouns are masculine, feminine, or neuter. It was not normally used either in the language of social sciences or nursing until after 1955, when the psychologist-sexologist John Money adopted the term to serve as an umbrella concept distinguishing femininity, or womanliness, and masculinity, or manliness, from biological sex (male or female). By using the word *gender* he believed he could avoid continually making qualifying statements about the hermaphrodites he was studying, such as "John was in a male sex role except that his sex organs are not male and his genetic sex is female" (Money, 1955). Sex, in his research, belonged more to reproductive biology than to social science, romance, and nurture, whereas gender belonged to both (Money & Ehrhardt, 1972). By using a new term to describe a variety of phenomena, Money opened up a whole new field of research. It was a field ripe for exploration because it appealed to the increasingly powerful feminist movement (Bullough, 1994).

Even as Money was putting forth his ideas about the influence of sociopsychological factors (nurture) during critical periods of child development, he was strongly criticized by Milton Diamond, another psychologist active in sex research. Diamond (1965) indicated that gender decisions for hermaphrodites, about whom Money had originally drawn his data, were perhaps not as clear-cut as Money implied. Diamond hypothesized that an individual hermaphrodite might be receiving mixed biological signals, which allowed him or her to conform to the assigned gender rather than change it. He charged that Money was in danger of deemphasizing biology, or nature, and overemphasizing nurture.

The argument over nature versus nurture continues although both sides recognize the influence of both factors and it remains an argument over degree. At their scientific best, most biologists and social or behavioral scientists agree that the coding of gender is multivariate, sequential, and developmental, reflecting a complex interaction across the boundaries of disciplines and across biological and social variables.

Ann Constantinople (1973) questioned the assumption that masculinity was the opposite of femininity and suggested that the identification of masculine traits might be independent from, rather than the opposite of, the identification of feminine traits. The "both/and" concept of psychological identification quickly replaced the "either/or" notion that had dominated thinking on the matter since Lewis Terman developed his scales of masculinity and femininity. Sandra Bem (1974) developed a gender identity measure, the Bem Sex Role Inventory, that treated identification with masculine traits independently of identification with feminine traits. Spence and Helmreich (1974) found wide variation in gender traits, although they also found that stereotypical masculine personality traits in males were correlated with self-esteem, which reflects just how much influence society and culture have on self-esteem. However, the difficulty remains because the scales are based on observable patterns without any attempt to evaluate whether there are behaviors that must be distinctly limited to males or to females.

Bonnie Bullough, a nurse theorist, held that the formation of gender identity and sexual preference included three steps: (a) a genetic predisposition, (b) prenatal hormonal stimulation that might follow or interfere with the genetic predisposition, and (c) socialization patterns that shape specific manifestation of the predisposition (Bullough & Bullough, 1993). This theory would allow for wider variations in gender behavior than those of some other theorists. For example, Nancy Chodorow (1978) noted out that infants, both males and females, generally have the most contact with their mothers and initially identify and form intense relationships with their mothers. For girls, this identification is never completely severed, but boys must relinquish their identification with their mothers as they take on masculine roles.

Chodorow maintained that this differing experience produced distinct coping strategies for males and females in dealing with the world. Specifically, women emphasize relationships *with others*, whereas men focus on their own individualism and independence *from others*. Gilligan (1982) pointed out that to hold this view limits personality development. A woman (or for that matter, a man) who views herself only in relationship to others (e.g., wife or mother but not an individual in her own right) may limit her own independent development. The man (or woman) who views himself only in terms of his own achievements and independence (boss, owner, director, sole author) may handicap his capacity for intimate connections with others. Obviously, conceptions of gender influence the way we think about what men and women can accomplish or achieve.

Probably most nursing theorists have followed Gilligan (1982), although a minority have emphasized the unique nature of being a woman. This is particularly true of some of the caring theorists. Dorothy Johnson (1959), who wrote before the concept of gender was fully developed, distinguished between caring and curing, and emphasized the caring aspects of nursing. This influenced Jean Watson in the establishing of caring centers. The concept of caring also became part of the basic educational mission of nursing.

The caring theory fits well into traditional concepts now associated with gender, but the problem is that one faction of nursing interpreted caring as a uniquely feminine quality and in the process ignored most of the mainstream research on gender to adopt a militant feminist extremist position. One male PhD student, D. Ross, in a 1995 letter to the *Skeptical Inquirer*, summarized this by stating that some nursing caring theorists held that

traditional science was paternalistic and male-oriented and thus suspect at all levels. They stated that men's and women's minds operated in dramatically different ways. "Men's science" dissected an event and attempted to empiricize it and in the process lost the gestalt that was essential to understanding the event. It was the feminists' contention that *only* women could understand a holistic viewpoint. (Ross, 1995, pp. 58–60)

Obviously, what some of the these theorists have said is historical fact. Science did develop as a male enterprise and remains male-oriented, but this does not mean that women cannot participate in it or even help change it. Still, the charges of Ross emphasize the importance of gender research to nursing development. It is a growing field, and the debate between nature and nurture and its influence on gender has to becomes a priority research area for nursing, which still remains a woman-dominated profession. Nurses are already involved in gender research, but only a few nurses have really done the quantitative studies needed to challenge the persistence of earlier stereotypes both within and outside of the profession.

VERN L. BULLOUGH

See also
CARING
FEMINIST RESEARCH METHODOLOGY
WATSON'S HUMAN CARE MODEL
WOMEN'S HEALTH RESEARCH

GENETICS IN NURSING RESEARCH

The Human Genome Project will complete identification of all of the approximately 100,000 genes in human DNA soon after the turn of the millennium (National Center for Human Genome Research, 1996), leading to revolutions in health care. It is now possible to describe definitely the genetic risk for some forms of breast, colon, and other cancers, some forms of Alzheimer's disease, several psychiatric disorders, and many other conditions affecting large segments of the population. In addition, conditions in which many genes interact with environmental factors (e.g., certain forms of heart disease, hypertension, and diabetes) are becoming understood in new, more accurate ways. Specific therapies that target gene sequences in early work with conditions such as sickle cell anemia, cystic fibrosis, and some forms of cancer are now possible. These sophisticated technologies extend a promise of pinpoint accuracy in diagnosis, treatment, and prevention of diseases.

The application of new genetic technologies in nearly all health care settings is growing rapidly. Somatic and germ cell gene therapies are being explored as soon as identification of genetic sequences is confirmed. Genetic screening in preconception counseling for childbearing couples is widespread, and families are being recruited for genetic diagnosis and linkage studies that determine risk for many conditions, leading to possible labeling and disenfranchisement in education, employment, and insurance benefits. Moreover, the ethical and legal ramifications of technology transfer for profit by the biotechnology industry call for careful examination and revision of health policy to protect the public, assure quality, and provide equity in access to care.

There is an urgency to explore the human experience with these advanced technologies. Nurses in clinical practice are witnessing increasing demands for genetic information by health care consumers and are challenged to transmit knowledge that is culturally sensitive and legally sound (Scanlon & Fibison, 1995). The commitment of nursing to placing clients at the center of health care decision making is a well-accepted standard of practice (American Nurses Association, 1985b). Applications of genetic treatment technologies hold great hope for prevention of illness and alleviation of suffering, yet they carry the potential for unpredictable mutational events and other undesirable effects. Many individuals and families, indeed communities of clients, with or at risk for genetic illnesses may face difficult dilemmas in choosing among diagnostic and treatment options and living with their outcomes. In addition to the experiential effects of these new approaches, the ethical and legal ramifications of advanced genetic technologies present important avenues of inquiry for nurse researchers.

Advances in nursing practice depend on discoveries in basic and clinical studies. Nurses are displaying a greater recognition of and respect and thirst for research-based clinical practice, resulting in democratization of scholarly work. Researchers in nursing have the responsibility to contribute to knowledge about the human experience with advances in genetic technologies because of their expertise in capturing the multilevel responses of individuals, families, and communities to health and illness. Nurses can examine the changes that clients and families experience over time as they confront the possibilities of inheriting risks for illness and passing them on to progeny. The body of nursing research devoted to clinical studies in genetics is still limited and depends on the acquisition of a knowledge base in genetics by nurse scholars and collegial relationships with other workers in this field for access to populations of interest.

The coming of the 21st century brings profound change in our basic assumptions about health and illness in the human condition and the uncertainties of sickness, suffering, and death. The Ethical, Legal, and Social Implications Branch (ELSI) of the National Human Genome Research Institute extends support for investigation of the impact of these developments in social arenas of community life, the education of health care personnel, and the philosophical foundations of human genetic research. The accomplishments of nursing research in understanding responses to health and illness will serve as valuable templates in future examinations of genetic advances in health care. No less attention must be paid to adequate preparation of nurses to deliver care in genetics and to participate in inquiries that foster understanding of genetic testing and gene-based therapy as these affect human lives.

The National Institute of Nursing Research has made a commitment to support inquiry that examines advances in genetics in nursing and health care. Beginning in 1996, opportunities for nurse scientists collaborating with genome investigators, mental health researchers, and scholars in the social sciences, law, ethics, and education were offered by the National Institute of Nursing Research, the National Human Genome Research Institute, and the National Institute of Mental Health. There is a distinct directive for interdisciplinary study of genetics in the context of the human experience from the many research-funding support streams in the public and private sectors. These developments portend a dawning era of scholarly cooperation for the advancement of nursing as a practice discipline.

RITA BLACK MONSEN

See also
BREAST CANCER
ETHICS OF RESEARCH
PREGNANCY

GERIATRICS

Geriatrics evolved from the Greek word *geras*, "old age," and it refers to the branch of medicine that covers the diagnosis and treatment of the diseases and syndromes that occur in old age. A board-certified medical practitioner of geriatric medicine is called a geriatrician. In the lay press the term has sometimes been overgeneralized to include comprehensive health care and preventive services for older adults, but this obfuscates the precise original meaning of the term.

In the specialty of nursing devoted to care of the aged, there has been considerable overlapping of words and definitions, linguistic confusion, and philosophical controversy. These problems led to attempts to clarify and specify terminology and make the terms fit the consensual philosophy and goals of practitioners within the specialty. The debate about proper terminology will continue into the next century and may become even more heated as the absolute numbers and subsequent health care needs of older adults escalate through at least 2030.

A specialty referred to as geriatric nursing was first suggested in an anonymous 1925 editorial, "Care of the Aged," in the *American Journal of Nursing*, and the first nursing textbook on the topic was published in 1950 (Burnside, 1988). However, the actual birth of the specialty occurred in 1962, when the American Nurses Association (ANA) formed the Conference Group on Geriatric Nursing Practice. In 1966 the ANA officially created the Division of Geriatric Nursing, and in 1976 the name was changed to the Division of Gerontological Nursing (ANA, 1982). The ANA published the first set of *Standards of Practice for Geriatric Nursing* in 1970. The *Journal of Gerontological Nursing* began operation in 1975, and *Geriatric Nursing* was first published in 1979. The titles of these two journals and the ANA division's name change reflect the ongoing debate about proper terminology for this nursing specialty.

Many people rejected the term *geriatrics* because it did not properly reflect nursing's interest in the entire continuum of health and disease, including health promotion, disease prevention, care of acute illness, and long-term care. Others rejected it on narrower terms, saying that it did not convey inclusion of the art of nursing.

Although the ANA division's name change to the Division of Gerontological Nursing pleased some nurses, others said it introduced a new error in terminology. The main criticism about this new label was that gerontology refers to the study of or science-work about the aging processes and the biological, psychological, sociological, and economic experiences of normal aging (Lueckenotte, 1996). Using an "ology" term did not logically lend itself to the name of a clinical specialty in a practice field. This problem led some leaders in the field to lobby for the term *gerontic nursing* to identify the specialty. Gerontic nursing as defined by Gunter and Estes (1979) is more philosophically palatable than geriatric nursing and more linguistically correct than gerontological nursing. Gerontic nursing was defined as a nursing specialty that includes the art and practice of nurturing, caring, and comforting older adults. Supporters of this term maintained that it included both the science and the art of nursing.

A review of the titles of the most popular clinical textbooks in the field today showed that the field of medicine clearly uses the term *geriatric medicine* in the titles of its textbooks, but nursing is more ambivalent. Nursing textbook titles include such terms as gerontological nursing, clinical gerontological nursing, gerontologic nursing, gerontic nursing, and geriatric nursing; however, the latter two are in the minority. Lueckenotte, in her 1996 textbook, goes so far as to say that geriatrics is a branch of medicine, that it has limited application to nursing because of its disease orientation, and that it generally is not used to describe nursing care of older adults. Gerontic nursing never became commonly accepted, and it now seems very dated in its conceptualization. As Gunter and Estes (1979) defined the term, it would not include health promotion, risk reduction, or disease prevention (primary and secondary prevention). So in today's reality it would not be inclusive enough to meet the health care goals and client needs of the 21st century.

An ideal term for this nursing specialty would cover the full range of knowledge needed and services to be provided in this practice field that has age of client as its sole parameter. The specialty is practiced at all levels of the health continuum, with persons who are aged 60+ to 115+, in any and all types of settings where older adults are to be found, and for periods of time that stretch from minutes to decades. Finding a fitting replacement for the term *geriatrics* or *geriatric nursing* has already challenged some of the best minds in the profession for over 30 years. The search for an ideal term is not likely to end soon.

JOANNE SABOL STEVENSON

See also
DEPRESSION AMONG OLDER ADULTS
ELDER ABUSE
FAMILY CAREGIVING TO FRAIL
   ELDERS
GERONTOLOGICAL CARE

GERONTOLOGICAL CARE

Gerontology emerged as a field of inquiry in the 20th century, but there is little agreement as to what gerontology is. According to the National Institute on Aging (NIA), scientists study aging from the broadest biological, medical, behavioral, and social perspectives in order to understand its fundamental processes and mechanisms (Achenbaum, 1995). This breadth of scope is both an asset and a liability because there is no single disciplinary perspective, few models and support for interdisciplinary work, and no common core of disciplinary knowledge to unify the field. Thus, the theory and practice of gerontology is often fragmented among multiple disciplines, each with its own traditions, theories, methods, and body of knowledge (Estes, Binney, & Culbertson, 1992).

The terms *gerontological/geriatric* nursing are often used interchangeably. In this section the former term is used, as it encompasses the study of aging, geriatrics (the medical treatment of old age and its disease), geriatric nursing, and research. Gerontological nursing practice standards were first published in 1967, and since then several reviews have assessed the state of gerontological nursing and research, including those by Adams, Basson, Brimmer, Gunter and Miller, Kayser-Jones, Rempusheski, Robinson, and Wolanin. These reviews and others in the *Annual Review of Nursing Research* and *Advances in Gerontological Nursing* indicated a steady increase in gerontological nursing research over the past 30 years. They also argued for more systematic investigations of interventions targeted to both older adults and the health care system that serves them.

Importance of Gerontological Nursing Research

Tripp-Reimer (1994) noted that interacting societal and professional factors create a current imperative for gerontological nursing research. The continuing growth of older adults (currently 13% of the U.S. population and estimated at 22.9% by 2050), the heterogeneous characteristics of the aging population, economic incentives to develop cost-effective interventions (elders account for 40% of health care expenditures), and national health objectives press for more gerontological research, especially on the effectiveness of interventions to address these diverse issues.

Early research was largely atheoretical, hindering development of a knowledge base. According to Murphy and Fenton (1991), only 59% of the 142 studies they reviewed evidenced an explicit theory-research link. Recently, nurses have used a number of conceptual models and theoretical frameworks to guide research. These include reactance (Meddaugh), behavioral theories (Whall & Boehm), basic need model (Nelson; Rossby, Beck, & Heacock), person-environment fit and interaction (Kayser-Jones; Maas and colleagues; Wyman), and stress and coping models (Archbold and associates; Hall & Buckwalter). Glick and Tripp-Reimer (1996) recently published an integrative model depicting the scope of gerontological nursing encompassing three spheres (elder, environment, and nursing) and designed to assist nurses to provide comprehensive and contextually relevant care.

Current reviews of research concentrate on single topics such as hypertension, caregiving, incontinence, confusion, sleeplessness, or dyspnea (Tripp-Reimer, 1994). Although most research has been descriptive, more nurses are using the existing knowledge base to identify and test interventions. The generalizability of gerontological research findings has been limited by methodological and measurement difficulties (i.e., inadequate sample sizes and sampling plans, lack of rigorous designs, insufficiently operationalized interventions, and inappropriate, ill-defined, insensitive, incorrectly timed or invalid outcome measures), but nurses have begun to address these methodological issues. It is important to note that there are recently issued clinical practice guidelines addressing common gerontological care issues such as pressure ulcers, cataracts, dementia, and incontinence.

Gerontological Nurse Researchers

Any compilation of this nature risks the omission of key topics, individuals, and studies. With this limitation in mind, selected nurse researchers and their areas of investigation are briefly highlighted. By no means exhaustive, these exemplars include caregiving, abuse, incontinence, confusion, and pressure ulcers—areas in which gerontological nursing research has made a significant difference in elder care.

Caregiving. Providing care for someone with a chronic illness can result in negative emotional, physical, financial, and social sequelae. The work of numerous gerontological nurse researchers (e.g., Given, Collins, Archbold, Wykle, Wright, Stewart, Hall, Farran, Davis, and others) in the areas of theory testing, interventions, outcomes, and ad-

vances in measurement has made a substantial contribution to our understanding of the caregiving experience and its multifaceted impact, particularly on family caregivers. In institutional settings, Chiverton, Burgener, Maas and associates, and Beck and colleagues have focused attention on the role of both professional and assistive personnel and its effect on care-recipient and family outcomes.

A related dimension of research in which nurses have played a key role is the etiology, identification, and intervention of elder mistreatment. The work of Fulmer, Phillips, and Rempusheski is notable in this area.

Urinary incontinence. Another common and costly gerontological condition is urinary incontinence. Nurse researchers such as McCormick, Wells, McDowell, Dougherty, Colling, and Wyman have increased our understanding and treatment of this condition in both community-dwelling and institutionalized elders. Their investigations to prevent, reverse, or reduce the negative physiological, psychological, and social effects of incontinence have ranged from the development of procedures testing pelvic floor muscle strength to nursing home staff interventions such as prompted voiding.

Acute and chronic confusion. Acute confusion can be caused by a variety of physiological, psychological, and environmental factors and is associated with high morbidity and mortality in older adults. Wolanin and Philips authored a seminal text on confusion, paving the way for others to study this pervasive condition in various patient populations. Champagne, Foreman, Neelon, Vermeersch, and M. Williams have elucidated the incidence and risk factors associated with acute confusion and developed methods to effectively capture this elusive phenomenon.

Most care needs of chronically confused elders, such as those with Alzheimer's disease, are met through nursing management strategies. Important advances have been made by Abraham, the Quayhagens, and Beck in the area of cognitive remediation; by Maas and colleagues, Mathew, and Hall in evaluating environmental designs; by Ryden, Snyder, Rader and associates, Beck, Burgener, Whall and colleagues, and Baldwin in diminishing disruptive behaviors; and by Beck and others in dressing behaviors. Gerontological nurse researchers have evaluated selected interventions to enhance sensory stimulation, such as music (Gerdner, Swanson, Abraham), exercise (Meddaugh), dolls and stuffed animals (Bailey), and animals (Baun, Kongable), and biobehavioral interventions for sundowning (Evans), wandering (Algase), and improved food consumption (Mion, Kayser-Jones), to name but a few.

Pressure ulcers. Nurse researchers also have made significant contributions to the etiology and treatment of pressure ulcers, a pervasive gerontological problem. Norton, Gosnell, Braden, and Bergstrom have been instrumental in developing risk assessment tools. Frantz evaluated prevention and treatment of pressure ulcers in a variety of settings, using transcutaneous electrical stimulation techniques, and developed measures to capture wound healing in elders.

Conclusion

As noted by Williams (1988), ''research and care require each other; they interact with each other; they benefit from each other . . . this applies to all aspects of care for older people, personal care, preventive and therapeutic health services, social services, and the organization and financing of care'' (p. 579). The scope of gerontology, a relatively new multidisciplinary field, is very broad. Nurses have made substantial contributions to research in the psychological, environmental, physiological, and sociological care of older adults, as supported by reviews of theory-research linkages (Murphy & Fenton, 1991), the usefulness of gerontological research for practice, and meta-analyses of gerontological research and theory. Nonetheless, Achenbaum (1995) cautions: ''Gerontology will continue to open new frontiers of knowledge as long as highly trained scholars are willing to cross the boundaries of their own scientific training and appreciate the rewards of broadening their fields of vision'' (p. 268).

KATHLEEN C. BUCKWALTER
SUSAN GARDNER

See also
CAREGIVER

COGNITIVE DISORDERS
GERIATRICS
PRESSURE ULCERS
URINARY INCONTINENCE

GRANTSMANSHIP

Grantsmanship is the knowledge and skill needed to prepare a grant application. It is the art behind the science. It cannot make bad science fundable, but poor grantsmanship can keep good science from receiving the favorable review needed for funding. Although good science is a necessary prerequisite for success in obtaining funding, good grant writing is what makes the good science shine. Indeed, many characterize good grantsmanship as a type of salesmanship.

Everything a grant writer does to make the grant reviewer's job easier is part of good grantsmanship. The grant writer wants to impress the reviewer with the soundness, importance, and perhaps even the creativity of the science of the proposal. At the same time, the grant writer must stimulate an excitement that turns the reviewer into an advocate or enthusiastic champion of the proposed project.

Achieving a balance between generating such enthusiasm and sticking with a somewhat rigid formula in the actual writing is an artful enterprise. Grant writing itself is not particularly creative. Rather, grant writing can be viewed as a type of formula writing. Good basic writing skills are essential. The grant writer must methodically walk the reader or reviewer through a well-constructed logical argument. The reviewer should have no question about where the grant writer is going. Moreover, a good grant writer anticipates the reviewer's questions and answers them before the question is raised.

Repetition of important content is a key aspect of good grant writing. An important point is worth repeating to ensure that a reviewer does not miss it. Repetition also is essential in the choice of words for key concepts. Once a concept is named and defined, the grant writer should stick with the identified word, term, or phrase. Altering a phrase or using alternative terms in order to provide some variety only serves to confuse a reviewer trying to follow the specific ideas presented.

Good grantsmanship also requires the ability to handle criticism. Many more grants are written and submitted than are actually funded. Therefore, a good grant writer will seek multiple reviews from colleagues before actually submitting a grant to the funding agency. It is wise to seek reviewers for a variety of purposes. Some should be familiar with the content area of the grant application to identify any important errors or gaps in content. Others should be unfamiliar with the specific content area to protect against assumed knowledge by insiders and to determine if the grant is written in a manner that convinces a knowledgeable but otherwise uninformed reviewer about the worthiness of the proposed project. Still others may be used for things such as grammar, editing, and typographical errors not found by computer spell-checks. The ability to handle criticism is needed to request and receive a brutal review and to respond to all concerns and criticisms without defensiveness. It is far better to acknowledge the concern from a colleague and be able to revise the grant application accordingly than to have the very same concern raised in the official review and result in a poor evaluation and no funding.

Although the specific proposal is the heart of the grant, grantsmanship involves much more than just writing the actual proposal. Good grant writers understand other aspects as well. For example, a cardinal rule is to follow the directions. It seems simple enough, but it is surprising how many would-be grant writers neglect to read carefully all instructions for a particular grant application and to follow them faithfully.

Most grant applications come with specific guidelines about such things as eligibility to apply, budget limits, allowable costs, page limits, margins, font sizes, section sequencing, the type of content expected, the number of references allowed, what may go into appendices (if allowed), who must sign where and what, and so on. It is imperative that the grant writer adhere to all the identified specifications. Some funding agencies will return grants unreviewed if the directions are not followed. Not following directions raises questions about the careful attention to detail needed to carry out most projects and thus may reflect poorly on the applicant.

Another basic element of good grantsmanship is to know and understand the goals and mission of the particular funding agency to which one plans to submit the grant. For example, each institute in the National Institutes of Health (NIH) has a specific mandate to fund certain types of research. Further, each institute generally sets priorities identifying specific areas in which they are seeking proposals. Prior to writing a grant, one should investigate and determine what funding agency would be the best match for the intended project.

The grant writer should specifically address the stated priorities and goals of the funding agency or foundation for support of the proposed project. This is particularly true for foundation grants. A helpful strategy when making these arguments is to use the exact language of the program announcement or the foundation's mission statement. It is rarely in the grant writer's best interest to try to convince a foundation or other funding entity of a worthwhile project not clearly within its mandate.

There are a number of references to assist a grant writer. One particularly useful book is the *Grant Application Writer's Handbook* by Liane Reif-Lehrer (1995). In addition to general information about writing and applying for grants, it contains extensive information about the grant programs of the NIH. Over half of the volume is devoted to appendices, with useful resources, references, and information about the NIH, the National Science Foundation, and applying to foundations. Although some of the specific information rapidly becomes dated, much remains valuable and timeless. The NIH also publishes a volume titled *Helpful Hints on Preparing a Research Grant Application to the National Institutes of Health* (NIH, 1991b) that contains several useful and informative articles and presentations. It is available free of charge.

LAUREN S. AARONSON

See also
FUNDING
MENTORING IN NURSING RESEARCH
NATIONAL INSTITUTE
   OF NURSING RESEARCH
NATIONAL INSTITUTES OF HEALTH

GRIEF

Definitions

Grief is the characteristic pattern of psychological and physiological responses a person experiences after the loss of a significant person, object, belief, relationship, body part, or body function. Grief includes the entire range of physical, psychological, cognitive, and behavioral responses to a loss. It is characterized by intense mental anguish and varies in duration from a few weeks to many years. Two major types of normal grief have been identified: conventional grief, which occurs after a loss, and anticipatory grief, which occurs in anticipation of a loss. Anticipatory grief is the characteristic pattern of psychological and physiological responses a person makes to an impending loss. Although there is little agreement on the exact nature of anticipatory grief, there is general agreement that anticipatory grief facilitates coping with a loss when the loss actually occurs.

Three terms related to grief should be defined: *loss*, *bereavement*, and *mourning*. Loss is defined as the experience of parting with an object, person, belief, or relationship that is valued; the loss necessitates a reorganization of one or more aspects of the person's life. Losses range from minor ones, such as the loss of a wallet, which necessitates only minor adjustments, to major ones, such as the death of a loved one, which necessitates major adjustments. Bereavement is the state of having experienced a loss, particularly the death of a significant other. Bereavement is usually but not always accompanied by grief. Mourning encompasses the socially prescribed behaviors after the death of a significant other. Such behaviors vary from culture to culture. Mourning behaviors are symbols or conventional outward signs of grief that are socially constructed and do not necessarily indicate the presence or absence of grief. Examples include wearing black clothing or a black veil or armband.

Throughout time nurses have had key roles in dealing with grief. Nurses in diverse settings are especially involved in dealing with anticipatory grief; however, little nursing research was conducted on grief until the late 1980s.

Researchers and Major Studies

Jeanne Quint Benoliel (1983) presented a review of nursing research on death, dying, and terminal illness at a time when few nurses were conducting research in those areas. Since then research on grief and bereavement has proliferated. Demi and Miles (1986) published a review of research on bereavement, and subsequently Opie (1992) published one on childhood and adolescent bereavement. Nursing interest in grief and bereavement flourished during the 1980s and 1990s and extended to grief and anticipatory grief related to hospice care. Martinson (1995) reviewed research on pediatric hospice care and addressed both anticipatory grief and grief following the death of a pediatric hospice patient; Corless (1994) in her critique of research on symptom control within hospice care reviewed research on coping with dying, strategies, and needs. All these reviews can be located in the specific *Annual Review of Nursing Research* volume, edited by J. J. Fitzpatrick et al. and published by Springer Publishing. A number of nurses developed research programs focused on grief, including J.Q. Benoliel, R. Constantino, A. Demi, M. Diamond, M. Miles, J. Saunders, and M. Vachon.

Researchers have used both quantitative and qualitative approaches to study grief. Standardized instruments such as the Texas Inventory of Grief, the Grief Experience Inventory, and the Bereavement Experience Questionnaire have been used to assess grief manifestations. The emotional distress that accompanies grief was often measured with instruments such as the Brief Symptom Inventory, the Profile of Mood States, the Impact of Events Questionnaire, or a depression scale such as the Beck's or Hamilton's. Children's and adolescents' grief was often measured by the Child Behavior Checklist.

Much nursing research on bereavement has been directed at describing the manifestations of grief among diverse samples: bereaved parents, children, siblings, and widows; suicide survivors; and people facing a life-threatening or terminal illness. Other researchers have described bereaved persons' responses to events such as the loss of a home by fire and a spontaneous or elective abortion. Still other researchers have focused on describing nurses' responses to caring for the dying or the bereaved. These descriptive studies have used diverse methods, including grounded theory, phenomenology, participant observation, semistructured interviews, survey questionnaires, structured instruments, and q-sort techniques. For example, Jacobs (1996) used grounded theory to describe the grief experience of older women whose husbands received hospice care during their final illness; Grossman, Clark, Gross, Halstead, and Pennington (1995) used interviews to describe children's bereavement process after paternal suicide; Feldstein and Gemma (1995) used the Grief Experience Inventory to describe oncology nurses' responses to caring for dying patients; McCowan and Davies (1995) used the Child Behavior Checklist to assess patterns of grief in young children following the death of a sibling; and Kerr (1994) used a qualitative approach to assess the meanings adult daughters attach to a parent's death.

Some nursing research on bereavement has focused on comparing different modes of bereavement (suicide vs. accident, expected vs. unexpected) or comparing bereaved persons with a non-bereaved group. For example, Kovarsky (1989) compared loneliness and grief manifestations of parents whose child died by suicide with those whose child died accidentally.

A number of nursing studies have investigated variables related to bereavement outcomes. For example: self-blame was associated with poorer outcomes after the death of a loved one (Weinberg, 1995); coping process was related to social support and adaptational outcomes in widows (Robinson, 1995); and a significant relationship was found between effective grief resolution and hope, coping styles, and death within a hospice setting among the elderly widowed (Herth, 1990).

A few studies have used quasi-experimental designs to investigate the effects of specific interventions to help the bereaved or to help nurses to better meet the needs of the bereaved. For example, researchers have studied the effect of a support group on bereaved parents whose child died from cancer, the effect of a support group on bereaved children and adolescents, and the effect of a grief workshop for pediatric oncology nurses.

Strengths and Limitations of the Studies

The descriptive studies have contributed greatly to our understanding of the grief process and the many forms it may take. The comparative and correlational studies have provided insight into variables related to good and poor bereavement outcomes. However, very little research has been done to assess the effects of bereavement interventions. More attention needs to be paid to intervention studies that address what helps people deal with anticipatory grief and grief due to a loss that has already occurred. Further, most of the participants in the studies reviewed were White Americans. With increasing cultural diversity in the United States, it is important that research address bereavement responses among diverse cultural groups. In addition, researchers should work on developing culturally relevant instruments to assess bereavement outcomes.

Ethical Issues

Grieving people are vulnerable and need special attention to protect them from studies that could increase their vulnerability. Although many grieving people find that participating in research that focuses on their grief provides them an opportunity to express their thoughts and feelings to a nonjudgmental researcher, there is the potential of increasing the participant's pain and distress. The researcher must have the skills to provide immediate support if this occurs and also should be prepared to refer participants for counseling if they need further support at a later time.

ALICE S. DEMI

See also
  COPING
  HOSPICE
  SUICIDE
  TERMINAL ILLNESS

GROUNDED THEORY

Grounded theory refers to an orderly, rigorous, constant comparative method for qualitative analysis to generate theory from data and the resultant conceptual schema. Grounded theory explains variation in social interactional and social structural problems and processes. According to sociologist originators Barney Glaser and Anselm Strauss (1967), grounded theories should be relevant and work to explain, predict, and be modified by social phenomena under study. Data are not forced to fit existing theories but rather are used to develop rich, dense, complex analytic frameworks. Unlike theory verifying research in which data collection and analysis are separate linear steps, data collection and analysis go on simultaneously, with concepts and propositions that emerge from the data directing subsequent data collection.

The grounded theory approach presumes the possibility of discovering fundamental patterns in all of social life, called core variables or basic social processes (Hutchinson, 1993; Wilson, 1993). Grounded theories are focused on what may be unarticulated social-psychological and social-structural problems and are integrated around the basic social process that is discovered in observational, interview, and document data (Wilson & Hutchinson, 1996). Properties, dimensions, categories, strategies, and phases of the theory are inextricably related to the basic social process. The researcher does not begin with a preconceived theory and experimentally prove it. Rather, the researcher begins by studying an area under natural conditions. What is relevant to that area is allowed to emerge and is refined into an integrated, dense, parsimonious, conceptual representation. Grounded theory may be context-bound to a specific substantive area (substantive theory) or may be at a more conceptual level and applicable to diverse settings and experiences (formal theory) (Glaser, 1978).

Grounded theory as an original mode of inquiry oriented to the discovery of meaning emerged from the social philosophy of symbolic interactionism and an intellectual tradition in social science called pragmatism. Both emphasize (a) the importance of qualitative fieldwork in data collection in order to ground theory in reality, (b) the nature of experience as a process of continuous change, and (c) the interrelationships among conditions, interpretive meaning, and action. Knowledge is viewed as relative to particular contextual circumstances. Such a worldview was in contrast to the dominant paradigm that emphasized stability and regularities in social life.

The grounded theory approach has resonated with a wide variety of social scientists and professional practitioners interested in human experiences with health and illness. Its influence has been particularly striking in the evolution of nursing research because Glaser and Strauss, who developed the method, were professors in the School of Nursing at the University of California, San Francisco, beginning in the 1960s. Consequently, many of the seminal methodological references and landmark publications of findings in the nursing literature can be traced to nursing doctoral students who studied and collaborated with them in the 1970s and 1980s. Subsequently, those early colleagues mentored cohorts of other nurse researchers. In addition, grounded theory as a qualitative, nonmathematical analytic process is particularly well suited to nursing studies that are conducted to uncover the nature of clinically relevant phenomena such as chronic illness, caregiving, and dying in real-world rather than laboratory conditions. The resulting theoretical formulation not only explains human experience and associated meanings but also can provide a basis for nursing intervention research and nursing practice.

Grounded theory as an approach to the generation of theory from data has undergone some major transformations since its introduction by Glaser and Strauss. Some of the changes that were designed to promote rigor in the method have been criticized as diverting the research from generating theory directly from data, for risking theoretical sensitivity in the investigator, and for eroding the method. Others are of the opinion that assuming that grounded theory was taught and conducted from a single unified perspective is erroneous and that the ongoing discourse among qualitative researchers is part of an intellectual movement essential to grounded theory's refinement and evolution. The hallmarks, however, continue to be data-theory interplay, making constant comparisons, asking theoretically oriented questions, conceptual and theoretical coding, and the development of theory.

Doing grounded theory research departs from the typically linear sequence of theory verifying research because data collection and analysis go on simultaneously. The investigator approaches a phenomenon without a preconceived theoretical framework, using only sensitizing questions to learn what is relevant in the situation under study. Sampling is not conducted according to conventions of probability, nor is sample size predetermined. Instead, purposive, theoretical sampling is used. Theoretical sampling is conducted so that concepts emerging from the data guide additional data collection. The sample is considered complete when saturation is achieved. Saturation refers to the point at which no new themes, patterns, or concepts appear in the data.

Data are usually derived from qualitative data sources—interviews, participant observation (field-work), and document analysis—although quantitative data can also inform the emerging analysis. The outcome of analysis is a dense, parsimonious, integrative schema that explains most of the variation in a social psychological situation. Data analysis proceeds through stages of in vivo (or substantive) coding in which themes and patterns are identified in the words of participants themselves, coding for categories in which in vivo codes are clustered together in conceptual categories, and theoretical coding in which relationships among concepts are developed. Memos are written detailing each of the codes and categories and linking them to exemplars from the data. Sorting memos (conceptual notes about codes and categories and their data exemplars) into an integrative schema provides an outline for integrating and then reporting the grounded theory discovered.

HOLLY SKODOL WILSON
SALLY A. HUTCHINSON

See also
DATA COLLECTION METHODS
PARTICIPANT OBSERVATION
PHENOMENOLOGY
QUALITATIVE RESEARCH
RESEARCH INTERVIEWS
  (QUALITATIVE)

H

HEALTH OF AFRICAN AMERICANS

Health problems confronting the African American (the terms *Black* and *African American* will be used interchangeably) community are staggering according to Braithwaite and Taylor (1992). Black men are nearly twice as likely to die from cancer as is the general population. Black infants are twice as likely as White infants to die before they are a year old. Young Black males (15–24) experience a homicide rate 700% higher than that for White males, and the rate of AIDS among Blacks is more than three times that among Whites. Thus, there are clear disparities in mortality rates between African Americans and White Americans. Since 1900 the life expectancy for African Americans has slowly but steadily increased until recently. During the past several years, however, there has been a decline in longevity for Blacks. African Americans have a life expectancy of 69.6 years, compared to 75.2 years for nonminorities—a gap of 5 years. Currently, there are close to 80,000 excess deaths among African Americans in this country (the number who would be alive if mortality rates were the same for both groups). Interestingly, the survival rate for Blacks, especially for women who reach age 75, is higher than that for Whites. This phase is often referred to as the "crossover"; however, more in-depth research is needed to understand this phenomena.

It is well known that African Americans suffer disproportionately higher morbidity and mortality rates for various illnesses, particularly cardiovascular disease, hypertension, cancer, diabetes, arthritis, asthma, and substance abuse. The decline in life expectancy of African Americans is largely due to poor health, poor health care, and a lower level of health promotion activities across the life span. For example, the infant mortality rate is higher in some parts of the African American community than in many third world countries.

Health professionals have largely neglected the health care problems of African Americans. This neglect of African American health can be traced to slavery, where racism led to an inequality in health care practices and a lack of knowledge regarding health care needs (McKinney-Edmonds, 1993). Many African Americans do not have access to culturally competent health care and health care programs; and when those are available, they are underutilized because of lack of trust.

There have been several studies that focused on African Americans' use of health care services. A study was done at the Henry Ford Healthcare System in Detroit, using administrative data and a diagnosis clustering program to assess health care needs of African Americans (Lamerato, Ye, & Tilley, 1996). Employing a descriptional, comparison design, the researchers found that utilization patterns for African Americans differed from those of White patients for care settings and reasons for visits. African Americans used the emergency department more frequently than outpatient services, and Whites used it less. Also, the rate of hospital discharges and hospital days were higher for African Americans in the adult and pediatric populations than for their White counterparts. After excluding routine medical examinations, the most frequent diagnoses associated with outpatient visits for adult African Americans were hypertension and uncomplicated (Type II) diabetes, followed by chronic renal failure. It is noteworthy that these conditions require lifelong management on the part of the pro-

vider and the client. For adult African Americans, a large number of high-volume diagnoses in the emergency department were related to injury, a minor infection, or asthma.

Physician-diagnosed health problems, by degree of problem severity, were examined in 581 Black elders (McKinney-Edmonds, 1993). The incidence of hypertension was highest (54.9%), followed by arthritis (52.8%). The highest reported severity was in circulation problems (37.5%), followed by arthritis (37.3%). Patterns of utilization among these same Black elders indicated highest use of private physicians and public health clinics ($N = 689$), compared to office visits with nurses and visiting nurses ($N = 67$).

Chronic diseases represent significant health problems for African Americans, causing substantial mortality and requiring the utilization of significant resources. As indicated in the report of the Secretary's Task Force on Black and Minority Health, the leading causes of death among elderly Blacks are cancer, heart disease, stroke, diabetes, and cirrhosis of the liver. Despite an overall decline in death rates in this country since 1960, the poor and poorly educated people (where a large percentage of Blacks are represented) still die at higher rates than those with higher incomes or better education, and this disparity increased between 1960 and 1986 (Pappas, Queen, Hadden, & Fisher, 1993).

According to some statistics, African Americans' illnesses are less likely to be treated aggressively than are those of Whites. Blacks were significantly less likely than Whites to be admitted to the hospital following cardiac arrest and half as likely to survive when admitted, even after controlling for recognized risk factors (Becker, Han, et al., 1993). Likewise, after adjustment for all potential confounders, including the absence of financial incentives, White veterans were more likely than Black veterans to undergo cardiac catheterization, coronary artery bypass surgery, and angioplasty (Whittle, Conigliaro, Good, & Lofgren, 1993).

Among patients infected with HIV, Blacks were significantly less likely than Whites to have received antiretroviral therapy or PCP prophylaxis when they were first referred to an HIV clinic (Moore, Stanton, Gopalan, & Chaisson, 1994). This disparity suggests a need for culturally specific interventions to ensure uniform access to care, including drug therapy and uniform standards of care. African Americans often delay seeking formal health care treatment until late in the disease process. Dismantling affirmative action programs, as is currently proposed, may threaten health care for poor people and members of minority groups. Alford-Smith (1997) argued that the impact of attitudes and understanding of health professionals about access to health care and health status, particularly for low-income Blacks, may become more significant as health professionals play the role of gatekeeper to the health care system.

The percentage of minority health care professionals is slim, and Blacks, particularly older African Americans, are reluctant to seek help from majority health care professionals because they are often viewed as being insensitive. The call for research on African Americans to learn more about their health care needs and illness interventions has been intensified (Wykle & Kaskel, 1991). Ironically, this comes at a time when there is a renewed lack of trust in health care researchers, given the increased notoriety from the recent exposé of the Tuskegee syphilis experiment.

A long history of suffering from systemic deprivation is known to have had a deleterious impact on the quality of health care for African Americans in this country (Braithwaite & Taylor, 1992). All nurses and health care providers should be aware of these disparities and the excess morbidity and mortality of African Americans. It is necessary to treat these concerns in the context of their relationship to the socioeconomic status of African Americans in the United States. Poor health status (including physical and mental health) is also thought to be the result of inherent qualities or racism that has limited African Americans' access to health care resources. Geronimus, Bound, Waidmann, Hillemeier, and Burns (1996) found important differences among impoverished communities in patterns of excess mortality. Many African Americans who live in poverty never reach an older age as a result of infant mortality, lack of access to preventive health care and advanced medical interventions, poor nutrition, and stress. A large number of African Americans work in labor-intensive or domestic settings that offer few protections to assure a safe workplace and impose higher risks of injury and disability; in addition, such jobs are less likely to have adequate retirement and health benefits. Most often there is a lack of health care services in areas where the majority of African Americans live. Poor transportation limits their ability to find services, along with unaffordable housing in neighborhoods where health services exist.

A critical dimension of nursing's role is assisting adults to move toward their maximum health potential, regardless of their socioeconomic status or cultural background. African Americans can be saved from excess morbidity and premature death caused by chronic illnesses through health education, better management of illnesses, and health promotion activities. To keep African Americans in good health, nursing's important role is to educate, rehabilitate, support, and counsel minority persons, using culturally competent preventive care. The multiple benefits of developing and maintaining healthy lifestyles cannot be overemphasized for African Americans. There is evidence to suggest that positive health behaviors not only extend life but reduce the risk of losing mobility and independence in later life. Even in late life, modifying certain risk behaviors into healthy ones can improve health and reduce the likelihood of disability.

Nurses can reinforce health behaviors in supportive social environments that promote exemplary emotional and physical health, through worksite health programs (e.g., smoking cessation, exercise, stress control), community groups, church-provided support, and self-help groups. Health facilities' screening and patient education are key to facilitating healthy lifestyle changes in African Americans. Research is needed to understand the uniqueness, similarities, and physical differences in ethnically diverse groups and to foster affordable, accessible, culturally sensitive health care. Well-designed, systematic nursing studies of African Americans' health care issues that reexamine, reevaluate, and promote the development of new nursing knowledge is mandatory. Thus, nursing research outcomes could have a positive influence on the nation's future health agenda for the care of African Americans in this country.

MAY L. WYKLE
PATRICIA McDONALD

See also
CHRONIC ILLNESS

CULTURAL/TRANSCULTURAL FOCUS
HYPERTENSION
RISK FACTORS

HEALTH CARE FINANCING ADMINISTRATION

The Health Care Financing Administration (HCFA) of the Department of Health and Human Services is the federal agency that administers the Medicare and Medicaid programs. It also regulates all U.S. laboratory testing (except research) through the Clinical Laboratory Improvement Amendments program (United States Health Care Financing Administration, 1997c). The HCFA's roles include purchasing health care services, conducting research on health care management, treatment, and financing; establishing reimbursement policies; and evaluating health care facility and services quality. The HCFA oversees about 17,400 nursing homes and 9,800 home health agency inspections each year (United States Health Care Financing Administration, 1997d). Title XVIII, Medicare, and Title XIX, Medicaid, of the Social Security Act were enacted in 1965. As of 1997 more than 74 million Americans receive health care through Medicare and Medicaid. Most of the care is provided through the fee-for-service delivery system, although many recipients receive care through managed care plans. The HCFA is important to nursing for health care service reimbursement, funding for nursing research, and monitoring for quality nursing and other health care.

Medicare is the nation's largest health insurance program, covering 38 million Americans. The HCFA expects to spend $210.9 billion for Medicare in 1997. Medicare provides insurance to people 65 years and older, the disabled (5 million), and those with permanent kidney failure (275,000). Medicare is hospital insurance (Part A) and medical insurance (Part B). Part A provides coverage of inpatient hospital services, skilled nursing facilities, home health services, and hospice care. Part B helps pay for the cost of a nurse practitioner, nurse midwifery, physician services, outpatient hospital services, medical equipment and supplies, and other health services and supplies. Part A is financed through a part of the Social Security payroll tax, although

Medicare beneficiaries must pay deductibles ($760 in 1997) and coinsurance. General tax revenues fund about 75% of Part B expenditures, although beneficiaries must pay monthly premiums for coverage ($43.80 in 1997) as well as deductibles and coinsurance (United States Health Care Financing Administration, 1997a).

Medicaid is a program that provides medical assistance for certain individuals and families with low incomes and resources. The program is jointly funded by federal and state governments and varies from state to state and within states over time as to eligibility and covered benefits. States provide medical care to eligible needy persons within broad federal guidelines. Each state ''1. establishes its own eligibility standards; 2. determines the type, amount, duration, and scope of services; 3. sets the rate of payment for services; and 4. administers its own program'' (United States Health Care Financing Administration, 1997b).

Title XIX requires that states provide specified basic services to the categorically needy population in order to receive federal matching funds. These services are

inpatient hospital services; outpatient hospital services; physician services; medical and surgical dental services; nursing facility (NF) services for individuals aged 21 or older; home health care for persons eligible for nursing facility services; family planning services and supplies; rural health clinic services and any other ambulatory services offered by a rural health clinic that are otherwise covered under the State plan; laboratory and x-ray services; pediatric and family nurse practitioner services; federally-qualified health center services and any other ambulatory services offered by a federally-qualified health center that are otherwise covered under the State plan; nurse-midwife services (to the extent authorized under State law); and early and periodic screening, diagnosis, and treatment (EPSDT) services for individuals under age 21. (United States Health Care Financing Administration, 1997c)

If states choose to provide Medicaid to the medically needy, they must provide the following additional services:

prenatal care and delivery services for pregnant women; ambulatory services to individuals under age 18 and individuals entitled to institutional services; home health services to individuals entitled to nursing facility services; and if the State plan includes services either in institutions for mental diseases or in intermediate care facilities for the mentally retarded (ICF/MRs), it must offer either of the following to each of the medically needy groups: the services contained in 42 CFR sections 440.10 through 440.50 and 440.165 (to the extent that nurse-midwives are authorized to practice under State law or regulations); or the services contained in any seven of the sections in 42 CFR 440.10 through 440.165. (United States Health Care Financing Administration, 1997c)

States may also provide optional services and receive federal funding for those services. Such services include "clinic services; nursing facility services for the under age 21; intermediate care facility/mentally retarded services; optometrist services and eyeglasses; prescribed drugs; TB-related services for TB infected persons; prosthetic devices; and dental services" (United States Health Care Financing Administration, 1997c)

Each state's Medicaid plan must allow recipients freedom of choice among health care providers participating in Medicaid. The waivers 1915(b) and 1115(b) allow states to pay for Medicaid services through managed care organizations. In 1995 about 25% of Medicaid recipients were in managed care organizations. The portion of the Medicaid program that is paid for by the federal government is based on each state's average per capita income and ranges from 50% to 83%.

The HCFA is the federal agency that manages the Medicare and Medicaid programs. Medicare is the national health insurance program for the elderly, the disabled, and those with permanent kidney damage. Medicaid pays for health care for people with low incomes and is jointly funded by the federal government and states.

CHRISTINE T. KOVNER

Se also
   HEALTH POLICY
   HEALTH SERVICES DELIVERY
   HOME HEALTH SYSTEMS
   MANAGED CARE

HEALTH CARE REFORM

As the American health care delivery system undergoes changes in the name of reform, there remain important issues and questions about the effect these changes have had and will have on patients and providers of care. Whereas most recognize the motivation for these reforms as primarily financial, there are two distinct problems generally recognized with the current system. One is that the overall cost for health care is too great, and continual growth in the system is not sustainable without significant negative consequences to the economy. The second problem is that the outcomes associated with the services provided are not optimal. Concerns about mortality rates and significant variation in treatment plans and costs with little difference in outcomes are examples of the latter problem.

Reforms are underway to address both of these problems. Reforms to decrease the cost of delivering care by reducing overhead expenses, by providing care in the least costly setting, and by changing the provider mix are attempts at reducing the overall costs of care. Reforms focused on the outcomes of care, on provider practice patterns, and on quality indicators are aimed at ensuring that the money is well spent—the second problem.

As these reforms go forward, there is little question that the changes significantly affect the practice of nursing and thus will have a significant impact on nursing research. First and foremost, these changes should influence and drive the questions that are asked. Within the first area, questions about how care is provided in the least costly manner are crucial, for example, What is the appropriate mix of professional and nonprofessional personnel? How is intensive nursing care provided in home settings in a safe and effective manner? In the second area there are questions not only about the outcomes of care but more fundamentally about what those outcome measures ought to be.

Research

Nursing research on issues relevant to health care reform is minimal. In the first area—overall reduction of cost—researchers have examined the use of advanced practice nurses, especially midwives and nurse practitioners, as a method of providing primary care at a lower cost (Bell & Mills, 1989; Feldman, Ventura, & Crosby, 1987). Studies examining changes in provider mix by using unlicensed personnel in inpatient settings are beginning. Research in the area of home care is beginning to describe issues of importance in delivering and paying for care in this setting (Shaughnessy et al., 1994).

Outcomes-oriented research in nursing is in its infancy, but there are a handful of studies that have examined cost and utilization markers as outcome measures (Brooten & Naylor, 1995), as well as various clinical studies (Brooten et al., 1994). Moreover, nursing has been active in the area of promotion of healthy lifestyles for some time. These studies provide a base for research, but much more is needed.

Research Issues in Health Care Reform

Nursing is faced with significant issues in implementing a research agenda for health care reform. These issues include the following:

1. The nature of the research is viewed as program evaluation rather than research.
2. A lack of consensus exists on the appropriate questions that need answers.
3. Conceptual and methodological problems abound in determining appropriate outcome variables.
4. There is a lack of adequate funding for systems-oriented proposals.

Nature of the Research. Research in the area of health care reform has generally been classified as health services research that is patient- or consumer-focused, not singularly focused on any discipline. Because this research frequently includes a significant component of evaluation in the design and because strict experimental study designs are impossible to implement, many do not believe these studies are research. Therefore, the role that nursing research ought to play in this area is not well determined.

Questions. The questions asked of the research on health care reform have been focused on the impact that these changes have on patients. A growing body of literature in the area of managed care for Medicaid-enrolled persons yields insights into the types of issues that government and insurers are interested in and willing to fund. As the reforms continue to emphasize health-promoting lifestyles as the cornerstone of health, examination into effective strategies for modifying health behaviors will be required.

Another problem that arises is that because this research is in some ways evaluative, it is driven by the needs of a particular system. Since the defeat of the Clinton health plan at the federal level, reform has become a local or state initiative, making the standardization of the questions difficult.

Outcome Variables. Cost has clearly been identified as one of the outcomes of interest, but nursing has never been able to articulate clearly the relevant costs of practice. Other outcome variables (e.g., utilization of services) are not specific to nursing care. Even inpatient utilization (length of stay) or home health visits cannot be used as "pure" markers because they are influenced by other disciplines. There are clinical indicators that theoretically could be used, such as infection rates, pain management, and complications associated with treatments; but method and collection issues must be addressed. Moreover, when examining outcome measures, methods must be available to adjust outcomes by severity of patient condition. Methodological work in this area is only beginning, and work specifically examining the relationship of severity to outcomes relevant to nursing has not been done.

Funding. Funding for research in the area of health care reform has been difficult to obtain. The only exception is research in the area of health behaviors and lifestyle modification. Systems-oriented research is generally not seen as a priority, for many of the above reasons—the questions cross multiple disciplines, are frequently program-oriented, and are local in interest.

Many of the current system reforms will have significant implications for how patients are cared for and how and where nursing care will be provided. For these reasons nursing must be a part of the research on health care reforms. Determining the best ways to deliver care and the best ways to measure these outcomes must be part of nursing research.

Pamela J. Salsberry

HEALTH CONCEPTUALIZATION

The concept of health is crucial for nursing because it informs the profession's goals, scope, and outcomes of practice. The goals of nursing are to restore, maintain, and promote health; the scope of nursing's concern is with problems of health. When nursing practice assists people back to a healthy condition, successful outcomes are correctly declared.

Health has been conceptualized in many ways in our society, including physical, emotional, mental, spiritual, and social well-being; what people in a culture value or desire; maximization of potential; high-level wellness; fulfillment of personal goals; successful performance of social roles; successful interaction with the environment; and proper functioning. Health has also been viewed as subjective or relative (self-report), objective (measured against an agreed-upon standard), comparative (a more-or-less condition viewed as a continuum or gradation), classificatory (a dichotomy), holistic (indivisible), a state (condition), and a process (continuous change over time). Thus, with such multiple, sometimes overlapping, sometimes redundant, sometimes contradictory conceptions of health, the term has to be understood in terms of the purposes to which it is being applied.

What is the meaning of health for nursing science, that is, for human responses to actual and potential health problems? Recent research in nursing regarding the concept of health has been dominated by two broad approaches. The first has been to provide a descriptive analysis. In this context, the intention is to understand the aims, goals, and criteria of success in current nursing practice. Investigators are trying to understand, systematize, and render coherent what nurses understand themselves to be doing and to clarify the different forms that disease or failures of health can take. Assessing the results of this approach amounts to determining which conception makes better sense of nursing practice and how the different parts of nursing practice fit together.

To most nursing clinicians and researchers, regardless of specialty area, the conception of health most applicable to practice is health as the absence of signs and symptoms of physiological malady and disability. Most nurses spend their careers observing, administering, modifying therapies, interpreting conditions, and treating people who are sick and need to be restored to health or teaching them how to stay free of those signs and symptoms. The theories that illustrate this approach include (a) Smith's (née Baigis) clinical, role-performance, and adaptive models of health (1981, 1983); (b) the conceptual models, including the self-care framework (Orem, 1991); and (c) those focused on stability, balance, and adaptation (e.g., Johnson, 1990a; Roy & Andrews, 1991).

The second approach goes beyond an analysis of actual nursing practice and presents a new vision of what the goals and practice of nursing should be. What currently passes for nursing is fundamentally inadequate; only by articulating a proper conception of health can we clearly explain what nurses should be doing. Assessing the results of this approach is much more difficult and controversial. In part, this is because some of the particular proposals reflect specific theories of human nature or philosophical orientations, like existential phenomenology, that have assessments that are a matter of dispute. In addition, these nondescriptive approaches disagree not only in their proposals for what nursing should be but also about what they identify as fundamentally wrong with current nursing practice.

Holistic theories of health are one type illustrating this second approach. Some of these are based on Rogers's (1990) science of unitary human beings. They are attempts to operationalize what Rogers meant by health as a state of continuous human evolution to ever higher levels. Examples are health as a process of becoming as experienced and described by the person (Parse, 1992); as the totality of the life process, which is evolving toward expanded consciousness (Newman, 1990); and as faster rhythms in a continuously developing life (Fitzpatrick, 1989). The concept of health as self-actualization is another type illustrating this approach, as in

Smith's (née Baigis) eudaimonistic model (1981, 1983) and Pender's (1996) definition of health in her health-promotion behavior model.

How are these theories applicable to practice? Within the context of these theories of health, there can be something wrong with a person even though the standard clinical concepts are not at issue. There are cases in the second approach where success in practice has not been achieved, yet success in practice implicitly determines what health is. If someone does not have any signs and symptoms of malady or disability and is still not actualized, the nurse has not done her job. Does this make the nurse's job unbounded? Is the nurse being set up for burnout? Does nursing practically and theoretically want to claim that its domain covers all of the actual and potential health problems inherent in all of these meanings of health? The profession must be clear about what a health problem is so that it can determine who has the problem and who does not.

Nursing is not the only profession analyzing the idea of health. Much work is also being done in the philosophy of medicine, public health, and public policy. For example, some theories of health care allocation rest on specific conceptions of health and disease—why there might be a right to adequate health care but not necessarily a right to convenient transportation (e.g., having a car) gets explained in terms of the details of what is health and why it is important. Nursing researchers should try to integrate these concerns into current theories or at least explore common themes in this work.

JUDITH A. BAIGIS

See also
FITZPATRICK'S RHYTHM MODEL
NEWMAN'S THEORY OF HEALTH
PARSE'S THEORY OF NURSING:
  HUMAN BECOMING THEORY
ROY ADAPTATION MODEL
WELLNESS

HEALTH MAINTENANCE ORGANIZATIONS

Historically, most physicians were paid on a fee-for-service basis. The physician received a payment for each patient encounter or other service from the patient receiving the care or from someone paying on behalf of the patient, such as an insurance company. Recently, health care has become "managed." Managed care systems integrate the financing and delivery of care and include financial incentives for people to use providers within the system. Health maintenance organizations (HMOs) are a type of managed care system.

Health maintenance organizations provide a defined set of health care services to persons for a predetermined periodic fixed prepayment unrelated to the actual services received and restrict their members to specific health care providers. In many cases the providers are paid a periodic payment unrelated to the services rendered. This payment method is called capitation. The providers receive a periodic fee whether or not they provide care. In HMOs there is a financial incentive to provide fewer health care services, and many people are concerned that the HMOs may not provide needed care. On the other hand, many traditional fee-for-service insurance plans have not reimbursed for preventive care. HMOs provide preventive care as part of the benefit package.

HMOs have a database on the health services the members receive. The database provides an opportunity for nurse researchers to study the health of people across settings. Many HMOs provide health promotion services, and studies could identify how these services are provided and the impact they have on people's health.

HMOs limit people's choice to a specific group of providers. Providers who are not part of these groups have few patients from HMOs. Nurses are anxious to become part of the group that is approved to provide care to HMO members.

HMOs provide a set of health care services for a fixed prepayment unrelated to the amount of health care services provided. This is beneficial to clients in need of extensive health care and clients involved in health promotion. Also, HMOs have given opportunities for nursing in the areas of research and health provider.

CHRISTINE T. KOVNER

See also
CAPITATION

HEALTH CARE REFORM
HEALTH SYSTEMS DELIVERY
MANAGED CARE

HEALTH POLICY

Health policy is a principle, plan, or course of action related to health care adopted by a government, organization, or individual. In a pluralistic society such as the United States, both public and private sectors play major and often interrelated roles in decision making about health care. Public policy focuses on decision making in the public sector, and all three branches of government—legislative, executive, and judicial—play roles in the development, implementation, and interpretation of health policy. In the private sector, professional associations, insurance companies, corporations, consumer organizations, and other interested parties set policy related to their membership and spheres of interest as well as influencing public policy through lobbying, serving as advisors, and other activities.

The discipline of health policy has developed since World War II, initially from the disciplines of economics, sociology, and political science, and is multidisciplinary in nature. Its development has accelerated during the past 30 years as the health care system has become more complex and costs have increased.

Health policy is concerned with three major issues: access, quality, and cost of health care. Although these three components of health policy are interrelated, the emphasis placed on each aspect and who determines the policy varies over time. For example, in the 1970s, as the amount of the Gross National Product spent on health care approached 10%, a major debate took place on how best to restrain the increase in costs. When various voluntary measures by the health care industry did little to hold down costs, the national debate in the late 1980s turned to how the federal government, working with the states and the private sector, could redesign the health care system to restrain costs and improve access to those Americans who are uninsured.

Although the Health Care Reform Act proposed by President Clinton in the early 1990s was not passed, health care has been transformed through the private sector. Multiple purchasers have experimented with new methods of buying health care, and providers of health care and insurers have responded with new approaches to organizing and paying for care. "This evolution, turned revolution, which has been underway for at least 25 years, is being driven by corporate purchasers and cost conscious consumers. It has created an extraordinary array of health plans aggressively competing with one another on price and quality" (Ellwood & Enthoven, 1995, p. 25).

The process by which policy is formed is complex and involves government representatives at federal, state, and local levels as well as representatives of multiple private groups. Increasingly, research and policy analysis are used by policymakers as a basis for their decisions. The increased emphasis placed on the need for research-based policy formation in health care was reflected in the establishment of the U.S. Agency for Health Care Policy and Research (AHCPR) in 1989. In the legislation establishing the agency, Congress indicated the need for continuing study of the organization, delivery, and financing of health care and added the need for attention to effectiveness and appropriateness of health care services and procedures.

Policy analysts review two or more alternatives for policy change, weighing the pros and cons in potentially meeting the goals to be achieved and the populations that will be affected. The analysis is presented to policymakers such as legislators in the public sector or executives of health care agencies in the private sector. An example of a policy analysis in the federal sector occurred when the director of the National Institutes of Health (NIH) commissioned a study of four different potential locations for an entity for nursing research within NIH. This analysis was done as nurses' professional associations were lobbying Congress to move the federal nursing research programs from the Division of Nursing in the Health Resources and Services Administration to the NIH, the mainstream of health science funding.

The Tri-Council of nursing organizations, comprising the American Nurses Association (ANA), the American Association of Colleges of Nursing, and the National League for Nursing, lobbied both the legislative and executive branches of the federal government regarding the location of the nursing research programs. The efforts were successful, and legislation establishing a National Center for Research (later changed to National Institute for Nursing Research) was passed in 1984. This example also illustrates the interplay between the public and private sectors, with nurses in the private sector trying to change federal policy regarding the location of federal nursing research programs.

Another example of health policy in relationship to nursing is the role of the nurse practitioner as established in the mid-1970s by Loretta Ford, a nurse, and Henry Silver, a physician, in response to the lack of access to health care for residents of inner cities and rural areas. Studies showed that access to care was improved and that the quality of care delivered was equal to or better than that provided by primary care physicians offering the same services (Office of Technology Assessment, 1986). An issue related to nurse practitioners is the cost of care delivered by nurses, who are paid less than physicians for delivering similar services, thus making nurse practitioners more cost-effective. A second cost issue has been direct reimbursement for services provided to patients or clients. Limited federal legislation has permitted nurse practitioners to be reimbursed for services to clients only in rural areas and in certain other settings, not in all settings. In August 1997, the U.S. Congress changed this payment policy with the passage of legislation expanding coverage to nurse practitioners and clinical nurse specialists in all settings, and the president signed the bill.

Health policy determines many functions. It outlines the standard of care and identifies who (a) receives health care services, (b) is permitted to do what in health care, (c) pays for the care, and (d) is paid for performing various services. In addition to determining which educational organizations can be accredited for educating health professionals, health policy sets guidelines for health care provider roles and for licensing and certification issues.

Nursing has focused on major nursing-specific areas of health policy. These issues have included (a) estimates of numbers and types of nurses needed, (b) reimbursement for nursing services, (c) accreditation of educational institutions, (d) salary and workplace issues that affect nurses, and (e) regulation of the practice of nurses by state boards of nursing, the ANA, and specialty organizations.

Additionally, nursing organizations and individuals attempt to influence policy related to the health and well-being of populations at risk for certain problems, such as prenatal women, infants, children, and older people. Organized nursing has lobbied to influence the establishment and expansion of public payment systems such as Medicare and Medicaid and has attempted to influence both public and private payment systems to emphasize health promotion and disease prevention.

A major effort of organized nursing was undertaken in the early 1990s, when the ANA and more than 60 other organizations worked together to establish a common framework for how nurses believed the health care system should be structured to assure access, quality and services at affordable cost. This was labeled *Nursing's Agenda for Health Care Reform* and was used to articulate nursing's interest in influencing health policy (ANA, 1991a).

ADA JACOX

See also
ACCESS TO HEALTH CARE
HEALTH CARE REFORM
HEALTH SYSTEMS DELIVERY
NATIONAL INSTITUTE OF NURSING
** RESEARCH**
ROLE OF GOVERNMENT

HEALTH SERVICES ADMINISTRATION

Definition

Health services administration (HSA) research is multidisciplinary and focuses on factors and issues affecting delivery of health services in a variety of settings from a systems perspective and on the effect of health care processes on the health and well-being of clients and populations. Issues such as access to care, development of tools to measure health status, effectiveness of treatment modalities, health policy, delivery systems, professional practice, outcomes of care, impact of managed care, financing of health care, and organizational change only partially represent the vast diversity of foci for HSA research. The breadth of issues, as well as the intent to affect care delivery are the hallmarks of HSA research.

Place in the Structure of Nursing Research

Health services administration research, by its multidisciplinary nature, must address nursing issues for full impact on systems affecting care delivery. Nurses, as the largest health care delivery professional discipline, are integrally involved in all aspects of the health care system. Nurse researchers in nursing administration, practice specialties, nursing health policy, and community health can lead or participate in HSA research. This type of research reflects the team concept by including all disciplines involved in a specific project and by reflecting those disciplines' perspectives in the study design and findings.

Relevance to Nursing

If quality of services is to be assured and improved, this type of research is necessary for improving care systems. Whether the research focus is smoking cessation or health policy, the HSA approach would be to investigate preferred systems for optimal client outcomes. Nurse researchers must shift their focus from studying individual adaptation to illness or disease to investigating the systems that facilitate maximizing such adaptation if participating in HSA research. The relevance to nursing comes in the ability to replicate such systems in practice settings and to extend the influence of research knowledge in practice.

In this age of multidisciplinary emphasis, nurses' participation in HSA research places them in a position to influence client outcomes on a larger scale than in the past. Many nursing research efforts have been hampered by not being able to account for the influence of other disciplines on client outcomes. The contribution of nursing to those outcomes is difficult to measure in isolation from medical and allied health treatments. There is tremendous potential for nursing's effect on client outcomes to be showcased by involvement in HSA research. Such research is presented in multidisciplinary forums that have potential to influence health policy beyond the discipline of nursing.

Effects on the Health Care Process

Donabedian's (1980) model of using a "structure, process and outcome" framework for evaluating the quality of medical care has been widely adopted for many HSA studies. Structure relates to the physical and organizational framework of the setting where care is delivered. Process refers to the "dynamic exchange" between provider and client that includes all interchanges that occur in support of care events. Outcomes are the dependent variables, the "measurable events" that occur as a result of the structure and process of care (Scott, 1996). The Joint Commission on Accreditation of Healthcare Organizations (JCAHO) has used this framework to evaluate health care organizations for decades. Recently, JCAHO has shifted emphasis, through its "Agenda for Change," to stress outcomes and to develop performance indicators that are less reliant on structure and process.

Health care delivery systems routinely engage in action research aimed at improving the quality of care. Quality improvement research has become ingrained in the very process of care delivery, and nurses are integrally involved in these studies. Although often not theoretically based, such studies have a direct impact on quality of care in our country and have potential to improve care broadly if the results are disseminated more widely, rather than serving solely as the basis for internal, proprietary improvement processes. Insurers are using the results of treatment effectiveness studies to determine which procedures to cover. Health maintenance organization (HMO) practices are evaluating the effect of their wellness plans on subsequent client illness patterns. Many of these studies examine cost-effectiveness.

The federal government routinely invests in HSA research. Agencies such as the Agency for

Health Care Policy and Research (AHCPR), the Center for Medical Effectiveness Research, the Health Care Financing Administration, the National Institutes of Health, the Health Resources and Services Administration, and the National Institute for Nursing Research, to name a few, are all engaged in funding and directing HSA research. The Medical Treatment Effectiveness Program was begun in 1989 by AHCPR to investigate clinical conditions that are costly, have high incidence, evidence variation in clinical outcomes, and affect Medicare or Medicaid programs. There are at present 100 projects directed by patient outcomes research teams (Foundation for Health Services Research, 1992). Such governmental support for HSA research directly influences health policy by making study results available to policymakers and caregivers. Information is available at governmental web sites (http://www.AHCPR.gov:8008) or (http://www.cdc.gov/.).

Private foundations actively fund HSA research. The Robert Wood Johnson Foundation is notable for its efforts to improve nursing care delivery. The Commonwealth Fund, the Henry J. Kaiser Foundation, and the Pew Charitable Trusts are among the most notable organizations that support HSA research on an ongoing basis.

Health services administration research can be found in almost every health care–related journal. Journals that concentrate on this multidisciplinary focus include the following: *Advances in Health Economics, Health Services Research, American Journal of Public Health, Frontiers of Health Services Management, Health Care Financing Review, Health Care Forum Journal, Health Policy, Health Services Research, Inquiry, International Journal of Health Services, Journal of Health Economics, Journal of Health Politics, Policy and Law*, and *Quality Review Bulletin*.

Future Directions

Health services administration research is engaged in investigating issues in improvement of health care delivery and in discovering ways to provide more effective and efficient care, both of which will have a great impact on the health care system.

Scarce resources can be more effectively utilized if we improve care delivery to "best demonstrated practices" levels. Of course, these levels continue to evolve and to be refined as knowledge expands. Thus, HSA research must expand understanding to maximize the potential of the health care system.

Health services administration research can provide a valuable check to the financial emphasis of our current managed care system. Outcomes research can demonstrate unanticipated effects of limiting access to care, limiting treatment options, and limiting care provider choice. Long-term outcomes can be monitored through systematic longitudinal studies to determine relative health status of client populations based on payer system, for-profit status, demographic variables, and treatment options. Health services administration research in needed to investigate these larger issues and to influence health policy for years to come.

MARY L. FISHER

See also
ACCESS TO HEALTH CARE
HEALTH POLICY
HEALTH SYSTEMS DELIVERY
MANAGED CARE
QUALITY OF CARE, MEASURING

HEALTH SYSTEMS DELIVERY

Health systems delivery is an organized approach in which health care services are provided to a defined population. The focus of the phenomenon is on the *processes by which* and the *places in which* care is delivered. Health systems delivery, by nature of its systems component, implies an integration of more than one person, department, or place. As a result, studies of health systems delivery generally use some unit level or aggregated unit of analysis.

Health delivery systems range along a continuum from discontinuous, or "haphazard," to fully integrated. Integrated health care delivery systems have the same overall goals: eliminate redundant systems, eliminate fragmentation, provide capital for clinical development, achieve a comprehensive medical (health care) record, and operate under a single management structure so that where or from whom a person receives care in the system becomes financially immaterial (Lewis, 1995). As Lewis notes, few of these systems currently exist.

According to McQueen (1995), integrated delivery systems differ from general health systems by their strategies for integration. General systems usually employ horizontal integration strategies to increase market share, whereas integrated systems use vertical strategies to create seamless experiences for clients. In today's health care environment most health delivery systems use a combined approach in which complementary organizations join together to provide more efficient services to a broader consumer population while at the same time redesigning internal departments to eliminate inefficiency and overlap.

Research concerning health systems delivery models is inconclusive and tends to focus on internal redesign initiatives (Ingersoll, 1996b). Most of these studies address unit level change in nursing professional practice models and rarely cover the complex systems redesigns that are occurring today. Designs of studies have been weak, and time frames for data collection have been inconsistent and often too close to the end of the intervention to measure long-term effect. Analysis of data also has suffered from inattention to issues associated with measuring data at the individual level and analyzing it at the unit level. Sample sizes have been small when health systems were measured at the unit level, and little generalizability was possible because of failure to address confounding variables in the subjects or the environments.

Determining costs and outcomes of health delivery systems have been particularly difficult. Many of the problems connected with these two indicators of system performance are related to lack of available data and inconsistency of measures. Costs of care delivery have been assessed by using charges for services as the primary source of data, with occasional attempts to identify indirect costs and other cost-effectiveness indicators of care delivery processes. This problem appears to be worsening rather than improving, with managed care systems in which the incentive for reporting fee-for-service information is reduced. Because reimbursement for

service is capped at a set rate, systems have less impetus for documenting and calculating charges associated with procedures and other subsumed interventions. Unless the delivery system is monitoring its own costs in relation to income, data are unavailable for comprehensive studies of systems delivery cost. Even when systems do record expenditures for care delivery operations, reporting formats and sensitivity of data may be suspect.

Outcome measures of health systems delivery are equally problematic. Considerable work has been done of late to identify and define common outcome indicators for various disease-focused activities. For nursing, this approach is wholly insufficient. Many of the indicators likely to be influenced by nursing care are not included in standard outcomes indicators packages. Furthermore, nurses have not defined and tested indicators sufficiently sensitive to detect differences in care delivery approach. Some initial work is underway to name potential outcome indicators, but formal studies of their usefulness are notably absent.

Health delivery systems research carries with it a number of methodological and measurement issues that make investigation of systems of care delivery difficult. Among these are the need for common indicators in systems where organizational characteristics and history may preclude introduction of new and different measurement approaches. Considerable time is spent determining what exists, whether it can be changed (and how much), and what the actual definitions for common terms are. For example, calculation of length of stay may or may not include day of admission or day of discharge. Without clear indication of the components of the measure, inaccuracy in data collection and report of findings is certain.

A second area of importance in measuring differences or change in health delivery systems is determining what actually *is* versus what is described in internal documents or other aging or philosophical documents. Use of written documents about health delivery systems is notoriously fraught with inaccuracies in data. Often what actually occurs is quite different from what is described in text or in reports from key informants in the system. To counter this problem, multiple data sources are required, and interviews with persons at all levels are needed. Nonparticipant or participant observation also is a useful addition, although both methods are expensive and require highly skilled observers.

A third issue pertains to change and its evolution over time. Within health systems, change occurs at varying speeds and variable degrees. Subdivisions within the system may appear similar at the outset and different over time. Or subdivisions may appear dissimilar when in fact their structures, processes, and outcomes are quite comparable. What differs may be their cultures or the climate in which work is done. Strategies implemented for measuring effect in one part of the system may fail in another, and enthusiasm of study participants will likely wax and wane at different times, making use of consistent approaches difficult or impossible. Frequent documentation of events and actions is essential for reconstructing and understanding what occurred. Modifications and compromise are usually necessary for investigators who study systems over time.

Sample size also is an issue. Health delivery systems studies usually measure effect at the organizational or system level. Because of this, large sample sizes (of systems or organizations within the system) are needed, and usually large effect sizes are chosen for estimates of power. These studies are expensive, complex, and lengthy, and many investigators avoid the hassles associated with this type of research. This is unfortunate in light of the multiple, dramatic changes that are occurring in health delivery systems today. Longitudinal, comprehensive studies are needed to determine whether or not the changes occurring result in the outcomes desired—namely, reduced cost with comparable or improved quality of care and outcomes.

GAIL L. INGERSOLL

See also
ADMINISTRATION RESEARCH
HEALTH MAINTENANCE
   ORGANIZATIONS
MANAGED CARE
ORGANIZATIONAL REDESIGN
QUALITY OF CARE, MEASURING

HEMODYNAMIC MONITORING

Definition

Hemodynamic monitoring is the use of advanced technology and application of physiological principles to clinically assess the cardiac function and circulatory system in critically ill patients and to guide therapeutic interventions. Since the pulmonary artery catheter was first introduced in 1970 (Swan et al., 1970), the catheter has been a frequently used tool in critical care to monitor and optimize the hemodynamic status of patients in the critical care setting. The catheter tip is positioned in the distal pulmonary artery and enables monitoring of the pulmonary artery systolic, diastolic, mean, and wedge pressure (when the distal balloon port is inflated) and mixed venous oxygenation blood sampling. Additional hemodynamic parameters and data are obtained from other ports and lumens of the catheter, such as right atrial pressure, blood temperature, and cardiac output measurements.

Using data obtained at the bedside from the pulmonary artery catheter and physiological concepts such as cardiac output, heart rate, preload, afterload, and contractility, critical care nurses and physicians are able to make rapid assessments and determinations about the clinical status of the critically ill patients. The catheter enables clinicians to assess ventricular function, diagnose complications following acute myocardial infarction, differentiate hypotensive states, differentiate cardiac and pulmonary disorders, manage high-risk cardiac surgical patients, and monitor unstable patients with complexities such as sepsis and major organ dysfunction who require interventions such as fluid management and vasoactive drips. The original balloon-tipped, flow-directed thermodilution catheter has evolved since 1970 and includes additional functions, such as mixed venous oxygen saturation (SvO_2), right ventricular volumes and ejection fraction, continuous monitoring of cardiac output, and intracardiac atrial ventricular sequential pacing.

Critical care nurses are responsible for continuous monitoring, interpretation, and trending of hemodynamic pressure data and for communicating this information within the medical team. The patient's vital signs are used in conjunction with the cardiac output and pulmonary artery pressures to obtain derived calculations such as systemic vascular resistance and pulmonary vascular resistance, which are physiological indexes reflecting the afterload of the left and right heart. Hemodynamic monitoring enables the critical care clinician to confirm a clinical diagnosis, identify complications, institute early intervention with the appropriate therapy, and monitor the patient's response to complex therapeutic interventions. It is for this reason that hemodynamic monitoring has great relevance to nursing, and clinical nursing research is critical to ensure positive patient outcomes.

Major Studies in Hemodynamic Monitoring

The majority of nursing research on hemodynamic monitoring has focused on the technical and clinical variables affecting accuracy of pulmonary artery pressure monitoring. This topic is particularly relevant for nurses caring for critically ill patients because of the many variables that affect accuracy in routine measurement. The standard in critical care has traditionally been to reference (level the air/fluid interface stopcock at the phlebostatic axis) and zero the catheter system a minimum of once per shift and at times more often, to offset zero drift and ensure accuracy. The results of a nursing study suggest that frequency requirements for zero-referencing disposable transducers may not be as frequent as the standard in most intensive care units. The author suggests that zeroing may be performed only once during hemodynamic monitoring, before initial readings are obtained (Ahrens, Pennick, & Tucker, 1995). Although replication studies are needed, these findings encourage practitioners to reevaluate a long-held nursing standard in critical care and demonstrate the value of keeping pace with new technology.

A major focus in nursing research has been to study hemodynamic pressures in various backrest elevations. Several studies have concluded that hemodynamic pressures can be accurately and reliably measured in backrest elevations of from 0 to 60

degrees if the air/fluid interface (zeroing stopcock) is leveled or referenced at the phlebostatic axis. Lateral positioning may be used if the air/fluid interface is leveled at the phlebostatic axis, but the patient must be at a 90-degree side position with the backrest flat to ensure accuracy. The phlebostatic axis in the right lateral 90-degree position is the fourth intercostal space at midsternum, compared to the fourth intercostal space at the left sternal border in the left lateral 90-degree position (Paolella, Dorfman, Cronan, & Hasan, 1988). Identification of the optimal reference point for lateral positions other than 90 degrees with backrest flat will require further study and validation. To ensure accuracy and reliability, all hemodynamic pressures must be read at end expiration in patients who are ventilated as well as those who are breathing spontaneously. Nursing research suggests that graphic readings of hemodynamic pressures (using a strip chart recorder) provide more reliable and accurate hemodynamic readings than do digital data (directly off the monitor) in both ventilated and spontaneously breathing patients (Johnson & Schumann, 1995).

The competency of critical care nurses in their knowledge of pulmonary artery catheters also has been a research focus. Mean scores of 48.5% to 56.8% were reported in two separate studies of critical care nurses (Burns, Burns, & Shively, 1996; Iberti et al., 1994). The results of these studies underscore the need to provide ongoing training and competency assessments of nursing staff to ensure safe and quality patient care. To ensure that appropriate interventions are based on valid hemodynamic data, accuracy as well as competency in hemodynamic monitoring is essential.

Future Directions in Research

Since the advent of the pulmonary artery catheter, technology in hemodynamic monitoring has advanced at a rapid pace. Future studies must continue to keep pace with the ever changing technology and be responsive to the clinical research needs of the nurses who work with critically ill patients. Technical difficulties in measurement, as seen in patients with severe respiratory variation, in ventilated patients on high levels of positive end expiratory pressure (PEEP), and in the presence of large "v" waves on the hemodynamic waveform, are examples of clinical issues that continue to confound critical care nurses. Additional studies that examine the effects of nursing care or interventions (e.g., cooling measures) on hemodynamic parameters, such as mixed venous oxygen saturation and intracranial pressure, would provide valuable clinical information for nurses caring for critically ill patients. Research that is meaningful and clinically relevant to nursing practice is essential to enhancing patient care.

Ethical Issues in Hemodynamic Monitoring

The potential risk versus benefit of pulmonary artery catheterization is an important ethical consideration in hemodynamic monitoring. Because of potentially serious complications, hemodynamic monitoring via pulmonary artery catheterization should not be undertaken unless clearly indicated. Although critical care nurses and physician intensivists have envisioned the pulmonary artery catheter as a critical tool for diagnosis and therapeutic decision making, questions have been raised within major medical journals and the media about the safety and efficacy of pulmonary artery catheterization. As a result of the controversy, organizations such as the Society of Critical Care Medicine have intensified efforts to examine and closely scrutinize the procedure of pulmonary artery catheterization. Large randomized controlled trials have been proposed to evaluate critically the safety and effectiveness of pulmonary artery catheters in critically ill patients.

The issue of clinical competency in hemodynamic monitoring also must be considered. For critical care nurses, ethical responsibility includes an understanding of indications for the use of pulmonary artery catheters and of the principles of hemodynamic monitoring, techniques of insertion, identification of potential complications, interpretation of hemodynamic data, and implementation of prescribed therapeutic interventions to ensure patient safety and desired therapeutic outcomes. Hemodynamic monitoring is a valuable tool if used judiciously by specially trained and competent medical and nursing professionals.

MAUREEN KECKEISEN

See also
CARDIOVASCULAR NURSING
CLINICAL NURSING RESEARCH
CLINICAL TRIALS
CRITICAL CARE NURSING
PHYSIOLOGICAL MONITORING

HENDERSON'S MODEL

Virginia Henderson wrote two important books that presented her thinking about nurses and nursing. The first was commissioned by the International Council of Nurses (Henderson, 1960/1997) and titled *Basic Principles of Nursing Care*. In this work, Henderson formally presented her ideas about the unique role of nurses and defined nursing. The second was called *The Nature of Nursing* (Henderson, 1966/1991) and expanded on the previous work to include consideration of the origin of her thinking as well as providing implications for how nursing so described could be practiced, researched, and taught. Henderson's model of nursing is most succinctly presented in these two works. In them she says:

> The unique function of the nurse is to assist the individual, sick or well, in the performance of those activities contributing to health or its recovery (or to a peaceful death) that the person would perform unaided given the necessary strength, will or knowledge. And to do this in such a way as to help the individual gain independence as rapidly as possible. (Henderson, 1997, p. 22)

Basic nursing care means helping the patient with the following activities or providing conditions under which the patient can perform them unaided:

1. breathe normally
2. eat and drink adequately
3. eliminate body wastes
4. move and maintain desirable postures
5. sleep and rest

6. select suitable clothes—dress and undress
7. maintain body temperature within normal range by adjusting clothing and modifying the environment
8. keep the body clean and well groomed and protect the integument
9. avoid the dangers in the environment and avoid injuring others
10. communicate with others in expressing emotions, needs, fears or opinions
11. worship according to one's faith
12. work in such a way that there is a sense of accomplishment
13. play or participate in various forms of recreation
14. learn, discover or satisfy the curiosity that leads to normal development and health and use the available health facilities. (Henderson, 1997, pp. 34–35)

Henderson (1997) also described conditions in persons that always affect basic needs:

1. Age: newborn, child, youth, adult, middle aged, aged and the dying.
2. Temperament, emotional state, or passing mood:
   a) "normal" or
   b) euphoric and hyperactive or
   c) anxious, fearful, agitated or hysterical or
   d) depressed and hypoactive.
3. Social or cultural status: A member of a family unit with friends and status, or a person relatively alone and/or maladjusted, destitute.
4. Physical and intellectual capacity:
   a) normal weight
   b) underweight
   c) overweight
   d) normal mentality
   e) subnormal mentality
   f) gifted mentality
   g) normal sense of hearing, sight, equilibrium and touch
   h) loss of special sense
   i) normal motor power
   j) loss of motor power. (Henderson, 1997b, pp. 34–35)

There are also pathological states (as contrasted with specific diseases) that modify basic needs, as follows:

1. marked disturbances of fluid and electrolyte balance including starvation states, pernicious vomiting, and diarrhea

2. acute oxygen want
3. shock (including "collapse" and hemorrhage)
4. disturbances of consciousness—fainting, coma, delirium
5. exposure to cold and heat causing markedly abnormal body temperatures
6. acute febrile states (all causes)
7. a local injury, wound and/or infection
8. a communicable condition
9. pre-operative state
10. post-operative state
11. immobilization from disease or prescribed as treatment
12. persistent or intractable pain. (Henderson, 1997, pp. 34–35)

The concept of the nurse as a substitute for what the patient lacks to make him "complete," "whole," or "independent," by lack of physical strength, will or knowledge, may seem limited to some. The more one thinks about it, however, the more complex the nurse's function as so defined proves to be. Think how rare is "completeness," or "wholeness" of mind and body. To what extent good health is a matter of heredity, to what extent it is acquired, is controversial but it is generally admitted that intelligence and education tend to parallel health status. If then people find "good health" a challenging goal, think how much more difficult is it for the nurse to help them reach it: the nurse must, in a sense, get "inside the skin" of each patient in order to know not only what the patient wants but also needs to maintain life and regain health. The nurse is temporarily the consciousness of the unconscious, the love of life for the suicidal, the leg of the amputee, the eyes of the newly blind, a means of locomotion for the infant, knowledge and confidence for the young mother, a "voice" for those too weak to speak, and so on. (Henderson, 1997, pp. 34–35)

Gladys Nite (Nite & Willis, 1964) explicitly tested this model of nursing in clinical experiments of effective nursing care of cardiac patients. Brooten and Naylor (1995) implicitly examined this model in their clinical research. The "nurse dose" they seek to measure may indeed be some quantified measure of this unique function. Similarly, other researchers seem to be addressing this model of nurses' function in their examination of the effectiveness of nurses in different roles and in different settings (Douglas et al., 1995; Landefeld, Palmer, Kresevic, Fortinsky, & Kowal, 1995; Olds et al., 1997).

Henderson went on from this work to prepare a critique of nursing research and an index of the English language nursing literature written between 1900 and 1960. When finished, she revised the textbook that she had twice previously redone. Remarkably, the textbook incorporated numerous citations from the professional literature and was the only edition written around her model of nursing. *Principles and Practice of Nursing* (Henderson & Nite, 1978/1997) not only synthesized much of what was known about modern nursing but organized a disparate literature around a model of nursing not appreciably altered in the nearly 20 years since her book first appeared. Rather than changing her mind based on her reading of the literature, Henderson synthesized the literature into a coherent reference document.

Three of Henderson's papers extend her model, two by validation and the other by contradiction. *The Concept of Nursing* (Henderson, 1978) specifically addressed her work as a model. "Preserving the Essence of Nursing in a Technological Age" (Halloran, 1995) extended her ideas to include services nurses provide in intensive care units and was organized on the basis of the professional functions first depicted in *The Nature of Nursing* (practice, research and education) and added material on how good administration could improve nursing. In "Nursing Process—Is the Title Right?" by Henderson (Halloran, 1995) she contradicted what had become the accepted alternative to the use of the word *nursing* by arguing that the phrase unnecessarily constrained professional vision and precluded experience, logic, and expert opinion as bases for practice.

The most complete exposition of Henderson's model of nurses' function and nursing practice is contained in the sixth edition of *Principles and Practice of Nursing* (Henderson & Nite, 1978/1997). The work is a modern book largely unknown to the American nurses who today struggle with many of the issues of professional practice elaborated on in the model and related documents.

EDWARD J. HALLORAN

See also
HEALTH CONCEPTUALIZATION
NURSING THEORETICAL MODELS

HERMENEUTICS

Historically, hermeneutics described the art or theory of interpretation (predominantly that of texts) and was prevalent in disciplines such as theology and law. German philosopher Wilhelm Dilthey (1833–1911) redefined hermeneutics as a science of historical understanding and sought a method for deriving objectively valid interpretations. Martin Heidegger (1889–1976) recast hermeneutics from being based on the interpretation of historical consciousness to revealing the temporality of self-understandings (Palmer, 1969).

Hermeneutics is an approach to scholarship that acknowledges the temporal situatedness of both the researcher and the participants. Time as it advenes, or time-as-lived, is central to the work of hermeneutics. The centrality of time is what differentiates hermeneutics from traditional forms of Husserlian phenomenology. The hermeneutic scholar works to uncover how humans are "always already" given *as* time. Hermeneutics has no beginning or end that can be concretely defined but is a *continuing* experience for all who participate.

Interpretation presupposes a threefold structure of understanding, which Heidegger called the fore-structure. The premise of the fore-structure is that all interpretations are based on background practices that grant us practical familiarity with phenomena. Heidegger called this sense of phenomena fore-having. Our background practices also form the perspective from which we approach understanding. Our interpretive lens, termed fore-sight, is constituted by background practices. Fore-conception describes our anticipated sense of what our interpreting will reveal. This too is shaped and framed by our background practices. Understanding is circular, and humans as self-interpreting beings are always already within this interpretive (hermeneutic) circle of understanding. Thus, "interpretation is never a presuppositionless grasping of something previously given" (Heidegger, 1927/1996, p. 141). Hermeneutic researchers do not attempt to isolate or "bracket" their presuppositions but rather to make them explicit. Hans-Georg Gadamer (1989), a student of Heidegger's, has extended hermeneutical research in this area. The essence of hermeneutics lies not in some kind of mystic relativism but in an attitude of respect for the impossibility of bringing the understanding of "Being" to some kind of final or ultimate closure. The way of hermeneutics is to allow oneself to be drawn into the complexity of the simple and overlooked (Heidegger, 1977/1993).

The work of interpretive phenomenologists moves beyond traditional logical structures to reveal and explicate otherwise hidden relationships. Calling attention to human practices and experiences, hermeneutics is closely related to critical social theory, feminism, and postmodernism. Unlike them, however, hermeneutics does not posit politically or psychologically determined frameworks as the modus operandi of the method, nor does the interpretive phenomenologist attempt to posit, explain, or reconcile an underlying cause of a particular experience. Rather, the description of the common practices and shared meanings is intended to reveal, enhance, or extend understandings of the human situation as it is lived.

The thinking that accompanies hermeneutical scholarship is reflective, reflexive, and circular in nature. However, describing the process of hermeneutical research may suggest a linearity and structure that belies the seamless, fluid nature of this approach to inquiry. On the other hand, not describing the process implies a thoughtless or haphazard approach that does not reflect the scholarliness of hermeneutical research. Therefore, although a brief summary of hermeneutical analysis is given here, the reader is referred to several authors (Benner, 1994; Gadamer, 1960, 1989; Grondin, 1995; Palmer, 1969) who discuss hermeneutical methodology in more detail.

Commonly, hermeneutical researchers work in teams and study areas of personal interest and expertise. Each interview, as text analogue, is read by team members to obtain an overall understanding. Members of the research team identify common themes within each interview and share their written interpretations, including excerpts from each interview, with the team. Dialogue among team members clarifies the analyses. As the team analyzes subsequent interviews, they read each text against those that preceded it. This enables new themes to emerge and previous themes to be continuously refined, expanded, or overcome. Team members clarify any discrepancies in their interpretations by referring to the interview text or reinterviewing participants. This is not to say that hermeneutic researchers reduce phenomena to differences or similarities. Rather, through dialogue, the team members explicate the practices of identifying the seemingly simple and overlooked.

Team members identify and explore themes that cut across interview texts. They reread and study interpretations generated previously to see if similar or contradictory interpretations are present in the various interviews. Though an underlying assumption of hermeneutical analysis is that no single correct interpretation exists, the team's continuous examination of the whole and the parts of the texts with constant reference to the participants ensures that interpretations are focused and reflected in the text. Whenever conflicts arise among the various interpretations of the interviews, team members provide extensive documentation to support their interpretations.

Reading across postpositivist, feminist, critical, and postmodern texts, team members hold open and problematic the identification and interpretation of common practices. Team members read across all texts and write critiques of the interpretations. The purpose is to conduct critical scholarship using other interpretive approaches to extend, support, or overcome the themes and patterns identified by hermeneutics. In this way analysis proceeds in "cycles of understanding, interpretation, and critique" (Benner, 1994, p. 116). Like the hermeneutic circle, interpretations are complete but never ending.

During the interpretive sessions, patterns may emerge. A pattern is constitutive, present in all the interviews, and expresses the relationships of the themes. Patterns are the highest level of hermeneutical analysis. The hermeneutic approach provides an opportunity for team members and researchers not on the team to review the entire analysis for plausibility, coherence, and comprehensiveness. In addition, participants in the study may be asked to read interpretations of their interviews as well as the interviews of other participants to confirm, extend, or challenge the analysis. Others, not included in the analysis but likely to be readers of this study, may review the written interpretations. This review process exposes unsubstantiated and unwarranted interpretations that are not supported by the texts.

The purpose of the research report is to provide a wide range of explicated text so that the reader can recognize common practices and shared experiences. The researcher writes the final report using sufficient excerpts from the interviews to allow the reader to participate in the analysis.

Hermeneutical research that draws on interpretive phenomenology was introduced to nursing by Patricia Benner in *Expertise in Nursing Practice: Caring, Clinical Judgment, and Ethics*. This study revealed nursing as a interpretive practice with skills, expertise, and practical knowledge (Benner, Panner, & Chesla, 1996). Viewing nursing as a practice rather than as an applied science presents a new approach to understanding that has implications for practice, research, and education. Hermeneutics deconstructs the corresponding relationship between theory and practice and reveals the practical knowledge and expertise that evolves overtime.

Following the Benner study, hermeneutics emerged as a significant area of scholarship in nursing. Christine Tanner, through hermeneutical analyses of the narratives of nurses, has recast clinical judgment making and clinical thinking as interpretive practices. Martha MacLeod is exploring the nature of experience in nursing and nursing education, and Philip Darbyshire uses hermeneutics to investigate the ways children and their families experience hospitalization. Nancy Diekelmann is utilizing hermeneutics to describe the concernful practices of teaching and learning. These shared practices of students, teachers, and clinicians offer a view of schooling, teaching, and learning as interpretive practices to transform conventional nursing education.

NANCY DIEKELMANN
PAMELA MAGNUSSEN IRONSIDE

See also
NARRATIVE ANALYSIS
PHENOMENOLOGY
QUALITATIVE RESEARCH
RESEARCH INTERVIEWS
   (QUALITATIVE)

HISTORY OF NURSING RESEARCH

In the 19th century, Florence Nightingale was the first nurse to do research in connection with nursing when she used statistics in analyzing her data. Nightingale did her work alone and not until after World War II was there an organized, continuing effort to conduct further nursing research.

1920. Josephine Goldmark, under the direction of Haven Emerson, conducted a comprehensive survey that identified the inadequacies of housing for nursing students and instructional facilities.

1922. The New York Academy of Medicine in a time study of institutional nursing showed wide discrepancies in the costs of nursing education and services.

1923. The Committee for the Study of Nursing Education conducted the first comprehensive study of nursing schools and public health agencies. The final report was published as *Nursing and nursing education the United States*.

1926. May Ayres Burgess was commissioned by the Committee on the Grading of Nursing Schools to ensure that nursing service provided adequate patient care. The result was the classic report, *Nurses, patients, and pocketbooks*.

1934. The second project of the Committee on the Grading of Nursing Schools was job analysis reported in *An activity analysis of nursing*. The grading of nursing schools was not realized until the establishment of the National Nursing Accrediting Service in 1950.

1935. The American Nurses Association (ANA) published *Some facts about nursing: A handbook for speakers and others*, which contained yearly compilations of statistical data about registered nurses.

1936. The ANA scrutinized the economic situation of nurses by studying incomes, salaries, and employment conditions; it excluded public health nurses.

1940. Pfefferkorn and Rovetta compiled basic data on the costs of nursing service and nursing education.

1941. The United States Public Health Service (USPHS) conducted a national census on nursing resources in cooperation with state nursing associations as World War II loomed.

1943. The National Organization of Public Health Nursing surveyed needs and resources for home care in 16 communities. The work was reported in *Public health nursing care of the sick*.

1948. The publication of the Brown Report identified issues facing nursing education and nursing services for the first half of the century. The recommendations led to much research during the next ten years, for example, studies on nursing functions, nursing teams, practical nurses, role and attitude studies, nurse technicians, and nurse-patient relationships. Other studies rooted in the Brown Report were on the hospital environment and economic security as well as the report *Nursing schools at mid-century*, from the National Committee for the Improvement of Nursing Services.

The Division of Nursing Resources (now the Division of Nursing) of the USPHS conducted statewide surveys and developed manuals and tools for nursing research.

1949. The ANA conducted its first national inventory of Professional Registered Nurses in the United States and Puerto Rico. An Interim Classification of Schools of Nursing Offering Basic Programs was prepared with classifications I, II, and III according to specific criteria.

1950. The National Nursing Accrediting Service, established a system for accrediting schools of nursing.

1952. The journal *Nursing Research* was published in June 1952. It was the ANA's first official journal for reporting nursing and health research.

1953. Leo Simmons and Virginia Henderson published a survey and assessment of nursing research which classified and evaluated research in nursing during the previous decade. Teachers College, Columbia University, established the Institute of Research and Service in Nursing Education under Helen Bunge.

1954. The ANA established a Committee on Research and Studies to plan, promote, and guide research and studies relating to the functions of the ANA.

1955. The ANA established the American Nurses' Foundation (ANF), a center for research to receive and administer funds and grants for nursing research. The foundation conducts its own programs of research and provides consultation to nursing students, research facilities, and others engaged in nursing research. *Twenty Thousand Nurses Tell Their Story* was published. The Nursing Research Grants and Fellowship Programs of the Division

of Nursing, USPHS, were established to stimulate and provide financial support for research investigators and nursing research education.

1957. Department of Nursing, established at Walter Reed Army Institute of Research, provided opportunities for growth in military nursing research. The Western Interstate Commission for Higher Education (WICHE) sponsored the Western Council on Higher Education for Nursing (WICHEN) to improve the quality of higher education for nursing in the western U.S., to focus on preparing nurses for research, and to develop new scientific knowledge and communicate research findings. Other such groups were the Southern Regional Education Board (REB), New England Board of Higher Education (NEBHE), Midwest Alliance in Nursing (MAIN), and Mid-Atlantic Regional Nurses Association (MARNA).

1959. The National League for Nursing Research and Studies (later the Division of Research) established to conduct research, provide consultations to NLN staff, and maintain information about NLN research projects. Publications: *NLN Nurse Career Pattern Study* (1975) and *The Open Curriculum Study* (1974, 1975, 1976). Abstracts of Studies in Public Health Nursing, 1924–1957 was published in *Nursing Research*.

1963. The Surgeon General's Consultant Group on Nursing reported on the nursing situation in the U.S. and recommended increased federal support for nursing research and education of researchers. Nursing Studies Index, Volume IV, 1957–1959 was completed as a guide to analytical and historical literature on Nursing in English, from 1900–1959. Volume I, 1900–1929 was published in 1972; Volume II, 1930–1949 was published in 1970; and Volume III, 1950–1956 was published in 1966.

1964. Nursing research: A survey and assessment provided a review and assessment of research in areas of occupational health, career dynamics, and nursing care.

1965. ANA Nursing Research Conferences (1965–1973) provided a forum for critiquing nursing research and opportunities for nurse researchers to examine critical issues.

1966. International Nursing Index was published.

1968. The *ANA blueprint for research in nursing* and *The nurse in research: ANA guidelines in ethical values* were published.

1970. ANA Commission on Nursing Research established and prepared position papers on human rights in research. Papers included: *Human rights guidelines for nurses in clinical and other research* (1974), *Research in nursing: Toward a science of health care* (1976), *Preparation of nurses for participation in research* (1976), and *Priorities for nursing research* (1976). *An abstract for action* made recommendations for changes in nursing such as increased practice research, improved education, role clarification and practice, and increased financial support for nursing. Overview of Nursing was supported by the Department of Health, Education, and Welfare, 1955–1968, to assess nursing research, knowledge available, gaps, and future needs.

1971. ANA Council of Nurse Researchers established by the ANA Commission on Nursing Research to advance research activities and published *Issues in research: Social, professional, and methodology* (1973). The Secretary's Commission, Department of Health, Education and Welfare (DHEW) published *Extending the scope of nursing practice* as a position of the health professions to support the expansion of the functions and responsibilities of nurse practitioners.

1973. The American Academy of Nursing was founded with 36 charter fellows to advance new concepts in nursing and health care, to explore issues in health care; the profession and society as affected by nursing; to examine dynamics of nursing; and to propose resolutions for issues and problems in nursing and health.

1977. Nursing Research became the first nursing journal to be included in Medline, the computerized information retrieval service. *An overview of nursing research in the United States* offered a historical perspective on the development of nursing research. *U.S. Public Health Services' contribution to nursing research: Past, present, future* by Faye G. Abdellah traced the Public Health Services' (PHS) role in development of nursing research.

1979. Healthy People, the Surgeon General's report on health promotion and disease prevention, was published.

1980. Promoting health, preventing disease: Objectives for the nation was published. ANA published *A social policy statement,* which defined the nature and scope of nursing practice and characteristics of specialization in nursing.

1981. Strategies for promoting health for specific populations was published by the Department of Health and Human Services (formerly Department of Health, Education, and Welfare).

1983. The 1981 White House conference on aging: Executive summary of technical committee on health maintenance and health promotion and *Report of the mini conference on long-term care; Report of the technical committee on health services: Nursing and nursing education—Public policies and private actions.* Report of the Institute of Medicine, National Academy of Sciences that defined nursing research and delineated its direction. *Magnet hospitals: Attraction and retention of professional nurses,* by the American Academy of Nursing. Report of the Task Force on Nursing Practice in Hospitals. New legislation established reimbursement policies for hospitals based on prospective payment of diagnosis-related-groups (DRGs) that determined amount paid for Medicare patients.

1983. First volume of the *Annual Review of Nursing Research* series published by Springer Publishing Company.

1984. ANA formed ANA Council on Computer Applications in Nursing to focus on computer technology pertinent to nursing practice, education, administration, and research. ANA Cabinet on Nursing Research published *Directions for nursing research: Toward the twenty-first century.*

1985. The National Center for Nursing Research (NCNR) was established in the PHS. Programs would work to enlarge scientific knowledge underlying nursing services, administration, and education. The Center is located in the Division of Nursing, Bureau of Health Manpower, Health Resources and Services Administration. In 1993, the NCNR was renamed the National Institute of Nursing Research.

1988. The Agency for Health Care Policy and Research (AHCPR) within Department of Health and Human Services (DHHS) was established to focus on the development of clinical practice guidelines, outcome measures, and effectiveness research.

1992. Congress appropriated initial funding of $1 million to establish TriService Nursing Research Program to support targeted research by military nurses. The program is located at the Uniformed Services University of Health Sciences (USUHS) in Bethesda, MD.

1997. Institute for Nursing Research in the Uniformed Services (INRUS) was established at USUHS, Graduate School of Nursing.

FAYE G. ABDELLAH

See also

AMERICAN ACADEMY OF NURSING
AMERICAN NURSES ASSOCIATION
JOURNALS IN NURSING RESEARCH
NATIONAL INSTITUTE OF NURSING
RESEARCH
NATIONAL LEAGUE FOR NURSING

HIV/AIDS: CARE AND TREATMENT

In 1981 the world became aware of an acute health problem that seemed to be targeting gay men and injected-drug users. Although that time now seems rather remote, the uncertainty surrounding what is known as the HIV epidemic persists. First responses were extreme: some nurses cared for the afflicted, and others refused to touch them. Both gay men and drug users were marginalized members of society; thus, beliefs and values about these groups often shaded the caregiver's response. People seemed to die quickly and dramatically, often with incredibly high fevers, profuse diarrhea, and strange skin lesions; and caregivers would identify with them because AIDS patients were usually young.

Larson (1988) reviewed the literature published during the period January 1983 to April 1987 and was unable to locate any nursing research articles addressing AIDS. In January 1987 the National Center for Nursing Research (forerunner of the National Institute for Nursing Research) at the National Institutes of Health issued a request for nursing proposals in seven priority areas: (a) etiology of HIV; (b) nursing care of AIDS patients at various stages of the disease; (c) comparative therapeutic benefits and cost-effectiveness of nursing interventions in the home, nursing home, and institutional settings; (d) knowledge, attitudes, and practices of AIDS patients and the effect of AIDS on family functioning; (e) ethical issues related to diagnosis

and treatment strategies; (f) public policy issues such as methods of early screening; and (g) integration of patients in community settings. Subsequent to that request for proposals, the National Center for Nursing Research convened an expert panel on HIV and nursing (Larson & Ropka, 1990). This panel identified five priority areas: (a) physiological issues, (b) psychological issues, (c) prevention of transmission, (d) care delivery systems, and (e) applied ethics.

The initial body of nursing research examined attitudes toward persons with AIDS and the effect of those attitudes on the provider's willingness to care for infected persons. This was perhaps a reflection of the ambivalence of nurses and other health care providers to respond to the needs of a new group of patients. Study after study explored nurses' and nursing students' attitudes toward caring for persons with AIDS. The second wave of nursing research related to HIV/AIDS patients examined psychosocial issues such as depression, stigma, and coping. Larson and Ropka (1991) did a follow-up review of nursing research during the period April 1987 to June 1990 and identified 54 articles; 20 of those articles addressed areas targeted by the National Center for Nursing Research. Client, rather than provider, needs were gaining importance as areas for study.

After the National Center on Nursing Research expert panel recommendations, attention shifted toward the physiological needs of persons living with the virus. Nursing experts identified five focus areas, but they put special emphasis on the physiological needs of persons living with HIV/AIDS. The allocation of federal research dollars has reflected those priorities, and nursing researchers responded by focusing on clinical issues such as fever, diarrhea, exercise, sleep pattern disturbance, and nutritional needs of persons living with HIV/AIDS.

Although disease severity measures such as CD4 cell counts and viral loads have been developed to determine the impact of HIV disease on the infected person's immune system, nursing researchers had to develop clinical indicators to determine the effectiveness of nursing intervention. A number of nursing researchers developed instruments such as the Quality Audit Marker (Holzemer, Henry, Stewart, & Janson-Bjerklie, 1993), the HIV Assessment Tool (Nokes, Wheeler, & Kendrew, 1994), and the

Living with HIV tool (Wilson, Hutchinson, & Holzemer, 1997). These instruments can detect subtle changes in health status, and they depend on the clients' perceptions of their health-related quality of life rather than on biological markers. Nurse researchers have also used standardized instruments such as the Medical Outcomes Study (MOS) scales, and the Center for Epidemiologic Studies Depression Scale (CES-D) (Radloff, 1977). Although most nurse researchers focused on secondary and tertiary care of persons with HIV/AIDS, a few developed primary prevention interventions.

Millions of dollars have been spent in clinical trials to develop medications to halt HIV or prevent opportunistic infections. Nursing researchers have not been particularly involved in the drug clinical trials other than as study nurses. These nurses learned valuable skills, but the research often did not contribute to the body of nursing knowledge. It is hoped that attention will be directed toward the development of theory-based nursing research to enhance the lives of persons living with HIV/AIDS and their support systems. Multidisciplinary research to support the investigation of questions for nursing solutions is a priority. Collaboration among teams of nurse researchers throughout the world would foster cross-cultural comparisons along with generating sample sizes with adequate power to detect intervention effects. Established nurse researchers could assist in the development of the research trajectory career of less experienced colleagues by permitting secondary analysis of their existing data sets so that data are used to the fullest extent possible.

Unfortunately, HIV seems to be an issue that is following us into the 21st century. Nursing researchers can respond to society's need by adding to theory-based knowledge, which will not only enhance the lives of persons with HIV/AIDS but also build our understanding of a variety of theories. HIV-related nursing research must move from description to evaluation of the effectiveness of a variety of nursing interventions to improve the health-related quality of life for persons living with HIV/AIDS and the many others who have been affected by this epidemic.

KATHLEEN M. NOKES

See also
CHRONIC ILLNESS

HOSPICE
INFECTION CONTROL
REDUCING HIV RISK ASSOCIATED
  SEXUAL BEHAVIOR AMONG
  ADOLESCENTS
TERMINAL ILLNESS

HOME CARE TECHNOLOGIES

Technology is defined in *Webster's New World Dictionary* (1990, p. 606) as "a science of the practical or industrial arts and applied sciences." The Office of Technology Assessment, in a 1987 memorandum to the U.S. Congress, described a technology-dependent person as one who needs both ongoing nursing care and a medical device to compensate for loss of a vital body function. Home care technologies include mechanical ventilation; apnea detection; oxygen assist; continuous positive airway pressure; nutrition or hydration via central venous infusion; hemodialysis and peritoneal dialysis; spinal infusion for pain; infusion for chemotherapy, insulin, or antibiotics; automatic internal defibrillation; and other systems that avert death or further disability. With home care technology a family member provides nursing care, makes complex decisions, and learns skills in managing machines and alarm mechanisms. Studies verify the additive length, quality of life, and cost-effective outcomes from use of various home care technologies (Smith, 1995).

Research with home care technologies should be systems-oriented on a variety of levels: machine reliability and safety, compensated physiological systems, family caregiving, community support, health care providers, and third-party payers' reimbursement. The most extensive research has been at the machine level, where manufacturers' studies of the mechanical system has led to Food and Drug Administration (FDA) approval for clinical trials conducted by nurses. Government regulation also has called for research on the manuals accompanying devices to determine readability and effectiveness of instructions for laypersons.

In 1996 the National Academy of Science presented a report to Congress from manufacturers, regulators, health professionals, families, and patients regarding findings from research on safety and issues of home technologies and family care. Problems to be studied included the impact of family caregiver quality of life (Smith, 1996), ethical decision making in use of technologies, costs of safety regulations for manufacturers, and quality control measures for home care.

Nursing research has contributed study findings in several areas. Smith (1995, 1996) has a series of studies on families, caregivers, and patients dependent on technology for lifelong survival (Smith & Kleinbeck, 1996). Studies on home care of technology-dependent children have identified parental stressors and the need for social support (Williams, Williams, & Griggs, 1990). The ethical issues in technological home care were summarized and research questions posed in a Hastings Center report (Arras, 1994).

Major conclusions from research are that home care technologies do enhance and extend quality of life for those who would otherwise succumb to illness, frailty, or disability. Further, family members are very capable and desirous of home care for their technology-dependent loved one. Direct physical care and indirect costs (reduced income, innumerable expenses, transportation fees) are shifted to the family (Barkauskas, 1990), and evidence of emotional and physical strain occurs in family caregivers. Delivery of technology services in home care is costly and uncoordinated, although cost savings and quality improvements occurred when models of comprehensive care were followed. In some communities and states and in some populations of patients (e.g., ventilator-dependent), coordinated services do exist (Brooten, Brown, Hazard-Munro, et al., 1988).

Future directions for research include the need for continued study of systems of delivery and family interventions for technology home care in culturally diverse populations (Smith, 1994a). Policy, ethical, professional, and interdisciplinary areas of authority issues should be studied to reduce duplication and to enhance resource availability. In addition, predicting costs and outcomes of care should be compared to patients' and families' desired quality of life. Consumer demand and technological advances will continue, with, one hopes, nursing research verifying theoretical frameworks that guide effective home care technology.

CAROL E. SMITH

See also
CAREGIVER
HOME HEALTH SYSTEMS
QUALITY OF LIFE
TRANSITIONAL CARE

HOME HEALTH CARE CLASSIFICATION SYSTEM

Overview

The Home Health Care Classification (HHCC) system is a decision-support system designed to assess and document home health care, using its standardized nomenclature. Its documentation method tracks home health care over time and across settings, whereas the nomenclature is used to code and classify the care. The HHCC system is based on a conceptual framework using the nursing process to access a patient holistically.

Background

The HHCC system was developed by Saba and colleagues at Georgetown University School of Nursing, Washington, DC (Saba, 1992a, 1992b; Saba & Zuckerman, 1992). It was developed from the Home Care Project research study (1988–1991) funded by the Health Care Financing Administration (HCFA; Cooperative Agreement No. 170C-98983/3; Saba, 1991) to develop a method to assess and classify home health Medicare patients in order to predict their need for nursing and other home care services as well as their outcomes of care. A national sample of 646 home health agencies (HHAs) randomly stratified by size, type of ownership, and geographic location participated in the study. The HHAs collected retrospective data on 8,961 newly discharged cases for the entire episode of home health care, from admission to discharge. This landmark study, which represents the largest sample of HHA data in the United States, provided new knowledge for the home health care industry.

The Home Care Project produced several materials, including the *HHCC of Nursing Diagnoses and*

Nursing Interventions nomenclature. The HHCC nomenclature was created empirically from computer processing of approximately 40,000 textual phrases representing nursing diagnoses and/or patient problems and 72,000 phrases depicting patient care services and/or actions collected on the study cases. The textual phrases were processed by computer, using key word sorts from which the standardized labels were developed. The labels were also grouped into 20 care components providing the framework for classifying, coding, and indexing the textual phrases for the nomenclature.

Scope and Structure

The HHCC nomenclature is used to assess and document the six steps of the nursing process, its conceptual framework for documenting nursing practice. The standards of nursing practice recommended by the American Nurses Association (ANA, 1991b) comprise the nursing process. They represent six phases: assessment, diagnosis, outcome identification, planning, implementation, and evaluation.

The nomenclature consists of six data dictionaries: (a) 20 home health care components to assess and classify care; (b) 145 home health nursing diagnoses (50 major categories and 95 subcategories); (c) three expected outcome goals that modified nursing diagnoses with one of three qualifiers—improved, maintained, and/or deteriorated; (d) 160 home health nursing interventions (60 two-digit major categories and 100 three-digit subcategories); (e) four types of nursing intervention action using four qualifiers—assess, care, teach, and/or manage; (f) three actual outcomes that evaluate the care process using one of three qualifiers—improved, maintained, and/or deteriorated (Saba, 1994).

Assessment: 20 Care Components

The HHCC nomenclature uses the 20 clinical care components as the standardized structure for implementing the nursing process as well as providing a holistic approach to assessing patient care and documenting clinical practice. Each of the 20 clini-

cal care components consists of a cluster of elements that represent a behavioral, functional, psychological, or physiological care pattern. They include (a) activity, (b) bowel elimination, (c) cardiac, (d) cognitive, (e) coping, (f) fluid volume, (g) health behavior, (h) medication, (i) metabolic, (j) nutritional, (k) physical regulation, (l) respiratory, (m) role relationship, (n) safety, (o) self-care, (p) self-concept, (q) sensory, (r) skin integrity, (s) tissue perfusion, and (t) urinary elimination. The care components are used to link and map the six data dictionaries as well as track the nursing care protocols.

Diagnosis: 145 Nursing Diagnoses

The HHCC nursing diagnoses data dictionary consists of 145 home health nursing diagnoses (50 two-digit major categories and 95 three-digit subcategories). A nursing diagnosis is defined as a "clinical judgement about individual, family, or community responses to actual or potential health problems/life processes. Nursing diagnoses provide the basis for the nursing interventions selected to achieve outcomes for which the nurse is accountable" (approved at the Ninth Conference of the North American Nursing Diagnosis Association [NANDA, 1992]).

Outcome Identification: Three Expected Outcome Goals

The data dictionary consists of three modifiers: (a) improvement, (b) stabilization, and (c) deterioration. Each nursing diagnosis requires an outcome identification to predict the expected outcome goals of care being performed as interventions. A modifier/qualifier expands the nursing diagnosis and provides the outcome goal for each diagnosis.

Planning: 160 Nursing Interventions

The HHCC nursing intervention data dictionary consists of 160 home health nursing interventions (60 two-digit major categories and 100 three-digit subcategories). These services are mapped and linked to the nursing diagnoses they address. A nursing intervention is defined as a single nursing action (treatment, procedure, or activity) performed to achieve an outcome for a diagnosis (medical or nursing) for which the nurse is accountable.

Implementation: Four Nursing Intervention Actions

The type action uses a data dictionary consisting of four modifiers/qualifiers: (a) assess/monitor, (b) care/perform, (c) teach/instruct, and (d) manage/coordinate. Each nursing intervention requires one or more type of intervention action to identify the specific type of care that is used to implement it. The four modifiers/qualifiers expand the number of nursing interventions fourfold, resulting in 640 possible patient interventions and/or services.

Evaluation: Four Actual Outcomes

The data dictionary consists of three modifiers: (a) improved, (b) stabilized, and (c) deteriorated. The outcome identification goal for each diagnosis is evaluated on discharge and/or discrete time periods during an episode of care as an actual outcome of care. The actual outcome for each diagnosis is used to evaluate and measure the outcome of care.

Coding Structure

The coding framework for the *HHCC of Nursing Diagnoses and Nursing Interventions* is structured according to 20 care components. Each is structured hierarchically and coded according to *ICD-10* (World Health Organization [WHO], 1992), using a five-character alphanumeric code: (a) first position—an alphabetic character for the care component; (b) second and third positions—a two-digit code for a core data element (major category) followed by a decimal point; (c) fourth position—a one-digit code for a subcategory (if needed); and (d) fifth position—a one-digit code for a qualifier.

This structure facilitates the design of critical care protocols and/or pathways as well as other applications that make the nomenclature useful. It is also critical for the development of decision support and/or expert systems. The *HHCC of Nursing Diagnoses and Nursing Interventions* has been "recognized" by the ANA as a valid and useful nursing language that can be used not only to classify nursing practice but also to document nursing care of patients in the computer-based home health systems. Additionally, the HHCC nomenclature has been incorporated in the metathesaurus developed by the National Library of Medicine for its Unified Medical Language System (UMLS).

Advantages

The system provides the coding strategy and methodology for tracking clinical patient care for decision support, offers standardized assessment data for mapping and predicting health care resources, and provides information for quality management and evaluation of various care protocols. The clinical information allows for the aggregation of gathered data to provide meaningful cross-population comparisons as well as administrative decisions for allocating human resources. Further, the Electronic Clinical Care System can be used in home health and ambulatory care settings to (a) improve the efficiency of assessing and documenting care by computer, (b) develop patterns of care, (c) develop a cost-effective methodology for evaluating quality and outcomes of care, and (d) develop a costing method for reimbursement and payment.

Summary

The HHCC nomenclature and system make it possible not only to assess and document but also to code, index, classify, link, and map the nursing process according to the 20 care components. This innovative nomenclature provides the structure and coding strategy for a computer-based patient record, identifies a nursing minimum data set, and tracks the nursing care process across time, different settings, and geographic locations, whereas the HHCC system facilitates the documentation of patient care by computer at the point of care instead of by the traditional paper-based method. The data once collected can be used many times, which allows for better documentation and more efficient analysis.

The HHCC system is free-standing and can be integrated into any home health system and linked electronically to any system designed to collect the data required for professional and/or federal home health care reporting. It can be used to (a) improve the efficiency of assessing and documenting home health nursing care, (b) develop clinical care protocols and/or pathways, (c) provide the strategy for evaluating quality and measuring outcomes of care, and (d) develop a costing method for reimbursement and payment. A complete description of the *HHCC of Nursing Diagnoses and Nursing Interventions*, together with the 20 care components and their definitions, is available on the Internet at http://www.dml.georgetown.edu/research/hhcc.

VIRGINIA K. SABA

See also
HOME HEALTH SYSTEMS
INTERNET
NANDA
NURSING MINIMUM DATA SET
UNIFIED LANGUAGE SYSTEMS

HOME HEALTH SYSTEMS

Home health systems are computer-based information systems designed to support care of the sick in the home. Home health systems primarily support home health and hospice programs provided by home health agencies (HHAs). Home health is more than "care in the home." It focuses on the continuity of care from the hospital to the community, public health concepts of disease prevention and health promotion, and out-of-hospital acute illness services. Home health care is defined as "a broad spectrum of health and social services offered in the home environment to recovering, disabled, or chronically ill persons" (Stanhope & Lancaster, 1988, p. 806).

Home Health Care

Home care is the oldest form of health care and yet the newest. Home health nursing, previously called care of the sick in the home, is one of the earliest developments in the field of public and community health. Care of the sick at home traditionally has been provided by voluntary nonprofit agencies, such as visiting nurse associations (VNAs), organized to provide out-of-hospital services (Saba & McCormick, 1996).

In 1966, with the introduction of Medicare and Medicaid legislation, home health programs emerged from hospital-based ambulatory care, health maintenance organizations, and proprietary home health agencies. The programs and providers increased in number and size. They increased faster than all other organized providers in the health care industry because Medicare primarily addressed the health care needs of the aging population. As this population group grew, more health services were required, resulting in an increase of health care costs that required cost containment. As a result, health care began to shift from acute short-term hospital care to community home-based and chronic long-term care. Patients began to be discharged "sicker and quicker" and required more health care services in the home.

Home Health Systems

Home health systems were initially introduced as management information systems designed to manage the flow of information in the proper time frame and to assist in the decision-making process. The early home health systems were introduced in large visiting nurse associations and other nonprofit HHAs as billing and financial systems. They were developed for the sole purpose of improving cash flow, holding down costs, and addressing the federal regulatory needs for HHAs. They were designed to furnish the information required for payment by Medicare, Medicaid, and other third-party payers for reimbursement for services (Health Care Financing Administration, 1980).

Home health systems were generally developed by commercial vendors who obtained the computer system hardware and developed the software to process the services data provided by the HHAs. The computer vendors owned the home health system and were responsible for maintaining and updating them. Home health computer vendors were usually contracted by the HHAs to provide billing services and financial management, without the HHAs having to develop their own system. With the introduction of the microcomputer and on-line communication systems, local area networks (LANs) and wide area networks (WANs) were introduced, designed to advance and enhance the home health systems. They were used to link state and local units, to share hardware and software, and to integrate data (Saba & McCormick, 1996).

Scope of Home Health Systems

Home health systems are designed not only to collect and process home health data required by the federal government and third-party payers for reimbursement of services but also for the efficient management of the HHA. They focus on billing and financial applications, such as general ledger, accounts receivable, accounts payable, billing, reimbursement management, and cash management. They also may include other management applications, such as scheduling, patient census, visit tracking, cost statistics, utilization reports, accounting statements, and discharge summaries.

Newer home health systems have emerged that are designed to focus on the patient encounter and visit during an episode of care. They include clinical applications used to assess and document the care process, to generate care plans, and to prepare critical pathways, or protocols that outline the critical events. These newer systems are using the electronic information superhighway to communicate patient information for continuity of care from hospital to the home, to the community, and back to the hospital. The systems also offer other applications that focus on decision support, evaluation of care, and measurement of outcomes across settings, time, and geographic locations. The systems are considered part of the lifelong longitudinal record containing patient-specific health-related data.

Home Health System Research

The home health care classification (HHCC) system researched at Georgetown University School of

Nursing is an example of a home health system designed to assess and document home health care by means of its standardized HHCC nomenclature. The documentation method tracks home health care over time, whereas the HHCC nomenclature is used to code and classify the care. The HHCC system is based on a conceptual framework, the nursing process to access a patient holistically and systems theory to process patient data (Saba, 1992a, 1994; Saba & McCormick, 1996). The HHCC system nomenclature consists of six data dictionaries: (a) 20 care components, (b) 145 nursing diagnoses, (c) 3 expected outcomes, (d) 160 nursing interventions, (e) 4 nursing action types (creating 640 nursing interventions), and (f) 3 actual outcomes. It also includes 20 medical diagnoses and surgical procedure categories and 10 sociodemographic variables. The HHCC system is being implemented in many home health systems.

Home Health System Trends

HHCC systems are being used to identify care needs in terms of care components and their respective nursing diagnoses and interventions and to determine resource use in terms of nursing and other health providers. They are being designed to document the clinical care pathways and record protocols for an entire episode of care. Further, they are being used to determine care costs and provide a payment method for managed care organizations offering home health care services.

VIRGINIA K. SABA

See also
HOME HEALTH CARE
  CLASSIFICATION SYSTEM
HOSPICE
MANAGED CARE

HOMELESS HEALTH

Prevalence of Homelessness in the United States

Since the 1980s homelessness has been a growing national problem. The number of homeless individuals is estimated at between 350,000 and 2.5 million (Clark, Williams, Percy, & Kim, 1995). Every day an unknown number of individuals move into the state of homelessness due to personal crises (illness, loss of job, loss of transportation, domestic violence, eviction) and other conditions (release from prison, substance abuse, mental disorders). At the same time, others move out of the defined ranks by "doubling up" with relatives or friends or attaining employment, welfare approval, or low-income housing. Because membership in this group is continuously changing, obtaining a precise number of the homeless is impossible.

In 1987 the Stewart B. McKinney Homeless Assistance Act (PL 100-77) defined the homeless person as (a) an individual who lacks a fixed, regular, and adequate nighttime residence or (b) an individual who has a primary nighttime residence that is a shelter, including welfare hotels, congregate shelters, and transitional housing for the mentally ill; an institution that provides a temporary residence for individuals intended to be institutionalized; or a public or private place not designated for nor ordinarily used as a regular sleeping accommodation.

The profile of the homeless has changed dramatically in the past 30 years, from the stereotypical elderly alcoholic transient male to the current one of young White men and women from 25 to 39 years of age. Nationally, single men make up approximately 75% of the homeless. Although women represent only 25% of the homeless population, they generally enter homelessness accompanied by their preschool children. Women with children are the fastest-growing subgroup of the homeless nationally (Clark et al., 1995).

In large metropolitan areas, many homeless live on the street, in abandoned cars, or in cardboard "homes" because of insufficient numbers of shelter beds, fear of bodily harm in shelters, or mental disorders. Many urban homeless also reside in shelters operated by public and private agencies that serve various subgroups of the homeless, such as battered women, substance abusers, single males, families. These shelters have varying residency rules regarding clientele served, length of stay allowed, requirements for program participation, and daytime lockout. They offer a variety of social services in addition to shelter and food. Few shelters offer on-site access to health care.

Homeless Health

The state of homelessness affects health in three major ways: health problems, such as schizophrenia, may contribute to becoming homeless; homelessness may contribute to becoming ill or may exacerbate chronic illness; and being homeless may make any illness almost impossible to treat (Institute of Medicine, 1988). The homeless environment predisposes residents to a variety of health risks, including trauma, communicable and weather-related disorders, and mental health and substance abuse problems (Lindsey, 1995). Traumatic and weather-related injuries (frostbite, sunburn) are most common in the homeless living on the street. Communicable respiratory, dermatological, and gastrointestinal health problems are common due to crowded living conditions in shelters, irregular mealtimes, and questionable personal hygiene practices. Hypertension, increased incidence of mental health disorders, and high rates of tobacco, drug, and alcohol abuse are also reported in studies of shelter residents (Vredevoe, Brecht, Shuler, & Woo, 1992).

Obtaining adequate food and shelter are daily challenges for the homeless. Many spend their days walking from a nighttime shelter to a soup kitchen and then wait for the nighttime shelter to open in order to find a bed. The food available at soup kitchens and shelters is generally nutritionally adequate but high in fat and low in various minerals such as iron and calcium. Mineral deficiencies are particularly important when considering preventive health practices for women and children.

Compared to the general population, homeless males have been reported to have more respiratory ailments, skin disorders, infectious diseases, dental problems, and mental health and substance abuse problems than the general population. Homeless women have greater prevalence of mental illness, unwanted pregnancies, adverse birth outcomes, and histories of domestic abuse. Homeless children exhibit increased incidence of physical, mental, emotional, behavioral, learning, and immunization delays (Aday, 1994).

Health Care

Lack of insurance, transportation, and finances are barriers the homeless encounter in seeking health care. They generally seek health care, from emergency rooms and free clinics, for acute conditions after they have become severe. The care they receive is episodic, delivered by a variety of practitioners, and focused on the immediate acute problem. Secondary health problems and chronic problems do not receive attention or necessary routine surveillance. Because of the lifestyle of the homeless and their lack of addresses, follow-up is difficult if not impossible.

Medications prescribed for homeless individuals are often unobtainable due to costs. Many free clinics dispense donated medications or samples, which may not be the drug of choice but will provide some pharmacological assistance for the problem. The homeless have special problems in complying with prescribed medication regimens. They may not understand the directions for appropriate medication use because of their limited reading levels or their mental status. They may not have access to food at required times to accompany the medication or may discontinue medications (e.g., antibiotics) as soon as they feel better and save them for a future illness. They may also use them to trade for drugs, money, or cigarettes. Their medications are often lost or stolen because there is no safe place to store them, or they may be rendered inactive due to lack of refrigeration.

Monitoring and tracking the health and health care of the homeless are very difficult. Homeless clients generally do not have a stable source of health care, one record, or any personal record of their health care visits, treatments, or prescriptions. They may seek health care from a variety of providers for a variety of problems and may use several different names on records. They must rely on their memories or the interviewing skills of a practitioner to elicit their health and medication histories at each health visit.

Research

Studies about the health and health care of the homeless are increasing (Lindsey, 1995). Nurse practitioner– and nurse-managed clinics have been in the forefront of delivering health care for the homeless and initiating research studies of this population (Stanhope, 1990). However, most of the reported research on the homeless and their health problems, concerns, and care has been descriptive, with data gathered from clinics or emergency room record reviews, convenience sample interviews, on-site surveys, and self-reports from clinic visits. Few studies have used comparative groups, been theory-based, or used standardized instruments. Intervention studies using control groups have not been widely reported (Lindsey, 1995). Research in the areas of health promotion and disease prevention with this population are not reported.

Directions for Future Research

For research to add substantively to the body of knowledge related to homeless health and health care, researchers must design interventions studies that use the same theory or conceptual base and accepted standardized instruments. Studies should also be intervention- and outcome-focused. The same conceptual, theoretical base will allow researchers to build on knowledge gained in previous studies.

Due to the great heterogeneity of this population, intervention studies should focus on particular subgroups of the homeless (e.g., battered women, women with children, single males, families, substance abusers, pregnant women, adolescents, or new homeless vs. chronic homeless) or on other common factors, such as length of homelessness (marginal, new, chronic). This would improve the homogeneity of the groups.

Research designs to yield more generalizable results should include random selection of subjects. Because of the transient nature of the homeless, this may require the development and coordination of projects at multiple sites in order to attain sufficient numbers of subjects. Intervention studies of a longitudinal nature could add valuable information about the health problems and outcomes of the homeless and provide guidance for future interventions. Qualitative studies identifying the important themes related to health in this population could add substantively to our knowledge about this group. Research focused on health promotion and disease prevention strategies, though difficult in this population, is needed. To obtain adequate follow-up with this population, research designs that incorporate creative incentives to motivate the homeless to participate and to continue participation will be required.

MARY J. MCNAMEE
ADA M. LINDSEY

See also
CHRONIC MENTAL ILLNESS
NURSING CENTERS
URBAN HEALTH RESEARCH: NURSING
    RESEARCH IN URBAN
    NEIGHBORHOODS
VIOLENCE AS A NURSING AREA
    OF INQUIRY
VULNERABLE POPULATIONS

HOSPICE

Definition

Hospice has been defined as a concept of care, a program of care, and a place for care. Hospice as a concept of care

> espouses: choice with regard to the place of one's dying; attention to the comfort of the individual; a consideration of spiritual, social, and psychological concerns, as well as the physiological and functional manifestations of the disease process; a focus on the family as well as on the patient; an emphasis on dying, death, and the bereavement that follows; the provision of interdisciplinary care (not simply the attention of professionals from multiple disciplines); and the implementation of coordinated care across settings. (Corless, 1995, p. 78)

As a program of care, hospice care is provided in a variety of settings, including the home, hospital, extended care facility, or designated hospice or palliative care beds. Hospice as a place for care is setting-defined and is either free-standing or part of another facility.

History

Arising from the research of Florence Wald and her colleagues (see Terminal Illness) and the model of St. Christopher's Hospice in England and inextricably bound to the death awareness movement, the first hospice programs developed in the United States in the late 1970s and early 1980s. Dame Cicely Saunders, nurse, social worker, and physician, was one of the founders of the modern hospice movement. She emphasized the importance of research as a part of hospice care. Her focus and that of Melzack, Ofiesh, and Mount (1976) was on the alleviation of pain. The concern with symptom control was part of the research focus of the Royal Victoria Hospital's Palliative Care Unit (PCU), founded by Balfour Mount and his colleagues.

The PCU's research team included Mary Vachon (Vachon, Lyall, & Freeman, 1978), who studied the stress that caring for the dying created for the caregiver. Vachon (1987) expanded her focus to examine the issue of occupational stress, discovering in her research that caring for the dying was not the major problem for caregivers. Rather, such issues as poor communication, lack of continuity, and conflicts between units were more significant sources of stress for caregivers.

Areas of Research

Support for caregivers and the prevention of burnout has continued to be of interest in hospice care but is not currently a primary area of research endeavors. Concerns about burnout have been superseded by an interest in spirituality, that of caregivers and of patients. Highfield and Cason (1983) investigated whether the spiritual needs of patients were being met. The paucity of attention to this area, in the United States, was likely due to the confluence of three factors. First, the emphasis in hospice care initially was on program development, referral of patients, and funding. Second, a number of the early hospice programs were started by psychiatrists or those with a psychosocial bent. Thus, psychiatrists were utilized both for patients and their families and to provide staff support. A third factor that had an influence is the historic division between church and state, a division not found in England. So devotions are incorporated in the life of St. Christopher's Hospice in a way that has not occurred in American hospices. That is not to say that the integration of spirituality is not an area of continuing concern for hospice programs.

Initially, however, most of the emphasis was on demonstrating the efficacy of the hospice intervention. The problems of effecting improvement in symptoms and quality of life in what is inevitably a downward trajectory, together with a concern about the research burden for dying persons and their family members, makes this a challenging area for investigators. Much of the more recent research has utilized hospice as a site for symptom control research rather than for evaluating whether hospice programs are more skilled in symptom management than nonhospice sites.

Economic and Regulatory Issues

The comparison of hospice programs with hospital and home care programs that served as controls was initiated by the federal government as a demonstration program to assess the cost savings of a hospice benefit. The benefit, however, was written into law prior to the completion of the research. As a result of the legislation and accompanying regulations, hospice funding is on a capitated basis rather than on a per visit basis. In addition, visits could be made by hospice personnel for psychosocial and other reasons that did not meet the "skilled care" requirements of traditional home care.

The emphasis in the regulations is on home care. Hospice programs are penalized if the yearly quota of home care is not met. This quota is determined by the 80/20 cap, which specifies that 80% of the care of hospice patients as a totality must be provided in the home if financial penalties are to be avoided. The hospice benefit provides for four levels of care: routine home care, continuous home care, inpatient respite care, and general inpatient care. The low level of reimbursement for respite

care means that this approach to providing some rest for caregivers is not utilized. It would cost the hospice program more money to secure this care than they would receive in compensation from the government.

Reimbursement is dependent on level of care received but is also financially capped. The constraints of the financial cap and the 80/20 cap have limited both the amount of care provided and the type of person accepted into the program. Consequently, individuals without a caregiver may not be accepted in many hospice programs unless the program has some other mechanism for keeping a dying person safely at home.

The advent of HIV/AIDS (human immunodeficiency virus/acquired immunodeficiency syndrome) has resulted in a change in the federal hospice requirements for persons with HIV disease. The 80/20 cap is not applied to these individuals. Nonetheless, some hospice programs have been slow in opening their programs to HIV-infected persons. At the same time, hospice was not an option readily selected by individuals dying as result of AIDS. The emphasis on dying was not congenial to these individuals, who were still looking for further treatment. And appropriate treatment often could cure an illness resulting from an opportunistic pathogen; consequently, meaningful life was still an option. With the advent of the protease inhibitors many AIDS hospice patients have been discharged and are resuming their former activities.

Hospice programs have been challenged with the opening of beds for palliative care, a term popular in England and Canada. Palliative care focuses on symptom control as well as psychosocial care and is more acceptable as a consultation service to many physicians practicing in major medical centers. Hospice care also can be offered as a consultation service but has been identified with home care and limited inpatient beds as a result of the government's reimbursement mechanisms for hospice care. Another term, supportive care only, is used to indicate that care is no longer directed at cure or invasive procedures but at helping the patient be comfortable in the dying process. Supportive care and palliative care may incorporate hospice principles of care and thus meet the goal of the early hospice pioneers, namely, that mainstream medicine and nursing incorporate hospice principles in the care of all patients.

INGE B. CORLESS

See also
CAREGIVER
HIV/AIDS: CARE AND TREATMENT
NURSING OCCUPATIONAL INJURY
 AND STRESS
PAIN MANAGEMENT
TERMINAL ILLNESS

HYPERALIMENTATION

Hyperalimentation is the enteral or parenteral infusion of a solution that contains sufficient protein, carbohydrate, fat, electrolytes, vitamins, minerals, and water to sustain life, maintain normal growth and development, and provide for needed tissue repair in the patient who cannot ingest sufficient nutrients orally. Common conditions for which hyperalimentation may be used include major anomalies of the gastrointestinal (GI) tract, necrotizing enterocolitis, short bowel syndrome, idiopathic intestinal pseudoobstruction, inflammatory bowel disease, bowel fistulas, intractable diarrhea, extensive body burns, abdominal tumors, immune deficiency, very low birthweight neonates (<1000 g), and renal or hepatic failure.

If the patient cannot or will not eat and malnutrition is supervening, an initial trial with enteral nutrition should be instituted before preserving lean body mass with parenteral nutrition. Basic and clinical research suggests that use of the GI tract provides physiological benefits that exceed the nutritional value of the feeding. Nutrition delivered enterally is better utilized and prevents gut mucosal atrophy, thereby maintaining barrier function, mass, normal gut flora, and immunocompetence, as well as supporting hepatic protein synthesis.

If enteral feeding is chosen, gavage tubes are commonly used for short-term supplementation, whereas endoscopically or surgically placed gastrostomy tubes are used for long-term enteral feeding. Patients may be fed either intragastrically or intraintestinally by bolus, intermittent, or continuous feedings. If fed intraintestinally, they must receive continuous feedings. Feeding into the small intestine may be safer in patients at risk for aspiration because both the lower esophageal and pyloric sphincters act as gates, decreasing the risk of regurgitation. Other indications for intestinal feeding include the presence of nausea or vomiting, poor gastric emptying, and nutritional support in the immediate postoperative period. Postoperative ileus affects the stomach for 1 to 2 days and the colon for 3 to 5 days but does not affect the small intestine (Hoover, Ryan, Anderson, & Fischer, 1980). Thus, the distal duodenum/jejunum can be used for fluid and nutrition on the first postoperative day if gastric decompression is also used. Jejunal feedings can be given in the absence of propulsive peristalsis such as occurs in intestinal pseudoobstruction because nonpropulsive contractions and the hydrostatic pressure of the feeding solution will move the enteral solution along the intestinal tract (Grant, Curtas, & Kelvin. 1983).

Patients receiving only total parenteral nutrition (TPN) over time will eventually develop liver abnormalities. In contrast to adults, pediatric patients can develop hepatobiliary dysfunction in the form of cholestasis with conjugated hyperbilirubinemia. If this happens, TPN should be discontinued and enteral feeding started if at all possible because it is curative. In adults the hepatic complications of TPN are usually confined to hepatic steatosis. It is hypothesized that hepatic steatosis results from an abnormal portal insulin-to-glucagon ratio, as glucagon is responsible for the mobilization of hepatic fat and insulin results in hepatic lipid deposition (Archer, Burnett, & Fischer, 1996).

Hyperalimentation therapy involves intravenous infusion of highly concentrated solutions of protein (as crystalline amino acids), carbohydrate (as glucose), fat (as fatty acids), electrolytes (potassium, sodium, chloride, calcium, phosphorus, and magnesium), vitamins (water- and fat-soluble), and trace minerals (zinc, copper, iodide, and manganese). A solution of glucose, lipids, and other nutrients can be mixed together in a bag and delivered through a volumetric pump. The highly concentrated solutions require infusion into a vessel (superior vena cava, innominate or intrathoracic subclavian veins) with sufficient volume and turbulence to allow for rapid dilution.

Long-term home TPN is needed by some patients. Vargas, Ament, and Berquist (1987), reporting on 102 patients, stated that the average patient received TPN for nearly 2 years; 8 had received TPN for more than 5 years and 4 for a decade. Bowel transplantation may eventually obviate the need for lifelong use of TPN.

Nursing Care

Nutrition support nursing may trace its beginning to Florence Nightingale. In her book, *Notes on Nursing: What It Is and What It Is Not* (1969/1860), she observed that thousands of patients starved to death in the midst of plenty. She emphasized the need for high-quality food and the nurses's responsibility to make accurate observations of the patient's daily oral intake. The involvement of nurses in nutrition support facilitated the early research in this area and was instrumental in developing a strong nursing role. For example, in Philadelphia in the 1940s, Marie Barnes assisted with studies on patients using oil emulsions, and Eina Goulding assisted with trials that force-fed preoperative patients in an attempt to prevent negative nitrogen balance (Grant & Kennedy-Caldwell, 1987).

Nursing Research

Most of the nursing studies deal with enteral feeding. Examples of physiological response research conducted by nurse researchers using animals include examining the effect of formula temperature on gastric motility and intragastric temperature and the effects of TPN on gastric motility and appetite in nonhuman primates. A rat model was used to examine GI and adrenocortical responses to modes of diet administration and dietary constituents.

Researchers found that nausea was reported to affect approximately 12% of patients receiving hyperalimentation. Such subjective responses as nausea and fullness were reported more frequently in response to the infusion of cold formula than with formula infused at room or body temperature. Other researchers studying patients receiving long-term home enteral feeding found that the most common

psychosensory complaints were related to the deprivation of favorite foods. Patients who experienced greater GI symptoms had the greatest restriction in their activities of daily living.

Many studies have been conducted to determine the prevalence of pathophysiological responses to enteral nutrition. For example, Cataldi-Betcher, Seltzer, Slocum, and Jones (1983) found that approximately 12% of hospital patients experienced GI, mechanical, or metabolic complications. Metheny, Eisenberg, and Spies (1986) found that approximately 6 of 105 (5.7%) nasogastric tube–fed patients had documented pulmonary aspiration, and an additional 7 patients had evidence of formula in secretions suctioned from the oropharynx. Patient characteristics such as decreased level of consciousness, vomiting, and altered swallowing mechanisms were found to contribute to pulmonary aspiration. Metheny's group had also shown that aspirating GI contents and testing pH was the most accurate bedside method of checking tube placement.

Kayser-Jones (1990) qualitatively investigated attitudes of patients, family members, nurses, and physicians toward the use of nasogastric tube feedings in three nursing homes. Fifty-three percent of the patients, 58% of families, and 70% of the nursing staff approved of the use of tube feedings. Diverse opinions characterized physicians' responses. Findings disclosed inadequate communication among health care providers, patients, and families. Some families perceived the tubes as being inserted for the convenience of nursing home staff.

In pediatrics, infants offered pacifiers during and following every tube feeding gained weight at greater rates and were discharged sooner than infants receiving routine care. Also, the use of regression equations incorporating height have been found to be the best method for predicting the insertion distance for feeding tube placement.

Nutrition support is a relatively new specialty area that has existed for approximately two decades. The American Society for Parenteral and Enteral Nutrition has published standards for nutrition support for hospitalized adult and pediatric patients as well as standards for nutrition support nurses. In 1995 the Joint Commission on Accreditation of Healthcare Organizations issued specific nutrition care standards.

In 1996 a study commissioned by the federal Nutrition Screening Initiative found that the use of medical foods (foods used for the specific dietary management of a medical disorder) as part of medical nutrition therapy could save the Medicare program $1.3 billion by the year 2002 through reduced hospital stays and lower complication rates. Savings would accrue by reducing medical complications, lengths of stay, and hospital readmissions.

Nutrition support teams are usually multidisciplinary, and the number of master's degree prepared nutrition support nurses is increasing; both should support nurse participation in multidisciplinary research. In the cost-conscious health care environment, nursing studies in the area of nutrition support are needed to focus attention on the patient and family perspective.

MARSHA L. ELLETT

See also
**CHRONIC GASTROINTESTINAL
    SYMPTOMS
NUTRITION**

HYPERTENSION

Definition

Hypertension is the term applied to sustained and elevated levels of systolic and/or diastolic blood pressure. The exact level at which hypertension poses a health risk has been arbitrarily and continually redefined; however, the importance of hypertension is based on a rational association between sustained, elevated levels of arterial pressure and the probability of increased risk for morbidity and mortality from cardiovascular disease. The Joint National Committee on Detection, Evaluation and Treatment of High Blood Pressure (1993) defined hypertension as systolic blood pressure ≥140 mm Hg and/or diastolic blood pressure ≥90 mm Hg or taking antihypertensive medication. The committee reclassified hypertension into four stages and introduced the high normal category for use in medical diagnosis, evaluation, and treatment (see Table 1).

Sustained and elevated systolic blood pressure is now considered as crucial a measure as the diastolic level in evaluating the risks for cardiovascular disease. Elevated systolic blood pressure accompanied by normal diastolic levels, known as isolated systolic hypertension, is common in older populations. Primary hypertension, formerly known as essential hypertension, occurs in as many as 95% of all individuals with high blood pressure, as opposed to secondary hypertension, which is due to an identifiable and usually treatable cause (Kaplan, 1994).

Prevalence in the United States

Hypertension affects approximately 43 million Americans, almost one fourth of the U.S. adult population. In the 1988–91 National Health and Nutrition Examination Survey (NHANES III), 32.4% of non-Hispanic Blacks, 23.3% of non-Hispanic Whites, and 22.6% of Mexican Americans had hypertension (Burt et al., 1995). Two thirds of hypertensive individuals were aware of their condition, and 53% reported being on drug therapy. In Mexican Americans, 35% of the hypertensive individuals were under treatment, but only 14% had controlled blood pressures; compared to 25% and 24% of the non-Hispanic Black and White populations, respectively, with controlled blood pressures. Given equal access to therapy, Black Americans, who are among the most affected population group, achieve similar blood pressure reductions. Almost 13 million people with normal blood pressures reported being told they were hypertensive on one or more occasions, and just over 50% of the 13 million reported self-compliance with lifestyle changes to maintain hypertension control.

Hypertension increases with age, is more common in Blacks, and is more prevalent among lower socioeconomic populations. Hypertension has a higher incidence in men throughout young adulthood to middle age. Thereafter, the incidence in women rises above that of men. The highest rates among women are found in non-Hispanic Black women and among men in non-Hispanic Black men. Among those with more severely elevated hypertension (DBP ≥115 mm Hg), Black men had four times higher incidence of complications than White men.

TABLE 1   Classification of Blood Pressure for Adults Age 18 Years and Older[a]

Category	Systolic (mm Hg)	Diastolic (mm Hg)
Normal[b]	<130	<85
High Normal	130–139	85–89
Hypertension[c]		
Stage 1 (mild)	140–159	90–99
Stage 2 (moderate)	160–179	100–109
Stage 3 (severe)	180–209	110–119
Stage 4 (very severe)	≥210	≥120

[a]Not taking antihypertensive drugs and not acutely ill. When systolic and diastolic pressures fall into different categories, the higher category should be selected to classify the individual's blood pressure status. For instance, 160/92 mm Hg should be classified as stage 2, and 180/120 mm Hg should be classified as stage 4. Isolated systolic hypertension (ISH) is defined as SBP ≥140 mm Hg and DBP <90 mm Hg and staged appropriately (e.g., 170/85 mm Hg is defined as stage 2 ISH).

[b]Optimal blood pressure with respect to cardiovascular risk is SBP <120 mm Hg and DBP <80 mm Hg. However, unusually low readings should be evaluated for clinical significance.

[c]Based on the average of two or more readings taken at each of two or more visits following an initial screening.

Note: In addition to classifying stages of hypertension based on average blood pressure levels, the clinician should specify presence or absence of target-organ disease and additional risk factors. For example, a patient with diabetes and a blood pressure of 142/94 mm Hg plus left ventricular hypertrophy should be classified as "stage 1 hypertension with target-organ disease (left ventricular hypertrophy) and with another major risk factor (diabetes)." This specificity is important for risk classification and management.

Detection and Measurement

Hypertension is not diagnosed by a single elevated reading but must be confirmed by multiple elevated blood pressure readings on several occasions. Standardized technique is strongly recommended to assure accurate and valid measurement (American Heart Association, 1993). Blood pressure is measured after 5 minutes of rest and without recent ingestion of alcohol, caffeine, or tobacco smoke, which can cause elevated readings. The blood pressure cuff must be the appropriate size for the patient and encircle the bare upper arm at heart level. The patient should be positioned with legs uncrossed, back supported, and feet resting flat on the floor. Systolic and diastolic readings should be measured by an accurately calibrated manometer. It is crucial that efforts be made to eliminate measurement errors, which result from observer bias, digit preference, and prior knowledge of patient blood pressure levels. At least two readings with a minimum of 2 minutes between measurements should be averaged.

Associated Factors

Hypertension seldom exists in isolation but most often occurs with other risk factors that potentiate the probability for cardiovascular disease. Factors commonly associated with hypertension that are nonmodifiable include low birthweight, older age, family history of high blood pressure, and history of diabetes mellitus, coronary heart disease, stroke, or end-stage renal disease. Modifiable confounders include smoking, alcohol consumption, high saturated dietary fats, excess dietary sodium, adiposity, and a sedentary lifestyle, as well as recreational and over-the-counter drugs. In addition, psychosocial and environmental factors create life stressors that may influence hypertension as well as care and management. Target-organ disease as a consequence of sustained, uncontrolled elevated blood pressure includes arteriosclerosis, heart failure, transient ischemic attacks (TIA), stroke, peripheral vascular disease, aneurysm, and end-stage renal disease.

Treatment

The ultimate goal for treatment is to prevent morbidity and mortality by the least intrusive means. The treatment regimen is determined by evaluating the severity of the blood pressure elevation, the presence of target-organ disease, and the effects of other coexisting risk factors. The inability to adhere to treatment recommendations is a major barrier in attaining and maintaining goal blood pressure levels in long-term management, evidencing the need for planned patient education programs. Traditional treatment strategies targeted to the general population lack cultural sensitivity, neglect active involvement of the patient in decision making, and fail to motivate and keep the patient in care. More individually oriented treatment methodologies that address the patients' concerns, including their social support system, employment status, health insurance, and barriers in daily life to meeting compliance goals, are required. Nursing can provide the training, education, and support to design planned health programs to increase the efficacy of interventions and improve overall compliance.

Lifestyle modification, formerly termed nonpharmacological therapy, includes interventions targeted toward healthier lifestyles and reducing the risks for cardiovascular complications at the family, community, and population levels. Lifestyle modifications for blood pressure control include reduction in weight, increased physical exercise, and dietary decreases in sodium, saturated fats, and alcohol consumption. Smoking, although not directly related to hypertension, is a major cardiovascular risk and should be avoided.

Pharmacological intervention is indicated in stages 1 and 2 hypertension only when blood pressure levels remain elevated for longer than 6 months despite lifestyle modifications (Joint National Committee, 1993). In stages 3 and 4 hypertension, it may be necessary to add a second or third agent if blood pressure levels remain uncontrolled. Hypertension management should include the simplest well-tolerated regimen and plans to gradually reduce dosages or the number of agents prescribed while vigorously incorporating lifestyle modifications into the treatment regimen.

The first preferred line of drugs used in initial therapy includes diuretics and beta blockers, followed by calcium antagonists, angiotensin converting enzyme (ACE) inhibitors, and alpha-1 receptor blockers. Factors such as side effects, effects of therapies on concomitant disease, and cost of therapy must be considered in selection of pharmacological treatment. As much as 80% of the total cost for hypertension treatment can be attributed to drug therapy. Newer classes of drugs are more costly than traditional and older pharmaceutical agents. Despite the costs involved, the reduction of blood pressure by using pharmacological treatment reduces the incidence of cardiovascular events and hospitalization.

Primary Prevention

Nonpharmacological therapy for treatment of hypertension is an evolving strategy in line with the objectives of Healthy People 2000 (U.S. Department of Health and Human Services, 1990). It represents a prevention area ideally suited for nursing practice and research. Public health prevention strategies focusing on lifestyle modification at the community and practice setting will help achieve an overall downward shift in the distribution of blood pressure levels in the general population. Interventions should target high dietary sodium, fats, alcohol, and low intake of potassium, as well as physical inactivity. Although these intervention strategies show promise in prevention of high blood pressure, societal barriers, such as the lack of satisfactory food substitutes, lack of access to care, and absence of economic resources, constrain compliance and achievement of intervention goals.

Gaps in Knowledge and Practice

Hypertension is a major independent risk factor for coronary artery disease and stroke, the first and third causes of mortality in the United States, yet its importance is not emphasized satisfactorily in research and practice. The individuals hardest to reach and at the highest risk are often not in care or are uninsured. Medical and behavioral intervention approaches lack cohesiveness and cultural relevance, therefore failing to achieve the strength of their impact as a combined intervention. Additional research is required to evaluate multidisciplinary strategies with a team approach to increase entry into care, remaining in care, and long-term compliance with prevention and treatment recommendations. Research also is needed to increase understanding of cost-benefit of interventions and the effects of self-monitoring and titration, including pharmacological vacations.

Nursing Practice and Research

Nurses can play leading roles in achieving improved health outcomes through lowering the rate and severity of hypertension and encouraging primary prevention. Nurses in all settings can provide case finding, referral, tracking and follow-up, and education and monitoring of patients with hypertension (Hill & Becker, 1995). Further important nursing interventions include developing more tailored patient-centered strategies to promote adherence by encouraging patient skill building and self-monitoring and using community outreach workers (Hill & Becker, 1995). Home visits and telephone contact strengthen understanding of the patient's environment and surrounding community, providing more insight into social, cultural, and psychosocial issues, including poverty, alcoholism, and substance abuse. Nursing research offers unlimited opportunities to improve hypertension prevention and care.

Testing multidisciplinary approaches to patient-centered care allows for resource sharing, team building, and community partnerships to strengthen the supportive network among hospitals, local clinics, health agencies, and community providers. Finally, new discoveries in genetics and pharmacology promise exciting developments in the prevention of hypertension and cardiovascular disease.

MARTHA N. HILL
SUSAN DALE TANNENBAUM

See also
**CARDIOVASCULAR RISK FACTORS,
    CHOLESTEROL
CEREBROVASCULAR DISORDERS
DIABETES MELLITUS
OBESITY AS A CARDIOVASCULAR
    RISK FACTOR
RISK FACTORS**

I

IMAGES

Images represent an important type of clinical data that permit visualization of the structure and function of the human body. Image types familiar to nurses include X rays, computerized axial tomography (CT) scans, magnetic resonance images (MRI), still photographs, and sketches. Images provide adjuncts to other clinical information about patients, allowing clinicians to diagnose, plan, and evaluate treatment. Images can serve as components in a clinical record as well as primary research data.

Existing Images: Where Do They Come From?

Still photographs and drawings are the most common forms of images; however, their use in nursing practice and research is informal rather than formal. These images serve as records of significant events and observations, functioning as communication tools and occasionally as benchmarks of wound repair and skin lesions. Plain film radiographs (X rays) depict body structures as shaded areas on special media. CT scans generate images of internal organs from computerized analysis of absorption of radiographic beams caused by passing X rays through body tissue (Gates & Brooks, 1991). MRIs result from the change in polarization of tissues caused by stimulating body parts with radio waves. Positron emission tomography (PET) scans map the differential uptake of certain ions in specific organs, thus depicting both structure and function. Many images are enhanced by exposing the index body part with radiopaque or radioactive substances.

Integration of image composition and display characterizes most images familiar to nurses. Radiographic images (X rays) are composed by passing radioactive ions through body tissue onto film. Thus, the image is both composed and displayed on the same physical medium—film. Photographs are composed by exposing special media to light and then treating the media with chemicals. The picture that is composed (the image) and the physical paper used to display it (e.g., paper, slide, film) are one. The image exists because the physical medium is altered. The only persons capable of viewing the image are those who actually possess the physical media. The image and its physical medium for display are one, and to store the image one stores the medium.

Computer technology has improved the construction of images in several ways. CT scans are feasible because of the computer programs that compose a new, intact image from thousands of smaller, sequenced images of slices of body tissue. Digital cameras now store on computer disks the types of images once available only through exposed film. Compact disks provide efficient, compressed storage for images that once required hundreds of feet of film.

To understand how computer technology markedly enhances the ability to use images for clinical practice, it is necessary to comprehend the separation of image construction from image display. Computer-generated images are composed not by altering physical media but by recording changes in light density as a series of coordinates in a computer file. To display the image simply requires creating a computer image that matches the series of coordinates. Image composition becomes the development of files of numerical coordinates, and image display involves recreation of the image, as many times as desired and at as many points as necessary. Additionally, because the display of the image is computerized, the image itself can be manipulated (i.e., turned, sliced, altered, or erased) much in the same way that the now familiar word processor allows manipulation of text in papers and manuscripts

Once images can be composed electronically, they can be transmitted anywhere in the world for display on remote computer screens. Picture archiving and communication systems (PACS) allow images acquired in a radiology department or cardiac catheterization laboratory to be transmitted to computer screens and terminals throughout a hospital or health care system, as well as to remote experts for consultation and interpretation. Transfer of images to and from remote sites ensures that telemedicine initiatives become clinically meaningful, since the simultaneous transmission of voice, video, and data provides a comprehensive view of the patient.

On the Horizon: The Visible Human and Virtual Reality

The Visible Human Project created, for the first time, a computer record of the structure and function of the entire human body (Spitzer, Ackerman, Scherzinger, & Whitlock, 1996). Using MRI, CT, and anatomical images obtained from a single human cadaver, this project constructed a large computer file that permits three-dimensional visualization of every part of the human body. Enhancements to the Visible Human Project data set labeled key anatomical structures and provided the computer tools necessary to segment out selected organs, examine cross-sections of body parts, and rotate structures. Future developments will link anatomical information with functional data.

Virtual reality is the term applied to a computer-generated experience within which the participant perceives an environment that appears to be real but in fact exists only as projections of computer-generated images and sound. Wearing special glasses and gloves, a participant can not only see this constructed environment but move and interact with features of it. Virtual reality tools, when connected to robotics devices, allow a participant at one location to force actions to occur at another. For example, remote surgeries are possible in that these tools allow a surgeon at one location to ''see'' a patient at a remote location and, using computer-generated images, guide a scalpel or laser to the precise point at which a cut must be made. Virtual reality may have important benefits for nursing in that it will allow remote examination and visualization of patients, as well as provide simulated environments in which nurses can practice assessment and intervention skills.

Imaging and Nursing Research

There are two key nursing research issues related to imaging. The first addresses clinical practice issues and includes such aspects as appropriate preparation of patients for imaging studies, actual interpretation of images in patient care, and appropriate utilization of images in patient management. The second addresses the use of images as essential nursing data. Little formal research exists for either issue.

Research addressing the clinical practice issues regarding the use of images for patient care focuses on the accuracy and acceptability of imaging tools in the clinical arena. Zelickson and Homan (1997) determined that a teledermatology consultation service led to improved diagnosis and treatment for patients experiencing dermatological problems in a nursing home. Reiner and colleagues (Reiner et al., 1996) investigated the acceptability of PACS-delivered images to surgical nurses and physicians and found benefits in the increased accessibility to images offered by the PACS systems. However, ensuring staff access to the training needed for proper interpretation of images remains a major challenge (Protopapas et al., 1996). Special computer programs that rapidly display CT and MRI scans facilitate interactive, stereotactic neurosurgical procedures (League, 1995) and challenge surgical suite nurses to integrate image-guiding systems into perioperative nursing care routines. Most of the recommendations for care of patients undergoing imaging studies is grounded in the wisdom of clinical practice rather than empirical research (see Gates & Brooks, 1991).

Recently, investigators have begun examining images, particularly still photographs, as primary data for nursing research. McGinnis and Axford (1997) evaluated the utility of still photographs of wounds as both a tool for the clinical record and as an aid in patient teaching. Computer programs that facilitate image manipulation have the potential to enhance the planning of nursing care by enabling nurses to determine the impact of clinical interventions, such as posturing, on internal organs. The long-term value of this level of patient information on clinical practice decisions remains an unanswered question in nursing research.

PATRICIA FLATLEY BRENNAN

See also
TELEHEALTH
TELENURSING/TELEPRACTICE
TELEPRESENCE
VIRTUAL REALITY

IMMIGRANT WOMEN

Immigration is a process of movement of people from one country to another. Immigrants experience a transition that begins with preparation for immigration and includes the act of immigrating, the process of settling in, and over time, identity transformation. Throughout this transition process, individuals and families experience both euphoric and highly stressed responses. These experiences increase the vulnerability of immigrating populations to health risks. The effects of marginalization and barriers to health care access, resources, and support are magnified for immigrant women.

The uniqueness of women's health care needs is well established and has led to several women's health care centers. Immigrant women share unique characteristics that require special gender-sensitive research and clinical efforts. Immigrant women share the vulnerabilities and the marginalization of minority women in general. Immigrant women face constraints associated with being new in the United States, such as language, transportation, and role overload. Another constraint is maintaining home country heritage and developing new values and beliefs to integrate themselves and their families into the host culture. These variables influence immigrant women's health and health care, and many of the variables have not been adequately studied.

Foreign-born or immigrant women tend to work in environments that increase their health risks. They are more likely to work at home or in family businesses that provide them with limited benefits. When employed outside the home, they often work in low-income jobs such as work in garment shops or domestic work. Women often accompany male family members in immigrating to the United States rather than obtaining their own visas. Therefore, their status is insecure, and they are more vulnerable and less likely to disclose battering, harassment, or abuse.

A nursing perspective focusing on immigrant women and their health includes research on gender and health, culturally influenced explanatory models of illness, transitions and health, and marginalization and health (Meleis, 1995; Meleis, Lipson, Muecke, & Smith, in press). Immigrant women's gender relates to their ability to access and receive quality care. They are expected not only to cook, do housework, care for children, and often to contribute income but also to act as family mediators and culture brokers. Health care professionals have limited knowledge of the demands and the nature of immigrant women's multiple roles and their health care needs, nor has research adequately uncovered the contextual conditions that influence their health-seeking strategies, the nature of their illnesses, and compliance with treatment (Anderson, 1991b). How immigrant women express their symptoms and what meaning they attach to health care encounters also determine their health outcomes. Describing their explanatory models of illness may improve provision of care and ultimately their health (Reizian & Meleis, 1987).

Conceptualization of immigration as a transition allows researchers to focus on the process, timing, and critical points in the process of becoming an American. Lipson (1993) described the traumatic experiences of Afghan refugees before leaving Afghanistan, during transit, and while settling in the United States. Knowledge of the traumatic experiences of the immigrants and refugees helped to explain their responses to the immigration transition and provided a context in which to identify their health care needs. During transitions there is loss of support and networks. In addition to these stressors, women in particular are expected to take responsibility for family health and to mediate between the demands of the new social structure and members of their families for health care, schools, and social services.

Several strategies have been developed to provide care for immigrant women. Some of the most effective models are groups that focus on women's strengths (Meleis, Omidian, & Lipson, 1993; Shepard & Faust, 1994), the use of cultural interpreters (Jezewski, 1993), and feminist participatory models, such as group discussion of dreams to deal with psychosocial issues (Thompson, 1991). However, there is a need for further research to capture the transition experiences of such neglected populations as women immigrants from South America, Eastern Europe, and the Middle East, as well as studies that address issues of language, symbolic interpretation, and cultural competence in health care. In particular, there is need to develop and test nursing interventions that decrease structural barriers to health care as well as those that support culturally appropriate preventive and health-promoting behaviors (Lipson & Meleis, in press).

Future areas for scholarship include methods for defining populations, developing culturally competent research tools, using appropriate theoretical frameworks, and uncovering the critical markers in the transition process that render immigrants more vulnerable. Developing and testing culturally competent models of care is of top priority with the increasing diversity of populations and the backlash against women and immigrants.

AFAF IBRAHIM MELEIS
JULIENE G. LIPSON

See also
CULTURAL/TRANSCULTURAL FOCUS
GENDER RESEARCH
TRANSITIONS AND HEALTH
VULNERABLE POPULATIONS
WOMEN'S HEALTH RESEARCH

INFECTION CONTROL

The infectious process depends on the interaction between an infectious agent, a susceptible host, and the environment. Essential to this interaction is a means of transmission of the agent from an infected host to a susceptible host. This occurs through direct contact, airborne droplet transmission, and indirect contact. Airborne transmission involves the dissemination of particles suspended in air that contain infectious microorganisms. When replication of the infectious agent occurs in the tissues of the host, causing local cellular injury, secretion of toxins, and/or an antigen-antibody reaction that produces signs and symptoms, infectious disease is present. Communicable diseases are infectious diseases that may be transmitted from one person (or animal) to another. Not all infectious diseases are communicable.

Infection control occurs both in the community and within institutions. However, since 1980 increasing emphasis has been placed on hospital-acquired infections. The excess cost for this complication of hospitalization can prolong hospital stay by approximately 6 days or more, resulting in extra charges that averaged $5,683 per hospital day in 1992 (Centers for Disease Control and Prevention [CDC], 1992).

Regulatory Bodies

The CDC has long been involved in the development of guidelines for infection control programs. The Joint Commission on Accreditation of Healthcare Organizations (JCAHO) sets standards for practice and requires infection control committees to recommend and approve surveillance programs based on previous nosocomial infection statistics. In addition, the Occupational Safety and Health Administration (OSHA) has published a regulatory document titled *The OSHA Bloodborne Pathogen Standard*. This document requires that all employers of health care workers provide employees with an environment safe from exposure to blood-borne pathogens (U.S. Department of Labor, 1991). The American Public Health Association has published a classification system for reporting communicable diseases that is used by state and national public health services (Benenson, 1995). The National Nosocomial Infection Surveillance system collects data from a variety of hospitals nationwide. Reports of findings are published periodically.

Surveillance

The purpose of infection control surveillance is to establish and maintain a data base that describes the endemic rates of nosocomial infections. Knowledge of endemic rates allows recognition of increased rates of nosocomial infection resulting in clusters or outbreaks. These data also can be used to prioritize infection control activities and identify trends such as shifts in prevalent pathogens or outcomes of hospital-acquired infections. The surveillance process includes definition of nosocomial infections, systematic gathering of case findings, and tabulation, analysis, interpretation, and reporting of relevant data to individuals or groups for appropriate action.

There are three major types of surveillance. Total house surveillance detects and records all nosocomial infections that occur anywhere in the hospital. It is expensive because of the time and personnel required. Priority-directed or targeted surveillance concentrates on specific areas, patient populations, or procedures, depending on the characteristics of the hospital. Problem-oriented surveillance is conducted to measure the occurrence of specific infection problems, such as outbreaks in specific areas of the hospital. Other surveillance programs may include prevalence surveys or a focus on the identification of risk factors associated with nosocomial infections (Harkness, 1995).

Sites of Nosocomial Infections

Urinary tract infections are the most common nosocomial infections. Approximately 80% are associated with urinary tract manipulations, including catheterization. Nosocomial pneumonia is the second most common hospital-acquired infection and has the highest case-fatality ratio. Intubation that bypasses host defense mechanisms is the most common risk factor. Surgical wound infections are the third most common nosocomial infection. Incisional wounds account for 60%–80% of surgical wound infections. The remainder is classified as deep infections. Primary nosocomial bacteremia is related to intravascular devices. Secondary nosocomial bacteremia is related to infection at other sites. Common risk factors and infectious organisms for the top four nosocomial infections are outlined in the accompanying Table 1.

Prevention and Control

Prevention of nosocomial infections is predicated on identifying the combination of patient risk factors that are associated with the development of infection prior to the emergence of clinical signs and symptoms. Preventive interventions remain the most effective way to reduce morbidity and mortality. More research is necessary in this area.

Control of nosocomial infections entails interruption of the interactions between the infectious agent, the susceptible host, and the environment. Because many pathogenic organisms are transmitted to susceptible patients by the hands of health care workers, handwashing is paramount in infection control. There are several systems that have been established for carrying out infection precautions in hospitals: category-specific, disease-specific, body substance isolation, and universal precautions. Reverse isolation is designed to protect the susceptible patient from environmental sources of infection. The CDC has recommended standard precautions for all patients, plus transmission-based precautions for airborne, droplet, and contact transmission (CDC and Prevention, 1994).

Control of infectious diseases depends on interrupting the interaction between an infectious pathogenic agent, a susceptible person, and the characteristics of the environment. The characteristics of transmission of the organism through direct contact, airborne droplets, and indirect contact are important considerations. Nosocomial infections are iatrogenic, costly complications of hospitalization. In order of incidence, the top four nosocomial infections are urinary tract infections, pneumonia, surgical wound infections, and bacteremia. Preventive interventions for high-risk patients are the most effective measures to prevent morbidity and mortality.

GAIL A. HARKNESS

See also
CRITICAL CARE NURSING
ENDOTRACHEAL SUCTIONING
EPIDEMIOLOGY
HIV/AIDS: CARE AND TREATMENT

TABLE 1   Common Risk Factors and Infectious Organisms Associated With the Leading Nosocomial Infections

Infection	Risk Factors	Microorganisms
Urinary tract	Debilitation	*Escherichia coli*
	Chronic disease	*Klebsiella*
	Presence of	Protei
	periurethral	Enterococci
	pathogens	*Pseudomonas*
		Enterobacter
		Serratia
		Candida
Pneumonia	Intubation	Aerobic gram-
	COPD	negative bacilli:
	Cancer	*Pseudomonas*
	Central nervous	*aeruginosa*
	system	*Klebsiella*
	depression	*Enterobacter*
	Electrolyte	*E. coli*
	imbalances	*Serratia*
		Gram positive:
		Staphylococcus
		aureus
Surgical wound	Advancing age	Gram-positive:
	Obesity	*S. aureus*
	Severe	Aerobic gram-
	malnutrition	negative bacilli
	Infection at	
	other sites	
	Extended	
	preoperative	
	stay	
Bacteremia	Intravascular	*S. aureus*
	devices	Aerobic gram-
	Infection at	negative bacilli
	other sites	

INFORMED CONSENT

Background

Informed consent is the process by which a potential subject or a legal representative is given explanations about the purpose of the research and the risks, inconveniences, costs, potential benefits, and right to withdraw from the study without repercussions. This must occur prior to obtaining written or verbal consent for enrollment. The use of informed consent for research and the process for obtaining it have evolved over the past 50 years. The major impetus for increased attention to the issues of informed consent was a series of studies involving unethical actions on the part of researchers toward their subjects. These studies involved human rights violations in which subjects were neither informed nor had the ability to refuse participation. Highly publicized examples included experiments conducted on Nazi prisoners in concentration camps; withholding treatment for a group of poor Black men with syphilis in Tuskeegee, Alabama, to determine the course of the untreated disease; and not informing elderly patients at the Jewish Chronic Disease Hospital in New York that they were injected with live cancer cells (National Commission for the Protection of Human Subjects, 1979).

The Nuremberg Code, which outlined ethical standards for research, was adopted in response to the human rights violations in Nazi prison camps. This was followed by the Declaration of Helsinki, adopted by the World Medical Assembly in 1964. In the United States the National Commission for the Protection of Human Subjects of Biomedical and Behavioral Research (1979) developed a code of ethics for the protection of human subjects, specifying guidelines for research sponsored by the federal government. The basic principles of beneficence, justice, and respect for persons were the guiding ethical principles. This was followed by federal regulations (U.S. Department of Health and Human Services [USDHHS], 1983, 1996), specifying in greater detail the conditions under which humans could be used in research sponsored by the federal government. Professional organizations then issued their own guidelines. In 1975, the American Nurses Association published *Human Rights Guidelines for Nurses in Clinical and Other Research.*

Today research involving human subjects requires that, prior to giving consent, the subject or legal representative be informed of the purpose, duration, and procedures of the study; risks or discomforts; potential benefits; alternatives to participation; confidentiality; compensation; person to contact for questions; and a statement that participation is voluntary. There are special provisions when subjects are fetuses (in and ex utero), children, pregnant women, or prisoners (USDHHS, 1983).

Issues for Nurses to Consider

Not all research involving humans requires informed consent. The local institutional review board (IRB) is the authority for determining the need for informed consent. Criteria for exemption from informed consent are found in the *Code of Federal Regulation* (1983), title 45, part 46 (USDHHS, 1983). Issues about informed consent debated in the literature include understandability of the consent form, research in emergency or critical care situations, genetic research, and use of blood cell line development.

Understandability of the consent form has two components: the subject's ability to understand the information in the consent form and the reading level. The subject must be legally competent to give informed consent. Competency to give consent can be affected by the age of the potential subjects (child vs. adult); mental ability (Alzheimer's patients or mentally retarded adults); medical condition (unconsciousness, sedated, incubated); or ability to read, speak, and understand English. The researcher has to ensure that the consent form is written at a level that can be understood by the subject. Articles on wording of consent forms and determining reading levels are available (Grossman, Piantadosi, & Couchey, 1994; Philipson, Doyle, Gabram, Nightingale, & Philipson, 1995).

Until the fall of 1996 the ability of researchers to conduct studies in emergency and critical care situations, when the potential subject was not able to give informed consent and the legal representative was not available, was severely limited. A change in federal regulations (USDHHS, 1996) allows the exemption from informed consent requirements for emergency research under very specific conditions: (a) the subject's condition is life-threatening, (b) available treatments are unproved or unsatisfactory, (c) consent cannot reasonably be obtained prior to the initiation of the intervention, (d) there is the potential for direct benefit to the subject, and (e) the community is aware of the research prior to the initiation of the study. Although somewhat controversial, the major debate on this new regulation pertains to the process of notification of the community about the research (Federal Register, 1996). Details on how this will be implemented in practice will evolve as IRBs use different approaches and share their experiences with the scientific establishment and the community.

Ethical issues continue to arise with advances in technology. Should subjects be informed that the blood taken from them may be stored indefinitely and used for other research purposes, such as the establishment of cell lines that may be commercially profitable? Should subjects who have genetic testing done as a part of the research be informed that although the results are confidential, there is a theoretical risk for discrimination if a medical disorder or condition is found? As part of the medical record, this discrimination may affect their ability to obtain life or health insurance or employment. Should health care practitioners who want to enhance their emergency skills be allowed to use the newly deceased for practice without obtaining consent from the legal representative of the individual (Burns, Reardon, & Truog, 1994)? These and other ethical dilemmas associated with informed consent will continue to challenge the nursing and medical community.

Nursing Research on Informed Consent

Nursing research on informed consent primarily has addressed the issue of patient advocacy, with emphasis on the patient's ability to understand the informed consent document. Susman, Dorn, and Fletcher (1992) investigated how much information 44 subjects, aged 7 to 20 years, retained about the research protocol in which they were enrolled. They found that over 50% of the subjects understood that they could ask questions about the research study, knew how long they would be in the study and what the benefit of the study would be, and were aware that they could withdraw at any time. However, less than 3% knew the purpose of the study, 9% knew the risks associated with the study, and 14% knew what procedures were associated with the study.

A second study focused on what subjects understood of the words used in research consent forms. Lawson and Adamson (1995) interviewed 86 adults on research protocols and found that over 80% understood the following commonly used terms: *efficacy, lesion, orally, benefits, adverse reactions, placebo, compensation, ineligible,* and *withdrawal of consent.* Conversely, less than 50% of the subjects understood words such as *protocol, open label,* and *nonsteroidal antiinflammatory drugs.*

Future Directions

How can we be sure that subjects understand the risks and procedures associated with the research? Dupont et al. (1995) used an innovative strategy for ensuring that potential subjects were informed of the risks of the study in which healthy volunteers ingested *Cryptosporidium parvum* oocysts. "Eligible volunteers were required to score 100 percent on a 10 question examination that tested their comprehension of salient features of the study, including the fact that they might become ill, that no effective treatment for the illness was available and that the organism could be spread to household contacts" (p. 856). Other techniques for improving subject understanding of the research include giving a copy of the informed consent form to the subject, viewing a videotape of the research procedure, and calling subjects after they have signed the consent to an-swer questions or concerns. Clearly, additional research is needed in the area of informed consent.

BARBARA S. TURNER

See also
ETHICS OF RESEARCH
GENETICS IN NURSING RESEARCH
RIGHTS OF HUMAN SUBJECTS
SCIENTIFIC INTEGRITY

INSTRUMENTATION

Instrumentation is a general term for the activities involved in developing, testing, and revising measures of concepts important to nursing. The term is usually applied to these processes as they relate to psychosocial or self-report measures of attitudes and behaviors. However, instrumentation also refers to the validating of measures for physiological parameters or laboratory devices. The goal of instrumentation is to create measures that reduce error in research through consistency, accuracy, and sensitivity of measurement. For self-report instruments, consistency is analogous to reliability, and accuracy is analogous to validity. With laboratory instruments, validity is also used to describe the accuracy of the measures, but precision refers to the instrument's consistency in measurement. Sensitivity is directly applicable to both types of measurement and refers to the instrument's ability to finely discriminate in individual differences and changes in the concept under study. Control of measurement error is achieved by assuring that as much response variability as possible is due to the subject's relationship to the concept under study rather than to inconsistent or systematic extraneous factors.

The term *psychometrics* is often used to refer to the results of testing self-report measures and to the statistics that are utilized in that examination. Self-report measures generally fall into the categories of norm-referenced and criterion-referenced. With norm-referenced instruments the goal is to obtain a spread of scores across a wide range for the purpose of discriminating between subjects. Criterion-referenced measures are constructed for the purpose of determining whether a subject has or has not achieved a predetermined set of target behaviors. Steps in instrumentation for these two categories differ; however, the majority of attitudinal and behavioral measures applicable to nursing are norm-referenced, and their construction and testing is emphasized. Information on construction and testing of criterion-referenced instruments may be found in Waltz, Strickland, and Lenz (1991).

Instrumentation for self-report measures involves three general phases: development, testing, and revision. Instrument development involves concept clarification, developing a theoretical definition, operationalizing the concept, and generating items. Walker and Avant (1988) propose three approaches to concept clarification. Concept analysis involves a careful review of literature with attention to consistencies and inconsistencies in the use of the concept. Concept synthesis uses clinical observations to explore the phenomenon of interest. Concept derivation consists of moving a concept from one field or discipline to another. After the concept to be measured is clarified, a theoretical definition is formulated that delineates the dimensions of the concept to be measured based on the result of concept clarification. Operationalization is the process of moving to an operational variable that is isomorphic with the theoretical definition. Item generation involves decisions about concept dimensionality and scaling methodology.

When the phenomenon of interest is a highly abstract concept, the theoretical definition will include a number of conceptual aspects. Less abstract concepts can often be indexed with items that tap only one, more finite aspect. For each aspect of the concept, items must be developed in a manner that assures homogeneity within that conceptual dimension. Thus, the instrument may have to be multidimensional or unidimensional, depending on the concept of interest. Typically, multidimensional concepts will be measured with instruments that have a subscale that relates to each dimension.

Decisions about scaling involve whether the model is meant to scale stimuli or people. Methods used for scaling stimuli are paired comparisons, constant stimuli, successive categories, and psychophysical methods. Common approaches to scaling people are cumulative (e. g., Guttman-type), differential (e. g., Thurstone-like), and summated (e. g., Likert-type) instruments. Nunnally (1978) provides an excellent overview of these scaling procedures. Other decisions in item generation include factors involved with instrument formatting. These factors relate to levels of measurement, scaling responses, and the appearance of the scale to the respondent.

Instrument testing for self-report measures involves two aspects. Initially, the content of the instrument is examined to assure its relationship to the theoretical definition of the concept. The procedures include estimates of whether the concept has been sufficiently indexed by the instrument's items and whether the format is clear and promotes response consistency. Evaluation of the link between the concept and items is primarily performed by a panel of content and instrument experts. Once it is determined that the concept is adequately indexed, a second phase of testing involves the use of the instrument with a sample from the target population. This testing results in a quantitative examination of reliability and validity measures (see "Reliability" and "Validity").

Instrument revision for self-report measures includes a critical examination of testing results and individual items. Options for items are (a) inclusion as is, (b) alteration to clarify or meet theory, and (c) elimination. Once the instrument has been revised, it must be tested again with another sample from the target population.

Instrumentation for laboratory measures involves the similar phases of development and testing. However, the development phase typically focuses on the establishment of procedures for the use of the device. Testing evaluates the precision, accuracy, and sensitivity of the device, given the procedures established. Examination of precision must include calibration of the device and evaluation for inconsistency in readings, given repetitive use. Assessment for accuracy includes not only the meeting of established standards but appraisal of appropriate theoretical specification of results to the concept of interest. Revision of procedures may be needed when results of testing do not meet established standards for precision and accuracy.

JOYCE A. VERRAN
PAULA MEEK

See also
MEASUREMENT AND SCALES
PHYSIOLOGICAL MONITORING
RELIABILITY
THEORETICAL FRAMEWORK
VALIDITY

INTERNATIONAL CENTER FOR NURSING SCHOLARSHIP

The Center for Nursing Scholarship is a concept, a place, and a program. The idea for a center for nursing scholarship evolved from the founding vision of Sigma Theta Tau. It was given shape when the society adopted its 10-year plan in 1981. In this plan the development and dissemination of nursing knowledge was identified as the essential contribution that nursing can make to the improvement of people's health. The center is conceptualized as a catalyst, a global communication network, an international data base of nursing scholarship and research, a repository of nursing knowledge, a link to the great collections and libraries of the world, and the home of nursing scholarship. The Center for Nursing Scholarship is also a think tank and a meeting place for scholars, researchers, educators, and clinicians. It welcomes not only members but all who share in and support the organization's mission to improve the health of people worldwide by increasing and broadening the scientific base of nursing.

The Center for Nursing Scholarship was dedicated in 1989 as the official headquarters of Sigma Theta Tau International (STTI), the international honor society for nursing. Sigma Theta Tau International ranks as the second-largest nursing organization in the United States and is one of the five largest nursing societies in the world. Its annual budget exceeds $4 million. Persons are invited to membership through one of the 356 honor societies that are located in colleges and universities in the United States, Puerto Rico, Canada, South Korea, Taiwan, and Australia. The center is located at 550 West North Street, Indianapolis, IN 46202; http://www.stti.iupui.edu/.

In pursuit of its knowledge-based agenda, STTI promotes a program to expand the intellectual base of nursing. This includes a small research grants program (more than 250 since 1936), the Virginia Henderson International Nursing Library, an international registry of nursing research, an on-line catalog of nurse researchers with their studies and their findings, an on-line *Journal of Knowledge Synthesis*, a leadership institute, international and regional research conferences, and research monographs and publications such as *Image: The Journal of Nursing Scholarship*. The society also sponsors an awards program that recognizes scholars, researchers, and the media; philanthropists and foundations support the work of the center and the advancement and dissemination of nursing knowledge throughout the world.

ROSEMARY DONLEY

See also
JOURNALS IN NURSING RESEARCH

THE ONLINE JOURNAL
OF KNOWLEDGE SYNTHESIS
FOR NURSING
VIRGINIA HENDERSON INTER-
NATIONAL NURSING LIBRARY

INTERNATIONAL CLASSIFICATION FOR NURSING PRACTICE

The International Classification for Nursing Practice (ICNP) is a classification of nursing phenomena, nursing interventions, and nurse-sensitive outcomes that describes nursing practice and provides a unifying framework into which terms from other nursing classifications may be cross-mapped.

The International Council of Nurses (ICN) initiated and developed the ICNP in order to have a common system for tracking nursing data. Other health professions track data through systems such as the *International Classification of Diseases and Related Health Problems* (ICD-10) and the *Diagnostic and Statistical Manual for Mental Disorders* (DSM-IV). The ICN vision for the ICNP is to have nursing information readily available and used in the health care information systems worldwide.

Significance and Relevance

As the uses of automated information systems expand, the lack of a common system to describe and record nursing threatens to obscure nursing contributions to health and to invalidate studies of the effectiveness of interdisciplinary and nursing interventions. The ICNP would provide a common language to describe and record nursing and is thus critical to the future of nursing. The significance and relevance of the ICNP to nursing research are great. Optimal development of nursing knowledge requires global collaboration, with recognition of the influence of culture and other contextual variables on nursing phenomena. The ICNP would provide the comparable data for the development of nursing knowledge across countries, cultures, and languages. For example, the prevalence of specific nursing diagnoses worldwide or the use and effec-

tiveness of specific nursing interventions could be studied.

Historical Overview

The ICNP has been built on the foundation of the nursing minimum data set (Werley & Lang, 1988) and the considerable nursing classification work done in several countries. The ICN decided to pursue the ICNP in 1989 (Clark & Lang, 1992) and approved a proposal to fund work, starting in 1991 with a survey of the National Nursing Association members of ICN on the need for an ICNP. From 1991 to 1995, the core ICNP project team included Fadwa Affara, June Clark, Norma Lang, Randi Mortensen, Margaret Murphy, Gunnar Nielsen, and Madeline Wake. In 1996, Alice Baumgart and Amy Coenen joined the team. Their work demanded international collaboration.

Nursing terms for nursing diagnoses, interventions, and outcomes were collected worldwide from nursing classifications and from literature, including journals referenced on computer databases and the proceedings of conferences on nursing classification and nursing informatics (Wake et al., 1993). These terms and the plan for developing an ICNP were reviewed during a meeting with nurses from Chile, Jamaica, Japan, Kenya, Israel, and Nepal. The scarcity of primary health care terms emerged as a major finding. Following that meeting, an ICNP working paper (International Council of Nurses, 1992) was published, and efforts were begun to obtain funding for work on community health terms.

The W. K. Kellogg Foundation funded an Advisory Meeting on the Development of an Informational Tool to Support Community-Based and Primary Care Nursing Systems, in Mexico in 1994. Nurses from Botswana, Brazil, Chile, Colombia, Mexico, South Africa, Swaziland, the United States, and Zimbabwe worked to identify terms. A similar meeting, supported by the Taiwan Nurses Association, was held in Taiwan for nurses from Japan, Korea, Malaysia, New Zealand, Philippines, Singapore, Taiwan, Thailand, and Western Samoa.

The expanded lists of terms were placed in a terms database according to a preliminary taxonomical structure (Coenen & Wake, 1996). Using principles of classification and of international standardization, comprehensive architectures for nursing phenomena (defined as phenomena that nurses diagnose) and nursing interventions were designed (Nielsen & Mortensen, 1996). These evolved to the alpha version of the ICNP, which was published by the International Council of Nurses (1996). In the European Union–funded Telenurse project, Mortensen, Nielsen, and associates are developing nursing prototypes for electronic patient records. With these prototypes, they will conduct European field tests of the alpha version of the ICNP with translation into 12 languages. Kellogg has funded some country-level applications of the ICNP in Latin America and Africa. Nurses in these countries and in other countries are participating, through national nurses associations, in validation studies of selected terms. Information from validation studies, field tests, and other feedback on the alpha version will be used to develop the Beta Version, targeted for completion in December 1998.

Future Directions

Current efforts of the ICNP project team are focused on outcomes, coding, and refining the classifications of nursing phenomena and interventions. Ongoing challenges include resolving conflicts between classification principles and nursing science as well as those between technical language and that easily translated. Work remains to be done on the terms and definitions in the areas of scientific basis, language clarity, and clinical relevance. In addition to the project team, involvement of nurse researchers from many countries is essential to ongoing development and usefulness of the ICNP, a tool for the global nursing community.

MADELINE MUSANTE WAKE

See also
**INTERNATIONAL NURSING RESEARCH
NURSING INFORMATICS
NURSING MINIMUM DATA SET
WORLD HEALTH ORGANIZATION**

INTERNATIONAL NURSING RESEARCH

International nursing research represents comparative research on nursing phenomena and on nursing issues conducted in more than one country. This includes research that is conducted cross-nationally to examine issues of global interest to nurses and to test and develop theories. The research is usually conducted by a nurse who resides in one country and studies phenomena in another country. The purpose is to compare the findings with the results of similar research obtained in other countries. Such research provides opportunities to clarify scientific values, explore assumptions, and develop shared frameworks.

International research in nursing is growing with the increased opportunities for travel, networking, and collaboration. The increasing abilities of nurses to study abroad, to attend international conferences, to visit international institutions, and to communicate through electronic mail systems, enhance comparative and collaborative research projects. International scholarship has focused on the use of U.S. nursing theories and the evaluation and testing of their utilities and appropriateness to the different nursing cultures. There are many descriptive and analytical dialogues related to theory in the international literature. These dialogues have resulted in scholarly publications related to the introduction and analysis of U.S. theories in many countries, such as in Ireland, Germany, Switzerland, Finland, and Australia (Greenwood, 1996; Mckenna, 1994).

Human resources analyses and investigations led to several international projects. Questions related to the image and status of nursing, shortage of nurses, and distributions of nurses in urban and rural settings were examined. The results were compared and contrasted among and between countries and regions. There is general agreement among researchers in many countries on the perception of nursing and the difficulty in recruitment of students and retention of nurses in the workforce (Meleis, 1987, 1994).

There are commonalities in nurses' reasons for leaving the countries and seeking employment in other countries or regions. Nurses emigrate to seek better job opportunities, to secure a better future for their children, to improve their skills, and to complete their graduate education. Research on nurses' adjustment to living and working in host countries is still in its infancy (Meleis, 1994).

Other research areas that received the attention of international nurses were the caring practices of nurses and the relationship between nurses' cultural heritage and language and patients' cultural heritage and their primary language of communication. There is beginning evidence that nurses of multicultural heritage who speak more than one language tend to provide more culturally competent care.

Other areas of comparative and collaborative research were focused on women's health and quality of life. Questions about women's health were considered within a sociopolitical context, with attention to health and health care in the overall development of women through better options, more education, and higher status. Other research examples were in ethical and clinical decision making, pain management, and the management of the care of the elderly.

Future international research requires the development of culturally competent methods, analysis of ethical issues in conducting collaborative international research, development of guidelines for international collaboration, and a framework for decisions related to data ownership, authorship, and culturally sensitive rules for data dissemination.

The International Council of Nursing, in collaboration with the U.S. Institute for Nursing Research, developed a list of priorities for international research, which addressed the urgency for preparing researchers internationally and providing international strategies to support nursing research. A future direction for priorities in substantive research questions has to be identified to enhance international collaboration and provide nurses with shared goals.

AFAF IBRAHIM MELEIS

See also
CULTURAL/TRANSCULTURAL FOCUS
ETHICS OF RESEARCH
IMMIGRANT WOMEN
INTERNATIONAL CLASSIFICATION
FOR NURSING PRACTICE

WORLD HEALTH ORGANIZATION COLLABORATING CENTERS

INTERNET

The Internet is a catch-all term used to describe the massive worldwide network of computers. The term *internet* literally means "network of networks." It was originally developed in 1969 in the United States as a system of communication in the event of war. The Internet was then adopted by universities as a means of communication among researchers. The Internet is composed of thousands of smaller regional networks scattered across the globe. On any given day it connects approximately 20 million users in over 50 countries.

With a network connection (either direct or via modem), the Internet can be accessed in a number of different ways. Currently, the most talked about method is the World Wide Web. Other methods include Gopher, Telnet, FTP, E-mail, and newsgroup utilities.

Nobody "owns" the Internet. There are companies that help manage different parts of the networks that tie everything together, but there is no single governing body that controls what happens on the Internet. Networks within different countries are funded and managed locally according to local policies. Access to the Internet usually means access to a number of basic services: electronic mail, interactive conferences, information resources, network news, and the ability to transfer files.

Nursing and the Internet

Nursing research of the Internet is primarily descriptive (Halstead, Hayes, Reising, & Billings, 1995; Masten & Conover, 1990) and related to use of the Internet. Recently, nurse researchers have begun to take advantage of the Internet for data collection in terms of survey completion time and user anonymity (Fawcett & Buhle, 1995; Murray, 1995).

Nurses are using the Internet in increasing numbers. Early nurse use of the Internet was via bulletin board services (BBs) and listservs (computer programs to distribute information to persons who belong to the same electronic group). Susan Sparks

(E.T.Net), Gordon Larrivee (NRSING-L), Linda Thede (NurseRes), and Judy Norris (NURSENET) were among the early adopters of this specific Internet technology (Fickeissen, 1995; Sparks, 1993). Currently, nursing research of the Internet includes Yensen's (1996) Virtual Nursing College, a unique approach to nursing education using the Internet as a tool to conduct classes and coursework for students.

The Internet contains tremendous potential for health care professionals as a tool that can and will be employed in many different roles. Some of these roles include communication among nurses, distance education, nursing knowledge access in distant sites by bedside nurses, promotion of real-time patient education, and increased interactions of nurses and homebound patients for health education and promotion.

W. Scott Erdley
Susan M. Sparks

See also
ELECTRONIC NETWORK
INTRANET
NURSING INFORMATICS
WORLD WIDE WEB

INTRANET

An intranet is the application of Internet technologies within an enterprise. Although Internet technologies are used, there is no external connection to the global Internet, making intranets "private" networks. An intranet is deployed and maintained to transparently distribute and share extensive information resources wherever needed in the enterprise and only within the enterprise.

Intranets use the infrastructure and standards of the Internet and the World Wide Web (WWW or Web). However, intranets are protected from external access by the public Internet through software programs known as "firewalls." An intranet is a private computer network that has the same look and feel as the graphic interface of the WWW, or browser, currently supporting the following hypermedia (the capability to link from one medium to another): text, graphics, audio, and still images.

WWW technologies are inexpensive, powerful alternatives to other types of protected internal communications such as wide area networks (which usually link multiple offices together) and groupware products (which allow multiple user access to a single document). Because Web browsers operate nearly all brands of computers, the same electronic information may be viewed by any authorized user and is not dependent on the kind of computer used. Thus, all kinds of documents, such as procedure manuals, training materials, forms, and internal lists, can be converted to electronic forms on an intranet and constantly updated with minimal cost.

By the time this entry is published, there will have been many enhancements that facilitate the practical use of additional hypermedia, such as moving images and live multimedia. These next-generation intranet web sites will incorporate technologies such as dynamic data bases to present the user with specific information based on the request, as well as multimedia objects.

Nursing and Intranets

Intranets are new, having been developed or "discovered" about 1995. Research investigating nursing and intranets is limited. Reports generally are anecdotal in nature (Claridge, 1996) and address related areas such as groupware or local area networks (Chapman et al., 1994; Skiba, 1993). Intranets hold tremendous potential for nursing, not only in terms of information dissemination among staff members but also for continuing education, patient education, and clinical information retrieval. It is easy-to-use technology, inexpensive, rich with media possibilities, and currently one of few options for secure, confidential networking within an enterprise. Thus, it is an ideal technology for patient and health care clinical research applications.

W. Scott Erdley
Susan M. Sparks

See also
ELECTRONIC NETWORK
INTERNET
NURSING INFORMATICS
WORLD WIDE WEB

J

JOB SATISFACTION

Job satisfaction represents the degree to which individuals like their jobs. Researchers study job satisfaction from varied perspectives, most commonly either as a dependent variable in assessing the impact of organizational innovations or as an intervening variable within complex multistaged models of employee turnover, retention, or absenteeism. More recently, nurses' job satisfaction has been examined as part of the organizational context that affects outcomes of health care, such as client satisfaction and compliance, length of stay, and mortality.

As general attitudinal constructs, job satisfaction reflects a positive affective orientation toward the organization and work, whereas job dissatisfaction reflects a negative affective orientation. Subconstructs distinguish attitudes toward specific dimensions of the job, such as the work or task, pay and benefits, co-workers, status, administration, or, for nurses, quality of care. Researchers choose measures of job satisfaction based on the nature of the investigation and the response burden for subjects. For instance, in examining the impact of a professional practice model innovation for nursing, one might be interested in changes in employee satisfaction related to quality of care, status, pay, and relationships with management. If, however, the focus is outcomes of rehabilitation care provided to individuals with stroke across several different settings, a short, general job satisfaction measure would impose less burden for subjects, who also could be responding to multiple measures of organizational and clinical variables.

In early studies of organizations, workers' liking or disliking their jobs usually was labeled morale. Midway through the 20th century, researchers began to develop both general (e.g., Brayfield & Rothe, 1951) and dimension-specific (e.g., Smith, Kendall, & Hulin, 1969) measures of satisfaction-

dissatisfaction. Disagreement arose about whether job satisfaction and dissatisfaction were opposite ends of a single continuum or were two separate constructs. Although job satisfaction currently is reported most often in the research literature, the one-or-two-constructs issue has not been resolved; the terms are used inconsistently and sometimes interchangeably. A more recent concern is the possibility that positive and negative affectivity, which are mood-dispositional personality traits, contaminate effects of determinants (e.g., autonomy, stress) on strain-related variables such as job satisfaction.

Registered nurse (RN) staff in acute care hospitals has been the population of greatest interest in studies of nurses' job satisfaction, and less is known about the dynamics of job satisfaction among RNs who work in other settings or among other nursing personnel. Commonly used measures have been influenced by or adapted from instruments developed in the organizational research field. Subsets of Brayfield-Rothe items frequently have been used as general measures of job satisfaction. Prominent in the measurement of dimension-specific job satisfaction among nurses has been the work of Hinshaw and Atwood (1983–1985), who assembled a battery of scales to assess organizational and professional job satisfaction that encompassed their original work on satisfaction with quality of care as well as other published items (Brayfield & Rothe, 1951; Slavitt, Stamps, Piedmont, & Haase, 1978). Use of other measures also is reported, for example, the Mueller and McCloskey (1990) Satisfaction Scale and the Nursing Work Index (Kramer & Hafner, 1989). Meta-analyses of the accumulated research (Blegen, 1993; Irvine & Evans, 1992) reveal that autonomy, stress, commitment to the organization, and intent to stay in the job demonstrate the strongest, most consistent correlations with job satisfaction; autonomy and stress usually are examined as antecedents and the other variables as outcomes.

Clarifying the relationship between nurses' job satisfaction and client outcomes is a high priority for future research. Investigators who probe that relationship face several challenges. First, clients have extended contact with nurses in the community, at home, and in nursing homes; and extension of research about nurses' job satisfaction to include those settings will facilitate utilization of the findings to improve client outcomes. Second, more information is needed about the degree to which nurses' positive and negative affectivity confound relationships between work characteristics such as autonomy or stress and job satisfaction. Third, given the beginning support in the literature for a relationship between nurses' job satisfaction and client satisfaction with nursing care, the possibility of that association being confounded by client positive and negative affectivity merits consideration. Finally, the unresolved question about whether job satisfaction and dissatisfaction are separate constructs warrants attention. Nurses' satisfaction and dissatisfaction may associate differently with client satisfaction and other outcomes of care.

ROMA LEE TAUNTON

See also
JOB STRESS
NURSING STUDIES INDEX
NURSING WORKLOAD
   MEASUREMENT SYSTEMS
PATIENT SATISFACTION WITH
   NURSING CARE
WORKFORCE

JOB STRESS

Results of a 1995 survey conducted by the American Nurses Association indicated that nurses considered stress to be their number-one occupational hazard. The nursing literature is replete with opinion articles on factors in the work setting that make situations conducive to stress for nurses; however, few articles report research results. It was during the 1970s that nurse researchers as well as sociologists and psychologists became interested in studying job stress for nurses. Early research on job stress for nurses centered on the disruptive effects of changing shifts on circadian rhythms and subjective sense of well-being. In large measure as a result of research on the effects of frequent shift changes, the practice of changing shifts more frequently than every 2 weeks ceased during the 1980s. Research to identify other factors that contributed to job stress focused on intensive care nurses, neonatal intensive care nurses, and hospice nurses.

One of the first studies concerning the experience of stress by staff nurses was conducted by Gray-Toft and Anderson (1981). They developed a measure of stress for nurses called the Nursing Stress Scale (NSS). The NSS contains 34 potentially stressful events divided into seven categories: death and dying, workload, uncertainty concerning treatment, conflict with physicians, conflict with other nurses, lack of staff support, and inadequate preparation to deal with emotional needs of patients. In 1983, Jacobson and McGraw published *Nurses under Stress*, which included a summary of their research on stress experienced by neonatal intensive care nurses as well as the work of other nurse researchers on stress experienced by nurses. During the 1980s and early 1990s much of the research on nurses and stress was conducted by nurse researchers in England. In response to dramatic changes in the health care delivery system and the resultant efforts of hospitals to restructure, redesign, and cut RN positions, there has been a resurgence of interest in studying stress experienced by nurses and nurse administrators in the United States since the mid 1990s (Moore, Kuhrik, Kuhrik, & Katz, 1996).

Among the studies focused on nurses and stress there have been consistent findings that the following factors make situations conducive to stress for nurses: work overload, staff shortages, lack of autonomy, equipment failures, conflict with physicians, conflict with administration or perceived lack of support from administration, lack of communication, ethical issues concerning patients on life support, high personal expectations for performance, and caring for high-acuity patients. Several factors have been examined as possible buffers to job stress experienced by nurses, including hardiness (Wright, Blache, Ralph, & Luterman, 1993) and social support (Cronin-Stubbs & Rooks, 1985). There is a fairly consistent finding in research reports that social support acts as a buffer to stress experienced by nurses in all settings.

Future directions for job stress research will include (a) studies to evaluate the person-environment fit model (French, Rodgers, & Cobb, 1974) or the job demand model (Karasek & Theorell, 1990) to explain factors that contribute to job stress for nurses; (b) intervention studies to evaluate the effectiveness of stress management strategies, including cognitive restructuring to bolster resistance resources such as hardiness and reducing job stress; and (c) longitudinal studies to evaluate the effectiveness of stress management strategies taught to students in nursing by following them to job sites.

BRENDA L. LYON

See also
JOB SATISFACTION
NURSING OCCUPATIONAL INJURY
    AND STRESS
NURSING WORK REDESIGN
NURSING WORKLOAD
    MEASUREMENT SYSTEMS
STRESS

(DOROTHY) JOHNSON'S BEHAVIORAL SYSTEM MODEL

Johnson's behavioral system model views the person as a behavioral system (Johnson, 1980, 1990a). Seven behavioral subsystems carry out specialized functions needed to maintain the integrity of the whole behavioral system and to manage its relationship to the environment. Each subsystem is able to fulfill its functions when the environment provides nurturance, stimulation, and sufficient protection from noxious influences. Behavioral actions associated with each subsystem are motivated by a particular drive and reflect the person's predisposition to act in certain ways, which is referred to as set, as well as all of the choices for actions that are available to the person.

The function of the attachment or affiliative subsystem is the security needed for survival, as well as social inclusion, intimacy, and formation and maintenance of social bonds. The function of the dependency subsystem is the succoring behavior that calls for a response of nurturance as well as approval, attention or recognition, and physical assistance.

The ingestive subsystem is concerned with the function of appetite satisfaction in terms of when, how, what, how much, and under what conditions the person eats, all of which is governed by social and psychological considerations as well as biological requirements for food and fluids. In contrast, the eliminative subsystem is concerned with the function of elimination in terms of when, how, and under what conditions the person eliminates wastes.

The functions of the sexual subsystem are procreation and gratification, with regard to behaviors dependent on the person's biological sex and gender role identity, including but not limited to courting and mating. The function of the aggressive subsystem is protection and preservation of self and society. The function of the achievement subsystem is mastery or control of some aspect of self or environment, with regard to intellectual, physical, creative, mechanical, and social skills, as well as the skills needed to take care of children, partner, and home.

Nursing research focuses on the description of and explanation for behavioral system disorders that arise in connection with illness. The ultimate purpose of research is to determine the effects on behavioral system balance and stability of nursing actions, including (a) provision of protection, nurturance, and stimulation; (b) temporary imposition of external regulatory or control mechanisms; and (c) fostering changes in set, choice, or behavioral actions.

JACQUELINE FAWCETT

See also
BEHAVORIAL RESEARCH
NURSING THEORETICAL MODELS

JOURNALS IN NURSING RESEARCH

Advances in Nursing Science
Peggy L. Chinn, RN, PhD, FAAN, Editor.

School of Nursing, University of Connecticut,
231 Glenbrook Rd., U-26,
Storrs, CT 06040.
FAX: (860) 486-0001;
E-mail: plchinn@uconnvm.uconn.edu.

The primary purposes of Advances in Nursing Science are to stimulate the development of nursing science and promote the application in practice of emerging theories and research findings. Quarterly (September, December, March, and June). Peer reviewed. Indexed in CINAHL. Special issues covered focus on a particular topic.

Annual Review of Nursing Research

Joyce J. Fitzpatrick, Editor.
Frances Payne Bolton School of Nursing,
Case Western Reserve University,
10900 Euclid Avenue,
Cleveland OH 44106-4904.
FAX: (216) 368-5050;
E-mail: jjf4@po.cwru.edu.

Purpose of the series is to critically analyze and synthesize the research pertinent to nursing and health, and systematically assess knowledge development in nursing. Published annually. Invited chapters of this publication are externally reviewed. Indexed in CINAHL and Index Medicus. Issues covered are clinical nursing research, research on nursing care delivery, and international nursing research.

Applied Nursing Research (ANR)

Joyce J. Fitzpatrick, Editor.
Frances Payne Bolton School of Nursing,
Case Western Reserve University,
10900 Euclid Avenue,
Cleveland OH 44106-4904.
FAX: (216) 368-5050;
E-mail: jjf4@po.cwru.edu.

Purpose of the journal is to bridge the gap between research and practice in nursing. Published six times per year. Chapters are externally reviewed. Indexed in CINAHL and Index Medicus. Issues covered are clinical applications of research and clinical research methods.

Clinical Nursing Research

Patricia Hayes, RN, MHSA,
and Marilynn J. Wood, RN, DrPH, Co-Editors.
Peggy Pilgrim, Journals Assistant.

Faculty of Nursing,
3-107 Clinical Sciences Building,
University of Alberta,
Edmonton, Alberta T6G 2G3, Canada.
Phone: (403) 492-1037;
FAX: (403) 492-2551;
E-mail: peggy.pilgrim@ualberta.ca.

Clinical Nursing Research (CNR) is a refereed journal that publishes research articles focused on clinical practice in nursing. It provides an international forum to encourage discussion among clinical practitioners, to enhance clinical practice by pinpointing potential clinical applications of the latest scholarly research, and to disseminate research findings of particular interest to practicing nurses. CNR also publishes Research Briefs and Replication studies. CNR is published 4 times each year. February, May, August, and November. 1998 is the 7th year in publication. CNR manuscripts are peer reviewed. CNR is indexed in Applied Social Sciences Indexes and Abstracts, CINAHL, Literature, English National Board of Health Care Database, International Nursing Index, Linguistics and Language Behavior Abstracts, Nursing Abstracts, Nursing Citation Index, PsycINFO, PsycLIT, Psychological Abstracts, RNdex Top 100, Sage Family Studies Abstracts, SocialPlanning/Policy & Development Abstracts and Sociological Abstracts. No special issues at present. For information about the Departments in Western Journal of Nursing Research (WJNR), and the various Dept Editors, please check our Web site: http://www.ualberta.ca./~fonjrnls/

Computers in Nursing

Leslie H. Nicoll, PhD, MBA, RN, Editor-in-Chief.
University of Southern Maine,
96 Falmouth Street,
PO Box 9300,
Portland, ME 04104-9300.
Phone: (207) 780-4568;
FAX: (207) 780-4953;
E-mail: lnjcoll@maine.maine.edu.

Computers in Nursing (CIN) is designed as a forum for communication among nurses who use computers. As a refereed journal, CIN is a vehicle for the publication of high-quality, relevant, and timely articles on a variety of topics related to the use of computers in and application of computer technology to contemporary nursing practice, education, research, and administration. Articles in *Computers in Nursing* are selected to reflect the diversity of computer hardware, software, and applications that nurses use in their work to provide current and useful information to a broad audience of readers. Bimonthly, 6 issues per year. Peer reviewed. Indexed in CINAHL, International Nursing Index, Index Medicus, MEDLINE, and Social Science Citation Index. Will publish supplements periodically, for example, Computerized Patient Record, March/April 1997.

IMAGE: Journal of Nursing Scholarship
Beverly Henry, RN, PhD, FAAN, Editor.
University of Illinois at Chicago,
College of Nursing (m/c 802),
845 S. Damen Avenue,
Chicago, IL 60612.
FAX: (312) 996-0680;
E-mail: imagebh@uic.edu.

As the official journal of Sigma Theta Tau International, Honor Society of Nursing, Inc., *IMAGE* is intended to provide a forum for the publication of superior nursing thought in the general areas of clinical scholarship and policy. Research reports, reviews of literature, and discursive pieces are desired. Published quarterly. Double-blind peer reviewed. Indexed in CINAHL and MEDLINE. Special issues covered: research, theory, state of the science, education, international scholarship, clinical cases, book reviews. The Journal is not "themed."

Journal of Nursing Administration
Suzanne Smith Blancett, EdD, RN, FAAN, Editor.
4301 32nd Street West,
Suite C12,
Bradenton, FL 34205-2748.
Phone: (941) 753-5662;
E-mail: ssblancett@aol.com.

The Journal of Nursing Administration (JONA) is designed for nurse leaders in hospitals, home healthcare agencies, and other healthcare organizations. JONA provides information on management and leadership development; human, material, and financial resource management; staffing and scheduling systems; staff development; research and innovations; labor-management relations; policy, legislation, regulations, and economics related to healthcare and program development; legal, ethical, and political issues; interdisciplinary collaboration; organization-wide projects; and professional trends. Published monthly. Peer reviewed. Indexed in Index Medicus, International Nursing Index, CINAHL, Hospital Literature Index, Current Contents/Social and Behavioral Sciences, The Social Sciences Citation Index, Nursing Abstracts, and RNdex Top 100. The May issue is devoted to research articles related to nursing administration.

Journal of Nursing Measurement
Ora L. Strickland, PhD, RN, FAAN,
and Ada Sue Hinshaw, PhD, RN, FAAN, Editors.
Nell Hodgson Woodruff School of Nursing,
Emory University,
531 Asbury Circle,
Atlanta, GA 30322.
Phone: (404) 727-7941;
FAX: (404) 727-0536.

Purpose is to serve as a forum for the dissemination of information regarding nursing-related instruments, tools, approaches or procedures developed or utilized for the measurement of variables for nursing practice, education, and research, and to encourage further development. Published twice yearly. Peer reviewed. Indexed in CINAHL, MEDLINE, and Index Medicus.

MCN The American Journal of Maternal/ Child Nursing
Barbara Bishop, MN, RN, FAAN, Editor.
555 West 57th Street,
New York, NY 10019-2961.
Phone: (212) 582-8820 ext 421;
FAX: (212) 586-5462.

MCN is a clinical practice journal for maternal and child nursing that is geared toward the seasoned and/or advanced practice nurse. While committed to accuracy and scientific integrity, MCN tries to maintain a reader-friendly style of writing. Published bi-monthly. Peer reviewed. Indexed in CINAHL, International Nursing Index, Index Medicus, Allied Health Literature, and RNdex Top 100.

Nurse Educator.
Suzanne Smith Blancett, EdD, RN, FAAN, Editor.
4301 32nd Street West,
Suite C12,

Bradenton, FL 34205-2748.
Phone: (941) 753-5662;
E-mail: ssblancett@aol.com.

Purpose: *Nurse Educator*, edited for faculty and administrators in schools of nursing, provides information on both the theories and practice of nursing education, including: educational philosophy, policies, and procedures; organizational, program, curriculum, and course development; instructional methods and materials; testing and measurement; research; faculty development; and administration. Published bimonthly. Peer reviewed. Indexed in International Nursing Index, CINAHL, Hospital Literature Index, Current Index to Journals in Education, and RNdex Top 100.

Nursing Management
Leah L. Curtin, Editor-in-Chief.
672 Neeb Road,
Cincinnati, Ohio 45233.
FAX: (513) 347-7022.

Nursing Management strives to be the leading source of practical education and cutting edge information for the management of health service delivery across the continuum of care. "The independent voice of leadership in health service delivery." Published monthly. Peer reviewed. Indexed in International Nursing Index, Cumulative Index to Nursing & Allied Health Literature, Hospital Literature Index, Nursing Abstracts, and RNdex Top 100. Special issues covered are financial, technology, law, and subacute care.

Nursing Research
Molly C. Dougherty, Editor;
Valerie Parham, Editorial Assistant.
School of Nursing,
CB#7460,
University of North Carolina,
Chapel Hill, NC 27599-7460.
Phone: (919) 966-9415;
FAX: (919) 966-9736;
E-mail addresses: mdougher.uncson@mhs.unc.edu,vparham.uncson@mhs.unc.edu.

The editorial purposes of *Nursing Research* are to report research, both completed and that which is in progress, that contributes to the knowledge base of the discipline of nursing and that provides a better understanding of human responses to illness and the promotion of health; serve an educational function through presenting reports and critiques of methodology and research design; and serve as a medium for the stimulation of ideas and exchange of information about nursing research and practice. Selection of articles for publication is based on their contribution to knowledge, value of method, significance of findings, and relevance to contemporary nursing. Published every two months (six issues a year). Peer reviewed. Indexed in CINAHL and MEDLINE.

Research in Nursing and Health
Madeline H. Schmitt, PhD, RN, Editor.
University of Rochester,
School of Nursing,
601 Elmwood Avenue,
Rochester, NY 14642.
Phone: (716) 275-8889;
E-mail: lpage@wiley.com.

Research in Nursing and Health is a general research journal devoted to publication of a wide range of research and theory that will inform the practice of nursing and other health disciplines. The editors invite research reports on nursing practice, education, administration, and history; on health issues relevant to nursing; and in the testing of research findings in practice. Published 6 times a year. Peer reviewed. Indexed in CINAHL, Current Contents/Social and Behavioral Sciences, Hospital Literature Index, Index Medicus, International Nursing Index, Nursing Abstracts, Psychological Abstracts, Research Alert (ISI), Social Sciences Citation Index (ISI), and Sociological Abstracts.

Scholarly Inquiry for Nursing Practice
Harriet R. Feldman, PhD, RN, FAAN,
Audrey G. Gift, PhD, RN, FAAN,
Ruth Bernstein Hyman, PhD,
Barbara Kos-Munson, PhD, RN, CS, NPP,
and Pierre Woog, PhD, Editors.
Pace University Lienhard School of Nursing,
861 Bedford Road,
Pleasantville, NY 10570.
FAX: (914) 773-3480;
E-mail: rhyman@liii.com.

The purpose of *Scholarly Inquiry for Nursing Practice* is to facilitate the integration of theory, research, and practice and to provide a forum for original manuscripts concerned with the development and testing of theory and research relevant to nursing practice. Each article is accompanied by an invited response from a renowned scholar who constructively examines the paper's relevance to practice. Published quarterly. Double-blind peer reviewed. Indexed in CINAHL, MEDLINE, Index Medicus. Open to new ideas about special issue topics. Past special issues: Chronic Illness Trajectory Framework, Who Gets Health Care?, Measures of Family Functioning, Nursing Care in a Violent Society, Concept Development in Nursing.

Western Journal of Nursing Research
Pamela J. Brink, RN, PhD, FAAN, Executive Editor; Peggy Pilgrim, Journals Assistant.
Faculty of Nursing,
3-107 Clinical Sciences Building,
University of Alberta,
Edmonton, AB T6G 2G3, Canada.
Phone: (403) 492-1037;
FAX: (403) 492-2551;
E-mail: peggy.pilgrim@ualberta.ca;
website: http://www.ualberta.ca/~fonjrnls/.

The *Western Journal of Nursing Research* is a bimonthly journal devoted to the dissemination of research studies, book reviews, discussion and debate, and meeting calendars, all directed to a general nursing audience. WJNR is published every two months. February, April, June, August, October, and December. 1998 is the 20th year of publication for the WJNR. WJNR manuscripts are peer reviewed. WJNR is indexed in Applied Social Sciences Indexes and Abstracts, Behavioral Medicine Abstracts, CINAHL, Current Contents/Social and Behavioral Sciences, Health Instrument File, Human Resources Abstracts, Index Medicus, International NursingIndex, Nursing Abstracts, Nursing Citation Index, Psychological Abstracts, PsycINFO, and RNdex Top 100. WJNR has published the following Special Issues: WJNR 16(5), Feminist Research Methods in Nursing Research, Betty Mitsunaga, Guest Editor, and WJNR 17(1), Physiological Nursing Research, Patsy Perry, Guest Editor. WJNR Special Issues in Press: WJNR 20(1), Weight Research Across the Lifespan, Janet D. Allan, Guest Editor, and WJNR Themed Issue, Scheduled for 20(3), Living with HIV/AIDS in the '90s.

See also
   CUMULATIVE INDEX OF NURSING
      AND ALLIED HEALTH LITERATURE
   INTERNATIONAL CENTER FOR
      NURSING SCHOLARSHIP
   THE ONLINE JOURNAL
      OF KNOWLEDGE SYNTHESIS
      FOR NURSING
   VIRGINIA HENDERSON INTER-
      NATIONAL NURSING LIBRARY

K

KANGAROO CARE

Most nurses working in an intensive care nursery have witnessed parents expressing their intense need to hold their ill preterm infants. A new method that addresses this need is called kangaroo care, a term derived from its similarity to the way marsupials mother their immature young. During kangaroo care the mother simply holds her diaper-clad preterm infant skin-to-skin and upright between her breasts. In complete kangaroo care she allows self-regulatory breastfeeding. In developing countries the method is called kangaroo mother care (KMC) because the mother is often the central figure responsible for care. Relevant theoretical paradigms include stress, mutual caregiving, and self-regulation (Anderson, 1977, 1989) and Fitzpatrick's rhythm model, Levine's energy principles,

Nightingale's model of nursing, Orem's self-care model, Rogers's energy fields, and Roy's adaptation model (Fitzpatrick & Whall, 1989). Kangaroo care is widespread in Scandinavia; proliferating in Africa, Europe, Latin America, and North America; and beginning in Australia, Asia, and the Pacific Islands. The method, which originated in Bogotá, Colombia, represents a blend of technology and natural care.

To facilitate description, five categories have been developed, based primarily on how soon kangaroo care begins. Late kangaroo care, the most common category in the United States, begins when the infant is considered stable in room air and approaching discharge. Infants given intermediate kangaroo care have completed the early intensive care phase but usually still need oxygen and probably have some apnea and bradycardia. Also included in this category are infants placed at the breast during gavage feedings if they are too weak to nurse and infants who are stabilized with the aid of a ventilator. Early kangaroo care is used for infants who are easily stabilized. It begins as soon as an infant becomes stable, usually during the first week and perhaps even on the first day postbirth. The idea is that the mother can help maintain the stability by giving kangaroo care. Very early kangaroo care begins in the delivery or recovery room, between 15 and 60 minutes postbirth. The thinking here and in the next category is that the mother can help to stabilize her infant. With birth kangaroo care the infant is returned to the mother immediately following birth. These categories are described in greater detail in Anderson (1995).

Scientific research has provided broad support for the safety of kangaroo care and has also documented health benefits (for reviews, see Anderson, 1991a, in press; Bell & McGrath, 1996; Ludington-Hoe, Thompson, Swinth, Hadeed, & Anderson, 1994a). In the United States most of this research has been done by nurses. Findings show that infants are warm enough and conserve energy. They have regular heart rate and respirations, a fourfold decrease in apnea, adequate oxygenation, more deep sleep and alert inactivity, less crying, less cranial deformity, no increase in infections, fewer days in incubators, greater weight gain, and earlier discharge. Lactation increases and lasts longer, and

more mothers breastfeed. Fathers also give kangaroo care effectively. Mothers feel more fulfilled, and parents become deeply attached to their infants and feel confident about caring for them, even at home. Kangaroo care parents benefit from anticipatory guidance, and they merit broad social services to facilitate and extend their caregiving. Cost-effectiveness and improved long-term outcomes surely exist but have been documented in only one study, a randomized clinical trial in Quito, Ecuador. This trial and one other have been published, one is in press, and three World Health Organization (WHO)-sponsored trials have just been completed; all but one of these trials were done in developing countries.

The National Institute of Nursing Research has funded nurses to conduct three trials in the United States: one trial with incubator infants is completed and two trials are in progress; one of those trials is with small intubated infants. The second trial is with 32–36-week infants who are healthy at birth; kangaroo care begins at 10 minutes following birth and continues thereafter. In pilot studies for the second trial, 34–36-week infants who began kangaroo care by 30 minutes postbirth had remarkable behavioral organization and began breastfeeding correctly by 2 hours postbirth, becoming competent breastfeeders within 24 hours. Importantly, some of these infants had developed respiratory distress (grunting) by the time kangaroo care began, but this disappeared quickly when the infants stayed in kangaroo care and were given warmed and humidified oxygen by oxyhood.

Trends in kangaroo care include increased backing by UNICEF and WHO, more rigorous research, federal funding, publication of detailed guidelines, conferences devoted to kangaroo care, kangaroo care for sicker infants and for full-term infants, kangaroo care opportunities for selected family members or friends, consumer awareness of and desire for kangaroo care, and increased use of kangaroo care to facilitate lactation and breastfeeding as new benefits of human milk continue to be documented. The new realization that very early kangaroo care can help stabilize some preterm infants and prevent Neonatal Intensive Care Unit (NICU) admission is leading to interest in beginning kangaroo care as soon as possible postbirth. Nursing research is needed to document the great potential that kangaroo care in its various forms has for quality care, improved outcomes, parent satisfaction, and cost reduction.

GENE CRANSTON ANDERSON

See also

CHILDBIRTH EDUCATION
MOTHER-INFANT/TODDLER
 RELATIONSHIPS
NICU PRETERM INFANT CARE
PREGNANCY
SOCIETY FOR RESEARCH IN CHILD
 DEVELOPMENT

(IMOGENE) KING'S GENERAL SYSTEMS FRAMEWORK

King's general systems framework focuses on the continuing ability of individuals to meet their basic needs so that they may function in their socially defined roles and on individuals' interactions within personal, interpersonal, and social systems (Frey & Sieloff, 1995; King, 1981, 1986, 1992). Each individual is regarded as a personal system that is rational, sentient, and social. Concepts related to the personal system are (a) perception, (b) self, (c) growth and development, (d) body image, (e) time, (f) space, and (g) learning.

Perception is a process of organizing, interpreting, and transforming information from sense data and memory that gives meaning to the individual's experience, represents his or her image of reality, and influences behavior. Self is viewed as a composite of thoughts and feelings that constitute the individual's awareness of his or her existence, of who and what he or she is. Growth and development, including cellular, molecular, and behavioral changes, are a function of genetic endowment, meaningful and satisfying experiences, and an environment conducive to helping individuals move toward maturity. Body image is defined as the individual's perceptions of his or her body. Time is defined as the duration between the occurrence of

one event and the occurrence of another event. Space is defined as the physical area or territory that exists in all directions. Learning is defined as the gaining of knowledge.

Two, three, or more individuals interacting in a given situation are collectively regarded as an interpersonal system. The concepts associated with the interpersonal system are (a) interactions; (b) intrapersonal, interpersonal, verbal, and nonverbal communication; (c) transaction; (d) role; (e) stress; and (f) coping. Interactions are the acts of two or more individuals in mutual presence and a sequence of verbal and nonverbal behaviors that are goal-directed. Intrapersonal, interpersonal, verbal, and nonverbal communication are viewed as vehicles by which human relations are developed and maintained. Transaction encompasses the process of interaction in which individuals communicate with the environment to achieve goals that are valued, as well as goal-directed human behaviors. Role is defined as a set of behaviors expected when occupying a position in a social system. Stress is regarded as a dynamic state whereby an individual interacts with the environment to maintain balance for growth, development, and performance and which involves an exchange of energy and information between the individual and the environment for regulation and control of stressors. Coping is viewed as a way of dealing with stress.

Social systems encompass organized boundary systems of social roles, behaviors, and practices developed to maintain values and the mechanisms to regulate the practices and rules. The concepts related to the social system are (a) organizations, (b) authority, (c) power, (d) status, (e) decision making, and (f) control. Organizations are composed of individuals with prescribed roles and positions who use resources to accomplish personal and organizational goals. Authority is described as a transactional process characterized by active, reciprocal relations in which individuals' values, backgrounds, and perceptions play a role in defining, validating, and accepting the authority of other individuals within an organization. Power is defined as the process whereby one or more individuals influence other individuals in a situation. Status is the position of an individual in a group or a group in relation to other groups in an organization. Decision making is defined as a dynamic and systematic process by which goal-directed choice of perceived alternatives is made and acted on by individuals or groups to answer a question and attain a goal. Control is defined as being in charge.

Nursing research focuses on the description of and explanation for actual or potential disturbances in the ability to function in social roles. The ultimate purpose of research is to determine the effects of mutual goal setting and nursing interventions on attainment of goals related to social role functioning.

JACQUELINE FAWCETT

See also

COPING
NURSE-PATIENT COMMUNICATION
NURSING THEORETICAL MODELS
SOCIAL SUPPORT
STRESS

L

LEININGER'S TRANSCULTURAL NURSING MODEL

Over 40 years ago, Dr. Madeleine Leininger began her pioneering work in creating transcultural nursing as a new area of nursing. Her sunrise model to depict theory of culture care diversity and universality stemmed from experiences as a young staff nurse caring for people from other cultures. Her keen observations led her to reflect on the influence of culture and care in explaining human behavior.

According to Leininger, the sunrise model serves as a cognitive map to guide the nurse in holistically examining the forces that influence care patterns and expressions and health and well-being for the individual, family, group, and community. In her model, cultural and social structure factors and worldview, in the context of environment, language, and ethnohistory, are critical dimensions operating in folk (generic) and professional health systems. The three major modes that guide nursing judgments and actions and lead to culturally congruent care are cultural care preservation (or maintenance), cultural care accommodation (or negotiation), and cultural care repatterning (or restructuring) (Leininger, 1991).

A major goal of the Leininger cultural care theory is to improve and advance the quality of nursing care through the deliberate and creative discovery and use of transcultural nursing knowledge that reflects the values, beliefs, and lifestyles of people from diverse cultures. According to the theory, culturally derived nursing care, based on transcultural human care knowledge, is predicted to maintain client health and well-being or to help clients face death in culturally appropriate ways (Leininger, 1991).

Leininger (1991) proposes several essential tenets and assumptive premises in her theory. The following selected examples have been refined through time by nurses in their discovery of culture care phenomena:

Care is essential for health, human growth, and survival.

Care is the essential unifying focus of nursing.

There can be no curing without caring.

Culture care values, beliefs, and practices are embedded in worldview, sociocultural dimensions, language, and environmental context. Culturally congruent nursing care occurs when cultural care values, beliefs, and expressions are known. Culture care conflict and stress occur when nursing care fails to reflect the client's care values, beliefs, and life ways.

In keeping with the theory, Leininger (1991) advocated the qualitative research paradigm to discover epistemic and ontological dimensions of human care transculturally. The ethnonursing method that she supports has guided the study of culture care phenomena in over 80 cultures, resulting in the identification of close to 200 caring constructs. Several doctoral dissertations and master's theses have contributed to the refinement of the assumptive premises of the theory. The theory has been developed further through dissemination of research in the *Journal of Transcultural Nursing* and discussion of research findings at conferences devoted to transcultural care phenomena.

Leininger's theory has guided a number of ethnocare studies, some focused on the following areas: caring practices in a large-scale general hospital, the influence of extended caregiving on the health status of elderly Canadian wives, care and cure meanings and experiences of those dying in hospice and hospital settings, values and practices of Mexican American and Philippine American nurses, and well-being and humor in Lithuanian Americans.

Evolution of the theory of cultural care diversity and universality is continuing. Leininger (1991) has succeeded in establishing the cadre of nurses with transcultural nursing knowledge and research skill that initially prompted her to withhold her theory from the public domain. She has instilled in nurses a passion for sensitivity and a plea for humanity in caring for those who come from all corners of the global village.

CYNTHIA F. CAMERON

See also
CARING
CULTURAL/TRANSCULTURAL FOCUS

LEVINE'S CONSERVATION MODEL

In 1963, Myra E. Levine, then chair of the Department of Clinical Nursing, Cook County School of Nursing, began work on the conservation model of nursing (Levine, 1991). Initially, the conservation model was devised to provide beginning nursing students with a framework for thinking about and interpreting all possibilities of patient care situations. Not until the late 1980s did Levine (1989) start to think about her model as a theory of nursing.

In developing the conservation model of nursing, Levine (1989) sought to provide students a structure that would enable them to integrate basic scientific knowledge and clinical skills while simplifying the complex nature and processes of human organisms and health. Levine was convinced that broad generalizations would unite independent and inexplicable concepts into a structure that would permit the individual examination and solution of specific nursing problems.

Throughout the development of the model, Levine (1988) acknowledged the antecedents to her thinking. Critical to the formulation of the ideas found in the conservation model were Bates, Beland, Dubos, Erikson, Feynman, Gibson, Goldstein, Hall, and Sherrington, among others.

The heart of Levine's model is the notion of conservation. Citing Feynman, Levine (1988) indicated that conservation is a natural law regulating all animate matter in the universe and promoting the unity and integrity of the individual. Conserving the integrity of the individual is critical because the crux of human existence is the enduring and dynamic struggle to preserve the integrity, the unity, the wholeness of the human being. This struggle emanates from the interaction between the individual and the specific environment in which the individual exists. The environment, both internal and external to the individual, yet open and fluid with the individual, completes the wholeness of the individual (Levine, 1989). Individuals cannot be defined outside the context of their predicament of time and space (Levine, 1991). This struggle or interaction between the individual and the environment Levine referred to as adaptation. Adaptation is a multidimensional process of change that has direction, purpose, and meaning. It is the individual's integrated and unified response, directed toward maintaining congruence, or the "best fit," between the person and the environment. This congruence conserves the integrity of the person—integrity that is the result of adaptation and the goal of nursing (Levine, 1989).

Having nurses examine or analyze the complex and dynamic process of adaptation for the purpose of designing patient-centered plans of care was the goal of Levine's work. The four conservation principles were proposed (Levine, 1967) as a means for isolating specific patient care problems while maintaining the unity and integrity of the individual within the context of this adaptive process. The four conservation principles focus nursing efforts on defending, sustaining, or restoring the integrity of the person:

1. Conservation of energy refers to the balance of energy output and energy input. Nursing activities to conserve energy include ensuring adequate rest, nutrition, and exercise.
2. Conservation of structural integrity refers to the structure and function of the body. Nursing activities for conserving structural integrity focus on supporting anatomical and physiological functions.
3. Conservation of personal integrity refers to the person's sense of identify, self-worth, and individual uniqueness. Nursing activities conserving personal integrity would include, for example, safeguarding patient autonomy and promoting patient independence and competence through patient education.
4. Conservation of social integrity acknowledges that the person is a social being with an ethnic, cultural, and religious heritage. Nursing activities conserving social integrity would emphasize the critical nature of human relationships.

Superficially, this categorization or compartmentalization of the complex nature and processes of human existence and health has led many critics of the conservation model to conclude that Levine has taken a reductionist view of the human organism. However, it must be remembered that the nursing problem is reduced to its constituent parts, not the individual human. The intent of this reduction is simplification for examination, analysis, and eventual design of a plan of care.

The value of the conservation model as a framework for examining, analyzing, and understanding specific patient care problems has been supported by numerous studies, publications, and personal anecdotes. Examples include (a) energy consumption during bathing in patients who recently experienced an acute myocardial infarction (Winslow, Lane, & Gaffney, 1985) and in preterm infants (Deiriggi & Miles, 1995), (b) acute confusion in elderly hospitalized patients (Foreman, 1989), (c) bearing-down techniques during the second stage of labor (Yeates & Roberts, 1984), (d) wound healing (Cooper, 1990), and (e) fatigue (Schaefer & Potylycki, 1993), among others. Although the preponderance of the work to date has focused on hospitalized individuals with various disease states, the conservation model is a model for health of individuals in any setting (Levine, 1991).

Levine (1989) reminds us that

> the Conservation Principles do not, of course, operate singly or in isolation from each other. They are joined within the individual as a cascade of life events, churning and changing as the environmental challenge is confronted and resolved in each individual's unique way. The nurse as caregiver becomes part of that environment, bringing to every nursing opportunity his or her own cascading repertoire of skill, knowledge, and compassion. It is shared enterprise [between the individual and the nurse], and each participant is rewarded. (p. 336)

MARQUIS D. FOREMAN
BARBARA E. BERGER

See also
FATIGUE
HEALTH CONCEPTUALIZATION
NURSING PROCESS
NURSING THEORETICAL MODELS

LONGITUDINAL SURVEY

In longitudinal study designs the variables of interest are measured at several points in time for the same individuals. A value of longitudinal designs is the ability to shed light on trends and the temporal sequencing of phenomena (Polit & Hungler, 1983). As discussed by Woods and Catanzaro (1988), most health-related phenomena of interest in nursing science are dynamic in nature. Describing patterns of change in phenomena and evaluating the outcomes of nursing interventions over time often are the focus of nursing research. Topics such as sense of well-being, family coping in chronic illness, adaptation to parenthood, and recovery from life-threatening illness are appropriate for longitudinal investigation. Nursing intervention outcomes are often measured during the course of the intervention and at several follow-up points—for example, changes in quality of life following a telecommunications nursing intervention or improvement in parents' ability to discipline children after participating in a series of parenting classes. A variety of longitudinal designs are employed in nursing research, such as time series design with repeated measures on a single entity or a number of entities at a relatively large number of time points. Panel designs may be used for making observations on many entities but at relatively few times (Woods & Catanzaro, 1988). Although the relationship of the selected variables to the appropriate timing of measurement is critical in longitudinal research, nurturing a longitudinal sample is an art that researchers often underestimate.

Attrition of the sample is a serious compromise to meaningful study outcomes. Despite a precise sampling strategy, the population of interest will be represented inadequately if a large proportion of the sample fails to respond to the questions. Motzer, Moseley, and Lewis (1997) observed that once a sample is accrued, retention is essential because attrition is financially costly and threatens the internal and external validity of results. They reviewed accrual and retention issues identified in their 3-year randomized trial of a nursing intervention and suggested 24 specific strategies to maximize sample size in clinical trial studies. Weinert and Burman (1996) noted that there were many reasons for sample attrition, including loss of interest, loss to follow-up due to address changes, burden of participation, and exacerbation of the illness.

Social Exchange

Obtaining an adequate response rate for cross-sectional surveys requires careful attention. A more challenging task is maintaining the response rate from participants who are repeatedly answering the same set of questions over several test points, extending for months or even years. Dillman (1978) established techniques that have been shown to facilitate the process of engaging respondents and enhancing the quality and quantity of responses. The total design method (Dillman, 1978) is based on the process of getting potential participants to complete questionnaires honestly and return them. The process can be viewed as a special case of social exchange. Classic social exchange theory asserts that the actions of individuals are motivated by the return these actions are expected to bring (Blau, 1964; Homans, 1961). The assumptions are that (a) people engage in any activity because of the rewards they hope to reap, (b) any activity incurs some costs, and (c) individuals attempt to keep their costs below the rewards they expect to receive. In the case of research there are three things that must be done to maximize survey response: minimize the costs of responding, maximize the rewards, and establish trust that rewards will be delivered (Dillman, 1978).

Minimize Costs

Costs to participants in survey research include tangible costs, such as envelopes and postage, which can be easily addressed by the researcher. The intangible costs of time and effort take more creativity and thoughtfulness. A questionnaire that is attractive, distinctively identified with the project, easy to read and complete; reduces perceived cost. Techniques for reducing the effort in completing the questionnaire include (a) stapling the booklet in the centerfold, thus allowing it to open out flat; (b) using clip art throughout the booklet to reduce boredom; (c) constructing response choices so that a simple mark is required, thus reducing error and mental effort; and (d) using adequate "white space" to give the image of being easy to complete.

Maximize Rewards

Thibaut and Kelley (1959) noted that being regarded positively by another person has reward value. Techniques to increase intangible rewards include (a) frequent expressions of positive regard in all correspondence; (b) expressions of the importance of participation; (c) personal salutations and real signatures; (d) a consultative approach, including an open-ended question asking for information that the respondent thinks would be important for the study; (e) holiday greetings and birthday cards; (f) newsletter every 6 months; and (g) handwritten notes in response to those who share personal information. Tangible rewards such as money or gifts should be carefully considered. Such rewards for children have included a certificate of appreciation for completion of an interview and the opportunity to choose from the "treasure chest" filled with small inexpensive toys (Weinert & Catanzaro, 1994).

Establish Trust

Identification of the research with an agency with a good reputation may increase the sense of trust. Respondents may return their questionnaires to the researcher, not so much because of any feelings of obligation to the researcher but because they feel that they have received past benefits from the university or health care agency (Dillman, 1978). Over the course of a longitudinal study, carrying out promises for a newsletter with updates on the progress of the study and brief reports of results is critical for engendering trust. Sensitivity to the needs of particular groups may also increase trust. For example, calling the post office in a small rural town before sending a mass mailing, to express concern about the additional work load, can engender trust with a key person in the community. This trust and interest in the study will be translated to the community at large. Exchange relationships must be nurtured throughout the course of the study. For example, as the project unfolds, members of the research team often come to be viewed as experts. When phone calls are received asking for advice about a specific disease or a new treatment or requesting information about the availability of sup-

port groups or educational programs, the response should be friendly and accurate; and a referral is made when appropriate. Dealing with phone calls and mail in a manner that is respectful and helpful is critical to the maintenance of the study sample.

Follow-up

Attention to follow-up is critical to a good response rate. The total design method contains a detailed routine for prompting nonresponders that has been very effective. An important aspect of follow-up is a personalized, signed thank-you letter after the return of the questionnaire. In a 5-year study in which questionnaires were completed annually, a systematic follow-up routine was used. A response rate of 89% for usable data for the 5th year was reported (Weinert & Catanzaro, 1994).

Conclusions

Undertaking longitudinal research requires a skillful and creative research team. Attention to issues related to costs and rewards, engendering trust, and maintaining interest are essential elements of success. Nonresponse and loss to the study cannot be totally eliminated, but careful attention must be paid to techniques designed to increase response rates and engage participants in the activities of the research project. Successful longitudinal research is truly an art form. Although careful attention to minor points may appear to be overly labor-intensive, they can lead to sustaining the sample for long periods of time and obtaining higher quantity and quality of data.

CLARANN WEINERT

See also
DATA COLLECTION METHODS
EPIDEMIOLOGY
SAMPLING
TIME SERIES ANALYSIS

M

MANAGED CARE

Managed care, a shorthand term for managed care health plans, describes a broad array of health insurance plans that integrate the financing and delivery of health care. These plans are distinguished by the following features: (a) each plan contracts with a selected panel of providers to render a comprehensive set of benefits for a predetermined monthly premium or negotiated fee, (b) the contracting providers agree to accept utilization and quality controls, (c) there are financial incentives for subscribers to use the providers on the panel, and (d) the contracting providers assume some degree of financial risk for the type and cost of services provided (Iglehart, 1992).

The origins of managed care plans, that is, organized prepaid health care delivery models, date back to the mid to late 1800s. They were pioneered by employers and providers as an efficient way to provide needed health services in less accessible areas and as a vehicle to attract workers to those areas (Friedman, 1996). The 1940s witnessed the emergence of a number of large and small cooperatives—organized groups, usually employer- or community-based, that owned or operated facilities such as hospitals and employed their own providers. Notable among them were Group Health of Puget Sound and Kaiser Permanente. These cooperatives were actively opposed by organized medicine, despite enjoying public support in many communities, and consequently were stymied in their development (Starr, 1982).

The escalation in health care costs in the late 1960s and early 1970s engendered a new look at cooperatives and organized models of care, which had experienced lower growth rates in health costs than traditional fee-for-service indemnity health insurance plans. Coincident with this newly peaked interest in cooperatives was the appearance of Paul Ellwood, a physician from Minnesota who advo-

cated the creation of health maintenance organizations (HMOs). These organized care models encouraged the use of preventive health services as a way to defer the use of later and more costly hospital care. The Health Maintenance Organization Act of 1973 provided the structure and the start-up funds to develop HMOs, a process that began slowly and only began to accelerate by 1990.

Most managed care plans can be grouped under two broad headings: HMOs and preferred provider organizations, or PPOs. There are essentially two types of HMOs: (1) group- or staff-model HMOs in which groups of physicians contract to provide services and (2) independent practice associations, or IPAs, in which doctors remain in their offices but agree to see patients who are enrolled in a health plan. Both types of plans provide comprehensive care for a fixed fee, control the numbers and types of providers with whom they contract, and enforce a strict primary care gatekeeping role. Independent practice associations have been the fastest-growing form of HMO. Two other HMO variants that have appeared in increasing number are network-model HMOs and mixed-model HMOs (Employment Benefit Research Institute, 1994). Another popular HMO-type plan is the point-of-service plan. These plans offer optimal coverage when using a panel provider while permitting out-of-plan service use at a somewhat higher out-of-pocket cost.

Preferred provider organizations, like IPAs, have grown rapidly. A PPO contracts with a network or panel of providers that agrees to provide medical services and be paid according to a discounted fee schedule. There is minimal use of primary care physicians as gatekeepers, and enrollees receive optimal coverage if they see a preferred provider. Costs are managed in the ways similar to that of HMOs: limiting provider panels, negotiating fees, and employing utilization review mechanisms.

The founding concept of managed care has evolved from seeking an efficient means of organizing and providing care to explicitly controlling the costs of health care. The goal of managed care today is to reduce the rate of growth in health spending. The principal mechanism through which this goal can be achieved is that of altering the choices of providers and consumers of health care services. For consumers the choice of provider is constrained by price; it will cost more to use a provider that is not on the chosen panel. For providers the choice of services is altered by attaching a cost to those choices; if the care one provides is more costly than the plan estimates it should be, the provider's remuneration may subsequently be reduced or the provider may be dropped from the plan.

Research in managed care has been largely dominated by analyses of the impact of these plans on utilization and cost of health care. In theory, managed care is designed to eliminate waste and consequently reduce overall spending in several ways: (a) reducing inappropriate care through the use of gatekeepers and strict utilization controls; (b) promoting health through the provision of preventive health services, hopefully leading to less service use; and (c) lowering the demand for services to reduce the supply of unnecessary services (e.g., hospital beds). Although the findings are still somewhat equivocal, there has been an increasing number of studies suggesting that managed care has an ameliorating effect on health costs. For instance, areas with high managed care penetration appear to have a slower rate of growth in health costs than areas with lower penetration (Robinson, 1996). These lower costs appear to be the result of lower utilization of services and lower fees negotiated with providers.

Assessments of the impact of managed care on quality of care and patient outcomes have had mixed results. For example, Ware and colleagues (Ware, Bayliss, Rogers, Kosinski, & Tarlov, 1996) found worse physical health outcomes for elderly and poor, chronically ill patients in HMOs compared to similar patients in fees-for-service plans. However, Yelin and others (Yelin, Criswell, & Feigenbaum, 1996) found no differences in outcomes for rheumatoid arthritis patients among prepaid and fee-for-service plans. These equivocal findings and those from other studies seem to reflect unmeasured selection bias and different and rapidly changing health plans, as well as true differences in the quality of care between managed and fee-for-service plans. Well-designed studies of the impact of managed care on access to quality care and patient outcomes is a critical area for future research.

The rapid growth in enrollment in managed care and the more recent proliferation of for-profit interests in managed care offerings have generated contentious debates between managed care plans and the provider and patient communities. Consumers and health care providers, expressing concern over denial of services that they feel results from an increased profit-making orientation in managed care plans, have galvanized lawmakers to introduce a number of regulatory bills in the area of consumer protection. These regulations would require managed care plans to publish their treatment options, eliminate provider "gag rules," assure clear documentation of guidelines for rejecting coverage for services, allow direct access to medical specialists, and guarantee minimum hospital stays for maternity care and mastectomies. Advocates for the poor have raised similar concerns regarding the adequacy of managed care plans offered to Medicaid recipients. In many areas nurse practitioners have struggled to attain independent status on provider panels as primary care providers. In response, managed care plans have argued that changes are required in the way health care is sought and delivered if the goal of reducing spending while maintaining quality is to be achieved.

JULIE SOCHALSKI

See also
ACCESS TO HEALTH CARE
CAPITATION
HEALTH CARE REFORM
HEALTH MAINTENANCE ORGANIZA-
   TIONS
HEALTH SYSTEMS DELIVERY

MATERNAL EMPLOYMENT

Maternal employment is defined as the labor force participation of women who are acting in the parental role and are responsible for the care of a dependent child or children (newborn to 18 years of age). The term *mother* generally refers to biological and adoptive female parents. However, sometimes other family members, such as grandmothers, are included if they are taking the place of the biological or adoptive mother in parenting a child under 18 years of age. The operational definition of mother varies with the focus of the study or discussion.

Employment can occur outside or inside the woman's home. The distinction is that employed women are paid for their efforts. Although nonemployed women (housewives or "stay-home mothers") work in their homes, they are not paid directly for that work. Variables that characterize the many aspects of maternal employment have been considered: status (employed or not employed), intensity (number of hours per week or part-time vs. fulltime), time during the day or week of the employment (e.g., day, evening, or night shift; weekends only), timing of return to employment after a child's birth, employment history (continuous vs. intermittent), and change in intensity of employment over time. Related aspects include consistency between the mother's attitudes about employment and her employment status, characteristics of the job, attitudes of the mother's partner/spouse, and quality and type of alternative child care.

Incidence

Labor force participation of mothers in the United States increased substantially during World War II because of the market's need for workers and the relative shortage of men to fill those needs. Once in the labor force, many mothers continued their employment, although a married woman's employment was often viewed as evidence that the husband could not provide adequately for his family. Employment rates for women have increased considerably since 1960 for both single and married women (U.S. Bureau of the Census, 1996). These rates vary with age of the youngest child, marital status, and race. By far, the largest increase has been for married mothers with young children. Employment rates for Black married mothers have been 10% to 20% higher than for White married mothers, controlling for age of the youngest child. Although

employed married women often cite economic need for their employment, other factors exist, such as desire to work for self-fulfillment, adult conversation, financial autonomy, or increased power in the marital relationship. Threats of instability in the spouse's job and the rising divorce rate, with associated financial hardships, also have an important effect on women's decisions to be employed.

Effects of Maternal Employment

Maternal employment and its effects for the mother, her children, and the family system is a complex phenomenon, although its conceptualization in research has usually been very simplistic. The conflicting nature of the results across studies is probably related to this simplistic conceptualization and lack of statistical and design controls for important family system variables. For example, single-parent and two-parent families often are included in the same sample without separate analyses or statistical control for family form despite likely differences in practical aspects of the mother's employment and the meaning of the mother's work to the family. In addition, characteristics of the child, especially health status, are rarely considered.

Research on the effects of returning to employment on postpartum recovery after full-term delivery revealed that at 4 months postpartum, one quarter to one third of employed women reported illness-related work absences or decreased job performance resulting from poor health (Killien, 1993). However, at 6 months more employed than nonemployed mothers reported having regained their usual level of physical energy, although they reported similar levels of functioning in their various roles (Tulman & Fawcett, 1990). These results are based on return to employment by 6 months postpartum. However, many women who experience preterm delivery return to work soon after the birth while their infant is hospitalized in the neonatal intensive care unit, saving their maternity leave until the infant is discharged. The implications of this employment pattern for the woman's physical recovery and its possible buffering effects on the stress associated with the preterm infant's critical condition are not known.

Research on effects of maternal employment on women's mental health generally takes one of three approaches: employment is a stressor or an added burden, employment may enhance performance of other roles, contextual variables are more important than employment itself. Contextual variables include support from spouse or a significant other, consistency between the mother's attitudes about her employment status and her actual employment status, commitment to worker and parent roles, quality of worker and parent experiences, and division of labor at home. Empirical support for the importance of these contextual variables for women's stress levels and psychological well-being is growing.

Research focused on the effects of maternal employment on children emanates primarily from a maternal absence framework, arguing that the mother's absence and the repeated mother-child separations necessitated by that absence will have a negative impact on the child. Although the results of this body of work are conflicting, studies that control for mother, child, and family factors generally find no effects of maternal employment on the child's development. However, maternal employment often has a positive effect on a variety of behavioral and cognitive outcomes for children in low-income or single-parent families.

Researchers operating within a stress framework focus on the quality and stability of the alternative child care situation and the degree of consistency between the mother's attitudes about employment and her employment status. As expected, higher quality child care (lower staff:child ratios, more responsive caregivers) and fewer different child care arrangements result in better child outcomes. When mothers' attitudes and behaviors are consistent, children benefit cognitively and behaviorally (Youngblut, 1995).

Implications for Nursing Practice and Research

Based on historical trends in employment rates, economic and lifestyle factors, and lack of strong empirical evidence of negative effects, employment rates for mothers are likely to remain high. The impact of this likelihood on nursing is pervasive and indirect, and it is most apparent when considered from a family systems perspective in conjunction with changes in health care delivery. Women traditionally have been responsible for the care of ill or disabled family members; however, high employment rates mean that fewer women are able to assume this role easily. To provide for the ill member, employed women must either quit their jobs, take a leave of absence, hire someone to provide the care, or place the disabled person in a long-term care facility. Each option results in increased cost to the family from lost wages, perhaps lost health care insurance, and added expenses. The family's decision about which option to choose may affect its ability to follow the recovering member's recommended treatment regimen, and the health of that member will suffer unless nurses consider the woman's employment situation in their treatment plans.

Intermittent labor force participation will affect women's lifetime earning power and subsequent retirement income, especially critical with public concerns about the solvency of the Social Security program. This puts older women at increased risk for poverty and its negative effects on health related to poor nutrition, diminished ability to pay for needed medications, and inadequate or delayed health care.

In summary, the effects of maternal employment on children, families, and the mothers themselves are important to consider in both research and practice. Research about its impact after preterm delivery and for families with other than healthy children is needed. Considering this influence in research and practice will provide a more complete picture of the family's situation, making more timely and effective interventions possible.

JoAnne M. Youngblut

See also
FAMILY THEORY AND RESEARCH
MOTHER-INFANT/TODDLER RELA-
   TIONSHIPS
PARENTAL RESPONSE TO THE NEONA-
   TAL INTENSIVE CARE UNIT
POSTPARTUM CARE: DEPRESSION

MEASUREMENT AND SCALES

The focus of measurement is the quantification of a characteristic or attribute of a person, object, or event. Measurement provides for a consistent and meaningful interpretation of the nature of an attribute when the same measurement process or instrument is used. The results of measurement are usually expressed in the form of numbers. Measurement is a systematic process that uses rules to assign numbers to persons, objects, or events which represent the amount or kind of a specified attribute (Pedhazur & Schmelkin, 1991b; Waltz, Strickland, & Lenz, 1991). However, measurement also involves identifying and specifying common aspects of attributes for meaningful interpretation and categorization, using a common conceptual perspective. Ambiguity, confusion, and disagreement will surround the meaning of any measurement when it is undefined. The measurement relevancy can be determined only when an explicit or implicit theory structures the meaning of the phenomenon to be studied. "Theory not only determines what attributes or aspects are measured but also how they are to be measured" (Pedhazur & Schmelkin, 1991b, p. 16). Qualitative assessments apply measurement principles by providing meaning and interpretation of qualitative data through description and categorization of phenomena. Thus, measurement may not result in scores per se but may categorize phenomena into meaningful and interpretable attributes. Therefore, measurement is also basic to qualitative analysis (Strickland, 1993b).

Measurement is a crucial part of all nursing settings. Nurses depend on measuring instruments to determine the amount or kind of attributes of patients and use the results of measurements such as laboratory and physical examination results to determine patient needs and their plan of care. Nurse researchers use a large array of clinical laboratory, observational, and questionnaire measures to study phenomena of interest. Nurse educators depend on measurement instruments and test scores to help determine a student's mastery. Measurement is central to all that nurses do. We cannot understand or "study well what we cannot measure well" (Strickland, 1993a, p. 4).

The rules used for assigning numbers to objects to represent the amount or kind of an attribute studied have been categorized as nominal, ordinal, interval, and ratio. These types of measurement scales are common in nursing. Measurements that result in nominal-scale data place attributes into defined categories according to a defined property. Numbers assigned to nominal-level data have no hierarchical meaning but represent an object's membership in one of a set of mutually exclusive, exhaustive, and unorderable categories. For example, categorizing persons in a study as either female or male is measurement on the nominal measurement scale. In ordinal-scale measurement, rules are used to assign rank order on a particular attribute that characterizes a person, object, or event.

Ordinal-scale measurement may be regarded as the rank-ordering of objects into hierarchical quantitative categories according to relative amounts of the attribute studied. The categorization of heart murmurs in grades from 1 through 6 is an example. In this ordinal measure, a Grade 1 murmur is less intense than a Grade 2, a Grade 2 less intense than a Grade 3, and so forth. The rankings in ordinal-level measurement merely mean that the ranking of 1 (for first) has ranked higher than 2 (for second) and so on. Rankings do not imply that the categories are equally spaced nor that the intervals between rank categories are equal.

Interval-scale measurement is a form of continuous measurement and implies equal numerical distances between adjacent scores that represent equal amounts with respect to the attribute that is the focus of measurement. Therefore, numbers assigned in interval-scale-measurement represent an attribute's placement in one of a set of mutually exclusive, exhaustive categories that can be ordered and are equally spaced in terms of the magnitude of the attribute under consideration. However, the absolute amount of the attribute is not known for a particular object because the zero point is arbitrary in an interval scale. The measurement of temperature is a good example of an interval-level measure because there is no true zero point. For example, the zero point is different based on whether the Fahrenheit or Centigrade measurement approach is used, and one cannot say that an object with a temperature of 0° F or 0° C has no temperature at all. Ratio-level measures provide the same information as interval-level measures; in addition they have absolute zero points for which zero actually represents absence of the attribute under study. Volume, length, and weight are commonly measured by ratio scales.

There is controversy about the level of measurement scales and the type of statistical procedures that may be appropriately used for data analysis. There are researchers and statisticians who believe that only nonparametric statistical procedures can be used for data analysis when data are nominal or ordinal and that inferential statistics can be properly applied only with interval and ratio data. There is controversy about whether Likert scaling (which is often used in nursing with measures of attitude or opinion) is in actuality ordinal-level measurement for which only nonparametric statistics should be used. Likert scaling involves having subjects rank their responses to a set of items on a range of numbers, such as "1" to represent lack of agreement to "5" to represent complete agreement. It has been the accepted practice for investigators to use scores generated with Likert-type scales as interval-level data.

Nurses have typically borrowed many measures from other disciplines. This reflects the fact that nursing is a field that considers the biological and psychosocial aspects of care and is based on knowledge generated by many fields of inquiry. Therefore, many instruments developed by other disciplines are consistent with nurses' measurement needs. However, the heavy dependence on borrowing instruments from other disciplines reflects the trend in the 1970s for nurses to pursue doctoral education in related fields, such as education, psychology, sociology, and physiology. Nurses became familiar with instruments from other fields during their graduate studies and were encouraged to use them in the nursing context.

By the mid 1970s nurses became more cognizant of some of the limitations in borrowing certain instruments from other disciplines. It is not unusual for instruments developed to measure psychosocial variables in other fields to be cumbersome and inefficient for use in the clinical settings of nurse researchers. Often the instruments needed by nurses to measure attributes in populations such as children, frail patients, the elderly, and the culturally diverse, instruments that measure important variables from the nursing perspective, do not exist. Nursing studies of families, communities, and organizations and systems have been hampered by the lack of effective measures to address group and system variables from the nursing perspective (Strickland, 1995).

The movement in nursing to develop more rigor in the use and development of measurement instruments gained prominence in the 1970s. In June 1974, a contract was awarded to the Western Interstate Commission for Higher Education by the Division of Nursing, Bureau of Health Manpower, and Health Resources Administration to prepare a compilation of nursing research instruments and other measuring devices for publication. With Doris Bloch as project officer, a two-volume compilation of instruments, titled *Instruments for Measuring Nursing Practice and Other Health Care Variables*, was published in 1978. Priority was placed on compiling instruments dealing with nursing practice and with patient variables rather than nurse variables. This was an important milestone for nursing measurement because it was the first effort that placed a large number of clinically focused instruments developed or used by nurses in the public domain.

During the late 1970s and early 1980s, two groups of nurse scientists focused their work on developing measurement as an area of special emphasis in nursing. At the University of Arizona–Tucson, Ada Sue Hinshaw and Jan Atwood focused their efforts on refining and further developing instruments for clinical settings and for clinically focused research. The first postdoctoral program in nursing instrumentation and measurement evolved at the University of Arizona, and annual national conferences on nursing measurement were offered. These conferences provided nurses a forum in which to discuss measurement issues and problems and to present information on instruments used in studies.

Ora Strickland and Carolyn Waltz at the University of Maryland at Baltimore focused on defining measurement principles and practices to build rigor in nursing research. Careful assessments of nursing research published in professional journals were conducted. The assessments revealed that nurse investigators were not giving adequate attention to reliability and validity issues when selecting and developing instruments. In addition, nurse investigators tended to rely too heavily on paper-and-pencil self-report measures and did not give adequate attention to selecting biological measures as indicated by the conceptual frameworks of the studies (Strickland & Waltz, 1986). The Maryland group published the first measurement textbook for nurses, *Measurement in Nursing Research*, and developed and implemented a measurement project funded by the Division of Nursing of the Department of Health and Human Services. This project prepared over 200 nurse researchers in clinical or educational settings to develop and test instruments for use in nursing and resulted in an award-winning four-volume series of books, Measurement of Nursing Outcomes, which compiled instruments developed by project participants.

In 1993, Ora Strickland initiated and edited the *Journal of Nursing Measurement* with Ada Sue Hinshaw as co-editor. This journal brought nursing measurement to a new level of focus, responding to the need for continuing development and dissemination of nursing measurement instruments and providing an identifiable forum for the discussion and debate of measurement concerns and issues of interest.

The nursing profession has developed nursing measurement to a great degree between the late 1970s and mid 1990s. Nurses have developed and tested instruments for use in a variety of settings. In addition to creating new instruments, nurses have further developed instruments designed in other disciplines for use in nursing studies. Although much has been done, much remains to be done in nursing measurement.

> As in the past, many existing instruments are too long and cumbersome for use in clinical settings. Reading levels of self-administered instruments are often too high for clinical populations most in need of study. Psychometric assessments of existing instruments are often limited and frequently are not available for minority and low socioeconomic populations. Nurse investigators still tend to rely heavily on paper and pencil self-administered instruments for the measurement of nursing variables when other approaches, such as observation or biologic measures, could render better data. Issues still remain regarding appropriate selection and uses of instruments, timing of measurements, conceptualization of variables for

measurement, use of appropriate measurement frameworks, and quality control procedures for the enhancement of clinical measurements. (Strickland, 1993a, p. 4)

ORA L. STRICKLAND

See also
DATA COLLECTION METHODS
INSTRUMENTATION
RELIABILITY
STATISTICAL TECHNIQUES
VALIDITY

MENOPAUSE

Medical and Biological Concepts

Menopause refers to the natural cessation of ovarian function and menstrual periods at the completion of the reproductive years, usually defined clinically after 12 consecutive months of amenorrhea. Reproductive aging is a continuum that begins with a decline in fertility after age 35, long before the final menstruation occurs, on average at age 51. During these later reproductive years (known in the past as the climacteric), there is a gradual elevation in the pituitary hormone follicle stimulating hormone (FSH), progressive loss of regular menstrual cyclicity, and depletion of responsive ovarian follicles capable of undergoing ovulation and fertilization. The perimenopause usually encompasses the immediate transition interval of the premenopause, when menstrual cycle irregularities commence, through the first year or two of the postmenopause, when signs of estrogen withdrawal may be most pronounced.

Despite the inevitability of this process in all women who live long enough, the time course of the perimenopause transition is highly variable in duration and magnitude from woman to woman, thus contributing to the wide range in age at menopause (ages 45 to 55). Some of this variation may be due to genetic, familial, nutritional, health, and behavioral factors. For example, smoking, exercise, and obesity are known to indirectly influence estrogen production and in turn the menopause experience. Premature menopause (ovarian failure) before age 40 is considered to be a medical disorder; it occurs in 1 in every 100 women. In the United States the number of women entering menopause is expected to rise sharply over the next decade as a result of the aging baby boom generation. Thus, a large and growing proportion of the population will be postmenopausal by the year 2000.

The precise physiological changes that precede the cessation of menstrual cycles are not well understood. The prevailing view is that menopause results from the gradual depletion of ovarian follicles over time, with consequent changes in the hormonal feedback systems governing the hypothalamic-pituitary-ovarian axis (see Menstrual Cycle). As the overall pool of follicles diminishes (ovarian reserve), the ovarian production of inhibin is reduced, resulting in a subtle loss of negative feedback and enhanced FSH secretion. In response to the heightened FSH, follicular maturation is at first accelerated, as evidenced by higher estrogen levels and shorter menstrual cycles in older ovulatory women. As the ovarian reserve declines further, the remaining follicles are resistant to gonadotropin stimulation, resulting in further rises in FSH. Now the cyclicity of follicular development, ovulation, and menstruation is lost, resulting in unpredictable waves of estrogen exposure and withdrawal and in turn, acyclic uterine bleeding.

With further reductions in the ovarian pool, the secretion of luteinizing hormone (LH) is no longer restrained by ovarian feedback and becomes magnified as well, resulting in long intervals of reduced estrogen and amenorrhea. Other signs of estrogen withdrawal may include hot flashes, night sweats, vaginal dryness, and the remission of cyclic breast pain. Finally, uterine bleeding ceases altogether. Although fertility ends, the ovaries continue to produce small amounts of hormones throughout life, which may be important for health. Compared to other organ systems, the female reproductive system is unique in that it undergoes spontaneous cessation at a relatively young age, thus making it an excellent model for the study of the aging process free of chronic disease.

Nursing Perspective

The biomedical model has led to the view of menopause as a treatable endocrine disease state, similar to diabetes, requiring hormone replacement therapy. Nurse-scientists have taken a much broader perspective of menopause, choosing to view it as a developmental milestone of continuing maturation, with a range of health and illness experiences (Barnard & Reame, 1996; Woods, 1994a). Considerable evidence exists to support the assumption that menopause is a complex phenomenon constructed within a sociocultural context (Woods, 1994a). The use of a feminist framework to guide studies of the menopause has been a prominent feature in nursing research (MacPherson, 1981; Voda & George, 1986). Moreover, nurses have joined with social scientists and women's health advocacy groups to voice concern about the medicalization of menopause and the rationale for treating an entire population of healthy, aging women with carcinogenic steroids designed to mimic the hormonal profiles of childbearing-age women.

A major nursing contribution to the body of work on menopause has been the application of biobehavioral research strategies to better contextualize the biology of menopause within a woman's lived experience. For example, Ann Voda (1997) developed self-coloring body diagrams for use in multicultural studies to capture both quantitative and qualitative characteristics of the hot flash. As an extension of her work on perimenopausal symptoms, Nancy Woods and colleagues (Woods & Mitchell, 1996) have conducted longitudinal studies examining the change in symptoms within the context of aging as well as life transitions, stressors, and conflicts in a multiethnic population of middle-aged women. Nancy Reame and colleagues (Reame et al., 1996) found subtle aging effects on hypothalamic secretion (inferred from pulsatile LH secretion) in healthy volunteers over age 40 that were not found in women aged 20–35 years despite similar menstrual cycle characteristics and symptoms. Marilyn Rothert and colleagues (Rothert et al., 1990) have provided important insights into the decision-making behaviors of women considering hormone replacement therapy.

Recently, the National Institute for Nursing Research, in conjunction with the National Institute on Aging, cosponsored a 5-year longitudinal observational study of the perimenopause transition in women of diverse ethnic and racial backgrounds at seven sites around the country. Known as the

SWAN (survey of women across the nation) study, this epidemiological investigation will for the first time examine an array of physical, emotional, social, and behavioral characteristics of nearly 3,500 participants on a yearly basis as they proceed through the menopause. The goal is to understand better the disparities and scope of the menopause experience in healthy women, especially as it is influenced by socioeconomic, cultural, and ethnic factors.

Nurse scientists have provided prominent leadership to the North American Menopause Society and the Society for Menstrual Cycle Research, as well as to the first National Institutes of Health invitational conference on the menopause in 1993. These research organizations have recognized the shortcomings in the field and are committed to providing a more balanced, woman-centered approach to the study of the menopause. Such approaches include the adoption of less biased medical jargon, research tools that ask about positive menopause symptoms, and the inclusion of research participants on advisory boards and as consultants for data interpretation.

Future Research Directions

As is true for the bulk of women's health research, future nursing studies should move toward the definition of the menopause experience for previously invisible populations such as women of color, lesbians, and disabled women. Given the fear and ambivalence associated with the use of hormone replacement therapies, nurse scientists are in a pivotal position to test alternative, nonpharmacological therapies for coping with menopause-related symptoms such as hot flashes (Voda, 1997), sleep dysfunction, fatigue (Shaver, Giblin, Lentz, & Lee, 1988; Wilbur, Holm, & Dan, 1992), and heavy menses (Voda & Mansfield, 1993). Until now, the emphasis has been on menopause-related pathologies and symptoms, with little attention to a better understanding of factors that mediate a positive menopause experience and robust health well into the postreproductive years. Additional studies are needed to span the traditional disciplinary boundaries and create a more complete account of menopause and health (Woods, 1994a).

NANCY E. REAME

See also
**FEMINIST RESEARCH METHOD-
OLOGY
MENSTRUAL CYCLE
PREMENSTRUAL SYNDROME
WOMEN'S HEALTH RESEARCH**

MENSTRUAL CYCLE

Biomedical Definition and Terminology

The menstrual cycle is the reproductive biorhythm in healthy women produced by a synchronized pattern of hormone signals between the ovary and brain that gives rise to the cylic production of a fertilizable egg from the ovary. Derived from the Latin *mensis* (month), the menstrual cycle is marked by the shedding of the uterine lining—a menstrual "period"—approximately every 28 days if a pregnancy fails to occur.

The hormones of the neuroreproductive axis govern the menstrual cycle through a highly synchronized interplay of negative and positive feedback systems that are sensitive to moment-to-moment fluctuations in pulsatile secretion. These hormones are gonadotropin releasing hormone (GnRH) from the hypothalamus; the pituitary hormones, luteinizing hormone (LH) and follicle stimulating hormone (FSH); and the ovarian sex steroids, estradiol and progesterone. Under the direction of GnRH, the gonadotropins (LH and FSH) are released from the pituitary in a coordinated fashion to stimulate the ovary to produce a developing egg for potential fertilization. In turn, increasing amounts of estrogen are followed by progesterone, the sex steroids needed to transform the uterus and breast in preparation for pregnancy.

A number of behavioral and cognitive phenomena, such as excessive exercise, compulsive dieting, depression, or other psychological stress can interfere with menstrual cycle regularity, disrupt the normal ovulatory process, and lead to states of hypoestrogenism with subsequent bone thinning and infertility. These environmental influences are believed to be mediated by inhibitory stimuli from higher brain centers interacting with the GnRH neurons via neuromodulators such as opioids, dopamine, serotonin, and norepinephrine. The hormones of the stress axis also suppress the function of the reproductive system. Thus, the menstrual cycle serves as an elegant example of a complex biobehavioral phenomenon responsive to both internal and external environmental stimuli.

Based on the functional changes in the ovary, the menstrual cycle is typically divided into the *follicular phase* (cycle days 1–12, when rising estrogen is produced by the growing follicle), the *ovulation phase* (days 13–14 in response to a midcycle LH surge), and the *luteal phase* (cycle days 15–28, when progesterone is produced by the corpus luteum of the ovary). The *menstrual phase* refers to the days of menstrual bleeding; cycle day 1, or the first day of menses, is considered the beginning of the next cycle.

The secretory patterns in blood, urine, and saliva of the sex steroids across the follicular, ovulatory, and luteal phases of the menstrual cycle have been well characterized, allowing researchers to link various behavioral or physiological phenomena with specific cycle phases. Further, the sequential and synergistic effects of estrogen and progesterone on the breast, reproductive tract, and body temperature are used by clinicians, researchers, and women themselves to monitor signs of fertility or reproductive health problems.

Nursing Contributions to Menstrual Cycle Research

The medicalization of women's menstrual function has predominated in biomedical research, with little attention to the interaction of psychological, sociocultural, lifestyle, and health factors. Nursing science has focused on defining these influences on the range and diversity of menstrual cycle experiences, moving beyond those of gynecological patient populations to the broader spectrum of healthy community samples. Data collection sites have included the home, place of work, athletic events, community centers, college campuses, outpatient health care settings, and clinical research centers. Nurse investigators also have examined the salience and characteristics of the menstrual cycle experience in populations seldom studied, such as disabled women, elite runners, nurses working night shifts, and oncology nurses working with antineoplastic drugs.

Perhaps the most important nursing science contribution to menstrual cycle research has been the explication of the effects of the woman's lived experience on menstrual symptomatology. Angela McBride (McBride & McBride, 1981) was one of the first nurse scholars to embrace feminist theory as a research paradigm, calling for a reframing of symptoms and disease within the greater context of a woman's everyday life. Formed in 1976, the Society for Menstrual Cycle Research, a multidisciplinary organization with strong nursing leadership, has been at the forefront of the movement away from a reductionist perspective to a more comprehensive approach to the study of women's health (Dan, 1994).

This paradigm shift has expanded the scope of explanatory models and methods for menstrual cycle research. Since the early 1980s, Nancy Woods and colleagues have systematically examined how symptoms synchronized to the menstrual cycle are influenced by the context of social class, education, race, marital status, self-esteem, occupation, and menstrual attitudes (Woods, Most, & Longenecker, 1985). They have documented the dynamic nature of symptom formation across and within individuals in response to their changing social environments.

A by-product of nursing studies has been the development of improved designs and methods for the biobehavioral assessment of menstrual cycle phenomena (e.g., Taylor, 1990; Woods, Most, & Dery, 1982). Such methods have included the measurement of menstrual flow absorbency, assessment of perimenstrual symptom patterns and cluster types, statistical methods for handling the detection of LH pulsatile secretion, and the comparison of daily menstrual symptoms across cycles of the same individual (Shaver & Woods, 1986). The Washington Women's Daily Health Diary is a refinement of earlier menstrual cycle symptom questionnaires that includes both positive and negative symptoms. It has been used by several nurse researchers to define a variety of menstrual cycle symptom patterns, including premenstrual syndrome, in their respective study samples.

Future Directions

In keeping with the challenge of Lentz and Woods (1989) for nursing research to consider the dynamic and multidimensional nature of women's health phenomena, there is a need to move away from the concept of the menstrual cycle as a static construct, employing single-occasion measures that fail to address it as an interactive process with evolving symptom patterns. To better define the complete spectrum of menstrual cycle health, future studies should examine the effects of seasonality, social rhythms, sexual preference, occupational stressors, and transition periods (e.g., divorce) in women across the reproductive life span.

Although steadily evolving, most nursing research on the menstrual cycle has been descriptive or correlational in nature, with little replication of prior work to confirm hypotheses. Furthermore, studies are only beginning to incorporate biomarkers of ovarian function into their design to confirm ovulatory status and anchor symptom reports to menstrual cycle phase (Estok, Rudy, Kerr, & Menzel, 1993). Recently, nurse scientists turned their attention away from the menstrual cycle characteristics of White women to the experiences of those from diverse ethnic backgrounds and other countries (e.g., Iceland, Japan, China). In keeping with a feminist view of "doing science," future studies should actively engage study subjects as co-researchers in all phases of the investigative process, with special emphasis on data interpretation and conclusions drawn from the findings.

Nurses also have begun incorporating the menstrual cycle as a study variable into research on the severity and management of chronic illness. This work has revealed menstrual cycle effects on irritable bowel symptoms, sleep disorders, depression, metabolic control in diabetic patients, and binge drinking in recovering alcoholics. These new directions hold promise for improving nursing interventions, not only for menstrual health problems but for a variety of illnesses specific to women.

NANCY E. REAME

See also
CULTURAL/TRANSCULTURAL FOCUS

FEMINIST RESEARCH METHODOLOGY
MENOPAUSE
PREMENSTRUAL SYNDROME
WOMEN'S HEALTH RESEARCH

MENTAL HEALTH IN PUBLIC SECTOR PRIMARY CARE

In the then Soviet community of Alma Alta in 1978, primary health care was delimited by the World Health Organization to meet the challenge of low life expectancy and high childhood mortality in many countries. Primary health care was determined to be low-cost, universally accessible, essential health care. This definition of primary care has been adopted throughout the international community, but in the United States primary care has become synonymous with service delivery because of the capitalist economic system that underlies health care. Unfortunately, community-based health status goals often are lost when emphasis is placed on service over care.

Primary care service delivery is housed in multiple organizational types that offer diverse services. Organizational structures mostly can be differentiated along the lines of the ability of the client to pay for services. Public sector clients, those who are publicly insured or uninsured, typically are cared for in tax revenue–supported agencies that must care for all who present themselves for health care. The effect of this dual primary care system is a real inequity in health care.

Disadvantaged persons clustered in low-income communities often have more immediate and pressing needs than obtaining formal health services. These include substandard housing, poor nutrition, environmental exposure, and crime. When they do use primary care services, public sector clients often find them to be inaccessible, not easy to use, and culturally insensitive. Many of these clients do not have a regular primary care physician, and they often delay seeking needed health care. Public sector clients are more likely to be hospitalized, for longer periods and for otherwise easily treated health care problems, than are privately insured individuals. The health of individuals within these relatively impoverished communities would be better served through public health modalities of intervention.

How primary care services evolved in this country is relevant to the provision of public sector mental health care. There is a growing movement in this country to reintegrate physical and mental health care within primary care. One factor motivating the move to integrated care is high prevalence rates of psychiatric disorders, estimated at 20% or more of primary care clients. Reintegration of physical and mental health care into primary care also is motivated by inadequate detection and treatment of psychiatric disorders by primary care physicians.

The service-based definition of primary care has led to two service-based models of psychiatric care. In for-profit settings serving the privately insured, the consultation-liaison model of psychiatric care has emerged: the primary care provider assumes responsibility for clients' mental health care. Staff psychiatrists and psychologists support primary care physicians in provision of mental health care. The specialty model of psychiatric care has been implemented in primary care clinics associated with tertiary care settings that serve many public sector clients. Specialty mental health providers assume responsibility for individual clients either collaboratively or as a referral from the primary care physician.

The efficacy of these models for mental health outcomes has been evaluated in randomized clinical trials. Results show that mental health services offered in primary care can be effective in detecting and treating depressive disorder under controlled conditions. Intervention seems less successful for persons with comorbid anxiety disorders or those who show symptoms of personality disorder. Findings demonstrated some support for integrating mental health with primary care.

Despite three generations of controlled studies of mental health care in primary care, including several randomized clinical trials, there are few findings that are applicable to public sector primary care. One reason is that there are few investigators examining mental health service delivery in primary care, and those tend to be clustered in a few sites. Because of this, most trials of mental health treatment have been limited to urban settings with samples containing mostly middle-class, middle-aged women. In many such studies treatment subjects fared no better in mental health outcomes than did controls. Attrition of subjects was high in many studies, especially among public sector clients. These findings have led some investigators to speculate about the cost-effectiveness of detection and intervention programs for psychiatric disorder in primary care.

With one notable exception there has been little evaluation of the efficacy of mental health interventions in the context of the organization in which they are provided (Katon & Gonzales, 1994). Research designs do not account for the pattern of health services use by disadvantaged groups, nor do they acknowledge that patterns of mental health services use are different from those for more conventional primary care services. Because the constituencies of public sector clients and the mentally ill overlap, mental health services delivery in primary care must be designed to encourage the use of services by these related disenfranchised groups.

There is growing recognition that the public health definition of primary health care chosen at Alma Alta must be adopted here if there is to be a significant impact on the health of the most vulnerable Americans (Barnes et al., 1995; Fowler & Padgett, 1994). This is especially true for those with psychiatric disorders, who appropriately fear the consequences of being labeled mentally ill (Neighbors & Jackson, 1996). Stigma, coupled with cultural insensitivity, often combines with monetary and resource concerns to keep disadvantaged public sector patients from accessing care until well into an illness episode. Models of mental health identification and detection must move into the community, be combined with other kinds of health care services, and be based in homes and community facilities. In these settings disadvantaged persons can seek health care without fear of being labeled "crazy," attend to multiple health care needs within the confines of one visit, and not expend significant personal resources in obtaining care.

Herein lies the test for nursing research and practice. Nursing already has provided considerable leadership in implementing public health models of care, as both practice and research evaluation models (Olds & Kitzman, 1990). Many of these models targeted at-risk, pregnant, adolescent, and young women and had improved child outcomes as the primary intervention target (Hauenstein, 1992). There is little evidence that these intervention research and practice programs have integrated mental health care into their treatment paradigm. This is a crucial omission, often cited by the researchers as a reason for less than optimal outcomes in their studies.

Many university-based schools of nursing have begun to initiate academic-community partnerships that aim to increase clinical training sites, provide settings for community-based research, and improve the health care of selected disadvantaged populations, with care provided in community settings. These linkages form an ideal setting for testing integrated models of health care that simultaneously and systematically address physical and mental health concerns. It is crucial, however, that they be designed and evaluated so that mental health care is within the mainstream of the client's physical health care. In this type of intervention model, health status outcomes for well-child care include the reduction of depression and anxiety in the mother and enhanced parenting. Outcomes for young men with abdominal pain include reduction in alcohol and nicotine abuse.

Process outcomes evaluated in these public health models include the degree to which services are actually used by the community, what settings are most effective, and the extent to which services are provided in a holistic fashion. This latter point would include the degree to which psychiatric and physical health care are integrated within and across settings of care. Outcomes measured by research evaluation designs accompanying these intervention paradigms must include measures of both physical and mental health, cost-effectiveness of services, and determination of what interventions are most effective in achieving health status goals.

Primary care nursing interventions aimed at reducing documented psychiatric disorders in specific communities and integrating mental and physical health care will need significant research attention to document their utility. Because they represent a variation in health care, careful documentation of their impact on community health status goals must be evaluated. Moreover, because public health models of primary care generally, and mental health in primary care specifically, are new, they will have to be modified and reevaluated in a variety of primary care organizational types and community settings. Nursing research has much to contribute to this process of returning holistic, truly primary health care to the community.

EMILY J. HAUENSTEIN

See also
**COMMUNITY MENTAL HEALTH
HEALTH SYSTEMS DELIVERY
MENTAL HEALTH SERVICES RE-
    SEARCH
PRIMARY CARE
PRIMARY HEALTH CARE**

MENTAL HEALTH SERVICES RESEARCH

Mental health services research (MHSR) is a relatively new body of research that focuses on issues of access to care, quality of care, outcomes of care, and cost of care. This field of research has gained recognition and increased federal grant funding in the past 10 years, sparked by the nation's interest in accountability and cost-effectiveness of health care. Mental health services research is a specialty area of health services' research and gains methodological strength from the growing knowledge base created by general health services research.

Mental health services research, as interdisciplinary research, benefits from the integration of disciplinary knowledge from clinical, administrative, and social sciences disciplines. Researchers from the clinical fields of psychiatric nursing, psychiatry, psychology, and social work and counselors and primary care providers often join with scientists from the fields of sociology, economics, statistics, business/health administration, and public health to combine clinical knowledge and methodological expertise in order to design the complex studies necessary to measure access, quality, and cost of care. Collectively, the results of MHSR are used to influence and improve the mental health delivery system.

The National Institute of Mental Health (NIMH; 1991) recognized the need to prepare more researchers as mental health service researchers and suggested that researchers need solid research training in their primary discipline (usually obtained through doctoral education) and proposed MHSR training through a postdoctoral fellowship program. Psychiatric nursing's contribution to outcome research provided a building block for the profession's contribution to interdisciplinary MHSR. Merwin and Mauck (1995) determined that most psychiatric nursing outcome research focused on clinical outcomes, but studies also addressed provider outcomes and rehabilitation public welfare and humanitarian outcomes based on NIMH's classification of mental health outcomes.

Increased numbers of doctorally prepared nurse researchers with postdoctoral training in MHSR are needed in order to include a nursing perspective within the rapidly developing interdisciplinary MHSR arena. Only one of the NIMH-funded MHSR centers is housed in a school of nursing (University of Virginia) and directed by a nurse. Examples of MHSR conducted by nurses includes the work of Hauenstein (1996b) on in-home intervention with depressed women, Merwin (1995) and Merwin, Goldsmith, and Manderscheid (1995) on rural mental health human resources, and Fox, Merwin, and Blank (1995) on rural mental health services.

JEANNE C. FOX

See also
CHRONIC MENTAL ILLNESS
COMMUNITY MENTAL HEALTH
MENTAL HEALTH IN PUBLIC SECTOR
  PRIMARY CARE
SCHIZOPHRENIA NURSING RESEARCH
YOUNG WOMEN AND DEPRESSION

MENTORING

The concept of mentoring, a unique type of developmental and support relationship, has attracted growing attention in the nursing discipline. It was not until the 1970s that mentoring was pinpointed as an area for discussion, study, and implementation in nursing. Although the terms *role model* and *preceptor* had been used extensively in nursing practice and education, the use of the term *mentor* is a relatively recent phenomenon. A mentor is someone who serves as a career role model who advises, guides, and inspires another person, the protégé, during an extended period of time. The mentor connection has been defined as a developmental, empowering, nurturing relationship extending over time, in which mutual sharing, learning, and growth occur in an atmosphere of respect, collegiality, and affirmation (Vance & Olson, 1998). Mentor-protégé relationships provide developmental support and socialization at every stage of a professional person's career, from the student level through the leadership stage. Both career and personal assistance are ingredients of the mentor relationship.

The first formal investigation of mentor relationships in nursing was conducted with American nurse-influentials (Vance, 1977). These leaders reported a strong presence of mentoring activity, 83% reporting one or more mentors in their career and 93% reporting the mentorship of others. The types of mentoring assistance in their careers and life stages included that of parent-sponsor, intellectual guide, sociocultural role model, visionary-idealist, promoter-coach, peer-colleague, and mentor emeritus (Vance, 1982, 1986). These varieties of mentoring help have been consistently reported in the literature of many disciplines. Nursing studies of mentoring are being conducted in every career level and specialty area of the profession. The research in the field has been summarized by Jowers and Herr (1990), Vance and Olson (1991), and Olson and Vance (1993, in press).

Studies reveal that there are two varieties of mentor relationships: (a) informal, or unplanned; and (b) formal, or assigned. Informal mentoring consists of the traditional expert-to-novice relationship as well as peer-to-peer mentoring. Unplanned mentoring occurs when two people are drawn together through shared interests and goals, mutual attraction, and a desire to help and be helped. Work and educational settings are places where potential mentors and protégés meet and establish mentor connections. Formal mentoring is an organizational application of this personal phenomenon. Many educational and work organizations, as well as professional associations, are establishing programs that incorporate mentoring in their everyday working structures and relationships. There is usually some assigned matching of mentor-protégé dyads and encouragement of informal and formal mentor networks. It has been demonstrated that benefits of mentoring accrue to both mentors and protégés as well as to the workplace and the profession.

Regardless of which theoretical approach is used to explore the mentor concept, it is clear that there are two major developmental outcomes of mentoring for persons in a supportive mentoring relationship: success and satisfaction. Persons whose talents and abilities have been nurtured and promoted by caring mentors experience professional success easier and faster. They are equipped to realized their "dream" and accomplish their goals as they move through various life and career stages. Future possibilities are articulated and doors are opened by the mentor's intentional assistance and guidance and the mentor's belief in the protégé. Personal satisfaction and self-development also are promoted by the mentor relationship. The two major developmental outcomes of success and satisfaction provide the background for the specific benefits of mentor connections in the new paradigm. These are documented through analysis of studies, anecdotal accounts, stories, and self-reports and include career success and advancement, personal and professional satisfaction, enhanced self-esteem and confidence, preparation for leadership roles and succession, and strengthening of the profession (Vance & Olson, 1998).

The female-dominant discipline of nursing provides a mirror of an emerging model of development and support that reflects the female experience and women's unique personal and career challenges. Empirical and anecdotal investigation has shown that mentoring in nursing exhibited a divergent pattern from the traditional model of mentoring that is found predominantly among men in the older professions and corporate world. For example, in contrast to the exclusive model of expert-to-novice mentoring, many women and nurses have multiple mentors and experience a variety of developmental relationships. These relationships frequently last for long periods, through many cycles of change and growth, and evolve into collegial collaboration and friendships. Peer colleagues, as well as senior professionals, serve as important mentors. Studies of nurses' mentor relationships reveal the creation of a new paradigm of mentoring that is androgynous, embodying both traditional and evolving patterns of help and support. This new paradigm will provide a more holistic, diverse, and satisfying mentoring experience for both women and men. It is characterized by inclusion, diversity, peer-to-peer connections, long-term and cyclic mentoring, affiliation, and empowerment (Vance & Olson, 1998).

The mentoring concept presents conceptual, definitional, and methodological challenges for researchers. The complex interactional, emotional, and longitudinal nature of this human phenomenon are difficult to capture fully. The application of a variety of research methods is essential to describe the complexity and diversity of the mentor connection throughout the life-career cycle. Qualitative research methodologies, including in-depth interviews, autobiographies and diaries, story-telling, case studies, and observational methods, will be particularly helpful in illuminating the essence and multiple dimensions of this unique developmental relationship. Careful sampling methods, appropriate instrumentation, use of comparison groups, and longitudinal and in-depth examination of subjects will assist in the development of conceptual and operational clarity of the characteristics, functions, and limitations of the mentor connection. Mentor research in nursing will yield greater insight into and acknowledgment of women's unique personal and professional developmental issues, particularly the extent and dimensions of mentoring influences at various personal and professional transition points.

CONNIE VANCE

See also
ADMINISTRATION RESEARCH
EDUCATION: NURSE RESEARCHERS
**   AND ADVANCED PRACTICE NURSES**
MENTORING IN NURSING RESEARCH
RESEARCH CAREERS

MENTORING IN NURSING RESEARCH

Definition

Although definitions of mentoring vary, analysis of the literature demonstrates that mentoring, along with mentoring in nursing research, includes the following attributes: a teaching-learning process, a reciprocal role, a career development relationship, a knowledge or competence differential between participants, a duration of several years, and a resonating phenomenon (Stewart & Krueger, 1996).

Trends and Issues

The need for mentoring in nursing research has increased over the past decade in response to an increased number of doctoral programs in nursing and a need to document how nurses improve health outcomes in an increasingly managed care environment.

Although research is integrated in nursing education at all levels, nurses are prepared to conduct research by a doctoral education. In doctoral education, research mentoring is necessary for development of grantsmanship, knowledge of and participation in the conduct of research, and introduction and incorporation of doctoral students into the scientific community (Fitzpatrick & Abraham, 1987). Research mentoring is fostered in an environment with strong interactions between faculty and students, where faculty are engaged in research and students are immersed in the process. Nursing faculty who are engaged in research are the best mentors for students (Lowery, 1991).

Mentoring for nursing research is unique compared to mentoring for nursing education and nursing practice because of the limited number of research mentors and the length of time needed to produce an independent investigator. The Institute of Medicine (1994) report *Careers in Clinical Research* noted that there were approximately 9,000 doctorally prepared nurses in this country. Of this limited number, only 20% to 25% were actually conducting research. The report indicated that the frequent lack of administrative support and undervaluing of research, combined with the availability of lucrative administrative, clinical, and consultative positions, reduced the number of individuals drawn to and retained in research. The report concluded that the number of doctorally prepared nurses was insufficient to meet the demand in academic and clinical settings for research and research training.

Producing a successful independent investigator is a lengthy process. In nursing education and in nursing practice, individuals can be successful with less than doctoral preparation. For a researcher to be competitive for major research funding at the National Institutes of Health (NIH) or elsewhere, a doctoral degree is essential. Additionally, the individual may have to demonstrate beginning to build a program of research and having the support of seasoned investigators as well as organizational support in order to secure major research funding. Similar support is needed for the conduct and publication of the research.

Attributes of Research Mentoring

Research mentoring involves both teaching and learning. Some authorities believe mentoring accelerates the process of learning because the protégé benefits from the research experiences of the mentor and can avoid many of the pitfalls involved in the research process. It is not yet clear, however, which research mentoring activities most enhance learning (Stewart & Krueger, 1996).

To produce an independent investigator, research mentoring requires reciprocity in which a sharing of perspectives, values, and goals and an energizing of each other occurs. The protégé gradually shifts from initial dependence on the research mentor to independence and autonomy with his or her own line of investigation. At the beginning of the research mentor relationship a knowledge or competence differential exists. As the protégé develops, this differential is reduced and over time may even be reversed.

Data on the mean number of years required to mentor an investigator to independence are not clear. Mentoring for nursing service executives has been reported to range between 1 and 5 years (Holloran, 1989). Mentoring for academic nurse administrators is reported at a mean of 8 years (White, 1988). Many authors also report a resonating phenomenon: those researchers who have been mentored then mentor younger investigators.

Career development, a part of mentoring, is a necessary component of research mentoring (Brooten, in press). Scientific maturing without development of the characteristics associated with and essential to career success limit dissemination and adoption of the protégé's research findings in both clinical practice and in the public policy arena.

Choosing a Mentor

Protégés should look for mentors who posses personal characteristics of integrity, self-discipline, openness, availability, and commitment to the work of the protégé. Mentors should have active and credible programs of research, publish their work regularly in well-respected peer-reviewed clinical and research journals, and present their findings regionally, nationally, and internationally. It is essential that protégés explore the investment and comfort a potential mentor has with the protégé's need to be mentored and yet recognized as an investigator in need of an independent line of research (Brooten, in press).

Choosing a Protégé

Because research mentorship is a significant investment of time and resources, protégés should be chosen very carefully. Mentors should look for characteristics such as intelligence, honesty, persistence, an analytic approach, problem-solving ability, verbal and writing skills, eagerness to learn, and compatibility with the mentor. The mentor should also be comfortable with the protégé's motivation for pursuing research. The protégé should have identified a credible program of research that is potentially fundable and fits with the mentor's knowledge, skills, and ongoing research.

Measures of Successful Research Mentorship

Objective measures of successful research mentorship include the number and quality of the protégé's publications in peer-reviewed journals, the number of national and international research presentations, research recognition awards, number of grants awarded, and level of external research funding. Later measures of success include the number of successful individuals mentored by the protégé.

Implications

Currently, the number of research mentors is insufficient to meet the demand for research and research training in academic and clinical settings. In addition, mentorship to produce an independent investigator takes many years. This combination of factors may serve to limit opportunities for both development of nursing's knowledge base and its next generation of researchers.

DOROTHY BROOTEN

See also
DOCTORAL EDUCATION
MENTORING
RESEARCH CAREERS

META-ANALYSIS

Meta-analysis is a quantitative approach that permits the synthesis and integration of results from multiple individual studies focused on a specific research question. Meta-analysis was first introduced in 1976 by Glass, who referred to it as an analysis of analyses. A meta-analysis is a rigorous alternative to the traditional narrative review of the literature. It involves the application of the research process to a collection of studies in a specific area. The individual studies are considered the sample. The findings from each study are transformed into a common statistic called an effect size. An effect size is a measure of the magnitude of the experimental effect on outcome variables.

Once the results from each study have been converted to a common metric, these findings can be pooled together and synthesized. The most common effect size indicator is r, which is the Pearson product moment correlation. Another effect size indicator is the d index. Cohen's d is the difference between the means of the experimental and control groups divided by the standard deviation. Cohen (1988) has provided guidelines for interpreting the magnitude of both the r and d effect size indicators. For the r index, Cohen has defined small, medium, and large effect sizes as .10, .30, and .50 or more, respectively. For the d indicator an effect size of .2 is considered small, .5 is medium, and .8 or more is large.

Approaches are available to examine and reduce bias from operating within a meta-analysis. Some ways that biased conclusions can occur in a meta-analysis are effects of a bias toward publishing positive but not negative results, giving each study an equal weight in the meta-analysis despite the fact they differ in sample size or quality, inclusion of multiple tests of a hypothesis from an individual study, and not ensuring an acceptable level of agreement or reliability among raters in coding the study characteristics.

The possibility that unknown, unpublished studies may exist, whose results fail to support the pattern illustrated by the published findings, is referred to as the file drawer problem (Rosenthal, 1979). The conclusions of the meta-analysis can be distorted if the retrieval of studies yielded only published studies in which a publication bias in favor of significant results may occur. Rosenthal developed a technique to assess the magnitude of the file drawer problem by calculating the minimum number of unpublished studies with nonsignificant results that would be necessary to change the conclusion reached by the meta-analysis.

It can be argued that not all studies synthesized in a meta-analysis should be given equal weight. Some studies may be poorly designed and have small unrepresentative samples, whereas other studies use randomized control group designs with large sample sizes. To remedy this problem, studies can be evaluated and assigned a quality score. The meta-analysis can then be calculated with studies weighted by their quality scores.

A source of nonindependence in a meta-analysis can result from using multiple hypothesis tests based on multiple variable measurements obtained from a single study (Strube & Hartman, 1983). One suggested remedy when selecting findings obtained from multiple measures of the hypothesis tests located within a single study is to collapse the various findings into a single, global hypothesis test.

One assumption that should be met before specific studies are quantitatively combined in one meta-analysis is that each study provides sample estimates of the effect sizes that are representative of the population effect size. Homogeneity tests can be calculated to identify any outlier studies. If outliers are identified, they can be removed.

Meta-analysis first appeared in the nursing literature in 1982, when O'Flynn published her article describing meta-analysis in the "Methodology Corner" of *Nursing Research*. A meta-analysis of the effects of psychoeducational interventions on length of postsurgical hospital stay (Devine & Cook, 1983) was the first meta-analysis published in nursing. Since then meta-analyses have been conducted and published in a wide variety of areas, such as patient outcomes of nurse-practitioners and nurse-midwives, job satisfaction and turnover among nurses, relationship between postpartum depression and maternal-infant interaction, effects of educational interventions in diabetes care, quality of life in cardiac patients, and nonnutritive sucking in preterm infants.

The outcome of this quantitative approach for reviewing the literature has tremendous potential for a practice-based discipline such as nursing. One example of a meta-analysis that has consequences for nursing practice integrated the research on predictors of postpartum depression. Beck's (1996a) meta-analysis of 44 studies helped to clarify which variables were significantly related to postpartum depression; there had been conflicting findings reported in the literature. The following eight variables were revealed to be significant predictors: prenatal depression, history of previous depression, social support, life stress, child care stress, maternity blues, marital satisfaction, and prenatal anxiety. An instrument based on the findings of this meta-analysis can be designed to help detect women at risk for developing postpartum depression.

Meta-analysis of the abundance of research being conducted can benefit nursing practice. Not only will the use of meta-analysis further knowledge development in the discipline of nursing, but it also can help nurses in the clinical setting to decide whether to apply research findings to their practice based on the size of the difference an intervention makes. Meta-analysis can resolve issues in nursing where there are multiple studies with conflicting findings. In addition, meta-analysis highlights gaps in nursing research for future studies.

CHERYL TATANO BECK

See also

QUANTITATIVE RESEARCH METHODOLOGY
RESEARCH UTILIZATION
STATISTICAL TECHNIQUES

MIDDLE-RANGE THEORY

Middle-range theory is a term used by sociologists (Merton, 1957) in the 1950s and 1960s as they were considering the kinds of theory most appropriate for advancing the knowledge base of a discipline. It refers to a level of theory that is differentiated from other levels by scope and degree of abstraction and by the degree to which they are empirically testable.

The term *middle-range theories* describes those that lie between global (also called grand or general) theories and abstracted empiricism, or minor working hypotheses. Global theories are too broad in scope and too abstract to permit direct empirical testing. In sociology they refer to attempts to construct a broad unified theory, and in nursing they include theories developed by early nurse theorists such as Rogers, King, Roy, Johnson, Neuman, Levine, and others. Grand or global theories provide a disciplinary worldview and thus sensitize researchers to the phenomena of concern in their discipline. They also may be used as a basis for specifying middle-range theories whose scope is both less abstract and empirically testable. Abstracted empiricism, at the other extreme of abstraction, refers to detailed accounts of phenomena that have no theoretical basis that would allow them to be related to other phenomena or situations.

The term *middle-range theory* was brought into nursing by nurses studying sociology during the time when these ideas were being discussed in that field (Jacox, 1970). Suppe (1996, 1997) has described in a series of papers the parallel between sociology and nursing in their concern with theory and its place in their respective disciplines. Suppe elaborated on what makes a middle-range theory testable, emphasizing that it must be possible at present to measure or objectively code the theoretical terms in the theory. He further has shown how the concept of middle-range theory is applicable not only in earlier positivistic views of science but in other views of science, including the humanistic and critical or emancipatory.

During the 1970s and 1980s a concern with global theories or conceptual frameworks dominated the nursing literature. At the same time, little of the research reported by nurses used nursing grand theories. Moody and colleagues (Moody et al., 1988) found that fewer than 13% of 720 nursing practice research studies published between 1977 to 1986 linked a nursing grand theory with the research design. Thirteen studies used Orem's theory, six used Rogers's, and five used Roy's. Approximately half of the studies used theory from another discipline, most commonly Lazarus's coping theory, the health belief model, and locus of control. Other analyses of nursing clinical research also have documented the limited use by nurses of nursing grand theories to guide their studies.

A criticism of global nursing theories is that they are too abstract to test directly in clinical settings, although some nurses have derived middle-range theories from global nursing theories. Krieger (1975), for example, used Rogers's theory to derive a theory of therapeutic touch and tried to show empirically the relationship between therapeutic touch and healing. Recently, Frey (1995) used King's theory to derive a theory of families, children, and chronic illness. Some nursing studies have very little conceptualization of any kind. They more nearly approximate what Merton (1957) earlier called abstracted empiricism and report on details of clinical practice in ways that limit the usefulness of their findings to other patients and settings.

In the 1990s there was a resurgence of nursing interest in middle-range theories. Several conferences at Wayne State University and Case Western Reserve University took middle-range theory as their theme, and a 1997 issue of *Advances in Nursing Science* was devoted to middle-range theory. There are now examples of middle-range theory development in nursing, including the classification work on nursing interventions and nursing-sensitive patient outcomes being conducted by investigators at the University of Iowa (Iowa Outcomes Team), Mishel's (1988) work on uncertainty in illness, and the substantial amount of work being done on stress and coping.

Good and Moore (1996) identified clinical practice guidelines as a potential source of middle-range theories. They illustrated how this might be done by deriving a middle-range theory of achieving a balance between analgesia and side effects in adults, using the acute pain guidelines of the Agency for Health Care Policy and Research as their source. More recently, some nurses are using the term micro-theory to designate testable theories that have a scope more limited than middle-range theories.

In summary, middle-range theories are those located between broad global theories and empirical details in level of abstraction. Unlike global theories, middle-range (and micro) theories have a more direct correspondence with the reality they are intended to represent and can be tested empirically.

ADA JACOX

See also
EPISTEMOLOGY
MIDDLE-RANGE THEORIES OF DEMEN-
   TIA CARE
NURSING THEORETICAL MODELS
THEORETICAL FRAMEWORK

MIDDLE-RANGE THEORIES OF DEMENTIA CARE

Implications for Research

The nursing care of persons with dementia, historically a process of trial and error (Hall & Buck-

walter, 1987), has recently become the basis for the development of *middle-range theories* in nursing. These theories focus on a limited number of variables, are more amenable to empirical testing, and are positioned between grand theories and micro-theories embodied in care procedures (Fitzpatrick & Whall, 1996). Utilizing the criteria of publication and dissemination within nursing, the following middle-range theories were selected for review: need-driven, dementia-compromised behavior (Algase et al., 1996), progressively lowered stress threshold (PLST) (Hall & Buckwalter, 1987), individualized care for frail elders (Happ, Williams, Strumpf, & Burger, 1996), and decision-making process for level of assistance with activities of daily living (Beck, Heacock, Rapp, & Mercer, 1993). In addition, several other theories are cited but not reviewed due to space limitations.

Need-Driven, Dementia-Compromised Behavior

The need-driven, dementia-compromised behavior approach views the person with dementia as experiencing an unmet need or goal that results in need-driven behaviors such as aggression, wandering, or disturbing vocalizations. These behaviors reflect the interaction of salient background and proximal factors found either within the person or in his or her immediate environment or both. Background variables include neurological, cognitive, health status, and psychosocial factors. Proximal factors include personal characteristics and the physical and social environment. Need-driven, dementia-compromised behavior is evaluated on dimensions of frequency and duration. Nursing's role is to identify those at risk and to intervene with strategies under various sets of environmental circumstances. The theory has been applied to the study of aggression by Whall and to the study of wandering by Algase. Research efforts are focused on the identification of variables common to and different from each of the disturbing behaviors and the application of linear modeling to further build the theory.

Progressively Lowered Stress Threshold

Hall and Buckwalter's (1987) framework views the person with dementia as experiencing baseline anxious and dysfunctional states throughout the course of the disease. Anxious behavior occurs during stress, and if stress continues, dysfunctional states such as panic occur. Six principles guide nursing care: (a) maximize the level of safe function by supporting all areas of loss in a prosthetic manner, (b) provide unconditional positive regard, (c) use behaviors indicating anxiety to determine limits of stimuli and activity, (d) teach caregivers to "listen" and evaluate verbal and nonverbal responses, (e) modify environment to support losses and enhance safety, and (f) provide education, support, care, and problem solving for caregivers. Evaluation research at 13 long-term care facilities has utilized such designs as pre- and posttests and longitudinal experimental approaches. Research has also identified behavioral characteristics and interventions for four types of wandering and has led to the classification of factors influencing dysfunctional behavior.

Individualized Care for Frail Elders

The individualized care for frail elders approach (Happ, Williams, Strumpf, & Burger, 1996) embodies an interdisciplinary approach to care. It emphasizes four critical attributes: (a) knowing the person (life story and patterns of response), (b) the relationship (staff continuity and reciprocity), (c) choice (decision making and risk taking), and (d) resident participation (daily planning). Evans's (1996) cross-cultural observations in four European countries supported these propositions and delineated three factors that contributed to individualized care: congruent societal and health care values, commonalties of patient needs in all settings, and primacy of caring through knowing the person. Rowles and Dallas (1996) found that family involvement in nursing home decision making served to individualize care and provided a continuing link to the residents' personal history and preferences. Several studies supported cost-effectiveness linked to lowered medication costs and staff turnover. Further research concerning resident outcomes and refinements in definitions, goals, and critical attributes is indicated.

Decision-Making Process for Level of Assistance with Activities of Daily Living

This algorithmic framework (Beck, Heacock, Rapp, & Mercer, 1993) emphasizes that each elder has an individual pattern of cognitive deficits that must be assessed to improve the quality of life and interactions; these include attention deficits, language impairment, sequencing problems, and impaired judgment. Seven levels of assistance are defined: stimulus control, verbal prompt, modeling/ gesturing, physical prompt, physical guidance, occasional physical guidance, and complete physical guidance. The decision-making process of prescribing strategies is displayed in a flowchart algorithm that results in selection of the most appropriate level of assistance. The process is based on research to improve dressing behaviors in nursing home residents with cognitive impairment.

A number of nurse scientists have explicated some of the bases for middle-range theory work and have produced instruments to assess demented subjects. Most notable are Tappen and Barry's (1995) Dementia Mood Picture Test, Hurley's Discomfort Scale (Hurley, Volicer, Hanrahan, Houde, & Volicer, 1992), Ryden's Aggression Scale (Ryden, Bossenmaier, & McLachlen, 1991), and Burgener's Modified Interaction Behavior Measure (Burgener, Jirovec, Murrell, & Barton, 1992). Utilizing decision trees to clarify nursing strategies for disturbing behaviors is an important new approach (Richie, 1996).

The latter decades of this century have been characterized by the designing and examination of middle-range theories and models of dementia care. The nursing approaches described above have been at the forefront of this exploration and provide effective and humane approaches for behavioral disturbance in dementia. As these efforts are supported by multiple programs of research, they hold great promise for more effective dementia care in the decades ahead.

KATHLEEN BYRNE COLLING
ANN L. WHALL

See also
ALZHEIMER'S DISEASE

COGNITIVE DISORDERS
FAMILY CAREGIVING TO FRAIL
   ELDERS
FUNCTIONAL HEALTH
MIDDLE-RANGE THEORY

MINORITY POPULATIONS: ASIAN AMERICANS

Although nursing service should be based on knowledge developed through culturally sensitive research, there is a dearth of studies on Asian Americans. In recent years there has been increased interest in the study of health behaviors and health problems of minority populations; however, Asian Americans have received limited attention. Thus, there is little information on the prevalent health problems among Asian Americans and how they practice health care. Asian Americans share a core of common values and behaviors, including family values, views of health and illness, and attitudes and interaction styles with health care professionals. However, they are markedly different in their languages, religions, national history, epidemiological risk factors, health practices, and treatment of illness, as well as degree of acculturation. Most beliefs about Asian Americans are drawn from data on the general Asian population or the Japanese American population. Most studies are done in non-nursing disciplines—that is, medicine and sociology—and may represent data from one specific ethnic group of Asians that have been generalized to all Asian Americans. A MEDLINE search of journals in nursing and other relevant journals published since 1969 revealed 105 articles based on the identifying words *Asian*, *nursing*, *Pacific Islander*, and Asian country names (Cambodia, China, the Philippines, Indochina, Japan, Korea, Laos, Southeast Asia, Thailand, and Vietnam). Studies reported by nursing institutions or nurse researchers in the United States were reviewed.

Asian American Population

Asian Pacific Islanders are defined by the U.S. census (1992) as a set of U.S. population subgroups whose origins are in "the Far East, Southeast Asia or the Pacific Islands," and they are the fastest-growing ethnic groups as a result of immigration and fertility. The population increased from 3.7 million to 7.3 million during the 1980s, with most residing on the Pacific Coast. Among the diverse ethnic groups included in the Asian Americans category, the Chinese (1.6 M) are the most numerous and Filipinos (1.4 M), Japanese (.87 M), Koreans (.8 M), Asian Indian (.79 M) and Vietnamese (.6 M) follow. Although the Chinese, Filipino, Korean, and Vietnamese population in the U.S. has doubled in recent years, the Japanese American population grew only 20% (U.S. Bureau of the Census, 1992).

Historical Background and Research

The Asian Pacific Islanders population consists of 60 ethnic groups and subgroups. Within these groups there exist both commonalities and a wide range of differences. The history of immigration of each ethnic group is different; therefore the level of acculturation and language barriers also differ. The Japanese and Chinese immigration started in 1910, Filipinos and Koreans began to enter the U.S. in the 1940s, while the others came in the 1960s. The Southeast Asians, also known as Indochinese (Cambodians, Laotians, and Vietnamese), are the largest refugee group in the U.S., and they came to the U.S. soon after the fall of Saigon in 1975. Fewer than 20% of Japanese but over 81% of Cambodians speak a language other than English at home.

Of the 105 articles reviewed, 12 were categorized as clinical reports, 27 tutorials, and 56 were data based articles. Educational and clinical reports emphasized the importance of understanding the health beliefs and practices of Asian Americans. Along with an increased East Asian immigration, a massive influx of Southeast Asian refugees occurred in the 1980s and the majority of these refugees were relocated in low-income inner cities in California and Massachusetts. These settlers required special attention for their health problems which challenged nurse researchers and practitioners to understand and utilize cultural themes in intervening with these highly traumatized immigrants.

Research Topics

Migration and Stress. The majority of descriptive studies were comparative; Asian Americans' health problems were compared with those of Blacks, Whites, and Hispanic Americans. These studies revealed that Cambodians, Koreans, and Vietnamese often suffered from psychiatric problems, and researchers interpreted this phenomenon in light of acculturative and socioeconomic stress in the host country. Culture-specific somatic symptoms of psychiatric illness were reported in Koreans and Cambodians, and perhaps this is due to the negative attitude toward psychiatry in their cultures.

Culture, Health, and Illness. The majority of Asian Americans, especially those who were foreign born, use both Western medicine and traditional treatment. Educational and clinical reports indicated that although Asian Americans generally believe in and use Western medicine, especially for diagnostic purposes or acute illness treatment, they also use traditional treatments and home remedies like acupuncture, acupressure, herb medicines, massage or amma, moxibustion, cupping, and Qigong (medication). Evaluation of the treatment is based on the quality of the pulse, restoration of appetite, healthy appearance and voice, and the disappearance of symptoms. Studies indicated that Korean (Choi, 1986) and Vietnamese (Wadd, 1983) mothers have continued their cultural practices related to pregnancy, birth, and the postpartum period; for example, they avoid cold (drafts and showers), sexual intercourse, and activity, and encourage bed rest. One departure from traditional birth practices was related to infant feeding with the bottle rather than breast feeding. Jambunathan and Stewart (1995) reported that Laotian women delayed prenatal visits because of fear of miscarriage when touched by doctors and nurses.

A few articles examined the aging population of Japanese and Chinese, reflecting the immigration history of Asian Americans. Several studies revealed that the majority of Asian Americans (except for the Japanese) have language barriers that cause problems in health-seeking behavior and actual treatment. D'Avanzo's (1992) study of Vietnamese revealed that concern about not having a translator in health care facilities ranked as the top barrier to seeking treatment.

Administration and Management. Because of the shortage of nurses in the late 1980s and early 1990s, many foreign nurses were recruited to work in this country. Filipino nurses represent over 75% of these foreign nurses. Articles related to Filipinos have emphasized the importance of well-developed hospital orientation programs for newly recruited Filipino nurses and staff education about Philippine culture and nursing practices. Parallel with international trends in many disciplines, articles about nursing management and administration for Japan were often published after the middle of the 1980s.

Summary

Although the Asian American population doubled during the 1980s, far exceeding the increases seen in other ethnic groups, there are little data to document the physiopsychological conditions, health-seeking behaviors, and health barriers of various Asian Americans. Stereotypes of Asian Americans are pervasive; however, it is critical for nurses who care for Asian Americans to understand their diversity in culture, native language and ability to speak English, time and condition of immigration, educational and socioeconomic levels, and health beliefs. However, for most, knowledge of the health beliefs and practices and issues and problems in health care for Asian Americans was derived from educational reports, clinical experience, or other disciplines rather than from research. Moreover, the data that exist are often skewed in favor of more socioeconomically established Asian Americans or in favor of more traumatized Asian American communities. Because the level of acculturation and socioeconomic status influences differently the barriers and access to health care as well as interactions with health care professionals, these variations should be studied and compared among Asian Americans, Blacks, Whites, and Hispanics.

HAE-OK LEE

See also
CULTURAL/TRANSCULTURAL FOCUS

IMMIGRANT WOMEN
LEININGER'S TRANSCULTURAL NURS-
  ING MODEL
NONTRADITIONAL THERAPIES

MINORITY POPULATIONS: HISPANIC

Hispanics historically have been and will continue to be an important population group in the United States. Currently, Hispanics comprise 9% (22.4 million) of the U.S. population, and because of high fertility rates among certain Hispanic subgroups and continued migration, the Hispanic presence in the United States will continue to grow. Between 1980 and 1990, Hispanics accounted for 35% of the U.S. population growth and are expected to account for 57% of the growth between 2030 and 2050 (U.S. Bureau of the Census, 1993a).

Hispanics are not a monolithic group. The term *Hispanic* was derived by the U.S. Census Bureau to categorize persons of Spanish descent, including those from Mexico, Puerto Rico, Cuba, Spain, and Central and South America. Although Hispanics share many common elements, such as the Spanish language, core values of family, respect, a strong sense of spirituality, and explicit gender differentiation, each subgroup has unique characteristics. As an example, Hispanic subgroups have both a shared and unique history with the United States. The shared history consists of one of migration and conquered nation status. Migration into the United States has been fueled by U.S. labor needs and political and economic unrest in Latin America. The degree to which Hispanics are welcome in the United States is tenuously tied to economic prosperity in this country. It is important to recognize that Hispanics have not only "crossed the border" but, as in the case of Puerto Rico, Cuba, and Mexico, also have had the U.S. border cross over them. Differences in citizenship and refugee status among Hispanic groups are linked to differences in social, economic, political, and health outcomes.

Demographic Characteristics

There are several demographic characteristics of Hispanics that are important to consider. First, His-

panics are younger than the U.S. population, with a median age of 26 years, compared to 34 years among non-Hispanic persons (U.S. Bureau of the Census, 1993a). Second, the importance of the family is evident in family structure. Although the proportion of female-headed households among Hispanic families continues to increase, two-parent families still comprise the largest percentage of family structure type. Further, Hispanic families of all types are more likely to have their own children living at home than are non-Hispanic families (U.S. Bureau of the Census, 1993a). Third, indicators of income consistently show that Hispanics have a lower level of income than that of non-Hispanic families.

Of special significance is that two out of every five Hispanic children under the age of 18 (39.9%) are currently living in poverty, a rate that is two times higher than for non-Hispanic youth (19.5%) (U.S. Bureau of the Census, 1993b). Puerto Rican children living on the mainland have the highest proportion of children living in poverty (57.9%) among all Hispanic children (U.S. Bureau of the Census, 1993a). Unemployment and underemployment are major factors contributing to poverty among Hispanics; they have higher rates of unemployment and, when working in full-time yearlong jobs, are more likely to be living in poverty. Fourth, Hispanics continue to lag behind the U.S. population in educational attainment at all levels. Only 52.6% Hispanics, compared with 81.6% of non-Hispanics, reported that they had at least a high school diploma (U.S. Bureau of the Census, 1993a). A characteristic common to many Hispanics is language; Spanish speakers comprise 54% of all non-English speakers in the United States, with 8.3 million reporting that they do not speak English well or at all.

Health Issues and Priorities

Despite high rates of poverty, limited educational opportunities, and cultural and linguistic barriers to health care, the health issues and priorities of Hispanics are similar in many respects to that of the U.S. population generally. The development of acute and chronic health conditions and causes of death across the life span are similar to those of non-Hispanic Whites.

However, because of high rates of poverty and unemployment, Hispanics are vulnerable to health conditions associated with unsafe environments as well as having limited access to care. For example, there is a higher prevalence of asthma among Puerto Rican youth (Mendoza et al., 1991) and a homicide rate among Hispanic youth that is nearly five times as high as that of non-Hispanic White youth. Also, Mexican-Americans and Puerto Ricans in the United States have increased morbidity and mortality from non-insulin-dependent diabetes mellitus (Maurer, Rosenberg, & Keemer, 1990). Similarly, for some diseases, as in the case of cancer, the incidence of certain cancers may be similar to that of the general population; however, morbidity is higher among Hispanics because of barriers to early detection and treatment.

The incidence of AIDS has disproportionately affected all Hispanics but particularly women and children. The annual rate for AIDS among Hispanic women was 61.9/100,000, compared with 18.5/100,000 among White women, and the cumulative rate of pediatric AIDS cases was three times higher among Hispanic children than among White children (Centers for Disease Control, 1996c). Differential modes of transmission of HIV, as well as rates of infection among Hispanic subgroups, illustrate the importance of considering the unique characteristics, health needs, and resources of each Hispanic subgroup in order to design effective care.

To address the health issue and priorities of this emerging majority, a landmark work group was convened as part of the Surgeon General's National Workshop on Hispanic/Latino Health (1992). Areas identified in which critical action is needed include (a) health data, (b) development of a comprehensive research agenda, (c) access to culturally and linguistically appropriate care, and (d) parity of Hispanic representation in all the health professions.

In relation to data on Hispanic health there is a significant lack, and existing data are insufficient to examine differences among subgroups of Hispanics. For example, in a recent survey of 21 major national data systems of the U.S. Department of Health and Human Services (DHHS), only the U.S. vital statistics system is designed to provide data on all four of the major Hispanic subpopulation groups (Delgado & Estrada, 1993). Furthermore, six of the data systems do not contain sufficient data on Hispanics to permit adequate and meaningful analysis. The development of a comprehensive research agenda is concerned with devising strategies to ensure that research with Hispanics is conducted in a culturally competent manner and, further, that there is an infrastructure in place to develop and support Hispanic researchers. The lack of data on Hispanic health is a major reason Hispanics are omitted from significant health policy initiatives.

A common issue and priority among Hispanics is access to culturally and linguistically appropriate health care. Lack of insurance coverage, whether public or private, is a major barrier in accessing health care. The high proportion of working poor among Hispanics limits access to public or private health insurance. But health insurance is only one component of access. The lack of culturally sensitive and competent providers, lack of access to transportation, lack of linguistic access, and lack of community-based health services have been identified as significant barriers to health promotion and maintenance services. Another priority in improving access to health care concerns is increasing the number of bilingual and bicultural Hispanic health providers. As an example, less than 2% of the registered nurse population is of Hispanic origin, with no significant increase in the number of Hispanics employed in nursing in the past 10 years (*National Sample Survey of Registered Nurses*, 1997).

Implications for Nursing Research and Practice

Nursing has only tangentially begun to examine the health care needs of this growing population. First, nurses must first recognize and understand the political, historical, economic, and social contexts that affect the health of Hispanics. Second, descriptive research must be conducted in nearly all health areas, not only to understand disparities in health outcomes but to recognize the strength and protective factors employed by this population in the areas of health promotion and management of symptoms and disease. Finally, nurses must develop and test interventions that are culturally acceptable and effective.

ANTONIA M. VILLARRUEL

See also
ACCESS TO HEALTH CARE
CULTURAL/TRANSCULTURAL FOCUS
DIABETES MELLITUS
REDUCING HIV RISK ASSOCIATED
    SEXUAL BEHAVIOR AMONG ADO-
    LESCENTS
VIOLENCE AS A NURSING AREA
    OF INQUIRY

MOTHER-INFANT/TODDLER RELATIONSHIPS

The study of mother-infant/toddler relationships centers on knowledge related to the health and development of the mother-child dyad from birth to 3 years. This focus of inquiry is necessarily large because the mother-child system is an open one, responsive to genetic, biological, environmental, cognitive, and psychological influences.

The mother-infant/toddler relationship is influenced by genetic factors. Temperament, for example, is currently viewed as an inherited constellation of traits that affects the individual's behavioral reactions to environmental stimuli. Temperamental qualities in the child, such as high-intensity reactions, low adaptability to change, or shyness, are likely to affect his or her adjustment to day care or changes in daily routines. Similar temperamental qualities in the mother are likely to affect her ability to adjust her parenting behaviors to accommodate an unpredictable infant or a defiant 2-year-old (Gross & Conrad, 1995; Medoff-Cooper, 1995).

Biology plays an important role in parent-child behavior. Differences in infants' abilities to regulate their behavioral and affective responses to stimuli cause some to be irritable and difficult to soothe and others to have extraordinary self-soothing capabilities. Such differences place different demands on the parent, significantly affecting the quality of the mother-child relationship (Keefe, Kotzer,

Froese-Fretz, & Curtin, 1996). Biological influence also may cause toddler boys to be at greater risk than girls for poor physiological and behavioral outcomes (Gross, Conrad, Fogg, Willis, & Garvey, 1995). Infant/toddler disabilities and chronic health problems create additional demands on mothers that affect the nature of their relationships with their children (Holaday, 1987).

The relationship between parenting environment and the mother-infant/toddler relationship has been extensively studied, although the theory underlying cause-and-effect relationships remains underdeveloped. For example, there are many hypotheses to account for the significant associations found between parenting in low-income environments and poorer outcomes in very young children. As a result, interventions for promoting healthy parent-child relationships among low-income families simultaneously target many environmental risk factors (e.g., support, psychological guidance, education, nutrition, and facilitating access to community-based services). The complexity of the parenting environment and the problems inherent in measuring environmental variables make this a particularly difficult area of inquiry (Walker, 1992). Conceptual as well as methodological issues related to studying environmental effects on the mother-infant/toddler relationship are important for future study.

The psychological health of the mother and child has received much attention. Maternal stress, low social support, marital discord, and psychiatric illness have been viewed as important factors placing the young child at risk for poor developmental outcomes (Beck, 1996c; Hall, Gurley, Sachs, & Kryscio, 1991). Recently, researchers have shifted the focus away from unidirectional to bidirectional effects. For example, depressed mothers who are sad, preoccupied, and irritable may be unable to attend to their infant/toddler's needs or deal calmly and effectively with the child's demands for attention. However, it is also possible that behaviorally demanding children cause mothers to feel ineffective, fatigued, and ultimately, depressed. The clinical implications of viewing problems in the mother-infant/toddler relationship as bidirectional is that effective nursing interventions should focus on the mother-child dyad or the family unit rather than on the mother or child alone.

Finally, maternal cognitions affect how mothers interpret and respond to their children's behavior. For example, a mother's belief that it is appropriate to spank her 2-year-old for saying no may be based on a series of cognitions related to her values about child defiance and physical punishment, cultural expectations, perceived environmental dangers, and her general knowledge of child development and other discipline strategies.

Although many investigators have understandably narrowed their research to one or two conceptual areas of inquiry, the dyad is dynamically affected by all of these influences. That is, mothers identify parenting goals and devise child-rearing strategies that are consistent with their temperaments, biology, child-rearing environments, cognitions, and psychological capacities. Likewise, children's responses to parents are similarly tied to these same factors. Future research should refine how these influences transact within the parent-child relationship so that research methods can be clarified and cost-effective nursing interventions disseminated to populations in need.

DEBORAH GROSS

See also
FAMILY THEORY AND RESEARCH
MATERNAL EMPLOYMENT
NEUROBEHAVIORAL DEVELOPMENT
PARENTING RESEARCH IN NURSING
PRESCHOOL CHILDREN

MUSIC THERAPY

Music therapy is the use of a musical intervention to improve physiological and psychological health and well-being. For music to be therapeutic, there must be an interaction between the music and the person who desires a health outcome (Meyer, 1956). Music therapy may be provided by a registered music therapist; however, any member of the health care team may suggest to patients that music can be helpful for stress, pain, mood, or exercise. Nurses can assess musical preferences, offer a choice of selections, and encourage patient involvement in the music with the goal of achieving specific health outcomes.

Throughout history, music has been used for a variety of therapeutic purposes by primitive people—ancient Egyptians, Persians, Hebrews, Greeks, and Romans. Music has been used to ward off evil spirits, prevent or cure illnesses, relieve depression, modify emotions, and achieve inner harmony. Early cultures had little means to treat disease, so music and spirituality were used to provide comfort and help people cope. During the Renaissance, physicians became interested in the scientific basis of healing. Because many physicians were also musicians, they believed in the therapeutic value of music and incorporated it in their training and practice. From the 17th century onward, physicians studied the effect of music on physiology and psychology. During this time there was debate over the need to focus on what type of music was effective versus what type of person responded positively to music. At the beginning of the 20th century, the first laboratory studies of the physiological effects of music were conducted on animals and humans. These experiments demonstrated changes in vital signs and body secretions related to various types of music, but they are rejected by most investigators today because of the poor quality of measurement, analysis, and control. In the 1930s music began to be used in patients' hospital rooms, in surgery prior to general anesthesia, and during local anesthesia. It was used in obstetrics and gynecology to reduce the side effects of inhalation anesthetics. During the past 50 years music has been used to (a) reduce acute, chronic, and cancer pain; (b) reduce stress and anxiety; (c) potentiate the effects of analgesic medications in patients during and after surgery and during labor and delivery; and (d) promote exercise.

Music can stimulate, soothe, encourage, or give pleasure to patients. Music has been found to reduce muscle tension, reduce pain and anxiety, raise levels of beta-endorphins, and lower adrenocorticotropic stress hormones. Nursing reviews of research on the effect of music on health outcomes can be found in chapters by Buckwalter, Hartsock, and Gaffney (1985), Cook (1981), Guzzetta (1988), and Chlan (1998). The *Journal of Music Therapy* is another resource. Music has been found to improve the immune system, salivary cortisol, and cardiac autonomic balance. It has also been investigated for its effect on sleep disturbances, cancer pain, and acute and chronic pain during stressful or painful procedures (e.g., injections and lumbar punctures). Music has been generally found to reduce anxiety before and during surgery, with injections, in chronically ill patients, in intensive care patients, and after myocardial infarction. It has been studied in agitated elderly or psychiatric patients, in critically ill patients, and in those who are comatose or dying.

Music has been categorized into stimulative and sedative types. Stimulative music has strong rhythms, volume, dissonance, and disconnected notes, whereas sedative music has a sustained melody without strong rhythmic or percussive elements. Stimulative music enhances bodily action and stimulates skeletal muscles, emotions, and subcortical reactions in humans. Sedative music results in physical sedation and responses of an intellectual and contemplative nature (Gaston, 1951). Precategorization by the nurse, however, does not consider the kind of subject response.

To choose music that is therapeutic, the nurse should consider the nature of the music, the patient preferences and the health state. Variations in the music include the type of music and the intensity, tempo, rhythm, pitch, tone, timbre, blending, complexity, melody, familiarity, length, variety, and novelty. Variations in the patient include age, sex, cultural background, musical preferences, music training, participation in music, degree of auditory discrepancy, time available, and most of all, degree of liking for the music under consideration. Variations in the nature of the health state determine whether music is needed to cheer, encourage, and soothe or will be used to relax, distract the mind, stimulate exercise, or evoke emotions of joy, triumph, resolve, or peace.

Music is economical for patient use. Tapes, compact discs, and players are relatively inexpensive, and a small library can be maintained on any nursing unit. Music piped into patients' rooms also may be available. Nurses can suggest that patients and their families bring in favorite music from home that is likely to invoke healthy responses. They can refer patients to a music therapist if one is available.

Future research in music may include studies that determine the kinds of music that are effective for health outcomes in countries around the world, between cultures in each country. More work on comparing symptomatic response with physiological response is needed to generate theories of conditions in which music is effective, how it affects body processes, and what effect it has on recovery, immune function, and health.

Music brings an air of normalcy, entertainment, pleasure, and escape into a world where illness is often the enemy and both patients and caregivers are fighting back. Music is an integral part of most people's normal lives and should not be forgotten when they go to hospitals and other health care facilities. With the increased reliance on technology in health care today, music can add a humanistic touch. But beyond the humanistic value of music is the therapeutic value in reducing stress, pain, anxiety, and depression and promoting movement, socialization, and sleep.

MARION GOOD

See also
COPING
NONTRADITIONAL THERAPIES
PAIN MANAGEMENT
STRESS MANAGEMENT
WELLNESS

N

NANDA

Definition

NANDA refers to the classification system of nursing diagnoses developed and published by the North American Nursing Diagnosis Association (NANDA, 1996). Nursing diagnosis, as defined by the association, is a clinical judgment about individual, family, or community responses to actual and potential health problems and life processes. Nursing diagnoses provide the basis for selection of nursing interventions to achieve outcomes for which the nurse is accountable.

Classification, as described by Bailey (1994), is the grouping of entities according to their similarities; it is both a process and an end product. Classification can encompass at least three levels of analysis: the conceptual (where concepts are classified), the empirical (where only empirical concepts are classified), and the combined conceptual/empirical level, where a conceptual classification is first devised and then empirical examples are identified. A conceptual classification is labeled a typology and an empirical classification is a taxonomy. Taxonomies are usually hierarchical, and they are evolutionary.

The NANDA classification system has nine major patterns. Each is defined as a human response pattern and includes the following: choosing, communicating, exchanging, feeling, knowing, moving, perceiving, relating, and valuing. Diagnoses are classified within each pattern according to goodness of fit between the definition of the diagnosis and that of the pattern. As of 1996 there were 128 approved nursing diagnoses that could be used in any appropriate setting. Each diagnosis appears in the published classification with its label, definition, defining characteristics, and related factors.

Diagnoses may be actual or at-risk diagnoses; in the latter case risk factors are identified. The year of acceptance is noted and also the year of revision if applicable.

Development of the Taxonomy

The formal effort to identify, develop, and classify nursing diagnoses began in 1973 with the First National Conference for the Classification of Nursing Diagnoses (NANDA, 1996). Diagnoses were generated by invited conference participants using an inductive format. The participants could not agree on a conceptual basis for classification, so they listed the diagnoses alphabetically. During subsequent conferences a group of nurse theorists focused on development of a conceptual framework. They reviewed the alphabetic list for similarities and grouped the diagnoses into nine patterns, which they called the unitary patterns of man. They also observed that there were different levels of abstraction among the diagnoses.

At the Fifth Conference, in 1982, a special interest taxonomy group sorted the 42 diagnosis labels, approved at that time, using these nine patterns as a horizontal dimension and the levels of abstraction as the vertical dimension, to form an initial taxonomy. The resulting structure was sketched as nine branching or tree diagrams, one tree for each pattern. There were four vertical levels, the lower levels being recognized as the most concrete and clinically applicable and the upper levels as likely labels of category sets. The structure was incomplete, as evidenced by absence of branches necessary to trace a concept through all of its levels. Where obvious gaps existed, the committee suggested a term and placed it in parentheses or indicated a blank box. In the final structure, Level I categories were labeled alterations in human response and were classed under the nine patterns of unitary man. Also at the Fifth Conference, bylaws were adopted for the formation of NANDA.

At the Seventh Conference, in 1986, the term "human response patterns" was adopted to replace "patterns of unitary man." The nine human response patterns became the major category headings, with the second category level referring to alterations. This taxonomy, Taxonomy I, was endorsed by the association for further use and clinical testing. Taxonomy I, Revised, was adopted in 1988. It incorporated newly approved diagnoses and also listed the rules and guidelines for classification. A shortened modification of the rules with the entire taxonomy appears in the Tenth Conference proceedings (Carroll-Johnson & Paquette, 1994). Diagnoses are placed within the taxonomy according to their level of abstraction, consistency with theoretical views in nursing, and consistency with basic definitions within each pattern area. The classification was revised at the 11th and 12th conferences by the additions of further new diagnoses.

Numerical codes are attached to each of the approved diagnoses to indicate its placement within the taxonomy. Patterns are numbered from 1 to 9, with "exchanging" arbitrarily numbered 1. The next level of coding within a pattern reflects alterations. In "exchanging," 1.1 is altered nutrition; 1.2, altered physical regulation; 1.3, altered elimination, and so on. At the next lower level, altered elimination, for example, 1.3.1 is altered bowel elimination, and 1.3.2 is altered urinary elimination. Each lower level in the hierarchy reflects a more concrete concept, with numerical codes ranging up to six digits.

Changes have been proposed in this structure, and recommendations for Taxonomy II were presented at the Ninth Conference, 1990; however, no formal actions have taken place. With the exception of the addition of new diagnoses, the taxonomy has remained unchanged since 1988.

Other Developments

In 1989, NANDA and the American Nursing Association approved and submitted a translation of the taxonomy into code for the *International Classification of Diseases* (ICD). Collaboration has continued with the American Nurses Association (ANA) and others to articulate the taxonomy with other nursing databases and health care databases. NANDA is one of five nursing databases recognized by the ANA. The others are the Nursing Intervention Classification (NIC), the Nursing Outcomes Classification (NOC), the Omaha systems, and the Home Health Care Classification. Efforts to map concepts across these classifications is part of the ANA's goal to develop a Unified Nursing Language System (UNLS) (Lang, 1996). The NANDA diagnoses have been linked to the NIC and to the NOC. NANDA has been included in the metathesaurus for a Unified Medical Language System (UMLS) of the National Library of Medicine, the Systematized Nomenclature of Medicine (SNOMED), and the International Classification of Nursing Practice (ICNP).

Research and Development

Efforts to improve the research base for nursing diagnoses are evident in the proceedings of conferences and in journal publications. Still, there is a recognized lack of consistency in the conceptual and methodological bases of the nursing diagnoses. Different diagnoses have different levels of validity and reliability, and the clarity of the language is challenged. Disagreement exists concerning the conceptualization and utility of the taxonomic structure itself. Some of this doubtlessly reflects the voluntary nature of this work spread over a period of 20-odd years. A collaborative effort is currently underway between NANDA and a University of Iowa team of researchers to do a conceptual analysis, refinement, and validation of the approved diagnoses. The plan includes extension of the classification by addition of other diagnoses and development of a taxonomy using an inductive methodology.

Implications

Fitzpatrick (1990) provides an argument supporting nursing diagnosis as a conceptual approach for developing disciplinary knowledge. Blegen and Tripp-Reimer (1997) suggest that the taxonomies—diagnoses, interventions, and outcomes—provide the structure for the development of middle-range theory in nursing. The concepts within these three taxonomies provide the pillars for the structure, and linking the concepts across the pillars provides the latticework. Explicating the theory that explains the linkage, or relationship, is the substance of nursing knowledge. Such theory will describe the phenomenon of concern (nursing diagnosis) and predict the outcomes from a choice of nursing interventions. This will add to our disciplinary knowledge and guide nursing practice.

LOIS M. HOSKINS

See also
NORTH AMERICAN NURSING DIAGNOSIS ASSOCIATION
NURSING DIAGNOSIS
NURSING INTERVENTIONS CLASSIFICATION
NURSING OUTCOMES CLASSIFICATION (NOC)
TAXONOMY

NARRATIVE ANALYSIS

Narrative analysis is gaining popularity among nurse researchers as one of the representative modes of studying human experiences, of both clients and nurses, especially from the perspective of interpretivism. Narrative analysis is being used in many different disciplines: literary studies, linguistics, anthropology, psychology, sociology, theology, history, and practice disciplines such as nursing, medicine, occupational therapy, and social work.

All sorts of oral and written representations are considered narratives—fables, folktales, short stories, case histories, exemplars, news reports, personal stories, historiography, interview data, and so forth. Although there are controversies, the term *narrative* in narrative analysis refers to a story that contains two or more sequentially ordered units, with a beginning, middle, and ending, and represents structured meaning. Narratives are structured about a story plot or plots illustrated by characters (actors) and events. Narratives as stories are characterized by a sense of internal chronology (either temporal or thematic) and connectedness that brings about coherence and sense making. Narratives differ from discourse in that narratives contain descriptions of chronologically articulated events along with sketches of characters of that story.

As narratives are human linguistic products, their construction is closely tied to "story-telling," that is, the processes involved in producing them. Story-telling is often the object of analysis, along with narratives themselves, in narrative analysis.

The heterogeneity of narratives, representative disciplinary plurality, and the varieties in narrative theories have evidenced in various approaches and orientations in narrative analysis. There are at least three diverse orientations within narrative analysis: (a) structural orientation, (b) story-telling orientation, and (c) interpretive orientation (for other ways of categorizing narrative analysis and a typology of models, see Mishler, 1995).

Structural Orientation

Structural orientation can be identified with structuralists such as Barthes (1974) and sociolinguists such as Labov (1972) and Gee (1991). In this orientation, narratives are thought to be organized about a specific set of structural units that bring about coherence and connectivity in the narratives. Attention to narrative structures is analytically juxtaposed to such aspects as functions that different structural units perform—sense making in story, or narrativity.

Narrative analysis in the structuralist tradition within literary studies and linguistics focuses on structural-functional connections, as in Propp's (1968) morphology in relation to internal patterning and narrative genre and in Genette's (1988) three specific aspects of a story's temporal articulation (i.e., order, frequency, and duration). In this tradition, narratives subjected to analysis tend to be public material such as folktales, novels, short stories, and case histories.

Sociolinguists attend to "natural" or "situated" narratives, which are constructions produced in specific situations of social life. Labov (1972) identified six structural units for fully formed narratives: abstract, orientation, complicating action, evaluation, resolution, and coda. He suggested that these structural units are related to two functions in narrative: the referential function and the evaluative function. Gee (1991), on the other hand, identified structural properties of narrative as poetic structures of lines, stanzas, or strophes, which organize meaning constructions in telling a story. The structural orientation is primarily an examination of structural elements of story in relation to the narrative's form, function, and meaning.

Story-Telling Orientation

In story-telling, narratives are not viewed simply as products that can be taken out of the context of narrating but as process-oriented constructions that are enmeshed with linguistic materialization of cognition and memory, interactive structuring between the teller and listener, and contextually and culturally constrained shaping of experiences and ideas. From this standpoint, narrative analysis is closely aligned with discourse analysis, as in ethnography of communication in anthropology and ethnomethodology in sociology.

Narrative analysis in this orientation is differentiated into two schools: linguistic/cognitive and sociocultural. The linguistic/cognitive version focuses on how narratives are materialized in language from ideas and experiences. This construction is viewed to be accomplished by applying communicative and interactive functions of language and through scripting and schematizing of yet unorganized information into connected story-telling. In this version, story-telling is considered as the processing of nonlinguistic ideas, events, and actions into a series of connected and coherent representation of meanings.

On the other hand, narrative analysis in the sociological version within the ethnomethodological tradition is concerned with the interactive process of narrative making. Conversational narratives are of prime interest. The listener is an active part of story-telling as an interactive participant in the making of a story. From an anthropological perspective, story-telling is viewed as bounded by cultural conditions and cultural categories. Narrative analysis in this orientation carries out an analysis of narrative texts in terms of form and content, along with an analysis of the flow of story-telling, with the assumption that the nature of narrative text is integrally connected to the processes of construction.

Interpretive Orientation

Narratives in the interpretive orientation are chronological in a double sense: chronology in terms of temporal serialization of events and chronology in terms of temporality of story itself. Ricoeur (1984) specified episodic and configurational dimensions as the temporal dialectics that integrated plot in narrative. Hence, narratives are stories of individuals etched within the communal stories of the time and context. Narrative analysis thus involves interpretation of representation posed within the contexts in which the story is shaped and the story-telling occurs, reflecting on the worldviews that provide a larger contextual understanding. In this sense, the interpretative orientation is more concerned with meaning of narratives than with either the structure or the process.

Riessman (1993) offers five levels of representation in the research process of narrative analysis: attending, telling, transcribing, analyzing, and reading. Interpretation occurs at the levels of transcribing and analyzing by the researcher, whereas the level of reading implies additional interpretation that occurs in the readers of research reports. Riessman favors the use of poetic structures as the mode of structuring narratives as interpretive; however, the use of any specific structuring model is less critical for the analysis than interpretation.

Although there are distinct differences among these orientations, there are many hybrid forms of narrative analysis used in actual research practice. Hybrid forms often combine analysis of process or meaning with structural analysis. In nursing research, narrative analysis has been applied with various orientations and in different hybrid forms. Narratives of clients' personal experiences, such as suffering, being diagnosed with cancer, isolation, and dying, have been studied by applying Labov or Gee as well as within the story-telling orientation. Narratives of practice by nurses have been subjected to analyses in the interpretive orientation for understanding the meanings of their practice and their value orientations. In addition, the interpretive orientation from the feminist perspective has been used to study women's experiences, such as health care seeking, pregnancy with the history of drug abuse, and recovery. Research of narrative accounts of clients and nurses, as well as their interactions, can produce deep understanding of human experiences that are fundamental to nursing practice.

HESOOK SUZIE KIM

See also
DISCOURSE ANALYSIS
ETHNOGRAPHY
QUALITATIVE RESEARCH

NATIONAL INSTITUTE OF NURSING RESEARCH

The National Institute of Nursing Research (NINR) is one of 24 institutes, centers, and divisions that comprise the National Institutes of Health (NIH). The NIH is one of eight health agencies of the Public Health Service in the U.S. Department of Health and Human Services. Headquartered in 75 buildings on more than 300 acres in Bethesda, Maryland, the NIH is the steward of biomedical and behavioral research for the nation. Its mission is to improve the health of the American people through increased understanding of the processes underlying human health and the acquisition of new knowledge to help prevent, detect, diagnose, and treat disease. Approximately 80% of the annual NIH investment is made through grants and contracts to support extramural research and training in more than 1,700 universities; medical, dental, and nursing schools; hospitals; and other research institutions throughout the United States and abroad. About 10% of its budget goes to the more than 2,000 projects conducted in its own intramural laboratories.

Creation of the NINR

In 1996 the NINR celebrated the 10th anniversary of its establishment at the NIH. Originally designated as the National Center for Nursing Research by Public Law 99-158 in 1986, it attained institute status through the NIH Revitalization Act of 1993. Its budget of $16 million in 1986 had grown to $59 million in 1997. The original staff of 9 members has increased to approximately 50 people, including scientists, administrators, and support staff.

Nursing research is a relative newcomer to the scientific community. Unlike other health-related disciplines, nursing began as an occupation in hospital settings, not as a discipline in academic institutions. Although there is a history of nurses receiving advanced degrees in many different academic fields, it has been only within the past 25 years that doctoral preparation has been available in the field of nursing, paving the way for nursing research to grow and flourish at universities and research centers.

The mission of the NINR supports basic and clinical research to establish a scientific basis for the care of individuals across the life span—from management of patients during illness and recovery to the reduction of risks for disease and disability and the promotion of healthy lifestyles. With this broad mandate, the institute seeks to understand and ease the symptoms of acute and chronic illness, to prevent or delay the onset of disease or slow its progression, to find effective approaches to promoting good health, and to improve the clinical settings in which care is provided. The NINR supports research on problems encountered by patients' families and caregivers. It also emphasizes the special needs of at-risk and underserved populations. These efforts are crucial in translating scientific advances into cost-effective health care that does not compromise quality.

NINR Leadership

The first NINR director, Dr. Ada Sue Hinshaw, who held the position from 1987 to 1994, is widely recognized for her contributions to teaching, nursing research, and academic administration. Under her leadership the institute was established as an active participant within the federal research community and achieved national recognition for nursing research. The current director, Dr. Patricia A. Grady, an internationally recognized stroke researcher, was appointed in 1995, following positions as deputy director and acting director of the National Institute of Neurological Disorders and Stroke.

National Advisory Council for Nursing Research

The NIH employs a two-level system for reviewing grant applications. In the first level, panels of extramural experts evaluate the scientific merit of the proposed research. The second level of review is carried out by national advisory councils, which consider scientific merit as determined in the first level of review, program relevance, and appropriate allocation of resources. Councils also advise on policy development, program implementation, evaluation, and other matters of importance to the missions and goals of the NIH institutes and centers. Advisory councils are composed of scientific and lay representatives who are noted for their expertise or interest in issues related to the missions of the institutes and centers they serve.

The NINR's advisory council—the National Advisory Council for Nursing Research—is composed of 15 members. Ten are leaders in the health and scientific disciplines relevant to the activities of the NINR, and five public members are leaders in health care, public policy, law, and economics. The advisory council also includes six ex officio members: the secretary of the Department of Health and Human Services (DHHS), the NIH director, the chief nursing officer of the Department of Veterans Affairs, the assistant secretary for health affairs of the Department of Defense, and the director of the Division of Nursing, Health Resources and Services Administration, DHHS.

Mechanisms of Research Support

NIH award mechanisms are divided into three categories: grants, contracts, and cooperative agreements. The primary mechanism used by the NINR is the investigator-initiated grant. This mechanism supports research and research training projects for which the applicant develops the protocol, concept, method, and approach. It includes research projects (R01s), First Independent Research Support and Transition (FIRST) awards (R29s), and Research Scientist Development awards (K01s). In certain instances, the NINR may solicit applications for special mechanisms such as core center grants (P30s) and small research grants (R03s). The NINR uses the cooperative agreement mechanism, which supports the recipient's activities and provides for substantial involvement of the funding agency during the period of performance. The NINR also supports research training through individual and institutional National Research Service awards (F31s, F32s, F33s, and T32s).

Recent Research Accomplishments

The following scientific advances illustrate some of the contributions of nursing research funded by NINR that have led to improved health.

Risk assessment. Investigators have created a rating scale that optimizes prediction of pressure sore development in an older patient population. The ability to identify individuals at risk within a few days of nursing home admission permits timely intervention, limiting further deterioration in these patients and leading to major decreases in the enormous annual health care costs for long-term wound care.

Risk reduction. A study to test stroke patients' responses to intense exercise and aerobic training demonstrated that moderately disabled individuals could improve their aerobic capacity with exercise training. Aerobic training also reduced exercise systolic blood pressure levels. This result has implications for reducing the risk of future strokes in patients who respond to everyday activities and exercise with a significant rise in blood pressure.

Recovery from trauma. Using a canine model, researchers found that the preadministration of an antioxidant, deferoxamine, is effective in absorbing metabolic toxins that are formed when brain tissue and cells are deprived of sufficient oxygen after severe head injury. This study points to a potential target for therapeutic intervention following trauma to the brain.

Symptom management. A study was undertaken to determine whether symptoms associated with changes in gastrointestinal function during certain phases of the menstrual cycle are related to ovarian hormone activity or other factors. The results clearly demonstrated that ovarian hormones modulate gastrointestinal function. Because estrogen receptors exist along the length of the gastrointestinal tract, this research suggests that ovarian hormones may have a direct effect on gastric muscles or nerve elements within the gut wall, thus producing the intestinal symptoms associated with the menstrual cycle.

Transitional care from hospital to home. Researchers have designed a program to prepare patients for hospital discharge and provide support at home under the guidance of an advanced practice nurse. This versatile program, which can be tailored to diverse patient populations and types of hospital facilities, has demonstrated significant cost savings and patient satisfaction in several high-risk, high-cost, or high-volume patient groups. The program not only affords the benefits of early hospital discharge but also reduces the occurrence of rehospitalizations and increased physician visits.

Gender differences in response to treatment. Two kappa-opioids, nalbuphine and butorphanol, were found to produce significantly greater pain relief in women than in men, even though the women reported higher amounts of pain initially. In the past, studies suggested that kappa-opioids were less effective than mu-opioids in pain management. The discrepancy between the studies may result from the fact that previous experiments relied heavily on men rather than women and obscured evidence that kappa-opioids were a good analgesic for treating women's pain.

Areas of NINR Research Emphasis

As the NINR identifies new opportunities for research, nursing researchers are moving to the forefront of many innovative areas of scientific exploration. For example, the NINR is responding to the clinical implications of genetics discoveries with research programs in the clinical management of conditions associated with genetic disorders, including genetic screening and counseling, clinical decision making, and bioethical considerations. Nursing researchers are also taking the lead in the remediation of cognitive impairment, the prevention and control of pain, and the management of side effects associated with medical treatment. In addition, nursing research focuses on methods to stem microbial threats to health through improved approaches to prevention and adherence to treatment. NINR-funded research also links biological and behavioral approaches to health care. A further area of research interest is the role of cultural sensitivity as a factor in health research and health care.

The NINR research portfolio is broad, invites collaboration among many disciplines, and is co-sponsored by most of the other NIH research institutes and centers. The NINR supports research across six major areas: (1) neurofunction and sensory conditions; (2) reproductive and infant health; (3) immune, infectious, and neoplastic diseases; (4) cardiopulmonary and acute illnesses; (5) metabolic and other chronic illnesses; and (6) human development and health risk behaviors. Individuals who are interested in submitting applications for grants to conduct research in areas of interest to the institute are encouraged to contact the NINR program staff at the following address and telephone number to discuss research opportunities and proposed areas of investigation before embarking on the application process. Division of Extramural Activities, National Institute of Nursing Research, NIH, Building 45, Room 3AN-12, 45 Center Drive, MSC 6300, Bethesda, MD 20892-6300; telephone: (301) 594-6906. General questions regarding the NINR may be addressed to Office of Science Policy and Information, National Institute of Nursing Research, NIH, Building 31, Room 5B13, 31 Center Drive, MSC 2178, Bethesda, MD 20892-2178; telephone: (301) 496-0207.

PATRICIA A. GRADY

See also
FUNDING
GENDER RESEARCH
GRANTSMANSHIP

NATIONAL INSTITUTES OF HEALTH
TRANSITIONAL CARE

NATIONAL INSTITUTES OF HEALTH

Begun as the one-room Laboratory of Hygiene in 1887, the National Institutes of Health (NIH) today is one of the world's foremost biomedical research centers. Although the institution's roots extend back over a century, the "modern" NIH dates from the years following World War II, when growing awareness of public health needs converged with new scientific capabilities and an increased national investment in health-related science. As the federal focal point for health research, the NIH is one of eight health agencies of the Public Health Service, which, in turn, is part of the U.S. Department of Health and Human Services. The NIH is composed of 24 separate institutes, centers, and divisions, each focused on a particular aspect of health research. The NIH has 75 buildings on more than 300 acres in Bethesda, Maryland. From about $300 in 1887, the NIH budget has grown to nearly $14 billion as of 1997.

Since its inception the NIH has had 14 directors. The first was Dr. Joseph James Kinyoun, who was the founder and director of the Laboratory of Hygiene that later grew to become the NIH. Dr. Harold E. Varmus became the current director on November 23, 1993. The winner of the Nobel Prize in 1989 for his work in cancer research, he came to NIH from the University of California, San Francisco. He is a leader in the study of cancer-causing genes, called oncogenes, and an internationally recognized authority on retroviruses, the viruses that cause AIDS and many cancers in animals.

NIH Institutes, Centers, and Divisions

National Cancer Institute (NCI)

National Eye Institute (NEI)

National Heart, Lung, and Blood Institute (NHLBI)

National Institute on Aging (NIA)

National Institute on Alcohol Abuse and Alcoholism (NIAAA)

National Institute of Allergy and Infectious Diseases (NIAID)

National Institute of Arthritis and Musculoskeletal and Skin Diseases (NIAMS)

National Institute of Child Health and Human Development (NICHD)

National Institute on Deafness and Other Communication Disorders (NIDCD)

National Institute of Dental Research (NIDR)

National Institute of Diabetes and Digestive and Kidney Diseases (NIDDK)

National Institute on Drug Abuse (NIDA)

National Institute of Environmental Health Sciences (NIEHS)

National Institute of General Medical Sciences (NIGMS)

National Institute of Mental Health (NIMH)

National Institute of Neurological Disorders and Stroke (NINDS)

National Institute of Nursing Research (NINR)

National Human Genome Research Institute (NHGRI)

National Library of Medicine (NLM)

National Center for Research Resources (NCRR)

John E. Fogarty International Center (FIC)

Warren Grant Magnuson Clinical Center (CC)

Division of Computer Research and Technology (DCRT)

Division of Research Grants (DRG)

The NIH website at http://www.nih.gov contains links to each of the above organizations' websites, which contain information on their missions and activities in support of research (Office of Communications, 1996).

The NIH Mission, Goals, and Research Support

The NIH is the steward of biomedical and behavior research for the nation. Its mission is science in pursuit of fundamental knowledge about the nature and behavior of living systems and the application of that knowledge to extend healthy life and reduce the burdens of illness and disability. The NIH works toward that mission by conducting clinical and basic research in its own laboratories, supporting research institutions throughout the country and abroad, helping in the training of research investigators, and fostering communication of information on health improvement.

The goals of the agency are as follows: (a) to foster fundamental creative discoveries, innovative research strategies, and their applications as a basis to advance significantly the nation's capacity to protect and improve health; (b) to develop, maintain, and renew scientific human and physical resources that will assure the nation's capability to prevent disease; (c) to expand the knowledge base in biomedical and associated sciences in order to enhance the nation's economic well-being and ensure a continued high return on the public investment in research; and (d) to exemplify and promote the highest level of scientific integrity, public accountability, and social responsibility in the conduct of science.

In realizing these goals the NIH provides leadership and direction to programs designed to improve the health of the nation by conducting and supporting research in the causes, diagnosis, prevention, and cure of human diseases; in the processes of human growth and development; in the biological effects of environmental contaminants; and in the understanding of mental, addictive, and physical disorders. The NIH also directs programs for the collection, dissemination, and exchange of information in medicine, nursing, and health, including the development and support of medical libraries and the training of medical librarians and other health information specialists (National Institutes of Health, 1996).

The NIH invests more than 81% of the annual appropriation from Congress in grants and contracts supporting research and training in more than 1,700 research institutions throughout the United States and abroad. NIH grantees are located in every state and territory. Their grants and contracts comprise the NIH Extramural Research Program. Approximately 11% of the budget goes to NIH's Intramural

Research Programs, the more than 2,000 projects conducted mainly in its own laboratories. About 8% of the budget is for both intramural and extramural research support costs (Office of Communications, 1996).

Current Areas of Research Emphasis

Each year, after reviewing the state of scientific knowledge and opportunity, the NIH director identifies areas of research emphasis that show the most promise for addressing public health needs and yielding medical advances that will lead to improvements in human health. Accordingly, six areas of research emphasis have been identified for fiscal year (FY) 1998 (U.S. Department of Health and Human Services, 1997).

The Biology of Brain Disorders. The neurosciences continue to grow at an extraordinary pace, with strong support from the fields of molecular genetics, imaging, and cell biology and signaling. The NIH anticipates expanded activity in the areas of neural development; neurodegeneration, especially in Alzheimer's disease, Parkinson's disease, and eye disorders; the biological basis of autism; physiology of pain in adults and newborns; brain imaging during drug and alcohol abuse and behavioral change; traumatic injury to the brain and spinal cord; the use of mouse models to study disease, addiction, behavior, and the regulation of weight and appetite; and the genetic basis of neurological diseases, including hearing impairment.

New Approaches to Pathogenesis. A more precise understanding of genes, proteins, and cells is transforming traditional descriptions of disease processes. In FY 1998 the NIH anticipates expanded efforts directed to the following goals: developing improved animal models to study carcinogenesis; understanding the mechanisms that cause the heart to fail as a pump; developing new methods for integrating information about complex biological processes; and applying new and diverse methods to the study of osteoarthritis, birth defects and growth disorders, and infections of the liver, lung, and gastrointestinal tract.

New Preventive Strategies Against Disease.   New insights into pathogenesis are stimulating tests to develop methods for preventing disease in both animal models and human populations. The disorders that will receive increased attention in FY 1998 include cancers, diabetes mellitus, cerebral palsy, asthma, and alcohol and drug abuse. Infectious agents continue to be a major cause of morbidity; efforts will be made to develop new vaccines against a variety of pathogens, especially HIV, and to expand research on new and resurgent infections. Behavior-based preventive strategies against HIV also will be emphasized. Changes in national and global demographic profiles are occurring rapidly; the NIH will accelerate efforts to understand the significance of these changes with respect to prevention research. Increased emphasis also will be given to training health professionals to guide the use of new genetic information that can promote prevention of disease.

New Avenues for Development of Therapeutics.   Chemistry, structural biology, genetic information, and advances in cell biology are providing new means to design therapies for a variety of diseases. In this newly identified NIH area of emphasis, the NIH will expand efforts to discover and develop drugs to combat cancer and drug and alcohol addiction; to use methods of bioengineering to repair tissues; to use methods for treatment of neurological diseases, alcoholism, and drug addiction; to intervene in infectious disease; to treat sensory disorders and mental illnesses in both children and adults; and to improve care at the end of life.

Genetic Medicine.   The rapid progress of the Human Genome Project, a growing understanding of the genomes of other species, and new methods for the manipulation of genes are swiftly changing concepts of disease and possibilities for its control. Broadened efforts in FY 1998 to hasten the arrival of gene-based medicine include efforts to improve the efficiency of genetic analysis and distribution of gene maps and sequences; define the genetic damage in different types of cancer cells (the Cancer Genome Anatomy Project); and identify the inherited mutations that contribute to cancer risk, developmental abnormalities, immunodeficiencies,

and mental and neurological diseases (e.g., epilepsy, stroke, autism, alcoholism, ataxias, psychoses, and sensory and neurodegenerative disorders). In addition, by developing new markers to assess gene-environment interactions, efforts to address the impact of the environment on genetic integrity will be expanded.

Advanced Instrumentation and Computers in Medicine and Research.   Recent advances in basic biology, genetics, diagnosis, and health care have been closely linked to the development of new research instruments and computer hardware and software. In FY 1998 the NIH proposes to support new initiatives to improve detection of early cancers; to determine DNA sequences and analyze them more readily; to provide better communication links for research groups and physicians; and to visualize the central nervous system and the eye with greater accuracy, using a variety of sophisticated imaging methods.

NIH Impact on the Health of the Nation

NIH research played a major role in making possible the following achievements of the past few decades (Office of Communications, 1996):

1. Mortality from heart disease, the number-1 killer in the United States, dropped by 41% between 1971 and 1991.
2. Death rates from strokes decreased by 59% during the same period.
3. Improved treatments and detection methods increased the relative 5-year survival rate for people with cancer to 52%. At present, the survival gain over the rate that existed in the 1960s represents more than 80,000 additional cancer survivors each year.
4. Paralysis from spinal cord injury is significantly reduced by rapid treatment with high doses of a steroid. Treatment given within the first 8 hours after injury increases recovery in severely injured patients who have lost sensation or mobility below the point of injury.

5. Long-term treatment with anticlotting medicines cuts stroke risk by 80% from a common heart condition known as atrial fibrillation.

6. In schizophrenia, where suicide is always a potential danger, new medications have reduced troublesome symptoms such as delusions and hallucinations in 80% of patients.

7. Chances for survival have increased for infants with respiratory distress syndrome, an immaturity of the lungs, because of development of a substance to prevent the lungs from collapsing. In general, life expectancy for a baby born today is almost three decades longer than one born at the beginning of the century.

8. Those suffering from depression now look forward to returning to work and leisure activities, thanks to treatments that have given them an 80% chance to resume a full life in a matter of weeks.

9. Vaccines protect against infectious diseases that once killed and disabled millions of children and adults.

10. Dental sealants have proved 100% effective in protecting the chewing surfaces of children's molars and premolars, where most cavities occur.

11. Molecular genetics and genomics research has revolutionized biomedical science. In the 1980s and 1990s researchers performed the first trial of gene therapy in humans and were able to locate, identify, and describe the function of many of the genes in the human genome. Scientists predict this new knowledge will lead to genetic tests to diagnose diseases such as colon, breast, and other cancers and to the eventual development of preventive drug treatments for individuals in families known to be at risk. The ultimate goal is to develop screening tools and gene therapies for the general population, not only for cancer but for many other diseases.

PATRICIA A. GRADY

See also
ALZHEIMER'S DISEASE

FUNDING
GENETICS IN NURSING RESEARCH
HIV/AIDS: CARE AND TREATMENT
NATIONAL INSTITUTE OF NURSING
RESEARCH

NATIONAL LEAGUE FOR NURSING

Historical Perspective

Since its inception the National League for Nursing (NLN) has developed and conducted research studies to evaluate nursing education and practice. The NLN also serves as a repository for numerous historical documents such as *Schools of Nursing Accredited by the State Board of Nurse Examiners*, dating back to 1918, and journals such as *Public Health Nursing*, dating back to 1920.

The NLN was formed when three nursing organizations and four national committees joined together in 1952 (Jensen, 1955). These groups were the National League of Nursing Education, National Organization for Public Health Nursing, Association of Collegiate Schools of Nursing, Joint Committee on Practical Nurses and Auxiliary Workers in Nursing Services, Joint Committee on Careers in Nursing, National Committee for the Improvement of Nursing Services, and National Nursing Accrediting Service. The two main divisions of the newly formed NLN were the Division of Nursing Services, consisting of the departments of hospital nursing, public health nursing, and industrial nursing, and the Division of Nursing Education, consisting of the departments of diploma and associate degree programs and baccalaureate and higher degree programs (Fillmore, Sheahan, & Miller, 1953).

Research was an integral function for each division. The Division of Nursing Services was responsible for conducting studies to examine how nursing services could be organized for maximum effectiveness and to develop criteria to evaluate nursing services. For example, in 1953 the Department of Public Health Nursing conducted a study on public health nurses with a focus on salaries. The Division of Nursing Education was responsible for conducting studies on curriculum development, examining expected proficiency of graduates from practical and basic nursing programs, and also maintaining extensive record keeping on the schools of nursing. In 1953 the division conducted a study to examine the proficiency level of nurses and the purpose of the type of program that prepared them.

Although some research involved new initiatives, other projects built on the framework established by preexisting organizations. In 1951 the National League of Nursing Education examined whether criteria such as selection tests for practical nursing students and personal characteristics were related to performance in practical nurse programs and the licensing exam. The study continued after the reorganization, with the findings reported by the NLN (1954).

The precursor of the current annual survey of nursing education programs was conducted by the National League of Nursing Education, with the Department of Studies analyzing trends in nursing education. A review of student enrollments from 1935 through 1947 showed that historical events clearly influenced the trend. In discussing a 22% increase in student enrollment between 1941 and 1947, the Department of Studies staff concluded:

> Nearly every nursing school has enlarged its student body—the good school, the medium school, and the poor school. During the war period country-wide expansion was accepted as an emergency necessity. But is it not now time for schools to take stock of themselves? Should they not review their educational objectives and consider the extent to which they are able to put those objectives into effect? (National League of Nursing Education, 1947, p. 490)

Over the years, NLN research continued to examine issues related to both education and practice, such as (a) organization and activities of hospital nursing services (1964), (b) the student selection process in schools of nursing (1975), (c) accreditation policies and procedures for schools of nursing (1980), (d) salaries of full-time employees of community health services (1983), and (e) use and development of microcomputer software in nursing schools (1984).

Contemporary Focus and Issues

More recent research projects include the educational and demographic characteristics of foreign-educated nurses, experiences of "nontraditional" students in practical nursing programs, skills required by newly licensed registered nurses within the current health care system, and preparedness of nursing students to care for people with HIV/AIDS. On a biennial basis, NLN research has tracked demographic and employment characteristics of nursing faculty and newly licensed nurses for over 25 years.

The annual survey of nursing programs has been performed for over 60 years, documenting the number of programs and the direction of nursing education. In 1953 there were 1,017 diploma programs, 21 associate degree programs, and 198 baccalaureate programs (NLN, 1953). In 1995 there were 119 diploma programs, 876 associate degree programs, and 521 baccalaureate programs.

As the program types have changed, debates have ensued over the impact on both education and practice. In reporting the results from the 1975 annual survey, Dr. Walter Johnson of the NLN Division of Research stated that although there was little change in the total number of RN programs over a 3-year period, the distribution of programs changed with a decline in the number of diploma programs and an increase in the number of associate degree and baccalaureate programs. In his analysis, Dr. Johnson (1976) concluded:

> The real question is not whether a zero growth rate, coming at the end of this period of expansion, is good or not good for nursing education. Considering the current level of output of all types of basic programs, the significant question is: Is the current and projected mix of RN graduates (baccalaureate, associate degree, and diploma) and the number of practical nurses being graduated likely to match the requirements for beginning licensed practitioners? In other words, to what extent will the supply match the demand for nursing personnel over the next few years, assuming that current growth rates continue? (pp. 569–570)

After 20 years, Dr. Johnson's question is still an issue. In 1997, nurse faculty are reexamining their curricula to deal with hospital "reengineering" so that their graduates have the necessary skills to work in this changing health care environment. For example, do our graduates get enough learning experiences centered on health, community systems, collaboration, interdisciplinary teams, clinical outcomes, and informatics? In response,

NLN's Division of Research, now the Center for Research in Nursing Education and Community Health, is monitoring these efforts with the 1997 newly licensed nurse survey by asking nurses to indicate the skills required in their jobs and whether these skills were taught in their nursing education programs. To address Dr. Johnson's questions, data analyses will assess the match of current curricula with current health care settings and whether the match is found across the three types of basic nursing education.

SHEILA RYAN

See also
AMERICAN NURSES ASSOCIATION
NURSING EDUCATION

NATIVE AMERICAN HEALTH

Native American and *American Indian* are the most common terms for the pre-Columbian inhabitants of North America, exclusive of Alaska Natives and Aleuts. The definition of Native American (NA) is a politically and emotionally charged issue. The most common definitions for research purposes are enrollment in a federally recognized tribe, degree of Indian blood (blood quantum), and self-identification. Researchers should use the group term and criteria preferred by their study populations.

Native Americans have greater morbidity and mortality and lower quality of life than the dominant culture and other minorities in the United States. High rates of poverty, low levels of education and literacy, and long distances to health care facilities characterize many NA groups. Postneonatal deaths and deaths from sudden infant death syndrome are twice as common among NAs as in the general population. The NA death rate from alcoholism is four times higher than the national average; ramifications include very high rates of fetal alcohol syndrome, spouse and child abuse and neglect, accidents, homicide, and suicide. AIDS, secondary to intravenous drug use, is increasing rapidly among NAs, and drug-resistant tuberculosis is emerging. The prevalence of diabetes in many tribes of NAs ranges from 20% to 50%, and cancer

diagnoses and deaths are increasing as more NAs live longer. The population is young, with a median age of 24.2, compared to 32.9 for all races. The NA birth rate is nearly double that of other Americans. The number of NAs surviving to old age is also increasing rapidly.

Nurses represent an underused resource for research on NA health. Nursing's focus on the holistic understanding of human experience and cultural perspectives as a precondition for effective health care is often more consistent with traditional NA values than the biomedical perspective is. The Indian Health Service has called for increased emphasis on nursing research, particularly on the control of chronic disease, and for more qualitative research, which it considers especially appropriate to eliciting NA cultural perspectives.

A search of CINAHL and MEDLINE located 55 nursing studies of NA health since 1982. Of these, 10 were from Canada, where the health of "aboriginals" or "First Nations" is also of concern. Nursing research on NA health is more tribally diverse than that by other disciplines, which focused disproportionately on Southwestern tribes. Only 7 nursing reports were on the Navajo, whereas 19 other tribes were named. The remaining reports referred only to NAs or did not identify the tribe or village in conformity with tribal preferences. The most frequently studied topics were health beliefs and practices (9), diabetes (8), instrumentation (6), alcoholism (6), and prenatal and infant care (5).

Most studies of NA health are descriptive, using small convenience samples, interviews, or, less frequently, written questionnaires. Very few are multidisciplinary, and no multistudy programmatic research was identified. Intervention studies, particularly those with evidence of community participation or true adaptation for the cultures, are rare. Hagey's (1984) account of the use of Ojibway legends to teach about diabetes is an outstanding example of both.

The majority of studies are not conceptually based. Of those that are, the most frequently used frameworks are Leininger's culture care theory, health belief models, caring, marginalization, and illness representations. Qualitative methods such as content analysis, ethnography, and focus groups are widely used for exploration of cultural patterns, values, and lifestyles. They are appropriate for people with strong oral traditions and avoid the problem of inappropriate application of Western frameworks to non-Western cultures. Such methods are especially useful for the development of much needed community-based interventions, as they are closer to the experiential approach that Native communities use to identify and resolve local problems. They should not, however, be used uncritically. For studies driven by the mission of nursing rather than pure cultural knowledge, other designs and methods may be more appropriate.

Nurses are showing a commendable interest in the problems of instrumentation in NA research. For example, they have explored the meaning of social support among Navajo women and the appropriateness of the Nursing Child Assessment Satellite Training (NCAST) instruments for studying NA parenting.

A small nursing literature on research access to and collaboration with NA communities is developing. Jacobson (1994) summarized recommendations by NA authors and non-NA investigators for successful research with NAs. These recommendations include (a) investigators' comprehensive knowledge of the NA culture, (b) planning of research that meets the felt needs of the NA community, (c) use of paid NA advisors and fieldworkers, (d) use of NA homes as primary sites for data collection and education, and (e) sharing research results with NA communities in a style meaningful to them. Jacobson (1994) and colleagues described the process of learning about a Native culture and planning and conducting collaborative research with a NA community. A disturbing aspect of many research reports on NA health is the absence of evidence of cultural knowledge, of the need to build trust and rapport before beginning the research, and of the historic, social, and political histories of NAs that hinder open communication with external investigators.

Researchers from other disciplines have identified a number of difficulties that external researchers in NA communities may encounter. The turbulent history of NA–U.S. government relations has engendered profound distrust of outsiders. Researchers often experience a long period of appraisal, skepticism, and questioning of their purpose for being in the community, a process that John (1990) termed "running the gauntlet." Tribal approval of research often takes much longer than researchers expect; periods of up to 3 years are not uncommon. NAs often resist comparative designs or randomization to treatments ("If it's a good idea, then everyone should get it"). Random samples are rarely obtained because of the lack of lists to serve as a sampling frame. Both individuals and tribes have resisted evaluation of interventions on the grounds of intrusiveness or fears that the program might be stopped. Tracking NA subjects over time can be difficult because of distance, low literacy, low telephone saturation, and migration between rural and urban locales.

The first need in nursing research on NA health is for more of it. Given its small volume, no restrictions can be placed on topics; however, topics that are nearly untouched by nurses include home care, managed care, nursing home placement, and NA perspectives on ethical matters such as the requirements for advance directives. Urban NAs, now a majority, have been studied much less than rural and reservation NAs. More descriptive studies, informed by awareness of issues in research on culture, are needed. Investigators should then proceed to community-based intervention studies that are evaluated and that empower NAs to meet their own needs. Translation should be used to reach non-English-speaking NAs, who may be most immersed in traditional cultures and most at risk of cultural barriers to care.

Investigators of NA health should not focus on culture to the exclusion of biology, poverty, and political and social structures. This leads to cultural reductionism and stereotyping. Also, intragroup differences are often as striking as those between groups. Empirical knowledge of cultural patterns does not eliminate the need for individual assessment of NA clients when providing care.

SHAROL F. JACOBSON

See also
ALCOHOLISM
DIABETES MELLITUS
**LEININGER'S TRANSCULTURAL NURS-
ING MODEL**

NEONATAL INTENSIVE CARE UNIT

See
NICU PRETERM INFANT CARE

NEUROBEHAVIORAL DEVELOPMENT

Neurobehavioral development may be viewed as a genetically determined and environmentally influenced process by which primitive structure of the central nervous system achieves maturity in form and function. The process of neurobehavioral development begins early in the embryonic period with the infolding of the neural plate and continues until at least the mid 20s. There is a peak period from approximately the 5th month of gestation until 2 years after birth. During this peak period, the brain is undergoing a rapid period of neuronal migration, myelination, and brain organization in which neurons are moving from their places of origin in lower brain centers, connections between neurons are being formed, and selective elimination of excess connections and death of excess neurons is occurring. Neurological insults occurring during this period will affect not only lower brain centers but also the development of the cerebral cortex and thus, potentially, the child's later cognitive and motor abilities. Therefore, this period is one in which nurses have the greatest opportunity to identify infants at risk and conduct interventions to improve neurobehavioral status. As a result, most of the nursing research on neurobehavioral development has been on this peak period.

A number of theoretical frameworks are used by nurse researchers studying neurobehavioral development. Probably the most common is the synactive model of neonatal behavioral organization. As compared to full-term infants, premature infants are not able to reach the necessary balance among subsystems. It is critical to understand that in the synactive theory of behavioral organization, one subsystem is not independent of the others; and any immaturity or disorganization of one causes an imbalance or disorganization in the others (Lawhon, 1986).

Als (1991) suggested that newborn behavior, which includes sucking, is an infant's primary expression of brain function and the critical route of communication. Investigation of central mechanisms, which regulate the temporal organization of behavior, is essential to understanding the basic relationship between cerebral activity and behavior. From this knowledge of the central mechanisms, the relation between abnormal brain function and abnormal behavior is understood by inference (Solberger, 1965).

Another framework used is the perspective of developmental science, a multidisciplinary field that brings together researchers and theorists from psychology, biology, nursing, and other disciplines (Cairns, Elder, & Costello, 1996). In this perspective, the individual functions as a total integrated system and develops in a continuously ongoing, reciprocal process of interaction with the environment. Moreover, plasticity is assumed to be inherent in the infant, the family, and the environment. The family and environment are constantly changing, thus influencing the infant. From this perspective, prediction with absolute certainty is impossible because the interactions affecting development of human beings are too complex and numerous to be totally identified and because humans can achieve the same developmental outcomes through different processes.

Nutritive Sucking as an Index of Neurobehavioral Development

The idea of evaluating the vitality and central nervous system integrity of a neonate by assessing sucking is not new. Sucking behaviors are thought to be an excellent barometer of central nervous system organization. They can be quantified in detailed analysis and are disturbed to various degrees by neurological problems. Wolff (1968) described sucking rhythms to investigate serial order in behavior and development, which has remained among the most resistant to empirical investigation. Medoff-Cooper (1991) demonstrated a strong correlation between increasing maturation and organized sucking patterns. Furthermore, the study of sucking rhythms has been found to be useful clinically when it differs among infants with a history of perinatal complications but with no abnormal neurological signs and infants with a benign perinatal history (Medoff-Cooper & Gennaro, 1996).

Nutritive sucking is initiated in utero and continues to develop in an organized pattern in the early weeks after birth. It involves the integration of multiple sensory and motor central nervous system functions. Nutritive sucking is organized as continuous rhythmic patterns rather than alternating between unpredictable bursts of activity and rest periods. There are several subtle differences in the sucking activity patterns between nutritive and nonnutritive sucking. Mean rates of sucking are slower, with shorter periods of pauses, for nutritive sucking than for nonnutritive sucking (Wolff, 1968). Nutritive sucking also provides reinforcement to an infant, thereby motivating a steady level of behavior that allows comparison of sucking records between two infants and with the same infant over time.

There seems to be a link between nutritive sucking and potential future developmental problems. For example, much of the literature suggests the occurrence of abnormal sucking patterns in infants who have experienced various neurological insults. One study by Burns and colleagues (Burns et al., 1987) showed that infants with significant intraventricular hemorrhage were delayed in their ability to achieve a nutritive suck reflex. At Week 40, only 75% of the 110 infants demonstrated mature nutritive sucking patterns. Dubignon, Campbell, Curtis, and Partington (1969) reported that nutritive sucking patterns were adversely affected by length of labor, type of delivery (other than spontaneous or low-forceps), maternal anesthesia, lower birth weight, and lower gestational age at birth.

As the infant matures, there should also be characteristic changes in the pattern of nutritive sucking that can be used as hallmarks of neurological integration; that is, there should be a link between nutritive sucking and developmental progress. In a study of 49 full-term and 49 preterm infants, Medoff-Cooper and colleagues (Medoff-Cooper, Weininger, & Zukowsky, 1989) found that term infants had a higher frequency of sucking than did preterm infants. In general, preterm infants generated significantly less peak negative pressure and attained lower peak flows.

Patterns of nutritive sucking seem to change with increasing postconceptional age. Hack and colleagues (Hack, Estabrook, & Robertson, 1985) have shown in 6 preterm infants from 30 weeks postconceptional age an increase in burst per minute; duration of each burst was stable. The pause between bursts decreased and sucking pace within bursts increased with age, resulting in an increase in the overall rate of sucking. These results suggested the possibility of a temporal organization of sucking from 30 weeks.

Healthy full-term infants also demonstrate substantial individual differences in effectiveness of sucking in the first day of life, gradually improving this effectiveness in the first 24 hours (Ellison, Vidyasagar, & Anderson, 1979). Clinical experience has shown that full-term newborn infants on the first day of life are often more sleepy and less likely to suckle than on the second day. When examining the relationship between state and sucking in 56 full-term infants on the first and second day of life, Medoff-Cooper, Verklan, Meyer, and Kaplan (1996) reported a significant correlation for several sucking parameters, including the number of sucks generated over a 5-minute period, the time between bursts, and the initial state assessment. Significant differences between state from Day 1 to Day 2 were also found, with more infants in sleep states prior to sucking on the first day of life.

After many years of observing and measuring sucking behaviors, it seems evident that this one element of infant behavior has great potential as an index of infant status or well-being. The information compiled from measuring sucking patterns are multidimensional, ranging from basic information about the ability to nipple-feed and receive adequate nutrition to neurobehavioral maturation as assessed through increasing organization of the sucking. These data can assist in appraising infant feeding readiness and discerning when an infant can be safety discharged from hospital to home.

Sleep-Wake States

Sleeping and waking states are clusters of behaviors that tend to occur together and represent the individual's level of arousal, responsivity to external stimulation, and central nervous system activation. Three states have been identified in adults: wakefulness, non-REM (rapid eye movement) sleep, and

REM sleep. In infants, it is also possible to identify states within waking and states that are transitional between waking and sleeping. Because the electrophysiological patterns associated with sleeping and waking infants are different from those in adults, the sleep states are usually designated active and quiet sleep.

In infancy, electroencephalography (EEG) is less reliable for the scoring of state and should be combined with observation because of infants' neurological immaturity. EEG and behavioral scoring of state in preterm and full-term infants provide quite similar results. Thus, sleeping and waking states in infants can be validly scored either by EEG or by directly observing the infant and identifying behaviors that tend to occur together and reflect a similar level of arousal and responsiveness to the environment. Four standardized systems for scoring behavioral observations of sleep-wake states are currently being used by nurse researchers: (a) the 6-state system developed by T. Berry Brazelton, (b) the 10-state system of Evelyn Thoman, (c) the 12-state system from Heideliese Als's Assessment of Preterm Infant's Behavior (APIB), and (d) the system developed by Gene Anderson. These systems define states in very similar ways and are equally useful for clinical purposes. However, for research, the Brazelton system is the most limited as it is appropriate for use only with infants between 36 and 44 weeks postconception, and Thoman's is the most flexible; it has been used effectively with preterm infants 27 weeks postconception through 1-year-olds.

Sleeping and waking states have widespread physiological effects. The functioning of cardiovascular, respiratory, neurological, endocrine, and gastrointestinal systems differ in different states. Sleeping and waking also affect the infant's ability to respond to stimulation. Thus, infant responses to nurses and parents depend on the state the infant is in when the stimulation is begun. Timing routine interventions to occur when the infant is most responsive is an important aspect of current systems of individualized nursing care.

Finally, studies have indicated that sleep and waking patterns are closely related to neurological status (Thoman, 1982). The oscillation between sleep and waking originates in the brainstem, and

the manifestation of these states involves the coordinated functioning of all areas in the brain. Recent conceptualizations view sleep as the result of interactions among neuronal populations that stretch from the brainstem to cerebral cortex (Hobson, 1989).

In addition, infants exhibit developmental changes in their sleeping and waking states throughout the first year of life that parallel the development of the brain. Preterm infants as young as 24 weeks postconception have been found to exhibit sleeping and waking. However, prior to 30 weeks gestational age, the various behaviors associated with sleep and waking—eye movements, body movements, respiration, and muscle tone—are not well coordinated. Infants exhibit greater amounts of active sleep and indeterminate states during the preterm period and lower amounts of waking states than after term. The major developmental changes during the preterm period are a decrease in the amount of active sleep and increases in the amount of waking states and the organization of quiet sleep. During the first month after term, healthy full-term infants will spend more than half the day in sleep, the majority of this being active sleep. Over the first year, waking periods become longer and more consolidated, the amount of crying decreases, and total sleep time decreases due to a decrease in active sleep time. The amount of quiet sleep remains about the same from term age on. Thus, by about 6 months of age, the amount of quiet sleep exceeds the amount of active sleep. The number of sleep episodes also decreases and becomes consolidated primarily into nighttime. The sleep states also develop the EEG patterns typical of adults by about 3 months (Holditch-Davis, in press).

Sleep and wakefulness may have direct effects on brain development and learning. For example, because active sleep is less common in adults than non-REM sleep but is much more common in infants, it has been hypothesized to be necessary for brain development (Roffwarg, Muzio, & Dement, 1995). Sleep also fills a necessary role in memory consolidation and in cognitive and attentional tasks, at least in adults (Hobson, 1989).

State patterns of preterm infants with neurological insults differ markedly from those of healthy infants. Markedly abnormal neonatal EEG patterns are associated with severe neurological abnormalities and major neurodevelopmental sequelae during childhood. Also, preterm infants with severe medical illnesses exhibit patterns of sleep-wake states that differ from those of healthier preterms, although most of these differences disappear when infants recover (Holditch-Davis, in press).

Sleep-wake patterns can also be used to predict developmental outcome. Sleep-wake measures during the preterm period—including amount of crying (one of the neonatal waking states) during gavage feedings and increased duration of states at 36 weeks—predict Bayley mental scores during the first year, and sleep measures at term relate to developmental outcome at age 8. Developmental changes in the amounts of specific sleep behaviors during the first year are related to developmental and health outcomes in the second year. Further, the stability of sleep-wake patterns in the first month predicts later development. In healthy preterms, lower spectral EEG energies predicted lower neurodevelopmental performance at 12 and 24 months. Low levels of trace alternans on the EEG of term-aged premature infants were predictive of lower intelligence quotients (IQ), and delayed maturity of EEG patterns was associated with poor neurological outcome. Elevated amounts of intense bursts of REM are associated with later developmental problems in full-term infants.

Acoustic characteristics of infant cries have been used to predict developmental outcome in preterm infants and infants exposed to drugs prenatally. In apparently normal full-term infants, in premature infants, and in siblings of infants who died from sudden infant death syndrome, the stability of state patterns in the first month has been found to predict developmental outcome. In addition, the known EEG changes with age in sleep architecture and continuity, increasing spectral energies, and greater spectral EEG coherence are probably indicators of maturational changes in the brain, including synaptogenesis, evolution of neurotransmitter pools, and myelination (Holditch-Davis, in press).

In summary, sleeping and waking patterns appear to provide an excellent index of neurodevelopmental status in preterm and full-term infants that can be scored either behaviorally or by EEG.

BARBARA MEDOFF-COOPER
DIANE HOLDITCH-DAVIS

See also
KANGAROO CARE
NICU PRETERM INFANT CARE
NURSING SLEEP SCIENCE
**NUTRITION IN INFANCY AND CHILD-
  HOOD**

NEUROBEHAVIORAL DISTURBANCES OF THE OLDER ADULT: DELIRIUM AND DEMENTIA

Impairments in cognitive functioning from disturbances in the brain's physiology can easily occur in older adults. Disturbances in processing information and in behaving in socially adaptable ways can result from neurological changes in the brain and the mind's attempts to compensate for these changes. The most frequent causes of neurobehavioral disturbances in older adults are organic brain disorders, the most common are delirium and dementia. The most challenging behavioral disturbances to caregivers are agitation and aggression.

Delirium, or acute mental confusion, is transient, often abrupt and fluctuating, and typically reversible. Key symptoms include anxiety, incoherent or disoriented thinking and perceiving, reduced ability to sustain and shift attention, and agitated behavior. Precipitants are related to physical illness (e.g., cardiovascular disease), infection, hormone disorders, or nutritional deficiencies. Most frequent precipitants are metabolic disturbances, fluid and electrolyte imbalances, drug and alcohol toxicity, and unfamiliar and excessive sensory-environmental stimuli. Delirium may be life-threatening and is a medical emergency (Early Alzheimer's Disease Guideline Panel, 1996).

Dementia is a neurological brain syndrome that affects cognitive and functional abilities. Dementia is usually chronic and progressive; some dementias are reversible. Key symptoms include impairments in memory, language, judgment, and visual-spatial motor skills. Personality changes include lack of initiative, paranoia, and aggressiveness. Aggressive behavior is considered the most serious behavioral disturbance associated with dementia. Alzheimer's disease, the most prevalent form of irreversible dementia, proceeds in stages insidiously over months or years and results in functional dependence and death, usually from secondary causes. Genetic factors may be more important in the etiology of Alzheimer's disease than previously thought. Common to both delirium and dementia is depletion of older adults' already limited cognitive reserves, making adaptation to even minor changes in either health status or social environments challenging.

Nursing research historically has focused on identifying risk factors, developing assessment tools, and evaluating nursing interventions by using anecdotal or case study evidence. With increased sophistication in designing intervention studies, nurses are conducting research on the care of persons with delirium (for a review, see Cronin-Stubbs, 1996), dementia (for a review, see Maas & Buckwalter, 1991), and behavioral disturbances (for a review, see Taft & Cronin-Stubbs, 1995).

Early identification and prompt treatment of the causes of delirium prevent irreversible dementia and death, with nursing interventions targeted to reversing physiological disturbances and preventing sensory deprivation (Neelon & Champagne, 1992). Limited evidence suggests efficacy for reality orientation, perioperative management of hypoxia and orthostatic hypotension, postoperative pain management, and curtailment of excessive or meaningless stimuli (Cronin-Stubbs, 1996). Rehabilitation models and cognitive-behavioral principles have guided development of interventions for dementia, including cognitive retraining and skills training in activities of daily living (for a review, see Beck, Cronin-Stubbs, Buckwalter, & Rapp, in press). The Progressively Lowered Stress Threshold model targets minimizing stressful stimuli as a way of bolstering functional reserves in persons with dementia (Hall, Gerdner, Zwycart-Stauffacher, & Buckwalter, 1995).

Caregiver research to date has focused on global psychosocial and educational interventions delivered for brief periods of time (8–10 weeks) and targeted to reducing caregiver distress (for a review, see Light, Niederehe, & Lebowitz, 1994). Multifaceted programs that include long-term effects on caregivers' health status and institutionalization rates are beginning to be tested, with particular attention to the facets of the program that pertain to specific levels of service intensity (Knight, Lutzky, & Macofsky-Urban, 1993).

Agitation and aggression in persons with delirium and dementia have been studied cross-sectionally with correlational-descriptive designs (Taft & Cronin-Stubbs, 1995). Longitudinal studies are needed to map the natural history of behavioral symptoms, and experimental and quasi-experimental studies are needed to identify alternatives to chemical and physical restraints for persons with agitation and aggression. Low doses of haloperidol for treating neurobehavioral disturbances have demonstrated efficacy in recent clinical trials. Nutritional interventions are being tested for curbing aggressive episodes. Special care units that integrate behavioral, nutritional, and environmental interventions are beginning to demonstrate treatment efficacy.

One issue in the conduct of intervention studies of neurobehavioral disturbances is the match between the definition of the syndrome and the items included on the instruments to measure them. Studies of delirium and dementia and their behavioral sequelae have used assessment measures of varying degrees of psychometric rigor. Most mental status exams, for example, are measures of general cognitive function and do not distinguish types of cognitive impairment. Another issue in the conduct of these studies is the design and implementation of the interventions. Intensity, frequency, and duration of the intervention delivery requires standardization, and assessments must be made to determine if the intervention that was intended matches the intervention that was delivered.

Even when outcomes of the intervention study suggest efficacy, the mechanisms or the active ingredients of the intervention are not known. In testing multifaceted intervention packages, for example, the relative efficacy of each component must be matched to specific outcomes if results are to be replicated and cost-effective generalizations to diverse patient care situations are to be made.

Future research directions include establishing the efficacy of interventions for eventual generalization to diverse settings. However, research has not advanced to the development and testing of standardized protocols in randomized clinical trials. Nor has efficacy of interventions been determined in subgroups of older adults (young-old vs. old-old, men vs. women, Blacks vs. Whites). Commonly used methods to control behavioral disturbances are known to either intensify target behaviors (physical restraints) or further impair cognition and active involvement in treatment programs (neuroleptic medications).

Future directions also include the continued development of interventions that promote rehabilitation and recovery. Combinations of pharmacological, behavioral, and environmental approaches warrant testing, and algorithms for individualizing and dosing interventions are needed. Methods for educating caregivers about managing behaviors associated with delirium and dementia also are needed. Nurses are challenged to develop, systematically evaluate, and use nonrestrictive strategies for responding to the behaviors associated with cognitive impairment experienced by older adults in all settings.

DIANE CRONIN-STUBBS

See also
ALZHEIMER'S DISEASE
ALZHEIMER'S DISEASE: SPECIAL
    CARE UNITS IN LONG-TERM CARE
CAREGIVER
COGNITIVE DISORDERS
MIDDLE-RANGE THEORIES OF DEMEN-
    TIA CARE
RELAXATION TECHNIQUES

NEWMAN'S THEORY OF HEALTH

Margaret Newman is an eminent, visionary nurse theorist whose contributions to nursing science and nursing practice span 30 years of sustained scholarship on the theory of health as expanding consciousness. Newman's theory of health exemplifies her focus on a unitary-transformative paradigm for the discipline of nursing and on research as praxis methodology.

Health as Expanding Consciousness

Newman's conceptual framework of health was introduced in her book *Theory Development in Nursing* (1979) and was expanded and refined in two editions of her book *Health as Expanding Consciousness* (1986, 1994) as the theory of health as expanding consciousness. Her work was published at a time when less abstract theories of nursing, based on current practice, were emphasized. Rather than being viewed as a visionary, with a creative, and futuristic conceptualization of health, Newman's highly abstract grand theory, as well as other grand theories of nursing, was dismissed by the majority of nurses as far removed from the real world of everyday practice. As scientists in other disciplines revolutionized their former mechanistic worldviews to align more closely with a unitary-transformative paradigm, Newman's theory of health has achieved greater acceptance by nurse scholars and practitioners, particularly holistic nurses and case managers.

Newman's (1986, 1994) theory of health was influenced by Rogers's science of unitary human beings, Bentov's evolution of consciousness, and Prigogine's theory of dissipative structures. She reconceptualized health as a manifestation of underlying unitary field pattern rather than a health-disease dichotomy. Health was defined as a dynamic evolving process of expanding consciousness, which occurs within a multidimensional matrix of movement, time, space, and consciousness. She utilized Young's theory of human evolution and Bohm's theory of undivided wholeness of reality to support the relationships in the matrix and the importance of unitary field pattern. Nursing practice was defined as a process of nurse-client attunement during which the client's underlying pattern is identified, and both client and nurse are transformed.

Unitary-Transformative Paradigm

Newman was an early, eloquent advocate for nursing to identify, develop, and differentiate a paradigm that addressed the unique knowledge of nursing embodied in practice and in scholarly inquiry. In collaboration with Sime and Corcoran-Perry (Newman, Sime, & Corcoran-Perry, 1991), she defined the focus of nursing as "caring in the human health experience" (p. 3) and articulated the differences between the prevailing particulate-deterministic and interactive-integrative paradigms, which had previously shaped nursing education, research, and practice, and a unitary-transformative paradigm for the discipline of nursing in the future. Clear articulation of nursing's paradigm in Newman's theory of health was logically extended to a differentiated nursing practice model that she based on both education and paradigm. She also proposed that nursing diagnoses should recognize patterns of person-environment interaction, in contrast to the North American Nursing Diagnosis Association (NANDA) diagnoses, which reflect a static client in isolation from the environment.

Research as Praxis

Newman (1990) identified the lack of conceptual fit between conventional quantitative research methods and the unitary-transformative paradigm of her theory of health. She posited that nurse researchers should use "research as praxis," a hermeneutic method of inquiry in which the client and nurse are co-researchers in identifying, describing, and verifying the client's pattern of expanding consciousness from narrative data about the most meaningful events in the client's life. Persons with coronary heart disease, women with breast cancer, adults with cancer, and persons with HIV/AIDS have been studied. Patterns were identified for individual study participants, with qualitative comparison of patterns across study participants. Research as praxis is both a research method and a transformative intervention and may be best suited for nurses who have the ability to identify patterns, have the time to evaluate the client, and have clients who are able to comprehend and communicate their meaningful life events in primary care settings (Engle, 1996).

Research Using Newman's Theory

Early research emphasized testing propositions derived from Newman's (1979) conceptual framework of health, focusing on the concepts of movement, time, space, and consciousness and establishing criterion-related validity by means of conventional quantitative methods. Nurse researchers included Engle, Guadiano, Mentzer, Newman, Schorr, and Tompkins. Healthy adults were studied in community and laboratory settings with predominantly small, nonprobability samples of male college students, female college students, older adults, and older women. Study results were equivocal.

Subsequent elaboration and refinement of Newman's (1986, 1994) theory of health shifted the focus of research to health as expanding consciousness, recognition of unitary field pattern, and research as praxis (Engle, 1996). Nurse researchers included Lamendola, Moch, Newman, Schorr, and Schroeder. Small convenience samples of adults with and without health problems were studied in community and health care settings, including adults who exercised regularly, women with rheumatoid arthritis, women with breast cancer, adults with cancer, adults with coronary heart disease, and persons with HIV/AIDS. Although results may have limited application to current nursing practice, they may be relevant in the future as the paradigm of nursing changes over time. Holistic nursing interventions using various energy modalities, such as light, sound, and touch, may be conceptually consistent with Newman's theory of health and provide direction for future research.

VERONICA F. ENGLE

See also
HEALTH CONCEPTUALIZATION
HERMENEUTICS
NONTRADITIONAL THERAPIES
ROGERS' SCIENCE OF UNITARY HUMAN BEINGS

NICU PRETERM INFANT CARE

Modern intensive care nurseries have been in existence since 1970. Life in an intensive care nursery, or neonatal intensive care unit (NICU), is characterized by patterns of stimulation that preterm infants would not have in the womb or at home with their families. The impact of this environment is the source of speculation, controversy, and research, especially because the focus of interventions has changed from applying generic infant stimulation techniques to assessing individual infants for growth and developmental needs (Burns, Cunningham, White-Traut, Silvestri, & Nelson, 1994). Limited nursing developmental assessment and intervention research has shown short- and long-term health and developmental benefits for low birthweight (<2500 g) and preterm (<37 weeks gestation) infants as a result of using individualized behavioral and environmental NICU interventions (Becker, Grunwald, Moorman, & Stuhr, 1993). However, as Blackburn and Barnard (1985) point out, appropriate preterm infant caregiving activities and types of stimulation in the NICU as they specifically coincide with modulating preterm levels of arousal have yet to be determined.

The ultimate goal of NICU intervention strategies is to promote significant positive growth and development and prevent negative alterations from normal growth and development. Establishing physiological homeostasis is necessary for survival and is enhanced by a sensitive, responsive NICU environment. Hospitalized preterm infants, especially those experiencing prolonged stays, can exhibit classic signs of institutionalized infants or infants suffering from maternal deprivation, as well as signs of sensory bombardment. It is the goal of neonatal nursing to prevent maladaptive behavior, outcomes, and growth and developmental delays by modifying the NICU to be more responsive and appropriate to infants' needs.

Perinatal History and Neonatal Assessment

The first step in the caregiving process that provides data for neonatal care and management decisions is the perinatal history. Information regarding the mother's prenatal care, medications the mother was taking, and any relevant prenatal tests that were done, together with their results, should be obtained. Traditionally, the first assessment of the neonate is the Apgar score. The Apgar score provides a rapid evaluation of a neonate's condition at birth and is a routine objective measurement for decisions about resuscitative and supportive measures. Repeated Apgar scoring can help evaluate the neonate's response to treatment and overall adaptation to extrauterine life. However, physical assessment, laboratory tests, and radiographs will provide a better picture of the neonate's clinical status.

Once immediate-life threatening conditions have been managed, primary preventive interventions have been initiated (such as the administration of exogenous surfactant), and the neonate's condition has begun to stabilize physiologically, a complete physical examination is necessary. Neonates also need a gestational age evaluation, growth measurements with graphic plotting, and a neurobehavioral developmental assessment. Using the perinatal history and results from the physical examination, laboratory tests, radiographs, and the birthing room measures employed, decisions are made about the intensity of care and whether to transport to another setting. Nursing research regarding the optimum pieces of information for various treatment decisions, the best methods for newborn physical and neurobehavioral assessments, and nursing algorithms for assessment has not been completed.

Routine Caregiving

Peters (1996) leads the way in examining the need for and effectiveness of routine NICU procedures with preterm neonates in her research on bathing. According to Peters, "no routine for the care of the critically ill infant should be regarded as immutable and above criticism" (p. 71). She stresses that the most critically ill and immature neonate typically requires aggressive care and frequent interventions, involving direct handling and manipulation in addition to meeting basic needs of oxygenation, ventilation, warmth, nourishment, and protection from harm. Peters found that tactile stimulation, using warm water, soap, and a washcloth leads to significantly increased compromise in terms of oxygenation, demonstrating the negative effects of sponge bathing. Nonetheless, most other routine interventions have never been subjected to critical testing for potential adverse effects or evidence supporting their effectiveness. Critically ill preterm neonates require individualized, supportive care based on a careful assessment of the infant's needs, with procedures completed only as needed.

Intervention Strategies

Infants' sensory capabilities and abilities to self-regulate are two guidelines for determining the appropriateness of nursing interventions (Barnard & Bee, 1983). Intervention strategies are grounded in tactile/kinesthetic, auditory, visual, olfactory/gustatory, and communication skills because neonates appear to experience their environment through sensory capabilities. Infants feel best when they perceive that they are in control of what they are doing and what is happening to them; therefore, caregiving interventions should be individualized to each infant's ability to self-regulate based on physiological status, motor status, state status, sensory threshold, and approach/avoidance behavioral capabilities. Each infant's ability to self-regulate can differ significantly, depending on whether the infant is being assessed prior to, during, or following a caregiving episode, and this will further determine caregiving interventions.

A comforting effect on recovering preterm infants and their mothers was detected by using kangaroo care, or placing diapered infants upright between their mother's breasts for skin-to-skin contact (Ludington-Hoe, Thompson, Swinth, Hadeed, & Anderson, 1994b). In addition to physiological benefits to infants, kangaroo care appeared to empower mothers while in the NICU.

Assessment of the Environment

According to Thomas (1990), determining how the NICU environment contributes to developmental disabilities is crucial now that more preterm infants are surviving but are exhibiting neurological abnormalities, intellectual impairments, attention deficit hyperactivity disorders, information processing deficits, sensory deficits, reading and writing difficulties, and growth delays. A kinder, gentler NICU atmosphere must be engendered, with perhaps the first step being active prevention of long-lasting high-intensity and high-frequency sound levels. Thomas admits that although safety standards for sound exposure have not been established for infants, when the NICU is seemingly quiet at 50 to 80 decibels (dB), the sounds exceed the 40-dB threshold for 28- to 34-week gestation infants.

Typically, NICUs are lit with fluorescent lights to enable immediate and ongoing observation of infants. After studying the hazards of using bright lights—for example, 40–100 foot candles (Glass, 1990)—developmental researchers are increasingly advocating dimming lights to prevent the occurrence and severity of retinopathies. Using incandescent bedside lights with dimmer switches, draping incubators, and tenting warmer beds with blankets are ways in which bedsides can be dimmed while still providing for immediate maximal illumination when the infant's condition requires such visibility.

Normalizing the NICU Environment

Normalizing the NICU environment begins with an assessment of the stimulation to which the individual infant is exposed. The type, amount, and timing of stimulation should be evaluated. To decrease inappropriate stimuli, even when basing care on critical paths, no infant should be given "routine" care but should have individualized care based on assessments of health and developmental status.

Specific aspects of the NICU caregiving environment will relate to maturation; different aspects of each environment will influence specific aspects of the infant's development, and the impact of the environment on the infant will be mediated by individual infant characteristics. By providing opportunities for infants to explore, learn about environmental predictability, and relate their behavior to environmental circumstances, the nurse can contribute to the infant's growth, development, and well-being (Blackburn & Barnard, 1985). Although the appropriateness of caregiving environments will vary among infants, the exact mechanisms and parameters that describe these individual response differences remain to be determined.

JANA L. PRESSLER

See also
**KANGAROO CARE
NEUROBEHAVIORAL DEVELOPMENT
PARENTAL RESPONSE TO THE NEONA-
    TAL INTENSIVE CARE UNIT
PSYCHOSOCIAL EFFECTS OF CHILD
    CRITICAL ILLNESS AND HOSPITAL-
    IZATION**

(FLORENCE) NIGHTINGALE

Florence Nightingale, born on May 12, 1820 (died on August 13, 1910), is considered the founder of contemporary nursing. She is a legend, and around the world nurses celebrate International Nurses Day on May 12, the anniversary of her birth. During the late 1970s and early 1980s, in the time of the development and analysis of conceptualization of nursing models in the United States, there was a renewed interest and analysis of Nightingale's thinking and writings regarding the nature of nursing. Her most widely circulated publication is *Notes on Nursing*, first published in London in 1859 by Harrison. In 1992 a commemorative volume of this work, with comments by 11 contemporary nurse theorists and nurse leaders, was published by Lippincott (Nightingale, 1859/1992).

Key components of Nightingale's conceptualization of nursing included an understanding of the laws of nature, described as both the prevention of disease and the use of personal power. Nightingale's science was epidemiological in its foundation; she used statistics to describe morbidity and mortality, and she considered the nurses' observational skills most significant to nursing practice. Other important concepts within Nightingale's understanding of nursing included her view of persons as both physical and spiritual beings, her emphasis on the environment as a key factor in promoting health and wellness, and her focus on caring for the patient, not the illness. Although not explicitly antagonistic to her medical colleagues, Nightingale saw nature as healer and medicine as primitive. Oliver Wendell Holmes (1860) agreed and saw the emetics, purges, and bloodletting used by her contemporary physicians as inferior to the nature lauded by Holmes as emanating from Hippocrates and his "noblest daughter Miss Florence Nightingale . . . in her late volume [*Notes on Nursing*, 1859/1860]."

Florence Nightingale entered service to her country in 1854 at the request of the Secretary of State for War when reports of negligence in hospital management during the Crimean War appeared in the *Times* of London. She embarked for hospitals in Scutari with a small band of women who, under Nightingale's direction, applied principles of sanitary science that had been recommended (and ignored) by a royal commission. In spite of opposition from the ranking medical and military hierarchy, Nightingale is credited with reforms that substantially reduced hospital mortality. Reports of her effectiveness reached London and conferred worldwide fame on her before she reached home in 1856.

For more than 10 years after her return from the war, Florence Nightingale produced a vast body of writings. Most notable were her notes on matters affecting the health, efficiency, and hospital administration of the British army, an 800+-page tome specifying every ill that befell the British army, with specific recommendations to ameliorate them (Nightingale, 1859/1860). She stimulated the appointment of a royal commission that published four volumes of reforms that had the effect of halving peacetime mortality rates among army troops (Nightingale, 1862). These reforms, including the introduction of female nurses in the military, were adopted by the United States during the American Civil War, and disease mortality was reduced to less than a third of that experienced by the British only a decade earlier (Duncan, 1905/1987).

Nightingale proposed a system of education for nurses at a time when they were uneducated. Although she is credited with founding contemporary nursing education, she learned practical nursing in Kaiserworth, Germany. Henley's poem, "In Hospital," shows the profound effect of the 1872 introduction of the new (Nightingale-trained) nurses into the Edinburgh Infirmary at the same time Lister was using antiseptic surgery there (Henley, 1888).

Notes on Hospitals, third edition (Nightingale, 1863), became a classic book on the building, organization, and management of civilian hospitals that was used throughout the world for more than 70 years. In it Nightingale recommended that nurses, physicians, and hospital administrators be in a perpetual rub with one another, with the threat of publicity keeping each at his or her assigned task and acting in the best interests of patients. Absolute authority in a hospital, she reasoned, compromises good patient care.

Bishop and Goldie (1962) cataloged Nightingale's writings, which they organized by subject and year. Nursing, the army, Indian and colonial welfare, hospitals, statistics, sociology, religion, and philosophy were the topics she wrote on in depth. In addition she corresponded with hundreds of persons in tens of thousands of letters. Many of these have been cataloged, summarized, and indexed—again, by Goldie and Bishop (1983).

It is remarkable that the infusion of nurses into hospitals throughout the Western world took place at a rate faster than the acceptance of the germ theory. It is quite possible that the application of cleanliness (asepsis), nutrition, rest, order, and warmth from nurses was more important in the treatment of disease than were the technological innovations developed from 1860 to 1950. Only after the widespread use of antibiotics did these natural ministrations lose their potency in the amelioration of disease. It is also possible that there will be a return to the principles of nursing (and asepsis) as mainstays of effective care and treatment for disease. For the 20th-century equivalent of Nightingale's writings, see Virginia Henderson.

There can be no mistake in attributing profound changes in health care to Florence Nightingale and the modern profession she established. That she and her successors functioned for more than 140 years without benefit of dominant educational, social, and economic institutions has been a remarkable achievement. It will be interesting to see what will be accomplished in a century of more equal access to these institutions. If the legacy of Florence Nightingale is any indication, health care led by nurses may advance well-being even more in the next century.

EDWARD J. HALLORAN
JOYCE J. FITZPATRICK

See also
EPISTEMOLOGY
HENDERSON'S MODEL
HISTORY OF NURSING RESEARCH

NONTRADITIONAL THERAPIES

Definitions

Nontraditional therapies encompass a broad spectrum of practices and beliefs. Consequently, descriptions and definitions of the collective philosophy vary according to one's professional or occupational perspective. Historically, and from the point of view of some within the biomedical community, nontraditional therapies are defined as practices that are not correct, proper, or appropriate or are not in conformity with the beliefs and standards of the dominant group of health care practitioners in a society. To this definition others add that nontraditional therapies collectively are those interventions that are neither taught widely in schools of nursing and medicine nor provided generally by hospitals. In some cultures, alternative modalities refers to therapies that are offered in place of orthodox health care practices, some of which are far outside of the realm of accepted health care theory and practices in the United States.

Complementary medicine/therapies, a term introduced in 1976 in the United Kingdom, encompasses many of the modalities categorized as nontraditional and in that country refers to linking the most appropriate modalities to serve the patient physically, mentally, emotionally, and spiritually. A recent and similar definition for nontraditional therapies is "those interventions for improving, maintaining and promoting health and well-being, preventing disease, or treating illness" (Jacobs, 1995).

One problem that arises with the terms *nontraditional*, *complementary*, and *alternative* is that these are judgmental terms that inhibit dialogue about the therapies, and they are in conflict with the nursing perspective and tradition of providing care that includes noninvasive and naturalistic therapies (Watson, 1995). Therapies that have traditionally been an integral part of nursing have begun to appear within the newly emerging field of alternative and complementary medicine. Nursing does not consider therapies related to caring, comfort, pain reduction or relief, and other means of symptom control as alternative but rather as therapies that nurses have traditionally provided and that are considered the foundation of caring, holistic nursing practice. Consequently, the terms *nontraditional*, *alternative*, and *complementary* are controversial within the field of nursing today.

Societal Value of Nontraditional Therapies

Today's emphasis on health promotion mandates education, personal responsibilities, and empowerment of individuals, which encourages use of these therapies. There are those in society who desire nontraditional therapies as adjuncts to conventional care or, in some instances, in place of invasive, painful, or unsuccessful therapies that lead to pain, suffering, and lengthy hospital stays.

One in three adult Americans in 1990 reportedly used some kind of nontraditional therapy and paid for them mostly out-of-pocket (Eisenberg et al., 1993). Most often these individuals were searching for modalities that could fight the major chronic diseases and conditions that were reducing their quality of life.

In response to the increase in the public's interest in nontraditional therapies, Congress, in late 1992, established the Office of Alternative Medicine (OAM) within the Director's Office of the National Institutes of Health (NIH). Reorganization in 1996 placed the OAM within the Office of Disease Prevention. The OAM's classification scheme of alternative therapies includes more than 200 modalities with more than 10,000 uses and categorizes these under the headings of diet, nutrition, lifestyle changes, mind-body control, manual healing, pharmacological and biological treatments, bioelectromagnetic applications, and herbal medicine. The OAM (1992) fosters research on nontraditional therapies and seeks to reduce barriers that keep promising therapies from emerging. To promote research in nontraditional therapies, OAM established 10 research centers across the country, one of

which is directed by a nurse. A Public Information Clearinghouse Database and Evaluations Section of the OAM is scheduled to be operational in 1998. It will be a resource to interested persons seeking state-of-the-science information on selected nontraditional therapies.

Researching Nontraditional Therapies from the Nursing Perspective

Theory-based nursing practices and the emerging "holistic nursing movement" (Watson, 1995) reflect a body of knowledge that includes therapies developed from the distinctive perspective of the nursing discipline. It is from the nursing perspective that nurse scholars and their students select from the phenomena of interest to the discipline those specific phenomena needing further development. Therapies such as aromatherapy, guided imagery and other forms of visualization, therapeutic touch, massage, acupressure, music listening, meditation and relaxation techniques, yoga, and support groups, although labeled nontraditional therapies, are and have been within the domain of nursing practice and research.

Good programs of research involving any of these therapies can begin with very basic questions: What's going on with a particular therapy in the investigator's target population? How do individual differences, as assessed by a given measurement tool, influence what happens or does not happen in the use of a particular therapy for management of a specified symptom? From general questions such as these, coupled with extensive literature reviews and consultation with experts, more specific questions about the use of these therapies in patient care evolve to guide the investigator's research.

Because nursing takes the position that patients' perceptions, thoughts, and feelings are an important part of their reality, these influence the nature of inquiry and the choice of outcome measures. Focusing on individual differences among patients when assessing use, efficacy, and effectiveness of nontraditional therapies permits the investigator to analyze disparate patient care findings and synthesize them into questions that will add to the body of knowledge about these therapies. Findings resulting from research studies testing the efficacy of nontraditional therapies may lead to knowledge that can be useful in making reliable predictions and linking appropriate therapies to a person for promotion of health or symptom management.

Certain problems may arise when researchers try to use conventional research techniques without adaptation for the evaluation of some nontraditional therapies. For example, use of placebo controls and double blinding may not be feasible in testing therapies such as massage, therapeutic touch, and acupressure. A variety of different study designs are appropriate to answer questions important to the evaluation of particular therapies. Existing nursing literature provides numerous examples of rigorous qualitative research as well as examples of studies without blinding or an active control. Solving methodological problems in testing nontraditional therapies is a matter of following simple guidelines that take into account the special features of the nontraditional therapy and research question being investigated. Each question raised by the researcher and the type of research implemented can play a role in developing a fuller understanding of the efficacy, effectiveness, and safety of nontraditional therapies within professional nursing practice.

Significant Issues for Future Research

Nursing knowledge development is driven by new questions and new conceptual frameworks. Reconceptualizing research problems with a new paradigm or framework may provide new insights into these therapies. Research efforts on nontraditional therapies should include additional efficacy and effectiveness studies, cost-effectiveness studies, and replication of existing studies. Research is needed to answer relevant questions about the use of complementary and nontraditional therapies in the nursing care of all persons. Attention should be given to the following:

- Outcome measures that are reliable, valid, and standardized for each specific therapy so that studies can be compared and combined;
- Qualitative research studies to determine patients' experiences with using particular non-

traditional therapies in the management of their specific conditions;
- Research that includes examination of consequences or outcomes of not integrating a potentially useful nontraditional therapy as part of the treatment regimen for a condition or symptom and treating a symptom or condition with a combination of pharmacological and nontraditional therapy;
- Investigations that build on advances in neurobiological sciences and psychoneuroimmunology to understand mechanisms of action of the less understood nontraditional therapies;
- Research that assesses individual differences in outcomes for nontraditional therapies, including cross-cultural applicability and efficacy;
- Research that examines nontraditional therapies for different populations and conditions, giving consideration to the influence of age, race, gender, religious beliefs, and socioeconomic status on the treatment efficacy; and
- The most effective timing for the introduction of a nontraditional therapy in the course of conventional treatment.

Conclusions

Some therapies referred to as nontraditional are integral to professional nursing practice, and others are seen as important to emerging holistic care developments. These therapies have been studied less than other nursing phenomena, yet there is research to support the effectiveness of selected nontraditional therapies, such as the use of relaxation techniques, as well as to provide a foundation for further research. The challenge and crucial step toward recognition and acceptance by the biomedical community is to continue to engage in conceptual work toward explanatory theories and to investigate these therapies in the context of the nursing perspective.

ANN GILL TAYLOR

See also
CULTURAL/TRANSCULTURAL FOCUS
MUSIC THERAPY

NORTH AMERICAN NURSING DIAGNOSIS ASSOCIATION

Beginnings

Bylaws were adopted for the formation of the North American Nursing Diagnosis Association (NANDA) in 1982 at the Fifth Conference for the Classification of Nursing Diagnoses. The idea for the series of conferences is credited to Kristine Gebbie and Mary Ann Lavin, who were both nursing faculty members in the School of Nursing at St. Louis University. In their work they encountered the dilemma of having automated record keeping made available to them in the hospital but not having a nursing language to capture what nurses do. They had nothing to put in the computer to distinguish their care from that of physicians. Realizing that they were probably not alone, they originated the idea of a national conference group to name the health problems that comprise the nursing domain and to classify them into a taxonomic system. The First Conference for the Classification of Nursing Diagnoses was convened in 1973 in St. Louis with 100 invited participants. This was the starting point for the formal effort to identify and classify nursing diagnoses.

Purpose

The purpose of the association as stated in the by-laws is "to develop, refine and promote a taxonomy of nursing diagnostic terminology of general use to professional nurses" (Rantz & LeMone, 1997, p. 481). Research has focused on the identification, validation, and refinement of nursing diagnoses.

Issues Emphasized in the Organization

The major issues emphasized in the organization flow from the purpose: the continuing research to promote and validate the taxonomy and continuing activities to educate and promote the use of nursing diagnosis. With changes in the health care delivery system and in computer technology, more emphasis has been placed on being a partner in the development of health care databases for the computerization of health care information.

Other Information

The organization is voluntary, and licensed registered nurses are eligible for membership. The address is NANDA, 1211 Locust Street, Philadelphia, PA 19107.

Lois M. Hoskins

See also
NANDA
NURSING DIAGNOSIS
TAXONOMY

NURSE ANESTHETISTS AND RESEARCH

From the beginning of the successful demonstration and use at the Massachusetts General Hospital in 1846 through the end of the 19th century, anesthesia, the new modality for relieving the pain of surgery, was plagued with significant morbidity and mortality worldwide. Surgeons in the United States, believing that much of this was due to the utilization of "occasional" anesthetists, turned to the professional nurse, prepared in the Nightingale model of education, as the provider who should specialize in and make anesthesia sufficiently safe for continued use. Not only did the nurses prove capable in this task, but they were often involved in the development of anesthesia techniques, procedures, and equipment. As in the nursing profession's earliest days, practice took precedence over research, even though the practitioners held and often acted on personal theories and resulting hypotheses. Perhaps the best research efforts by a nurse anesthetist at the turn of the 19th century were those of Alice Magaw.

At Mayo Clinic in Rochester, Minnesota, nurses had been recruited by the Doctors at Mayo to learn the art and the available science of anesthesia and to serve as their anesthetists during surgery. Alice Magaw, later called the "Mother of Anesthesia" by Dr. Charles Mayo, mastered this new field, documented her practice, and published her findings in the medical journals of the day. From 1899 through 1906, she reported on more than 14,000 anesthetics that she administered—all without a death attributable to anesthesia (Magaw, 1899, 1906).

Magaw was documenting anesthesia outcomes as well as reporting on the anesthesia techniques and procedures she was developing. Other nurse anesthetists, including Alice Hunt, Agatha Hodgins, Helen Lamb, and Hilda Soloman, also were involved in the early stages of development in anesthesia, but often their labors and accomplishment were published in their surgeons' writings. Considering the state of the art of the biophysical sciences, research methodology, and technology, these were significant studies.

The period between the turn of the century and World War II was one of refining anesthesia procedures and equipment rather than developing new drugs (Thatcher, 1953). Nurse anesthetists, physicians, and engineers were involved in this work. Two drugs, pentothal and curare, were studied and introduced into practice in the late 1930s and early 1940s, achieving notice during World War II. Florence McQuillen, CRNA, the executive director (1948–1970) of the American Association of Nurse Anesthetists (AANA), along with John Lundy, MD, Section of Anesthesiology at the Mayo Clinic, started a journal club and publication entitled *Anesthesia Abstracts* in 1937. When the journal club meetings were discontinued, *Anesthesia Abstracts* became the sole responsibility of McQuillen, though published under the Lundy and McQuillen names with the physician name taking precedence until 1965. Lundy characterized McQuillen as "the best-read person on the literature of anesthesia. Her contribution to the development of the literature on anesthesia is not excelled and probably will not be" (Bankert, 1989, pp. 152–153).

The war served as a major impetus for an increasing number of physicians entering the field. The announced plans by the American Society of Anesthesiologists to eliminate nurse anesthetists and make this an all-physician specialty came when less than one third of the anesthesia providers, nurses or physicians, were qualified by formal education. Thus, the AANA initiated manpower studies

to assess needs for anesthesia providers. The first three studies were reported in the *AANA Journal* in 1955, 1965, and 1971.

Because of the lack of qualified anesthesia providers to meet the needs of this country, the few physicians who entered the field, along with basic scientists in biophysics and pharmacology, performed much of the pharmaceutical and physiological research; nurse anesthetists carried the practice load and sometimes collected data for the studies. Furthermore, the nurse anesthetists' education, being hospital-based, concentrated on practice. It was not until the 1950s and 1960s, after AANA accreditation was well established, that the educational programs were extended to 12 and then 18 months and the performance of small studies was made a part of the students' experiences. Many of these studies related to topics of preoperative preparation for anesthesia and means of preventing postanesthesia nausea and vomiting, that is, problems of concern to nurses.

Goldie Brangman and Ira P. Gunn were notable for their efforts in fostering research for and by nurse anesthetists in the 1960s. Brangman's research efforts and those of her students were published in the *AANA Journal*. Gunn was the first certified registered nurse anesthetist (CRNA) to attend the military nursing and research course at the Walter Reed Army Institute of Research; she studied under Harriet Werley and Phyllis Verhonick, noted nurse researchers. Gunn, with Betty Lewis, a nurse anesthetist and public health nurse, published research findings on the impact of a nursing procedure for oxygen administration on respiratory resistance in tracheotomized patients, utilizing laboratory models (Lewis & Gunn, 1964). An additional article concerning the study was published in the *Journal of the American Medical Association* by adding two physician colleague names as coauthors (Gunn, Jenecik, Lewis, & Meyer, 1965). Gunn and research associates (Gunn, Sullivan, & Glor, 1966) also published an article on the efficacy of blood pressure measurements as a quantitative research criterion.

Gunn (1974) advocated the incorporation of an orientation to research methodology as a part of the nursing anesthesia educational curriculum. She also stated, "The primary role for which nurse anesthetists should be prepared is . . . that of clinical practitioner. However, as with all professionals, they must also have a capability to function as a teacher, a consultant, an administrator, and as a researcher'' (p. 34).

Some educators in nursing anesthesia were advocating moving that subject into degree programs within institutions of higher learning by the mid 1960s, though the movement did not get major impetus until the mid 1970s. By 1985 a BSN or other appropriate baccalaureate degree was required for admission. As of January 1998, all such programs were required to offer a master's degree.

As education moved into institutions of higher learning, research in anesthesia practice became a priority for the profession. With the advent of more master's and doctorally prepared CRNAs and an increase in institutional requirements for research by faculty, the incorporation of research requirements in the nursing anesthesia curriculum established a greater research initiative. Studies predominantly have been practice-based and have not been organized within encompassing theoretical frameworks.

The AANA Foundation was established in 1981 to support both education and research. Funding for nurse anesthesia research has come from traditional funding sources for nursing research, from pharmaceutical and equipment manufacturing firms, and the AANA Foundation. A research-in-action program for students and CRNAs, with an annual award for the best research, is administered by AANA and from 1984 to 1995 was sponsored by Critikon Corporation. Research areas encompass basic science, clinical practice, credentialing, manpower and manpower delivery models, and international studies.

In 1990 the Centers for Disease Control and Prevention (CDC) proposed research on morbidity and mortality in anesthesia. After review of preliminary data, the CDC concluded that the morbidity and mortality rates in anesthesia were too low to warrant a multimillion-dollar study. In a telephone conversation on June 5, 1990, between John Garde, CRNA, MS, Executive Director of AANA and Douglas Klaucke, MD, Assistant Director for Science, Division of Surveillance and Epidemiological Studies of the Centers for Disease Control, Dr.

Klaucke stated that "the expected benefit of this multimillion dollar study is clearly not justified." However, anesthesia outcome studies at the local level must be undertaken by CRNAs as a means of improving practice and demonstrating accountability to the public.

CRNAs have been avid consumers of practice-oriented research. Although CRNAs and the AANA have not been a major source of modern-day research in the 20th century, they are positioned to produce significant research in the 21st century.

JOHN F. GARDE
IRA P. GUNN

See also
**CLINICAL NURSING RESEARCH
EDUCATION: NURSE RESEARCHERS
    AND ADVANCED PRACTICE NURSES
HISTORY OF NURSING RESEARCH
PHYSIOLOGICAL MONITORING**

NURSE-MIDWIFERY

According to the American College of Nurse-Midwives (ACNM), "a Certified Nurse-Midwife (CNM) is an individual educated in the two disciplines of nursing and midwifery, who possesses evidence of certification according to the requirements of the ACNM" (ACNM, 1978). Nurse-midwifery practice is the "independent management of women's health care, focusing particularly on pregnancy, childbirth, the postpartum period, care of the newborn, and the family planning and gynecological needs of women. Nurse-midwives are educated in programs that are accredited by the ACNM Division of Accreditation (DOA), which is recognized by the U.S. Department of Education as an accrediting agency for basic certificate, baccalaureate, and master's degree programs in nurse-midwifery.

The ACNM DOA requires that an education program require a baccalaureate degree upon admission or offer no less than a baccalaureate degree on completion of the program. The majority of nurse-midwives (68%) have master's degrees, and an additional 5% have earned doctorates (ACNM,

1996). All accredited nurse-midwifery education programs are associated with an institution of higher learning and have an educational curriculum that is consistent with the *Core Competencies for Basic Nurse-Midwifery Practice* (ACNM, 1993) as developed by ACNM. The purpose of nurse-midwifery education is to prepare safe, beginning practitioners who are eligible for certification by ACNM or its designate. The national certification examination for nurse-midwives is administered by the ACNM Certification Council, Inc. (ACC). The multiple choice examination is criterion-referenced to the *Core Competencies* and based on a task analysis of current midwifery practice.

Historically, midwifery is the commitment of women to be with women during childbirth and is practiced worldwide. Nurse-midwifery was established in the United States in 1925, when Mary Breckenridge committed her significant knowledge, talent, and financial resources to send public health nurses to England to be trained as midwives. With these nurse-midwives she started the Frontier Nursing Service (FNS) in Hyden, Kentucky. Today the FNS has the largest education program, the Community-Based Nurse-Midwifery Education Program (CNEP), that is also associated with Case Western Reserve University in Ohio. Since 1925 and especially in the past 20 years, there has been a rapid growth in the number of nurse-midwifery education programs and practicing nurse-midwives. A number of publications and research have documented the contributions nurse-midwives are making to the health of women.

A recent national study, funded by the Robert Wood Johnson Foundation, documents the quality and scope of nurse-midwifery practice (Scupholme, Paine, Lang, Kumar, & DeJoseph, 1994). Of all visits to CNMs, 90% are for primary, preventive care. Of these visits, 70% are for care during pregnancy and after birth, and 20% are for care outside the maternity cycle. One third of the time CNMs spend with patient is in education and counseling. Of the women and newborns seen by nurse-midwives, 70% are considered vulnerable by virtue of age, socioeconomic status, education, ethnicity, or place of residence.

The majority of research done by or about nurse-midwives has addressed the nature and outcomes of nurse-midwifery practice (Thompson, 1986). Nurse-midwives have consistently been well-received by women and highly effective in achieving desired pregnancy and birth outcomes. Studies indicate low rates of preterm and low birthweight infants; low cesarean section rates compared to the national rates; lower use of interventions and technology, such as episiotomy and electronic monitoring; high return rates of care and lower costs (Brown & Grimes, 1995). The practice of nurse-midwives is characterized as highly skilled and collaborative in that CNMs are well educated and able to detect complications in a timely manner and consult appropriately with a physician. They also provide emotional support and continuity of care that make a major difference in pregnancy and birth outcomes.

In addition to descriptive and epidemiological research about nurse-midwives and practice outcomes, some investigators have addressed specific clinical practices, such as maternal position (Joyce Roberts) and posture to assist labor and alter the position of the fetus prior to birth (Claire Andrews), hydrotherapy for pain relief in labor (Laraine Guyette and Rebecca Benfield), strategies to avoid episiotomy or lacerations and preserve the integrity of the perineum (Nancy Fleming and Leah Albers), and various approaches to assist women with bearing down in the second stage of labor (Linda Bergstrom, Joyce Roberts, Deborah Woolley). Judith Fullerton has conducted elegant research in the development and validation of the nurse-midwifery certification examination. The methodologies used include experimental designs, case study, retrospective and prospective cohort analysis, and psychometric evaluation (Fullerton & Wingard, 1990.)

In addition, CNMs have addressed the site of practice and environment for birth, including out-of-hospital birth centers and home. Twelve percent of CNMs practice in birth centers. A national study of birth centers by a team of CNMs documented the safety of this setting for low risk women (Rooks et al., 1989). Home births are carried out by 8% of CNMs, and a current study is in progress by Pat Murphy that is a prospective analysis of the outcomes of birth in the home by CNMs. These studies are limited by the nonexperimental nature of the prospective analyses, but respect for women's birth options has made random assignment to birth settings objectionable. Clinical studies are needed to address the effectiveness of such practices as perineal massage and herbal remedies for comfort and for enhancing labor and of innovations in prenatal care.

The process as well as the content of nurse-midwifery care has been addressed, including the model of practice associated with midwifery (Oakley et al., 1996). The components of this model are self-determination of the persons seeking care; collaboration between the midwife, the woman and her family, and other health professionals; use of minimal technological or pharmaceutical interventions; and the organization of care in a way that promotes or preserves continuity. It is imperative that CNMs continue to address the cost-effectiveness of their practice as the health care system and payment patterns change and interdisciplinary models of care emerge.

JOYCE ROBERTS

See also

CHILDBIRTH EDUCATION
PREGNANCY
PRENATAL CARE: COMMUNITY APPROACH
PREVENTION OF PRETERM AND LOW-BIRTHWEIGHT BIRTHS

NURSE-PATIENT COMMUNICATION

Communication is an essential component of nursing intervention, and in some cases it is the intervention itself. As a result, there has been considerable focus on understanding communication as it occurs between nurses and patients. Although communication has been defined in many ways, common features include the transfer or sharing of information in a dynamic process that involves a common set of rules. Depictions of this process typically illustrate messages being sent back and forth between two separate and discrete entities—the sender and the receiver using both verbal and nonverbal channels of communication. This conceptualization of communication has dominated discussion, theorizing, and research on nurse-patient communication, with few exceptions. However, with the emergence of caring theory in nursing, the assumption that communication takes place from a position of distance and from within discrete boundaries has been questioned. Montgomery (1993) suggested that overlapping circles may represent a more appropriate communication model, reflecting nurses' incorporation of the other's subjective experience during caring encounters.

The terms *nurse-patient communication* and *nurse-patient interaction* have sometimes been used interchangeably in the literature. However, it appears that nurse-patient interaction is increasingly being used to refer to the complex dynamics that occur between nurses and patients, of which communication is a key component. The study of communication between nurses and patients appears to be increasingly reserved for the examination of specific verbal or nonverbal behaviors that may be important in nurse-patient encounters.

In the study of nurse-patient communication, most attention has been focused on nurse-initiated verbal and nonverbal behaviors, such as touch, empathetic verbal responses, and blocking statements. Researchers have attempted to describe how nurses use specific communication behaviors, factors that influence the use and interpretation of these behaviors, and their effect on desired patient outcomes. However, research efforts have been hampered by inadequate conceptualizations of the communication behaviors under study. Touch, for example, has been the topic of much research. Primarily viewed as a channel of communication that can function independently of others, it has been studied in isolation from other verbal and nonverbal behaviors. Recent investigations of touch have indicated that a broader concept may be necessary. Eye contact, tone of voice, body position, and purpose of the interaction may all influence the meaning of a touch gesture. The potential value of inductive approaches, such as grounded theory, ethnoscience, and qualitative ethology in developing a more complex understanding of specific communication behaviors such as touch (Bottorff, 1993; Estabrooks, 1989) and in identifying new patterns of communication, such as the comfort talk register (Proctor,

Morse, & Khonsari, 1996), has been demonstrated. Using these approaches, the situated nature of communication is taken into account.

The effect of nurses' communication behavior on patients has been a subject of considerable study. Dependent variables have been measured in a number of ways, including investigator-developed questionnaires, standardized questionnaires, interviews, observational measures, and physiological indices. Yet methodological problems associated with lack of clear or consistent communication interventions, small sample sizes, inadequate attention to reliability and validity of measurements, and lack of adequate control of extraneous variables, in addition to the use of a wide variety of settings, patients, and dependent measures, make it difficult to identify areas of coherence among findings. Inadequate control of other forms of communication that may be associated with the behavior that is the focus of investigation may influence outcomes and explain inconclusive findings. It may be that the most fruitful avenue for future research is to study specific communication behaviors of interest in the context in which they occur, rather than as isolated behaviors in contrived settings. Paying more attention to the perceptions of patients may also assist in determining which effects of nurses' communication behaviors should be addressed.

Recently, researchers have begun to focus on patient verbal and nonverbal behaviors in an attempt to identify behaviors that have particular significance for nursing practice. The underlying assumption is that patient behaviors communicate important information that can be used to guide clinical decision making. For example, detailed analysis of videotaped behaviors of postsurgical neonates has lead to the identification of observable pain responses (Coté, Morse, & James, 1991). Using similar methods of analyses, the examination of maternal sounds and verbalizations during second-stage labor revealed differences between adaptive and nonadaptive sounds, providing important cues to guide caregiver behavior (McKay & Roberts, 1990). Moreover, these findings are important because they indicate that evoking a ''no noise'' rule during second-stage labor is contraindicated.

Although expert nurses often intuitively recognized the meaning of behavioral cues, they were not able to clearly identify the behaviors they were responding to. Microanalysis of videotaped patient behaviors, using approaches like ethology help to explicate clinically relevant patterns of behaviors that can be used as a basis for enhancing the nurse's sensitivity to subtle changes in patient behavior or appearance. In addition, identification of clinically significant behavior patterns also can provide a foundation for the development of outcome measures to evaluate the efficacy of particular nursing interventions. By observing patients in the emergency room, behavioral indicators of escalating levels of distress were identified and provided researchers with the outcome measures to evaluate the efficacy of nurse-initiated interventions such as those aimed at comforting patients (Intrieri, Cerdas, & Morse, 1994). If the interventions are effective, changes in levels of patient distress in the hypothesized direction should be observed.

Methods of data collection that record the actual communication behaviors of nurses and patients, such as audiotape and videotape recordings, are essential to expanding our understanding of communication behaviors although they are time-consuming, expensive, and often intrusive. Taking advantage of advancing technologies to record and analyze physiological indices and communication behaviors simultaneously is an important future direction. Much work remains in identifying and describing important communication concepts that are the foundation of effective nursing interactions and interventions.

JOAN L. BOTTORFF

See also
   CARING
   COMFORT
   NURSE-PATIENT INTERACTION
   NURSE-PATIENT RELATIONSHIP

NURSE-PATIENT INTERACTION

Nurse-patient interaction refers to the dyadic reciprocal interactions that occur between nurses and patients in the context of providing and receiving nursing care. Early nursing theorists such as Peplau,

Orlando, Travelbee, and Widenbach, who drew attention to the process of interaction in nursing practice, prompted researchers to describe, operationalize, and measure the efficacy of nursing interactions. In 1977, Diers and Schmidt classified the rapidly expanding research on nurse-patient interaction as descriptive or correlational studies, studies that measure the indices of nursing by using hypothetical interactions, and studies that describe or evaluate nursing interactions using conception or interaction frameworks borrowed from other disciplines (e.g., counseling psychology). These initial research efforts were largely focused on single channels of communication (e.g., nurse conversation or touch) and produced only partial information about the interaction. Resulting failures to capture relevant clinical data prompted the redesign of instruments and studies specifically for examining nurse-patient interactions. As one example, the Nurse Orientation System developed by Diers was used by researchers to examine the effect of nursing on patient experiences of pain (Diers, Schmidt, McBride, & Davis, 1972).

Researchers continued to study those aspects of the nurse-patient interaction that were quantifiable, using predominantly deductive approaches; and despite the use of increasingly sophisticated techniques, the results of many studies raised concern about the quality of nurse-patient interactions. Some researchers attempted to explain their findings in terms of nurses' lack of communication skills or their busy workloads; others pointed to problems inherent in the research, citing a lack of attention to the patient's role in nurse-patient interaction, unsubstantiated assumptions about the nature of nurse-patient interactions, and failure to take into consideration important contextual factors that influence nurse-patient interactions as major issues (Jarrett & Payne, 1995; May, 1990). In addition, in the absence of adequate definitions of nurse-patient interaction or its components (e.g., touch) researchers used narrow and simplistic conceptualizations. As a result, in deciding a priori what behaviors were important to study, researchers risked missing important behaviors or focusing on insignificant behaviors; as a consequence, they ended up with incomplete or invalid descriptions.

As support for "caring" in nursing developed in the 1980s, theorists drew attention to the complexities inherent in the process of providing nursing care, stimulating a resurgence of interest in examining nurse-patient interactions with a variety of new approaches, such as grounded theory, conversational analysis, ethology, and discourse analysis. By using inductive approaches, researchers identified nurse and patient behaviors that were important to study (rather than deciding this a priori), explored interaction patterns from the perspective of the nurse and patients, and considered important factors of context and relationship. Studies completed by researchers such as Carl May, Maura Hunt, Jocalyn Lawler, and Janice Morse are representative examples. Using these new approaches, researchers identified exceptional nursing interaction skills, such as "tactics," "comfort talk," "minifisms," and other previously unrecognized interaction strategies that nurses typically used in clinical settings—skills that were rarely part of communication courses and often devalued.

One of the most important developments in the study of nurse-patient interactions is the use of video technology. Videotaping observations preserves the observational context, verbal content, nonverbal behaviors, and interactive processes for analysis and coding. Of particular advantage is the ability to repeatedly review videotapes, both in real time and in slow motion. This facilitates in-depth study of a wide range of simultaneous behaviors, including rarely occurring events and subtle or rapid changes in behavior. Videotaped observations are particularly useful when studying interactions with patients who are preverbal, unconscious, or otherwise unable to recall interactions with sufficient detail.

When videotaped observations of naturally occurring nurse-patient interactions are used as data for qualitative studies, new patterns of interaction have been revealed. For example, by use of qualitative ethology (Morse & Bottorff, 1990), an analysis of videotaped interactions of cancer patients and their nurses led Bottorff and Morse (1994) to suggest alternative ways of looking at and structuring nurse-patient interactions to capture the unique styles of interaction that are characteristic of nursing practice. The four types of attending identified in this study captured the dynamic nature of interaction between nurses and patients from a more global perspective than did previous sentence-by-sentence analysis. This facilitated the identification of subtle changes between and within interactions that were not possible using previous dichotomous descriptions of interactions (e.g., therapeutic/nontherapeutic) and took into account more than just the component of verbal communication.

Although these new lines of research show promise and appear to be unraveling some of the unique complexities inherent in nurse-patient interaction, much work remains to understand nursing interactions as they occur in health care settings, including patients' homes or other community settings. Far more attention has been given to identifying and describing components and patterns of nurse-patient interaction than studying the efficacy of different types of interactions in relation to patient outcomes. It appears that some patterns of interaction may be powerful therapeutic tools, yet more systematic investigation is needed to demonstrate these effects. Furthermore, negative or undesirable psychological and physiological sequalae associated with interaction patterns should be documented.

Although the definition of nurse-patient interaction has not received careful attention, the focus has been on the verbal and nonverbal behaviors of the nurse. Yet increasingly, patients are being encouraged to take an active role in decision making and their nursing care. To develop innovative and supportive strategies to foster collaboration in care and involvement in decision making, a sound understanding of the nature of interactions between nurses and patient, with a strong focus on the role of patient behavior in these interactions, is necessary. In addition, the links between nurse-patient interaction and types of nurse-patient relationships must be explored.

JOAN L. BOTTORFF

See also
   CARING
   NURSE-PATIENT COMMUNICATION
   NURSE-PATIENT RELATIONSHIP
   PARTICIPANT OBSERVATION
   PEPLAU'S THEORETICAL MODEL

NURSE-PATIENT RELATIONSHIP

The interpersonal relationship between nurses and patients has become an important subject of discussion, theorizing, and research since Peplau and Orlando introduced the concept of the nurse-patient relationship as an essential component of nursing practice. Recognition of the need for individualized nursing care, the introduction of new approaches to care delivery (e.g., primary nursing), increasing concerns about dehumanization related to advances in technology, and the emergence of theories delineating caring as a pivotal concept in nursing have reinforced the centrality of the nurse-patient relationship in contemporary practice. The nurse-patient relationship is now viewed as essential content in nursing curricula, and clinicians value the development of therapeutic relationships with patients as a significant part of their work. Yet despite the overwhelming endorsement of the importance of the nurse-patient relationship, the practical difficulties associated with developing relationships remain unresolved. Of importance are issues related to balancing personal involvement and professional detachment. Other important issues concern building relationships in contexts where the organization of nurses' work limits involvement or where reporting practices undermine the development of trust. Issues also arise from challenges related to renegotiating relationships in response to changes in patient dependence and vulnerability.

Nurses have attempted to identify the unique characteristics of the nurse-patient relationship through their conceptualizations, although to date there is little evidence to support this assumption. The nurse-patient relationship has been described as a therapeutic instrument with levels or types of involvement and as an interactive process requiring the active participation of both patients and nurses. Important components of the nurse-patient relationship include concepts such as empathy, trust, respect, knowing the patient, commitment, advocacy, and social control. Nursing writers critiquing current conceptualizations of the nurse-patient relationship have pointed out the failure to consider the collective nature of nursing work and other realities of everyday practice such as the provision of bodily comforts (May, 1990; May & Purkis,

1995). Theorists such as Sally Gadow and Jean Watson have attempted to explain the nature of the links between nurse-patient relationships and positive health care outcomes, and there is some empirical evidence that supports these assertions.

Although researchers have begun to explore the complex dynamics involved in nurse-patient interactions and their therapeutic potential, there is relatively little empirical data related to what takes place in everyday clinical settings to support current conceptualizations of the nurse-patient relationship. Early investigations of nurse-patient relationships were influenced by definitions from the social sciences and the traditions of logical positivism. However, explanations of the relationship proved difficult to quantify. With increasing acceptance of qualitative research methods in nursing, researchers have turned to a variety of new approaches to examine patterns of relationships in nursing, including grounded theory and narrative analysis. For representative examples, see Carl May (1991), Janice Morse (1991), and Joan Liaschenko (1997). These studies have revealed important new information about nurse-patient relationships, some of which has contradicted professional rhetoric surrounding the development of these relationships. For example, Morse's (1991) grounded theory analysis revealed that nurses used several strategies to increase the level of involvement, including sharing personal information. This strategy often is not condoned in nursing textbooks.

The complexities inherent in the nurse-patient relationship demand that the research agenda be augmented by micro-level approaches (such as sociolinguistics, ethnomethodology, and in-depth videotape analysis), advances in interpretive methodology (e.g., using a feminist perspective), and triangulation (e.g., triangulating conversational analysis with data from ethnographic research), as well as by taking advantage of constructionist, critical, and postmodern theory to understand the dynamics of nurse-patient relationships (Lowenberg, 1994; May, 1990; May & Purkis, 1995). For example, observational studies of the development of nurse-patient relationships as they occur in everyday clinical settings would augment nurses' narratives of memorable relationships. Some researchers are exploring the potential value of using video recorders to capture the development of relationships over time. Detailed analysis of videotaped patient and nurse behaviors at the interaction level have produced some encouraging results.

For the most part, researchers have focused on the affective dimensions of nurse-patient relationships by interviewing nurses, particularly those who were able to provide exemplar cases. Other dimensions of the nurse-patient relationship should be examined, as well as outcomes, as they relate to different phases and types of relationships. Attention must be given to the patient's perspective and role in shaping relationships. Morse's (1991) research was a beginning step in unraveling the strategies that patients used to increase or decrease the rate and level of the developing relationship. Finally, assumptions related to the consistency of nurse-patient relationships across clinical settings require empirical examination. Most research efforts have been concentrated in acute care settings. Nurse-patient relationships in other contexts also should be studied, including community health and home care nursing.

JOAN L. BOTTORFF

See also
**FEMINIST RESEARCH METHOD-
    OLOGY
NURSE-PATIENT COMMUNICATION
NURSE-PATIENT INTERACTION
PEPLAU'S THEORETICAL MODEL
TRIANGULATION**

NURSE RESEARCHER IN THE CLINICAL SETTING

The term *nurse researcher in the clinical setting* is used to denote nurses who have research as one of their responsibilities or their sole responsibility and are at least partly supported by salary from a clinical setting, inclusive of hospitals, clinics, and other agencies providing health care to patients. Such nurses are usually prepared at the doctoral level but sometimes at the master's level. The additional responsibilities of these individuals may include education, quality improvement, evaluation in the clinical facility, and the requisite administration accompanying those duties. The position in the clinical setting can be either line or staff. The individual also may be jointly appointed to a school or college of nursing or another health-related institution for a percentage of their time.

The specific responsibilities for these individuals include conducting research and assisting others in conducting, applying, and utilizing research. Although those are the explicit role responsibilities, the nurse researcher in a clinical setting is expected to affect the nursing staff positively in several indirect ways. The nurse researcher is an educator, teaching about the research process, guiding critiques of completed research for application and utilization, and developing research days for sharing of research. The researcher is involved in the professional development of staff, facilitating staff to present and publish their data-based projects under the tutelage of the researcher. Nurse researchers in clinical agencies usually have the responsibility to represent the agency with outside researchers using the agency as a data collection site. In the role of change agent, the researcher helps to make practice research-based. The change agent role and the researcher role are often combined with the quality control role, where pre- and postmonitoring or longitudinal monitoring around a change are needed.

To carry out these responsibilities, the researcher must possess several attributes. Knowledge and skills in the research are the most obvious, but equally important are people skills (e.g., motivating, confirming, guiding professional development) and conceptual skills. The latter set of skills comes into play in several ways, for example, identifying a researchable problem and reworking complaints and questions into a basis for finding solutions.

A major difference between the academic researcher and the nurse researcher in the clinical setting is the mission of the employer. The university has a societal responsibility for knowledge advancement. The health care institution has a responsibility for health care. Mission is a key work environment characteristic, and the work environment has a profound impact on the outcomes of one's work. This is especially true for nurse researchers in clinical settings, whose outcomes are influenced by their environment. Research productivity (conducting, using, and communicating research) has been shown to be associated with the agency's work environment (Martin, 1988, 1993). Within clinical agencies the following have been associated with research productivity: (a) research culture (policies and procedures indicative of a consistent commitment to nursing research, such as the presence of research in the agency's mission); (b) resources for research activities (e.g., library holdings, funding of research activities, presence of other nurses with advanced nursing education); (c) attitudes (e.g., belief that the public and other professional colleagues value nursing research; and (d) esprit, a positive group work morale. Clearly, these nurse researcher roles are complex and not an insignificant addition to any staff.

One of the first tasks for the nurse researcher new to a setting is to assess the work environment, including the resources available. In particular, the nurse researcher cannot function well if isolated from others with research skills. Baccalaureate graduates with a foundation in research, master's-prepared nurses who have completed a thesis or have had strong intermediate research instruction, and doctorally prepared nurses with advanced research preparation are important resources. The last may not be part of the researcher's organization but available through an affiliated university. The availability of university-educated nurses is both an indication of the education programming needed and whether the environment has a "critical mass" of nurses for research activities.

The initial national survey of these individuals was conducted by Knafl, Bevis, and Kirchhoff in 1987. At that time there were 34 nurses who were employed at least 50% of the time and had been in that position for 6 months or more. They and their corresponding chief nurse executive were interviewed by phone about the development of the relatively new role. Additionally, strategies for success were identified: (a) promoting interest of the nursing staff in nursing research, (b) increasing the researcher's autonomy and control over position and activity, (c) demonstrating the contribution of nursing research to the organization, and (d) conveying acceptability as an individual. These 34 researchers were involved in more than 200 projects at the time of the interview. This national study and reports of single programs in hospitals or across a few settings are summarized by Kirchhoff (1993) in an *Annual Review of Nursing Research* chapter.

A second national follow-up using a mailed questionnaire was done 10 years later by Kirchhoff and Mateo (1996). At that time there were 142 nurses in research positions, usually employed solely in the clinical setting (56%). They spent about 50% of their time on research which is the same as that found by Knafl, Bevis, and Kirchhoff (1987). They also had responsibilities for education (55.7% of respondents), administration (80% of respondents), and quality assurance (37.7%).

Karin T. Kirchhoff
Patricia Martin

See also
ADVANCED PRACTICE NURSES
CLINICAL NURSING RESEARCH
DOCTORAL EDUCATION
EDUCATION: NURSE RESEARCHERS
   AND ADVANCED PRACTICE NURSES
RESEARCH CAREERS

NURSE STAFFING

Nurse staffing refers to the number and types of workers employed by an agency to provide nursing care to the persons served by the agency. Nurse staffing numbers are typically given in full-time equivalent (FTE), which represents 52 40-hour weeks, or 2,080 hours, the typical amount paid to a full-time individual. The hours that individuals actually work would be fewer and would depend on paid benefit hours (e.g., vacation, holiday, sick, etc.) that are included in each FTE-paid 2,080 hours. Hours are reported in the type of worker used or needed, and those are classified as registered nurses (R), licensed practical (or vocational) nurses (L), and aides (A), variously called attendants, technicians or assistants.

Analyses of nurse staffing are performed retrospectively (essentially a count of the workers who were present and the patients they cared for) and prospectively. Nearly all reported nurse staffing research is prospective in that studies attempt to predict the number and types of workers needed to care for specified patient groups. Nurse staffing has been examined in detail, and anthologies of the studies have been prepared (Aydelotte, 1973; Young, Giovanetti, Lewison, & Thoms, 1981). In addition, research critiques and recommendations for further study have been advanced (Halloran & Hadley-Vermeersch, 1987; Wunderlich, Sloan, & Davis, 1996). New techniques have been developed for estimating the need for nurses (Murphy, 1978), but these tend to lack connection to professional knowledge.

Implicit in the study of nurse staffing is an expectation that research will yield results that are generalizable—that is, others in the specified universe can safely apply the findings from valid and reliable studies and experience comparable results. To date few such generalizable findings have been made. It may be unreasonable to expect a high degree of standardization among the individuals (patients) who use nursing services and those (nurses) who provide them. Yet it seems worthwhile to understand the reasons for the one consistent finding in nurse staffing analyses: some hospitals (where nurse staffing has been studied most) provide twice as much nursing care for their patients as do similar institutions (Dartmouth Medical School, 1996).

The three different perspectives from which to study nurse staffing are (a) by task, procedure, intervention, or work analysis; (b) by disease and treatment; and (c) through nursing viewpoints. Nurse staffing studies based on task or work analysis emanate from Taylor's (1911) *Principles of Scientific Management*. These were first applied to hospital work in the 1920s and have been in use since that time. The most important development of work analysis methods applied to hospitals was the linkage Connor (1960) established between nurse staffing and variability in patient types and numbers. Patients are classified on the basis of the type of work they generate, and the classifications are mapped to an unstandardized number and mix of nursing staff. It is uncommon to find reports that compare patient classification done in one institution to that of another.

A great deal of attention has been directed to the reliability of patient classification techniques, with few reports to validate patient classification beyond the face validity established in the agency using the instrument. Two nurses classifying the same patient at the same time and in the same way achieve perfect reliability. Because of differences in nurses, it is not infrequent that ratings of the same patient differ. To bypass this reliability concern, prototype patient classification instruments have been developed. Prototype instruments cumulate time-weighted factors (items from a list of procedures done or a list of patient conditions for which interventions are needed) into scores that two nurses can agree on but that may have been derived from different factors. The result is to refer to the classified patient as a member of classes I, II, III, or IV, rather than as a patient who needs assistance with toileting, feeding, and/or ambulating. Further validity is lost because psychosocial aspects of care, long described as essential to effective care, have never been associated with weights reflecting the time nurses spend with patients.

Failure to specify intended results and measure the capacity of different patterns of work and worker to achieve those results is the most common problem with work analysis techniques for the study of nurse staffing. Few have studied the appropriateness of either the task or the performer in achieving a specified end result. Work analysis methods are criticized because they result in standards of care that are inconsistent with clinical research results, qualitative studies of nursing care, and nearly all concepts or theories of nursing. In one concept of nursing work, nurses assist individuals to perform their own tasks, procedures, or interventions through encouragement and education as a means to their independence (Henderson & Nite, 1978/1997).

Nurse staffing research has been linked to the diseases and treatments afforded patients on hospital specialty units. Most hospital inpatient wards care for specific patient groups organized by the physicians who admit the patients. Common groupings include orthopedic, cardiological, oncological, neurological, respiratory, gynecological, psychiatric, obstetric, pediatric, geriatric, and many others. The earliest nurse staffing studies differentiated medical from surgical units, and many recent reports are addressed to even more specific patient disease groupings, for example, HIV-AIDS.

The assumption that underlies the representation of patients' disease as the basis for nurse staffing is that the care rendered is homogeneous for the members of the patient group, different from other groups, and associated with a specific mix and number of nursing staff. Also implicit in the use of disease and treatment classification for the prediction of nursing staff is that nursing care is prescribed by physicians. The diagnosis-related group (DRG) is the most common representation of the medical approach to nurse staffing. Medical methods for computing staff needs should be used with caution, as much nursing literature addresses the differences in individual human beings even if they are suffering from the same disease (Henderson & Nite, 1978/1997).

A clear exposition for the representation of time in nurse staffing research is needed. In nurse staffing research, time can be represented in three ways: (a) by nurse (or nursing) hours per patient day, (b) by nursing hours per case, and (c) by length of hospital stay (LOS). The association between nurses' time and length of patients' stays raises questions of causality: Are physicians and medical care responsible for variability in LOS (and thus nursing hours per case)? Development and use of LOS norms (including care maps) established by physicians suggest that doctors control LOS and nursing hours per case. But because DRGs are a poor predictor of LOS, another perspective on nurse staffing is needed to explain and predict case time measured by day or stay.

Length-of-stay variability within DRGs has been explained and predicted from nurses' classifications of patients (Rosenthal, Halloran, Kiley, & Landefeld, 1995; Rosenthal, Halloran, Kiley, Pinkley, & Landefeld, 1992). The classification used to explain variation in patients' use of nurses' time, as well as variations in their hospital stays, were derived from literature describing nurses' unique contributions in terms of patients' human functions (Henderson, 1960/1997; Henderson & Nite, 1978/1997). Nurses' classification data have been variously described in terms of patients' problems, needs, symptoms, conditions, syndromes, factors, intensity, and severity. Common to all these is a concern for the following basic needs: respiration, eating and drinking, elimination, posture and movement, rest and sleep, clothing and dressing, temperature, cleanliness and hygiene, protection, communication, morals and religion, work, recreation and learning, and the personal and social conditions that always affect basic needs, as well as the pathological states that may modify them.

Research on staffing should be intrinsically linked to concepts and theories of nursing as well as to the scientific and expert opinion literature on nursing. Existing methods for studying nurse staffing that employ work measurement methods or assume that nursing care is derived from medical care should be viewed with caution. Much more study of nurse staffing is required for generalization. Needed research should take place on two levels. First and foremost, differences in nursing care and their effects on patients should be examined at the bedside (Brooten & Naylor, 1995). Second, comparisons should be made among institutions using standardized methods that capture valid, reliable, and retrievable data from nurses about patients. These institutional comparisons should also incorporate data about nurses (e.g., education, experience, assignments, etc.) so that inferences can be drawn about nurses' contributions to the end results of patient care.

EDWARD J. HALLORAN

See also
  **COST ANALYSIS OF NURSING CARE
  NURSING INTENSITY
  NURSING WORKLOAD MEASURE-
    MENT SYSTEMS
  PATIENT CLASSIFICATION**

NURSING ASSESSMENT

Assessment is widely recognized as the first step in the nursing process. Nurses use assessment to determine patients' actual and potential needs, the assistance patients require, and the desired outcomes to evaluate the care provided. There is widespread consensus that nursing assessment is crucial as the starting point for establishing relationships and for determining how patients and nurses will subsequently interact. Assessment begins with the initial nurse-patient encounter and continues as long as the nurse and patient interact. Assessment involves collecting information to plan care and is an important basis for determining which interventions can be delegated to other providers. Information collected can be classified as either social and health history data, which come directly from patients, or physical assessment data, which are derived from physical assessment techniques and diagnostic studies.

The purposes of assessment are to begin to establish a therapeutic relationship and to identify the patients' strengths and problems in order to determine appropriate interventions. Both the process and the content of assessment are important. Process includes using communication and physical assessment skills to establish a relationship and to gather needed information. The important content will vary with the patient but generally includes physical assessment, other diagnostic data, and assessment of the meaning of the health experience, quality of life, and symptoms. It is important to consider cultural features that may affect health.

Historical Perspective

Florence Nightingale was among the first to discuss nursing assessment (Nightingale, 1860/1969). She believed that the process of observation was essential, and she provided very specific guidance about both the process and needed content of nursing assessments. Nightingale outlined the best process for interactions. "Always sit down when a sick person is talking business to you, show no signs of hurry, give complete attention and full consideration. . . . Always sit within the patients' view" (pp. 48–49).

Assessment must be complete and detailed. Nightingale (1969) noted that "leading questions" are "useless or misleading" (p. 107). Rather than asking for evaluation (e.g., asking if a night's sleep was good), details should be asked for (e.g., the number of hours the person slept). These details, rather than the opinions derived from them, must be reported. Nightingale attributed the fact that physicians did not believe nurses' assessments to nurses' failure to provide such details. Nightingale also gave examples of information that was misleading because it was incomplete or was based on incomplete observations (e.g., the difference between "how often the bowels acted" and the number of times the "utensil" was emptied, p. 107).

Nightingale (1860/1969) discussed the content needed in assessment, which included individualization, as "taking averages" is misleading (p. 120). She noted the need to understand "all the conditions in which the patient lives" (p. 121), including lifestyle factors, social conditions, and hygiene. Among the areas that ought to be observed she noted the patient's dietary intake, symptoms and their meaning, changes in patterns (such as physical abilities) and "idiosyncracies" of patients. She noted that "peculiarities might be observed and indulged much more than they are" (p. 117).

Process of Assessment

Considerable research has been conducted on factors that influence interpersonal relationships. Several classic works in nursing have dealt with the process of establishing relationships and the role that nursing plays at various phases of relationships. Observation and communication, including the use of self-disclosure and empathy, are important in establishing relationships (e.g., Peplau, 1952). The assessment is the beginning of the relationship and will determine how nurses and patients will work together.

Literature on communication is important in informing nurses about the appropriate process for assessment. Communication is essential in assessment; it is the means for nurses and patients to influence each other and the process that leads to therapeutic and supportive influences on patients' health. Patients' successful communication of their needs to nurses is vital to individualized care. Individualized patient care has been found to produce more favorable outcomes and to reduce the cost of health care (Gardner, 1991).

Although assessment and communication skills have been taught for decades, many studies have found that nurses had difficulty in facilitating communication, and the patients' analysis of communication is often omitted. A variety of factors have been related to low facilitation of communication, including management in some health care settings, increased patient volume, the value placed on tasks, and not having attitudes and desires to communicate (May, 1990). Nurses also have been found to be confused about the purpose of nursing assessment. Observations indicated that nurse-patient interactions are superficial, routinized, and task related and that it is the nurse who creates barriers in communication.

Surveys of nurses revealed that most had received training in communication skills. They felt that they were fairly effective in using these skills and that the skills were important to their jobs. However, they also thought they needed additional training in communication and were willing to receive such training. Communication training programs have been studied with mixed results, including benefits that did not persist, changes that were limited, and programs that did not improve nurses' ability to elicit and identify patient concerns despite increased use of the skills learned.

Content of Assessment

Physical assessment skills are routinely included in nursing curricula. They include (a) a general survey of the patient's appearance and behaviors; (b) assessment of vital signs, temperature, pulse, respirations, and blood pressure; (c) assessment of height and weight; and (d) physical examination to assess the patient's structures, organs, and body systems.

Physical assessment can be complete, assessing all of the persons' organs and body systems, or modified to focus on areas suggested by the health history or symptoms. Perceptions of symptoms and quality of life are important areas for assessment. Both symptoms and quality of life are primarily subjective experiences, influenced by many factors but knowable primarily through the patients' descriptions of the experiences. Moreover, symptoms that are not properly managed can be life-threatening.

Nurses should explore meaning of illness from the patient's perspective to help patients mediate between the medical role of fighting disease and the patients' perspective (Dougherty & Tripp-Reimer,

1990). The link between meaning making and the experience of illness and treatment may help elucidate important nursing interventions that can assist patients in ways helpful to coping with the experience and symptoms.

Understanding the experiences of illnesses and treatments of minority individuals is important but currently limited. Many have argued for the need to understand clients' lived experiences and their interactions in order to provide quality nursing care (Sawyer, Regev, Proctor, et al., 1995). Producing unbiased and culturally appropriate knowledge is both important and complex. The experiences of those in minority groups may differ in ways that profoundly affect assessment.

Despite consensus about the importance of understanding the patient's perspective, patients' descriptions show a consistent and persistent discrepancy between views of their health care experiences and professionals' understandings of these experiences. The meanings that patients attribute to their experiences help determine what needs they have and how these needs can best be met. Because action is based on meanings, common meanings for both nurses and patients will provide the most effective base for helpful nurse-patient relationships. Research indicates that nurses must understand the patient's perspective in order to deliver effective nursing care, but often nurses assume that they know what their patients need without eliciting actual patient concerns. Effective assessment is the essential basis for providing effective nursing care.

MARLENE ZICHI COHEN
ANITA J. TARZIAN

See also
(FLORENCE) NIGHTINGALE
NURSE-PATIENT COMMUNICATION
NURSE-PATIENT INTERACTION
NURSE-PATIENT RELATIONSHIP
NURSING PROCESS

NURSING CENTERS

Definition

Nursing centers, also known as nurse-managed centers, nursing clinics, or community nursing organi-

zations, provide nursing services to individuals, families, and communities and serve as sites for nursing research and education (Riesch, 1992). The types of services provided usually are ambulatory and of a health-promotion, risk-reduction, or illness-prevention nature. The Council for Nursing Centers within the National League for Nursing serves as the official source of information on the number, types, and locations of nursing centers.

History

Historically, the nursing center idea originated in the early 1900s with the establishment of district and public health nursing. Later examples were the Kentucky Frontier Nursing Services and the New York City Loeb Center. During the 1970s storefront clinics, independent nursing practices, and community nursing center demonstration sites represented the nursing center concept. During the 1980s many schools and colleges of nursing, as well as hospitals, clinics, and public health agencies, established nursing clinics. With increasing emphasis on primary, managed, and interdisciplinary care in the 1990s, nursing centers entered into partnerships and business agreements. Though fiscal gain was never a primary goal, fiscal management has emerged as a survival skill (Frenn, Lundeen, Martin, Riesch, & Wilson, 1996).

Conceptual Models

Nursing centers may be classified by the types of services they provide. The first model, community health and institutional outreach programs, generally focuses on the delivery of primary care services in underserved areas with interdisciplinary collaborative practice partnerships. Funding is diverse, provided by the sponsoring institutions, fees for service, grants, and gifts. An example of this type of nursing center is the Silver Spring Neighborhood Center in Milwaukee, Wisconsin. Partnerships with health and social service agencies, a consumer advisory board reflecting the community served, and a nurse executive director distinguish this type of center.

Nursing centers based on wellness and health promotion are the second type of model and commonly are located where people gather—in workplaces, schools, meal sites, neighborhoods, and homeless shelters. Services provided are based on aggregate needs. Creative use of private and public funding sources is necessary to establish and maintain these services. The following are examples of wellness and health promotion models: (a) the Pine Street Inn of Boston, supported by city and county funds and serving homeless persons, and (b) the Minnesota Block Nurse Program funded as a community nursing organization (CNO) demonstration project of the federal Health Care Financing Administration (HCFA) and serving Medicare beneficiaries who are homebound elders.

Faculty practice, independent nursing practices, and entrepreneurship models are the third type of model and often follow a business model of ownership, funding, and operations while providing specialized care such as home health care or midwifery services. Examples include (a) the Carondolet Health Network based in Tucson, Arizona, which is an HCFA-funded CNO group of case-managed health and preventive services, including community and inpatient settings; (b) the Maternity Center in New York City, which has provided prenatal, perinatal, and postpartum care since its inception in 1975; and (c) the Penn Nursing Network, a group of 10 community-based nursing practices whose mission, beyond direct patient care, is to utilize and test nursing research in practice. Each Penn Nursing Network site has co-directors who are affiliated with the University of Pennsylvania School of Nursing faculty.

Research

Most of the research on or in nursing centers has used quantitative approaches to describe phenomena of concern or to test nursing interventions for specific outcomes. The utilization of research in the development of patient care protocols is often reflected in the philosophy or mission statements of nursing centers.

Early studies documented the concepts that define a nursing center, such as (a) direct access by patients and families to professional nurses for holistic health promotion and disease prevention strategies that are reimbursable and based on theory and research; (b) operating as part of a larger system of health care delivery for the purposes of collaboration and referral; (c) nurse administration; and (d) serving as a site for research and student learning. Other early studies included surveys of the location of centers, services provided, differentiation of nurse and physician role, patient outcomes, client satisfaction, and documented student learning outcomes.

A number of more recent single, unreplicated studies have documented improvements in client and family health status, client satisfaction, cost-effectiveness, and quality of care. Knowledge, attitudes, and behavior outcomes that improved as a result of care received in nursing centers included parental ability to deal with and understand childhood asthma; parents' compliance with recommended immunization schedules; elders' increased participation in hypertension, glaucoma, diabetes, and cancer screening activities; and childbearing couples' increased self-care. Outcomes indicating improved client health status have included Apgar scores, birthweight, and prevalence of breastfeeding; communication between parents and young teens; control of blood sugar and healing of leg ulcers in older persons with diabetes; reduced incidents of seeking medical attention for minor complaints among persons with chronic illness; and weight loss among persons with Type II diabetes.

Patients and families who receive care in nursing centers overwhelmingly are satisfied with the care. They learn about disease processes and progression (referred to as "what is wrong"), as well as about side effects of treatments and pain management. They are pleased with the amount of attention received, the limited waiting periods to see the nurse, and the comprehensiveness of the care received. Though limited in amount, data on cost-effectiveness and quality of care are promising. Early studies demonstrated that costs were within the same range as similar services in the community. However, visits were longer and fewer, indicating that utilization potential was not met. The HCFA-funded CNOs have demonstrated that comprehensive quality care can be delivered successfully within a capitated system.

Future

With the introduction and implementation of nursing information systems linked to larger health care data sets, major multisite studies of nursing processes and outcomes will become feasible, and implications for policy will be substantiated. However, the care and outcomes should include the patient and family perspective in care delivery and research design. Utilization of the Nursing Minimum Data Set and classifications systems for nursing diagnoses, interventions, and outcomes has assisted practitioners and scholars in nursing centers to define and refine the diagnosis and treatment of human responses to actual and potential health problems.

The concept of a single discipline demonstrating its capabilities has outlived its usefulness. Accessible, comprehensive, interdisciplinary care delivered across multiple settings, with specific aspects sensitive to nursing diagnosis, intervention, and outcome, is where the discipline should focus its education, research, and practice resources.

SUSAN K. RIESCH

See also
ACCESS TO HEALTH CARE
COMMUNITY HEALTH
HEALTH SYSTEMS DELIVERY
HOMELESS HEALTH
WELLNESS

NURSING DIAGNOSIS

A nursing diagnosis is a condition or response of patients and clients that involves nursing care. It is the clinical judgment made by professional nurses based on an assessment of objective and subjective patient responses.

In 1953 the term *nursing diagnosis* was introduced by V. Frey as a step in the development of a care plan. For 20 years the nursing community virtually ignored nursing diagnosis. Then, in 1973, Gebbie and Lavin sponsored a conference on the classification of nursing diagnosis at the University of St. Louis. They organized the conference in response to a need for a standardized language for nursing. This standardized language was necessary for the computerization of nursing activities for automated record keeping. More than 115 nurses attended the conference and participated in the identification and description of 100 health problems or conditions that nurses diagnosed and treated in patients and clients. The nurses identified the diagnoses through recall of clinical conditions or problems in their patients by body systems to generate nursing diagnosis (Gebbie & Lavin, 1975).

Between the first and second conference, from 1973 to 1975, a national task force based at the University of St. Louis formed and conducted the first validity study of nursing diagnoses. This was a multisite research project involving 28 agencies and 588 patients. The task force asked nurses in acute care and long-term care hospitals, community health and home nursing agencies, and nursing homes to identify clinical problems in their patients. The results showed that 81% of the patient problems or conditions were related to diagnoses identified at the first conference, and the other 19% were disease-specific. The most frequent patient conditions were related to pain, mobility, anxiety, and impaired skin integrity (Gebbie, 1976).

The original list of diagnoses was ordered alphabetically. In 1977, Sister Callista Roy suggested that a theorist group form to categorize the diagnoses into an organizing framework. There was general support for a taxonomy or classification system of nursing diagnoses. A taxonomic structure should improve utility of diagnoses by clinicians and researchers, facilitate interface with other classification systems, assist in the evaluation of the impact of practice, provide a universal vocabulary used by nursing, and identify phenomena of concern to nurse researchers. In 1978, 14 individuals accepted the invitation to participate in a theorist group to form a framework for the first nursing diagnosis classification system. This theorist group, chaired by Sr. Roy, along with input from clinicians and graduate students, was a historic event for convening the leading nurse theorists. The theorists identified 60 potential methods for categorizing the diagnoses, and they presented a classification system consisting of nine patterns of unitary man: acting, exchanging, feeling, choosing, communicating, knowing, perceiving, relating, and valuing. Since that time this taxonomic structure has been revised and updated, and additional classification systems, such as the Omaha system (see "Formal Languages") and the Saba system (Saba et al., 1991), have been developed.

In the 1970s the American Nurses Association (ANA) published the first set of professional standards, including a standard on nursing diagnosis. Each specialty organization replicated this diagnosis standard as professional standards were developed within respective specialty areas. As each of these sets of standards has been revised, the standard referring to nursing diagnosis has been strengthened. The ANA social policy statement (1995b) strongly mandated the inclusion of nursing diagnosis as a component of nursing practice, with nursing diagnoses directing the goals for nursing care. The ANA maintains a Steering Committee on Databases to Support Clinical Nursing Practice, which has the responsibility for recognizing nomenclatures and classification systems on behalf of the profession.

In 1982 the initial task forces formed the organization North American Nursing Diagnosis Association to continue to identify, review, refine, classify, and disseminate information about nursing diagnosis. Over the next 15 years nursing diagnosis and its taxonomic structure sparked immense scholarly debate and controversy relative to its validity, syntax, organizing structure, and clinical utility. In particular, discussion and work centered on the inclusion of all patients and clients (individuals, families, and communities), the designation of health promotion and wellness conditions as nursing diagnosis, the impact of growth and development on diagnosis, the question of specialty-focused diagnosis, and the effect of diagnoses across cultures.

The North American Nursing Diagnosis Association adopted the following definition for nursing diagnosis in 1990: "Nursing diagnosis is a clinical judgment about an individual, family, or community response to actual or potential health problems/life processes. Nursing diagnoses provide the basis for the selection of nursing intervention to achieve outcomes for which the nurse is accountable."

In 1990 the ANA, in association with the North American Nursing Diagnosis Association, submitted an adapted list of nursing diagnoses, "Conditions That Necessitate Nursing Care," to the World Health Organization for inclusion in the *International Classification of Diseases*, version 10 (ICD-10). The list was adapted from multiple taxonomic structures used within nursing (Fitzpatrick, 1991b). Although the list was not included in the ICD-10, the action stimulated international work on classifications (Lang, 1995). In 1989, the International Council of Nurses (ICN) passed a resolution that resulted in the development of the *International Classification for Nursing Practice*. An alpha version of this classification was published in 1996 (International Council of Nurses, 1996).

The ANA forwarded four nursing classification systems to the National Library of Medicine for inclusion in the Unified Medical Language System (UMLS). The entry of this set of terms was completed in 1997. The goal of ANA is a unified language of nursing, and the ICN is working to develop a global unified nursing language system (McCormick et al., 1994).

Since the initiation of the first conference on nursing diagnosis, biannual national conferences as well as regional meetings have been held to support the identification, review, refinement, and dissemination of nursing diagnoses and taxonomic structure. Energy and enthusiasm for the generation of nursing diagnosis reached a peak in 1988, after which the generation of new nursing diagnoses decreased. As of 1997, 12 national conferences have been held, including the first conference in 1972. Research on the validity of individual nursing diagnoses and the classification system continues with strong international support by representation of nursing from more than 20 countries at the national conferences. Current challenges to the continued utilization of nursing diagnosis as a basis for practice involve the integration of nursing diagnoses into a managed care environment and the expanded role of the nurse practitioner. Celebration of the 25th anniversary of nursing diagnoses will occur at its founding location, St. Louis, Missouri, in the spring of 1998.

MARY E. KERR

See also
NANDA

FORMAL LANGUAGES
INTERNATIONAL CLASSIFICATION
  FOR NURSING PRACTICE
OMAHA SYSTEM
UNIFIED LANGUAGE SYSTEMS

NURSING EDUCATION

History

In 1873 three hospital training programs, modeled on Florence Nightingale's work in the United Kingdom, were established in the United States. In 1907 a Department of Nursing and Health was initiated at Teachers College, Columbia University, to provide graduate-level leadership for the preparation of nurse tutors, faculty, and administrators (Dock, 1912). Not until 1923 did nursing education enter the university with the establishment of programs at Yale University and at Western Reserve University. These were the country's first schools of nursing to have an independent status among the schools and colleges of a university. These early developments led to nursing education both as a training program controlled by the hospitals and an academic program within the university setting.

As early as 1915 the National League of Nursing Education called for university-level education, a demand reinforced by the Committee for the Study of Nursing Education, in the Goldmark (1923) report and other important reports on nursing education (Brown, 1948). However, Mildred L. Montag's (1959) writing on the potential role of nursing education at the community college level has had the greatest impact on nursing education today. From these early writings arose the distinction between the professional nurse, educated at the baccalaureate level or above, and the technical nurse educated at the community college level. In 1971 the first nursing program at a community college opened in Middletown, New York. Today community colleges prepare the largest number of nurses for practice.

From the turn of the century until the 1960s nursing leaders often obtained their graduate preparation in schools of education. Consequently, most major developments that took place in schools of education were rather quickly transferred to nursing curricula. The University of Chicago's influence, through Ralph Tyler, had a major impact on nursing education, with focuses on learner objectives and curricular structure. However, in the 1980s there was a backlash against the objectives-based curriculum and a renewed focus on the nursing curriculum as a humanistic endeavor, where "caring" and not behavioral objectives formed the core of the content (Watson, 1988).

Licensure is required to practice nursing in each state, and until 1944 each state developed its own testing mechanism to license nurses. Today the National Council of State Boards of Nursing (NCSBN) has jurisdiction throughout the United States and its territories. The NCSBN sets standards for requirements and regulations for schools of nursing and licensure of new graduates. However, authority for requirements and regulations rests at the state level. All the states have agreed to use the same licensing examination to facilitate the mobility of the nursing work force in the United States.

Types of Programs

Currently, three main types of educational programs prepare students for licensure as registered nurses (RN): diploma, associate degree (ADN), and baccalaureate degree (BSN) programs. In 1989 there were 1,457 basic RN programs in the United States: 488 (33.5%) BSN, 812 (55.7%) ADN, and 157 (10.8%) diploma (NLN, 1991). These programs enrolled 201,458 students, including 74,865 (37.2%) BSN, 106,175 (52.7%) ADN, and 20,418 (10.1%) diploma. There were 212 master's degree programs in 1989 enrolling 22,587 students and 47 doctoral programs enrolling 2,417 students (NLN, 1991).

In 1989 there were 16,723 full-time faculty positions in schools of nursing and 6,187 part-time faculty positions (NLN, 1991). The faculties were 8.5% minority and 2.5% male (Gothler, 1988).

There are currently 2,239,816 RNs in the United States, and these nurses are 96% female, 90% White (non-Hispanic), and 82.7% employed (Moses, 1992). Their level of education is as follows: 33.7%

diploma, 28.2% associate degree, 29.9% BSN degree, 7.5% master's degree, and 0.5% doctorate (Moses, 1992).

Professional Organizations

Nursing has many professional organizations, yet it has successfully developed a unified position in dealing with federal issues that affect nursing education and patient care. The vehicle for cooperation is the Tri-Council, made up of representatives from three major nursing organizations; the American Nurses Association (ANA), the National League for Nursing (NLN), and the American Association of Colleges of Nursing (AACN). The AACN, headquartered in Washington, DC, is an organization composed of collegiate schools of nursing. It conducts annual surveys of faculty salaries, faculty workload, and similar topics of primary interest to deans and directors of programs.

The ANA provides a voluntary credentialing mechanism that recognizes both RNs who are involved in advanced practice and those who are generalists practicing in a specialty area; more than 30,000 RNs have been certified to date. Other specialty organizations, such as the American Association of Critical Care Nurses, have certified an additional 46,000 RNs.

Continuing Education and Relicensure

Smith (1979) defined continuing education as post-registered learning activity designed to increase knowledge or skill or to challenge attitudes. Several states now require varying amounts of additional education for relicensure. Moreover, some states (including Michigan, Idaho, Utah, and Minnesota) require competency-based continuing education.

Nursing Education Research

Research on topics related to nursing education has been comprehensive and have examined many different areas, including quality of education, care planning, clinical judgment, clinical decision mak-

ing, clinical teaching, learning styles, performance on licensure examination, faculty productivity, computer-assisted instruction, socialization processes, teaching learning processes, competencies, and others.

WILLIAM L. HOLZEMER

See also
**AMERICAN NURSES ASSOCIATION
CLINICAL DECISION MAKING
CLINICAL JUDGMENT
DOCTORAL EDUCATION
NATIONAL LEAGUE FOR NURSING**

NURSING INFORMATICS

Nursing informatics is a branch of informatics concerned with all aspects of the nursing profession's use of computer technology. It is a new nursing specialty that expands computer systems to include nursing information. Nursing informatics enhances and facilitates the legitimate access to and use of data, information, and knowledge. It is integrated in nursing practice, administration, education, and research programs and activities. It is incorporated in the design and development of computer-based patient records and other health-related systems (Saba & McCormick, 1996).

Definition

In 1992 the American Nurses Association (ANA) designated nursing informatics as a new nursing specialty. They defined it as

> the specialty that integrates nursing science, computer science, and information science in identifying, collecting, processing, and managing data and information to support nursing practice, administration, education, and research; and the expansion of nursing knowledge. It supports the practice of nursing specialties in all sites and settings of care, whether at the basic or advanced practice level. (ANA, 1994a, p. 3)

Historical Background

Informatics is derived from the French word *informatique*, which refers to all aspects of the computer milieu. Informatics emerged in the 1960s with the introduction of computers in the health care industry. As the industry advanced and expanded, computer applications and information systems emerged for health care facilities, specialties, and professions. During the past three decades several nursing initiatives also have advanced the progress of nursing informatics for the profession. During this period the ANA made several recommendations designed not only to advance the development of nursing practice but also nursing data standards for computer-based systems.

As early as 1970 the ANA recommended that the nursing process be used as the standard for documenting clinical nursing practice. In 1988 the ANA recognized the Nursing Minimum Data Set (NMDS) as those 16 minimum data elements designed to document nursing care of patients and their families in any delivery setting. The four nursing care data elements—nursing diagnoses, nursing interventions, nursing outcomes, and intensity of nursing care in the NMDS—were envisioned as essential for computer systems and designed to compare nursing data across health care facilities, clinical population groups, and geographic areas (Werley & Lang, 1988).

In 1992 the ANA also recognized four classification schemes or vocabularies as meeting nursing data standards and clinical practice standards. They included NANDA Taxonomy I, Home Health Care Classification (HHCC) System, the Omaha System, and Nursing Intervention Classification (NIC). The ANA indicated that each of these schemes addresses one or more of the data elements in the NMDS, and they are professionally recognized as the data standards essential for computer-based nursing information systems. These four schemes were subsequently included in the National Library of Medicine's (NLM) Unified Medical Language System (McCormick, Lang, Zielstorff, Milholland, & Saba, 1994; Saba & McCormick, 1996).

Another national nursing initiative was instituted by the National Institute for Nursing Research (NINR), National Institutes of Health (NIH), Public Health Service (PHS), and Department of Health and Human Services (DHHS). In 1988 the NINR convened an expert panel, "Priority Panel E: Nursing Informatics," to investigate the scope of nursing informatics. In 1993, the NINR Panel E report recommended seven research priorities that must be addressed to advance research in the field of nursing informatics. For effective use of nursing informatics they recommended research and development for a common nursing language and standardized data elements. The panel indicated that research should be conducted to determine the data and information needed by nurses for the computer-based patient record systems that affect nursing practice. They also recommended that methodologies focus on designing decision support systems, evaluating nursing information systems, and developing other applications to improve patient care.

Scope of Nursing Informatics

Nursing informatics focuses on the information management and processing of nursing data. It provides the framework for nursing data, information, and knowledge processed by the computer. Nursing informatics concepts require nursing classification schemes and vocabularies to provide the structure and framework for the data. Applications of nursing informatics are needed to standardize nursing documentation, to improve communication, to support the decision-making process, and to develop and disseminate new knowledge. They also are needed to enhance the quality, effectiveness, and efficiency of health care; empower clients to make health care choices; and advance the science of nursing (ANA, 1994a).

Basic to the understanding of nursing informatics is an understanding of nursing data, data standards, and practice standards. Nursing data form the basis and foundation of nursing informatics. They are essential for the documentation of nursing care and management of clinical nursing practice. Nursing data refers to the atomic-level data elements, or the unstructured raw facts. These data, once processed with other data elements, are transformed by the computer into information; and information, once aggregated and synthesized, creates new knowledge. Nursing knowledge forms the basis of knowledge-based systems, expert systems, and decision support systems that advance the science of nursing (Saba & McCormick, 1996).

Research Trends

Nursing informatics is critical to the conduct of research of nursing practice problems. Computer hardware and software are being used to design research tools, collect and process research data, and analyze and retrieve research information. The nursing vocabularies and data standards are being used to research the critical data elements for the computer-based patient record (CPR) systems, including the lifelong longitudinal health care record. The data elements also are being used for nursing information systems designed to document patient care, measure outcomes, and determine quality indicators. Nursing informatics is becoming an integral component in nursing administration, practice, education, and research as well as the nursing profession and health care industry.

VIRGINIA K. SABA

See also

**COMPUTER-BASED DOCUMENTATION
    OF PATIENT CARE
NANDA
NURSING INFORMATION SYSTEMS
NURSING MINIMUM DATA SET
UNIFIED LANGUAGE SYSTEMS**

NURSING INFORMATION SYSTEMS

A nursing information system (NIS) is the application of nursing informatics to a computer-based information system. An NIS is encompassed in the broad field of nursing informatics and focuses on processing nursing data into information; it is described according to its purpose, focus, usage, or service. An NIS is used to administer hospital and community nursing services and manage the delivery of nursing practice, as well as support nursing education and nursing research.

Definition

An NIS has been defined by several experts. Saba and McCormick (1996) defined it in their second edition as follows:

> The use of technology and/or computer system to collect, store, process, display, retrieve, and communicate timely data and information in and across health care facilities that
>
> • Administer nursing services and resources
> • Manage the delivery of patient and nursing care
> • Link research resources and findings to nursing practice
> • Apply educational resources to nursing education. (p. 226)

Historical Background

In the 1960s, with the introduction of computer technology in the health care industry, computer developers of the early hospital, medical, and patient care information systems began to expand their systems to include subsystems that addressed the documentation of nursing care. They focused on computerizing the existing paper-based methods of documenting nursing in health care facilities. The developers began to computerize the standardized nursing care protocols or plans that focused on medical diagnoses, surgical procedures, or disease conditions. With the introduction of the microcomputer, NISs emerged as stand-alone systems for a specific nursing application for different aspects of nursing administration, practice, education, research, and community health. Such systems were designed by nurses who were becoming proficient in their design.

Models

Many NISs have been illustrated, using different concepts that were developed as frameworks for NISs and nursing informatics. One model, developed by Graves and Corcoran (1989), focused on the design of an NIS as the framework that represents the management processing of data, information, and knowledge. Another is the linked model developed by Gassert (1991), which defines the requirements for an NIS as consisting of five elements. Still other models have been designed that depict the four major types of nursing information systems, namely, nursing administration, practice, education, and research.

Scope of NISs

Nursing information systems can be found in all areas where nurses function and in all settings where nurses provide patient care: hospitals, community health agencies, managed care organizations, ambulatory care facilities, and other settings where services are provided. NISs are generally configured as stand-alone microcomputer systems, subsystems, or components of a larger minicomputer or mainframe system. The systems also are applications that address a specific nursing problem.

The NISs in nursing administration are used primarily for the administration of nursing services and the management of nursing units. For the administration of nursing services, NISs are designed to generate information focusing on budget, personnel, and resource management. The NISs focus on the specific applications needed to run a nursing department effectively and efficiently, such as staffing, scheduling, utilization, productivity, quality assurance, and discharge planning. The NISs designed for the management of nursing units focus on the patient care services. They address nursing intensity, patient classification, acuity, decision support, and patient outcomes. These systems are used to track the care process during an episode of illness as well as measure the impact and outcomes of the care.

In the area of nursing practice, NISs are designed to document care planning and patient care services. They focus on the computer-based patient record (CPR). The major applications are order entry, results reporting, medication protocols, care planning protocols, patient education, quality assurance, and discharge planning systems. The system utilizes the point-of-care computer terminals to capture direct patient care and can support the care process with decision support systems (Chang & Hirsch, 1991).

NISs focus on the integration of information and care by all providers. They also can be used for discharge planning and referral to community health agencies and home health care services for follow-up.

In the area of nursing education, NISs address the technology that supports the education process, such as computer-assisted instruction (CAI), interactive video (IVD) programs and also the management of educational programs, that is, students, faculty, and courses. NISs in education have addressed the hardware and software requirements for computer resource centers and distance learning centers. They include a wide range of educational strategies that enhance and integrate nursing informatics into the educational process (Saba & McCormick, 1996).

In the last area, nursing research, NISs support the research process. Without such systems, nursing research cannot be accomplished on large-scale data bases and population groups. NISs are needed to process and analyze research data that only a computer application can perform. Nursing research applications include searching the literature by using bibliographic retrieval systems containing nursing-related material. Other applications include classification systems needed to code, classify, process, and analyze nursing research data, as well as the instruments and tools used to conduct research: data-base management systems, file managers, spreadsheets, and statistical software designed to process research data. Other applications, such as graphic displays, text preparation, and editors, are designed to disseminate and communicate research findings and conclusions via on-line data bases or the Internet.

Nursing information systems represent the nursing informatics applications. They are described by the focus of the specific application, which varies according to the focus of the nursing activities supported. NISs address several major areas of nursing, namely, nursing administration, practice, education, research, and community health.

VIRGINIA K. SABA

See also
**BIBLIOGRAPHIC RETRIEVAL SYS-
TEMS**

COMPUTER-AIDED INSTRUCTION
COMPUTER-BASED DOCUMENTATION
    OF PATIENT CARE
NURSING INFORMATICS

NURSING INTENSITY

The concept of intensity of nursing care, or *nursing intensity*, was formally developed during the 1970s as nurses sought ways to assure that adequate nursing resources were provided to hospitalized patients. There is not yet a universally accepted definition for nursing intensity. In the research literature it is often operationally defined as patient acuity because nursing resources ought to be based on patient needs for care (Phillips, Castorr, Prescott, & Soeken, 1992; Prescott, 1991; Prescott, Ryan, et al., 1991). In a report submitted to the American Nurses Association's Database Steering Committee, McHugh (1994) conceptually defined nursing intensity as an integration of the following critical attributes: Time frame to be represented by a single ''instance'' of intensity (the instance of intensity is the context in which the following variables are to be considered), hours of nursing care provided to a patient or set of patients, educational level of nurses, years of nursing experience, years of experience in the specialty, and years of experience in the particular setting in which the instance of intensity is addressed.

Measurement of Nursing Intensity

Measures of nursing intensity have not addressed the critical attributes because such measurement is difficult. However, the desired result of a measure of nursing intensity has always been recognized to be an adequate supply of nursing service to the patient. Patient census and acuity are more readily measured. Thus, the concept has always been linked with patient acuity and was first formally measured by Connor (1960), who noted that demand for nursing services (required nursing intensity) was linked not only to census but also to the illness level (acuity) of the patients. He developed a three-level measure of degree of patient dependency on nursing

and a staffing algorithm based on that measure. Although Connor did not use the term *nursing intensity*, he did specifically discuss the importance of matching nursing resources to patient needs. Thus, nursing intensity was indirectly measured by gauging patient care requirements. Currently, most published measures of nursing intensity actually quantify patient characteristics. However, the two concepts, nursing intensity and patient acuity, are not the same, and a distinction must be made between these concepts for the purposes of research.

This approach carries an unfortunate assumption: Nursing resources will be provided to match patient care needs. To the extent that the number of adequately educated and experienced nurses are readily available, the assumption is probably true in most cases. However, when adequate numbers are not available or when financing for adequate nursing is not provided, that assumption may not be true. Clearly, patient numbers and acuity should drive nursing intensity. This is not always the case in a health care delivery system in which cost reduction may take precedence over quality of care. Nurses assume that higher nursing intensity will be associated with better patient outcomes. This has not been conclusively demonstrated in the literature. Research on propositions about the relationship between nursing intensity and patient acuity and their joint and individual effects on patient outcomes is needed. The first step in developing a research protocol to test those types of propositions is development of a valid and reliable measure of nursing intensity.

Nursing Intensity as an Item in the Nursing Minimum Data Set

At the Nursing Minimum Data Set (NMDS) Conference in Milwaukee, Wisconsin, in 1985, intensity of nursing care was identified as one of 16 variables to be included in a national nursing minimum data set (Werley & Lang, 1988). In papers from that conference, ''nursing intensity'' and ''patient classification'' are treated as virtually synonymous. Reitz (1988) described a patient classification measure and named it the Nursing Intensity Index. Reitz defined nursing intensity as ''a measure of the degree, complexity, or magnitude of nursing input into patient care in response to patient need'' (p. 314). However, her measure of nursing intensity, like many others in the literature, consisted of a collection of measures of patient characteristics.

The NMDS conference's Nursing Intensity Task Force advanced the concept of intensity by relating various characteristics of the nursing staff to an individual patient. They identified the following variables as components of nursing intensity: ''(b) the total amount of nursing resources, direct and indirect, consumed [by an individual patient] per episode; . . . (d) the skill level of the care giver'' (Werley & Lang, 1988, p. 394). In the writings of the task force, it would seem that the concept became inextricably intertwined with the purpose for which they thought it should be used.

In their recommendations, the task force also added the concept of skill mix. Nurse staffing is generally an inclusive term that encompasses unlicensed nursing personnel, practical nurses, and all levels of registered nurses. However, the nursing literature reflects the concerns many nurses have expressed about numbers of nurses, about differing experience levels of nurses, and about the putative expertise of nurses prepared at different levels (i.e., MSN, BSN, ADN, diploma). All of these variables may have to be tested for their impact on patient outcomes and for their validity for inclusion in an index of nursing intensity.

Number of nurses, as a variable, is also problematic. In inpatient settings, the nurse-to-patient relationship is usually a many-to-many relationship; that is, a team of nurses is assigned to a number of patients. It is also common for each patient to have one RN each shift who assumes primary responsibility for the patient's care during that shift. Each RN may hold primary responsibility for several patients. Nurses prioritize care requirements, and thus different patients receive different amounts of time from both the responsible nurse and the other members of the nursing care team. As the number of nurses appears to be of interest primarily as it relates to amount of nursing time delivered to each patient, the complexity of measurement of this concept is of concern.

Another factor to consider is the time frame during which a particular level of intensity is deliv-

ered. The question is, what constitutes a single instance of intensity? This factor complicates the measurement of nursing intensity. For example, should a single instance of intensity encompass the entire length of stay for hospital inpatients? Should intensity be measured for outpatients for each encounter or for an episode of care or for some other time span?

Nursing intensity is a variable in the NMDS for which there is great interest and concern. There is no universally accepted conceptual definition; therefore, it is understandable that there is no one measure of nursing intensity that has achieved wide acceptance in the nursing community. The importance of this concept and the dearth of information on its impact on patient care outcomes lead to the conclusion that this is an important topic for further research.

MARY L. MCHUGH

See also
  COST ANALYSIS OF NURSING CARE
  NURSE STAFFING
  **NURSING WORKLOAD MEASURE-
    MENT SYSTEMS**
  PATIENT CLASSIFICATION
  QUALITY OF CARE, MEASURING

NURSING INTERVENTIONS CLASSIFICATION

Definition and Overview

The *Nursing Interventions Classification* (*NIC*) is a standardized language of treatments that nurses perform. The first edition of *NIC* was published in 1992 by the Iowa Intervention Project, with 336 direct care interventions; the second edition was published in 1996 with 433 direct and indirect care interventions. A nursing intervention is defined as ''any treatment, based upon clinical judgment and knowledge, that a nurse performs to enhance patient/client outcomes. Nursing interventions include both direct and indirect care, both nurse-initiated, physician-initiated, and other provider-initiated treatments'' (Iowa Intervention Project, 1996, p. xvii).

Each *NIC* intervention is composed of a label, a definition, and a set of activities that a nurse does to carry out the intervention. The interventions are grouped in 27 classes and 6 domains for ease of use. Each *NIC* intervention has a unique four-digit number that facilitates computerization. *NIC* interventions have been linked with the North American Nursing Diagnosis Association (NANDA) nursing diagnoses and the Omaha System problems. They are in the process of being linked with *Nursing-sensitive Outcomes Classification (NOC)* outcomes (Johnson & Maas, 1997). There are a form and a review system for submitting suggestions for new or modified interventions.

The *NIC* is comprehensive, containing all interventions used by all nurses irrespective of their specialty or work setting. *NIC* interventions include both the physiological (acid-base management, airway suctioning) and the psychosocial (anxiety reduction, home maintenance assistance). There are interventions for illness treatment (hyperglycemia management, ostomy care); illness prevention (immunization/vaccination administration, fall prevention); and health promotion (exercise promotion, smoking cessation assistance). Interventions are for individuals or for families (family integrity promotion, family support). Indirect care interventions (emergency cart checking, supply management) and some interventions for communities (environmental management: community) are also included.

Purpose and Uses

The classification assists professional nurses to communicate with colleagues and clients. The researchers who developed the classification identified eight uses:

1. Standardize the nomenclature of nursing treatments. Prior to the development of the *NIC*, there was little conceptualization of how discrete nursing actions fit together to form interventions or treatments. Long, wordy care plans and nursing information systems with thousands of nursing actions resulted. In contrast, the *NIC* intervention labels are concepts implemented by a set of nursing activities (actions) directed toward the resolution of patients' actual or potential health care problems. A nurse can describe the care given to a patient with only a few labels.

2. Expand knowledge about the links between diagnoses, treatments, and outcomes. Nursing knowledge about the effectiveness of nursing care is limited. When nurses systematically document the diagnoses of their patients, the treatments they perform, and the resulting patient outcomes using a common standardized language, researchers will be able to determine which nursing interventions work best for a given diagnosis or population. The relationships among diagnoses, interventions, and outcomes using the data bases generated by the classifications will help build prescriptive theory for nursing science.

3. Develop nursing and health care information systems. Computerized documentation of nursing care requires a standardized system for describing the treatments that nurses perform. Without use of a standardized language, data cannot be compared across agencies or within agencies from one unit to another. The *NIC*, in conjunction with those of nursing diagnoses and patient outcomes, provides the discipline of nursing with the clinical data elements for an automated patient record.

4. Teach decision making to nursing students. Defining and classifying nursing interventions is useful for teaching beginning nurses how to determine a patient's needs and respond appropriately. Curricula of the future will emphasize two major foci: the information contained in the classifications and the process of making clinical decisions. A classification of nursing interventions makes it easier to distinguish among interventions requiring beginning preparation from those requiring higher knowledge and skill levels.

5. Determine the costs of nursing services. Reimbursement to nurses is a key issue in the reduction of health care costs. Physician classifications are not adequate to capture all of the work of nurses. A classification of nursing interventions provides the essential framework for a reimbursement system for nursing care. The ability to identify the interventions that are delivered to a particular population enables contracting for services in a managed care environment.

6. Plan for resources needed in nursing practice settings. Identification of costs for specific nursing interventions will allow evaluation of the cost-effectiveness of nursing care. Currently, resource use is based mostly on tradition; however, knowing the cost and the effectiveness of specific interventions will facilitate the distribution of staff and other resources to maximize cost reduction and quality care delivery. After identification of the interventions that nurses perform, the time for delivery, the cost, and the effectiveness of these interventions can be studied. Nursing administrators can use this information to plan more effectively for staff and equipment required to deliver the interventions.

7. Communicate the unique function of nursing. Despite the fact that nurses are the largest group of health care providers and that nurses spend the most time with patients, the work of nurses is largely invisible. A classification of nursing interventions describes the uniqueness of nursing as well as its similarities with other health professionals. In an interdisciplinary environment, the contributions of each discipline must be identified and clearly communicated.

8. Articulate with the classification systems of other health care providers. For purposes of reimbursement and research, the federal government, insurance companies, and medical community have been collecting standardized health information for a number of years. Several health data sets and medical classifications have been developed for making health policy, but these do not include nursing. The inclusion of NIC and other nursing standardized languages in regional, state, and national health data sets will help to demonstrate the contributions of nursing care to patient outcomes.

Research

The NIC is part of the Center for Nursing Classification at the University of Iowa College of Nursing. Research methods used to develop the classification include content analysis, expert survey, focus group review, similarity analysis, hierarchical cluster analysis, multidimensional scaling, and field testing. More than 40 national nursing organizations have reviewed the NIC and assisted with intervention development and validation and taxonomy construction and validation. The details of the methods and results and related issues are described in multiple publications over the past 7 years. (An anthology of publications 1990–1996 is available from the Center for Nursing Classification at Iowa.)

Ongoing Work and Issues

The ongoing research by a large team at the University of Iowa includes (a) the development of interventions that are used with whole populations or communities, (b) continued refinement of existing interventions and additions of new interventions from user feedback, (c) development of additional strategies to facilitate the use of the NIC in practice and education, (d) completion of the linkages of NIC interventions with NOC outcomes, (e) revision of the linkages with NANDA diagnoses and Omaha System problems, (f) determination of average times to perform each intervention, (g) construction of mechanisms to facilitate nursing data base development and effectiveness research, and (h) determination of the use rate of particular interventions for selected patient populations and settings. Current issues include (a) how the NIC language can be incorporated into multidisciplinary critical paths; (b) to what extent the activities in the NIC can be changed to meet the needs of a particular patient or agency and whether each NIC intervention has "core activities;" (c) how to assure that an NIC intervention has been delivered if only the NIC label is documented; and (d) whether there can be one rather than three organizing structures for nursing diagnoses, interventions, and outcomes. There are also issues related to copyright, licensure, and the funding of the Center for Nursing Classification at Iowa to continue the research and to update the classification.

Relationships and Recognitions

The NIC is endorsed by the American Nurses Association as one classification to be used in a unified nursing language. It was added in 1993 as one of the first two nursing languages in the National Library of Medicine's *Metathesaurus for a Unified Medical Language*. Both the *Cumulative Index to Nursing Literature (CINAHL)* and Silver Platter have added the *NIC* to their nursing indexes. The *NIC* is included in the Joint Commission on Accreditation for Health Care Organizations (JCAHO) as one nursing classification system that can be used to meet the standard on uniform data. Users of the *NIC* include health care agencies, nursing education programs, authors of major texts, and researchers. Interest in the *NIC* has been demonstrated in several other countries. Several translations of the *NIC* are in progress.

The *NIC* is intended as the classification of nursing interventions that can be used to implement the Nursing Minimum Data Set (Werley & Lang, 1988). It can be used in conjunction with other nursing languages, and the linkages with Omaha System problems and NANDA nursing diagnoses facilitate this; linkages with *NOC* outcomes will be completed by 1998. The *NIC* also can be used in conjunction with classifications of other providers: the future inclusion of the *NIC* in federal, state, regional, and network data bases will allow for the identification of nursing impact on patient outcomes and cost.

JOANNE COMI MCCLOSKEY

See also
NANDA
NURSING MINIMUM DATA SET
**NURSING OUTCOMES CLASSIFICA-
TION**
OMAHA SYSTEM
UNIFIED LANGUAGE SYSTEMS

NURSING MINIMUM DATA SET

The Nursing Minimum Data Set (NMDS) is defined as "a minimum set of items of information with uniform definitions and categories concerning the specific dimension of professional nursing, which meets the information needs of multiple data users in the health care system" (Werley, 1988, p. 7).

This definition is consistent with and indeed adapted from the definition of a uniform minimum health data set created by the Health Information Policy Council of the U.S. Department of Health and Human Services in 1983, and it represents the gold standard for the development of all health related-data sets. Before the terminology of NMDS was used, Murnaghan (1978) described, defined, and identified two purposes for uniform basic data sets: "First, it defines the central core of data needed on a routine basis by the majority of decision makers about a given facet or dimension of the health services system: and second, it establishes standard measurements, definitions, and classification for this core" (p. 263).

Although credit for early work in "comparative reporting systems . . . based on uniform minimum data" has been given to Nightingale (McPhillips, 1988, p. 233), more contemporary work in this area began with a 1969 conference on hospital discharge abstract system cosponsored by the U.S. Department of Health and Human Services and the Johns Hopkins University (McPhillips, 1988).

Werley (1988) described several benefits for the profession and discipline of nursing from the development and implementation of a NMDS. These benefits included the accumulation of nursing and patient data that will facilitate the identification of trends and guide the formation of subsequent research questions. "The research on this kind of investigative practice will be the basis for further development of nursing knowledge [and] will be the impetus for advancing nursing practice, health care delivery, and the profession of nursing" (pp. 11–12). Subsequent benefits from this research will enrich other related sectors, including nursing administration, nursing education, and health policy.

The development of an NMDS has been a major focus for nurse scholars in several countries, notably, the United States, Canada, United Kingdom, and Belgium. In the United States three broad categories of data elements were defined: those related to nursing care, including nursing diagnosis, nursing interventions, nursing intensity, and outcomes; patient demographics and selected service items such as admission and discharge dates; and principal nurse provider (Werley & Lang, 1988). Considerable effort toward the identification of data elements and consensus among U.S. nurses have occurred over the past two decades. The text by Werley and Lang (1988) represents a valuable compilation of the papers and discussions that resulted in the data set identification. Subsequently, major work has proceeded on the development of classification schemes for nursing diagnosis, nursing interventions, and outcomes, as well as field testing on the availability and reliability of the proposed NMDS (e.g., see Kim, 1989).

The Canadian effort began in early 1990, and following a national conference on the topic, an NMDS was proposed. The unique data elements selected matched those identified in the United States, with the notable exception of nursing diagnoses. As an alternative the Canadian Nurses Association in 1992 selected the phrase *client status.* Further, the Canadian proposed data set is referred to as *Health Information: Nursing Components,* in keeping with a national initiative on the subject of health information. Of note, neither the U.S. nor Canadian nursing data sets have been mandated in spite of the considerable dialogue that has taken place by nurses and other supporters. Both countries have a relatively long history of the routine collection and retrieval of selected hospital data through their respective hospital discharge data sets; however, the data abstracted largely represent the care and domain of medicine and are focused on acute care.

In the United Kingdom, the Korner data set implemented in 1988 is one of only two data sets that contain elements unique to nursing (National Health Service, 1982). In this United Kingdom system, however, the nursing elements are limited to a few items within the service items, reflecting that the data set is used for both acute care settings and for the delivery of services in the community by home (nurse) visitors. Perhaps the greatest achievement in the application an NMDS comes from Belgium. By royal decree, the NMDS was implemented in all general hospitals with compulsory monitoring in 1988. The variables monitored include a selected list of 23 nursing activities, selected patient variables, selected variables that deal with the nursing staff in the nursing unit, and nine variables that monitor the patients' activities of daily living, although the latter are not mandatory (Ministère de la Santé Publique, 1988).

PHYLLIS B. GIOVANNETTI

See also
NANDA
NURSING INFORMATICS
NURSING INTERVENTIONS CLASSIFICATION
NURSING OUTCOMES CLASSIFICATION

NURSING OCCUPATIONAL INJURY AND STRESS

Health care environments are high-risk work settings with numerous exposures that can result in worker illness and injury (Rogers & Travers, 1991). Exposures in these settings pose a significant threat to the health of health care workers. Stress related to the work, work load, interpersonal relationships, and shift work contribute to illness, injury, and fatigue. The impact of these events is of concern for worker health risk and effects on health care delivery. The U.S. Bureau of Labor Statistics expects nearly 11 million workers employed in this country by the year 2000, with approximately 50% in hospital settings; 30% in offices, laboratories, and outpatient facilities; and 20% in nursing homes and related settings. The bureau reports that the 1993 nonfatal occupational illness and injury incidence rates per 100 full-time workers were 11.8% for hospitals and 17.3% for nursing and personal care facilities, compared to a private industry rate of 8.5%, thereby emphasizing work-related risk in the health care sector.

Hazard exposures act independently or interactively with other agents to create actual or potential avenues for illness and injury. Hazard exposures are classified into five areas: biological, chemical, environmental/mechanical, physical, and psychosocial (see Table 1). Although concern exists for exposure to several biological agents, the greatest contemporary concerns are for exposure to human

TABLE 1 Categories of Potential or Actual Occupational Hazards

Biological-infectious hazards: Infectious-biological agents, such as bacteria, viruses, fungi, or parasites, that may be transmitted via contact with infected patients or contaminated body secretions or fluids

Chemical hazards: Various forms of chemicals that are potentially toxic or irritating to body systems, including medications, solutions, and gases

Environmental-mechanical hazards: Factors encountered in work environments that cause or potentiate accidents, injuries, strain, or discomfort (e.g., poor equipment, lifting devices, or slippery floors)

Physical hazards: Agents within work environments, such as radiation, electricity, extreme temperatures, and noise, that can cause tissue trauma

Psychosocial hazards: Factors and situations encountered or associated with the job or work environment that create or potentiate stress, emotional strain, interpersonal problems

From *Occupational Health Nursing: Concepts and Practice* (p. 96), by B. Rogers, 1994, Philadelphia: Saunders. Copyright © 1994 by Bonnie Rogers. Reprinted with permission.

immunodeficiency virus (HIV) and the hepatitis B and C viruses (HBV, HCV). Studies indicate that percutaneous exposure is the primary route for HIV and HBV, with incidence rates for needlestick injuries ranging from 10% to 34% (Linneman, Cannon, DeRonde, & Lanphear, 1991). Approximately 800,000 needlestick injuries occur to health care workers annually in the United States, and about 16,000 have a potential risk for HIV/HBV transmission. Recapping of needles is the primary source of exposure.

According to the Centers for Disease Control and Prevention (CDC), 47 health care workers in the United States have been documented as having HIV seroconversion following occupational exposure (CDC, 1996a). Although the rate of HIV seroconversion from an HIV-contaminated needle is only about 1 in 300, the HBV infection rate from an HBV-contaminated needle is about 1 in 6. The CDC estimates that between 15% and 30% of health care workers with frequent blood contact have one or more serological markers of HBV infection and that 1%–2% of these persons are chronic carriers of HBV (CDC, 1996b). In 1994 the CDC estimated

the number of HBV infections in health care workers to be 1,000, with an alarming 150 deaths per year (CDC, 1996b).

Hepatitis C virus is of relatively new concern, with an estimated 35,000 infections and 4,470 reported cases (CDC, 1996b). The number of occupationally related cases is unreported; however, percutaneous exposure is the principal route for transmission. The concern rests with the potential for chronic hepatitis in the exposed individual. Preventive monitoring and surveillance procedures are essential for all types of exposures (Jagger, 1994).

Chemical agent exposures in the health care work environment can be irritating and toxic to tissues, mostly through inhalation or skin contact. The most common exposures include disinfectants, sterilizing agents, chemotherapeutic agents, and latex. Disinfectants can result in airway symptoms and skin problems, and ethylene oxide, used to sterilize equipment, has mutagenic and carcinogenic properties, as demonstrated in animal studies (Rutala & Hamory, 1989).

Health care workers exposed to antineoplastic agents have been found to have a significantly greater risk of urine mutagenicity and adverse symptoms common to specific agents, including lightheadedness, nasal sores, nausea, hair loss, depressed leukocytes, skin rash, and higher fetal loss. Those most at risk for toxicological effects will have regular cumulative exposure in practice settings such as hospital oncology floors, oncology units, private physicians' offices, and outpatient clinics (Rogers & Emmett, 1987).

Latex allergy, a growing problem for health care workers, with 10% prevalence rates reported in heavy glove users, can occur through direct skin contact or inhalation of the allergen. The allergen is usually a protein that binds to the glove powder as part of the manufacturing process (Beezhold, Koystal, & Wiseman, 1994). Inhalation occurs when the powder is expelled into the air during glove donning or removal. Reactions can range from contact dermatitis to systemic reactions or anaphylaxis.

Environmental or mechanical agents relate to exposures resulting from poorly designed or inadequate equipment or devices, work stations, or situations that can result in worker injury. Back injuries are cited as the most costly worker's compensation problem today. Although back injuries are highly prevalent in the health care industry, the actual incidence is thought to be underestimated. Several studies implicate lifting techniques, poor staffing, lack of ergonomic design, and constitutional factors as contributory (Larese & Fiorito, 1994). Garg, Owen, and Carlson (1992) observed nursing assistants in their lifting behavior and found that lifting devices were used less than 2% of the time. In addition to the aforementioned factors, the authors cited lack of accessibility, physical stress, lack of skill and training, increased patient transfer activities, and solo lifting. Poor nurse-patient ratios have also been linked to back injuries (Larese & Fiorito, 1994). The impact of these injuries is enormous in terms of worker pain and safety, disability, lost work time, absenteeism, medical care costs, personnel replacement costs, and decreased productivity. Better use of equipment, training, and improved work conditions and staffing could help prevent this disabling problem.

Shift work is a long-standing issue, as it creates body burden demands that can lead to both psychosocial and physical health problems. Sleep deprivation, lowered sense of well-being, decreased socialization, fatigue, and family problems are reported (Gold et al., 1992). Clockwise shift rotation, as well as shift work management programs emphasizing appropriate sleep, exercise, and nutrition, is imperative (Todd, Robinson, & Reid, 1993).

Physical agents are probably the least important hazard in health care environments; however, exposures do occur. Radiation is a common hazard in medical therapeutics, and exposure can occur during diagnostic x-rays and radioactive implants and from patient body fluids with metabolized therapeutic nuclear radiation (National Safety Council [NSC], 1996). Lasers emit nonionizing radiation and can cause eye or skin injury from a point of impact. Care must be taken to avoid exposure.

Psychosocial agents or stressors and their effects are reported in nursing literature (Fielding & Weaver, 1994). Although many highly stressful areas in nursing have been studied, intensive care, hospice, emergency nursing, and oncology nursing have been studied the most (Boumans & Landeweerd, 1994). Factors cited most frequently as con-

tributory to workplace stress in nursing include (a) death and dying, (b) inadequate staffing and resources, (c) interpersonal conflicts, (d) dealing with family needs, (e) work overload, (f) organizational politics, and (g) poor communications. The quality concern stressor created the most job stress and resulted in increased depressive symptomatology, increased role conflict, and decreased job satisfaction.

Burnout continues to be a serious problem and is associated with shift work, lack of autonomy, floating, and lack of administrative support (Kandolin, 1993). Many of the same factors that contribute to stress also lead to burnout, resulting in decreased job satisfaction and increased absenteeism and turnover.

Preventive and control strategies necessary to reduce work-related health risk include the following:

1. Engineering controls and designs to modify or eliminate the exposure source; examples include provision of a needle disposal container, rooms with ventilation, high-efficiency fibers, and elimination of toxic substances

2. Work practice controls to enhance worker safety and alter practice behaviors that are risky; examples include good hygiene, good housekeeping, and utilization of assistive devices or nonrecapping needles

3. Administrative controls to relate to policy and assurance mechanisms for worker risk reduction; examples include job rotation, workplace monitoring, vaccination, and training programs

4. Personal protection is the last resort for workplace hazard control, as it places emphasis on worker management or exposures. Examples include glove and eye goggle use and utilization of hearing protection. This method should be used in concert with other strategies when hazardous conditions cannot be eliminated through other control mechanisms.

In summary, nurses and other health care workers must be cognizant of work-related hazards and must work with management to eliminate or substantially reduce associated risk. Applicable standards and guidelines can provide measured approaches to occupational health and safety at work.

BONNIE ROGERS

See also
CRITICAL CARE NURSING
EMERGENCY NURSING RESEARCH
JOB STRESS
NURSE STAFFING
NURSING WORKLOAD MEASURE-
    MENT SYSTEMS

NURSING OUTCOMES CLASSIFICATION (NOC)

The *Nursing Outcomes Classification* (NOC) is a standardized taxonomy of nursing-sensitive client outcomes developed by a research team at the University of Iowa. The outcomes describe individual patient or family caregiver states and behaviors, including perceptions and subjective states. They are developed for use across the care continuum to provide a consistent measure of patient and family caregiver status. Each outcome contains an outcome label and definition, outcome indicators, and a 5-point scale for measuring patient status in relation to the outcome. For example, energy conservation is defined as the extent of active management of energy to initiate and sustain activity. The 5-point scale used to measure patient status uses the following anchors: not at all, to a slight extent, to a moderate extent, to a great extent, and to a very great extent. A sample of the indicators used to assess patient status for extent of energy conservation includes the following: balances activity and rest, recognizes energy limitations, uses energy conservation techniques, and has endurance level adequate for activity. Each of these indicators can be measured on the same scale as that used for the outcome.

The published classification (Iowa Outcomes Project, 1997) contains 196 outcomes, but additional outcomes have been developed since the work was published. All of the current outcomes are classified in a taxonomy that contains six domains: (a) Functional Health, (b) Physiologic Health, (c) Psychosocial Health, (d) Health Knowledge and Behavior, (e) Perceived Health, and (f) Family Health. Each domain has a number of classes that contain the outcomes. For example, Functional Health has the following classes: Energy Maintenance, Growth and Development, Mobility, and Self-Care. The outcomes in the Energy Maintenance class include endurance, energy conservation, rest, and sleep. Each of the domains and classes in the taxonomy are defined to facilitate the placement of new outcomes as they are developed. The entire taxonomy, including the outcomes, indicators, and scales, is coded for implementation in computerized clinical information systems.

Methodologies used to develop the classification included inductive and deductive methods and qualitative and quantitative methods (Iowa Outcomes Project, 1997). The first step in development was the extraction of outcome statements from nursing textbooks, clinical information systems, and nursing research studies. The majority of outcomes from these sources were written as goal statements that are measured as met or not met. A number of exercises were used to group the outcomes taken from the literature into like categories for further analysis. Eight focus groups were established to develop the outcomes, including the definition and indicators for each outcome. Each group was chaired by a doctorally prepared investigator and included members of the research team and practicing clinicians. A modified concept analysis was used for each outcome to establish face validity as the focus groups developed their assigned outcomes.

Content validity was established by submitting the outcomes to master's-prepared nurse experts using a survey questionnaire. The questionnaire asked the respondents to rate the importance of each indicator for determining the outcome on a 5-point scale from "never important" to "always important." To ascertain sensitivity to nursing interventions, the respondents were asked to rate each indicator on a 5-point scale from "no contribution" to "contribution is mainly nursing." Fehring's (1986) methodology, using ratios identified by Sparks and Lien-Gieschen (1994), were used to evaluate importance and sensitivity of the indicators and outcomes. The importance of the indicators and the contribution of nursing were supported by the survey results, although there was more variation in the nursing contribution, particularly with some of the physiological indicators. In some cases, respondents suggested additional indicators, and these were evaluated by the focus groups and included if supported in the literature. Following completion of the surveys, the outcomes were pilot-tested with favorable results in a tertiary care setting, a community hospital, and a nursing home.

The taxonomy was developed in two steps. In the first step, three groups of nurse experts sorted the outcomes into categories. Following this sort, outcomes were grouped into 5, 10, 15, and 25 tentative categories, using hierarchical clustering techniques. Using the 25-category clustering scheme as a framework, 24 categories were identified as classes and given a name and a definition. The classes were then sorted by the same three groups of nurses and analyzed by using the same clustering techniques. This sort resulted in the six domains discussed earlier.

A standardized language for nursing practice is essential to capture both nursing interventions and outcomes for evaluation of quality and for sharing information with policymakers. The *Nursing Outcomes Classification* is the most comprehensive classification of nursing-sensitive patient outcomes currently available for use with individual clients across the care continuum. A number of outcome classifications have been developed for use in the home care setting but do not capture outcomes important in other clinical settings, a disadvantage in developing integrated health care systems in which patients receive nursing assistance in several settings during a single episode of care (Head, Maas, & Johnson, 1997). The American Nurses Association has identified a Nursing Care Report Card for acute care settings; however, the outcomes identify adverse incidents and complications reported as ratios or occurrence rates rather than as individual patient outcomes.

The work of the research team is ongoing. Individual client outcomes continue to be developed for inclusion in the classification, and work is beginning on the development of family outcomes. Outcomes for community or public health nursing also are needed to complete the classification. Maintaining the usefulness of the taxonomy requires consistent reevaluation of current outcomes and development of additional outcomes to keep pace with changes in practice. Additionally, measurement methodologies must be implemented to evaluate the measurement scales, and sensitivity of the outcomes to nursing interventions requires further evaluation in the clinical setting.

This research was funded by Sigma Theta Tau International and NIH, National Institute of Nursing Research, No. 1 RO1 NR03437-01.

MARION JOHNSON
MERIDEAN MAAS

See also
EVALUATION
NURSING INTERVENTIONS CLASSIFICATION
TAXONOMY

NURSING PRACTICE MODELS

Definition

A nursing practice model can be described as a guide, a road map, or a framework that provides a structure for the organization and the delivery of care. Practice models have been developed by administrators and managers in response to changes in health care. Over the years, practice models used within organizations have resulted in various outcomes, including decreased cost and increased quality of care. Several practice models have incorporated dimensions such as interdisciplinary practice, differentiated practice, and communication as integral components of the framework.

Discussion and Research

The goal of most nursing practice models focuses on decreasing cost, improving quality outcomes, increasing nurse satisfaction, autonomy, financial compensation, and impact on patient satisfaction with care. Models developed during the past decade have focused on shared governance, professional practice, collaborative governance, theory-based practice, and transitional models of care.

Shared governance is designed to increase nursing's presence in the health care system by differentiating responsibilities of providers based on education and experience while compensating expert practitioners financially. This model provides opportunities for shared decision making and organizational participation through committee work. Evaluation of successful implementation of the model has varied. Cost and commitment to the governance process have became issues, although evaluation reports indicate satisfaction with staff participation in decision making and teamwork. Some continue to use the model, whereas others have abandoned it for other structures.

Use of professional practice models and collaborative governance is a more recent practice model and builds on some aspects of shared governance. The model focuses on the contribution of all professionals within the organization, including nurses and other providers. Collaborative governance is used to implement many of the components of the professional practice model. A committee structure is developed to involve staff from across disciplines to participate in the leadership of patient care services. Interdisciplinary team building is used to bring about change. Emphasis is placed on communication among caregivers and respect for each discipline's contribution to quality patient care. The model offers individuals who deliver patient care at all levels a voice in decision making through a committee structure and open forums. The goal of the model is to work toward increased recognition of all providers and as a result improve the work environment and patient care outcomes. "Collaborative governance is a communication and decision making model that involves the placement of authority, responsibility and accountability for patient care with the practicing clinician" (Erickson, 1997, p. 2).

Theory-based practice models incorporate nursing and theoretical perspectives outside the discipline to guide practice. For example, Bhola's configuration theory of planned change (Swartz & Tiffany, 1994) has been used as a model to facilitate the redirection of practice and care delivery. Other models have implemented midrange theories (e.g.,

pain and stress) to direct practice. Community-based practices have focused on prevention and risk reduction (Suarez, Nichols, Pully, Brady, & McAlister, 1993) to decrease mortality related to smoking. Nursing theories also have been used as practice frameworks. For example, advanced practice nurses in managed care setting structured nursing practice around the Neuman system model. The framework used in a community nursing center provided a structure for costing out nursing services in primary, secondary, and tertiary care settings (Walker, 1994). Nursing practice models have been found successful in directing resource utilization and staffing. In addition, nursing models have been used with high-risk populations in rural communities to demonstrate the impact of nursing interventions (e.g., teaching) on decreasing cost while improving and maintaining health across populations and settings.

Transitional models of care have been developed to focus on care outcomes such as cost, length of stay, and patient satisfaction. Models using advanced practice nurses as case managers or clinical specialists enable patients to move rapidly from the acute care settings to a less costly care site, such as the home. Studies using master's-prepared clinical nurse specialists (CNS) to promote early discharge to home have been demonstrated as successful with populations such as low-birthweight infants (Brooten, Brown, Munro, et al., 1988), women having unplanned cesarean sections, pregnant women with diabetes and hypertension, the elderly with multiple health problems, and HIV infants and families. The use of CNSs as case managers with high-volume Diagnosis Related Group admissions resulted in earlier discharge and decreased health care costs (Anderson-Loften, Wood, & Whitefield, 1995). Evaluation of this particular nursing practice model suggests improved quality care outcomes; better symptom management, including improved pain management; increased patient perception of quality care; and overall decreased cost, length of hospital stay, and hospital readmissions (Walker, 1994).

Relevance to Nursing

Use of various models to guide nursing practice help to foster the philosophy, values, and beliefs of an organization. A nursing practice model can serve as a structure for the planning and direction of nursing and health care and help guide resource distribution. Strategic planning is improved as participation from all providers in organizational decisions can occur when nurses and have a shared vision about health care. Through the use of nursing practice models, practitioners from beginner to expert can be recognized for unique contributions to care and for their educational and clinical expertise.

Organizing care around a nursing practice model also can create a stronger patient-centered environment, where providers can come to know the patient and use nursing knowledge to improve care outcomes. A professional practice model can help to expand nursing's leadership for patient care and foster those behaviors associated with patient, family, and community health. Through practice models, new strategies and nursing interventions can be generated and tested to expand nursing knowledge and inform clinical practice.

Future

With the continued emphasis on health care reform, cost savings, and quality, it is essential that practice be implemented within a framework that is realistic and useful. Within nursing, the continued creation of practice models will promote quality care and facilitate the articulation of nursing's contribution to care outcomes. Emerging practice models that are patient-centered and respectful of the contribution of all providers will foster quality health care for all and initiate creative approaches to practice that can maintain and sustain individuals in less costly environments. Through teamwork, cooperative planning, and increased participation in decision making, system members can move the organization toward a shared vision and new directions in care delivery.

DOROTHY A. JONES

See also
   COST ANALYSIS OF NURSING CARE
   HEALTH SYSTEMS DELIVERY
   ORGANIZATIONAL REDESIGN
   QUALITY OF CARE, MEASURING
   TRANSITIONAL CARE

NURSING PROCESS

Nearly all authors define the nursing process as a problem-solving process composed of the elements of assessment, planning, implementation, and evaluation. Many a priori assumptions have been identified and studied concerning the nursing-process approach to patient care that includes decision making as a characteristic of the process. These assumptions are that the nursing process is a holistic, scientific, individualized, problem-solving approach with an emphasis on diagnosing. The concept emerged as early as the 1950s from Lydia Hall and was more directly described by Orlando (1961).

Interest in the type of systematic identification of a nursing process spread rapidly, as evidenced in many proceedings, position statements, and policies from groups as influential as the American Nurses Association and the Joint Commission on the Accreditation of Hospitals. By the mid 1970s there was widespread implementation underway. Early writings began to emerge in the literature at this time. Although little research appeared in publications, writings in journals and textbooks were abundant, promoting the process as a useful tool for teaching and understanding nursing. It was commonly held that full implementation of the nursing process would bring about radical changes in nursing education and nursing practice. In the late 1970s the World Health Organization (WHO, 1977) endorsed the use of the nursing process. With this support the United Kingdom quickly adopted the approach throughout nursing.

A review of the research on nursing process in the past 15 years has focused less on the merits, processes, and structure of the nursing process and more on the study of the implementation of the nursing process. A large amount of the research conducted on this concept has come from the United Kingdom. However, studies on the implementation of the nursing process in both the United States and the United Kingdom reveal that nursing process has not been implemented. Researchers have attempted to identify and study what barriers exist to the full use of the nursing process as identified by educators and clinicians in both countries. Studies focused on the attitudes of nurses, environmental factors, educational preparation, strategies to promote and encourage use, and instrument development to measure the concept more empirically. The reports were very consistent in finding that nurses placed a high value on the nursing process as a vehicle to provide quality, individualized, patient care, although they did not implement the nursing process regardless of their preparation and knowledge of the process or their educational level or years of experience. The data indicate that even those novice nurses recently educated within the nursing process did not use it in actual patient situations when providing independent nursing care.

There are problems with the evaluation and study of such a multidimensional concept as the nursing process. A review of the literature reveals few objective indicators or criteria to measure this concept. A variety of research designs and methodologies have been described in the literature primarily aimed at investigating the implementation or lack of implementation. Instrument development to measure the nursing process has been reported in the literature. Authors have designed quantitative studies using such strategies as attitudinal questionnaires with complex analyses, intervention studies intended to compare group outcomes, retrospective studies, and questionnaires assessing documentation. Other research strategies to study implementation issues have been inductive in nature. Researchers have used extensive literature analyses on the subject, grounded theory approaches, action research, direct observation with field recording, and cooperative inquiry to describe and understand these phenomena.

There is a considerable amount of unpublished dissertation work in the United States addressing issues and concerns about educational variations, environmental impact, and barriers in attitude and structure to the full implementation of the nursing process. Intervention studies have attempted to influence attitude and behavior with motivational therapy, increased education through innovative teaching strategies and on-site inservice, and skills-reinforcement strategies.

Throughout the reported studies a clear theme emerges. The profession of nursing holds a high value for the nursing process. There seems to be a convergence of thinking that it is the best vehicle to individualize patient care. Nurses verbally articulate this commitment and value on behalf of the profession and practice of nursing, but consistently the data support the reality that nurses do not use the nursing process in practice and that the assumptions and characteristics of the nursing process are not supported as tested in a myriad of research approaches.

Researchers interested in this field in the future might take some direction from this review as well as from clinical judgment. There are strong indications that a scientific, analytical, systematic approach to patient care is of value to the novice student who experiences the complexities of the human condition in early training. However, equally supportive research indicates that more advanced students and practicing nurses revise and adapt the nursing process within the realities of practice. Some nursing process researchers, as well as those that study clinical judgment (decision making), call for a new model that reflects a more holistic approach to analyzing patient situations and arriving at individualized care that is open to multiple ways of knowing and the evolving contexts of the environment and the patient. One future direction might be generating theory-based practice models for individualized patient care and testing the effectiveness of these new process models. This research may contribute greatly to the new outcomes-focused initiatives shaping nursing for the 21st century.

SALLY PHILLIPS

See also
CLINICAL DECISION MAKING
CLINICAL JUDGMENT
NURSING EDUCATION
NURSING PRACTICE MODELS

NURSING SLEEP SCIENCE

Sleep is a behavior oscillating on a regular basis (every 24 hours) with waking; and compared to waking, it represents a series of distinguishing brain and somatic state changes, not the least of which is the loss of conscious awareness. Sleep can be measured physiologically by using somnography such as the electroencephalogram (EEG), the electromyogram (EMG), and the electrooculogram (EOG) to reveal a series of stages or by using activity monitors, which distinguish sleep from waking less precisely. Sleep can be assessed behaviorally by direct observational judgment or by self-reported perceptions of retrospective recall, global impressions such as histories, or concurrent reports in the form of diaries or logs. Physiological measurement is time-consuming and expensive, and it can interfere with natural sleep because of the necessary instrumentation. Behavioral observations are tedious, time-consuming, and potentially inaccurate. Self-report methods are subject to preferred answers and the propensity to report negative impressions indiscriminately. People's impressions of their sleep do not always match physiological documentation.

In brain wave analysis by EEG, sleep is recognized by signs of a transitional stage (Stage 1) that progresses into a light stage (Stage 2) and progressively descends into slow-wave sleep (SWS) or deep (delta) sleep (Stages 3 and 4). Brain waves progressively change from mixed-frequency and low-amplitude waves to slower frequency and higher amplitude as sleep progresses through these stages of nonrapid eye movement sleep. The deepest stage of sleep is followed by a period of rapid eye movement (REM) sleep to complete one sleep cycle, taking about 60 to 90 minutes. Consequently, a night of sleep consists of three to six cycles of sleep depending on sleep duration.

The study of sleep is a highly transdisciplinary enterprise. Biological scientists seek to understand the regulation of sleep of sleep/wake cycles. Behavioral scientists seek to understand the function of sleep, normative patterns across age groups or species, the need for sleep, and why affective disorder is closely associated with sleep disorder. Abnormal behaviors during sleep, such as apneas and large-muscle movements, claim the interests of some clinical scientists.

We are only beginning to understand the ways in which sleep is basic to health and survival. Poor sleep results in impaired performance, is a precursor to many injury accidents, impairs tissue healing, alters the immune system, and in some cases may herald early onset of psychiatric impairment. Therefore, the development of sleep science is relevant to nursing science. Nursing scientists most often seek to understand how sleep—or more precisely, sleeplessness—is related to health and illness, what can be done to promote sleep, and how sleep is affected by environments and life contexts. The last often include care environments such as critical care units and longer-term care centers and the context of enduring pain, injury, diseases, or major transitions.

Out of 50 recently reviewed studies done by nursing scientists, most involved adults (about 80%) and the remainder, infants or children. Almost one-third of these studies were focused on sleep associated with disorders or illness, about one-quarter were intervention studies, and in about three-quarters self-report or behavioral observation was used.

The depth of science generated by nursing scientists is rudimentary but built on the premise that personal stress has an impact on sleep/wake cycles. The notions that illness and disease interfere with normal sleep/wake behavior and that the hospital environment constitutes a stressful environment are prominent. Interventions are individually or environmentally focused. Environmental manipulation is a likely intervention for infants and children. For example, one group tested the effect of recorded bedtime stories on the time to fall asleep in hospitalized children (White, Williams, Alexander, Powell-Cope, & Conlon, 1990). Results implied that the use of the parental voice might prolong falling asleep. Another has looked, before and after a staff training program for reducing environmental stress factors, for an effect on infant behavior, including sleep/wake (Becker, Grunwald, Moorman, & Stuhr, 1993). In a research program related to intensive care unit (ICU) noise and sleep, a sound conditioner failed to have an effect on somnographic sleep (Topf, 1992). Other intervention studies have used standardized rest periods for preterm infants to produce better behaviorally measured sleep; ocean sounds, with evidence of better perceived sleep in post–coronary artery bypass graft (CABG) surgery; and progressive muscle relaxation in seniors, with evidence of better perceived and somnographic sleep variables.

Lee's group studied sleep in times of transition, in women during the menstrual cycle, in pregnancy and postpartum, and in nurses working shifts, using somnography and self-report (Lee, 1992; Lee & DeJoseph, 1992; Lee, Shaver, Giblin, & Woods, 1990). In the menstrual cycle luteal phase, time to REM sleep was shorter compared to the follicular phase, and women with premenstrual negative affect symptoms had less deep sleep during both menstrual cycle phases. Women in transitions of pregnancy have been found to have sleep problems, both prenatal and postpartum. Primigravidas experienced significantly more disturbed sleep than do multigravidas. In a descriptive study of registered nurses working and not working day shifts, shift work was associated with more sleep disturbances and sleepiness; but age and family factors, more than alcohol and caffeine intake, contributed to the differences in types of sleep disturbances.

Two groups of investigators have developed research programs focused on individuals with sleep problems. Rogers's group has a program of research investigating subjects with narcolepsy (Rogers & Aldrich, 1993; Rogers, Aldrich, & Caruso, 1994). They found that those with narcolepsy have disturbed sleep and nap more; memory is not measurably affected, although concentration is, and timed naps can improve time to fall asleep. Shaver's group has ongoing work describing sleep in midlife (perimenopausal) women, particularly those with insomnia (Shaver, Giblin, Lentz, & Lee, 1988; Shaver, Giblin, & Paulsen, 1991). Those researchers have found that menopausal status is not profoundly linked to somnographic sleep unless hot flashes are manifest, but midlife women reporting insomnia can be classed as two types. One group of women reporting insomnia had high life strain and expressed high psychological distress, but they exhibited little abnormality in somnographic sleep patterns and few classical symptoms of menopause, such as hot flashes. Another group with insomnia reported hot flash activity but had less overall distress and life strain than the other group. Implications are that interventions to manage hot flashes and menopausal symptoms are more warranted in the latter, and life and stress management skills might be more efficacious in the former group.

Besides these program studies, other studies have involved assessment of sleep in conjunction with health threats, for example, postabdominal sur-

gery, post-CABG surgery, renal dialysis, chronic fatigue and fibromyalgia in women, Parkinson's disease, and cancer, as well as in hospitalized adults and children. Sleep issues associated with pregnancy, mostly the postpartum phase, have been studied by other investigators. Sleep issues also have been reported in midlife women and in preteen and teenage individuals.

In synchrony with a central focus for nursing practice, the repertoire of studies by nursing scientists mainly represents understanding sleep in relation to health and illness. Such study has been diverse, and sustained work has been done by only a few investigators. The majority of studies have used descriptive methodology and were limited to self-reports of sleep. It is imperative to the development of nursing sleep science that more sustained study is done on vulnerable populations, that is, those that are acutely ill, chronically ill, or suffering from sleep disorders for which behavioral treatments are prominent (e.g., insomnia, narcolepsy) and those that are in high-risk environments (e.g., hospitals, high stress factors). Within these populations and environments, sustained intervention studies that reveal dose response elements, titration, timing, individualized responses, and the factors affecting behavioral choice and adherence are needed. Furthermore, the application of biobehavioral methods that involve combined physiological and perceptual measures will do much to develop future knowledge that will be important to symptom management, illness and disease prevention, and health promotion.

JOAN L. F. SHAVER

See also
CRITICAL CARE NURSING
FATIGUE
MENSTRUAL CYCLE
NICU PRETERM INFANT CARE
STRESS

NURSING STUDIES INDEX

The *Nursing Studies Index* (Henderson & Yale University School of Nursing Index Staff, 1963–1972,

1984) is a four-volume annotated guide to literature on nursing published in English from 1900 through 1959. The literature indexed was cumulated in a broad and systematic search of periodical and non-periodical sources and the indexing of everything in those journals, books, and pamphlets of an analytical or historical nature that involved nursing or nurses. The *Index* was designed to serve a public with widely different interests and educational backgrounds, and therefore the indexing staff developed an inclusive policy. Historical and biographical articles and monographs were included, as were articles believed to involve nurses or nursing. No effort was made to index publications of interest to nurses, and the *Index* did not supplant *Index Medicus, Hospital Literature Index, the Education Index,* or other essential library tools.

The *Nursing Studies Index* filled a void in the development of the modern nursing profession. The professional literature was scattered and inaccessible to those who desired to review a topic systematically. This was especially true for nurses involved in research but also concerned practitioners and teachers. Virginia Henderson, director of the indexing project, was aware of the challenge in accessing nursing literature because of her involvement in two related activities: textbook writing and review and critique of nursing research. The latter project was performed under the direction of Leo Simmons, and together they published a volume entitled *Nursing Research: A Review and Assessment* (Simmons & Henderson, 1964). Henderson had previously prepared two editions of the textbook *Principles and Practice of Nursing* (Harmer & Henderson, 1939; 1955).

The *Index* is organized chronologically, with Volume 1 covering the years 1900 through 1929, 2 covering 1930 through 1949, 3 covering 1950 through 1956, and 4 covering 1957 through 1959. They were published inversely, Volume 4 first in 1963 followed by volumes 3, 2, and 1 in 1966, 1970, and 1972. The entries are arranged using the first edition of *Medical Subjects Headings* (MeSH) (National Library of Medicine, 1960). MeSH was employed in the hope that doctors and nurses would access each other's professional literature when searching topics of mutual interest. Contemporary automated library database literature searches make

this hope more remote, as a keystroke now divides the medical and nursing literature, even when the topics generate results applicable to both fields.

The first volume of the *Index* (Volume 4) contains a classification system for nursing studies that was not used in the work. The classification scheme is instructive and timely now that the proliferation of professional literature has made it challenging to place articles and studies in context and into mutually exclusive and exhaustive categories.

The *Nursing Studies Index* is the direct forerunner of the *International Nursing Index* (American Journal of Nursing, 1966), the standard reference to nursing literature. There is a 6-year gap between the *Index* and the 1966 beginning of the *International Nursing Index.* The gap was filled through the *Cumulative Index to Nursing Literature* (Seventh Day Adventist Hospital Association, 1961–1967). The four-volume index was initially published by Lippincott and reprinted by Garland Publishing and is now used primarily for historical research. Henderson went on from the indexing project to write a sixth edition of her text, *Principles and Practice of Nursing*, co-authored with Gladys Nite (1978/1997). It is the only edition that capitalized on her exhaustive knowledge of the professional literature and, as such, is perhaps the most important book written on nursing in the 20th century.

EDWARD J. HALLORAN

See also
BIBLIOGRAPHIC RETRIEVAL SYSTEMS
CUMULATIVE INDEX TO NURSING
  AND ALLIED HEALTH LITERATURE

NURSING THEORETICAL MODELS

A nursing theoretical model is a conceptual representation of nursing phenomena. It consists of concepts that are defined and related in ways that are relevant and representative of the discipline of nursing. Theoretical models present basic assumptions, boundaries, content, and context associated with the substantive focuses of the discipline. Nursing theoretical models provide a framework, unique to nursing, for understanding the nature of human beings, their health, and their environments and for understanding the methods by which nursing is studied and practiced.

Theoretical Models and Nursing Knowledge

Theoretical models are an essential dimension in the structure of nursing knowledge, part of a hierarchy of abstractions about nursing phenomena. The most abstract conceptual structure is the metaparadigm, which presents a global perspective on phenomena of interest to the discipline.

Conceptual models consist of concepts that are less abstract than those in the metaparadigm but more abstract than those found in other theoretical models. Conceptual models are not directly testable in research nor directly applicable in practice, because of the abstractness of the concepts and the lack of specificity in defining concepts and in describing relationships among the concepts.

Theoretical models referred to as middle-range theories consist of less abstract concepts, with definitions and interrelationships specifically described. These theories are more directly applicable to research and practice.

In nursing, the term *theoretical model* is often used to refer to theories at the level of abstraction and scope of conceptual models, whereas the term *theory* is reserved to refer to theories of middle range. Noted sociologist Thomas Merton originated the term *middle range*. Theory texts, such as those by Dubin (1978) and by Walker and Avant (1995), typically focus on the development and critique of middle-range theory. In nursing, classic texts by Fitzpatrick and Whall (1996), Fawcett (1995), and Riehl-Sisca (1989) focus on the evaluation and application of conceptual models. Fawcett (1993, 1995) proposed a distinction between nursing conceptual models. She classified the models of Leininger, Newman, Orlando, Parse, Peplau, and Watson as theories and identified the models of Johnson, King, Levine, Neuman, Orem, Rogers, and Roy as conceptual models. All of these models may be considered theoretical models at varying levels of abstraction, scope, and specificity.

The distinction between levels of abstraction of theoretical models is important. Each abstraction stimulates and validates nursing knowledge as it evolves through the processes of research, practice, and theory development. Theoretical models are mechanisms for (a) framing and making sense of the world, (b) submitting ideas about practical nursing application, (c) eliciting critiques, and (d) advancing the discipline.

Nursing theoretical models must meet four general criteria: (a) conceptual adequacy fosters development and refinement of theoretical ideas and theories and displays logical consistency and comprehensiveness in concept definition and use; (b) empirical adequacy supports and serves as a conceptual resource for research endeavors designed to generate or test theories; (c) pragmatic adequacy provides congruence with contemporary societal needs and supports nursing's professional obligations in health policy, practice, and education; and (d) isomorphism ensures representativeness of nursing reality. Nursing reality is identified broadly by this metaparadigm: a holistic perspective of human beings, human health, human environments, and the nursing processes that sustain them.

Theoretical Models and Research

Theoretical models are integral to the process of nursing research. They provide perspective and guidance in (a) identifying meaningful and relevant areas of study, (b) proposing plausible approaches to health problems to examine empirically, (c) developing or reformulating middle-range theory linked to research, (d) defining the concepts and proposing relationships among concepts, (e) interpreting research findings, and (f) developing clinical practice protocols and generating nursing diagnoses based on research findings.

Theoretical models provide direction regarding the syntax and the substance of the discipline. They are useful in selecting the research design, approaches to measurement, and methods of data analysis and in specifying criteria for acceptability of findings as valid.

The nature of nursing knowledge is such that theoretical models do not exist nor are they developed independent of the contexts of research and practice. Theoretical models both derive from and inform nursing knowledge, conceptual, ethical, clinical, personal, and empirical. The models support the research process and may be used in reference to the more abstract structures of nursing knowledge. Theoretical models may be used to further clarify nursing philosophies and develop nursing's metaparadigm.

Past, Present, and Future Directions

Viewing the theoretical models across time provides insight into the history of nursing and the changes and enduring patterns that are evident in nursing's substance and syntax. The theoretical models are repositories of nursing's beliefs, ideas, philosophies, and pragmatic concerns of practice and research.

Historically, theoretical models were critical to the emergence of nursing as a learned profession. The inception of professional nursing was associated with Nightingale, who in the mid 19th century articulated a view of nursing regarded as nursing's earliest theoretical model. Nightingale's systematic observations and formal education abstracted a view of nursing's role in managing the environment so as to facilitate the human reparative process.

Knowledge development resumed after a lapse during the early 1900s, as theorists such as Peplau, Orlando, and Henderson in the 1950s and 1960s explicated their theoretical ideas about nursing. The 1970s brought forth several new theoretical models. During the 1980s and 1990s, further refinement of extant models occurred, influenced in part by nurses' increased sophistication in theory development and by the shift in worldviews from modernism to postmodernism.

Nursing currently espouses a number of theoretical models, each of which offers a distinct view of nursing reality. A sampling of key concepts across nursing theoretical models demonstrates the following unique and diverse perspectives: (a) adaptation and expanding consciousness; (b) human becoming and conservation; (c) behavioral system and unitary being; (d) interpersonal process, transactional process, and reparative process; (e) pattern recognition and tertiary prevention; (f) transpersonal caring and self-care; (g) universal environmental stressors and cultural care diversities; (h) normal and flexible lines of defense and human rhythmic patterns.

In the future, theoretical models will likely hold an essential place in the structure of nursing knowledge and research activities. Some will be supplanted by new models, others will be reformulated as influenced by the philosophical and pragmatic need of the discipline, and a few will endure. Theoretical models that are less abstract and more specific in defining and relating concepts are more amenable to a critique and testing and therefore are more likely to undergo transformation or replacement.

The theoretical models that become part of the evolution of knowledge will be effective in linking the practical to the theoretical and in making the "concept-ual" "act-ual." The presence of theoretical models in the future will help elevate nursing as a discipline by providing an organized perspective for nursing researchers, theorists, and practitioners to use in ways that clarify nursing's unique contributions to an increasingly complex society.

PAMELA G. REED

See also
  EPISTEMOLOGY
  HEALTH CONCEPTUALIZATION
  MIDDLE-RANGE THEORY
  SCIENTIFIC DEVELOPMENT
  THEORETICAL FRAMEWORK

NURSING WORK REDESIGN

Nursing work redesign is defined as the restructuring of work roles or revising of work processes performed by nursing personnel for the purposes of improving the efficiency and effectiveness of the patient care delivery system and the quality of patient care services. There are a variety of synonyms for nursing work redesign: work/job redesign, work/job restructuring, redesigning nursing practice or patient care systems, nursing role redesign, and workplace restructuring. The term *reengineering* is sometimes synonymous with redesign efforts although reengineering implies a radical, comprehensive, "start from scratch" approach, whereas redesign implies an incremental, process-improvement approach. Organizational restructuring, characterized by downsizing or mergers, is not considered work redesign, although organizational restructuring and work redesign efforts often are undertaken concurrently. There is considerable lack of conceptual and methodological clarity regarding both the purposes of nursing work redesign or the expected outcomes of such efforts (Redman & Ketefian, 1995).

The total quality management (TQM), or continuous quality improvement (CQI), movement that was infused into the health care delivery system in the late 1980s also had an impact on work redesign efforts. The focus on process improvement and customer requirements, hallmarks of any TQM/CQI effort, is closely aligned with the goals of many work redesign efforts. Conceptually, work redesign and TQM/CQI are distinct. However, TQM/CQI efforts frequently result in work process redesign, and in this regard the approaches often may be related in nursing practice settings.

Approaches to nursing work redesign may begin at the top levels of the organization and disseminate down to the individual production or patient care unit levels. This macro-level approach tends to be driven by cost or organizational integration goals. Redesign efforts also may begin at the individual nurse or patient care unit level and move outward in the organization. This micro-approach generally focuses on goals to improve the quality of service and professional standards for nursing roles and responsibilities.

The goals of work redesign efforts may be similar, whether approached from a macro- or micro-level perspective. Although there are a variety of reasons for redesign, the majority of redesign projects are driven by the need to decrease operating costs in health care organizations. In addition to decreasing costs, organizations undertake these efforts to increase operational flexibility, improve efficiency, improve quality of service, and strengthen organizational integration. Any particular redesign effort may address a primary goal or a combination of goals. Whether a macro- or micro-level approach is used, redesign efforts often have far-reaching effects beyond the particular roles and departments that may be directly involved in redesign.

In an examination of nursing work redesign strategies, two distinct approaches were identified: patient-focused care models and operations improvement models (Greiner, 1995). In the patient-focused care models, new multiskilled workers are used to reconfigure the patient care team and reduce the number of different types of workers who come into contact with the patient. This model emphasizes quality service from the patient's perspective. In the operations improvement model, nurse extenders are used to shift some basic nursing care tasks from the registered nurse to nursing assistants, changing the ratio of registered nurses to ancillary staff on the nursing care team and emphasizing cost reduction. Greiner (1995) reports that research on both redesign approaches remains very limited. The impact on quality of nursing care remains inconclusive as the data related to clinical quality are either mixed, nonexistent, or methodologically flawed.

Many work redesign efforts have resulted in staff substitutions for registered nurses and reductions in the overall proportion of registered nurses to other nursing personnel in acute care institutions. The decrease in the average length of stay and the rising level of severity of illness and comorbidity of acute care patients present increased complexity of care requirements for registered nurses across all nursing practice settings in the 1990s.

Changes in the composition of nursing and patient care teams have raised concerns from professional nursing. The American Nurses Association (ANA) has developed several initiatives to address the impact of nursing work redesign on nursing practice and patient care. In 1995 the ANA supported the development and inclusion of nursing care indicators in quality assessment report cards, which measured the safety and quality of health care in hospitals (ANA, 1995d). The ANA also has developed a formal position statement on the impact of workplace restructuring and work redesign on nursing practice and issues of safety in the workplace (ANA, 1995c).

In response to these concerns about the transformation taking place in the health care delivery system, the U.S. Congress and the Department of Health and Human Services commissioned the Institute of Medicine to undertake a study to determine how changes in nurse staffing in hospitals was affecting the quality of patient care (Wunderlich, Sloan, & Davis, 1996). The Institute of Medicine concluded that there was a paucity of research on the definite effects of staffing ratios and models of nursing care on the quality of patient care. In addition, the report called for the development of a research agenda to examine the relationships among nurse staffing, workplace and role restructuring, and quality of patient care. When this proposed agenda is developed, it will lay a foundation for rigorous examination of the effects of nursing work redesign on both patients and nurses.

RICHARD W. REDMAN

See also

NURSE STAFFING
NURSING INTENSITY
NURSING WORKLOAD MEASURE-
   MENT SYSTEMS
ORGANIZATIONAL REDESIGN
WORKFORCE

NURSING WORKLOAD MEASUREMENT SYSTEMS

Nursing workload systems refer to the array of methods and procedures designed for the determination and allocation of nursing personnel in both inpatient and outpatient settings. Some of the systems are based on the concept of patient classification, yielding a specified number of hours of care for each patient category. Others identify a unique care-time requirement for each patient. In general, the systems have become a major component of the management of nursing resources.

Nursing resource management is not a new concept. Florence Nightingale addressed not only the question of how many nurses were needed for her many exploits but gave serious thought to the larger question of human resource planning. From a historical perspective, Giovannetti (1994) has identified three major perspectives for addressing the questions related to nurse staffing. First, staffing decisions were made primarily on the basis of the

perceived requirements of recognized leaders in the field, employing both personal and professional sources of power. This approach was employed by Nightingale and remained dominant until about the mid-1930s. Possibly driven by rapid growth in both the size and complexity of institutional care, this gave way to a more scientific approach, resulting in the development of global staffing standards. Fixed staff-to-patient ratios in terms of hours per patient-day became the norm. This approach assumed that the basis for staffing was the number of occupied beds.

The work of Connor, conducted at the Johns Hopkins Hospital in the 1960s, was instrumental in bringing about a shift in focus from occupied beds to the varying needs of patients who occupy the beds (Connor, Flagle, Hseih, Preston, & Singer, 1961). This was the beginning of the third stage, the development of workload measurement systems. Connor developed a three-category patient classification scheme using criteria from observational studies of direct nursing care that were deemed to reflect a significant proportion of nurses' time. The criteria for assigning patients to categories included physical needs (based on activities of daily living), emotional needs, selected treatment needs such as oxygen and suctioning, and certain patient states such as unconsciousness and impaired vision. Following the work of Connor, there was a proliferation of nursing workload measurement systems, developed by both individual nurse investigators and vendors. A number of sources are available for the reader interested in the historical development in the United States, Canada, and the United Kingdom (Baar, Moores, & Rhys-Hearn, 1973; Giovannetti, 1978).

The terminology employed in reference to nursing workload measurement systems varies widely and, according to Edwardson and Giovannetti (1994), has contributed to both misunderstanding and misuse. The term *patient classification systems* is frequently used, leading to confusion with many other types of patient classification systems such as diagnostic related groups (DRG), case mix groups (CMG), and medical severity of illness systems. Further, many nursing workload measurement systems do not employ the grouping or classification of patients. The terms *nursing severity* and *nursing acuity* systems have also been widely used, suggesting a purpose or intent beyond the assessment of nursing care time. In addition, nursing intensity and patient dependency have been used to label nursing workload measurement schemes, although the preferred (and more accurate) term in North America appears to be that of nursing workload measurement systems.

A variety of approaches to the measurement of nursing workload has been developed; and although substantial differences exist among the approaches, they all aim to estimate the total hours of nursing care, including both direct and nondirect time required to care for patients. Most employ a prospective approach to the assessment of patients' nursing care needs; however, as the systems are increasingly used for costing out nursing care, retrospective assessments are common. Edwardson and Giovannetti's (1994) integrative review of systems is the most comprehensive source for the research base of the systems, whereas Lewis (1989) contains a comprehensive volume of examples of many of the systems used in North American hospitals.

The proliferation of systems attests both to the numerous issues that surround the use of nursing workload measurement systems and to the complexity of the task of determining the appropriate level of nurse staffing. The nursing literature is replete with advice on implementation strategies as well as techniques for measuring and monitoring both reliability and validity. Recent work by O'Brien-Pallas, Cockerill, and Leatt (1991) and Phillips, Castorr, Prescott, and Soeken (1992) highlighted concerns about the comparability of different systems and thus raised new concerns about their inherent validity. The systems tested by these investigators revealed a high degree of correlation, yet evidence of comparability was not obtained. This finding has major implications for multiple hospital organizations and for any widespread application of cost comparisons.

PHYLLIS B. GIOVANNETTI

See also

COST ANALYSIS OF NURSING CARE
NURSE STAFFING
NURSING INTENSITY

PATIENT CLASSIFICATION
QUALITY OF CARE, MEASURING

NUTRITION

Nutrition as a research area crosses a variety of disciplines, including biochemistry, pharmacology, nutrition science, public health, medicine, and nursing. From a nursing research perspective, nutrition has been studied for its role in health promotion and disease prevention and its use as a therapeutic intervention. In addition, nurse investigators have long been concerned with the impact of disease and therapeutic treatments (e.g., chemotherapy) on nutritional intake. Thus, nutrition studies run the spectrum, from studies of subcellular mechanisms to epidemiological surveys of large groups of individuals. Clinical nutrition studies have focused on patients at risk (e.g., the elderly, pregnant and lactating women, low-birthweight infants), those with specific diseases, and age-related nutritional needs.

There is a sizable body of data supporting the link between diet and common health problems, the most notable of which is coronary artery disease. This relationship is complicated by the addition of genetic factors that place the individual at risk for problems related to lipid metabolism and body fat accumulation. Nurse scientists have participated in the study of this relationship, from molecular bench research to epidemiological studies. These studies provide important insights into our understanding of the pathophysiological and sociocultural mechanisms linking diet to blood vessel changes. There is also a need to increase the number of individual and community-based intervention studies to reduce dietary fat intake and decrease the risk for coronary artery disease.

Specialized nutrition therapies, including total parenteral nutrition, enteral feedings, and supplemental oral feedings, also have been the focus of research for nurse scientists. In these studies, nurses have examined strategies for delivering nutrition, including amounts, constituents, and timing, as well as strategies to reduce adverse consequences (e.g., diarrhea, hyperglycemia, catheter infection). In the early to mid 1970s nurse scientists began to describe the current practice of enteral nutrition support as well as the frequency of complications associated with this therapy in the acute care setting. The ongoing improvements in patient assessment techniques, commercialized diets, and diet delivery technology such as tubes and surgical techniques require nurses to collect descriptive information on the frequency of complications and the adequacy of nutritional intake. In addition, nurses should continue to conduct intervention studies focused on reducing complications (e.g., aspiration). With the trend for more patients to receive total parenteral nutrition and enteral nutrition in the home setting, descriptive research related to types and frequency of complications is needed. Also, patient and family education strategies, as well as providing support for family members, must be examined.

Another important nutrition-related problem in the United States is obesity. Obesity, or excessive body fat, is a complex phenomenon involving a multitude of factors, including genetics, lifestyle, and nutrition. Research has informed the public about the adverse outcomes such as mortality and morbidity. Again, nurse researchers working with animal models have provided insights into the links between heredity and metabolism. Clinical therapeutic studies have focused on the role of exercise, diet counseling, and psychological support in weight reduction in adolescent and middle-aged groups. Issues of compliance, self-efficacy, cultural variations, and individual physiology variations are often considered in examining patient responses.

Undernutrition states can be produced by a number of conditions, including anorexia nervosa, anorexia, wasting diseases, and symptoms such as nausea, pain, and fatigue. Of recent importance are studies linking tumor growth and inflammation to suppression of appetite. Nurse scientists working with animal models have shown that specific cytokines—interleukin-1 (IL-1), interleukin-6 (IL-6), and tumor necrosis factor (TNF-α)—decrease food intake. Such studies are likely to increase our ability to develop therapeutic strategies to enhance nutritional intake in select patient groups.

Other nurse scientists have focused on strategies to improve the caloric intake of patients undergoing chemotherapy for cancer treatment. Of particular significance is the previous work in instrument development and identification of patient groups most

at risk for nausea and vomiting and thus for inadequate nutrition. Therapeutic interventions such as relaxation therapy, guided imagery, and music therapy have been tested to determine their utility in reducing nausea and vomiting with therapy. The results of these studies are, for the most part, inconclusive because of the heterogeneity of the small samples, but they do suggest that they may be useful adjunct therapies along with antiemetics. More work is needed to examine biobehavioral strategies to enhance nutrient intake in select patient groups. Similarly, dietary intervention studies are being conducted in patients with compromised immune function (e.g., AIDS patients). The role of high fiber and low dietary fat intake in reducing diarrhea and thus improving nutritional status also is being studied in dietary intervention research.

Lactose intolerance is another common nutritional problem that has received some investigation by nurse scientists. Individuals with lactose intolerance have a decrease in lactase enzyme, the small intestine enzyme that is necessary for the breakdown of milk sugar lactose. In these individuals the consumption of lactose results in symptoms of bloating, increased flatus, and abdominal discomforts. Nursing research has focused on identifying patients at risk and testing strategies to enhance compliance with a low-lactose diet.

Nurse scientists also have studied problems related to phenylketonuria (PKU). This is an inherited defect caused by defective metabolism of the amino acid phenylalanine. If not treated, PKU can result in severe mental retardation. The intervention is a restriction in dietary phenylalanine intake. Women with PKU are at extremely high risk for bearing children with multiple congenital anomalies as well as mental retardation. Areas for nursing study include identifying individuals at risk, testing strategies to improve dietary compliance, decreasing risk of complications in offspring of women with PKU, and describing the coping strategies of individuals with PKU.

Cystic fibrosis is another condition that poses particular challenges for maintaining optimal nutritional balance. Growth failure and malnutrition are common clinical features of this condition. In cystic fibrosis the resting energy expenditure as well as the total energy expenditure are elevated from infancy. In addition, patients with cystic fibroses also exhibit pancreatic insufficiency, which places them at risk for malabsorption. Research should be focused on testing strategies to enhance dietary compliance and describing outcomes of nutritional interventions with regard to functional ability, quality of life, and morbidity.

MARGARET HEITKEMPER
ELEANOR BOND

See also
CARDIOVASCULAR RISK FACTORS, CHOLESTEROL
HYPERALIMENTATION
NUTRITION IN INFANCY AND CHILDHOOD
OBESITY AS A CARDIOVASCULAR RISK FACTOR
WEIGHT MANAGEMENT

NUTRITION IN INFANCY AND CHILDHOOD

Background and Definition

Nutrition in infancy and childhood refers to dietary intake necessary to support optimal growth and developmental processes from birth through the school-age years. During the past two decades substantial research attention has focused on the role of nutrition in health promotion and disease prevention across the life span. Dietary intake has emerged as a major environmental determinant of numerous chronic diseases, including hypertension, osteoporosis, insulin-dependent diabetes mellitus (IDDM), some forms of cancer, and coronary heart disease. Accumulated data suggest that many of these disease processes begin early in life and are influenced over time by patterns of dietary intake. Obesity, the most prevalent nutritional disorder in childhood and adolescence, is linked with many of these chronic conditions. Nutrition has always been a cornerstone of pediatric primary health care; however, these collective diet-disease observations, primarily of adult populations, have placed increasing emphasis on preventive interventions beginning early in life.

Infant Nutrition: Current Status and Recommendations

Infancy is a time of rapid growth and developmental change in all domains, including physical, cognitive, and psychosocial processes. Energy requirements during this period of the life span exceed others and approximate 90 to 120 kilocalories per kilogram (kg) of body weight per day. Because of its caloric density and role in myelination of the central nervous system, fat is an important macronutrient and normally comprises 40%–50% of the daily caloric intake during infancy. The Food and Nutrition Board of the National Research Council (1989) has defined recommended daily allowances (RDAs) for individuals (by developmental phase) across the life span. RDAs are neither minimal requirements nor necessarily optimal levels of intake; however, they are considered safe and adequate levels reflecting the state of knowledge concerning a nutrient, its bioavailability, and variations among the U.S. population (National Research Council, 1989). The RDA for protein intake is 1.38 g/kg of body weight per day for the first 6 months of life and 1.21 g/kg/day for the second 6 months. To date, no RDAs have been defined for carbohydrates or fats for this same time period.

The American Academy of Pediatrics Committee on Nutrition (AAP-CON) (1993) recommends human milk as the ideal source of nutrition for the first 4 to 6 months of life. In situations where breastfeeding is not practical nor desired, commercial formulas are recommended as the alternative form of infant nutrition. The Infant Formula Act of 1980 (revised in 1986) established human milk as the compositional model for formulas and specified the minimum levels of micronutrients to be included. Recent AAP-CON recommendations reaffirm human milk or commercial formula as the primary milk source throughout the first year of life and discourage cow's milk, reduced-fat milk, and evaporated milk.

In addition, breast-fed infants should receive 400 international units (IU) of vitamin D daily and iron supplementation at 4 months of age. Accumulated data indicate that the age of introduction of supplemental foods should not be rigidly specified; however, 4 to 6 months of age appears to be optimal for the majority of healthy term infants. AAP-CON emphasizes the introduction of single-ingredient foods, started one at a time at weekly intervals, to allow for the identification of food intolerance. Progression of feeding practices beyond this point may vary as a function of individual, family, cultural, and economic factors. Achievement of individual growth and developmental milestones, however, is universally recommended as a major determinant of nutrition throughout the first year of life (AAP-CON, 1993).

Although significant advances in the art and science of infant nutrition have been made in the past two decades, many challenges remain. The American Academy of Pediatrics (1997) issued a policy statement designed to address some of the major issues in infant nutrition. A continuing focal point for pediatric health care professionals is increasing the proportion of women who breast-feed in the early postpartum period. Breastfeeding has increased in some segments of the population; however, national goals, as indicated in *Healthy People 2000 Review* (U.S. Department of Health and Human Services, 1996) are far from realized. The prevalence of iron deficiency has decreased in the past several decades; however, data indicate that low-income, ethnically diverse infants continue to be a population at risk. In this regard, the American Academy of Pediatrics (1997) and other child health professionals acknowledge the contributions of the Special Supplemental Nutrition Program for Women, Infants and Children (WIC) and advocate for its continuation.

Recent research attention has focused on several controversial areas in infant nutrition, including supplementation of commercial formulas with polyunsaturated fatty acids (PUFA), the relationship of infant nutrient intake and risk factors for adult-onset cardiovascular disease (CVD), and gene-diet interactions early in life. Answers to questions raised in each of these areas will assist in defining guidelines for preventive interventions relevant to dietary intake in early life.

Nutrition in Early Childhood and the School-age Years: Current Status and Recommendations

The national emphasis on the role of nutrition in health promotion and disease prevention has prompted several recent surveys of dietary intake in children and youth. Methodological differences make cross-study comparisons difficult to interpret; however, accumulated data indicate that dietary patterns of U.S. children are not consistent with recent recommendations. In a recent population-based study using the Food Guide Pyramid, which defines recommended servings for each of the five major food groups, Munoz, Krebs-Smith, Ballard-Babash, and Cleveland (1997) observed that only 1% of children (2–19 years of age) met all current recommendations, whereas 16% did not meet any. Compared with their White counterparts, ethnically diverse children were less likely to meet the recommendations for grains and dairy; the percentage of children meeting the requirements for fruit and dairy was larger in the higher-income categories (Munoz et al., 1997).

Particularly noteworthy and consistent across all age, ethnic, and income groups was the excessive intake (35% of daily caloric intake) of dietary fat. Recent recommendations for all children 2 years of age and older indicate that fat should comprise 30% or less of daily caloric intake. These results are consistent with data from the National Health and Nutrition Examination Survey (NHANES III) (Lenfant & Ernst, 1994). Other surveys, however, report that African American and low-income children consume diets that are higher in total and saturated fat and least consistent with dietary recommendations (Bronner, 1996). Collectively, these observations point to the importance of both high-risk and population-based preventive interventions focused on adherence to dietary recommendations.

Numerous agencies have advanced dietary recommendations for children and youth. Recent recommendations reflect the state of knowledge regarding diet-health relationships and place emphasis on prudence and moderation in macronutrient consumption, particularly fat intake. Although specific RDAs vary as a function of age and other individual factors, recent guidelines also emphasize increased consumption of soluble and insoluble fiber and decreased consumption of sucrose and sodium. The American Academy of Pediatrics (1993) and the American Heart Association are consistent in recommending that children's diets should provide calories to support growth and developmental processes and maintain desirable body weight and should include a variety of foods (as suggested by the Food Pyramid). In addition, daily food intake should provide 30% or less of total calories from fat, less than 10% from saturated fat, and less than 300 mg of cholesterol.

Pediatric health care professionals are faced with both challenges and opportunities in implementing these guidelines across health care settings. Translating provider-oriented dietary guidelines and recommendations for consumers of varying developmental, educational, and cultural backgrounds is a particular challenge. In the pediatric population numerous factors influence dietary intake, including the contexts of family, school, and community. Traditional, individualized approaches to dietary behavior change in children and youth have yielded varying results. Recent data suggest an ecological approach to improving the nutritional status of U.S. children, with efforts that extend beyond the individual level to the school and community environments. By definition, such ''interventions'' will be multicomponent, require a multidisciplinary team approach, and involve formulation and implementation of health policies on both local and national levels. With knowledge of nutritional science and human behavior, as well as experience and expertise across the continuum of health care, nurses and nursing are particularly well qualified to participate in these efforts.

Nursing Research and Practice

Programs of nursing and multidisciplinary research focus on feeding practices and dietary intake in infancy and childhood; results to date have contributed to the existing body of knowledge in these areas of pediatric health care and have influenced clinical practice. As Kennedy (1997) observed, nursing research has contributed substantial information relevant to neonatal and preterm infant feeding. Nurse-initiated research focused on infancy and childhood has been primarily descriptive in

design; however, nurses have contributed in various roles in multidisciplinary research that incorporated dietary interventions. A particularly relevant program of research, conducted by Dr. Lindin Brown and colleagues at the University of Pennsylvania, is designed to examine factors associated with the initiation and maintenance of breastfeeding in diverse populations and interventions to increase breastfeeding in term and preterm mother-infant dyads. As part of a longitudinal twin-family study, Hayman, Cleves, and Meininger (1997) examined diet-lipid associations in school-age twins. Consistent with other results from this multidisciplinary program of research (Hayman, Meininger, Coates, & Gallagher, 1995; Meininger, Hayman, Coates, & Gallagher, 1997), findings emphasize environmental determinants of risk for CVD and point to the importance of heart-healthy nutrition beginning early in life.

As part of a multidisciplinary, school-based cardiovascular-risk-reduction project, Harrell and colleagues (Harrell et al., 1996) have employed dietary interventions in both rural and urban classroom settings. As in other school-based intervention studies, Harrell et al. observed that population-based classroom approaches can positively influence CVD risk profiles in elementary school children. A major challenge for all school-based and other nutrition interventions is maintenance of behavioral change over time. From a health-promotion and disease-prevention perspective, dietary adherence continues to be a viable area for nursing and multidisciplinary research.

LAURA L. HAYMAN

See also
CHILD FAILURE TO THRIVE
KANGAROO CARE
NEUROBEHAVIORAL DEVELOPMENT
**OBESITY AS A CARDIOVASCULAR
   RISK FACTOR**
VULNERABLE POPULATIONS

O

OBESITY AS A CARDIOVASCULAR RISK FACTOR

Definition and Prevalence

For decades, cardiovascular disease (CVD) has been the leading cause of mortality and premature morbidity among midlife and older men and women, with obesity as the primary risk factor. Characterized by the storage of excess fat, obesity is defined as 20% or more over desirable weight, based on the midpoint of the range of weights for a medium frame from the 1983 Metropolitan Life Insurance height and weight tables. The body mass index (BMI) normalizes body weight for height so that relative degrees of obesity can be evaluated among individuals; it correlates highly with weight and is nearly independent of height. A BMI (weight in kilograms / height in meters)^2 of 27 or higher also defines obesity.

Based on four separate national surveys conducted since 1960 (National Health and Nutrition Examination Surveys), the prevalence of overweight in America increased 9%, from 24.3% in the 1960–1962 survey to 33.3% in the 1988–1991 survey. This occurred despite accelerated national emphasis on and awareness of healthy nutrition, as well as a marked increase in the availability of low-fat foods. Using the World Health Organization Expert Commission obesity cutpoint as a BMI of 25, the National Center for Health Statistics estimated that the prevalence of obesity in America has soared to over 50%.

Empirical Evidence

Although there is little short-term relationship between obesity and morbidity or mortality, the long-term relationship is strong for both men and women. The Framingham Study included more than 5,000 men and women living in Framingham, Massachusetts, who were initially examined between 1948 and 1950 and reexamined at 2-year intervals thereafter. Even controlling for age, cholesterol level, systolic blood pressure, cigarette smoking, left ventricular hypertrophy, and glucose tolerance, higher BMI was significantly associated with the development of coronary heart disease (CHD) in these men and women, and in women it also was associated with an elevated risk of stroke. Moreover, weight gain was associated with increased blood pressure and increased serum levels of cholesterol and glucose. Weight gain after the young adult years increased the risk of CVD in both sexes. Data from the Nurses' Health study, established in 1976 with 121,770 female registered nurses and continuing to the present, corroborate and extend these findings (Manson et al., 1990). After adjusting for age and smoking, the risk of both nonfatal myocardial infarction and fatal coronary disease among women in the heaviest BMI category (≥ 29) was more than three times higher than that in women with a BMI of 21 or less. Moreover, cardiac disease in women with a weight gain of more than 20 kg in the preceding 4 years was twice as high as in women whose weight was stable.

Even more important than adiposity per se is its distribution, with central obesity and its intermediary mechanisms shown to be related to CHD incidence (Larsson et al., 1984). In women as well as men, an upper body distribution of fat indexed as waist:hip ratio is an independent risk factor for ischemic heart disease, diabetes, stroke, and premature mortality. In middle-aged women, an upper body fat distribution was associated with significantly higher systolic blood pressure, total cholesterol, low-density lipoprotein cholesterol, triglycerides, and lower levels of high-density lipoprotein cholesterol, even after the data were statistically adjusted for BMI (Wing, Matthews, Kuller, Meilahn, & Plantinga, 1991). Nevertheless, the strong relationships between waist:hip ratio and degree of obesity make it difficult to ascertain whether obesity per se or the distribution of body fat is the major determinant affecting risk factors for CVD.

Analyzing data by both BMI and waist:hip ratio in women pre- and post–weight loss, Dennis and Goldberg (1993) reported that an upper body fat distribution in women worsens lipid risk factors for CVD posed by obesity, and weight loss is an effective intervention to improve lipid profiles in these women. Although weight loss reduced CVD risk factors regardless of BMI or waist:hip ratio, the magnitude of the increase in plasma high-density lipoprotein cholesterol and decrease in triglycerides in women with upper body fat distribution suggests that weight loss in these women has the greatest potential to reduce their risk factors for CVD.

A persistent argument is whether or not obesity is an independent risk factor for CVD. Although the uniform relationship between the degree of overweight and CVD holds in simple univariate analysis, obesity often fails to emerge as an independent risk factor in multivariate analysis. However, the failure of obesity to emerge in a regression equation that also includes its component risk factors may be more an issue of multicollinearity than of physiological processes.

Insulin has been identified as an important physiological mechanism underlying obesity as a CVD risk factor, for the insulin levels in both the fasted and postprandial state are elevated in obese individuals. Hyperinsulinemia secondary to insulin resistance impairs glucose tolerance, increases triglycerides and cholesterol, and lowers high-density lipoprotein cholesterol. Increased insulin secretion that ensues to compensate for insulin resistance and glucose intolerance increases production of hepatic very low density lipoprotein triglyceride; impairs the catabolism of triglyceride-rich lipoproteins by adipose tissue lipoprotein lipase; increases small, dense low-density lipoprotein particles; and reduces the synthesis of HDL_2 particles. Insulin resistance also raises blood pressure through its effects on sodium retention and peripheral vascular tone (Bierman, 1992).

Numerous studies (Dennis & Goldberg, 1993; Wing & Jeffery, 1995) regarding the beneficial impact of weight loss on CVD measure its metabolic risk factors (e.g., cholesterol, triglycerides, insulin sensitivity, blood pressure) rather than "hard" disease end points, presumably because the small sample sizes in these tightly controlled clinical trials are not likely to reach epidemiological proportions large enough to make statements about subsequent disease incidence in the population. Nevertheless, a consolidation of studies establishes causal links of obesity to CVD risk factors and then to CVD end points.

Nursing Research

Despite the overwhelming prevalence of obesity and its profound physiological, psychological, and sociological sequelae, consuming more than $50 billion annually, only a few nurse investigators have focused on this major health problem, and fewer have examined obesity as a cardiovascular risk factor. Using qualitative research methodology, Allan (1988, 1989) explored weight management practices among women, including how women interpret and use health information in weight management, their strategies for maintaining their weight, and the factors that influence the complex self-care activities for dealing with weight gain and values of thinness. Using triangulation methodology and a sensitivity to cultural diversity in weight management, Walcott-McQuigg (1995) examined the dynamics and relationships among stress and weight control in African American, European American, Mexican, Mexican American, and Puerto Rican women. Brink identified the characteristics of successful weight management and evolved a new definition of "success" from the construction of weight history based on changes in BMI as an adult.

Purfield and Morin studied the impact of weight gain during the pregnancy of previously normal-weight primigravidas on length of second-stage labor and mode of delivery. Although Morin noted that obesity was a significant predictor of pregnancy-induced hypertension, hypertension was conceptualized as an obstetric complication rather than a risk factor for CVD. The only nurse investigators who have studied obesity and its relationship to CVD risk are Hansen, Bodkin, and colleagues, who worked with nonhuman primates, and Dennis and colleagues, who examined obesity and metabolic risk factors for CVD in women. None of these nurse investigators, with one exception (Dennis & Goldberg, 1996), have as yet translated their findings into intervention studies that implement and evaluate strategies to help obese individuals reach their uniquely personal, weight-related health goals and reduce their risk for CVD.

Supported in part by 1 R01 NR03514 from the National Institute of Nursing Research, National Institutes of Health and the Geriatric Research Education and Clinical Center at the Maryland VA Health Care System, Baltimore.

KAREN E. DENNIS

See also
**CARDIOVASCULAR RISK FACTORS,
    CHOLESTEROL
DIABETES MELLITUS
NUTRITION
RISK FACTORS
WEIGHT MANAGEMENT**

OBSERVATIONAL RESEARCH DESIGN

Observational designs are nonexperimental, quantitative designs. In contrast to experimental designs in which the investigator manipulates the independent variable and observes its effect, the investigator conducting observational research observes both the independent and the dependent variables. In observational studies, variation in the independent variable is due to genetic endowment, self-selection, or occupational or environmental exposures. Because of the myriad sources of bias that can invalidate naturally occurring events, rigorous designs and methods are required to minimize bias. Observational designs should not be confused with observational methods of data collection.

Observational designs are used when there is not enough knowledge about a phenomenon to manipulate it experimentally. Sometimes research involving human subjects is restricted to observational designs because of the nature of the phenomenon; that is, experimental research is precluded for ethical reasons.

Observational designs include quantitative, descriptive studies as well as analytical studies that are designed to test hypotheses. Descriptive, observational studies provide a basis for further study by describing and exploring relationships between variables, informing the planning of health services, and describing clinical practice for individual clients or groups of clients. In contrast, analytic research is designed to test specific hypotheses in order to draw conclusions about the impact of an independent variable or set of variables on an outcome or dependent variable under scrutiny. Observational designs are classified as longitudinal or cross-sectional. In a cross-sectional study, all the measurements relate to one point in time; in the longitudinal approach, measurements relate to at least two points in time.

A cross-sectional study, sometimes referred to as a correlational study, is conducted to establish that a relationship exists between variables. The term *correlational* refers to a method of analysis rather than a feature of the design itself. Cross-sectional studies are useful if the independent variable is an enduring or invariable personal characteristic, for instance, gender or blood type. Cross-sectional studies are also useful for exploring associations between variables.

Longitudinal comparative designs are usually undertaken to explain the relationship between an independent variable and an outcome. One type of longitudinal, comparative design is referred to as a cohort study. Although the investigator does not manipulate the independent variable, the logic and flow in a cohort study is the same as the logic of an experiment (Meininger, 1989). Subjects are measured or categorized on the basis of the independent variable and are followed over time for observation of the dependent variable. In a cohort study it is established at the outset that subjects have not already exhibited the outcomes of interest (dependent variable). Thus, the time sequencing of events can be established. In other words, it can be demonstrated that the independent variable preceded the occurrence of the dependent variable.

Another type of longitudinal, comparative design is a case-comparison study. In this design the flow is the opposite of a cohort study. Subjects are selected and categorized on the basis of the dependent variable (the outcome of interest). The purpose of the study is to test hypotheses about factors in the past (independent variables) that may explain the outcome. Although case-comparison designs are not prevalent in the nursing research literature, they have great potential for studies of outcomes that occur infrequently. Furthermore, this design is very efficient because it is possible to achieve greater statistical power with fewer subjects than in other types of observational designs.

Longitudinal comparative designs are also classified according to the time perspective of the events under study in relation to the investigator's position in time. A study is retrospective if, relative to when the investigator begins the study, the events under investigation have already taken place. A study is prospective if the outcomes that are being investigated have not yet taken place when the study is initiated. Various hybrid designs are also possible; referred to as ambidirectional studies, they combine features of both designs (Kleinbaum, Kupper, & Morgenstern, 1982).

As in experimental research, observational research designs and methods are selected with the aim of minimizing bias. Bias refers to distortion in the result of a study. A biased study threatens internal validity if the distortion is sufficient to lead to an erroneous inference about the relationship between the independent and dependent variable. Potential sources of bias that can threaten the internal validity of observational studies are those related to selection, measurement, and confounding.

Selection bias is a distortion in the estimate of effect resulting from (a) flaws in the choice of groups to be compared; (b) inability to locate or recruit subjects selected into the sample, resulting in differential selection effects on the comparison groups; and (c) subsequent attrition of subjects who had initially agreed to participate, which changes the composition of the comparison groups.

Measurement bias occurs when the independent variable or outcome (dependent variable) is measured in a way that is systematically inaccurate and results in distortion of the estimate of effect. Major sources of measurement bias are (a) a defective measuring instrument, (b) a procedure for ascertaining the outcome that is not sufficiently sensitive and specific, (c) the likelihood of detecting the outcome dependent on the subject's status on the independent variable, (d) selective recall or reporting by subjects, and (e) lack of blind measurements when indicated.

Because of the lack of randomization in a nonexperimental study, uncontrolled confounding variables are a major threat to internal validity. Unless confounding factors are controlled in the design of the study or in its analysis, distortion in the estimate of effect will result. A confounding factor operates through its association with both the independent and the dependent variables. It can distort the results in either direction; that is, it can lead to an overestimation of the relationship between the independent and dependent variables by producing an indirect statistical association, or it can lead to an underestimate of the relationship between the independent and dependent variables by masking the presence of an association between the independent and dependent variables. A distinction between confounding bias and other types of bias is that confounding is correctable at the design or analysis stage of the study, whereas bias due to selection and measurement problems are usually difficult or impossible to correct in the analysis. Confounding can be controlled or minimized at the design stage of the study by restricting the study sample or by matching the comparison groups. At the analysis stage confounding can be controlled or minimized by using a multivariable approach to the statistical analysis to adjust for the confounding factors or by examining the independent-dependent variable relationship within specified levels or categories of the confounding factors (stratified analysis). Confounding variables should not be confused with mediator and moderator variables.

In summary, observational designs are prevalent in nursing research because they are used to describe phenomena in early stages of knowledge development and provide a basis for designing experimental interventions. Additionally, they are the only feasible approach to hypothesis testing when it is unethical to manipulate the independent variable. In the absence of randomization and manipulation, myriad sources of bias can influence observations and conclusions drawn from naturally occurring events; thus, rigorous observational designs and methods are essential.

JANET C. MEININGER

See also
ETHICS OF RESEARCH
RELIABILITY
VALIDITY

OMAHA SYSTEM

The Omaha System is a research-based taxonomy. It is a structured and complete approach to practice, documentation, and information management. The system is organized from general to specific and includes the *Problem Classification Scheme*, the *Intervention Scheme*, and the *Problem Rating Scale for Outcomes*. The architecture is flexible and allows for additions or revisions consistent with established taxonomic rules and a research environment (Martin & Scheet, 1992).

The Omaha System is one of the four vocabularies recognized by the American Nurses Association. Between 1975 and 1993 four research projects were conducted to develop and refine the Omaha System and to establish its reliability, validity, and usability (Martin & Scheet, 1992; Martin, Scheet, & Stegman, 1993). The first three projects were Division of Nursing, U.S. Department of Health and Human Services, contracts, and the fourth was a National Institute of Nursing Research RO-1 grant. Funding during the 13 years of research approximated $1.4 million. Because of this funding the Omaha System exists in the public domain. Numerous faculty and master's and doctoral students are conducting Omaha System research and extending the body of knowledge. Research has expanded to include acute care settings. Several studies have demonstrated the ability to describe resource utilization patterns and severity or case-mix variables using the data elements of the Omaha System.

As vertical integration and the shift to community-focused care continues, the Omaha System is used across increasingly diverse settings (Elfrink & Martin, 1996; Frenn, Lundeen, Martin, Riesch, & Wilson, 1996; Martin & Martin, 1997; Martin & Norris, 1996). It is used in home care, public health, clinic, case management, school, nursing center, hospital, and other practice settings. Changes in health care delivery also prompted college of nursing faculty to revise their curricula. The first undergraduate-graduate program that revised its curriculum to one based on the Omaha System did so in 1997. In addition to use in the United States, the Omaha System is used internationally. It has been translated into Danish, Dutch, Chinese, Japanese, Swedish, and other languages. Additional known Omaha System users reside in Canada and Australia.

KAREN S. MARTIN

See also
FORMAL LANGUAGES
NURSING INFORMATION SYSTEMS
TAXONOMY

THE ONLINE JOURNAL OF KNOWLEDGE SYNTHESIS FOR NURSING

The Online Journal of Knowledge Synthesis for Nursing (OJKSN) is a full-text peer-reviewed electronic journal published by Sigma Theta Tau International. The journal began publication in January 1994 and was the first peer-reviewed electronic journal in nursing. There is no paper version; it is completely electronic.

The purpose of the journal is to publish timely, synthesized knowledge to guide nursing practice and research. Knowledge synthesis is the gathering of research studies on a topic, assessing the validity of the findings, and asserting implications for practice from the valid findings. The process includes identifying gaps in the knowledge base that would provide direction for future research on the topic. OJKSN provides critical reviews of research pertinent to clinical practice and research situations that nurses can access and use immediately. The journal does not have articles that are reports of a single study, such as you would find in other nursing research journals.

An on-line electronic journal delivers articles across commercial telecommunications to a computer terminal at a workstation or a personal computer. Transmission is through the Internet. The OJKSN is accessible on the World Wide Web through Sigma Theta Tau International's web site (http://stti-web.iupui.edu). It is available through subscription, which may be either individual or institutional. A combined subscription with the *Registry of Nursing Research* is also available.

All articles include a statement of the practice problem, a summary of the research, annotated critical references, practice implications, directions for future research, search strategies used, and references. Features of the journal include full-text searches, access to graphical displays such as tables and charts, links to referencing in external bibliographical databases such as *Cumulative Index to Nursing and Allied Health Literature* (CINAHL) and MEDLINE.

"Statement of the Practice Problem/Issue" is a brief statement explaining the scope of the article. "Summary of the Research" contains the review, analysis and synthesis of the research on the topic. The review is a state of the science for the topic. The extensiveness of the review depends on the depth and breadth of the research on the topic. The summaries differ from a literature review in that there is an assessment of the validity of the information contained in the research reports. It may include a meta-analysis, the statistical manipulation of findings from multiple research studies. The narrative is used to make summary statements about the research as a whole, and tables are used to describe the individual review of studies and the significant variables and findings. "Annotated Critical References" contains an abstract of the most significant research publications on the topic. A maximum of seven are annotated.

In "Practice Implications," the specific implications for practice based on the research are presented and discussed. This section delineates what practitioners can or should do as a result of the research on the topic. The research references are cited for all practice directives so that the clinician can refer to them if desired. "Research Needed" discusses the various directions for future research and the questions that remain unanswered. Knowing about the knowledge that does not exist is often as important as knowing what exists. This section is a good guide for directing master's theses and doctoral dissertations, as well as for clinical research studies. "Search Strategies" describes how the research cited was identified, the citation bases searched, the search terms that were used, and the years that were searched. References cited are listed in the American Psychological Association format. Each reference listed in MEDLINE or CINAHL has a hypertext link so that the entire citation, including abstract, can be accessed.

There are many advantages to an on-line journal. These include faster publication, immediate access, continuous publication, hypertext links, and instant access. Once a manuscript for a paper journal is accepted and revised, it may be anywhere from 6 to 24 months before it is out in print. With the electronic journal, articles are brought on-line generally within weeks after final acceptance and editing. The journal is available on-line 24 hours a day, 7 days a week. Although it may take weeks or months for an international journal to come through the mail, with a computer journal there is instant access.

Unlike a traditional print journal, where there are numerous issues a year with a varying number of articles per issues, an electronic journal has continuous publication. As an article is finalized, it is brought on-line. Articles are identified by the year and the article number for that year (e.g., 1997, No 11). Uniform standards are being developed for citing electronic publications.

Hypertext links allow direct access to the database of a reference (e.g., MEDLINE) for scanning the abstract of the reference. Once the abstract is read and perhaps printed, the reader is able to click back into the article at the same spot. There is instant access to all previously published articles in the journal; keeping paper copies of back issues is unnecessary.

Subscription information is accessed through the Sigma Theta Tau International web site at http://stti-web.iupui.edu or by requesting subscription information through the international headquarters. Once a subscription is processed, the user is sent a user guide, authorization, and password.

There is a tremendous amount of knowledge available for use in nursing practice. The key is accessing, synthesizing, and having it organized to readily make clinical decisions. The OJKSN greatly increases nursing's opportunities for knowledge-based practice, education, and research.

JANE H. BARNSTEINER

See also
INTERNET
JOURNALS IN NURSING RESEARCH
WORLD WIDE WEB

OREM'S SELF-CARE DEFICIT THEORY OF NURSING

Orem's self-care deficit theory of nursing provides a comprehensive framework for defining and describing nursing and is one of several nursing theories often called grand theories. Orem describes nursing as a specialized helping service in which the nurse provides assistance to an individual, family, or community with existing or potential self-care deficits (Orem, 1995).

Development of Orem's Theory

Dorothea Orem developed her ideas about the nature of nursing over four decades, beginning in the period from 1949 to 1957 when she was a consultant with the Indiana State Board of Health. She became aware that nurses were able to engage in nursing practice but unable to adequately describe what nursing was. The awareness of the need to articulate the nature of nursing increased in the late 1950s when Orem served as a consultant to the U.S. Department of Health, Education and Welfare, developing a curriculum for vocational nurses. This job necessitated that she delineate the scope and boundaries of technical versus professional nursing. These and other experiences convinced Orem of the importance of a comprehensive framework of nursing as a foundation for practice, teaching, and research within the discipline (Hartweg, 1991).

The work of developing the theory continues to involve many scholars, students, practitioners, educators, administrators, and researchers in nurs-

ing and other disciplines. Although there are monographs, papers, and books from earlier work on Orem's theory, the first publication of the entire theory was in her first edition of *Nursing: Concepts of Practice* in 1971. Subsequent editions have been published approximately every five years, with the most recent, fifth edition in 1995. Each new edition has reflected the evolution of the theory based on conceptual work of Orem and others, along with results of testing the theory in clinical, educational, administrative, and research arenas. Forums in which development has occurred include the biannual conferences at the University of Missouri beginning in 1992, international conferences beginning in 1989, and most recently, conferences and newsletters of the International Orem Society.

Components of Orem's Theory

As noted above, Orem's theory describes nursing as a specialized helping service needed when persons are unable to "provide continuously for themselves the amount and quality of required self-care because of situations of personal health" (Orem, 1995, p. 8). Orem chose the term "deficit" theory deliberately to reflect the idea that nursing is needed only if a self-care deficit exists. A deficit reflects the relationship between the abilities of individuals to care for themselves compared to the self-care needs or demands that exist at a particular point in time. If individuals, families, or communities are unable to meet these demands for self-care because of various kinds of limitations, then a need for nursing exists.

Orem's self-care deficit theory of nursing is a general theory of nursing, consisting of three interrelated theories: (a) the theory of self-care, (b) the theory of self-care deficit, and (c) the theory of nursing systems. Each of these theories has a central idea, a set of propositions and presuppositions. The reader is referred to the primary source, Orem (1995) or Hartweg (1991), for descriptions of the propositions and presuppositions.

The central idea of the theory of self-care is that self-care is a learned behavior that requires deliberate action. Self-care is defined as "the voluntary regulation of one's own human functioning and development that is necessary for individuals to maintain life, health, and well-being'' (Orem, 1995, p. 95). Orem emphasizes that self-care is not simply reflex or instinctual but is performed thoughtfully when a need is recognized. Within this subtheory is also the complementary notion of dependent care, or caretaking provided by other adults to those who are not mature or are unable to care for themselves. Nursing may be needed to assist those who provide care to their dependents.

The theory of self-care deficit reflects the central idea that individuals at times are unable to meet their self-care needs because of a great variety of limitations that may interfere. One key action of nursing is to determine the ability of the patient, family, or community to meet existing or predicted self-care needs.

The relationship between nursing actions and role as well as patient actions and role are explicated by the theory of nursing systems. In this component, Orem describes what nurses do when they ''nurse'' and the outcomes or results sought by nurses (Hartweg, 1991). The main idea is that nurses possess capabilities for designing a system of care that is appropriate to the individual's needs for self-care and nursing assistance.

In summary, the three interrelated theories of self-care, self-care deficit, and nursing systems comprise Orem's self-care deficit theory of nursing, answering the core questions ''What is self-care?'' ''When is nursing needed?'' and ''How do nurses provide nursing care?''

The components of Orem's theory consist of six basic concepts and one related or peripheral concept. The six core concepts are (a) self-care, (b) self-care agency, (c) therapeutic self-care demand, (d) self-care deficit, (e) nursing agency, and (f) nursing system. The related or peripheral concept of basic conditioning factors consists of factors that influence all of the central concepts, for example, self-care needs, capabilities of persons to engage in self-care, and capabilities of the nurse to provide nursing care. The basic conditioning factors are age, gender, developmental state, sociocultural orientation, socioeconomic factors, health state, family system factors, patterns of living, environmental factors, and resource availability and adequacy (Orem, 1995).

These six core concepts and the related concept of basic conditioning factors are best understood in relationship to one another. Self-care is the focal point of nursing, and the role of the nurse is seen in relation to the other concepts. The nurse determines the totality of actions that need to be performed by a person to meet self-care needs at a particular point in time (therapeutic self-care demand). Subsequently, the nurse assesses whether the person has the knowledge, judgment, decision-making skills, and action capabilities (e.g., self-care agency) to meet specific therapeutic demands. If deficits exist in the capabilities of the person to meet self-care demands, the need for nursing is clear and the capabilities of the nurse (nurse agency) are mobilized to provide necessary assistance and to promote increased self-care capabilities over time.

In summary, Orem's self-care deficit theory of nursing is a general theory of nursing that has been under development for approximately 40 years by Orem and others. The theory is currently used in clinical settings, in educational programs, and by nurse administrators. Nurse researchers have utilized the theory as a framework for research (Aish & Isenberg, 1996; Utz & Ramos, 1994) and have conducted research testing components of the theory (Hartley, 1988; Silva, 1986). Currently existing organizational structures, such as the International Orem Society at the University of Missouri School of Nursing, exist to promote the further development and testing of Orem's theory.

SHARON WILLIAMS UTZ

See also
ACTIVITIES OF DAILY LIVING
NURSING ASSESSMENT
NURSING THEORETICAL MODELS

ORGANIZATIONAL CULTURE

Although definitions vary within the broad range of studies that explore organizational culture, nursing studies define organizational culture as the workers' norms, beliefs, or values or as the ways of thinking, believing, and behaving that members of a unit share (Cooke & Rousseau, 1987). Nursing literature focuses on the culture of an organization as a means of clarifying relationships within the health care system, as well as between the system and other health care features. Of special concern intraorganizationally are those characteristics of the health care system that enhance the work of nursing personnel in the delivery of care, including the administration; concerns interorganizationally are for those features and the relationships that are established, which in turn enhance the patient's care. From a research perspective, these foci are not mutually exclusive.

The organizational culture is an important research focus because the nursing system comprises a significant proportion of the organization's budget. Another research issue is the ability of the organizational culture to be altered through additional education or improved leadership. Studies employing the organizational culture as a variable provide a direct measure of the culture as indices of the opinions employees have as well as an index of the organization. These various perceptions can be used to target areas for potential change or improvement. The measures may be applied to the individual, to the subunit, or to the system as a whole (McDaniel, 1995). The results can be compared, and baseline measures may be ascertained and used to reflect change due to intervention or to education. Other studies link the culture to work satisfaction, leadership, positive ethics, work satisfaction, and high performance, with tentative links to enhanced patient outcomes (Cooke & Rousseau, 1987; McDaniel, 1995; McDaniel & Stumpf, 1993; Shortell et al., 1994).

One of the reasons that culture is receiving increased attention in nursing research is its relationship to nursing practice and patient care outcomes and the fact that it is measurable. Instruments are available that produce high-quality results through valid and reliable assessments; they are cost-effective, and they require a realistic time investment. From a methodological perspective the need is to clarify whether the culture of the organization is measured among individuals reflecting the individual as the unit of analysis or measured within the organization and thereby reflecting the system as the unit of analysis. Significant error is introduced with confusion about these two approaches, resulting in flawed interpretation of the results. Most of the studies in nursing have focused on intraorganizational dimensions and have measured the individual as the unit of analysis. Measure at the aggregate level requires additional methodological adaptation and thus differing interpretations of the data.

A significant proportion of nursing research examining organizational culture focuses on the administration or the characteristics of the health care system and is conducted by researchers who are centrally interested in the improvement of patient care outcomes. Exploration of organizational culture assists in establishing models of health care system research and offers links with other dimensions of the nursing system that are a challenge to measure. As nursing research advances, organizational culture provides an avenue for more complex and interrelated models of health care services and systems analysis that involve nursing personnel and reflect measures applicable to nursing. As with most nursing research, the ultimate aim is the enhancement of health care delivery and the improvement of patient care.

CHARLOTTE MCDANIEL

See also
ADMINISTRATION RESEARCH
HEALTH SERVICES ADMINISTRATION
HEALTH SYSTEMS DELIVERY
ORGANIZATIONAL REDESIGN

ORGANIZATIONAL REDESIGN

Organizational redesign, or restructuring, as some experts refer to the phenomenon, is a "redoing" of the architecture of the organization. It is broader than reengineering, which involves a revamping of the processes by which work is accomplished, and job redesign, which entails changing who will do what, where, and for how long (Curtin, 1994). More than 75% of health care nurse executives report that they are involved in some form of organizational redesign, with more than 50% of the redesign efforts driven by the need to reduce costs (Gelinas & Boston, 1995).

Extent of organizational redesign has been categorized into first order and second order by Meyer, Goes, and Brooks (1993). Ingersoll (1996b) added an additional level, third order, when she reviewed the state of the science concerning organizational redesign and its effect on outcomes. First order redesign is associated with efforts directed at subsystems within an institution in which the overall organizational structure remains the same. Second order redesigns are those in which the fundamental properties or states of the organization are changed; third order redesigns involve interconnected, or integrated, health care systems.

Organizational redesign falls within the overarching framework of change, and a number of investigators prefer to use terminology associated with this model when describing and measuring what happens when organizations evolve. The benefit of the term *restructuring* is its focus, which implies planned, intended action; whereas change involves both intended and unintended activities. Although restructuring efforts invariably result in unanticipated outcomes and the need for revamping along the way, the intent is always deliberate; with change it is not. Nonetheless, some research relevant to organizational redesign has been conducted by using a change framework. Glick, Huber, Miller, Doty, and Sutcliffe (1990) conducted a study that focused on both "design (organizational redesign) change" and "nondesign (random, unanticipated) change." They were interested in the types of changes that occur in organizations, the antecedent conditions for change, its causes and its consequences, and how these varied according to organizational forms, contexts, and internal processes. Their overall goal was to build theories of change in organizational design that could be tested through empirical means.

The investigators of this study (Glick, Huber, Miller, Doty, & Sutcliffe, 1993) identified several issues of importance to researchers interested in organizational redesign. One relevant issue pertains to the identification of true causal determinants of organizational redesign, which is difficult because of the number of competing and overlapping events that often occur. Moreover, these determinants change over time and may play a more important role at one point or with one group of organizational and leadership characteristics and play a lesser role at another. In addition, data pertaining to what caused the redesign usually are gathered retrospectively and often require recollections by key players. These recollections may be influenced by a number of factors, including the individual's role and placement in the organization, the number of events that have occurred during the period of recollection, the number of changes occurring simultaneously that distract from the focus on the redesign (e.g., internal departmental restructuring while an overall organizational merger is occurring), and the social desirability of one antecedent over another. Although cost and external policy decisions routinely drive organizational restructuring efforts, common responses to questions about reasons for undertaking redesign initiatives pertain to the institution's desire for improved care delivery access or care delivery process. A focus on quality of care is much more socially acceptable to consumers than is a focus on cost reduction.

Glick et al. (1990) suggest that two approaches can be taken to address this problem. The first is to emphasize the context-dependent processes that contribute to the change; the second is to treat all causal explanations as probabilistic rather than deterministic. With the first approach, generalizability is limited. With the second, large samples are required to measure effect. Each of these approaches has its limitations and requires trade-off and consideration based on resources available and overall intent of the study.

An additional measurement issue common to organizational redesign is the difficulty associated with collecting true baseline, pre-redesign data. Because organizational redesign is fluid and may or may not have a clearly defined implementation date, collecting preintervention data may be impossible, particularly if some new measurement instrument will be used to measure change post-redesign. This issue reinforces the desirability of ongoing monitoring of organizational outcomes using reliable, valid indicators. Efforts to establish minimum data sets that track nursing indicators, patient outcomes, and organizational performance should partially alleviate this concern. Because this process is in its infancy, however, the problem is likely to continue for a number of years.

A third, serious issue with organizational redesign studies pertains to the quality of the research conducted in this field. Comprehensive, methodologically sound investigations of the effect of organizational redesign on anticipated outcomes are few. Moreover, the ones conducted thus far have been of an insufficient duration to adequately assess effect. Most postimplementation measurements have occurred within less than 1 year of redesign, and most have been collected at less than 6 months. Many reports of organizational redesigns include anecdotal statements about effect, and few contain sufficiently clear descriptions of the designs, methods, and instruments used to measure impact. Rarely is attention paid to confounding factors in the environment, such as characteristics of the work force, environment, or organization; and little effort is made to quantify the extent to which the intended redesign is implemented (Ingersoll, 1996). These limitations make analysis across studies difficult and seriously restrict the utility of the findings.

Future investigations of organizational redesign should focus on both the processes used to implement the redesigns and the outcomes they are expected to improve. Without an indication of what was done, as identified through the process component, no cause/effect determination can be made about the changes in outcomes. Studies also must control for confounding factors associated with the environments and individuals studied. Reliable, valid instruments developed according to some theoretic framework and used in more than one investigation are needed before any cross-comparison studies can be done. Even with the use of knowledge synthesis techniques for comparing outcomes of different studies, using different methods and measurement tools, the assumption in these approaches is that the instruments used to measure the effect are reliable and valid and the methods used to collect the data are reasonable for the phenomenon of interest.

Longitudinal studies are urgently needed, as are multisite studies using large data sets. This focus on large data sets should not consume researchers. The state of the science is such that small, well-done investigations using samples large enough to detect differences will be extremely helpful for extending theory and providing direction for other,

broader based investigations. Interdisciplinary efforts should be the standard rather than the exception in studies of organizational redesign. In light of nursing's integral role in health care delivery systems and organizations undergoing redesign, the need for nursing involvement and leadership in this field of research is paramount.

GAIL L. INGERSOLL

See also
EVALUATION
HEALTH SYSTEMS DELIVERY
ORGANIZATIONAL CULTURE
OUTCOMES MEASURES
QUALITY OF CARE, MEASURING

OSTEOARTHRITIS

Signs and Symptoms

Osteoarthritis, the most common of the rheumatic diseases, is characterized by progressive loss of articular cartilage and by reactive changes at the margins of the joints and in subchondral bone. Clinical features can include pain in the involved joint, which is typically worse with activity and relieved by rest; stiffness after periods of immobility; enlargement of the joint; instability; limitation of motion; and functional impairment. Depending on the absence or presence of an identifiable local or systemic etiological factor, osteoarthritis has been classified into idiopathic (primary) and secondary forms. Classification of the disease is based on various combinations of clinical, radiographic, and laboratory parameters (Schumacher, Kippel, & Koopman, 1993).

Epidemiology

The prevalence of osteoarthritis is strikingly correlated with age; it is uncommon in adults under 40, but it is the number-one chronic disease in late life, with more than 80% of those over the age of 75 being affected. Osteoarthritis is a major cause of disability in older adults, and knee osteoarthritis is more likely to result in disability than osteoarthritis of any other joint. However, the prevalence of osteoarthritis at all joint sites increases progressively with age, which is the most powerful risk factor for the disease. Women are about twice as likely as men to be affected, and African American women are twice as likely as Caucasian women to have knee osteoarthritis. The pattern of joint involvement also differs with sex: women have a greater number of joints involved and more frequent complaints of morning stiffness, joint swelling, and nocturnal pain. Factors that appear to be associated with osteoarthritis, based on cross-sectional and longitudinal studies, include obesity, bone density, trauma and repetitive stress, and genetic factors (Schumacher et al., 1993).

Impact of Osteoarthritis

The impact of osteoarthritis on function and costs of care are substantial. Patients with osteoarthritis are more likely to be limited in the amount and kind of major activities they can perform, have more restricted bed days, and are more likely to report disability. When disease prevalence figures were applied to estimates of health care utilization and disability for both rheumatoid arthritis and osteoarthritis, an aggregate economic impact some 30-fold greater was found for osteoarthritis than for rheumatoid arthritis (Kramer, Yellin, & Epstein, 1983). In addition to the functional disability and economic impact of osteoarthritis, older people with this disease experience an inordinate amount of suffering, depression, and diminished quality of life (Daltroy & Liang, 1993).

Treatment and Management

Treatment approaches to patients with osteoarthritis have been mainly pharmacological, usually combined with physical therapy and sometimes surgery. Although these interventions are useful, they often fail to control disease progression, and symptoms may be associated with high costs and many toxicities. In addition, they frequently fail to address important issues of patient concern, such as psychological stress, quality of life, and autonomy. Because of the chronicity of the disease, patients must learn to manage and cope with osteoarthritis on a day-to-day basis. The ability to succeed in this task differentiates those who are incapacitated from those who continue to lead full and active lives in the face of equal disease severity. For this reason, health education has a potentially important role.

One of the most common educational interventions used for chronic disease is self-management. Self-management has been described as the day-to-day tasks an individual must undertake to control or reduce the impact of disease on health status; it includes all the tasks for handling clinical aspects of the disease away from the hospital or physician's office. For persons with osteoarthritis this may include using medications, managing acute episodes and emergencies, maintaining adequate exercise and activity, using relaxation and stress-reducing techniques, seeking information, using community services, adapting to work, managing relations with significant others, and managing emotions and psychological responses to the illness. Studies of self-management programs for patients with osteoarthritis have shown that subjects gained an overall increase in knowledge, self-efficacy, management behaviors, functional ability, and overall health status. In addition, subjects showed an overall decrease in pain, depression, visits to physicians, and health care costs (Hawley, 1995).

Practice and Policy Implications for Nursing

The population is aging, and the number of aged is expected to increase from 33.2 million in 1994 (12% of the U.S. population) to 65 million (22%) in 2030. By the year 2020, this group will account for approximately half of the nation's health care expenditures (Feldstein, 1994). This "graying of America" and its concomitant increase in the prevalence of osteoarthritis poses problems for an ever spiraling health care budget. Incurable by definition, management of osteoarthritis extends over time, creating continuous costs to both patient and provider. It is important that we examine innovative ways to deliver high-quality care for older adults with osteoarthritis in as efficacious and economical a manner as possible. Advanced practice nurses are in a unique position to help patients with osteoarthritis adjust to living with this chronic disease by educating them in the use of self-management skills. The use of advanced practice nurses in various settings has been shown not only to improve patient outcomes but also to decrease costs (Brooten, Naylor, York, et al., 1995). Randomized controlled clinical trials of self-management programs conducted by advanced practice nurses are needed to provide documentation of quality and cost-conscious health care delivery for older patients with osteoarthritis.

CAROL E. BLIXEN

See also
CHRONIC ILLNESS
FUNCTIONAL HEALTH
GERIATRICS
QUALITY OF LIFE

OUTCOMES MEASURES

Outcomes of nursing and health care encompass changes in both client variables and organizational variables as a consequence of specific processes. Examples of client outcomes include satisfaction and preferences, disease- or problem-specific indicators, functional status, and quality of life. Examples of organizational outcomes include internal customer satisfaction (i.e., nurse or physician satisfaction), personnel safety (i.e., injuries from needles and other "sharps"), and cost-effectiveness. Client-focused variables that cross multiple diseases and conditions, such as mortality, nosocomial infections, falls, skin integrity, and medication errors, have been reported as both client and organizational outcomes.

The national thrust toward outcomes management and research emanates from studies of medical practice variation, which became a priority research agenda in the 1980s. Outcomes management is an ongoing, research-based quest to meet specified quality goals. Outcomes research seeks to deter-

mine whether specific interventions or practice models are beneficial in naturalistic environments. It is aimed at broad-based populations and includes service settings other than academic medical centers or large urban environments. In addition to randomized clinical trials, investigators attempt to link information about client outcomes with large administrative and clinical databases. Given an impetus to improve the outcomes of nursing care, investigators must solve various puzzles around appropriate target populations, the right outcome variables, and the associated process and structure variables.

Outcome measures incorporate intermediate clinical variables, such as blood pressure, as well as more extended outcomes, such as return to work. Researchers and managers are challenged to select or design outcome measures and establish their reliability and validity by issues related to sensitivity, specificity, situational contaminants such as severity of illness, and response set and other biases. Variations in definitions, formulas, and data collection procedures frustrate between-group comparisons, particularly for researchers who work with the large databases available from government agencies and organizations within the health care industry. Contextual factors influence client outcomes, including organization ownership (public/ private, profit/not for profit), involvement in teaching, case mix, volume of patients treated, organization size, and the extent to which the organization engages in high-tech procedures. Still to be determined is the impact on client outcomes of the integration of health care providers into complex networks.

Projects to develop standardized measures abound. For example, John Ware Jr. and colleagues (Medical Outcomes Trust, 1993) published the *SF-36 Health Survey*, which investigators are using with increasing frequency to assess health status and quality of life from the client's point of view. The SF-36 measures eight concepts: (a) limitations in physical activities because of health problems, (b) limitations in social activities because of physical or emotional problems, (c) limitations in usual role activities because of physical health problems, (d) psychological stress and well-being, (e) limitations in usual role activities because of emotional problems, (f) bodily pain, (g) vitality, and (h) general health perceptions.

Prominent among efforts to standardize measures for outcomes research is the ongoing project conducted by McCloskey and Bulechek (1996), Johnson and Maas (1997), and their colleagues at the University of Iowa College of Nursing to develop and maintain taxonomies of nursing interventions and outcomes. In a different arena, the Joint Commission on the Accreditation of Healthcare Organizations (1997) has initiated a program that will require organizations seeking accreditation to report patient outcomes. Under that program, *Oryx Outcomes: The Next Evolution in Accreditation*, hospitals choose two clinical performance indicators for reporting from among 60 measurement systems; the selected outcomes must relate to at least 20% of the hospital's patient population. The Agency for Health Care Policy and Research (AHCPR) and the president and fellows of Harvard College have released a computerized compendium of approximately 1,200 clinical performance measures developed by public and private sector organizations to examine the quality of health care. *CONQUEST 1.0* (*CO*mputerized *N*eeds-Oriented *Qual*ity *M*easurement *E*valuation *System*) can be accessed and downloaded from the AHCPR World Wide Web home page at (http://www.ahcpr.gov/).

ROMA LEE TAUNTON

See also
NURSING OCCUPATIONAL INJURY AND STRESS
NURSING OUTCOMES CLASSIFICATION (NOC)
PATIENT SATISFACTION WITH NURSING CARE
QUALITY MANAGEMENT
QUALITY OF CARE, MEASURING

P

PAIN IN CHILDREN

Definition

The definition of pain of the International Association for the Study of Pain (IASP; 1979) is widely accepted. "Pain is an unpleasant sensory and emotional experience associated with actual or potential tissue damage, or described in terms of such damage. . . . Pain is always subjective" (p. 250). For children, however, pain is often simply defined as "the hurt we feel." These perceptual approaches, although appropriate for verbal children, are insufficient for a great number of children who are unable to express their pain verbally. Included in this group are young children who lack adequate skills to convey their perception of hurting and older children who may be unable to vocalize their hurt. The reasons for inability to vocalize pain may be (a) medical status (e.g., children on respirators, the comatose child, or the child in severe pain), (b) cognitive impairments, (c) developmental delays, (d) cultural background (e.g., speaking another language or cultural constraints on expressing feelings of pain), and (e) personality factors (e.g., shyness or fear). A widely accepted definition for these children has yet to be generated.

Historical Perspectives

Nurse researchers pioneered pain research in children in the 1970s. Eland and Anderson (1977) exposed several myths regarding children and pain, documented the undertreatment of pain in children, and developed the Eland Color Tool. Hester (1979) developed the Poker Chip Tool and the Behavioral Observations of Pain Scale for measuring pain in children. Savedra (1976) identified pain as a major component of burn care in children. These researchers still continue their work, addressing the ongoing issue of undertreatment of children's pain.

In the 1980s the cadre of nurse researchers increased, including other names commonly found in the literature, such as Abu-Saad, Beyer, Broome, Denyes, Foster, Fowler-Kerry, Fuller, Gedaly-Duff, Grunau, Johnston, Stevens, Tesler, VanCleve, Villarruel, and Wong. Researchers (primarily anesthesiologists and psychologists) from other disciplines also began to contribute to the field. By the end of the 1980s, research was focused on multiple aspects of pain, including the development of numerous measurement approaches, descriptions of children's experience with pain, use of pharmacological and nonpharmacological approaches for management of pain, exploration of the safety and appropriateness of high-tech devices for administration of medications to children, and description of provider knowledge, attitudes, and practices concerning pain. During this decade, the first international research conference on children's pain was held.

In the 1990s the pain research community continued to expand, focusing on the themes of the 1980s and emergent areas such as quality assurance and models for changing clinical practice. Unfortunately, research still tends to be discipline- or specialty-specific rather than interdisciplinary. In 1990 the Agency for Health Care Policy and Research established an interdisciplinary panel to develop clinical practice guidelines for pain. This panel affirmed an interdisciplinary perspective of pain in their documents on acute pain (Acute Pain Management Panel, 1992) and cancer pain (Management of Cancer Pain Panel, 1994). Both of these documents include research-based clinical practice guidelines for children. In 1997 the fourth international research conference on children's pain was held.

Future Directions

Research on children's pain is in its infancy. There are many aspects of pain that have been inade-

quately addressed or not addressed at all. Only one area has been deemed sufficiently addressed, and that is the development of measurement tools for verbal children. In 1994 the National Institute of Nursing Research published a national research agenda for pain. The agenda for pain in children includes topics such as (a) exploring the consequences of invasive procedures on neural pathways; (b) developing appropriate tools to measure different types of pain; (c) specifying pain needs of children with special needs, such as those with disorders of sensory mechanisms and those who have been abused; (d) examining the roles and effectiveness of parents and other family members in caring for children with pain; (e) examining the link between physiological indicators of pain and behavioral and self-report responses; and (f) examining the synergistic effect of nonpharmacological strategies when used in conjunction with each other or with pharmacological strategies for managing pain.

Several of the research agenda recommendations concern the delivery of care. Examples include (a) examining attitudes and decision-making processes related to safe and effective analgesic management, (b) determining the effects of informal unit standards that guide pain management on clinical units, and (c) evaluating the effectiveness of pain management services on patient outcomes, satisfaction with care, and cost. An area not addressed by either the Agency for Health Care Policy and Research clinical practice guidelines or the National Institutes of Nursing Research agenda is chronic nonmalignant pain in children. Although there is some research in this area, little of it has been conducted by nurses. Hence, this must be an agenda for the future. Research methodologies to address these agenda recommendations may include traditional experimental and correlational research methodologies, qualitative approaches, and the combinations of various approaches. In addition to traditional methods of data collection, databases will become a common source for information. Research designs need to allow for more complexity, and use multiple units of analysis with quantitative and qualitative data. Models for analyses will need to address the complexity of these designs. They will need to facilitate the integration of findings across types of data, levels of units of analyses, and studies. Further, designs that preserve appropriate controls while enhancing generalizability are needed to facilitate more rapid linkage of research to clinical practice.

Relationship of Research to Nursing Practice

Research on children's pain should be informing nursing practice. There is, however, a great time lag between the availability of the research findings and integration into practice. For example, the first self-report tools for measuring pain in children were developed in the mid 1970s. For the most part, measurement of pain has yet to be satisfactorily integrated into nursing practice. A plausible explanation for this time lag is that research on pain in children has not been adequately integrated into nursing curricula or into continuing education programs. Hence, nurses receive inadequate education on one of the most common symptoms experienced by children. Further, most health institutions do not prioritize pain as an important aspect of care. To date, researchers have primarily emphasized the ethical perspective and humanistic value of pain treatment. Coupling the ethical perspective and the humanistic value with the economic value of pain care is a pressing challenge for researchers who wish to impact the care of children with pain.

NANCY OLSON HESTER

See also
> ADOLESCENCE
> CANCER IN CHILDREN
> CHRONIC CONDITIONS IN CHILDHOOD
> PAIN MANAGEMENT
> PSYCHOSOCIAL EFFECTS OF CHILD
>   CRITICAL ILLNESS AND HOSPITAL-
>   IZATION

PAIN MANAGEMENT

Pain is "an unpleasant sensory and emotional experience associated with actual or potential damage or described in terms of such damage" (International Association for the Study of Pain, 1986, p. 249).

This definition includes pain of pathophysiological and psychological origin. *Pain management* refers to the care and treatment of the pain. Pain is a common accompaniment of disease and illness and is the most common reason that people seek medical attention. It is the nursing diagnosis most frequently identified by nurses.

Pain generally is classified into two types: acute and chronic, with chronic further differentiated into pain associated with malignancy and pain not associated with malignancy. Acute pain subsides as healing takes place; it has a predictable end and is of brief duration, usually less than 6 months. Chronic pain most commonly is said to be that which lasts for longer than 6 months, although Bonica (1990) suggested that chronic pain is "pain that persists a month beyond the usual course of an acute disease or reasonable time for an injury to heal or that is associated with a chronic pathologic process that causes continuous pain or the pain recurs at intervals for months or years" (p. 19).

The undertreatment of pain has been well documented for at least the past 25 years (Marks & Sachar, 1973). Recent studies (Bookbinder, Coyle, & Thaler, in press; Miaskowski, Nichols, Brody, & Synold, 1994; Ward & Gordon, 1994) show that average present pain scores for hospitalized patients range from 3.6 to 4.3 (on a 0–10 scale), and worst pain in the past 24 hours scores range from 6.6 to 7.8. The undermanagement of pain has been particularly pronounced in children and in the elderly. Barriers to the effective treatment of pain include clinicians' lack of knowledge of pain management principles, clinician and patient attitudes toward pain and drugs, and overly restrictive laws and regulations regarding use of controlled substances.

The gate control theory published by Melzack and Wall (1965) provided a theoretical basis for showing how pain, transmitted peripherally to the brain, can be influenced by cognitive and affective as well as physiological factors. An understanding of the mind-body relationship exemplified in the experience of pain provides a basis for many of the strategies used to manage pain.

Nociception is the body's reaction to a noxious stimulus; pain describes the person's perception of that event. Tissue damage causes the release of pain-producing substances, such as serotonin, histamine, and bradykinin, which stimulate nerve endings called nociceptors. Nociception leads from the peripheral nervous system through the spinal cord to the central nervous system. Nerve fibers descending from the brain to the spinal cord can inhibit the perception of pain. Opiate receptors on the brain or spinal cord react both to opiates that are externally administered and to enkephalins and endorphins produced by one's own body to modulate pain.

Pain management includes pharmacological, cognitive-behavioral, physical, radiation, anesthetic, neurosurgical, and surgical techniques. Depending on the cause of the pain, one or more strategies may be used. Most pain can be managed by the use of analgesics administered orally or intravenously and by simple cognitive-behavioral techniques such as relaxation and distraction. More complex pain, such as that experienced by patients with reflex sympathetic distrophy or by cancer patients who have unrelieved pain from several origins, may require evaluation and treatment by a multispecialty pain management team. The successful management of pain depends on a careful assessment of the pain, including reassessment to determine the effectiveness of interventions used.

Pharmacological management of pain usually is treated by three types of drug: (a) aspirin, acetaminophen, and nonsteroidal anti-inflammatory drugs (NSAIDS); (b) opioids; and (c) adjuvant analgesics. Nonsteroidal anti-inflammatory drugs decrease the levels of inflammatory mediators generated at the site of tissue injury, thus blocking painful stimuli. They are useful in the management of mild pain and may be used in combination with opioids for moderate to severe pain. Opioids are morphinelike compounds that produce pain relief by binding to opiate receptors. They are used with moderate and severe pain and can be administered orally, subcutaneously, intramuscularly, intravenously, rectally, transdermally, epidurally, nasally, intraspinally, and intraventricularly. Patient-controlled analgesia (PCA) can be accomplished by mouth or by use of a special pump set to prescribed parameters to administer a drug intravenously, subcutaneously, or epidurally. Adjuvant drugs are used to increase the analgesic efficacy of opioids, to treat other symptoms that exacerbate pain, or to provide analgesia for specific types of pain (Jacox et al., 1994).

Physical modalities for pain management include use of heat and cold, counterstimulation such as transcutaneous electrical nerve stimulation (TENS), and acupuncture. Cognitive techniques are focused on perception and thought and are designed to influence interpretation of events and bodily sensations. Providing information about pain and its management and helping patients think differently about pain are examples of cognitive techniques. Behavioral techniques are directed at helping patients develop coping skills and modify their reactions to pain. Cognitive-behavioral techniques commonly used by nurses and other clinicians include relaxation, imagery, distraction, and reframing. Psychotherapy, structured support, and hypnosis also have been used successfully in pain management.

When the use of drugs, with or without physical and cognitive behavioral modalities, is not adequate to manage pain, other management techniques may be used. These depend on the cause of the pain and may be temporary or permanent. Radiation therapy is used to relieve metastatic pain and symptoms from local extension of primary disease. Nerve blocks include the injection of a local anesthetic into a spinal space and peripheral nerve destruction. Surgical procedures are used to remove sources of pain, such as debulking a tumor that is pressing on abdominal organs or removing bone spurs that are compressing nerves. Neuroablation techniques include peripheral neurectomy, dorsal rhizotomy, cordotomy, commissural myelotomy, and hypophysectomy.

It is difficult to know how frequently each of the above management strategies is used. Estimates of their frequency in the management of cancer pain are as follows: oral, transdermal and rectal drugs, 75% to 85% of patients; intravenous and subcutaneous drugs, 5% to 20%; epidural and intrathecal, 2% to 6%; and nerve blocks, palliative surgery, and ablative surgery, 1% to 5% (Jacox et al., 1994).

During the past 10 years, various agencies and organizations have published guidelines for the management of pain. These have included the American Pain Society's (1995) principles of analgesic use in acute and cancer pain and the Agency for Health Care Policy and Research guidelines for the management of acute pain, cancer pain, and low back problems (Bigos et al., 1994; Carr et al., 1992; Jacox et al., 1994). In addition to these, the American Pain Society Quality of Care Committee (1995) published guidelines for using quality improvement mechanisms in institutions to improve the management of acute and cancer pain. There is greater consensus regarding how to manage acute and cancer pain than for chronic nonmalignant pain.

ADA JACOX

See also
CHRONIC ILLNESS
HOSPICE
NONTRADITIONAL THERAPIES
PAIN IN CHILDREN
RADIATION THERAPY

PARENT-ADOLESCENT RELATIONSHIPS AND COMMUNICATION

Communication is defined as the expression of ideas and feelings assertively but unoffensively and the receiving of ideas expressed by others attentively and accurately. Among humans, communication is the cornerstone of interpersonal relationships. Aspects of adolescent and middle adult social, emotional, and physical development may alter the topics, styles, and perceptions of communication and influence the parent-adolescent relationship.

Nursing has not contributed in a significant way to knowledge development in parent-adolescent communication. However, several nurse researchers have conducted studies in the area, specifically, Brage, Lynam, Riesch, and Tenn. The disciplines of psychology, social psychology, and communications contribute significantly toward knowledge development. Investigative teams are led by Brooks-Gunn, Conger, Forehand, Olson, Robin, and Steinberg. Because of nursing's commitment to the provision of care that promotes well-being in indi-

viduals and families, particularly those undergoing life transitions, it is an area of importance.

Theoretical Context

Early studies were based on a stress-and-storm view of adolescence (Blos, 1979). The adolescent was expected to be impulsive, moody, influenced by peers, resistant to authority, and belligerent. Issues of power, sexuality, identity, and independence were thought to be hallmarks of this transitional period. There is little empirical evidence, however, to support this view, and it may have gained recognition from the generalization of findings of studies of troubled adolescents to all adolescents.

In the next phase of studies, investigators (Steinberg & Silverberg, 1986) identified adolescents' major issues as autonomy seeking and self-governance. Power struggles were diminished with appropriate family and community environments and boundaries. Researchers documented that adolescents sought parents' advice and support and desired a close, positive relationship, including participation in family activities.

Recent studies are framed with a view that parents and adolescents are active relational partners who embrace similar values and together negotiate and renegotiate new roles with regard to autonomy and individuation while remaining connected (Hill, 1987). Theoretically, communication that is perceived as open within this evolving relationship contributes to discussion of issues essential to identity formation, achievement of intimacy, and a stable sense of self.

Developmental Outcomes

Research demonstrates that communication perceived as open and allowing for the resolution of conflict is linked to positive adolescent outcomes, such as (a) improved decision-making skill and self-esteem, autonomy achievement, school achievement, ability to resolve difficult life issues, beliefs and intentions regarding condom use, sex education in the home, and knowledge on HIV/AIDS and (b) decreased loneliness and depression, substance abuse, and sexual experimentation and pregnancy. Alternatively, research demonstrates that negative adolescent outcomes such as drug and alcohol use, delinquency, suicide, and dropping out of school and running away are associated with communication perceived as closed or problematic (Olson, 1995).

Family Characteristics Influencing Communication

Cumulative evidence indicates that the relationship between the parents is fundamental to and reflected in the parent-adolescent relationship. Adolescents are accurate in their assessment of their parents' marital relationship. Discord between parents and coalitions among family members have potentially detrimental effects on child development that may be buffered if the parent(s) maintains a strong relationship with the adolescent (Hill, 1987).

The greater the education level and the higher the self-esteem of the parent, the more likely the perception that communication is open. Parental substance use is associated with poor problem solving between parent and adolescent. Financial difficulties affect the parents' emotional state and the quality of family interactions. Some effects attributed to economic hardship include increased alcohol use, emotional and behavioral problems, reduced social and academic competence, and diminished sense of self among adolescents. Extended family responsibilities, particularly among mothers, contribute to perceptions of poor communication.

Mothers tend to take on larger and wider-ranging roles in communicating with the adolescent than do fathers, and parents find communication with daughters to be more open and calmer than communication with their sons. Generally, mothers discuss socioemotional topics and sexuality and use self-disclosing techniques, whereas fathers discuss politics and engage in problem solving. Adolescents report that intimacy (defined as emotional closeness, affection, enjoyment, solidarity) was more likely with mothers than with fathers, but intimacy with fathers is an important predictor of adolescent functioning.

Studies of Parent-Adolescent Conflict

A predominant view of conflict is that it is inevitable and manageable and that families who communicate well do so noisily! Most conflicts occur around mundane topics, such as helping out around the house, sibling relationships, and doing chores or homework. Older adolescents, though, report family relations, career/education, living circumstances, and money/material items as sources of conflict. Parents generally perceive their role as guiding their adolescents toward societal conventions of behavior, whereas teenagers perceive their role as exploring and testing conventions of behavior.

Two salient areas of research on parent-adolescent conflict are (a) defining when conflict is problematic, requiring therapeutic intervention, and (b) testing of conflict resolution strategies. Conflict is considered problematic when it is perceived as too intense, too frequent, and too long-lasting, leading to aggression and disturbing personal functioning or relationships. Effective conflict resolution strategies usually include several steps, such as defining the problem, listing possible solutions, testing solutions, and evaluating the outcome. A number of coding schemes have been developed to reliably and validly measure parents' and adolescents' skills at conflict resolution (Robin & Koepke, 1990).

Promoting Parent-Adolescent Communication

Adolescents cite not being listened to as the major communication problem between themselves and their parents. Interventions to promote communication among parents and teenagers are available. They are (a) community based and delivered over a number of weeks, (b) targeted toward both the parent and the adolescent to emphasize the bidirectional aspects of the relationship, and (c) based on a number of concepts, including social learning, growth and development, problem solving, and family (Riesch et al., 1993). To measure communication effectively and thoroughly, both self-report and observational methods are employed. Significant outcomes include improved family satisfaction and skill in conflict resolution, increased perceived openness of communication, better social skills, improved decision making, and increased empathy.

Methods

Most studies use cross-sectional, quasi-experimental approaches. Randomization is difficult to achieve, leading a number of investigators to suggest randomizing entire schools or using wait list control strategies. Samples tend to be homogeneous, small, and confined to single ethnic groups. Participation in studies by families usually involves extensive commitment of time and effort. Variable measurement often involves technological strategies, a number of scales and tasks, and multiple data collection points, which may include visits to laboratories by families or visits to homes by investigative teams. Training research staff in the methods and maintenance of reliability and validity is expensive.

Future Directions

The major function left to the postmodern family is the care and nurturance of its members, accomplished chiefly through the emotional climate of the family based on communication among its members. Preparation for childbirth has demonstrated impressive outcomes and has become commonplace. Preparing for birthing an adult through communication skills training for families about to launch into adolescence is an inexpensive, nonintrusive strategy for families with children in middle school. Greater involvement of fathers in research, addressing the reciprocal nature of communication re fully, and more attention to adolescents, particularly from minority ethnic groups, as they negotiate situations of divorce, single parenting, and other significant life events merits consideration.

SUSAN K. RIESCH

See also
FAMILY THEORY AND RESEARCH
MATERNAL EMPLOYMENT
PARENTING RESEARCH IN NURSING

PARENTAL RESPONSE TO THE NEONATAL INTENSIVE CARE UNIT

Nurses involved in care of high-risk infants in *neonatal intensive care units* (NICUs) have long been concerned about the needs of parents. It has been recognized that parents play an important role in the lives of their infants both during hospitalization and after discharge. The recent emphasis on family-centered care in the NICU is a direct result of these concerns about parents.

Thus, a major focus of research in maternal-child nursing has been on parents of preterm infants. Research focused on the emotional responses of parents to the NICU was heavily influenced by the work of Caplan, who hypothesized in the 1960s that the birth and hospitalization of a preterm infant may constitute an emotional crisis for parents (Caplan, Mason, & Kaplan, 1965). It was also influenced by research conducted in other disciplines, such as medicine and psychology, that in the 1960s and 1970s were concerned about the possible deleterious effects of the birth and hospitalization of a preterm infant on parenting (Miles & Holditch-Davis, 1997). A major concern of researchers during this era and up to the present is the impact on parents of anticipatory grieving for a child who might die, the long separation from the infant, and the subsequent delayed opportunities to parent. Reflecting these concerns, nursing research related to parental responses to the NICU has focused on two broad areas: (a) the emotional responses of parents and (b) the sources of stress experienced by parents whose infants are hospitalized in the NICU. In addition, there is a small body of research related to social support as a mediator of parental responses.

Brooten, Gennaro, Brown, and their colleagues (1988) have reported extensively on the emotional responses of preterm mothers, particularly those of anxiety and depression, and Miles and her colleagues (Miles, Funk, & Kasper, 1992) have studied anxiety. Other emotional responses identified in small descriptive studies include shock, guilt, fear, sadness, disappointment, failure, helplessness, and detachment. A small group of researchers have viewed the experience of parents as a grief response. In general, the research on parental emotional responses suggests that parents, particularly mothers, have intense emotional responses to the birth and hospitalization of their prematurely born infant. The findings are inconclusive, however, regarding the level and type of emotional responses or the long-term implications of this distress (Miles & Holditch-Davis, 1997).

Another major focus of research has been on identifying the sources and amount of stress experienced by parents related to the hospitalization of their infant in an NICU. This work was facilitated greatly by the development of the Parental Stressor Scale: Neonatal Intensive Care Unit (PSS: NICU), designed to assess parental perception of stressors in the NICU (Miles, Funk, & Carlson, 1993). Using the PSS: NICU tool, Miles and colleagues (Miles, Funk, & Kasper, 1992) completed two studies of parent stress in an NICU. The appearance and behavior of the infant and the changes in the parental role were found to be the highest sources of stress. Parental role alterations included (a) separation; (b) feeling helpless in not being able to protect, help, and hold the baby; and (c) fear of holding the baby. Aspects of the infant's appearance that were most stressful included seeing the child in pain or experiencing apnea; perceiving that the child looked frightened or sad; observing the small size and limp, weak appearance of the infant; seeing needles and tubes put into the child; and watching the respirator breathe for the child.

Mothers reported more stress than fathers, particularly in regard to parental role changes. Parents also reported high uncertainty regarding their infant's health outcomes, particularly unpredictability, with mothers having higher scores than fathers. Parental perceptions of stress related to the NICU admission was significantly correlated with parental anxiety. Similar findings have been made by other researchers using the PSS: NICU tool and other approaches.

Findings from this body of research indicate that parents experience stress related to changes in the expected and desired parental role with the infant and to the appearance and behavior of the premature infant. It is unclear whether parents experience stress related to staff relationships and, if so, the specific sources of this stress. Current approaches to studying staff-parent interactions may be inadequate, as parents may have difficulty evaluating

staff while the infant is still dependent on the staff's care. Small retrospective descriptive studies suggest that parents may experience stress related to their interactions with nurses.

A small cadre of nurse researchers has focused on the amount and sources of social support received by these parents. Findings indicate that support from family and friends is important, but support from the NICU nurses is highly valued and influential in parents' overall response and adjustment. Much of this research was retrospective and descriptive, and almost all of the studies included only mothers. Thus, there is a need for more research related to social support, particularly its link to parental emotional responses and parenting of the infant.

In conclusion, nurse researchers have made contributions to the study of parental responses to preterm birth and NICU hospitalization of a preterm infant. This research has undoubtedly influenced nursing interventions with parents. NICUs generally have open visiting hours, recognize the important role of parents, and facilitate the development of the parental role even while the infant is critically ill. Still, the amount of research does not parallel the intense clinical interest and concern of staff in helping parents during this crisis and the quality of the research is variable.

Most of the research in this area is descriptive, sample sizes are small, and many studies are retrospective. As preterm infants often experience long hospitalizations and the assumption and attainment of the parental role with newborn infants is known to be a process that occurs over time, it is essential that we study parental responses over time to really understand the process and outcomes of this experience. Likewise, we must link parents and the infants conceptually or methodologically in the design of these studies in order to understand how parental emotional distress and other responses influence parenting behaviors in the critical care period and parenting and the parent-child relationship and interactions during childhood. Although there is another body of literature related to parent-infant interaction within the NICU (Holditch-Davis & Miles, 1997), this research is rarely linked to parental emotional responses.

There also is a need to study the interplay between the nurses and parents as they assume caregiving responsibility for the sick infant, and attention should be focused on critical decision making by parents and the link between decision making and parental responses. More information is needed on the response of fathers and on the unique and differing responses of parents from ethnic minority and low-income groups. Finally, research should focus on interventions aimed at reducing the distress of parents and enhancing the parental role with the infant.

The preparation of this article was supported in part by grants from the National Institute of Nursing Research, National Institutes of Health: Grant No. R01 NR02868—Parenting The Medically Fragile Child.

MARGARET SHANDOR MILES

See also
**MOTHER-INFANT/TODDLER RELA-
   TIONSHIPS
NICU PRETERM INFANT CARE
PARENTING RESEARCH IN NURSING
POSTPARTUM CARE: DEPRESSION
SOCIAL SUPPORT**

PARENTING RESEARCH
IN NURSING

Parenting has always been a major focus for nurses interested in child health, family, women's health, and community nursing. Currently, two parenting diagnoses are in the nursing diagnosis literature: altered parenting, which involves at-risk or problematic parenting, and parental role conflict, which describes the altered roles of parents when a child is ill (Kim, McFarland, & McLane, 1995). The diagnosis of altered parenting implies that parenting involves promoting the optimal growth and development of another human being. Parental role conflict suggests that parenting an ill child involves providing illness-related care, comforting and helping the child, teaching the child, and stimulating the child's growth and development in special ways because of the illness.

Recently, Miles, D'Auria, and Avant (1997), in their model of parental responsibility, described parenting as a process that involves a complex set of activities or responsibilities. These responsibilities include being present for the child, caregiving, teaching, protecting and encouraging the child, and advocating on behalf of the child. These parental responsibilities evolve over time and change as the child and parent mature. This occurs not only in response to the child's changing developmental needs but also in response to the context within which one parents a child, to the special needs of a child, and to the developing maturity of the parent.

An identifiable community of nurse researchers who study parents and parenting has emerged in the nursing research literature (Barnard, 1983; Holditch-Davis & Miles, 1997; Mercer, 1995). Nurse researchers share an interest in the phenomenon of parenting with researchers from a variety of disciplines who agree that parenting plays a critical role in the development of children (Bornstein, 1995).

The substantive focus of research on parenting in nursing is diverse and broad. Nursing research has focused on parental attachment, interactions and relationships, the impact of parenting on the child's health and development, and parental responses and needs in normal and at-risk situations.

The area that has probably received the most attention by nurse researchers is the parenting of infants during the transition to parenthood. This involves research focused on maternal identity and competence, adjustments to parenting a newborn infant, parent-infant interaction, and the effects of stressors such as an infertility or high-risk pregnancy. Although researchers are beginning to focus on fathers during this transition period, most of the studies have focused on mothers. A number of researchers have also studied the development of the parental identity during pregnancy by exploring concepts such as maternal identity, maternal-fetal attachment, and the emotional tasks of pregnancy.

A related area of research focuses on parents of prematurely born children. A number of descriptive studies have explored the emotional distress and the sources of stress experienced by parents during the infant's hospitalization in the neonatal intensive care unit. Of particular concern is the impact of parental distress and parent-infant separation on subsequent parent-child interactions and attachment. An important line of research has attempted to identify parental influences on child development in this at-risk population by longitudinally studying the relationship of parenting behaviors and the social environment provided by parents to child outcomes. Even though the situation for parents is similar, less research has focused on parents of infants with birth defects and other serious chronic conditions diagnosed at birth.

A number of researchers have focused on parents of older children with chronic illness and developmental delays. Although much of this research concentrated on the family, parents were identified as the most important element in family responses. Other studies have targeted the impact of the child's diagnosis and the stressors associated with treatments, surgery, and repeated hospitalizations on parents. Similarly, researchers have focused on responses and experiences of parents when a child is acutely ill. This research has included identifying the emotional responses of parents, parental participation in care, and parental stress during hospitalization, particularly in the ICU environment. Research with parents of acutely and chronically ill children has largely been limited to descriptive, cross-sectional studies done with small convenience samples of parents in one institution. There are no multisite studies, and few studies are longitudinal even within the period of hospitalization. There is a need for research that examines the impact of acute and chronic illness on the parent-child relationship and on parenting behaviors. Research on the influence of parenting on child health and developmental outcomes in this population is also needed.

There is a small but important body of knowledge about parents' relationships with nurses and other health care providers. This research is highly descriptive with small samples but stresses the powerful role nurses have in helping or hindering parents' responses and the development or maintenance of the parental role during an acute illness crisis. Very little research has focused on the nurse-parent relationship when a child has a chronic health problem. More research is needed to explore the nature of the interaction of health care providers and parents and how to strengthen those interactions. More knowledge should be obtained about what nurses can do to help parents with parenting in a variety of settings and situations.

A number of nurse researchers have studied parenting of normal, healthy children. Preschool children have been studied the most, with limited attention to parenting the school-aged, adolescent, and young adult child. Much of this research investigated parental perceptions of the child rather than parenting per se. The effects of stressors, such as maternal employment, and supports for parenting also have been examined. Some of this research has focused on issues of parenting after divorce or after the death of a spouse. In addition, researchers have begun to study ethnic differences in parenting

Problematic parenting has been another focus of research. This includes studies exploring the impact of maternal depression on parenting and studies of parents who are involved in physical and sexual abuse of their children. Both areas of study target very high risk groups, and further research is needed to develop and test interventions with these parents.

Several newer areas of research include studies of the relationship between parents and their adult children and research related to caregiving of parents by adult children. However, few authors have studied parenting as an adult developmental stage. We need to know more about how parenting affects adult development and particularly about how the diagnosis of acute or chronic illness in a child affects parental development.

Intervention studies have been conducted to improve parenting in a variety of at-risk groups, including parents of prematurely born children, teenage parents, and low-income parents. Many of these interventions are atheoretical. More theoretically based intervention studies aimed at improving parenting and removing situational or environmental obstacles to positive parenting are needed.

The theoretical models used as frameworks for nursing research on parenting are as diverse as the substantive foci. Researchers interested in the transition to parenthood often build on the concepts put forth by Rubin and adapted by Mercer and Walker: the emotional tasks of pregnancy, maternal identity, and maternal role development. These concepts have their bases in role attainment theory from sociology.

Another theoretical framework commonly used by nurse researchers interested in parenting is ecological systems theory, based in psychology and influenced by the work of Bronfenbrenner, Belsky, and Sameroff. This framework is used frequently by nurse researchers in the area of parenting infants. Within nursing, Barnard's theory follows in this tradition.

Other theories used in parenting research by nurses include attachment, cognitive, and stress theories. Attachment theory with has origins in ethology and is influenced by the work of Bowlby and Ainsworth. This framework is widely used in infancy and preschool parenting research. Cognitively based theories of parenting, developed by Pridham and Rubin, are used as the bases for studies of mothering during the prenatal and postpartal periods. Finally, stress models, influenced by Lazarus and his colleague Selye, have been used in research on the impact of acute illness on parents.

Despite this theoretical diversity, much of the research conducted by nurse researchers in the area of parenting is atheoretical and highly descriptive. Therefore, the findings in this area of research are fragmented, and nurse researchers often are not building a coherent body of science on parenting.

The major gaps in the parenting literature in nursing include a need for more information about fathering in all populations, including children with health problems. More emphasis should be placed on parenting during adolescent and young adult years. There is also a need for research that examines parenting from a cultural perspective. Nursing researchers must go beyond comparing and contrasting ethnic groups and move toward understanding what is effective and adaptive for parents from varying ethnic backgrounds. Identifying the unique needs of parents from differing ethnic groups in specific situations is also important. Likewise, nurse researchers, using longitudinal designs, should conduct more studies on parenting as a process that unfolds over time.

DIANE HOLDITCH-DAVIS
MARGARET SHANDOR MILES

See also
   **CHRONIC CONDITIONS IN CHILD-
     HOOD
   MATERNAL EMPLOYMENT
   PARENT-ADOLESCENT RELATION-
     SHIPS/COMMUNICATION**

**PARENTAL RESPONSE TO THE NEONA-
   TAL INTENSIVE CARE UNIT
TRANSITIONAL CARE**

PARSE'S THEORY OF NURSING: HUMAN BECOMING THEORY

Human becoming theory (Parse, 1992, 1995) was first entitled *Man-Living-Health: A Theory of Nursing* (Parse, 1981). The theory evolved from Parse's concern about the use of the medical model applied to the nursing discipline. Parse was dissatisfied with the mechanistic view of human beings and its lack of congruence with the focus and goals of nursing. The human becoming theory describes a theory of nursing that views the mysteries and uniqueness of humans as unitary beings in mutual process with a multidimensional universe. Human becoming is viewed as an evolving journey that is the co-created reality of an individual's lived experience. Knowledge of being is acquired through paradoxical processes that create an evolutionary, dialectic experience. The experience of the now includes what was, is, and will be all at once (Parse, 1997). The central ethic of the theory is to preserve the dignity of human beings by revering each person's perspective on quality of life. The uniqueness of the discipline within the context of human becoming theory is nursing's contribution to the quality of life of humankind. The focus of knowledge development for the discipline are universal lived experiences of all people, such as hope, joy-sorrow, grieving and persevering.

Humans are described as unitary living beings who have the freedom to choose their way of living and becoming (Daley, Mitchell, & Jonas-Simpson, 1996). One recognizes human beings by their unique patterns of relating (Daley et al., 1996; Parse, 1981, 1992). Each person co-creates reality in mutual process with the environment and therefore has a unique perspective on quality of life. Quality of life is health, and health is a manifestation of human becoming. The goal of nursing is to co-create an individual's becoming through a person-centered focus that affirms the person's capacity to know the way to live in health situations (Daley et al., 1996).

Human becoming theory is guided by nine philosophical assumptions about human beings and becoming that were synthesized from Rogers's Science of Unitary Human Beings and the writings on existential phenomenology by Heidegger, Merleau-Ponty, and Sartre. There are five assumptions about human beings:

1. Human beings coexist with the universe and simultaneously create evolving, rhythmical patterns.
2. Humans are open and have the capacity to freely choose the meaning of an experience.
3. Human beings are responsible for their decisions.
4. Humans are unitary beings who continually coconstruct their respective patterns of relating with the universe.
5. Human beings are capable of multidimensional transcendence as they evolve toward the possibles, what was, is, and will be.

Becoming is "unitary human living health; a rhythmically coconstituting human-universe process; the human's patterns of relating value priorities; an intersubjective process of transcending with the possibles; unitary human evolving" (Parse, 1997, p. 32).

In addition, three assumptions about human becoming were derived from the original nine assumptions. The assumptions are that human becoming is "freely choosing personal meaning in situation in the intersubjective process of relating value priorities; cocreating rhythmical patterns of relating in mutual process with the universe; and cotranscending multidimensionality with the emerging possibles" (Parse, 1997, p. 33). One can clearly identify the three themes in these assumptions, which are threads interwoven in the theoretical principles of human becoming. The themes include meaning, rhythmicity, and transcendence.

Three principles about human becoming constitute the theoretical structure. Principle 1 states "structuring meaning multi dimensionally is cocreating reality through the languaging of valuing and imaging" (Parse, 1981, p. 69). The major conceptual processes of this principle are imagining, valuing, and languaging (Parse, 1987). The para-

doxes inherent in Principle 1 are explicit-tacit knowing, confirming–not confirming, speaking–being silent, and moving–not moving (Parse, 1996). Principle 2 is that "cocreating rhythmical patterns of relating is living the paradoxical unity of revealing-concealing and enabling-limiting while connecting-separating" (Parse, 1981, p. 69). There are three paradoxes relevant to this principle: revealing-concealing, enabling-limiting, and connecting-separating (Parse, 1996). Principle 3 states that "cotranscending with the possibles is powering unique ways of originating in the process of transforming" (Parse, 1981, p. 69). The key conceptual processes for this principle are powering, originating, and transforming (Parse, 1987). The paradoxes include pushing-resisting, certainty-uncertainty, and familiar-unfamiliar (Parse, 1996).

Parse has developed a specific research methodology based on human becoming theory and phenomenological hermeneutic methods. It is a qualitative method that focuses on knowledge of universal human health experiences that emerge from the mutual human-universe process. The method focuses on four processes: participant selection, dialogical engagement (researcher-participant), extraction-synthesis (dwelling with the data), and heuristic interpretation (Parse, 1997). The method has been used, for example, to develop knowledge of the lived experiences of aging, AIDS, grieving, homelessness, recovery from addiction, suffering, and laughter. Several doctoral dissertations have been completed using the theory and research method. Currently, Parse is leading a multinational research project on the lived experience of hope in eleven countries (see Parse, 1997, for specific study references).

In addition, Parse (1996, 1997) has delineated a practice method that guides the practice of nurses who are living the human becoming theory and implementing the theory in practice settings. Three dimensions and three respective processes guide nurses in their commitment to a person's personal perspective of quality of life and knowledge of ways of health. The nurse lives human becoming through use of the dimensions and processes as the nurse engages and is engaged by the person. The artistic medium employed by the nurse is described as true presence, the basis of nursing practice. True presence is the "subject to subject interrelationship with the other to enhance quality of life" (Parse, 1987, p. 169). The nurse approaches engagement with the person by preparing and centering for the intention of "coming to be present," "being with," and listening (Parse, 1997). The nurse explicates meaning that is manifest through languaging, dwells with the other in the paradox of connecting-separating, and mobilizes transcending movement beyond what is now to what is not yet (Parse, 1997). Together the person and nurse co-create quality of life, the evolving becoming of the human being. The practice method has been implemented and evaluated in several health care settings. The settings include sites in the United States (centers in Kentucky and North Carolina), Canada, and Finland. (See Parse, 1997, for specific references about practice applications.)

Discussion and dissemination of the human becoming theory occurs through several means other than journal manuscripts. There are two Internet sites: Parse-L and Parse's home page. In addition, the International Consortium of Parse Scholars meets annually, and the Institute of Human Becoming offers summer sessions on the theory and research (Parse, 1997).

DIANA LYNN MORRIS

See also
FITZPATRICK'S RHYTHM MODEL
HEALTH CONCEPTUALIZATION
ROGERS' SCIENCE OF UNITARY HU-
    MAN BEINGS

PARTICIPANT OBSERVATION

Participant observation is an approach to data collection that is most often associated with naturalistic or qualitative inquiry, and it involves the researcher as a participant in the scene or observation that is being studied. The primary purpose is to gain an insider's, or emic, view of an event, setting, or general situation. The researcher focuses on the context of the scene along with the ways that individuals are behaving. Examples might include making and participating in observations in a busy emer-

gency room, observing the ways in which people carry out rites of passage, or participating in a special feast or occasion. The researcher attempts to make sense of the situation by interpreting personal experiences and observations and talking with individuals who are present, while simultaneously being fully involved in all of the experiences that occur in that setting. In this way participant observation enables the researcher to gain a view of a society but also serves as a way to validate verbal information that was provided by members of a society or group being studied. Another way in which participant observation may be used in research is with populations in which there is limited communication, such as very small children, the mentally impaired, or elderly stroke survivors. The challenge for the researcher is to combine the activities of observation and participation so that understanding is achieved while maintaining an objective distance.

To carry out participant observation the researcher needs to decide on (a) the role of the observer, (b) the degree to which the role is known to others, (c) the degree to which the purpose is known to others, (d) the amount of time that will be spent in conducting the observation, and (e) the scope of the observational focus. There is a continuum along which the role of the observer may be involved that ranges from involvement of the researcher in all aspects of the observational experience to only partial or minimal involvement. The researcher bases this determination on the research question and the nature of the research. For example, a researcher who assists in a homeless shelter may wish to be involved in all aspects of the daily routine; another researcher may wish only to conduct observations in a busy emergency room for which the routine is more complex. On the other hand, an invitation to participate in a special ceremony or ritual may involve only partial participation.

The degree to which the observer's role and the purpose of the observation are known to others also is related the intent of the research. In some cases the role of the researcher will be known to all, and in others it may not. If the purpose of the study is to know and understand a particular ritual or religious ceremony, for example, the role of the researcher may be known to all involved in the situation. In other cases the role of the researcher may be minimized, as in situations in which the informants may not fully understand the researcher's participation: observing children on a playground or in a children's unit in a hospital. However, ethical and moral issues arise when the nature and role of the researcher are not made known to all of the individuals being observed. The extent to which individuals are informed varies greatly, from full disclosure to no disclosure, and is often based on the researcher's estimation of how scientific truth can best be obtained.

The amount of time the researcher spends in observation and the scope or focus of the observation also depend on the purpose and intent of the research. In some cases the participant observation experiences are carried out for the length and duration of the research. In other research studies, participant observation may occur at only one point during the study. For example, sometimes a researcher may choose to enter the field and become a participant observer prior to conducting interviews. This gives the researcher time to learn about a community, group of people, or situation and then to use this knowledge to develop questions for subsequent interviews. In addition, the focus and intent of the observations may vary from making general observations of the entire situation, context, or event to very focused observations. For example, a focused observation might include personal interactions or a specific nursing or caring behavior.

One major concern in using participant observation is the degree to which subjects may become sensitized to the researcher's presence and may not behave as they normally would if the researcher were not present. The issue of subject sensitization can be addressed by increasing the duration of time the researcher spends in the observational experience. A longer time spent in observing can also enhance and strengthen the researcher's credibility, as well as any theoretical and empirical generalizations that are made.

In summary, participant observation is a commonly used approach to data collection that is used in naturalistic or qualitative research. It is an approach that allows the researcher to gain an insider's perspective on a social situation or event and can permit the researcher to be totally or minimally involved.

KATHLEEN HUTTLINGER

See also
DATA COLLECTION METHODS
QUALITATIVE RESEARCH

PATERSON AND ZDERAD'S HUMANISTIC NURSING THEORY

In the early 1960s, Josephine G. Paterson, and Loretta T. Zderad, psychiatric mental health nursing specialists with experience in institutional and community health settings, consultation, and education, began to come to the realization that empiricist science (formerly logical positivism) and its research paradigm could not answer all the questions that arose from the empirical realities of nursing practice. Inspired by philosophers such as Martin Buber, Gabriel Marcel, Teilhard de Chardin, and Viktor Frankl and through a process of dialectical dialogue, a nursing practice theory called humanistic nursing (Paterson & Zderad, 1976/1988) was gradually developed, taught, implemented, and published.

Flowing from and guided by the values and assumptions of existential philosophy and infused with its language, the theory incorporates three major components. The first component is the nursing act as a deliberate here-and-now existential encounter and intersubjective transaction between two persons: (a) the nursed, a person (client, family, group) who issues a call for help with health-illness needs, and (b) the nurse, who commits to a helping response to those needs. A second component is an approach to nursing as existential presence, awareness, and authentic dialogue. The third component is a phenomenological research method for nursing termed *nursology*. Existentialism is also recognized in the nurse's provision of opportunities for the patient to make responsible choices within the limits of safe and sound practice and support of the patient's maximum participation in care.

In humanistic nursing theory the person is viewed as unique, whole, independent, interdependent, and relational. Environment is not clearly defined, but it is recognized that the embodied (incarnate) person lives in an objective world of persons and things in space and in real and clock time. The person affects the world of others and things and is affected by them through the body, which changes in response to illness. The notion of angular view refers to the internalized worldview or angle of perception of the individual. Health also is not clearly defined, but it is said to go beyond the narrow concept of the absence of disease to being and becoming more (well-being and more-being) as is humanly possible in situations of living, suffering, or dying.

The goal of nursing is nurturance of well-being and more-being and the development and unfolding of the human potential of nurse and nursed. The meaning of humanistic nursing is found in the nursing act itself, which is always related to the quality of the human condition. Acts may be physical, manual, or technological; verbal or nonverbal; or solely authentic physical presence. Although physical care (doing with) is acknowledged as a component of holistic care and knowledge of science and technology is essential for the ''doing with'' that physical care entails, humanistic nursing goes beyond the biopsychosocial categorization of patients to focus on the person's angular view of the world and the uniqueness of being and becoming in the realities of health/illness situations. The ''being-with,'' or intersubjective relating between nurse and nursed, is enhanced by knowledge from the arts and humanities.

Three ways of relating are described as I-It, or subjective-objective, that recognizes the objectivity of nursing actions guided by science; the rarer but highly valued and rewarding subjective-subjective, or I-Thou, relationship, the authentic presence of the other with the self, wherein each becomes more; and the ''we'' type of relating that takes place with family, others, and community. The interhuman, or person-to-person, relating of the nurse and patient is complex, combining I-Thou and I-It relating that can be examined sequentially and retrospectively but actually occurs all at once.

The essence of nursing is the nurse-nursed relationship, the dialogue experienced, and the lived intersubjective experience of the shared ''between''

of the two (or more) unique beings. The between—that is, the intersubjective or interhuman element—is highly significant because therein are found phenomena such as loneliness, courage, hope or despair, and as yet undiscovered phenomena, as well as the processes such as comfort or nurturance that are the nursing responses to the patient's call. For example, when the nurse comforts and the patient is comforted, each experiences something, but they also experience something additional in the relation between them. The message or the meaning of the comfort–being comforted process is in the between.

The level of intersubjective transaction achieved in the variety of nurse-nursed experiences is one of degree and depends on the active involvement of the patient as well as the authentic nurse. Humanistic nursing theory expects that active clinical practitioners engage in clinical theorizing by describing as richly as possible and analyzing the nature and meaning of nursing acts as they experience them, articulating their findings, comparing them with similar experiences of other nurses, and bringing them to a higher level of conceptualization for the refinement of nursing care. Although experiencing, reflecting, describing, and articulating the between as a source of clinical knowledge may be overlooked in the fast pace of being and doing in nursing, the component of conceptualization of the between is inherent in humanistic nursing and at least must be held by the humanistic nurse as a goal or value.

The process of formally studying nursing as it is present in the subjective-objective world of the between is termed phenomenological nursology. Dominantly inductive, nursology leads to the development of concepts, constructs, or theoretical propositions grounded in the raw data of the nursing phenomena and processes that must be shared in durable form with colleagues.

Paterson and Zderad (1976/1988) developed and refined a five-phase phenomenological nursing practice research method based on humanistic nursing theory. The phases include the following:

1. Preparation of the nurse knower for coming to know or preparing the clinical nurse for the simultaneous research endeavor.

2. The nurse knowing the other intuitively (in the phenomenological sense) through the deliberate questioning of and response to the patient's unique lived experience, which corresponds to the transactional phase of nursing as it is practiced.

3. The nurse knowing the other scientifically, or the movement from intuition to analysis through comparing, contrasting, categorizing, interpreting, and synthesizing themes or patterns.

4. The nurse complementarily synthesizing known others, or the nurse researcher as a "knowing place" examining other similar realities and comparing and synthesizing them to arrive at an expanded view of the phenomenon.

5. The succession within the nurse from the many to the paradoxical one, or propelling nursing knowledge forward by development of an inclusive conceptualization or abstraction of the phenomena or process being studied. This systematic approach identifies the commonalities of nursing practice that become components of the science of nursing.

Humanistic nursing theory has relevance and significance for nursing practice, research, education, and administration. However, in each of these areas published literature related to use and specific output of humanistic nursing theory and its nursing practice research methodology have been sparse. The theory is abstract, and the existentialist language is uncommon parlance; but it is broad in scope, with the potential for intersubjective transactions wherever nursing is practiced. Paterson and Zderad (1976/1988) boldly identified the need in the[1] 1960s and 1970s for acceptance in the 1980s and 1990s of an essential paradigm for nursing research beyond traditional empiricism. The National League for Nursing supported Paterson and Zderad's 1976 work and its republication in 1988.

CAROL P. GERMAIN

See also
EPISTEMOLOGY
NURSING THEORETICAL MODELS
SCIENTIFIC DEVELOPMENT

PATIENT CLASSIFICATION

Patient classification is a generic term referring to the grouping or categorization of patients according to a predetermined set of characteristics. Until the late 1980s, this term was used almost exclusively to refer to the classification systems for grouping patients according to their requirements for nursing care and nursing resource determination and allocation. The exclusive use of the term to represent nursing systems became inappropriate with the widespread development of other patient classification systems (diagnostic related groups, case mix groups, and medical severity of illness systems) to capture medical resource use and complexity as the basis for hospital case costing.

With some peril, the terms *severity* and *acuity* systems were and continue to be used as equivalent terms. Connotations associated with these terms from the perspective of medical status led to misconceptions, as neither patient severity nor patient acuity correlates uniformly with nursing workload. In contrast, patient dependency and nursing intensity have been offered as more suitable labels to describe the intent of the patient classification systems designed for nursing. During the past decade, however, a shift in the use of terms has occurred. Those patient classification schemes that form the basis for the measurement of patients' requirements for nursing care for the express purpose of nursing resource determination and allocation are now referred to as nursing workload measurement systems (Edwardson & Giovannetti, 1994).

According to Sokal (1974), the process of classifying is defined as the ordering or arranging of objects or concepts into groups or sets based on relationships among the objects or concepts. The relationships can be based on observable or inferred properties. Classification theory also includes the distinction between monothetic and polythetic classifications. Monothetic schemes refer to those in which the classes established differ by at least one property that is uniform among the members of each class. In contrast polythetic schemes refer to those in which the classes share a large proportion of the properties but do not necessarily agree on any one property. Patient classification schemes for nurse staffing are recognized as polythetic, and their development coincides with the principles of this type (Giovannetti, 1978).

Work by Connor, Flagle, Hsieh, Preston, and Singer (1961) at the Johns Hopkins Hospital during the 1960s introduced the concept of classification into the study and measurement of nursing workload. The critical indicators or predictors of nursing care emanating from this work appear in most contemporary nursing patient classification systems.

Two types of patient classification systems, prototype evaluations and factor evaluations, were identified by Abdellah and Levine (1979). Prototype evaluations rely on the creation of several mutually exclusive and exhaustive patient categories. These are graded in terms of an ordinal scale in which the categories represent greater or lesser requirements for nursing care. The patient is classified into the category that most closely matches the profile or prototype description. Factor evaluation systems employ the selection of specific elements or indicators of care, representing either unique care activities or clusters of care activities. Ratings on individual elements are combined on the basis of a predetermined set of decision rules to provide an overall rating that determines the appropriate category.

The end product of the two types of evaluations is essentially the same. The difference lies in the method of rating; in prototype, the patient is rated on a number of characteristics simultaneously, whereas in factor, the characteristics are evaluated one by one. Edwardson and Giovannetti (1994) noted that many systems have been developed by vendors and consequently were not fully described in the published literature. More systems have been developed or modified at the institutional level and also not published. The interested reader may wish to consult two documents that contain numerous examples of nursing patient classification systems (Giovannetti, 1978; Lewis, 1989).

Transforming classification schemes for their ultimate use as resource determination and allocation methods requires an estimate of the nursing care time required of patients in each category. The literature is replete with techniques for doing so and discussions of the central issues of reliability, validity, and comparability (Giovannetti, 1984). Similar to nursing workload measurement system

research, research on patient classifications systems has much to offer nursing practice, nursing administration, health care administration nursing, and other institutional policy formation. Information on patient classification systems is available in professional, scholarly, management, and policy journals as well as in texts and government reports.

PHYLLIS B. GIOVANNETTI

See also
NURSE STAFFING
NURSING INTENSITY
**NURSING WORKLOAD MEASURE-
MENT SYSTEMS**

PATIENT CONTRACTING

Patient contracting is an intervention for promoting patient adherence in practice or research settings. Patient contracting provides an opportunity for patients to learn to analyze their behavior relative to the environment and to select behavioral strategies that will promote learning, changing, or maintaining adherence behaviors (Boehm, 1992). Patient contracting is relevant to nursing practice and research because it can assist patients to adhere to health care regimens, such as medication taking, meal planning, and exercise.

Research on the effectiveness of patient contracting in nursing has been reported for a variety of behaviors and in several settings. For example, patient contracting has been used to control serum potassium levels in patients on dialysis (Steckel, 1974); to increase knowledge and consistency in use of contraceptive methods by sexually active college women from a student gynecology clinic (Van Dover, 1986); to increase knowledge, keep appointments, and reduce diastolic blood pressure in hypertensive outpatients (Swain & Steckel, 1981); and to keep appointments, lose weight, and reduce blood pressure among outpatients with arthritis, diabetes, and hypertension (Steckel & Funnell, 1981). Patient contracting did not reduce blood glucose and glycosylated hemoglobin in patients with diabetes (Boehm, Schlenk, Raleigh, & Ronis, 1993; Steckel & Funnell, 1981).

Patient contracting is the process in which the nurse and patient negotiate an individualized, written, and signed agreement that clearly specifies the behavior and identifies in advance the positive consequences that will ensue when the patient has successfully performed the behavior (Steckel, 1982). The patient chooses the behavior and reinforcer in the contract with direction by the nurse. Patient contracting is based on the principle of positive reinforcement, which states that when a behavior is followed by a reinforcing consequence, there is an increased likelihood of the behavior being repeated (Boehm, 1992).

The nursing process provides the context within which to develop the patient contract. The nursing process provides the clinical data that can be jointly used by nurses and patients to establish priorities for adherence behaviors (Steckel, 1982). The adherence behavior is the ultimate complex behavior to be learned or changed. The adherence behavior is broken down into successive approximations or small steps. By performing small steps of the behavior, the patient gradually achieves performance of the adherence behavior. Over a series of patient contracts, the patient will specify a variety of behaviors, which include such behavioral strategies as self-monitoring, arranging and rearranging antecedent events, practicing small steps of the adherence behavior, and arranging positive consequences (Boehm, 1992).

The first several patient contracts are usually for self-monitoring to identify the successive approximations of the adherence behavior and the antecedents and consequences of the behavior. In later patient contracts, patients specify behavioral strategies related to arranging antecedent events, practicing a small step of the behavior, or arranging positive consequences. For example, a patient may substitute a piece of fruit for a bag of chips at bedtime three times each week for 6 weeks. Self-monitoring is ongoing throughout the behavior change process to provide data about the effectiveness of the new antecedents, the performance of the small steps of the behavior, and the new positive consequences.

The reinforcer in the contract is chosen by the patient and provided by the nurse in return for evidence that the behavior was successfully performed, such as the self-monitoring records. Reinforcers are unique to patients. The availability of reinforcers varies greatly by the practice or research setting. For example, patients may request more convenient appointments, magazines, lottery tickets, and so forth. Tokens or points can be collected and exchanged for a larger reinforcer (Boehm, 1992).

Behavioral analysis is the foundation of the patient contracting intervention. Behavioral analysis is the process by which the patient's behavior is observed, recorded, and analyzed in order to describe the successive approximations of the adherence behavior, the antecedent events that precede the behavior, and the consequences that follow the behavior. The behavioral data used in the analysis are obtained by the patient through self-monitoring (Boehm, 1992).

Behavioral analysis begins with the patient self-monitoring the adherence behavior. Self-monitoring provides baseline data that can be used to determine the effectiveness of the behavioral strategies implemented later in the behavior change process. By using the patient's self-monitoring records, the nurse can teach the patient to identify antecedent events that precede the behavior, small steps that comprise the behavior, and consequences that follow the behavior. Based on the behavioral analysis, behavioral strategies are specified that will assist in the behavior change.

An antecedent event precedes a behavior and prompts the behavior by identifying conditions under which a behavior will be reinforced or not (Boehm, 1992). Much behavior is under the control of antecedent events. When behavioral analysis demonstrates that the behavior the patient chooses to decrease or eliminate is cued by an antecedent event, the behavioral strategy is to rearrange, avoid, or eliminate the antecedent event. For example, the patient may take a different route home to avoid stopping at a fast-food restaurant after work. Conversely, when the patient chooses to increase a behavior, the behavioral strategy is to arrange an antecedent event in order to cue the behavior. For example, setting out jogging clothes and shoes at night may cue exercising the next morning.

Behavioral analysis can identify the multiple small steps that comprise the adherence behavior. When the small steps are identified, the behavioral strategy is to perform a small step of the adherence behavior for a designated period of time. When that small step is being successfully performed, the patient moves onto the next small step. Eventually, patients gradually achieve performance of the adherence behavior (Steckel, 1982). This behavioral strategy is effective because patients are often overwhelmed by expectations of a health care regimen, which can lead to nonadherence. For example, patients who are beginning stationary cycling can exercise for the shortest duration and the lowest frequency per week. Each week the stationary cycling is gradually increased until the designated level is achieved.

Positive reinforcement is the behavioral strategy in which a positive consequence is provided contingent on performance of the desired behavior, which results in an increase in the behavior. Behavioral analysis can identify positive consequences for behaviors and provide ideas for new consequences (Boehm, 1992). The behavioral strategy is to arrange positive reinforcement to acquire or maintain a desired behavior. For example, each small step of stationary cycling will be strengthened if followed by a positive consequence. Positive consequences can be pleasurable items and activities; social reinforcement, such as praise; and cognitive reinforcement, such as feelings of pride. Conversely, eliminating positive reinforcement can be used to decrease or extinguish an undesired behavior. For example, eating with selected companions may eliminate positive consequences for inappropriate food item selections.

There are several directions for future research in patient contracting. First, studies are needed to determine the frequency of contact with subjects needed to produce progressive changes in adherence interventions using patient contracting. Second, patient contracting during the maintenance phase of adherence interventions has not been studied. Third, studies could include multiple measures to verify performance of behaviors, such as self-monitoring records, electronic event monitoring of medication taking, and accelerometers of exercise routines.

This paper was supported in part by the National Institute of Nursing Research (5 P30 NR03924 03).

ELIZABETH A. SCHLENK

See also
ADHERENCE/COMPLIANCE
BEHAVIORAL RESEARCH
WELLNESS

PATIENT EDUCATION

Since the mid 19th century, patient education has been a fundamental cornerstone of health care and a well-established component of nursing care. Recently, patient education has been included in many professional standards of care promulgated by professional nursing organizations, in *A Patient's Bill of Rights* published by the American Hospital Association, and in the regulations of the Joint Commission on Accreditation of Healthcare Organizations.

Definition

Patient education has been defined as a planned learning experience using a combination of methods such as teaching, counseling, and behavioral strategies that influence the patient's knowledge and behavior (Bartlett, 1985). It is a critical component of health care because the well-being of patients with diagnosed disease and of individuals without diagnosed disease often is dependent on health-related actions those individuals take on their own behalf.

Research

Despite widespread belief in the importance of patient education, controlled clinical research on the effectiveness of patient education began in the early 1960s. Since that time there has been a growing body of research contrasting the effect on patient outcomes of a specific educational intervention with either "care as usual" or with a placebo control treatment.

Since the late 1980s many meta-analyses (quantitative reviews) have been published on the effect of patient education provided to adults or children with selected health conditions. Major researchers in this area and the patient population that was the focus of their reviews include the following: Bernard-Bonnin and associates (children with asthma), Brown (adults with diabetes), Devine and associates (adults having surgery, adults with hypertension, adults with cancer, adults with chronic obstructive pulmonary disease, and adults with asthma), Huestron and associates (women at risk for preterm birth), and Mullen and associates (adults with coronary disease, adults with arthritis, and pregnant women who smoke).

Most meta-analyses on the effectiveness of patient education indicated that it is beneficial for the patients receiving it (Redman, 1993). These beneficial effects have included not only increased patient knowledge but also positive effects on a wide range of disease-specific outcomes, for example, blood pressure control among individuals with hypertension (Devine & Reifschneider, 1995), pain and anxiety among surgical patients (Devine, 1992), and blood sugar control among adults with diabetes (Brown, 1990). In some instances cost-relevant outcomes have been affected as well, for example, in decreased use of emergency health services in adults with asthma (Devine, 1996).

However, statistically significant positive effects have not always been found. For example, there was not a consistent beneficial effect of patient education on morbidity among children with asthma (Bernard-Bonnin, Stachenko, Bonin, Charette, & Rousseau, 1995) or on pregnancy outcomes among women at risk for preterm labor (Hueston, Knox, Eilers, Pauwels, & Lonsdorf, 1995). The effect of patient education in adults with chronic obstructive lung disease was disappointing unless pulmonary rehabilitation exercises were also included as part of the intervention (Devine & Pearcy, 1996). Clinicians wanting to apply patient education research findings in their practice should review the research carefully to find research that matches their client group. Referring to the growing number of meta-analyses on the topic also should be of assistance.

Future Directions

Critical issues for the profession remain: What combinations of treatment components and modes of treatment delivery are the most effective? How do we make best use of newer computer-based technologies (e.g., the Internet)? How do we make sure that patient education is both sufficiently valued and provided with adequate resources so that health care practitioners can provide comprehensive patient education consistently? Who will pay for patient education?

Although many of the reviews of patient education research suggest that such education is beneficial for patients, the research is less clear about which specific types of patient education and which modes of treatment delivery are the most effective for which types of patients. This limitation arises from three problems. First, it is common for patient education researchers to contrast the experimental patient education program with usual health care for the setting and yet never to describe the patient education included in usual care. Second, very few studies contrast different types of patient education or different modes of treatment delivery in the same study. Third, many studies fail to provide detailed descriptions of the subjects included in their sample. Because of these limitations, it is difficult to make causal inferences about which types of content and which modes of treatment delivery are the most effective ones for which types of patients. More research in this area is needed. In the interim clinicians will have to use their best judgment, based not only on existing research but also on a needs assessment of their patient population. It is critical that clinicians assure that the patient education content is culturally appropriate for their target patient group and, if printed, that it is written at an appropriate reading level.

Clinicians and researchers interested in patient education will face many new opportunities and challenges as use of the Internet increases. Many patients from their homes or local libraries can use the Internet to access an almost limitless amount of health-related information (e.g., from literature searches, professional or consumer organizations, support groups, and disease-specific chat groups). This provides an opportunity for clinicians and researchers to provide patient education in innovative ways that allow the patient some control over the topic, the timing, and the pacing of the education. Some innovative educational programs also allow patients to submit questions via electronic mail and receive a response from their health care provider. The Internet will also provide many challenges to clinicians and researchers. Patients may receive inaccurate information over the Internet and be ill-equipped to judge its trustworthiness. In some situations patients may become aware of the latest research findings before their nurses and doctors are. At a minimum, clinicians and researchers should determine if their patients are using the Internet to seek health-related information and be prepared to help them make good use of this resource.

Knowing that some forms of patient education are effective in improving patient outcomes and having standards that say it should be provided may not be enough to ensure that patient education will be provided consistently in a comprehensive manner to all patients who may benefit from it. Although patient education is excellent in some settings, in the typical patient education study, the usual patient education for the setting was not withheld from patients in the control group and yet the new patient education program provided to the experimental treatment group often led to improved patient outcomes. This suggests that at least in some settings there is room for improvement in the patient education provided. Under the current system, improving patient education may be easier said than done. Nurses are under great pressure to provide comprehensive patient care. When time is limited, patient education may be judged to be less critical than interventions that address a patient's immediate safety or physiological well-being. If patient education were a specific reimbursable activity rather than subsumed under "nursing care" and billed as part of the room charge or the outpatient visit charge, it would be easier to ensure that health care providers had the time and other resources needed to provide comprehensive patient education.

ELIZABETH C. DEVINE

See also
ADHERENCE/COMPLIANCE
BEHAVIORAL RESEARCH
INTERNET
PSYCHOSOCIAL INTERVENTIONS

PATIENT SATISFACTION WITH NURSING CARE

The publication of the classic model of evaluation for health care services in the 1960s established the three criteria components for quality services (Donabedian, 1980). Of those three components—structure, process, and outcome—the last set the context for future generations of patient satisfaction measurement. Donabedian's assertion prevails. The consumers of health care need a voice in the assessment of the services and the care that are, at least theoretically, designed to meet their needs. Essentially, the thesis proposes that no health care services are complete in the evaluation of quality without including measure by the consumers of that care, the patients and, where appropriate, their families.

Nursing has long identified with the need to measure patients' perceptions of care, developing research and instruments to measure them. There are several reasons that patient satisfaction is so central to nursing, to nursing care, and to outcomes of nursing practice. The concept spans all areas of clinical or service delivery and all sociodemographic facets of the patient population. Recent developments in health care increase the importance of outcome measures, including the patients' perceptions. Many of these developments are influenced by a marketing or consumer orientation. Reimbursement is often tailored to quality of care reflected in the patient-as-consumer's perception. Regardless of the reasons, nursing has long recognized the complexity of measuring a patient's perception of the care that he or she receives while searching for sustained or improved health.

The challenges in measuring the multidimensional concept of patient satisfaction are myriad. One challenge is illustrated by the status of instrumentation in the field. The need for complex instruments that are valid and reliable yet reflective of the patient's clinical area are well documented (McDaniel & Nash, 1990). Instruments need multitesting and administration. They need application not only in the acute care hospital but in nonhospital, ambulatory, and community sites in order to identify the current changes in health care restructuring. These studies are continuing to emerge. Instruments also need adaptation to nonadult and non-English-speaking populations, which are the current foci.

A particular challenge is some acknowledgment of patients' prior experience with health care, their current status, and their expectation-set when entering the health care situation. The latter, especially, tend to influence the resulting rating of the care received. Not to be ignored is the overall issue of measuring the concept of health and health care, an issue recognized by nurses. Health itself is the most valued outcome but is a concept often difficult to articulate.

Research on patient satisfaction with nursing care includes the development and refinement of instruments as well as research using the instruments (Hinshaw & Atwood, 1982; La Monica, Oberst, Madea, & Wolf, 1986; Munro, Jacobsen, & Brooten, 1994). Research projects typically employ questionnaires, although telephone surveys, structured and semistructured personal interviews, and combinations of these (Wilcock, Kobayashi, & Murray, 1997) are frequently used. Researchers also articulate the need to include a measure of the patient's perception in research that assesses the service model, the delivery of care, or the outcomes of nursing care.

Current developments, however, include a more generic approach to the measure of patient satisfaction, referencing provider or multiproviders in health care, not just nurses. These developments highlight the need to evaluate the outcomes of clinical practice by nurses in various domains among their recipients. Earlier trends are giving way to a contemporary focus on the outcomes of practice and on the alteration of patients' health status.

Another change is expansion of patient's satisfaction to include a measure of the patient's perceived need and the patient's perception that the need is met (Thornton, 1996). The measure indicates the patient's perception of how well the health challenge is met. This expansion is not only more advanced and potentially more accurate but also more complex. It requires a broad yet targeted health measure of patients' perceptions. There are nuanced differences between measuring satisfaction and measuring needs met that are foundational to conceptual precision pertaining to satisfaction. Included, however, in the patient's perception of health status is a continuing emphasis on the recipient's expectation of care, the perceptions of care, and the satisfaction with care.

An important issue and continuing challenge for the future in nursing is a measure of the patient's care that reflects an alteration in the health status that is valid and reliable and that is tailored to an antecedent of that care. Here the major challenge is to measure the care of patients and the influence on health status alteration that is attributable to, or preferably effected by, nurses or nursing care. The challenge is finding a reference allowing nursing to tailor the concept to nursing care and to substantiate its antecedent influence on the outcomes of care. Indeed, this is the central and lingering issue for nursing as it pertains to patient care measures. The issue is advanced by more precise definitions of nursing practice, more precise and tailored constructs, and more quality instruments in the field.

The challenge to measure patients' perceptions of the influence that professional nurses have on their care and health status continues. Ironically, it is also complicated by an emphasis on a health care team, on a collaborative approach to health care delivery, and on an insistence, primarily by reimbursement parties, on the use of a generic term, "providers." This does not imply that nurses work individually or that nurses are not care providers but rather that increased attention should be given to measures that allow patients, as recipients of care, to identify the occupations of personnel who provide their health interventions. It suggests that attributable occupational identifiers be included in questionnaires, that nurses identify themselves to their patients, and that the measures be sensitive to the nuances of care.

Given the costs of testing and administration and the increasing acuity of patients in health care facilities, the measures must be realistic and inclusive regarding interventions and providers. Indeed, nurses should be included in decisions regarding the development of questionnaires, the specific items, the length of the questionnaires, and the use of the measures. Otherwise, the continuing satisfaction with nursing care and the quality of health care delivery to patients by nurses will be unexamined and therefore unreimbursed in tomorrow's outcome reports.

CHARLOTTE MCDANIEL

PEPLAU'S THEORETICAL MODEL

Peplau's theoretical ideas about interpersonal relations in nursing were formulated in the 1940s and
published in 1952 after a lengthy dispute with publishers about the ability of a nurse to author a book.
At a time when nurses were "doers" for patients
and "followers" of physicians' orders, Peplau's
theoretical work and teachings helped catapult nursing from an occupation to a profession. This precipitated a need for nurses to understand and establish
interpersonal relations with patients, as the significant context in which nurses facilitate patients'
health.

Through Peplau's therapeutic relationship, the
patient develops inner resources for healthy behaviors by actively participating with the nurse in the
change process. Peplau's interpersonal relationship
is also a process through which nursing knowledge
is developed and validated (Reed, 1996b). Peplau
(1992) purposefully linked her theory to practice
and research, as evidenced in her basic assumption
that "what goes on between people can be noticed,
studied, explained, understood, and, if detrimental,
changed" (p. 14).

Overview of the Model

Peplau's theoretical model was based on study,
observation, and analyses of nurses and patients
and derived from the work of Harry Stack Sullivan
and other psychodynamic perspectives. Peplau's
(1952) classic descriptions of nursing express the
nature and goals of the interpersonal process:
"Nursing is a human relationship between an individual, who is sick, or in need of health services,
and a nurse especially educated to recognize and
to respond to the need for help" (pp. 5–6). Nursing

is an "educative instrument, a maturing force, that
aims to promote forward movement of personality
in the direction of creative, constructive, productive, personal, and community living" (p. 16). Consistent with her earlier statements, Peplau (1988)
described nursing as an "enabling, empowering,
or transforming art" (p. 9). The interpersonal relationship was how nurses assessed and assisted people to attain healthy levels of anxiety and resume
mental health and development. The components
necessary for an interpersonal relationship were the
nurse, patient, professional expertise of the nurse,
and needs of the patient.

Peplau's (1952) four phases of the nurse-client
relationship are orientation, identification, exploitation, and resolution. Throughout these phases the
nurse functions cooperatively with the patient in
the roles of stranger, resource person, counselor,
leader, surrogate, and teacher. The nurse's range
of focus includes patient, family, and community
(Peplau, 1952).

During the phase of orientation, the patient has
a "felt need" and seeks professional assistance
(Peplau, 1952, p. 18). This is the first step in the
personal growth of the patient. The nurse and patient initially experience the role of stranger as the
patient seeks assistance from the nurse. During this
phase the nurse gathers observable data, recognizing that the power to accomplish the tasks at hand
always resides within the patient (Peplau, 1952).
The nurse and patient collaborate on a plan, with
consideration of the educative needs of the patient.

The focus during the identification phase is to
assist the patient to incorporate personal power to
address the problem. The relationship is flexible
enough for the patient to function dependently, independently, or interdependently with the nurse,
based on the patient's developmental capacity, level
of anxiety, and other needs. The nurse may assume
the role of surrogate, counselor, resource person,
and leader during this phase (Peplau, 1952).

The exploitation phase marks the time when
patients have identified their own resources and
strengths. They are enabled to derive full benefits
of the interpersonal relationship and other services
offered by the nurse to the patient (Forchuk, 1994;
Peplau, 1952).

The final phase in the interpersonal relationship
is that of resolution. Patients move beyond the ini-

tial identification with the helping professional and engage their own strengths to foster health, outside the therapeutic relationship.

According to Peplau (1952), health is a "word symbol that implies forward movement of personality and other ongoing human processes in the direction of creative, constructive, productive, personal and community living" (p. 12). Health is linked closely to successful management of anxiety, which ranges from pure euphoria to pure anxiety. Between these anxiety extremes, as determined by nurse and patient, is an optimal level of anxiety for healthy functioning. The nurse uses a complex set of strategies to assist the patient in using energy provided by the anxiety to identify and grow from a problematic situation (O'Toole & Welt, 1989; Reed, 1996a). Illness forces a "stock-taking by the sick person, which nurses can use to promote learning, growth and improved competencies for living" (Peplau, 1992, p. 13).

Research, Practice, and Education

Peplau's theoretical model can be categorized as a middle-range theory. It is narrower in scope than a conceptual model or grand theory. The model addresses a limited number of measurable concepts (e.g., therapeutic relationship, anxiety). The theory has a specific focus on the characteristics and process of the therapeutic relationship as a nursing method to help manage anxiety and foster healthy development. As such, the model is directly applicable to research and practice.

Peplau was explicit in promoting theory-based nursing practice and research-based theory. Research based on Peplau's theoretical model has addressed a variety of nursing problems, including (a) the work roles and practices of psychiatric–mental health nurses, (b) understanding specific phases and roles in the nurse-patient relationship, (c) recovery from depression, (d) working with patients infected with HIV, and (e) family systems nursing.

A major strength in Peplau's theory of interpersonal relations is its application to psychiatric–mental health nursing practice and to nursing wherein the nurse-patient relationship is relevant. Examples of this theory's application can be found throughout the literature on nursing research and practice.

Peplau's theory permeates all areas of nursing education. A philosophy of nursing curricula is belief in the value of a therapeutic nurse-patient relationship that focuses on needs, resources, and active participation of patients and supports collaboration between nurse and patient.

Future Directions

Peplau's theoretical model continues to be used by nurses who desire to advance nursing's knowledge base. Peplau's original contributions have become knowledge in the public domain and are not always acknowledged by researchers, clinicians, and educators. Nevertheless, the interpersonal relations theory continues to influence nursing theories, education, and practice (O'Toole & Welt, 1989). Peplau's philosophy of nursing and approach to knowledge development connect theory, practice, and research in creative ways (Reed, 1996b).

The reawakening of nursing by Peplau's ideas in the 1950s continues today through exploration, study, and use of the science-based practice of interpersonal relations in nursing. Through research and practice applications the theoretical model will continue to be refined and enhanced to meet contemporary needs of society. Peplau's theoretical ideas are expected to withstand the current health care crisis and to provide future nursing research for the cost-effective resources for health that exist within patient-nurse relationships.

NELMA B. SHEARER
PAMELA G. REED

See also
  HEALTH CONCEPTUALIZATION
  MENTAL HEALTH IN PUBLIC SECTOR
    PRIMARY CARE
  MIDDLE-RANGE THEORY
  NURSE-PATIENT RELATIONSHIP
  NURSING THEORETICAL MODELS

PHENOMENOLOGY

Phenomenology refers to both a philosophical movement and a research method. The philosophical underpinnings of phenomenology are first summarized to provide a backdrop for what this methodology aims to accomplish. One of the philosophical tenets of phenomenology is intentionality, which refers to the inseparable connectedness of human beings to the world (Husserl, 1962). Subject and object are united in being in the world. One cannot describe either the subjective or objective world but only the world as experienced by the subject (Merleau-Ponty, 1964). The observer is not separate from the observed. One can know what one experiences only by attending to perceptions and meanings that awaken conscious awareness. Phenomenologists hold that human existence is meaningful only in the sense that persons are always conscious of something. Meaning emerges from the relationship between the person and the world as the person gives meaning to experiences. Phenomenology focuses on lived experience, that is, human involvement in the world.

Perception is one's original awareness of the appearance of a phenomenon in experience (Merleau-Ponty, 1962). In phenomenology the process of recovering our original awareness is called reduction. Through phenomenological reduction one refrains from preconceived notions and judgments. Schutz (1973) described reduction as a process that is completed in degrees. Little by little, one's layers of preconceived meaning and interpretation are peeled away, leaving the perceived world. The layers of meaning provided by a researcher's knowledge and interpretation are preserved by being temporarily set aside—that is, bracketing. Through phenomenological reduction the world of everyday experience becomes accessible.

Edmund Husserl is considered the father of phenomenology. His is a descriptive phenomenology. He was interested in the epistemological question, How do we know about man? The goal of his phenomenology is the description of the lived world. Husserl's student, Martin Heidegger, took phenomenology in a different direction. Heidegger (1927/1962) was more interested in the ontological question, What is being? The goal of his phenomenology, called hermeneutic phenomenology, was understanding. This understanding is achieved through interpretation. Heidegger argued that it was not possible to bracket one's being-in-the-world.

The phenomenological philosophies of Husserl and Heidegger have different methodological implications for nurse researchers. Husserlian phenomenology focuses on the analysis of the subject and object as the object appears through consciousness. Bracketing is essential in this descriptive phenomenology. In Heideggerian phenomenology, bracketing is not used because this phenomenology views people as being in the world. This notion of being-in-the-world allows researchers to bring their experiences and understanding of the phenomenon under study to the research.

As a research method, phenomenology is inductive and descriptive. Phenomenology provides a closer fit conceptually with clinical nursing and with the kinds of research questions that emerge from clinical practice than does quantitative research. The goal of phenomenological research is to describe the meaning of human experience (Merleau-Ponty, 1964). In its focus on meaning, phenomenology differs from other types of research, which may, for example, focus on statistical relationships among variables. Phenomenology tries to discover meanings as persons live them in their everyday world. It is the study of essences, that is, the grasp of the very nature of something (Merleau-Ponty, 1962). Essence makes a thing what it is; without it, the thing would not be what it is. The phenomenological approach is most appropriate when little is known about a phenomenon or when a fresh look at a phenomenon is indicated.

As a research method, there are various interpretations of the phenomenological method available, from which nurse researchers may choose. Examples of descriptive phenomenology include Van Kaam's (1966), Colaizzi's (1978), and Giorgi's (1985) approaches. Van Manen's (1990) method is a type of hermeneutic phenomenology. Specific examples of how these different methods were used in nursing research are provided.

Van Kaam's (1966) phenomenological method of analysis was used by Beck (1992a) in exploring the meaning of nursing students' caring with physically/mentally handicapped children. The 36 nursing students' written descriptions of their caring experiences yielded 199 descriptive expressions related to the phenomenon under study. The next step in Van Kaam's method focuses on grouping these descriptive expressions into "necessary constituents," which are moments of the experience expressed either implicitly or explicitly in the majority of the participants' descriptions.

The following six necessary constituents of a caring experience between a nursing student and an exceptional child were revealed: authentic presencing, physical connectedness, reciprocal sharing, delightful merriment, bolstered self-esteem, and unanticipated self-transformation. In the final step in Van Kaam's (1966) analysis the necessary constituents are synthesized into one description of the experience being studied. In Beck's (1992a) study this description of caring between a nursing student and an exceptional child was as follows: "an interweaving of authentic presencing with physical connectedness and reciprocal sharing overflowing into delightful merriment, bolstered self-esteem, and an unanticipated self-transformation" (pp. 3–4).

An example of Colaizzi's (1978) phenomenological method is found in Beck's (1992b) study of the lived experience of postpartum depression. After reading and rereading the transcriptions of interviews with seven mothers, 45 significant statements that directly pertained to postpartum depression were extracted. Meanings were then formulated from each of these significant statements. Next in Colaizzi's method is the clustering of these formulated meanings into themes. Eleven themes describing mothers' experiences of postpartum depression emerged. These themes captured the women's unbearable loneliness, uncontrollable anxiety attacks and obsessive thoughts, haunting fear that their lives would never return to normal, consuming guilt, inability to concentrate, loss of control of their emotions, insecurity, lack of positive emotions and previous interests, and contemplating death. Finally, these 11 theme clusters were integrated into an exhaustive description of the experience of postpartum depression.

Bennett (1991) used Giorgi's (1985) method of phenomenological analysis to uncover the meaning of adolescent girls' experience of witnessing marital violence. Interviews with five adolescent girls who had grown up in violent homes were read and reread to identify what Giorgi labeled as "meaning units." These units were segments of the interviews that revealed some aspect of the phenomenon under study. These meaning units were then transformed into statements that expressed implicit or explicit meaning. Next, the transformed meaning units were synthesized into a summary of each adolescent's experience of witnessing physical violence directed toward her mother by her father. Giorgi refers to this synthesis as the "situated level description." The final phase of Giorgi's analysis called for an integration of each of these individual descriptions into one "general level description" that was composed of shared themes and meanings. Bennett's general level description of violence experienced included the following seven themes: (a) remembering, (b) living from day to day, (c) feeling the impact, (d) escaping, (e) understanding, (f) coping, and (g) resolving or settling.

Lauterbach (1993) used Van Manen's (1990) method of "doing" phenomenology to study the meaning of mothers' experiences of the perinatal death of wished-for babies. The following four concurrent procedural activities in Van Manen's method were incorporated in this study: turning to the nature of lived experience, existential investigation, phenomenological reflection, and phenomenological writing. Data analysis and interpretation of the data yielded the discovery of the essences in meaning of mothers' experiences. These essential themes included (a) the essence of perinatal loss; (b) reflective pulling back, recovering, reentering; (c) embodiment of mourning loss; (d) the narcissistic inquiry; (e) the finality of death of the body; (f) living through and "with" death; (g) altering worldviews; (h) death overlaid with life; and (i) failing and trying again.

Diverse clinical specialties of nursing such as maternal-child, gerontological, and medical-surgical nursing provide fertile ground for phenomenological research. These studies illustrate the breadth of applicability of this qualitative research method for nursing.

CHERYL TATANO BECK

See also
HERMENEUTICS
QUALITATIVE RESEARCH
RESEARCH INTERVIEWS (QUALITA-
  TIVE)

PHILOSOPHY OF NURSING

A philosophy of nursing lays the essential foundation for nursing research. Whether explicitly articulated or implicitly implied, all nursing research begins and ends with a philosophy of nursing. This relationship can be depicted as follows:

philosophy of nursing ↔ theory ↔ nursing research ↔ nursing practice ↔ philosophy of nursing

A philosophy of nursing is important because it represents the values, visions, and convictions of nurses about what ought to be nursing's central phenomena, that is, those phenomena that are both necessary and sufficient to provide a viable framework for the discipline and practice of nursing (Silva, 1997). Therefore, to conduct nursing research, nurse researchers must understand what are considered to be nursing's central phenomena and derive their research objectives, questions, and hypotheses from those phenomena. To better understand the underpinnings of nursing's central phenomena, nurse researchers must turn to the relationship between philosophy and philosophy of nursing.

Relationship between Philosophy and Philosophy of Nursing

Philosophy is a specific discipline that deals with ultimate or first-cause questions and phenomena that transcend other disciplines and cannot be answered by science or scientific investigation, for example, Is there a God? and What is reality? Koestenbaum (1968) states the nature of philosophy:

> Philosophy asks the very last questions which the human mind is capable of formulating, and it examines the ultimate foundations in our understanding of man, the world, and their connections. Specifically, philosophy lays bare all implicit assumptions, theories and methods in any belief whatsoever, and it systematically organizes, structures, and relates all the data and experiences that are available. (p. 21)

How, then, does the preceding definition of philosophy relate to a philosophy of nursing? First,

like philosophy, nursing is viewed as a specific discipline; thus, a philosophy of nursing should address ultimate questions about nursing and its phenomena. Examples follow:

> What ought to be the basic phenomena of the discipline?
>
> What are the metaphysical and ontological claims that underlie the phenomena of the discipline?
>
> What are the moral claims that underlie the phenomena of the discipline?
>
> What are the aesthetic claims that underlie the phenomena of the discipline?
>
> How can the basic phenomena of the discipline be known?
>
> How should the basic phenomena of the discipline articulate with basic phenomena of other human, helping service disciplines?

As health care professionals approach and enter the 21st century, distinct disciplinary boundaries are blurring rapidly and more interdisciplinary disciplines are emerging. As this trend continues, so too will the questions that constitute the essence of nursing philosophy. In summary, the preceding questions raised about nursing have metaphysical, ontological, moral, and aesthetic claims that emerge from philosophy but manifest themselves in phenomena related to nursing and ultimately to nursing philosophy.

Koestenbaum's (1968) definition of philosophy also challenges nurses to question the status quo and to lay bare all assumptions about nursing that ring intuitively or analytically false or that do not hold up in nursing practice. Only through such careful scrutiny can a philosophy of nursing remain current and provide a framework for nursing that is representative of the "truth" of nursing. Furthermore, Koestenbaum's definition of philosophy challenges nurses to develop a philosophy or philosophies of nursing that are cohesive, coherent, and complete.

Relationship between Philosophy of Nursing and Nursing Science and Research

Philosophy is not science, and nursing philosophy is not nursing science. But philosophy is the foundation of science, and nursing philosophy is the foundation of both nursing science (i.e., the body of nursing's scientific knowledge) and nursing research (i.e., the process of obtaining not only nursing's body of scientific knowledge but also the process of obtaining knowledge derived from scholarly critical analyses).

Implicit in most nursing research are assumptions about human beings (i.e., study subjects or participants), about selected phenomena of the discipline (i.e., variables), and about how the selected phenomena can be known (i.e., the research method). In addition, in qualitative research the meaning or artistry of the selected phenomena is often addressed (e.g., hermeneutics, photography). Finally, regardless of whether the research is quantitative, qualitative, or scholarly critical analysis, it must be ethical. Thus, all research grounded in nursing contains explicit or implicit philosophies of nursing that determine research approaches. The important point is that "research must be driven from a well-developed base of what nursing is—it should provide the foundation for the science" (anonymous peer reviewer, personal communication, February 24, 1997).

Relationship between Philosophy of Nursing and Philosophical Inquiry in Nursing

Philosophical inquiry in nursing—one type of nursing research *method*—is based on using the analytical powers of the mind to question and elucidate and then intellectually justify questions and issues related to nursing philosophy. According to Burns and Grove (1997), philosophical inquiry is a qualitative research approach that includes, but is not limited to, foundational inquiries, philosophical analyses, and ethical analyses. The investigative tool is the mind; the expression of the mind is through words.

Foundational inquiries in nursing are conducted prior to the development of nursing theory or nursing research programs and focus on critical analyses of nursing's philosophical underpinnings, theories, and concepts. An example of a philosophical foundational nursing inquiry would be to delineate the boundaries of nursing (Burns & Grove, 1997).

Philosophical analyses in nursing focus on critical exploration of language or concepts. Regarding concepts, the technique most commonly used is concept analysis, which, according to Morse (1995), consists of one or more of the following techniques: concept development, concept delineation, concept comparison, concept clarification, concept correction, and concept identification. An example of philosophical analysis using the concept clarification technique of concept analysis would be to clarify the concept of "spirituality" as used in nursing.

Ethical analyses in nursing focus on critical reasoning to examine assumptions, logic, strengths, deficits, and language usage in ethics. An example of ethical analysis in nursing would be a critical examination of a theory of nursing ethics, with logical and scholarly justification for why the theory or a part of it is either defensible or indefensible (Burns & Grove, 1997).

In summary, foundational inquiries, philosophical analyses, and ethical analyses in nursing must all be driven from a philosophy of nursing. The philosophy of nursing, then, becomes the foundation for the nursing knowledge derived through the research method of philosophical inquiry.

Future Directions

Future directions regarding philosophy of nursing and nurse researchers include the following:

1. Nurse researchers need greater knowledge about and appreciation for the discipline of philosophy.
2. Nurse researchers must interact regularly with nurse philosophers to grasp more fully that philosophy of nursing must provide a foundation for nursing science and other nursing knowledge.
3. Nurse researchers must commit themselves in greater numbers to philosophical inquiry as a legitimate method of nursing research.
4. Nurse researchers must prepare themselves for the blurring of distinct disciplinary boundaries as more interdisciplinary disciplines emerge.

MARY CIPRIANO SILVA

See also
CONCEPT ANALYSIS

EPISTEMOLOGY
RESEARCH IN NURSING ETHICS
SCIENTIFIC DEVELOPMENT

PHYSICAL RESTRAINTS FOR THE ELDERLY

A physical restraint is attached to or adjacent to a person's body, cannot be removed easily, and restricts freedom of movement. Physical restraints are applied primarily for three reasons: fall risk, treatment interference, and other behaviors (e.g., restlessness, agitation, confusion, etc.). During the 1980s several nurses called attention to frequency of the practice, suggesting it was understudied, poorly understood, and a worthy area for nursing research. Because of the serious sequelae associated with restraint use for frail elders in hospitals and nursing homes and the authority of nurses to determine whether or not a restraint is used, research on use of physical restraints is an important concern as nurses seek evidence-based, best practices.

The first thorough review concerning use of physical restraint for the elderly was published by Evans and Strumpf (1989). At the time, incidence and prevalence of restraint varied depending on settings and studies but was reported as 7% to 22% in hospitals and 25% to 85% in nursing homes. Ten studies on the subject of physical restraint were identified in the review, and all were descriptive. Although prevention of injury to self or others was the most frequently cited rationale for use, no scientific basis for efficacy of restraints in safeguarding patients from injury was found.

Somewhat paradoxically, literature existed from the 1980s onward noting safety hazards associated with physical restraints, along with numerous physical, physiological, psychological, and behavioral consequences of restraint and immobilization. Since 1990, documentation of consequences has intensified. Physical restraints are implicated in serious injuries and death. The negative impact of physical restraints on functional capacity has been demonstrated and includes (a) development of complications, (b) dependency and morbidity, (c) biochemical and physiological effects, (d) altered perceptual and behavioral responses, and (e) emotional desolation.

The persistent use of physical restraints is troubling given a wealth of empiric evidence against the practice. The history and the culture of restraint use in the United States suggests a practice based more on myth than science. Reports from several European countries indicate that despite cross-cultural similarities in disability and illness between hospital patients and nursing home residents, there are pronounced differences in therapeutic belief and style and in the assumptions made about managing and controlling behavior (Strumpf & Tomes, 1993). One study compared the differences in prevalence in three American and two comparable European homes. Prevalence in the United States was nearly 40%, and in the Scottish and Swedish homes less than 10%. Scores on a measure of functional status showed the European residents to be even frailer than residents of U.S. homes (Evans et al., 1993). Remarkably contrasting practices with regard to restraint use can be attributed to differences in philosophy and cultural style, perceptions concerning legal liability, staff mix, availability of knowledgeable professionals, limitations on use of catheters and feeding tubes, nonavailability of restraining devices, and modifications in equipment and architectural environment.

In view of differences in American and European homes and with no empiric evidence for the therapeutic value of restraints, deep-seated myths explain the prominence of restraint use in the United States. The myths are based on the following beliefs about restraints: (a) they prevent falls and injuries, (b) they eliminate perceived harms associated with various behaviors, (c) they limit legal liability, (d) they do not bother the restrained person, (e) they substitute for inadequate staffing, and (f) they remain the only intervention available (Evans & Strumpf, 1990). Shifting the paradigm from a risk focus aimed at controlling behavior to an individualized focus aimed at restraint-free care is part of a significant debate occurring between researchers and clinicians. Arguments for individualized care are being bolstered by clinical intervention studies that dispel myths and demonstrate that restraint practices can be changed.

A recent and still small body of research on restraint reduction or elimination suggests that restraint-free care is a transitional process facilitated by understanding and applying change theory to guide a program of education, policy change, and procedural innovation for all levels of staff. Changing the traditional and habitual practice of physical restraint depends on altering beliefs and increasing knowledge about appropriate practices and standards of care.

Although hundreds of articles have been written on the subject of physical restraints, the only research studies to emerge in the past decade have focused on compliance with regulations or efforts at reduction and elimination. In one clinical trial on restraint reduction in nursing homes (Evans et al., 1997), three homes were randomly assigned to restraint education (RE), restraint education with consultation (REC), or control. The RE and REC homes received intensive education by a master's-prepared gerontological nurse to increase staff awareness of restraint hazards and knowledge about assessing and responding to resident behaviors likely to lead to use of restraints. In addition, one nursing home also received 12 hours per week of unit-based nursing consultation to facilitate restraint reduction for residents with more complex conditions. Only the home receiving REC had a statistically significant reduction in restraint prevalence. This was achieved without increased staff, psychoactive drugs, or serious fall-related injuries, dispelling several of the above-mentioned myths that have plagued progress in restraint reduction.

Although education is useful, a far greater effect is achieved when education is combined with consultation to assist staff in providing individualized, high-quality care for clinically challenging patients and residents. In addition, a continuing focus on individualized care is necessary if changes in practice are to be implemented, maintained, and appropriately modified over time. The success of consultation and other "best practice" models supports the use of advanced practice nurses to improve quality of care and outcomes for frail older adults in nursing homes and other settings. Recently, interest in restraint reduction has intensified in hospitals, driven in part by warnings of restraint hazards by the Food and Drug Administration and guidelines from the Joint Commission on Accreditation of Healthcare Organizations (Sullivan-Marx & Strumpf, 1996).

Given the state of the science on restraint use, restraint reduction, and the emergence of restraint-free care as the standard of practice, ethical debate on the subject of physical restraints has also shifted. Until recently, this debate has been framed as the classic moral conflict between caregiver determinations of beneficence versus individual autonomy. Although physical restraint has long been viewed as an infringement of personal rights, the ethics literature has focused on three basic concerns: (a) mental competence, (b) patient wishes and duties of staff to protect from harm, and (c) the benefit-to-burden ratio. In these formulations, however, the choice to restrain is always an option. Protection of the patient, preventing harm to others, and the benefits of preventing a fall, keeping a tube in place, or controlling behavior outweigh any burdens.

Today an expanding empiric base and practices guided by a philosophy of individualized care are transforming our understanding of beneficent and autonomous care for frail elders. Beneficent care requires empirical knowledge, along with an appreciation of its uncertainties, and commitment to evidence-based practice. Autonomy means enabling independent function to the fullest extent possible given the circumstances, including frailty and physical and cognitive impairment. Thus, the classic beneficence and autonomy conflict has new meaning. Care that adheres to the principles of both beneficence and autonomy, in light of existing knowledge of physical restraints, must be restraint-free. Even if restraint-free care remains merely a goal or is held out as a gold standard, on purely ethical grounds, care without restraints is what patients and residents should expect and what professionals should provide.

In 1994 a priority expert panel report for the National Institute of Nursing Research included physical restraints in its research agenda for long-term care for older adults. The recommendations were to determine reasons for restraint use and clarify decision making; investigate care needs of the restrained patient; examine ethics, values, and attitudes as they affect use of restraints and quality of patient care; establish and evaluate standards of care; and test and evaluate alternative approaches with a view toward reducing or eliminating restraint use. Substantial knowledge now exists in all but the last of these areas. As no therapeutic value for physical restraints has been determined, the devices should be eliminated; the research clearly indicates this can be done safely and with positive outcomes. The emphasis for future research should be enhancement of care protocols for those behaviors and situations that have, in the past, resulted in the application of physical restraints. This means research directed toward specific nursing interventions aimed at minimizing falls and serious injuries, enhancing delivery of technological care (when necessary), and individualizing care approaches for a range of behaviors associated with cognitive impairment.

NEVILLE E. STRUMPF
LOIS K. EVANS

See also
**ALZHEIMER'S DISEASE: SPECIAL CARE UNITS IN LONG-TERM CARE
ELDER ABUSE
FAMILY CAREGIVING TO FRAIL ELDERS
GERONTOLOGIC CARE
NEUROBEHAVIORAL DISTURBANCES OF THE OLDER ADULT: DELERIUM AND DEMENTIA**

PHYSIOLOGICAL MONITORING

Physiological monitoring is a useful nursing approach to measure biological functioning in living organisms. Generally, it refers to data collected through an interface of technological instrumentation with a living organism. This technological instrumentation can be relatively simple, such as a thermometer, or as complex as combined hemodynamic and laboratory instrumentation used to measure oxygen utilization in the critically ill patient. Physiological monitoring can be used to examine both normative functions (e.g., homeostasis) and disordered responses (e.g., illness and related manifestations). Physiological monitoring occurs in vivo and in vitro, among animal models, in laboratory settings, and in clinical practice areas. Information about physiological parameters promotes understanding about the phenomena with which nurses are concerned: health-supporting and health-restoring human responses.

A variety of physiological variables are measured by nurses: (a) electrical potentials of the brain, heart, and muscle; (b) pressures in arteries, veins, lungs, mouth, esophagus, bladder, vagina, uterus, and brain; (c) sound (mechanical) waves in the ear and heart; (d) temperature and the concentration of gases in the lungs and blood; (e) physical symptoms such as size and color of bruising, stool, and wounds; and (f) serum levels of hormones and coagulation factors through biochemical analysis. The most common physiological measures reported in nursing research are blood pressure, heart rate, weight, and temperature (Lindsey, 1984). Note that monitoring of physiological measures can be either direct or indirect, can be utilized continuously or at a particular point in time, and include physical, electronic, and biochemical devices.

Although much of nursing practice is concerned with the physiological dimensions of health, physiological nursing research has lagged behind the study of psychosocial dimensions of nursing practice because of measurement and training issues. The recent upsurge of interest in research focusing on physiological phenomena may be attributed to nurses who in the 1970s and 1980s chose to pursue doctoral preparation in physiological sciences and to the explosion of technological monitoring used across clinical settings. Data on physiological dimensions of interest to nurses are more readily available to nurses and to nurse researchers. Physiological monitoring devices are found in the acute care setting, home health care settings, and outpatient and surgical environments and are often employed as a routine of care.

Further, nursing scientists are prepared with a strong theoretical and experiential base for designing physiological studies. One aspect of their work has been to evaluate the accuracy, selectivity, precision, sensitivity, and error (Gift & Soeken, 1988) of physiological measures so that reliability and validity are supported. Another important focus of physiological monitoring has been outcome measures. Examination of changes that occur as a consequence of nursing practice has produced a broad range of research, as evidenced by the variety of physiological variables studied in this decade alone (Burns & Grove, 1997). Finally, data about physiological measures have led to a wealth of integrated reviews that advance nursing science by describing and critiquing a coherent body of knowledge about physiological monitoring (e.g., Bliss-Holtz, 1995; Noureddine, 1995; Thomas & DeKeyser, 1996).

CHRIS WINKELMAN

See also
CRITICAL CARE NURSING
DATA COLLECTION METHODS
FETAL MONITORING
HEMODYNAMIC MONITORING
OUTCOMES MEASURES

PILOT STUDY

A pilot study is a smaller version of a proposed or planned study that is conducted to refine the methodology for a larger study. A pilot study uses subjects, settings, and methods of data collection and data analysis similar to those of a larger study (Burns & Grove, 1993; Polit & Hungler, 1995).

It is recommended that all large-scale studies have either pilot work or other preliminary work as evidence of feasibility of the project and to demonstrate the competence of the investigator with the area of study. Feasibility issues that might be addressed in a pilot study include the availability of subjects and estimating the time required for recruitment of subjects, the conduct of the investigation, and the cost of the study. Particularly when planning studies with populations that may not be easily available or accessible, a pilot study is an opportunity to develop or refine sampling methods and to evaluate the representativeness of a sample.

Preliminary work in the form of a pilot study provides an opportunity to identify problems with many aspects of study design (Burns & Grove, 1993). One important design issue that can be evaluated during the pilot work is determining the number of data collection points and the optimal time between phases of data collection. Pilot work can be used to develop, test, or refine a study protocol, including the treatment or intervention to be used in an experimental or quasi-experimental study. Sufficient pilot work is necessary to support the efficacy of an intervention prior to proposal submission for a large-scale intervention study. During a pilot study extraneous variables that had not been considered in the design may become apparent, and methods to control for them can be introduced when the larger study is designed.

Pilot work also allows the development or refinement of data collection instruments, including questionnaires and equipment. The performance of instruments with a particular sample under specific conditions also can be evaluated in the pilot project. When collecting quantitative data, the reliability and validity of instruments and the ease of operation and administration can be evaluated prior to data collection in a large-scale study. This is an important step whether the data collection instruments are interview schedules, questionnaires, computers data bases, or equipment to gather biophysical data. For example, during pilot work, questionnaires can be evaluated for clarity of instructions, wording of questions, reading level, and time required for completion. For qualitative studies, pilot work may be important for gaining experience in interacting with the sample and with aspects of data collection, coding, and analysis.

The results of a pilot study are likely to be significant for the larger proposed study. If the pilot study is of sufficient size, estimates about the relationships between variables and of effect sizes can be made. This is essential not only for statistical power analysis but for a better understanding of the phenomena under study. Pilot studies often provide important insights into the problem being investigated and may lead to reconceptualization of the problem or refinement of the research questions.

CAROL M. MUSIL

See also
DATA COLLECTION METHODS
INSTRUMENTATION
QUANTITATIVE RESEARCH METHOD-
  OLOGY
RELIABILITY
VALIDITY

POPULATIONS AND AGGREGATES

In a very broad sense the term *population* refers to a collection of entities that have one or more characteristics in common. According to Kendall and Buckland (1960), "in statistical usage the term 'population' is applied to any infinite collection of individuals. It has displaced the older term 'universe' . . . it is practically synonymous with 'aggregate' and does not necessarily refer to a collection of living organisms" (p. 223). The conception of population is basic to an understanding of inductive or inferential statistics. Stated succinctly by Blalock (1960), "the purpose of statistical generalizations is to say something about various characteristics of the populations studied on the basis of known facts about a sample drawn from that population or universe" (p. 89). In statistics, population characteristics are called parameters and are denoted by Greek letters; sample characteristics, called statistics, are denoted by Roman letters. According to Blalock, in inductive statistics "it is the population, rather than any particular sample, in which we are really interested." As a matter of convenience, a sample is selected but the goal is "practically always to make inferences about various population parameters on the basis of known, but intrinsically unimportant sample statistics" (p. 90). The underlying foundation for making inferences from samples to the population is the mathematical theory of probability.

Within the health field, particularly in public health, the disciplines of epidemiology and biostatistics, and the nursing specialization of public health nursing, the term *population* usually refers to biological entities such as people, animals, or microorganisms that hold characteristics in common. Population has a very prominent position in epidemiology. In discussing the classical understanding of epidemiology, Morris (1964) referred to it as "the study of the health and disease of populations" (p. 4). Recently, Mausner and Kramer (1985) defined epidemiology as "the study of the distribution and determinants of diseases and injuries in human populations" (p. 1).

Historically, public health specialists such as health officers focused on populations and subpopulations as the target for planning, service programming, and evaluation efforts. Although public health nurses provided clinical services in public health programs directed to target populations such as children under 6 years or prenatal clients, predominant focus was clinical, at the level of the patient or the family. The concept of using a population or aggregate approach to the practice of public health nursing first began to be seriously discussed in the literature in the 1970s (Williams, 1977). The conceptual shift from a focus on individual patients, the thrust in the clinical preparation of nurses, to a focus on populations, which is the concern of public health, can be difficult. However, it is necessary to understand public health and the specialization of public health nursing. "The basic notion in population-focused practice (the essence of public health practice) is that problems are defined (diagnoses) and solutions (interventions) are proposed for defined populations or sub-populations as opposed to diagnoses and interventions or treatment carried out at the patient or client level" (Williams, 1996, p. 25).

Taking a population approach to decision making in health care, that is, defining problems and proposing solutions for a population or aggregate, may facilitate health services and care delivery research and the utilization of research in practice for two reasons. First, such an approach involves obtaining data on each member of the population and summarizing it in meaningful ways. Adopting strategies and methods used by nurse researchers, epidemiologists, and others who study community-based or clinical populations may be used. This process may be sufficiently systematic and rigorous to make a contribution to the research literature. Second, a population approach to decision making is highly compatible with the empirical thinking of researchers.

Researchers study samples of populations with specific characteristics. The extent to which a finding in a sample from a particular population can be predicted in another can be assessed primarily by determining the comparability between the populations. If the individuals in a clinical or community-based program were identified as a population or subpopulation, with key characteristics in common, rather than unique individuals, the program population could be compared with another studied population. For example, if those working with very low birthweight infants view the infants as a population, they are in a strong position to relate to the work of Brooten and colleagues (Brooten et al., 1986), who worked with this population, and determine whether the intervention developed by Brooten et al. would work for their population. In a like manner, those serving urban adolescents at risk for unintended pregnancies would find of interest the multifaceted program (a school-linked clinic combined with free contraceptive services and curricular strategies) reported by Zabin et al. (Zabin, Hirsch, Smith, Streett, & Hardy, 1986) and cited by the U.S. Preventive Services Task Force (1996b) as one of the most effective programs directed to this population.

Although a population-focused approach has traditionally been central to public health practice, the spread of capitated managed care has precipitated a growing interest in the concept of populations and decision making at the population level throughout the health care industry. The population emphasis has many positive implications for health services and care delivery research and for a more systematic, rational, and data-based approach to decision making in the health care system.

CAROLYN A. WILLIAMS

See also
COMMUNITY HEALTH
EPIDEMIOLOGY
HEALTH SYSTEMS DELIVERY
STATISTICAL TECHNIQUES

POSTPARTUM CARE: DEPRESSION

Postpartum depression is a well-documented affective disturbance experienced by 10%–15% of women and generally occurring within the first 6 months to 1 year after childbirth. A majority of American and British women (70%–90%) experience a transient episode of "postpartum blues" in the form of tearfulness, feelings of sadness, increased irritability, and anxiety within 2–4 days after delivery. These mood disturbances have a pre-

sumed association with the rapid fall in progesterone and estrogen levels following loss of the placenta. Research findings suggested a relationship between more severe postpartum blues and an increased risk for the development of postpartum depression, particularly for primiparas. Postpartum psychosis is a rarer diagnosis (1–4 per 1,000 women), occurring within 1 to 2 weeks postpartum, accompanied by the more extreme symptoms of hallucinations and delusions, and usually requiring hospitalization and psychotropic medications.

Postpartum depression is distinguishable from the milder, short-term, and usually self-resolving symptomatology of postpartum blues and the debilitating illness of postpartum psychosis on the basis of severity of symptoms and a combination of other factors: later onset (2–6 weeks postpartum is common) and the insidious progression and often long-term duration of the illness—up to 1 year postpartum. Research reports are typically divided between these three childbearing depression categories. Not included in the research on postpartum depression is the relatively unstudied postdepression aftermath, including the unknown related effects of experiencing a traumatic illness during a critical period of family development. This could prove a fruitful area for nursing research by those interested in primary health care from either a systems- or family-based conceptual framework.

Risk Factors

Documented risk factors for the development of postpartum depression are numerous and include genetic predisposition and a history of previous psychiatric illnesses. Psychosocial indicators also have been studied; they include problems in the marital relationship, infant temperament, and low self-esteem as most prominent. Demographic predictors such as age and parity vary, based on a review of cumulative research findings. It is likely that combinations of psychosocial factors in the presence of heightened sensitivity to hormonal changes and difficulties encountered during pregnancy and postpartum, such as a complicated childbirth and breastfeeding problems, put women at risk for postpartum depression. For nurse researchers the study of the relationship of current limitations in health care availability to the increasing incidence of postpartum depression among American women is indicated. It is widely accepted that support for childbearing women during postpartum is inadequate, but the type and extent of needed additional care is still uncertain.

The obstetrical and medical perspective on this illness has provided insights on the biological significance of pregnancy as a stressful event and the potential influence of hormonal alterations that are normal and abnormal concomitants of pregnancy and postpartum (Affonso, 1992). Research has focused on the contribution of thyroid disturbances to postpartum depression, and influences of neurotransmitters (i.e., serotonin, dopamine) have been studied. Recent studies have centered on the potentially positive effects of administering prophylactic estrogen to women with a previous history of postpartum depression.

From the nursing perspective, mood and affective changes accompanying the childbearing period can be viewed as maternal responses to the interaction of complex psychosocial and physiological changes. Proponents of this perspective advocate examination of the symptoms of depression as cues to a developing pattern of difficulty along the continuum of coping and adaptation. Research with this focus requires longitudinal designs (rather than one-point cross-sectional assessments) to provide insights into the time boundaries of both the development and resolution of postpartum depression during early pregnancy and to 1 year postpartum (Affonso, Mayberry, Lovett, et al., 1993). Depression measurements required refinement for childbearing women to establish reliability and validity that could be differentiated from the nonpregnant samples evaluated to determine population norms. For example, it is known that the Beck Depression Inventory has symptom categories that overlap with normative postpartum changes, such as body image, sleep-fatigue, somatic preoccupation, and weight loss. More studies are needed to develop and test pregnancy-related stress and coping instruments for use in screening and for research purposes.

The goal of preventing even mild symptoms of postpartum depression through management techniques in health promotion is emerging as a priority among nurse researchers. This is based on research findings that revealed mild dysphoric symptomatology during pregnancy as a potential risk factor for subsequent postpartum depression. Another promising variable is the role of maternal self-esteem as a potential mediator of the effects of everyday stressors and social resources on depressive symptoms (Hall, Kotch, Browne, & Rayens, 1996). The investigators concluded that further study is warranted on interventions to decrease postpartum stressors and improve the quality of primary intimate relationships to reduce the likelihood of depressive symptoms.

Nurse researchers have begun to contribute to knowledge of the long-term effects of maternal depression on other family members. Research findings from a recent meta-analysis of 19 studies indicated a substantial negative impact of maternal depression on infants and children (Beck, 1996a). Mothers exhibited less affectionate behaviors toward their infants when depressed, and infants of depressed mothers can be more difficult and discontented. Thus, an asynchrony of behavioral states may exist within the maternal-infant dyad. Researchers in this field believe that problems occur because mothers exhibiting depressed behaviors have infants who tend to imitate those behaviors, or the infant may receive inappropriate stimulation during a critical period of development for interaction skills—or a combination of both.

Strategies were recommended to enhance interactions, to increase maternal sensitivity to infant cues, and to institute relaxation techniques. In terms of nursing research, the timing, format, and cultural context of these interventions require further study. For example, community-based home interventions have been described as helpful for some mothers. Cross-cultural studies to assess the varying symptom patterns, predictors, measurement issues, and health care needs of women experiencing depression are needed to understand the experiences of immigrant women and those living in other countries. On the other hand, comparisons between American and Mainland Chinese women are complicated by the fact that the term *depression* is not directly translatable into Chinese.

Because nurses in the United States and Canada are often involved in breastfeeding support and counseling, there is a need to collaborate in research targeting the effects of antidepressant treatment during breastfeeding. A recent report states that, although effects vary among antidepressants, extensive mother-baby serum level data and infant behavioral data associated with these medications are very limited (Wisner, Perel, & Findling, 1996).

In the experience of current clinicians, the diagnosis and treatment of postpartum depression could be improved if women with a previous history of postpartum depression or exhibiting early signs were recognized and supported earlier in the pregnancy and postpartum. Nurse researchers should focus on refining brief assessment tools for community-based screening by nurses and physicians, who can thus be alerted to early signs of adjustment difficulties following childbirth. Because these assessments will require close follow-up monitoring and supportive interventions for affected women, studies aimed at examining outcomes of basic protocols regarding management and referrals will have to be developed. Although a combination of pharmacotherapy and psychotherapy is considered generally successful in the treatment of postpartum depression, the ability to assess and provide early interventions could avoid the longer duration and the outcomes of a more severe illness when women's "cries for help" are overlooked (Hamilton & Harberger, 1992, p. 43).

LINDA J. MAYBERRY
DYANNE D. AFFONSO

See also
CULTURAL/TRANSCULTURAL FOCUS
MOTHER-INFANT/TODDLER RELA-
    TIONSHIPS
YOUNG WOMEN AND DEPRESSION

PREGNANCY

Nurses have conducted much research on pregnancy and the childbearing period. This research has paralleled national concerns and issues. The Association of Women's Health, Obstetric, and Neonatal Nurses (AWHONN) identified priorities for research drawing attention to prenatal care, low-birthweight infants, mothers and infants who are HIV-positive, adolescent pregnancy, substance abuse during pregnancy, the effect of stress on pregnancy, and the use of health care during pregnancy.

The practice of nursing has changed dramatically. The wide use of technology, the legal climate surrounding maternity care, shorter hospital stays, focus on the family, consumer demands, single room maternity care, and cross-training have been topics of research studies affecting the delivery of care. Couplet care (mother-baby) is another area of research. This type of care has been shown to increase maternal competence. Patient satisfaction also has been studied. The provider relationship was reported to have the greatest influence on the women's satisfaction with prenatal care (Omar & Schiffman, 1995).

Roles of nursing have expanded exponentially. There are women's health practitioners, midwives, perinatal practitioners, and nurses certified in ultrasound and monitoring. A specific nursing model for prenatal care was extensively studied by Affonso and colleagues (Affonso et al., 1992) in Hawaii. The use of nurses who make routine home visits and their positive effect on many maternal and infant outcomes has been studied by Olds and Kitzman (1993). Many studies examining the effect of advanced practice nurses on the cost and outcome of early discharge with extensive support in the home were published (Brooten, 1995). The use of midwives for special populations has been studied, and positive outcomes were reported when they served low-risk populations.

Childbearing Periods

Simple and advanced technologies have been evaluated. The use of tympanic thermometers was judged to be appropriate during pregnancy, and oscillatory blood pressure measurement was questioned when patients move during the actual measurement. Biophysical profiles were examined as to the degree of agreement between nurses and physicians. Auscultated acceleration testing also was examined as to its status in predicting poor perinatal outcomes. Maternal-fetal attachment was related to gestational age, and there was an association between prenatal and postpartal attachment. Exercise was associated with fewer discomforts, and regular exercise before conception did not adversely affect maternal or neonatal outcomes. Smoking cessation information given at the first prenatal visit was associated with better results than at other times during pregnancy. Women who gained more than 25% of their normal weight were reported to have a higher proportion of operative deliveries than those who gained less than 25%. Interpersonal care was found to be important in relieving stress during labor.

In adolescents, exercise was reported to decrease depressive symptoms and increase self-esteem, and attachment to the fetus began with quickening. Emotional and financial needs are paramount to teens; young teens and older teens use different support systems during pregnancy. Adolescents identified infant illness and pregnancy complications as particular topic areas to be learned.

Symptoms

Beck (1993) conducted significant qualitative and quantitative research in the area of postpartum depressive symptoms and developed a theory of postpartum depression that linked prenatal depression and postpartum depression. Postpartum depression has an effect on maternal-infant interaction, on infant temperament, and on a child's interaction. Other symptoms reported were nausea, fatigue, and pain.

Breastfeeding

Several descriptive and experimental studies were conducted on the topic of breastfeeding. Behavioral attitudes prenatally were shown to be a strong predictor for the initiation of breastfeeding among low-income women. Insufficient milk supply was associated with early weaning and with smoking. Measures to combat nipple soreness included warm compresses and the application of a moist dressing.

Culture

"In *no* culture is childbearing treated with indifference" (Callister, 1995, p. 327). Many cultures have been studied, including African, Alaskan Eskimo, American, Asian (specifically, Japanese and Taiwanese), Ethiopian, and Navajo. In addition, Americans who gave birth in Japan and Southeast Asians who gave birth in the United States were examined.

Fertility versus Infertility

Comparisons among fertile and infertile women were made (e.g., adaptation to pregnancy, physical and psychosocial symptoms). Both partners involved in infertility were compared on loneliness, social support, stress, and ways of coping.

Abuse

Several studies reported that the prevalence of abuse during pregnancy was 16%, and higher rates were reported for teens. Jealousy of and anger toward the fetus were reported by one study to be the reasons for this abuse. Anxiety, depressive symptoms, housing problems, inadequate prenatal care, and drug and alcohol use also were reported to be correlates of abuse during pregnancy.

High-Risk Pregnancy

Specific conditions such as diabetes mellitus, breast cancer diagnosed during pregnancy, arteriovenous malformation, and hypertrophic cardiomyopathy were studied. Preterm labor prevention and the needs of women who have preterm labor were examined in several studies. Numerous studies, among them Fawcett, Pollio, and Tully (1992), have examined functional status issues after childbirth and the women's response to cesarean delivery. The perception of women who have cesarean deliveries and those who have vaginal birth after cesarean deliveries were reported. The attitudes about cesarean delivery and concerns women have afterward were examined. The experience of having a high-risk pregnancy was examined, as was the treatment of bedrest at home (e.g., economic and physical hardship) and in the hospital (e.g., effect on muscle atrophy, weight loss, and dysphoria).

Substance Abuse

Drug use was reported to be 11% in urban populations and 3.9% in rural areas. Specifically, crack cocaine and alcohol were examined in regard to prevalence. Sexual risk taking, AIDS knowledge, and drug use were examined.

Summary

The amount of research conducted has been so significant that AWHONN has been able to sponsor three major research utilization projects. The most recent one has been for research-based practice during the second stage of labor. Practices that have sufficient empirical support include use of the upright position during labor and pushing when the parturient is ready (not when the health care provider is ready). Having research ready for practice is a powerful statement about nurses conducting significant research during pregnancy and the childbearing period.

LINDA C. PUGH

See also
  CHILDBIRTH EDUCATION
  NURSE MIDWIFERY
  POSTPARTUM CARE: DEPRESSION
  PRENATAL CARE: A COMMUNITY APPROACH
  PREVENTION OF PRETERM AND LOW-BIRTHWEIGHT BIRTHS

PREMENSTRUAL SYNDROME

Premenstrual syndrome (PMS) is the term used to describe the cyclic occurrence of a wide range of distressing physical, psychological, or behavioral symptoms in the final week of the fertile menstrual cycle that resolve with the next menses. Symptoms commonly include but are not limited to bloating, breast tenderness, depression, unexplained anger or irritability, fatigue, difficulty concentrating, and food cravings. Although symptoms can begin as early as ovulation (midcycle), central to the PMS definition is the disappearance of symptoms after menses. Thus, it is the timing, duration, and severity of symptoms, rather than the symptoms per se, that distinguish PMS as a distinct medical disorder, separate from other physical or psychological problems.

Although most experts support the idea of a hormonal trigger for the entrainment of symptoms to the menstrual cycle, the cause of PMS is unknown, and there is currently no way to detect it by physical examination, blood test, or x-ray. A major clinical and research problem of the past was the use of retrospective questionnaires for symptom charting, which was shown to favor the exaggerated recall of perimenstrual symptoms, perhaps because of cognitive prompting by menses, versus those at other times of the month. Guidelines have now been developed for the diagnosis of PMS that rely heavily on the prospective daily assessment of multiple cycles to confirm retrospective self-reports and the exclusion of other physical and emotional illness.

In the worst form, PMS results in significant interference with daily activities and personal relationships, requiring medical intervention. Because of the preponderance of debilitating emotional symptoms, severe PMS (affecting about 5% of childbearing women in Western countries) is considered a form of clinical depression by the American Psychiatric Association. Premenstrual dysphoric disorder, the psychiatric diagnosis for PMS, has recently been responsive to fluoxetine and other related serotonin reuptake inhibitors. This was the first time that any medication, hormone supplement, herb, or vitamin therapy has been consistently superior to placebos in clinical trials, suggesting that the severe form of PMS may be related to a biochemical disorder in the brain.

Nursing Contributions to PMS Research

The etiology of PMS symptoms has been the topic of particularly keen interest among nurse researchers. A number of nurse scientists, via funding by the NIH National Institute for Nursing Research, have helped characterize the biopsychosocial context of PMS, its impact on women's lives, and methods to distinguish it from other menstruation-related conditions (Sveinsdottir & Reame, 1991; Taylor, 1994). For nearly two decades, Nancy Woods, her students, and her colleagues have focused on the development of explanatory models that incorporate family, psychosocial, and cultural predictors of perimenstrual symptoms (Taylor & Woods, 1991). Using a daily health diary and symptom analysis method that have now been tested by nurse researchers in the United States and other countries, their body of work defined three types of menstrual cycle symptom patterns in healthy menstruating women: (a) low intensity, acyclic symptoms; (b) a PMS pattern; and (c) high-intensity symptoms that increase in severity during the premenstrual week (premenstrual magnification) (Mitchell, Woods, & Lentz, 1994). These symptom patterns are related to a number of psychosocial correlates, such as psychological stress level, years of education, and maternal symptom pattern, as well as age, laboratory-induced arousal, and stress responsivity (Woods, Lentz, Mitchell, & Kogan, 1994).

Given the diverse features of PMS, it is not surprising that nursing studies have been guided by a variety of theoretical underpinnings, including family systems theory, psychosocial concepts, health promotion paradigms, and hypotheses grounded in the psychoneuroendocrinology of stress. In general, these theories have served as the basis for studies that can be grouped into three categories, describing (a) incidence rates, symptom features, and distinguishing psychosocial traits of women with PMS; (b) biological characteristics such as physiological arousal and LH pulsatility patterns; and (c) the effects of nursing interventions, including self-care strategies, patient support groups, and marital counseling.

Current Methodological Pitfalls and Gaps

Despite the general acceptance among researchers of an association between endocrine factors and premenstrual changes, it is somewhat surprising that few studies of symptom patterns have adequately defined the hormonal status of the study populations. Endocrinologically diverse samples have included infertility clinic patients, college populations, perimenopausal women, and oral contraceptive users. Moreover, screening criteria have failed to account for the influence of aging, body weight, and fertility status as important predictors of adequate ovarian function. It is unknown to what extent these confounds have masked important nuances in the PMS phenomenon.

The biomedical literature has focused on the need for confirmation of ovulatory status of participating subjects by concurrent hormonal measures. Yet nursing studies of menstrual symptoms have frequently relied on cycle length and regularity as evidence of ovulation, using days before or after menses onset as reference points for estimating the follicular and luteal phases of the ovarian cycle. Thus, in many cases, conclusions have been drawn about a relationship between reproductive biology and symptom changes based on data from heterogeneous samples lacking hormonally defined cycle phases.

Future Directions

As in the case of menstrual cycle research in general, a major problem of PMS research has been the glaring absence of nursing studies focused on women of color. The typical PMS research subject has been a White, middle-class woman with few barriers to adequate health care. There is now a body of descriptive research available on the etiology and characteristics of women with PMS that begs for further scrutiny via the systematic application of meta-analysis. Such analysis could greatly enhance the integration and synthesis of this work into a more meaningful picture of the PMS syndrome and its impact on women's health. Given the existing theory-based data that supports the value of social support, self-care measures, peer support groups, and lifestyle modifications for other chronic health problems, the time is ripe for clinical trials of these same nursing strategies for the management of PMS.

To design rigorous clinical trials for testing nursing interventions for PMS symptoms, it will be necessary to solve several thorny methodological issues that have plagued PMS research for years.

A recognized weakness of menstrual symptom studies is the difficulty in blinding subjects to the purpose of the investigation and the well-known placebo effect, which frequently is as powerful as the experimental intervention. It may be important for future studies to evaluate the so-called placebo response as a therapeutic intervention, given the growing interest in understanding the neurocognitive underpinnings of the healing powers of faith.

In summary, there is a need for further refinement of PMS research methodologies, particularly with respect to sample selection, design considerations, and methods for monitoring menstrual symptoms in a nonintrusive way. Given the negative biases that exist in society about the influence of the menstrual cycle on women's health, attention should be paid to the researcher's own set of stereotypes and values about gender and race to effectively interpret research findings in this important area of women's health.

NANCY E. REAME

See also
FAMILY HEALTH
MENSTRUAL CYCLE
STRESS
YOUNG WOMEN AND DEPRESSION

PRENATAL CARE: A COMMUNITY APPROACH

Over 10 years ago, the Institute of Medicine (1985) released a report that described problems in the recruitment and retention of women into prenatal care. The report emphasized (a) making care more accessible to underserved women, (b) improving the content of prenatal care for hard-to-reach women, and (c) providing nontraditional approaches for recruitment and retention of women from disadvantaged, ethnic, minority, and rural backgrounds. Considerable research has shown the contribution of prenatal care programs in reducing low birthweight infant rates and other adverse newborn outcomes. However, women who need prenatal care the most do not always receive it, and standards by which this care is delivered and studied have been criticized by both providers and consumers.

Standard prenatal care in the United States consists of brief, periodic encounters with a physician, nurse practitioner, or nurse-midwife throughout pregnancy for the purpose of monitoring uterine fundal height, fetal heart rate, weight gain, and biochemical status through urine and blood samples. Early entry into prenatal care by late first trimester or early second trimester is recommended, although the actual frequency of visits is currently being questioned. The National Institutes of Health Expert Panel on Prenatal Care recommended a reduction in the number of prenatal visits for low-risk nulliparous women, and a recent study (Binstock & Wolde-Tsadik, 1995) showed no statistically significant differences in complications of pregnancy or neonatal outcomes between low-risk women receiving the standard frequency of prenatal visits and those receiving fewer. Studies to evaluate scheduling and content of prenatal visits are needed.

The problem is that the prevailing standard for obstetrical care provided in the United States is considered insufficient to improve overall birth outcomes (Thompson, Walsh, & Merkatz, 1990). Most medical complications of pregnancy affect only a small proportion of pregnant women. Also, some medical practices may actually increase the risk for preterm or low-weight births because induction of delivery as early as 34 weeks gestation is considered the way to treat complications of conditions such as diabetes and toxemia. From the perspective of women, particularly those from minority and culturally diverse backgrounds, current prenatal services are often considered unsatisfactory in terms of comprehensiveness, cultural sensitivity, and adequacy of time to ask questions and receive counseling.

It has been recommended that more emphasis be placed on the availability of nursing care services that focus on psychosocial issues and health promotion efforts related to pregnancy and postpartum adaptation to motivate women to increase healthy behaviors and to enhance maternal and infant outcomes (Augustyn & Maiman, 1994). In doing so, more women will choose to seek prenatal care earlier in pregnancy and will continue through the postpartum with appropriate newborn follow-up.

The goal for nurse researchers is to determine the optimal approaches for introducing and studying new models of prenatal care for short- and long-term effects on the mother and family.

In ethnically diverse communities, both urban and rural, cultural knowledge and values are a dominant influence on individual behaviors concerning motherhood and childbirth. However, a dilemma exists for various ethnic groups on how to make the health care system more responsive to beliefs and values centered on quality of life indices (Affonso, 1996). For nurse researchers, this requires conceptualizing the reorganization of a prenatal care system with related intervention protocols and evaluation outcomes designed for and with women and families in a specific community.

The formulation of these "community partnerships" for developing and evaluating health care endeavors is a relatively new concept that requires commitment on the part of scientists who "should be accountable for the practical efficacy of the information they produce" (Affonso, DeLeon, Raymond, & Mayberry, 1994, p. 14). In addition, "the obligation of academics is to bring their efforts, ideas and inquiries into partnership and engagement with the community before, during, and after their work is completed" (Affonso et al., 1994, p. 15). One recent prenatal care study conducted in a rural Hawaiian community serves to illustrate this model for practice and research. A nursing project called Malaya Na Wahine Hapai (Caring for Pregnant Women), funded by the National Center for Nursing Research, incorporated community participation and input at all key phases of the project. Multiple focus group data obtained in the initial needs assessment phase of the project were utilized (Affonso, Mayberry, Graham, Shibuya, & Kunimoto, 1993). The focus group participants resided in the community and included representatives from the targeted ethnic groups served by the program and local women leaders who were respected for their childbearing and child-rearing knowledge and skills. Data derived from the focus groups' content analysis were used to develop several nursing interventions, comprising a prenatal care program that was coordinated and implemented by specially trained public health nurses.

Common themes that emerged were used to design the care protocols for the program. Examples of these included (a) the need to talk about women's health issues and concerns in the local communication style known as "talkstory" for one-to-one encounters and group sessions with program nurses, (b) freedom to choose and access a variety of caregiving approaches deemed culturally sensitive by pregnant women, and (c) the promotion of local ethnic healing systems using support networks established for specific ethnic identities. In addition, based on input received from the women, the concept of "care giving without walls" was instituted, whereby women had the option of receiving care not only in clinic sites but also the workplace, home, and via telephone. Program content within the conceptual framework of promoting cognitive adaptation—that is, search for meaning, developing a sense of mastery, and enhancing self-esteem—included self-care management issues such as nutrition related to infant growth and stress reduction. The difference from standard obstetrical care was the focus on areas of health monitoring and education predicated on assessment of individual progress in pregnancy adaptation.

Focus group methodology was successful as a research approach in a community-level program because it produced an important data base at the beginning of the study for designing cultural and community-sensitive program mechanisms. The data base facilitated subsequent phases of the research project built on an initial contract of mutual decision making between researchers and consumers. For example, in the Malaya project the creation of the Neighborhood Women's Health Watch (NWHW) that evolved from the initial focus group experiences expanded on the typical community worker's role to sanction the partnership concept. Members were recruited on the basis of their reputation as local leaders of the designated ethnic groups and their prior experience as mothers. Expertise in the health field or maternity care was not considered necessary for membership, but the ability to communicate in culturally sensitive ways was important. Core NWHW leaders helped to recruit others and assisted with ongoing training regarding the prenatal program goals; however, their key role was as "cultural consultants" to the program nurses in modifying interventions.

Even though community-based prenatal care programs are directed primarily to women, access and retention issues are often directly or indirectly influenced by the presence of men in the community. Another strategy was employed to make the improvements in pregnancy health not only a women's issue but more focused on the community responsibility for the health concerns of childbearing families. The decision to promote the involvement of men who believed in the project goals was an effective strategy for marketing the program in the community. Local business leaders were enthusiastic about providing gift certificate incentives to women enrolled in the Malaya program, and other men in the community were willing to serve on the advisory council and to participate in marketing and evaluation activities. Whereas the preliminary focus group work set the tone for the ensuing practice and research project, outcomes testing has to include evaluation criteria for feasibility and consumer acceptability, which is assessed (involving members of the community, such as the NWHW) throughout the study.

Finally, there is a tendency among those who allocate resources to consider population-based preventive measures, such as nursing care, as less essential within the scope of health care costs. It is important that cost variables be included in nursing research studies designed to demonstrate prenatal outcomes effectiveness. Several perinatal interventions have shown health care cost-effectiveness in the United States, including prenatal smoking cessation interventions, food supplementation, enhanced public health nursing services, community-based prenatal care for adolescents, home visitation by nurses, and prenatal care visit adequacy. Justification for new models of prenatal care that incorporate essential nursing care services requires continued emphasis on cost-effectiveness. Studies also should include the significance of new patient care outcomes that target quality of life indices and community impact on long-term and even generational effects of interventions.

DYANNE D. AFFONSO
LINDA J. MAYBERRY

See also
**CULTURAL/TRANSCULTURAL FOCUS
CHILDBIRTH EDUCATION**

**PREGNANCY
POSTPARTUM CARE: DEPRESSION
PREVENTION OF PRETERM AND LOW-
    BIRTHWEIGHT BIRTHS**

PRESCHOOL CHILDREN

The ages 3 to 5 years of life represent the traditional preschool period of the early childhood years. Injuries are the single greatest cause of death among children over the age of 1 year (*Emergency medical services for children*, 1993). Automobile accidents are the major causes of death for preschool children. Although the mortality rate for preschool children is low, the morbidity rate is high. It has been suggested that the total number of illnesses that children experience during this period exceeds that of any other age. Most of the illnesses (80% or more) seem to be respiratory in nature. Respiratory conditions accounted for 701,000 hospitalizations, and injury caused 266,000 hospitalizations of children under 15 years of age in 1990 (*Emergency medical services for children*, 1993).

The organic system of preschool children is sufficiently mature. Desirable habits of eating, eliminating, sleeping, and breathing are fairly well established. In 1968, Erickson defined the developmental tasks of the preschool period as learning initiative versus guilt. Whether the child leaves this stage with a sense of initiative rather than with a sense of guilt depends to a great extent on how the parents respond to the child's self-initiated activities. Piaget described the preschool child as one indulging in preoperational thought, which he termed intuitive thought. Parents are critical to the healthy development of preschool children, as they provide the discipline and the security that is necessary for these children to develop appropriately. It is important that health and psychosocial conditions occurring during this period of life or undiscovered in infancy and toddlerhood be identified and treated to avoid adverse effects on development and learning.

Green (1994) noted that for many children and their families each new day is an opportunity for further self-realization, enhancement of good health, and the promotion of self-esteem. For millions of others, however, the future holds little promise. Their health status is poor, the risks to their health are many, and the prospects for them to overcome these problems are limited. Children deserve the attention, the encouragement, and the intervention of care providers from many disciplines to ensure that they develop the healthy bodies, minds, emotions, and attitudes to be competent and contributing adults.

Nursing Research and Research Relevant to Nursing

The nursing research literature on preschool children from 1979 through 1984 was focused primarily on delivery of care, development, health-illness state, communication and coping, and interactions among and perceptions of parents, children, and others. The study designs were usually descriptive or quasi-experimental. Few studies were done exclusively on preschool children; they often included other children of varying ages (Fleming, 1986).

Projective techniques in pediatric nursing research were used from 1984 through 1993 to study some preschool children who were in varying states of health. Over half of the studies reported involved ill children. Phenomena studied varied, but the largest number of studies were on pain, body-related knowledge, stress, and anxiety (Bellack & Fleming, 1996).

The *Cumulative Index Medicus* for the period 1986 through 1996 listed few studies on preschool children in any of the health or health-related disciplines. The Conference on Nursing Research Priorities held in 1992 resulted in the selection of five research priorities. Those that might include preschool children were community-based nursing models (1995), cognitive impairment (1997), living with chronic illness (1998), and biobehavioral factors related to immunocompetence (1999). The National Institute of Nursing Research (NINR) supports nursing research exploring the effects of radiation and chemotherapy in children, helping families with conduct problems and assisting children through video-based nursing interventions.

The Maternal and Child Health (MCH) Bureau of the Public Health Service identified broad categories as research priorities for preschool children: major morbidity and mortality problems, children with special health needs, child life course development, and fatherhood (Lamberty, Papai, & Kessell, 1996). Opportunities exist to seek funds for meritorious research on preschool children. Sources other than the NINR and MCH are possible, depending on what areas are being studied. Though the NINR does not specify preschool children in any of its priorities, some of the priorities are not specific to any age group. Further, only about one third of the NINR's total competing grant funds are awarded for the priority areas.

Future Directions

There is a need for longitudinal, intervention, and collaborative studies on preschool children within other disciplines. Delivery of care to preschool children in the managed care environment should be addressed. The complex health needs of some conditions that affect preschool children exceed the capability of any single discipline, and interdisciplinary research is sorely needed. Research to evaluate outcomes, particularly patient outcomes of interdisciplinary models of education and practice, was recommended by the American Association of Colleges of Nursing in 1996. The need for research on clinical aspects of care, severity and outcomes of illness and injury, costs, optimal system configuration and operations, and effective approaches to education was stressed by the Committee on Pediatric Emergency Medical Services (Emergency Medical Services for Children, 1993).

The Children's Action Network (CAN) and a coalition of business, health, government, child care, and community organizations launched a National Immunization Campaign in 1991. In 1994, CAN hosted a national conference that brought together 250 immunization activists from 33 states to highlight the experiences of individuals and organizations that were successful in helping families and service providers overcome barriers to immunization ("Immunizing America's children," 1995). However, there are still a number of children in society who have not been immunized by 2 years of age, as well as many preschool children (ages 3–5).

Research on the best community strategies may help resolve the problem of getting more children immunized before the age of 2. However, the belief that federal initiatives to lessen provider vaccine costs would increase the number of children with up-to-date immunizations was not confirmed by a study done by the Agency for Health Care Policy and Research in 1996.

By the year 2000 the United States will have a non-White population of 67 million—larger than the total combined populations of France, England, and Germany. One in every four Americans will be Black, Hispanic, Asian, or Middle Eastern. It is expected that a proportionate number of this population will be preschool children. Basic physiological requirements and needs for safety, belonging, love, and self-actualization are universal for all humans; but how, what, and when humans eat and how social needs are met are culturally determined. Without some means to ensure the inclusion of the cultural aspects of society in research, it is unlikely that the needs of many preschool children and their families will be met.

Cultural sensitivity offers many rewards; patients follow advice more readily when it matches and respects their cultural values. Cultural assessment may suggest interventions that speed recovery and result in fewer miscommunications and conflicts resulting from differences in values and cultural norms. The opportunity to enhance knowledge about preschool children through systematic study of culturally diverse groups will aid in the development of the art and science of the discipline of nursing. It is essential that society deal effectively with the changes emerging in the population.

JUANITA W. FLEMING

See also
CANCER IN CHILDREN
CHILD LEAD EXPOSURE EFFECTS
NUTRITION IN INFANCY AND CHILD-
    HOOD
PSYCHOSOCIAL EFFECTS OF CHILD
    CRITICAL ILLNESS AND HOSPITAL-
    IZATION
SOCIETY FOR RESEARCH IN CHILD
    DEVELOPMENT

PRESSURE ULCERS

Pressure ulcers are defined as any skin lesion caused by unrelieved pressure, resulting in damage of underlying tissue. Pressure ulcers usually occur over bony prominences and are graded from Stage 1 (nonblanchable erythema) to Stage 4 (full-thickness skin loss with tissue necrosis and destruction extending to muscle, bone, or supporting structures) (Panel for Prediction and Prevention of Pressure Ulcers, 1992). Pressure ulcers are a persistent, not a new clinical problem. It is difficult to estimate the incidence and prevalence of pressure ulcers, but one recent survey of 143 hospitals indicated that 11% of the patients had ulcers (Meehan, 1994). This problem is higher among critical care patients and elderly nursing home residents. The cost of treatment and the cost in human suffering, delayed rehabilitation, and an increased use of health care resources are difficult to determine, but one recent estimate suggested that $1.3–$6.8 billion may be spent on pressure ulcer treatment of hospitalized patients alone.

The goal of good patient care is to prevent pressure ulcers. This goal was supported by the Agency for Health Care Policy and Research (AHCPR) with the assistance of a multidisciplinary panel that created clinical practice guidelines (Panel for Prediction and Prevention, 1992) based on a comprehensive review and synthesis of scientific evidence and the judgment of clinical experts. In general, preventive measures recommended in this document include assessing risk of all bedfast or chairfast individuals on admission to a health care setting, reducing the amount and duration of pressure to which the tissue is exposed; keeping tissues clean, supple, and free from undue exposure to moisture or to dryness; and providing for adequate dietary intake.

Predicting pressure ulcer risk has been a goal of nurses for several decades. Early work by Phyllis Verhonick at Walter Reed Army Hospital and Doreen Norton in Great Britain focused on understanding the etiology of pressure ulcers with a view to predicting risk. This work in the late 1950s and early 1960s drew attention to the problem. The Norton Scale (Norton, McLaren, & Exton-Smith, 1962/1975), reported in 1962 and 1964, was the first tool tested for predictive validity. Attempts were continued in the early 1970s by Davina Gosnell (1973) and in the 1980s and 1990s by Barbara Braden and Nancy Bergstrom (Bergstrom, Braden, Laguzza, & Holman, 1987). The Braden Scale for Predicting Pressure Sore Risk© was introduced in 1987 and has been studied extensively since that time, proving effective in predicting who will develop pressure ulcers.

The Braden and Norton scales were recommended for use on all bedfast and chairfast individuals in the guidelines. The Braden Scale, now more commonly in use, is composed of six subscales (Mobility, Activity, Sensory Perception, Nutrition, Moisture, Friction, and Shear) that address major conceptual risk factors. The total of these scores indicates the level of risk. This tool has very good sensitivity and specificity; that is, it accurately identifies who is at risk and who is not at risk. Individuals known to be at risk receive care based on the specific factors placing them at risk.

The hallmark of an effective pressure ulcer prevention program is teamwork. It is important for a multidisciplinary team to put a systematic prevention plan in place. Staff education and participation is essential. Planning mechanisms that focus on the processes of care and mechanisms for ensuring that risk is assessed and preventive practices are delivered have been most effective. Susan Horn and colleagues (Horn, Ashton, & Tracy, 1994) from Intermountain Health System have demonstrated that computer-assisted decision support based on risk assessment and accompanied by risk reduction as recommended by the AHCPR guidelines can reduce pressure ulcer incidence among even the most severely ill. Cost savings have been documented to accompany this improved patient outcome.

When pressure ulcers develop, it is important to create a comprehensive plan of care and a mechanism for systematic delivery of care. A management program, suggested by the AHCPR guideline and based on best evidence synthesis (Bergstrom, Bennett, & Carlson, 1994), suggests including the following factors: assessment of wounds, selection of support surfaces to reduce the amount and duration of exposure to pressure, incontinence management, and selection of dressings, wound cleansing agents,

moisture barriers, and skin cleansing agents. Treatment plans must be written, communicated, and carried out regularly. Wounds should be evaluated at each dressing change and at periodic intervals to ensure that healing is occurring and the wound is not worsening. Signs of beginning healing are usually evident in 2 weeks for large ulcers. It is also important to monitor the patient for signs of complications, such as local and systemic infection and osteomyelitis.

A wound assessment guide developed by Barbara Bates-Jensen (1990) is useful for quantifying the size and depth of the wound and other wound characteristics. Another wound assessment schema is also under development by the National Pressure Ulcers Advisory Panel. Wound assessment serves as the basis for planning care and monitoring progress.

Pressure reduction, using specialty beds, has been shown to provide an environment for wound healing. Reducing exposure to pressure is central to the healing of pressure ulcers. Some support surfaces are more effective than others in achieving this objective, but even those that provide for lower interface pressures often have high interface pressures over the heels. It is important to provide for pressure relief by keeping the heels off the mattress surface, keeping in mind the fact that the support surface alone is not sufficient to heal wounds.

Wound care includes debridement, cleansing, and appropriate dressing. Pressure ulcers must first be debrided to reduce the bioburden and promote healing. This can be accomplished in a number of ways, depending on the condition of the wound and the condition of the patient. At each dressing change, the wound should be cleansed, using products that are not cytotoxic (usually normal saline) and mild pressure. Products such as betadine and other skin cleansers should be avoided. Dressings that provide for a moist (not wet) wound environment should be used. The moist environment can be achieved with gauze moistened with normal saline or with occlusive dressings. Occlusive dressings are more expensive but do not need the frequent changing required to keep saline gauze moist.

Skin surrounding the wound should be kept dry and supple. Wound contamination and damage to surrounding tissue are important issues for incontinent individuals. Skin cleansing, toileting, special collection devices, and moisture barriers for the skin are all important. Adequate nutrition is a key factor in wound healing. Provision of calories and protein sufficient to meet the individual's requirements should be ensured.

Perhaps the most useful concept to emerge from the pressure ulcer treatment guideline is the expectation that wounds make progress toward healing in 2 weeks. Clear expectations of healing, a comprehensive plan of care, and continuous monitoring of the effectiveness of the treatment plan can promote healing and prevent pressure ulcers from becoming chronic wounds.

NANCY BERGSTROM

See also
DIABETES MELLITUS
GERONTOLOGICAL CARE
INFECTION CONTROL
NUTRITION
URINARY INCONTINENCE

PREVENTION OF PRETERM AND LOW-BIRTHWEIGHT BIRTHS

Preterm birth occurs before 37 completed weeks of gestation. A low birthweight birth (LBW) is birth of an infant weighing less than 2500 g (5 lb, 8 oz). Preterm labor is labor between 20 and 37 weeks gestation in which there is documented cervical change. LBW is frequently used as an outcome variable in studies because it is more easily documented than gestational age. However, approximately 30% of LBW infants are born at more than 37 weeks gestation and are thus term LBW rather than preterm.

In the United States preterm birth is the major cause of perinatal mortality and morbidity, affecting more than 300,000 infants each year. Infants born prematurely represent a major health care cost. Although a great deal of attention has been focused on preterm LBW birth in the past two decades, the incidence has not declined. The overall rate of LBW birth is 7%, and rates for African American infants are twice as high as those of White infants.

There is no single proximal etiology for preterm birth; some infants are delivered early because of maternal or fetal health indications; some labor begins with preterm premature rupture of membranes; in other instances contractions with effacement and dilatation initiate the birth process.

The work of Papiernik in France in the 1970s led to research in the United States in the early 1980s focusing on risk assessment, nurse education of the pregnant woman that stressed early identification and appropriate response to the signs of preterm labor, and education of health care providers to respond promptly to a woman's reported symptoms. Herron, Katz, and Creasy (1982) reported a reduction in preterm birth using this protocol, but replications of their study provided mixed results. Subsequent research has focused on a number of issues deemed relevant to a reduction in the incidence of preterm and LBW births.

Risk Assessment

Although risk assessment has been considered a cornerstone of preterm birth prevention, a nursing study reported that the Creasy assessment identified only 31% of women experiencing preterm deliveries. A high risk score predicted preterm birth in only 44% of women identified at high risk (Edenfield, Thomas, Thompson, & Marcotte, 1995). One major limitation of many risk assessment instruments is their reliance on physiological parameters and past reproductive history; variables such as domestic violence and substance abuse, which have been linked to preterm birth, are not included.

Prenatal Care

Although it is clear that women who receive prenatal care, particularly care beginning in the first trimester, have a lower incidence preterm births, it is unclear if this is related to the prenatal care per se or to other differences in the women. A change in the content and timing of prenatal care, with increased emphasis on risk assessment, health education and promotion, and psychosocial as well as obstetric interventions was recommended by an

Expert Panel of the United States Public Health Service (Caring for our future, 1989). Two studies examined women's lack of information about pregnancy and preterm labor. Freda, Damus, and Merkatz (1991) found that one third of an inner-city population did not know that preterm infants could have health problems; one-half did not know the number of weeks in a normal pregnancy.

Libbus and Sable (1991) found a relationship between LBW births and lack of advice about calling a health care provider if preterm labor was suspected. Patterson (Patterson, Douglas, Patterson, & Bradle, 1992) reported that ambiguous symptoms, the lack of a meaningful label to attach to those symptoms, and the normal discomforts of pregnancy create diagnostic confusion, making it difficult for women to know what actions to take. She found that recourse to a professional was a strategy of last resort for the women she interviewed.

Nursing and Other Interventions

Enhancement of prenatal care through nursing care coordination, the use of paraprofessionals working under nursing supervision (maternal outreach workers, peer counselors) has been explored in a variety of sites, primarily with low income women. Specific nursing intervention to decreased preterm/LBW births have included home visits and nurse telephone intervention. Olds found that nurse home visits that included parent education enhancement of social support and linkage to community services reduced LBW births in adolescents under 17 and in smokers. In contrast, Moore reported that telephone calls from a nurse with a similar focus were most effective for African American women over 18 years of age and for nonsmokers.

Modification of lifestyle has long been associated with prevention of preterm LBW births. For more than 40 years, research has demonstrated a relationship between cigarette smoking and preterm LBW. Studies have demonstrated the efficacy of smoking cessation programs for pregnant women. Other significant lifestyle factors include the abuse of substances other than cigarettes and the importance of nutrition and a balance of exercise and rest. Three nursing studies have demonstrated the value of relaxation techniques in small samples.

Pharmacological intervention with tocolytic medications include beta-sympathomimetics (ritodrine, terbutaline), magnesium sulfate, and calcium channel blockers. In spite of more than a decade in which tocolytics have been widely used, there has been no decrease in preterm or LBW births.

Technological intervention by home uterine activity monitoring, accompanied by daily nurse telephone contact, was introduced in the 1980s. Several studies purported to show a reduced incidence of preterm births; methodological concerns in some led to questions about the results. In one study some women received monitoring plus the nurse telephone call and others received only telephone intervention; there was no difference in outcome between the two groups. A second device is a pump designed to deliver the tocolytic drug terbutaline.

The role of infection, particularly bacterial vaginosis, in both idiopathic preterm labor and preterm premature rupture of the membranes, has become an increasing focus of research. Evidence for the role of infection comes from studies that link a variety of organisms with increased rates of prematurity and studies showing decreased rates of prematurity in women treated with antibiotics.

Other Issues

Although domestic violence is rarely listed as a risk factor for preterm birth, it was first related to preterm birth in the work of Bullock and McFarlane (1989), who found that the relationship held when controlling for race, smoking, alcohol use, prenatal care, and other complications in a sample of 589 women. The role of psychosocial variables in preterm birth has been studied by nurse researchers and others. Unfortunately, although some studies have linked stress and anxiety with preterm and LBW birth, others have not.

The possible link between the work environment and preterm birth was suggested in the 1980s by Mamelle in France. In a study of nurses in the United States a 33% rate of preterm labor was found in nurses who worked in adult intensive care units, in contrast to a 7% rate among nurses on other units (Fraulo, Munster, & Pathman, 1991).

In addition to studies focusing on reducing preterm and LBW births, nurse researchers have investigated the perceptions of mothers and of nurses about the needs of women experiencing preterm labor and the experiences of women using the terbutaline pump. Mackey and Coster-Schultz (1993) used a naturalistic approach to identify the ways in which women describe, interpret, and manage preterm birth. May (1994) examined the effect of preterm labor on fathers. She found a high level of worry at the time of initial diagnosis; subsequently, fathers were distressed over child care, household management, maintaining a supportive environment for their partners, and lack of support for themselves.

Research aimed at reducing the incidence of preterm and LBW birth is complex. It is unlikely that a single strategy or set of strategies will be effective in all women.

Future research should address the following questions:

1. Can we develop better prediction of risk?
2. Is it reasonable to expect that a single intervention will be the most appropriate and effective in all instances of preterm labor?
3. What type or combination of nursing interventions are most effective for which women?
4. Why are rates of preterm and low birthweight birth so high in African American women?
5. Can better designed studies clarify the relationship between stress, social support, and preterm birth?

MARY LOU MOORE

See also
CHILDBIRTH EDUCATION
FETAL MONITORING
NICU PRETERM INFANT CARE
PREGNANCY
PRENATAL CARE: A COMMUNITY APPROACH

PRIMARY CARE

Primary care is prevention-oriented general wellness and illness care of individuals and families.

Primary care is characterized as being accessible, affordable, continuing, comprehensive, and coordinated. This form of personal health care delivery evolved to its contemporary state in the 1960s from earlier public health nursing and general medicine practices. Now primary care in the United States is seen as foundational and the gateway to secondary and tertiary care, especially in managed care systems. However, the present health care system and funding mechanisms have resulted in inequitable distribution of primary care to vulnerable populations, especially those residing in rural areas and inner cities.

Organizations and researchers have defined primary care according to the type of provider, the actual service, the level of acuity of the illness, the delivery setting, and the client-provider relationship (American Academy of Nursing, 1976; Marion, 1996; Starfield, 1992). The Institute of Medicine (Donaldson, Yordy, Lohr, & Vanselow, 1996) defined primary care as "the provision of integrated, accessible health care services by clinicians who are accountable for addressing a large majority of personal health care needs, developing a sustained partnership with patients, and practicing within the context of family and community" (p. 33).

The nursing perspective is largely congruent with that of the Institute of Medicine, except that the family as well as the individual is considered to be a primary care client. Also, nurses place primary care within the context of primary health care, a set of beliefs and principles concerning rights and responsibilities of individuals, communities, and providers as partners (World Health Organization, 1978). Finally, nurses emphasize their teaching/coaching and caring roles in providing primary care.

As a client-centered form of health care, primary care is based on a mutually trusting client-provider relationship. This form of health care delivery is continuing and therefore entails first contact care and care over time as the client experiences all types of health care demands. Continuity of care requires coordination of referrals to other sources of health care, such as health specialists, alternative providers, and delivery settings, as necessary. The clinicians collaborate with specialists to ensure quality care of complex illnesses, to avoid unnecessary referrals, and to maintain continuing protocols after specialty care.

Primary care is comprehensive because clinicians provide complete health assessments, health promotion and disease prevention, and diagnosis and treatment of common illnesses. Prevention includes not only disease-specific activities such as immunizations but also a belief or approach that extends to all levels of wellness and illness care. Finally, primary care encompasses care for the client who is dying and therefore the responsibility for assuring dignity and comfort until death.

Nursing and medicine have responded to the demand for general health care by developing advanced training programs for primary care clinicians (Marion, 1996). Nurses who deliver primary care include advanced practice nurses (APNs), that is, nurse practitioners, certified nurse midwives, clinical nurse specialists, and generalist nurses with basic nursing preparation. Primary care physicians are prepared in family and internal medicine, obstetrics and gynecology, and pediatrics. Health care specialists often provide primary care services to their clientele, and these specialists may or may not ensure that a full range of primary care services are delivered within the specialty system. The ideal primary care team is multidisciplinary, with nursing, medical, and other professionals collaborating in a mutually respectful way to capitalize on each member's individual strengths.

Primary care research can generally be categorized into health services delivery, effectiveness of diagnostic methods and care regimens for specific health needs, and client-provider interaction research. Primary care as a method of health service delivery includes health services access and utilization; cost; process and outcomes according to type of provider, health care system, setting, geographic region, and payment mechanism; client satisfaction; barriers to care; and continuity of care models. Defining primary care, determining essential primary care competencies, and identifying preferred providers for specific activities are topics for further research. Distance care, such as telecommunications support of self-care, is a health services modality that will require more attention from researchers. Related to health services delivery research is health care policy research. The effects of policy on primary care and the effects of primary care trends on policy are explored and described in this field of research.

Effectiveness among diagnostic methods and care regimens for client-specific health needs is a main focus of primary care research. Primary care client needs span most of the health continuum, from health promotion to palliative care. Various forms of effectiveness research encompass the development and evaluation of (a) screening protocols based on the epidemiology of the problem and the community; (b) diagnostic procedures; (c) pharmacotherapeutics; (d) exercise, nutrition, and other health promotion prescriptions; (e) alternative therapies; (f) comfort measures; and others. Effectiveness measures include benefits such as health/illness and functional status, quality of life, costs, and client (individual and family) satisfaction. A goal of this research is to establish evidenced-based practice guidelines that are acceptable to consumers and clinicians.

Client-provider interaction is of great interest to primary care researchers. Interaction is a vehicle to gain and deliver information, demonstrate caring and support, and plan health care on a mutual basis. Besides the development of a trusting relationship, interaction is largely directed at improving client health behaviors and supporting adherence to recommended regimens for specific health problems. Because the client is ultimately responsible for these activities, client-provider interaction is crucial to the health outcome.

Research on nursing within a primary care context has mostly centered on APN processes and outcomes in comparison to those of physicians or physician assistants using medical care models (Marion, 1996). Also, primary care APN data are often buried within physician and insurance data sets. However, these numerous APN studies together provide a convincing picture of competence and cost-effectiveness. In 1996 the American Academy of Nursing, with initial funding from the Agency for Health Care Policy and Research, U.S. Department of Health and Human Services, began to explore the possibility of a primary care research network. This network of primary care nurses would provide data to describe their practices, clientele, and health delivery systems. The data then would be merged with those of a large sample of nurses. The success of the research network will depend on the creation of data collection tools with reliable and valid measures that capture APN practice, the commitment of network nurses, and funding to initiate and maintain a large database. The National Organization of Nurse Practitioner Faculties (NONPF) is developing a nurse practitioner research issues paper and has begun to explore the research priorities identified by the membership. Other organizations and funding sources promote the study of primary care, especially for vulnerable populations.

LUCY N. MARION

See also

ADVANCED PRACTICE NURSES
HEALTH SYSTEMS DELIVERY
PRIMARY HEALTH CARE
TELENURSING/TELEPRACTICE
WELLNESS

PRIMARY HEALTH CARE

Definition

Primary health care (PHC) is based on an understanding of health as "a state of complete physical, mental and social well-being, and not merely the absence of disease or infirmity" ("Alma-Ata Conference," 1978, p. 428). The interdependence and complementary nature of health with social and economic development is a basic premise of PHC. A PHC approach emphasizes full development of human potential, community mobilization, and collaborative decision making between health professionals and community members.

The World Health Organization (WHO) and the United Nations Children's Fund (UNICEF) sponsored the International Conference on Primary Health Care held in Alma-Ata, USSR, in 1978. The Declaration of Alma-Ata, endorsed by member governments of the United Nations at the 32nd World Health Assembly in 1979, provided foundational explication and definition for PHC.

Primary health care is essential health care based on practical, scientifically sound and socially acceptable methods and technology made universally accessible to individuals and families in the community and through their full participation and at a cost that the community and country can afford to maintain at every stage of their development in the spirit of self-reliance and self-determination. It forms an integral part both of the country's health system, of which it is the central function and main focus, and of the overall social and economic development of the community. It is the first level of contact of individuals, the family and community with the national health system bringing health care as close as possible to where people live and work, and constitutes the first element of a continuing health care process. ("Alma-Ata Conference," 1978, p. 429)

Five basic principles for implementation of PHC are (a) equitable distribution ensuring accessibility of health services to all of the population, (b) maximum community involvement in the planning and operation of health care services, (c) focus on the prevention of disease and the promotion of health, (d) use of appropriate technology and local resources that are socially acceptable and sustainable, and (e) multisectoral approach that integrates health programs with social and economic development (WHO, 1985).

Implementation of primary health care is contextually grounded. The development of PHC policies and services is based on the predominant health concerns of communities and adapted to the cultural, political, and economic conditions of each country or community. Decentralization enables local community involvement in planning and implementation. Through collaboration, community members and health professionals shape programs and services to the particular sociocultural circumstances of the community.

Primary health care teams interact to coordinate community health activities. The composition of a primary health care team is determined by program needs, availability of health professionals, and local practices. Lay community health workers (CHWs) and traditional practitioners are often provided with basic health education. CHWs serve on health teams with nurses, midwives, social workers, physicians, or other appropriate multisectoral personnel. Although preventive and promotive activities are given priority, curative and rehabilitative services are provided within a referral network.

A predominant function of the health team is provision of education for communities and clients. Health education includes relevant information about common health concerns but goes beyond this to enable community mobilization for full participation in community-based health programs. PHC team members facilitate community involvement in the assessment process that identifies local resources and capabilities for community health and development. The PHC process promotes health through self-learning, self-determination, self-care, and self-reliance.

Primary care is a component of PHC. Although the terms *primary health care* and *primary care* are often used interchangeably, they have distinctive characteristics that have been elucidated in nursing literature (Barnes et al., 1995). Primary care concentrates on the individual users of health services within a PHC framework that focuses on the community as a whole (Marion, 1996).

The essence of PHC is community involvement in defining and addressing problems; practical understanding of the integral relationships among social, economic, and health conditions of a community; commitment to essential health services; and collaboration between community residents, health professionals, and a multisectoral network of other professionals. Therefore, PHC is an interactive approach to health care in which community residents are expected to be knowledgeable in health matters and to participate actively in their health care management. Moreover, PHC addresses self-care practices for physical and mental aspects of community health, as well as community social and environmental conditions. The basic goal of PHC is the attainment of optimum health for all.

PHC research is innately complex. An effect of the evolutionary nature of a community's identification of health priorities and planning is a lack of predetermined outcome measures. There is a need for longitudinal multisectoral studies that use research strategies consistent with PHC concepts and that accommodate community development and involvement processes. The nursing research literature on PHC is sparse and focused predominantly on conceptual development or descriptive analysis of PHC implementation.

Over the years various international and national nursing organizations have promoted PHC as a means for meeting the health needs of the public, with special attention to vulnerable and underserved populations. To this end, Dr. Halfdan Mahler (WHO, 1986), the director-general of WHO until 1988, recognized the potential for nurses to be a powerhouse for change if they mobilized around advancement of PHC ideas and convictions. An illustration of nursing leadership in PHC is the National Nursing Research Agenda for Community-Based Health Care (NINR, 1995). An NIH priority expert panel adopted PHC as a key concept for community-based health care and as a strategy for developing nursing knowledge for practice in urban and rural settings. Overall, PHC concepts offer a framework for constructing future directions for nursing within a rapidly changing health care environment.

BEVERLY J. MCELMURRY
GWEN BRUMBAUGH KEENEY

See also
ACCESS TO HEALTH CARE
COMMUNITY HEALTH
PRIMARY CARE
WELLNESS
WORLD HEALTH ORGANIZATION

PRIMARY NURSING

Primary nursing is a nursing care delivery system that places the nurse-patient relationship at its center. One nurse is accountable and responsible for planning, management, delivery, and evaluation of a patient and his or her family's nursing care. Primary nurses practice with a small group of associate nurses who care for the patient in their absence. Continuity between nurse and patient is essential. Primary nursing flourishes best in an environment that recognizes the unique contributions of the professional nurse and supports the various components of professional practice. Typically, a decentralized approach to nursing management featuring a clinical nurse manager, participation in professional committees, and strong systems of accountability are present. Autonomy and authority over nursing practice are emphasized.

Primary nursing was initially conceived in the early 1970s by Manthey, Ciske, Robertson, and Harris (1970). Giovannetti (1980) extended this work, and Clifford (Clifford & Horvath, 1990) is widely recognized for expanding a nursing care delivery system into a professional practice model. Historically, primary nursing has been anecdotally identified as a strong predictor of patient and nurse satisfaction. Research on primary nursing has been fraught with conceptual and methodological challenges (Giovannetti, 1986). Many studies lack conceptual and operational definitions, theoretical frameworks are not explicitly stated, instrumentation is frequently flawed, and research design less than rigorous.

Despite this lack of research rigor, primary nursing was widely implemented. Many of the original magnet hospitals, for instance, used a primary nursing model. Lack of cost-benefit analyses and measures of efficacy contributed to a building sense in many hospitals that primary nursing was no longer affordable, and many of the myths associated with primary nursing were promulgated. Many believed, for example, that a 100% RN skill mix was necessary for primary nursing.

Recent pressures to decrease the cost of inpatient hospital care and wide spread adoption of reengineering principles have resulted in new patient care delivery models. Many of the patient-focused care models herald a return to the team or functional nursing care delivery models of the past. Concepts such as the nurse-patient relationship, professional nursing practice, and continuity between nurse and patient are conspicuously absent in many of the new patient-focused care models. Rather than recognizing primary nursing as one of the earliest process redesigns in health care, elaborate new systems are being promoted that actually create numerous hand-offs between team members. Clinical nurses are in jeopardy of being pulled further from patients to coordinate an increased volume of support tasks. Interestingly, many of the methodological flaws present in the initial evaluation of primary nursing have returned to the evaluation of patient-focused care models. Instruments lacking validity and reliability, inappropriate sampling methods, and lack of operational definitions prevail. Once again, major decisions are being made about nursing care delivery without rigorous evaluation.

Those institutions that have reaffirmed a commitment to primary nursing and professional practice models offer another opportunity to scientifically assess the outcomes of this nursing care delivery system. Rigorous qualitative and quantitative methods are required in this important area of investigation.

MAUREEN P. MCCAUSLAND

See also
NURSE-PATIENT RELATIONSHIP
NURSING PRACTICE MODELS
PATIENT SATISFACTION WITH NURSING CARE

PSYCHOSOCIAL EFFECTS OF CHILD CRITICAL ILLNESS AND HOSPITALIZATION

Child critical illness is defined as a condition that requires hospitalization of the child (newborn through 18 years of age) in an intensive care unit (ICU). These conditions include surgical and medical diagnoses resulting in emergency or scheduled admission. Although specific criteria vary across hospitals, children admitted to an ICU generally require frequent monitoring and intensive nursing care; some are physiologically unstable and require ICU therapies to maintain one or more physiological functions.

Psychosocial effects include behavioral, emotional, cognitive, developmental, and social outcomes that occur either during hospitalization or after discharge. Both parents and children experience psychosocial effects. Indeed, most research in this area has focused on psychosocial effects for parents. Considerable research has been conducted on effects for critically ill newborns and their siblings, with much less research on critically ill children beyond the newborn period. This discussion will refer only to the effects on children beyond the newborn period who are critically ill.

Incidence

In 1993 there were about 328 pediatric ICUs (PICUs) in the United States, with an average of 528

($SD = 24$) critically ill children admitted to each PICU each year (Pollack, Cuerdon, & Getson, 1993), or more than 165,000 children annually. However, this number underestimates the real number of critically ill children, as some are hospitalized in adult ICUs. Mortality rates are low, about 5% in the United States (Pollack et al., 1993). Most PICU children require the use of invasive physiological monitoring and a 1:1 nurse:patient ratio during their PICU stay. Almost 95% of PICU children are developmentally normal prior to the illness event that necessitated their admissions, and fully 75% of PICU survivors achieve complete physical recovery (Fiser, 1992).

Effects of Critical Illness

Clinicians frequently express concerns about the effects of critical illness and PICU hospitalization for children. Studies of PICU children's responses have found anxiety, anger, apprehension, fearfulness, and regressive behavior. In one study, PICU children's responses were more severe than the reactions of acutely ill children hospitalized in a general care unit, and the PICU child's apprehension and degree of confusion or disorientation increased as severity of illness increased (Jones, Fiser, & Livingston, 1992).

After transfer to a general care unit, PICU children frequently remember painful, invasive procedures as well as monitors and other equipment, restraints, health care providers, and admission of other children to the PICU (Barnes, 1975). Indeed, almost half (44%) of the stressors that PICU children identified were invasive procedures causing pain and discomfort; another 26% were environmental factors (Tichy, Braam, Meyer, & Rattan, 1988). Separation from parents also was an important stressor (Gabriel & Danilowicz, 1978). Although transfer to a general care unit is a sign that the child's condition is improving, children and families often reported feeling more secure in the PICU because of the ready availability of nurses.

Studies of short-term effects of PICU hospitalization have indicated both positive and negative outcomes. PICU hospitalization was a growth experience for some children, resulting in greater physi-

cal and emotional maturity and greater self-confidence. Negative outcomes included sleep disturbances and regressive, apprehensive, fearful, or demanding behaviors for up to 1–2 months postdischarge (Gabriel & Danilowicz, 1978). However, the reactions of PICU children were not compared to those of children hospitalized on a general care floor. Indeed, when compared to published norms for posthospitalization behavior, ratings of child general anxiety by mothers of PICU children were lower, but ratings of separation anxiety, sleep anxiety, eating disturbances, aggression, and apathy or withdrawal were similar to ratings of mothers of general care unit children (Youngblut & Shiao, 1993).

The possibility of long-term negative outcomes for child survivors of critical illness was raised by a study of children who recovered from an illness that was expected to be fatal (Green & Solnit, 1964). For years after the illness, children demonstrated separation anxiety, sleep disturbances, infantilization, and school phobia and underachievement. Green and Solnit named this the "vulnerable child syndrome," believing that its occurrence resulted from the parents' perception of these children as considerably more vulnerable to illness because of the child's near-death experience. Because parents of PICU children often have the fear that their child might die, regardless of the child's prognosis (Youngblut & Jay, 1991), child survivors of a critical illness may be at risk for developing this syndrome.

Implications for Nursing Research and Practice

With so few recent studies, implications for practice are premature. However, recommendations for research are numerous. Contemporary studies of PICU children's experiences and short- and long-term responses are needed. Effects of factors such as age, sex, degree of sedation, and type and severity of illness or condition, which may dampen or heighten these responses, should be identified. Comparison of responses by PICU children and general care unit children is imperative to separate the effects of hospitalization and severity of illness.

Interventions to ameliorate any negative effects then can be designed and tested.

JoAnne M. Youngblut

See also

CANCER IN CHILDREN
CHRONIC CONDITIONS IN CHILDHOOD
PAIN IN CHILDREN
SOCIETY FOR RESEARCH IN CHILD DE-
    VELOPMENT

PSYCHOSOCIAL INTERVENTIONS

The health outcomes of clients may be improved through psychosocial or psychoeducational interventions. Psychosocial interventions include individual and group psychotherapies and educational interventions. An intervention may be defined as a programmatic attempt at altering the course of some life span developmental phenomenon. Interventions may be classified as concrete technologies involving such parameters as the goal: enrichment, prevention, or alleviation; the target behavior: cognition, social interactions, or attitude; the setting: family, classroom, community, or hospital; and the mechanism: training-practice, psychotherapy, or health delivery (Baltes & Danish, 1980).

Nurses are implementing psychosocial and psychoeducational interventions and testing the results of their efforts for many health problems and chronic illnesses. There are a number of integrative literature reviews, including meta-analyses conducted by nurse researchers. Meta-analyses will be reviewed to provide depth and breadth to this summary.

Surgical Patients

Devine and Cook (1986) evaluated 49 studics for the effect of brief psychoeducational interventions on the length of postsurgical hospitalization. The interventions consisted of information, skills training, and psychosocial support and were provided by nurses, physicians, psychologists, pastoral coun-

selors, and social workers. The results showed that these interventions had a positive influence on recovery, pain, psychological well-being, and satisfaction with care among hospitalized adult surgery patients. Not only did these patients have better outcomes; there were positive cost effects across a wide range of patients, treatment providers, and hospital settings. The interventions reduced the hospital stay on average by 1 1/4 days.

Hypertensive Patients

In a meta-analysis of 102 studies, Devine and Reifschneider (1995) evaluated the effects of psychoeducational care on blood pressure, knowledge about hypertension, medication compliance, weight, compliance with health care appointments, and anxiety. A nurse was the primary author in 23% of the studies. Three psychoeducational interventions—education, behavioral monitoring, and relaxation—had small to medium benefits for blood pressure. Usually, the nonrelaxation interventions were directed to promoting adherence and were conducted in outpatient health care facilities. The majority of participants were taking antihypertensive medications, and blood pressure measurement was part of the routine care. In studies with relaxation only and relaxation with biofeedback, the interventions occurred in lab-type settings, and subjects were not taking antihypertensive medications.

Cancer Patients

Devine and Westlake (1995) evaluated psychoeducational intervention studies provided to 5,326 adults with cancer by means of meta-analysis. In this review the results were analyzed to determine how educational and psychosocial care provided to adults with cancer affected seven outcomes: anxiety, depression, mood, nausea, vomiting, pain, and knowledge. A nurse was the primary author in 34% of the studies. The authors found a statistically significant beneficial effect for all seven outcomes. However, it was not possible to determine which type of psychoeducational care—for example, education, muscle relaxation, other relaxation, muscle relaxation with guided imagery, multiple behavioral interventions with relaxation, or education and relaxation—was the most beneficial.

Caregivers

Taft (1995) in a qualitative study interviewed 40 family and professional caregivers with the aim of describing and classifying the specific interventions that could be used as alternatives to physical and chemical restraints in dementia care. She found seven domains of caregiving approaches: (a) social (providing activities, relating, empathic caring, and supportive touching); (b) psychological (being responsive, seeing the world from the recipient's perspective, offering choices, following the recipient's lead, and reframing); (c) functional (assisting with activities of daily living, providing cues, providing supervision, providing rest periods, and assisting with instrumental activities of daily living); (d) behavioral (diversion, noninterference, going along, time-away, delaying, confrontation, and using fibs); (e) environmental (modifying stimuli, providing safety, limiting access, providing personal identification, and using signs); (f) medical (using psychotropic and other medications); and (g) cognitive (helping to remember and reorienting).

Relaxation Training

Hyman, Feldman, Harris, Levin, and Malloy (1989) reviewed 48 experimental studies of nonmechanically assisted, educational relaxation techniques to control a variety of clinical symptoms. Treatment interventions consisted of nonpharmacological methods, such as Benson's relaxation technique, Jacobson's progressive muscle relaxation, rhythmic breathing, Lamaze, autogenic training, hypnosis, transcendental meditation, yoga, Zen, and imagery. Biofeedback was included only when an alternative relaxation technique was used as an additional treatment in the study because biofeedback requires complicated technology not readily available to practicing nurses. Subjects suffered from chronic continuous or acute clinical symptoms, and the average age was 41. In summary, all treatments except Benson's relaxation technique demonstrated positive results for chronic problems such as insomnia, headaches, and hypertension.

Technology Interventions

The use of computers as a psychosocial intervention is a novel idea in nursing. The findings from studies in two populations of caregivers of the elderly with Alzheimer's disease and persons living with AIDS are innovative (Brennan, Moore, & Smyth, 1995; Ripich, Moore, & Brennan, 1992). A project nurse monitored each of the Computer Links and was seen as a group facilitator and a troubleshooter for the participants. The nurse read all public areas daily and maintained the currency of the electronic encyclopedia. In this role the nurse moderator interacted with users via typed messages by reviewing all public messages and also reviewed any personal mail and typed responses to individuals or to the group. There were 102 Alzheimer's disease caregivers, who averaged two encounters per week for sessions lasting an average of 13 minutes. The decision-making confidence of the caregivers was enhanced through this unique psychosocial intervention. There were 31 persons living with AIDS who used the network for catharsis and self-disclosure. They identified group cohesiveness with their new family as very important. Overall, persons living with AIDS with high rates of Computer Link use expressed high levels of satisfaction with the network.

Psychosocial and psychoeducational interventions are a primary method of improving the health of clients and patients entrusted to nurses' care. There is a beginning knowledge base, documented on the outcomes of these interventions to improve the health status of individuals. Nurse scientists and practitioners must continue to develop, test, and document the effects of these interventions and their impact on phenomena of concern to nursing.

GRAHAM MCDOUGALL

See also
BEHAVIORAL RESEARCH
COGNITIVE INTERVENTIONS

PATIENT EDUCATION
PSYCHOSOCIAL INTERVENTIONS DE-
  CREASE MORTALITY AFTER CORO-
  NARY ARTERY DISEASE
RELAXATION TECHNIQUES

PSYCHOSOCIAL INTERVENTIONS DECREASE MORTALITY AFTER CORONARY ARTERY DISEASE

Many studies have linked psychosocial distress with mortality in patients with acute myocardial infarction (Ahern et al., 1990; Frasure-Smith, Lesperance, & Talajic, 1993). Recently, Linden, Stossel, and Maurice (1996) published a meta-analysis of 23 randomized clinical trials studying psychosocial interventions for patients recovering from coronary artery disease. Mortality was measured in 12 of the trials. Patients with coronary artery disease who did not receive psychosocial interventions had a significantly greater risk of mortality during the first 2 years of follow-up, with log-adjusted odds ratio of 1.70; 95% confidence interval, 1.09–2.64. Interestingly, the 2,024 patients who received psychosocial interventions also showed greater reductions in psychological distress, systolic blood pressure, heart rate, and cholesterol levels.

A review of the literature by the Agency for Health Care Policy and Research (AHCPR; 1995) Cardiac Rehabilitation Guideline Panel led to the following recommendation: "Education, counseling, and behavioral interventions reduce cardiac and overall mortality rates and are recommended in the multifactorial rehabilitation management of patients with CHD" (p. 130). They reported the findings on eight randomized, controlled trials describing the effects of psychosocial interventions on mortality in cardiac patients (Frasure-Smith & Prince, 1985; Friedman, Thoresen, Gill et al., 1986; Haskell et al., 1994; Ibrahim et al., 1974; Karvetti & Hamalainen, 1993; Rahe, Ward, & Hayes, 1979; van Dixhoorn, Duivenvorden, Stall, Pool, & Verhage, 1987). Three of the randomized studies showed a statistically significant psychosocial treatment effect to reduce the risk of mortality (Frasure-Smith & Prince, 1989; Friedman et al., 1986; Karvetti & Hamalainen, 1993). Three randomized studies did not show a statistically significant difference

in mortality rates after psychosocial intervention (Ibrahim et al., 1974; Rahe et al., 1979; van Dixhoorn et al., 1987). Only two of the studies were consistent with the meta-analyses by Linden, Stossel, and Maurice (1996): Rahe et al., (1979) and Frasure-Smith and Prince (1989).

Most of the patients studied have had a myocardial infarction. The components of the psychosocial interventions varied greatly among the aforementioned randomized trials: cognitive-behavioral therapy, group psychotherapy, relaxation techniques, group education, individual "psychological support," breathing relaxation strategies, music therapy, social support with spouse, education about coronary risk behaviors and their modification, Type A behavioral counseling, progressive muscle relaxation, cognitive affect learning, exercise prescription, smoking cessation, nutritional education (i.e., decreased salt, decreased cholesterol, weight reduction), and case management by telephone calls and home visits.

Thus, the theoretical rationales for the therapies have been diverse, including (a) social learning theories for altering health beliefs, self-efficacy, and risk factor modification; (b) cognitive behavioral theories for alleviation of depression and anxiety and enhancement of positive coping; (c) relaxation and stress reduction for altered autonomic nervous system functions; and (d) standardized health education. The common element in all the treatments, however, is the underlying assumption that psychological distress contributes to poor prognosis in cardiac disease and that psychosocial interventions are beneficial in decreasing the risk of mortality as well as showing greater reductions in psychological distress, mostly depression and anxiety (Linden, Stossel, & Maurice, 1996).

The process of implementation of the therapies from the aforementioned clinical trials was also diverse. The length of the therapy ranged from 4 to 50 sessions; the length of the sessions ranged from 30 to 90 minutes. Both individual and group support sessions were effective. However, the data from the meta-analyses by Linden et al. (1996) suggest that lengthier interventions spread over a long time, especially when given individually, will lead to the greatest effects.

The type of person administering the therapy in the randomized clinical trials appeared to provide uniform positive effects (Linden et al., 1996). They included nurses, cardiologists, social workers, psychiatrists, psychologists, and physicians, alone and in combinations with each other.

Given the apparent overall benefit of psychosocial interventions to decrease mortality in cardiac patients and the lack of a clear explanation about how they work, more research is needed to identify which components of the multifactorial interventions are most effective in altering specific determinants of psychosocial distress. For example, depression may be more effectively treated with cognitive-behavioral therapy than with stress management. Treating major depression after an acute myocardial infarction is an urgent intervention, given the known negative impact of depression on 2-year mortality after myocardial infarction (Ahern et al., 1990; Frasure-Smith, Lesperance, & Talajic, 1993).

The benefits of psychosocial therapy for reducing mortality is evident during the first 2 years after an acute myocardial infarction, reflecting about a 41% reduction in all-cause mortality (Linden, Stos-

sel, & Maurice, 1996). At 3-year follow-up, all-cause mortality was 19% in the treatment group and 31% in the control group, a significant decrease of 12% (Karvetti & Hamalainen, 1993). At 5-year follow-up, the death rates did not differ significantly between groups (van Dixhoorn et al., 1987).

In summary, psychosocial interventions decrease risk of mortality in persons with coronary artery disease. The mechanisms by which the intervention affects mortality is not known. There is a wide diversity in the nature of the content, length, number of sessions, and the protocol of the psychosocial interventions.

MARIE J. COWAN

See also
BEHAVIORAL RESEARCH
CARDIOVASCULAR NURSING
DEPRESSION AND CARDIAC DISEASE
PSYCHOSOCIAL INTERVENTIONS
STRESS MANAGEMENT

Q

QUALITATIVE RESEARCH

Taken literally, qualitative research includes all modes of inquiry that do not rely on numbers or statistical methods. However, the terms *qualitative* and *quantitative* research are misnomers, albeit commonly used. The terms *qualitative* and *quantitative* actually refer to the forms of the data, not to specific research designs. It is more accurate to discuss naturalistic and positivistic designs during which qualitative or quantitative data may be collected. For this reason, the subject usually considered under the topic of qualitative research will be called naturalistic inquiry here.

Naturalistic approaches comprise a wide array of research traditions, most often in the categories

of ethnography, grounded theory, and phenomenology but also including ethnology, ethnomethodology, hermeneutics, oral/life histories, discourse analysis, case study methods, and critical, philosophical, and historical approaches to inquiry. Each tradition has a distinct set of undergirding philosophical or theoretical orientations, strategies for data collection and analysis, and forms of research products.

The ultimate purpose of all research is the generation of new knowledge. However, different modes of inquiry produce different kinds of knowledge. Knowledge developed from naturalistic methods is at the level of rich description or in-depth understanding. Naturalistic inquiry tends to be exploratory in nature and is particularly useful in identifying important contextual features of the phenomenon. Naturalistic approaches are called for when the purpose of the research is to obtain in-depth information about a phenomenon, when little is known about a topic, or when new perspectives are needed. Secondary purposes for naturalistic approaches include hypothesis generation, obtaining the range of possible items for instrument development, providing illustrative examples or cases, and delineating the context from which other data may be better interpreted.

There are several features that are common to most naturalistic studies. A basic tenet is that reality is socially constructed; as such, there are multiple realities for any phenomenon, given the multiple lenses through which different individuals perceive and experience a situation. Naturalistic approaches favor conducting research in the field setting (vs. an artificial laboratory) in order to observe phenomena as they are lived and to preserve the contextual elements of the phenomena. In contrast to positivist approaches, which use established instruments, in naturalistic inquiry the investigator is the instrument. However, investigators are aware that their own experiences, biases, and perceptual sets particularize both the data that they elicit from informants and ultimately the data analysis/interpretation. There are generally accepted standards for rigor in naturalistic approaches. These include the degree of intimacy of the investigator to the informants, the auditing of interviews and coding structures, trustworthiness, dependability, conformability, meaning-in-context, and saturation/redundancy.

Naturalistic approaches (also known as constructivist or inductive inquiry, Paradigm II, or field approaches) are often contrasted with positivist approaches (also called empiricism, Paradigm I, or experimental approaches). Naturalistic and positivistic modes of inquiry provide different types of data. However, these data sets are most fruitfully viewed as complementary rather than in opposition. Together they provide a more complete understanding than can be obtained by using either approach singly. Sometimes the methods can be employed simultaneously (methodological triangulation); at other times the methods must be applied sequentially in order to satisfy the requirements of each. The reciprocal interweaving of naturalistic and positivist research builds nursing knowledge as each contributes different but important information.

Historical Overview

Specific approaches to naturalistic inquiry were developed primarily in the social sciences and philosophy. For example, phenomenology as a method derived from phenomenological and existentialist philosophy, ethnography from anthropologists' study of culture, grounded theory, and ethnomethodology from sociology (specifically the school of symbolic interactionism).

In the discipline of nursing, there were several early reports of qualitative data without a specified naturalistic approach. In 1952 the first issues of the first volume of *Nursing Research*, articles report the qualitative results of unstructured interviews. Orlando (1961) used data from participant observation to describe case examples and advocated the use of open-ended interview techniques followed by validation to determine each patient's individual needs. Although not giving a formal name to this approach, she used data grounded in clinical nursing observations to inductively derive her theory concerning deliberative nursing practice.

In 1962 nurse scientist graduate training programs were initiated through the Division of Nursing for the purpose of increasing the number of nurse research scientists with doctorates in basic physiological or social sciences. As a result, many nurses completed programs that trained them in the qualitative methods developed in the social sciences. Many nurse anthropologists were trained during this period. Similarly, from 1962 to 1967, Benoliel served as a member of the three-person team (with Glaser and Strauss) studying dying and developing what was to be called grounded theory.

Over the decade of the 1960s the number and methodological specificity of naturalistic inquiry increased. By the end of the 1960s, *Nursing Research* had published articles specifically using grounded theory methods, ethnographic methods, and other naturalistic approaches. *Image: the Journal of Nursing Scholarship* was initiated in 1966 and also published research using naturalistic methods (although positivist approaches predominated in both journals). With the advent of the *Western Journal of Nursing Research* in 1978, edited by Brink, there emerged an outlet with a balanced representation of qualitative research. In 1976, Paterson and Zderad published a book based on phenomenological observations and Brink's (1976) book contained a series of methodological articles on conducting qualitative (largely ethnographic) research. Nearly a decade later two broad-based books on qualitative research were published (Field & Morse, 1985; Leininger, 1985). With the advent of the journal *Qualitative Health Research* in 1991, also edited by a nurse-anthropologist, Morse, an entire journal was fully dedicated to reporting naturalistic research.

Research conferences and societies also have been influential in fostering the development of naturalistic inquiry. The series Communicating Nursing Research, co-sponsored by the Western Interstate Commission for Higher Education and the Division of Nursing, and The Transcultural Nursing Care series organized by Leininger from 1977 to the present offered an opportunity for the presentation of naturalistic research. More recently, regional research societies such as the Midwest Nursing Research Society have added qualitative research sections that meet annually, sponsor symposia, and disseminate newsletters.

Variations across Methods

The selection of a particular naturalistic approach depends on the purpose of the research. For example, phenomenology is the method of choice when the purpose is to understand the meaning of the lived experience of a given phenomenon for informants; grounded theory is selected to uncover or understand basic social processes; and ethnography is selected to understand patterns and/or processes grounded in culture.

Although most qualitative approaches do not employ formal theoretical frameworks, they do rest on established philosophical assumptions. However, some naturalistic inquiry (particularly ethnography) is conducted in the context of theoretical orientations that reflect the training of the investigator and may focus attention on particular phenomena, relationships, data collection techniques, or research products.

In most forms of naturalistic inquiry, investigators typically use participant observation, informant interviews, and document analysis. However, the extent to which the investigator relies on any one strategy will vary. For example, phenomenology relies primarily on informant interviews, ethnography, and grounded theory and generally has a more even reliance on participant observation and interviewing, whereas ethnology relies primarily on observations.

Methods for data manipulation include strategies for taking notes, making memos, and coding and indexing systems. More recently, computerized software programs such as ETHNOGRAPH, NUD-*IST, and MARTIN have been fruitfully employed to aid in the management of data. Methods used in data analysis are inductive and include matrix, thematic, and domain analysis. Finally, the form of the final product may vary. In grounded theory, a substantive theory with a process model is common; in ethnoscience (a form of ethnography) a taxonomic structure is the product.

In summary, naturalistic inquiry most commonly occurs in field settings, with investigators collecting data through participant observation and unstructured interviews and analyzing data through thematic content analysis. It developed initially in the social sciences and began to be incorporated in nursing research in the 1960s and 1970s. Today it is an accepted scientific approach that complements knowledge derived from positivist inquiry.

TONI TRIPP-REIMER
LISA SKEMP KELLEY

See also
ETHNOGRAPHY
HERMENEUTICS
PARTICIPANT OBSERVATION
PHENOMENOLOGY
RESEARCH INTERVIEWS (QUALITATIVE)

QUALITY MANAGEMENT

Quality management is the process by which an organization mobilizes people to achieve quality goals (JCAHO, 1994); it is systems-focused, organizationally pervasive, and culturally supported. Although definitions and approaches to measuring quality vary, the important elements for assessment of health care in regard to quality goals are structure, process, and outcome. Over time, the health care industry and specifically the nursing profession have devoted significant resources and energy to a quality assurance process based on the development of standards of care and systematic evaluation of compliance with the standards. Contemporary total quality management (TQM) and continuous quality improvement (CQI) processes emphasize meeting and exceeding customer expectations rather than conforming to standards. Results of care are the focus when process and structure are examined for opportunity to improve outcomes. Critical pathways and statistical controls are important tools in assessing clinical processes, and cost-effective analyses inform choices related to the improvement of care.

Concern about the quality of care is part of nursing's legacy from Florence Nightingale, who systematically collected and analyzed information on differences in mortality rates across hospitals and evaluated the effects of improved nutrition and other innovations on the mortality of soldiers during the Crimean War. Historically, quality assessment has been a political issue driven by a variety of private and government agencies, whereas quality management focused on operations to demonstrate conformance to external standards and regulations. The beginning of formal efforts to address the quality of health care is marked by the establishment of the American College of Surgeons in 1913 to develop minimal standards of care for hospitals, and the Hospital Standardization Program implemented by that group is the precursor of the accreditation process provided by the Joint Commission on Accreditation of Healthcare Organizations (JCAHO). The American Nurses Association and nursing specialty organizations disseminate standards of care and other materials to support quality assurance. Federal regulators such as peer review organizations and the Health Care Financing Administration use data on costs and outcomes of care to develop changes in the system. Government units, for example, the Agency for Health Care Policy and Research, allocate funds for research related to the effectiveness of care. Consumers, particularly groups that focus on issues related to women and the elderly, have become important advocates for the evaluation of health care quality. The movement toward managed care and integrated health care delivery systems increased the emphasis on customer satisfaction and other quality indicators as providers competed for client service contracts, and quality management has emerged as a dominant corporate strategy.

Total quality management is an industrial phenomenon grounded in the turn-of-the-century scientific management movement that emphasized "management by facts." Although Deming is the best known proponent, Shewhart, Feigenbaum, Juran, and Crosby have made noteworthy contributions to the development of TQM. Health care organizations began to apply TQM methods as CQI in the mid-1980s, with leading work by Batalden, Hospital Corporation of America; Berwick, Harvard Community Health Center; and James, Intermountain Health System. Thus, TQM/CQI may be viewed as a continuum, with manufacturing at one end and health services at the other. Compared to the industrial model, the health care model places greater emphasis on the complexities of the client-provider relationship, the qualifications and characteristics of providers, and quality/cost trade-offs. Continuous quality improvement emphasizes clinical as well as administrative activities, and statistical controls may include comparisons to normative standards, comparisons within the organization over time, or comparison to similar institutions providing similar services. Both models avoid emphasis on personal blame. The principles of CQI have been incorporated into the JCAHO accreditation process.

Research related to quality management cycles as the technology changes. Generally, researchers pursue questions about the extent to which health care providers are adopting emerging approaches, the factors that influence their success, the costs associated with implementing the new technology, the impact of variations in the methods, and the effectiveness of quality management programs in improving patient outcomes. Donabedian's early publications (e.g., 1969) proposing structure, process, and outcome as a framework for examining the quality of health care have stimulated a continuing search by researchers for links among those constructs. Under conformance-to-standards goals, the relative merit of the three types of standards in assuring quality has been a primary issue. Under continuous-improvement goals, critical issues relate to identifying desirable outcome indicators for targeted client populations and demonstrating associations between those indicators and process and structure variables. Improvement opportunities surface around the structure and process variables that account for variability in outcomes. Nurse researchers are challenged to identify outcome indicators that are sensitive to nursing care.

Examples of recent research related to quality management include studies of the implementation of CQI/TQM (e.g., Carman et al., 1996; Shortell, O'Brien, Carman, et al., 1995), the effectiveness of interventions that incorporate CQI techniques in reducing ventilator-associated pneumonia among intensive care unit patients (Kelleghan et al., 1993), and hospital mortality rates among patients undergoing coronary artery bypass graft surgery (O'Connor et al., 1996). Improvements in nursing home resident dryness have been sustained for 6 months using an incontinence system that included a computerized quality management model (Schnelle, McNees, Crooks, & Ouslander, 1995).

ROMA LEE TAUNTON

See also
ADMINISTRATION RESEARCH
BENCHMARKING IN HEALTH CARE
OUTCOMES MEASURES
PATIENT SATISFACTION WITH NURS-
  ING CARE
QUALITY OF CARE, MEASURING

QUALITY OF CARE, MEASURING

Although attempts to measure nursing care quality are not new, the most vigorous activity occurred in the 1970s and again in the 1990s. The early activity was initiated when Donabedian's model of quality measurement, identifying the measurement

components of structure, process, and outcome, was published. Current activity is the result of an increasing expectation that health care providers must demonstrate the quality of the services they provide and the impact of these services on the health and welfare of patients.

An accepted definition of quality in health care remains elusive despite the multiplicity of books, articles, and speeches on the subject. Quality health care is difficult to define because quality reflects a judgment about the degree to which health care meets a standard of excellence. Who defines this standard in health care if the patient's perception of excellence is markedly different from the provider's? What aspects of care are included in the standard? Should quality include the appropriateness of care, the manner in which care is delivered, the amount of care, the cost of care, the outcomes of care? Although definitions of quality have focused on all of these aspects, there is agreement that quality is an attribute of the care process having to do with whether the right care was done (appropriateness) and whether it was done well. There is also agreement that quality health care achieves the most desired balance of benefits and risks; that is, the probability of desired patient outcomes outweighs the probability of undesired patient outcomes.

Measurement of nursing care quality requires the identification of elements essential for quality, psychometrically sound measures for these elements, and specification of the measurement process. Elements traditionally used to measure nursing care quality focus on human and financial resources and their organization (structure), technical and interpersonal activities of the clinician (process), and effects of nursing actions on patient health (outcome). The American Nurses Association has identified structure, process, and outcome elements for the evaluation of quality in acute care settings but has not specified measures for these elements. Identification of structure, process, and outcome criteria against which performance can be measured is critical for the measurement of nursing care quality but is no longer sufficient. Determination of how well customer expectations are met has become an essential element of quality measurement.

Although there have been numerous studies of nursing care quality, there are no universally accepted measures for structure, process, outcome, and patient satisfaction. Measures of structure have focused on financial resources and cost; human resource utilization, including staff mix and staff qualifications; patient classification variables that determine the intensity of nursing care; organization of nursing care delivery systems; interdisciplinary collaboration; and environmental factors, such as background hospital sounds, that affect patient outcomes. In general, tools used to measure care structure have varied between studies and have not been subjected to rigorous testing. One exception is the development and testing of patient classification instruments during the 1970s and 1980s; however, none of the instruments received wide use, and they are being replaced with measures such as Diagnosis Related Groups and nursing diagnoses to describe patient complexity. Another exception is the current use of financial tools based on economic models to measure resource consumption and service cost.

The development and testing of instruments to measure nursing process reached its peak in the 1970s. During this period the Phaneuf Nursing Audit, the Quality Patient Care Scale (QUALPACS), and the Rush-Medicus System, all of which measure nursing activities, were developed. Scales to measure nursing competency, such as the Slater Nursing Competencies Rating Scale, also were developed and tested. These instruments, or modifications, continue to be used in studies of nursing care quality although with less frequency. Currently, measures of care documentation and discharge management have received increased attention, as have criteria to monitor the appropriateness of nursing care. In addition to measuring the manner in which care is provided, process outcomes have measured nurses' role perception and satisfaction.

The identification of patient outcomes sensitive to nursing care and the development and testing of outcome measures is a priority if nursing is to demonstrate the impact of nursing care on the health and welfare of patients. Although considerable work was done during the 1970s and 1980s to identify outcome criteria and define ways of measuring these criteria, validation of the criteria was incomplete; and the criteria received minimal use in research and even less use in practice. Currently, a variety of instruments are used to measure patient

outcomes in nursing research studies. Tested instruments include those developed by nurses (Waltz & Strickland, 1988) as well as those developed in other disciplines. A number of outcome measures that have received little testing have also been used to measure patient outcomes (Rantz, 1995). Occurrence rates for undesirable patient outcomes also have been used as measures of nursing care quality. Although they serve to identify the risks associated with nursing care, they fail to identify the benefits. In practice settings patient outcomes are frequently stated as goals that are met or not met, a measurement insufficient for the determination of nursing care quality.

The majority of instruments currently available measure a specific outcome category, such as functional status, or measure outcomes of patients with specific medical or nursing diagnoses. A few research efforts (e.g., Iowa Outcomes Project) are underway to identify outcomes sensitive to nursing care that can be used with a variety of patient populations and in all settings in which nursing care is provided (Johnson & Maas, 1997; Ozbolt, Fruchtnight, & Hayden, 1994). The work by the Iowa Outcomes Project includes measures for each of the outcomes, but further work is needed to test the measures and to identify the risk adjustment factors that influence the level of outcome achievement.

Multiple measures of patient satisfaction with health care services, including nursing services, have been developed recently. Many of these have received minimal testing, but a few are undergoing more rigorous analysis. As with other measures of quality, the majority of instruments measuring satisfaction with nursing care were developed in the 1970s.

Measurement methodology has evolved as new statistical approaches have emerged and has become a distinct area of study beyond the scope of this article. In conjunction with new methods for analyzing data, processes for quality measurement such as benchmarking, quality assessment, total quality management, and performance improvement have emerged.

Measuring nursing care quality requires description and study of the causal relationships between nursing care structure, nursing process, patient outcomes, and patient satisfaction. This necessitates the development of clear descriptions and measures for each of the components and requires action to identify the essential indicators of nursing care quality, standardize measures and test for reliability and validity, code measures for use in electronic information systems, specify timing of data collection, identify and collect risk adjustment data, and determine the most accurate methods for the aggregation and analysis of data.

MARION JOHNSON

See also

BENCHMARKING IN HEALTH CARE
HEALTH SYSTEMS DELIVERY
NURSING OUTCOMES CLASSIFICATION (NOC)
PATIENT CLASSIFICATION
PATIENT SATISFACTION WITH NURSING CARE

QUALITY OF LIFE

Quality of life research is an extensive field, with scholars who have thought carefully about the parameters, indicators, diversity, and variability of the dimensions of quality of life (Benner, 1985; Spilker, Simpson, & Tilson, 1991). However, there is no universally accepted definition of quality of life. A consensus among researchers seems to be that its components should include a person's satisfaction with his or health and function, economic status, family life, and spiritual, occupational, and psychosocial well-being. The scope of the research typically includes a general assessment of perceived well-being and subsets of health-related components of quality of life. General overall assessment of quality of life typically gauges the health and functional abilities of the person; the health-related aspects are often measured as symptom experiences, disease management, economic effect of disease and treatment, and level of wellness.

Definitions of quality of life vary greatly. Early studies measured patient functional capacity, illness status, and longevity. Currently, components measured include impact of an illness and its treatment, socioeconomic status, and cultural or personal characteristics influencing a person's ability to have a fulfilling life. Many researchers now use a health-related framework that defines quality of life as measures of rehabilitation following disease or disability. Rehabilitation indexes often use measures of a person's ability to carry out routines of daily living and roles of life (e.g., homemaker, employee, student).

Numerous measures that represent quality of life have been developed, and many of the early definitions were unidimensional. Early definitions of quality of life were often measures or ratings of physical function made by the physician. Both the unidimensional and the outside rater approaches to measurement of quality of life have been criticized as too simplistic as well as inaccurate. Nurse researchers indicate that qualitative methods are preferable to questionnaires. However, the ability to follow changes over time by using quantitative methods is important for researchers (Jalowiec, 1992). Utilizing quantitative methods is also appropriate with large sample sizes. Discussions about the validity of using subjective versus objective measures of quality of life have ended in the notion that both are available but must be discussed in relation to the purpose of the research study.

In the 1980s the Adjusted Quality of Life Years Utility Index was developed (Torrance, 1987). This formula-oriented definition of quality of life included the cost of medical treatments over the expected number of years survival and patients' preferences for living with the treatment. This approach and definition added the economic factor and the individual's opinions to quality of life measures. The World Health Organization's 1995 position paper on quality of life assessment broadens the view of quality of life beyond health without illness.

The current regulations by the Food and Drug Administration requiring quality of life to be a component of drug studies have resulted in numerous specific and narrow measures of medication efficacy, commonly using single-item indicators and linear analog scales. Many instruments have been developed for specific populations of patients, resulting in illness-, functions-, and symptom-oriented measures that reflect treatment outcomes (Smith, 1993).

Nurse researchers and others have expanded the definitions of quality of life to include a person's satisfaction with health and function, economic status, family life, occupation, and psychosocial well-being (Padilla et al., 1983). In 1989 the Institute of Medicine staff published a monograph on the quality of life measures they recommended for use. Padilla's quality of life instrument for cancer patients was the only nurse-authored questionnaire in the monograph. Medical studies and clinical trials have often employed health-rating scales. Judgment analysis also has been used in assessing quality of life (McGee, O'Boyle, Hickey, O'Malley, & Joyce, 1991).

In a unique instrument, Ferrans and Powers (1992) measured not only a person's satisfaction with health, family, economic status, and psychospiritual well-being but also measured the importance of each of those areas to the person. This comparison between importance and satisfaction ratings by the person better reflects quality of life unique to each individual's life goals. Self-comparison of importance versus satisfaction also allows for following changes in a patient's quality of life over time. One conclusion common to all researchers, in the past and currently, is that quality of life for individuals with incomes below the poverty line will be low, regardless of health and family status or self-perceived well-being.

The paradigm has shifted to a multifactoral basis of measurement: multiple variables which obtain a variety of subjective perceptions of each patient that go beyond the physical aspects of life. There are differences in a single-person quality of life measure, which measures personal function, and a community-oriented concept, which reflects the person's ability to have an effect on the greater society. Nurses have also expanded the notion of quality of life beyond the individual and his or her disease state. Research with family caregivers and discussion of family and community quality of life are being formulated for further study by the authors.

CAROL E. SMITH
CAROL GASKAMP

See also
DECISION MAKING: ADVANCE DIRECTIVES

FAMILY HEALTH
FUNCTIONAL HEALTH
WELLNESS

QUANTITATIVE RESEARCH

Quantitative research consists of the collection, tabulation, summarization, and analysis of numerical data for the purpose of answering research questions or hypotheses. The term *quantitative research* is of recent origin and is distinguished from qualitative research in design, process, and the use of quantification techniques to measure and analyze the data. The vast majority of all nursing studies can be classified as quantitative.

Statistics

Quantitative research uses statistical methodology at every stage in the research process. At the inception of a research project, when the research questions are formulated, thought must be given to how the research variables are to be quantified, defined, measured, and analyzed. Study subjects are often selected for a research project through the statistical method of random sampling, which promotes an unbiased representation of the target population among the sample from whom generalizations will be made. Statistical methods are used to summarize study data, to determine sampling error, and in studies in which hypotheses are tested, to analyze whether results obtained exceed those that could be attributed to sampling error (chance) alone. The important role of statistical methodology in quantitative research should not obscure the fact that other methodologies and scientific disciplines play important roles in nursing research. These methods are used in the delineation of research questions and hypotheses, exposition of conceptual frameworks and hypotheses, design of data collection instruments and tools, and interpretation of study data, particularly determination of the clinical significance of the data and dissemination of findings.

Evolution

Much of the history of nursing research involves quantitative research. Florence Nightingale, who was a skilled statistician, used quantitative measures to describe and evaluate hospital performance (Nightingale, 1858). Studies of nursing in the United States, beginning in the 1940s, used quantitative techniques to survey and analyze nursing education and supply and distribution of nurses (Abdellah & Levine, 1986). In the 1960s, with support from the federal government, research in nursing began to use advanced research designs, such as controlled experiments, which made extensive use of quantitative tools, techniques, and processes (Hasselmeyer, 1961).

Scales for Collecting Quantitative Data

Quantitative data collected in quantitative research are obtained by the use of measurement scales. There are three distinct types of scales: nominal, ordinal, and continuous. Nominal scales consist of two or more ungraded or unranked categories of variables, such as eye color (green, blue, brown) or political affiliation (Republican, Democrat). Ordinal scales possess categories that are ranked or graded, from high to low, small to large, near to far. Graded scales, such as the Likert and Guttman scales, are commonly used in nursing research to measure intensity of opinions, attitudes, and other psychological variables. When nominal and ordinal scales are used, quantitative summaries of the data collected consist of aggregating the number of responses in each scale category, converting them to relative frequencies such as percentages, and if hypotheses are being tested in the research, applying one of many nonparametric techniques available to test the statistical significance of the data.

Continuous scales have continuous quantitative values rather than verbal categories, as in nominal and ordinal scales. These include the scientific measuring instruments widely used in nursing to measure variables such as temperature, weight, height, blood pressure. Continuous measurement scales have certain advantages over other scales because they yield more precise and sensitive data. Also, the statistical significance of continuous data can be analyzed by the more powerful parametric techniques.

Methods for Analyzing Data

Quantitative research is concerned with making generalizations from a study sample to a target population, a process called statistical inference. There are two categories of generalizations in quantitative research: (a) estimates of the quantitative value of selected characteristics of a target population and (b) results of tests of statistical hypotheses concerning relationships among variables in the target population. Studies in the first category are called descriptive studies; those in the second category are called analytical or explanatory studies. The focus of many early nursing studies was to describe nurses and nursing practice using questionnaire or interview techniques to collect data from large samples of respondents. Recent studies using conceptual frameworks from emerging nursing theories and models have tested hypotheses in controlled or semicontrolled settings.

Statistical techniques are used extensively in descriptive studies to compute summary measures, such as means, standard deviations, and coefficients of correlation, and to determine the sampling error of the measures. In explanatory studies statistical techniques are used to test whether there are significant relationships among study variables that are delineated in the hypotheses, meaning relationships that cannot be explained by random sampling error (chance). Widely used statistical techniques to test hypotheses include parametric tests such as the t test and analysis of variance and nonparametric tests such as chi-square and rank-order correlation.

Advantages

Quantification in nursing research has helped advance nursing as a scientific discipline (Abdellah & Levine, 1994). Quantification offers many advantages to nursing research. There is a rich set of statistical tools available for data analysis that can be applied to practically every research question to assist in summarizing the data and evaluating their statistical significance. The internal and external validity of the data of quantitative research can be readily verified by other researchers. Results of similar quantitative studies can be synthesized and analyzed by the meta-analysis technique to shed new light on the research questions. Dissemination of the results of quantitative research is facilitated by the clarity and objectivity possessed by quantitative data.

Limitations

Some studies in nursing tend to overquantify. Reports of these studies are dominated by statistical data and tests, with a minimum of narrative discussion, providing little interpretation of the clinical significance of results. Sometimes too little time is spent on evaluation of the quality of data used or on the appropriateness of the statistical tests. Qualitative research, with its focus on meaning and interpretation of data, can help to enrich the results of quantitative studies in nursing. The approach called triangulation, which utilizes and integrates methodology from quantitative and qualitative research in a single study, can help achieve the best of both worlds of research methodology.

Future of Quantitative Research

The history of nursing research reveals a trend from purely descriptive studies of nurses and nursing to the evaluation of the effects of nursing care. Properly applied quantitative research can advance the scientific basis of nursing as well as provide a potent tool for defining and evaluating the outcomes of nursing care. In the future, quantitative research will play an increasingly valuable role in nursing effectiveness studies. The randomized clinical trial (RCT) method, perhaps the most quantitative of all research methods, will find increasing application in nursing as attempts are made to determine the efficacy of nursing interventions (Abdellah & Levine, 1994; National Center for Nursing Research, 1992). The usefulness of the RCT method in nursing research was demonstrated by Brooten and colleagues (Brooten et al., 1986) in an evaluation of alternative methods of delivering nursing care to premature infants. Clinically oriented research using methods such as randomized clinical trials requires development of quantitative outcome measures of variables such as quality of care and quality of life. This will stimulate quantitative research to provide the needed measures and indicators. As more replications of quantitative nursing research become available, the research synthesis techniques of meta-analysis will be increasingly applied to expand nursing's knowledge base.

EUGENE LEVINE

See also
  DATA ANALYSIS
  DESCRIPTIVE RESEARCH
  **QUANTITATIVE RESEARCH METHOD-
    OLOGY**
  STATISTICAL TECHNIQUES
  TRIANGULATION

QUANTITATIVE RESEARCH METHODOLOGY

Research methodology is the term commonly used for the procedures employed to accomplish the specific aims of a research project. In other words, research methodology is the means by which we collect data to answer research questions or to test hypotheses.

The methods are derived from the research design and generally include sample, interventions (if applicable), instruments, data collection procedures, and plans for data analysis. A research design, according to Kerlinger (1986), "expresses both the structure of the research problem and the plan of investigation used to obtain empirical evidence on the relations of the problem" (p. 279).

There is no "best" design. The appropriate design is the one that fits the theoretical formulation underlying the research questions or hypotheses. Theory generation often requires qualitative approaches, whereas relation, association, and theory testing often require quantitative data.

Quantitative designs are often divided into experimental, quasi-experimental, or nonexperimental. We often think of experiments as having been around for a long time, but actually it was only in the 1930s that the first experiments were conducted. Sir Ronald Fisher's (1935) book *The Design of*

Experiments provided the first details of experimental techniques. The purpose of experimental design was to gain greater control and thus improve validity. The aim is to associate a treatment with its outcome by minimizing the effect of other variables on the outcome and reducing error introduced by extraneous or confounding variables. Random assignment to groups, manipulation of the independent variable, and control of extraneous variation are the key elements in experimental design.

Originally, experiments were conducted in laboratories; then the social sciences adopted the techniques, and other designs emerged, such as quasiexperimental designs. In quasi-experimental designs there is an experimental intervention, but one or more of the other elements of experimental design are missing. There may be no random assignment to groups. In such cases, the investigator should address the issue of group equivalence by comparing the groups on relevant variables. There may be no control group, as when a group of subjects is measured over time or under different conditions. This is usually referred to as a within-subjects design.

In nonexperimental designs there is no investigator-controlled intervention. Because the investigator does not control the independent variable, it is more difficult to test the direct effects of one variable on another. What is usually tested is the relationship between and among variables. This includes the testing of models through techniques such as path analysis and structural equation modeling.

One type of experimental design that is of special interest to health care professionals is the randomized clinical trial. In such an experimental design the intervention is tested in practice rather than in a controlled laboratory experiment. In the United States the first randomized clinical trial was reported in 1951 by Yale researcher Cadman (1994). He studied the effectiveness of penicillin in treating pneumococcal pneumonia. Another Yale researcher, Dumas (Dumas & Leonard, 1963), published the first report of the use of experimental design in nursing research. In 1963 she reported on nursing interventions to reduce postoperative vomiting.

In all designs, sample selection is crucial. Whether the sample consists of an *N* of 1, or of thousands, the sample must represent the population of interest. Additionally, the size of the sample must be adequate for subsequent analyses.

Sample designs are often divided into probability and nonprobability designs. Some form of random sampling is used in probability sampling. This enables the researcher to make use of probability theory to determine the accuracy of results through the computation of standard errors. The notion is that all potential subjects have an equal possibility of being included in the sample.

Nonprobability sampling includes several techniques, including selecting subjects based on some criteria (purposive or judgmental), taking those subjects that are available when the study is conducted (convenience or accidental), accruing a set number of subjects in various categories (quota), and advertising for volunteers.

The procedures for implementation of the study and for data collection are designed to maintain the integrity of the study. In experimental designs, methods for assignment to groups and implementation of the experimental conditions must be determined. Careful attention should be paid to ensuring that there is no contamination of experimental intervention across study groups.

Campbell and Stanley (1963) coined the phrases "internal" and "external" validity. Internal validity refers to the integrity of the study through which we can infer the relationships among the variables under study. External validity refers to how generalizable the results of the study are to other samples, settings, and so forth.

All variables included in the design must be defined and measured. Selection of psychometrically sound instruments and establishment of controlled methods for data collection are necessary for the integrity of the data. Data analysis is based on the questions being answered, the characteristics of the data collected, the size of the sample, and the assumptions underlying the statistical techniques.

Quantitative research methods from design through data collection and analysis must be carefully explicated prior to embarking on a study. Careful attention to all aspects of the methodology is necessary to produce valid results.

BARBARA MUNRO

See also
CLINICAL TRIALS

DATA COLLECTION METHODS
EXPERIMENTAL RESEARCH
QUASI-EXPERIMENTAL RESEARCH
STRUCTURAL EQUATION MODELING

QUASI-EXPERIMENTAL RESEARCH

Under "Experimental Research" in this encyclopedia, Cook and Campell's (1979) definition that experiments are characterized by manipulation, control, and randomization was cited. However, when conducting research in field settings, it is not always possible to implement a design that meets these three criteria. Quasi-experimental research is similar to experimental research in that there is manipulation of an independent variable. It differs from experimental research because either there is no control group, no random selection, no random assignment, and/or no active manipulation.

Quasi-experimental research is a useful way to test causality in settings when it is impossible or unethical to randomly assign subjects to treatment and control groups or to withhold treatment from some subjects. The main disadvantage of quasi-experimental research is the increased threat to internal validity (see "Experimental Research" for a review of types of design validity). Within quasi-experimental designs, a distinction is made between preexperimental, nonequivalent control group designs, and interrupted time series designs. Note also that the boundaries between experimental and quasi-experimental research have blurred. Often investigators like to define their study as experimental when in fact it is quasi-experimental.

Preexperimental Designs

Preexperimental designs are the weakest of the quasi-experimental designs. They may lack a control/comparison group, observation before the intervention (commonly known as pretests), or both. Their use is strongly discouraged because they do not permit even remote inferences about the direction and dynamics of change and causality.

Nonequivalent Control Group Designs

Nonequivalent control group designs refer to situations in which naturally occurring groups of subjects are used as control/comparison group or those in which it is impossible or unethical to withhold treatment from a given group. In spite of the absence of randomization, nonequivalent control group designs can be considered relatively strong designs. The use of a control group and a pretest significantly increase the strength of nonequivalent control group designs. Good pretest data will enable the researcher to improve the level of analysis. When subjects from different settings are used, a nonequivalent control group design may control some threats to internal validity, such as compensatory rivalry and demoralization of controls. When subjects in each group are naturally kept separate, it is less likely that they will have contact with each other, and it is often useful to minimize contact between treatment and control groups.

Interrupted Time Series Designs

In time series designs the researcher does not always use a control group and does not use randomization. An interrupted time series study uses several observations of subjects over time with a treatment given at a specified point (or longitudinally over time, with start and end time points). A time series study can be designed to study the same individuals at specified intervals or to study different individuals at some common point in time. When the researcher studies one group of subjects, the subjects act as their own controls, which provides the researcher with equivalent control groups. Time series designs are used when a control group population is not available. When only one group is available to the researcher, the time series design significantly increases the strength of the research.

Some Examples of Studies

Quasi-experimental studies can be found throughout research literature. Following are some examples of quasi-experimental design used by researchers. Atterbury, Groome, and Baker (1996) examined whether women who developed severe preeclampsia had a higher midtrimester main arterial pressure than a matched group of normotensive women. Gustafson et al. (Gustafson et al., 1991) tested the effects of oxygen therapy to reduce hypoxia in elderly hip fracture patients and reported a reduction in incidence and severity of postoperative acute confusion. MacVicar, Winningham, and Nickel (1989) found that aerobic exercise had a positive effect on fatigue experienced by cancer patients.

Ivo L. Abraham
Lynn I. Wasserbauer

See also
ETHICS OF RESEARCH
EXPERIMENTAL RESEARCH
QUANTITATIVE RESEARCH METHODOLOGY
TIME SERIES ANALYSIS
VALIDITY

R

RADIATION THERAPY

Radiation therapy is the use of ionizing x-rays in the treatment of cancer. Radiation oncology is the specialty within cancer care devoted to the care of patients receiving radiation therapy. The specialty of radiation oncology nursing is a well-defined, well-developed practice area within oncology. Radiation oncology nurses provide direct care for patients and their families through teaching, coaching, symptom management, and psychosocial support. In addition, they serve as coordinators of care and manage large radiation oncology facilities.

Radiation oncology nurses have traditionally participated in numerous clinical trials and served as data managers, research nurses, and co-investigators on research studies. They have increasingly focused on the challenge of studying problems related to the practice of nursing within radiation oncology, including symptom management and improvement of patient care outcomes.

Nursing research conducted within radiation oncology includes descriptive and correlational studies of informational needs during treatment, self-care management, patient and family education, symptom management, late effects, and cancer survivorship (Hassey Dow, 1997). These research areas rank high on overall research priorities within oncology nursing.

Informational Needs

Several studies were conducted that evaluated patients' informational needs during radiation therapy. For example, Dodd and Ahmed (1987) investigated patients' preference for type of information (cognitive vs. behavioral) in a longitudinal research design that included 60 subjects. Findings revealed that the majority of subjects ($n = 38$) preferred cognitive information over behavioral. Other findings showed that control and anxiety were associated with the type of preferred information when starting a course of radiation treatment.

Harrison-Woermke and Graydon (1993) evaluated informational needs of women receiving radiation therapy and breast-conserving surgery. Women were interviewed about information needs regarding diagnosis, investigative tests, treatment, physical and psychological functioning, family, and financial resources. Although the women desired information across all of these areas, they preferred highest in the need for information on treatment and physical side effects.

Education

Several studies described different approaches to educational needs (Israel & Mood, 1982; Llewelyn-

Thomas, Thiel, Sem, & Woermke, 1995; Padilla & Grant, 1987). These included the use of slide-tape program formats, newsletter formats, and interactive computer instruction. Israel and Mood (1982) used three slide-tape programs to educate patients about radiation side effects. Thirty-six subjects were included in this study. Patients were asked to respond to knowledge questions after viewing the tapes. Results showed that the tapes were effective in teaching information about radiation treatment and side effects.

Llewellyn-Thomas et al. (1995) evaluated the effects of two teaching approaches (audiotape and interactive computer instruction) in a hypothetical clinical trial. Patient satisfaction, understanding of information, and decisions to enter a clinical trial were assessed in 100 patients. Results showed that there were no significant differences between the two groups with respect to understanding or satisfaction.

Patient Experiences during Radiation Therapy

The vast majority of descriptive studies focused on patient experiences and side effect management during radiation therapy (King, Nail, Kraemer, Strohl, & Johnson, 1985; Margolin, Breneman, Denman, LaChapelle, & Weckbach, 1990). Studies included symptom experiences of skin changes, sleeping problems, nutritional changes (anorexia, nausea, vomiting, indigestion, dysphagia), diarrhea and constipation, and psychosocial studies of coping and comfort.

Fatigue is a high priority for research in oncology nursing. Graydon (1994) assessed quality of life in 53 women receiving breast-conserving surgery and radiation therapy for breast cancer. She found that women did not report significant emotional distress; however, they experienced fatigue. In a follow-up study, Graydon and colleges examined strategies that were most effective in relieving fatigue. They found that sleep and exercise were the two most common fatigue-reducing strategies. Mock et al. (Mock, Dow, & Meares, 1996) examined the effectiveness of a walking exercise program for women with breast cancer who were re-

ceiving radiation therapy. A convenience sample of 50 women were stratified into two groups (experimental or usual care groups). Results showed that women in the exercise group experienced better physical performance, decreased symptom intensity, and higher quality of life than the usual care group.

Intervention Studies

Intervention studies conducted within radiation oncology related to self-care behaviors during treatment and skin care management. Dodd (1984) conducted several self-care studies of patients receiving radiation therapy. She used a convenience sample of 30 patients to determine what self-care behaviors were demonstrated during radiation therapy. Patients reported an average of 3.3 side effects and initiated few self-care management activities of the side effects. Since this earlier study, Dodd has continued her program of research in self-care management of patients with cancer.

Studies of Late Effects of Radiation

Studies of late effects of radiation treatment and concerns in cancer survivorship include a study of cognitive functioning after treatment for leukemia (Moore, Kramer, & Albin, 1986) and pregnancy after radiation therapy for breast cancer (Hassey Dow, 1994).

Future Research Goals

Several multisite studies are in the planning stages. The Radiation Special Interest Group (SIG) of the Oncology Nursing Society is involved in a multisite collaborative endeavor to further evaluate skin care reactions and assess interventions to radiation therapy treatment. In addition, future research conducted in radiation oncology will extend our knowledge in the areas of symptom management, patient education, outcomes of care, and research utilization.

KAREN HASSEY DOW

See also
BREAST CANCER
CANCER SURVIVORSHIP
FATIGUE
PATIENT EDUCATION

REDUCING HIV RISK–ASSOCIATED SEXUAL BEHAVIORS AMONG ADOLESCENTS

Acquired immune deficiency syndrome (AIDS) is caused by infection with the human immunodeficiency virus (HIV) and continues to be a major, complex, and multidimensional public health crisis. One in 250 people in the United States is infected with HIV, with African American and Latino communities experiencing disproportionate rates of infection. Only 12% of the nation's population is Black, yet 31% of persons with AIDS are Black (Centers for Disease Control, 1991); 52% of patients are female and 52% pediatric. Only 5% of the nation's population is Hispanic, yet 17% of persons with AIDS are Hispanic. Hence, Blacks and Hispanics represent a total of only 17% of the nation's total population yet make up 49% of all the people with AIDS.

Currently, the epidemic in the United States is shifting to adolescents at an alarming rate, particularly those who are out of school, homosexual, and members of racial and ethnic minorities. Efforts to find a cure for HIV have been unsuccessful. However, the disease can be prevented, and interventions are urgently needed to reduce HIV risk–associated behaviors, particularly among adolescents. A description of effective cognitive-behavioral research intervention strategies and implications for nursing practice and research follows.

HIV Risk–Associated Sexual Behavior among Adolescents

Adolescents currently represent only 1% of all reported AIDS cases in the United States. However, this statistic may dangerously underestimate the potential for AIDS among adolescents. Young adults in their 20s constitute 20% of all reported AIDS cases. Because several years typically elapse between the time a person is infected with HIV and the appearance of clinical signs sufficient to warrant a diagnosis of AIDS, many young adults acquired the infection as adolescents.

Looking at newly diagnosed cases of HIV infection helps to clarify the risk of HIV infection among adolescents. Individuals 13 to 24 years of age comprised 16% of the new cases of HIV infection reported between July 1995 and June 1996 and 18% of the cumulative HIV infections reported as of June 1996. Unintended pregnancy and sexually transmitted disease (STD) rates also suggest an elevated risk of HIV infection among adolescents. Despite recent reports that the teenage birthrate dropped 5% between 1991 and 1994, the teen birthrate was still higher in 1994 than in any year during the period from 1974 to 1989, and it remains a national concern. The rates of gonorrhea and chlamydia continue to be higher among adolescents than in any other age group.

These statistics on pregnancy and STDs are consistent with data on adolescent sexual behavior. About 56% of adolescent women and 73% of adolescent men have had sexual intercourse by the time they are 18 years of age. The risks associated with unprotected sexual activity are especially great among inner-city Black adolescents (Jemmott & Jemmott, 1996). Although the use of latex condoms has risen substantially since 1982, far too many adolescents still fail to use condoms consistently and have sexual intercourse with multiple partners. The younger the adolescents are the first time they have sexual intercourse, the less likely they are to use condoms on that occasion. In addition, longitudinal studies suggest that among adolescents who ever used condoms the use declines as the individual gets older.

These data suggest that adolescents are at risk for STDs including HIV. HIV infection can be prevented by changes in sexual behavior, but the important question is how to create changes. Efforts to dissuade adolescents from engaging in risky sexual behavior may be most effective if based on a solid theoretical foundation. Theory can be used in the development of intervention procedures and also can drive the selection of variables to be assessed. By measuring the putative theory-based mediators of intervention-induced behavior change, a better conceptual understanding of risk behavior will emerge. In this connection, it is useful to consider theories such as (a) the social cognitive theory (Bandura, 1986; Jemmott, Jemmott, Spears, Hewitt, & Cruz-Collins, 1992; Jemmott & Jemmott, 1992); (b) the theory of reasoned action (Jemmott & Jemmott, 1991, 1992); (c) its extension, the theory of planned behavior (Ajzen, 1985; Jemmott, Jemmott, & Hacker, 1992; Jemmott, Jemmott, Fong, & McCaffree, 1997). These theories highlight the importance of beliefs, outcome expectancy, perceived norms, skills, self-efficacy, and intentions as determinants of HIV risk–associated behavior.

Effective Cognitive-Behavioral Interventions for Adolescents

A growing body of evidence indicates that well-controlled cognitive-behavioral interventions (Bandura, 1986) can reduce HIV risk–associated sexual behavior among adolescents and the theory-based determinants of such behavior. These interventions share a common approach based on social learning behavioral principles and use intensive, small-group risk reduction interventions. In addition, these interventions have been delivered in small-group programs with 5 to 18 hours of contact time, allowing participants to practice risk reduction skills and review successes and problems encountered in enacting these behaviors.

These interventions produce evidence of change in self-reported sexual risk behavior, usually on the order of 30% to 70% reduction in the frequency of unprotected sex. For instance J. B. Jemmott, L. S. Jemmott, and Fong (1992) reported successfully reducing HIV risk behaviors at a 3-month follow-up session with a culturally sensitive intervention tailored for African American male adolescents. Measured against a control group receiving a career opportunity workshop, the experimental group reported less sexual activity, fewer partners, and less frequent sexual intercourse after 3 months. Additionally, the experimental group reported more consistent condom use and decreased frequency of anal intercourse. The authors reasoned that teaching adolescents to eroticize the use of condoms might help remove attitudinal barriers to condom use but also would be a formidable normative barrier to condom use.

HIV risk–reduction interventions for runaway and street youth are also effective in changing behavior. A study implemented at two runaway shelters (one intervention and one nonintervention site) in New York City for African American and Latino adolescents reported a significant behavior change at 3 and 6 months following a small-group intervention averaging 11 sessions (Rotheram-Borus, Koopman, Haignere, & Davies, 1991). Those youth who attended a higher number of intervention sessions showed significant increases in consistent condom use and decreases in high-risk behaviors.

Two studies demonstrated effective behavior change results among adolescents in clinical settings. The first study was designed to test the effects on condom-use intentions of an AIDS prevention intervention based on social cognitive theory among sexually active African American adolescent women recruited from an inner-city family planning clinic (J. B. Jemmott, L. S. Jemmott, Spears, et al., 1992). The participants who received the intervention reported greater intentions to use condoms, and scored higher in perceived self-efficacy and favorable hedonistic expectancies than did those in the two control conditions. These results highlight the value of a social-cognitive approach to AIDS risk behavior: outcome expectancies regarding the effects of precautionary practices on sexual enjoyment and perceived self-efficacy to implement such practices play an important role in decisions about condom use.

The second study (St. Lawrence et al., 1995) tested a theory-based intervention to reduce risk of sexually transmitted HIV infection. The study examined whether behavioral skills could be increased and behavior change could be sustained at a long-term follow-up among African American adolescents at a comprehensive health center. The adolescents in the cognitive-behavioral skills intervention scored significantly better on behavioral skills measures, HIV knowledge, response efficacy, and perceived self-efficacy postintervention than did those in the control condition. The skill-trained participants also reported reduced unprotected intercourse, with fewer adolescents in the intervention group initiating intercourse. These effects on behavior were sustained through the 12-month follow-up.

In a study with young middle school–aged adolescents in a community setting, Jemmott, Jemmott, Fong, et al. (1997) addressed the important question of whether it is possible for a theory-based, culture-sensitive HIV intervention to be effective when the race and gender of participants and facilitators are not matched or when the groups are not homogeneous on gender. The study revealed several important findings. The participants in the cognitive-behavioral HIV intervention had greater HIV knowledge, more favorable behavioral beliefs about condoms, greater perceived self-efficacy, and stronger condom-use intentions; and they reported less HIV risk–associated sexual behavior, including unprotected sexual intercourse, than did their counterparts in the health promotion intervention. The effects of the HIV intervention were about the same irrespective of the race or gender of the facilitator, the gender of the participants, and the gender composition of the intervention group.

In a school setting, Walter et al. (1993) tested effects of an HIV risk–reduction intervention implemented by regular classroom teachers in public high schools in New York City. Three-month follow-up data collected on 72% of the original participants revealed significant effects of the intervention. The students who received the intervention scored higher in HIV risk–reduction knowledge, perceived susceptibility, beliefs about benefits of condom use, normative support for condom use, and self-efficacy; and they reported significantly less HIV risk–associated behavior than did those who did not receive the intervention. They reported fewer high-risk partners, more monogamy, and more consistent condom use.

In a study using collaborative strategies with a community based organization, Jemmott and Jemmott (1992) studied the effects of a culturally sensitive, theory-based AIDS risk–reduction intervention implemented by community agency staff. Analyses revealed that the adolescent women scored higher in intentions to use condoms, AIDS knowledge, outcome expectancies regarding condom use, and self-efficacy to use condoms after the intervention than before the intervention. Although increased self-efficacy and more favorable outcome expectancies regarding the effects of condoms on sexual enjoyment and sexual partner's support for condom use were significantly related to increased condom-use intentions, increases in general AIDS knowledge and specific prevention-related beliefs were not. Outcome expectancies regarding the effects of precautionary practices on sexual enjoyment and self-efficacy to implement such practices played an important role in decisions about condom use.

This body of research supports the view that effective interventions (a) are tailored to the study population or culture, (b) are based on formative research with members of the study populations, and (c) have an explicit theoretical basis. A strength of this research is that it not only considers whether the interventions are effective in changing behavior but also considers theoretical mechanisms, the variables hypothesized to mediate intervention effects. This research suggests that the significant behavioral effects are due to changes in HIV risk–reduction knowledge, outcome expectancy, self-efficacy, skills, and behavioral intentions induced by the interventions.

Disseminating Effective Interventions

As effective HIV infection interventions are identified, an important concern that arises is whether those interventions are disseminated to likely end-users. There is always the possibility that successful interventions will remain buried in the pages of scientific and public health journals, unavailable to those who might be in the best position to apply them. Unfortunately, the ideal of translating research results into community-based programs is seldom realized; however, there has been progress along these lines. One example is the curriculum dissemination project of the Division of Adolescent and School Health (DASH) of the Centers for Disease Control and Prevention, entitled ''Research to Classrooms: Programs That Work.'' The project identifies HIV infection–prevention curricula that are user-friendly and have credible evidence of effectiveness in changing the behavior of youth, and then it brings them to the attention of educators and others concerned with the welfare of youth. One of the four curricula selected is entitled "Be Proud! Be Responsible! Strategies to Empower Youth to Reduce Their Risk for HIV" (Jemmott, Jemmott, & McCaffree, 1995). This model curriculum is currently being nationally disseminated, and 26 states are implementing it.

Implications for Nursing Practice

Reports of adolescents' sexual behavior indicate that most youths engage in unprotected acts that place them at risk for contracting HIV. The present review of the literature suggests that interventions to increase African American adolescents' use of condoms must address hedonistic beliefs regarding the consequences of safer sex practices for sexual enjoyment. Thus, nursing interventions should attempt to weaken the common belief that sexual enjoyment is curtailed if condoms are used. Quite apart from adolescents' beliefs about condoms, HIV risk–reduction interventions should address the reactions of adolescents' sexual partners, particularly the sexual partner's approval or disapproval of safer sex practices, including abstinence. Nursing interventions should address skills and perceived self-efficacy. Perhaps the most widely recognized type of skill or perceived efficacy is negotiation or resistance skill—the ability of the individual to persuade a sexual partner to use a condom and/or to resist partner pressure to practice unprotected sexual intercourse. Technical skill in condom use also is important, particularly skill at using condoms without ruining the mood.

Implications for Research

Research suggests that carefully designed, theory-based interventions that take into account the behaviors and the characteristics of a particular population or culture can curb HIV risk–associated sexual behavior among adolescents in a variety of set-tings. Behavior change is the best and perhaps only means of preventing HIV infection. Our success in preventing new HIV infections throughout the new millennium will depend on how well we learn from, adapt, and expand on the prevention lessons of the first decade of AIDS.

Nevertheless, several issues merit investigation in future studies. There is a need for (a) more studies on the long-term effects of interventions on early adolescents and preadolescents, (b) studies comparing the effects of different intervention strategies, and (c) studies on the generalizability of intervention effects when the interventions are implemented by people other than university-based researchers—for example, community-based organizations. Because cultural factors may affect the ability of individuals to change behavior, there is also a need for culturally appropriate strategies to understand values, attitudes, behaviors, and factors such as socioeconomic status in different communities. Researchers from different ethnic or cultural backgrounds may help to address this issue. Language and cultural barriers to delivery of interventions must be addressed, with special consideration for individuals whose physical or other impairments limit access to most programs.

Conclusion

Research conducted with adolescents demonstrate that interventions to prevent HIV infection can significantly affect HIV risk–associated sexual behavior, including condom acquisition, condom use, unprotected sexual intercourse, frequency of sexual intercourse, and number of sexual partners. As we know, success in preventing HIV infection often requires helping people make and maintain highly consistent behavior changes, often with very little margin for error or lapses—a challenge virtually unprecedented in the behavioral sciences. Nurses are confronted with unique challenges and opportunities in the prevention of HIV infection.

Although nurses have long been called on to improve the quality of human life, the HIV epidemic challenges us—perhaps more urgently than any other issue in nursing history—to quickly develop better approaches that can save lives. We have always played an important role in the area of health promotion and primary prevention. Therefore, we are a very important link in the chain of HIV infection prevention in this country. Today, with no cure for HIV or AIDS available, it is crucial that we focus on prevention. Nurses can play an integral part in the battle against HIV infection. We have the expertise, opportunity, and philosophical basis on which to design and implement effective HIV/AIDS prevention interventions that will save many lives. Our increased involvement as nurse researchers will help answer these research questions and enhance the quality of research for HIV infection prevention. We urge all nurse researchers to work together to do it.

LORETTA SWEET JEMMOTT
JOHN B. JEMMOTT, III

See also
ADOLESCENCE
CULTURAL/TRANSCULTURAL FOCUS
HIV/AIDS: CARE AND TREATMENT
SELF-EFFICACY
SEXUALITY RESEARCH

RELAXATION TECHNIQUES

A relaxation technique is any intervention that produces the relaxation response. This response is characterized by decreases in blood pressure, pulse, respiratory rate, muscle tension, anxiety, and increases in skin temperature. Recent developments in the field of psychoneuroimmunology and society's renewed attention to holistic approaches to health care are expanding the parameters being examined as outcomes of relaxation techniques. Indices such as T lymphocyte and natural killer cell (NK) counts are being used to measure outcomes of relaxation interventions. In the past, nurses tended to measure only psychological outcomes, such as anxiety, as outcomes of relaxation training interventions. However, an increasing number of stress management studies conducted by nurse researchers are measuring both psychological and physiological parameters (Hyman, Feldman, Harris, Levin, & Malloy, 1989; Snyder, 1997).

Since the pioneering work of Edmund Jacobson on progressive muscle relaxation in the 1930s, numerous interventions that produce the relaxation response have been identified. Commonly used relaxation techniques include autogenic therapy, biofeedback, humor, imagery, music, massage, progressive muscle relaxation, sensation information, and therapeutic touch.

Nurses, along with researchers in the biobehavioral sciences, have conducted research about the efficacy of many of these techniques. Although an increasing number of studies using relaxation interventions are being conducted by nurses, few programs of research have evolved. Sensation information (Johnson, Rice, & Endress, 1978) and therapeutic touch (Quinn, 1984) are examples of interventions for which programs of research have evolved. Explorations by nurse researchers on the efficacy of imagery, massage, and music in reducing stress are increasing (Snyder, 1997). Eight studies on imagery were published in nursing journals during the 1991–95 time span, as well as seven studies using massage and four studies using music.

Despite the increase in the number of published reports, many studies continue to be characterized by small sample sizes and lack of methodological sophistication. Thus, a sound scientific basis to guide practitioners in selecting specific relaxation techniques for use with a client is lacking. Attention also must be given to other variables that may have an impact on study results. For example, in several studies on massage the results differed for male and female subjects (Snyder, 1997).

Another factor that impedes the development of a scientific basis for relaxation techniques is the widespread use of the term *relaxation training* without authors specifying the technique being tested. Because numerous techniques can be used to produce relaxation, it is important that descriptions of the techniques be provided to inform other researchers and practitioners of the outcomes from specific relaxation techniques. When multiple interventions are included, study designs should provide for the examination of each intervention.

Complementary therapies, which encompass many of the relaxation interventions, are being more widely accepted and used. Findings from well-constructed studies are needed to guide the use of such interventions. Nurse researchers can play a key role in furthering the scientific basis for relaxation interventions.

MARIAH SNYDER

See also
BIOFEEDBACK TRAINING
MUSIC THERAPY
NONTRADITIONAL THERAPIES

RELIABILITY

Reliability refers to the consistency of responses on self-report, norm-referenced measures of attitudes and behavior. Reliability arises from classical measurement theory, which holds that any score obtained from an instrument will be a composite of the individual's true pattern and error variability. The error is made up of random and systematic components. Maximizing the instrument's reliability helps to reduce the random error associated with the scores, although the validity of the instrument helps to minimize systematic error (see "Validity"). The "true" score or variance in measurement relies on the consistency of the instrument as reflected by form and content, the stability of the responses over time, and the freedom from response bias or differences that could contribute to error. Error related to content results from the way questions are asked and the mode of instrument administration. Time can contribute to error by the frequency of measurement and the time frame imposed by the questions asked. Error due to response differences results from the state or mood of the respondent, wording of questions that may lead to a response bias, and the testing or conceptual experience of the subject.

There are generally two forms of reliability assessment designed to deal with random error: stability and equivalence. Stability is the reproducibility of responses over time. Equivalence is the consistency of responses across a set of items so that there is evidence of a systematic pattern. Both of these forms apply to self-report as well as to observations made by a rater. For self-report measures, stability is examined through test-retest procedures; equivalence is assessed through alternative forms and internal consistency techniques. For observational measurement intra- and interrater techniques assess the two forms of reliability respectively.

Stability reliability is considered by some to be the only true way to measure the consistency of responses on an instrument. In fact, stability was the primary manner in which early instruments were examined for reliability. Stability is measured primarily through test-retest procedures in which the same instrument is given to the same subjects at two different points in time, commonly 2 weeks apart. The scores are then correlated, or compared for consistency, using some form of agreement score that depends on the level of measurement. Typically, data are continuous; thus, correlation coefficients and difference between mean scores are usually assessed. A correlation tells the investigator whether individuals who scored high on the first administration also scored high on the second. It does not provide information on whether the scores are the same. Only a test that looks at the difference in mean scores will give that information.

The problem with stability is that it is not always reasonable to assume that the concept will remain unchanged over time. If the person's true score on a concept changes within 2 weeks, instability and high random error will be assumed—when, in effect, it is possible that the instrument is consistently measuring change across time. Knapp (1995) points out that reliance on a 2-week interval for measuring stability may be faulty. The time interval chosen must directly relate to the theoretical understanding of the concept being measured.

A special case of stability occurs with instruments that are completed by raters on the basis of their observations. Intrarater reliability refers to the need for ratings to remain stable across the course of data collection and not change due to increased familiarity and practice with the instrument. The same assessment procedures are used for intrarater reliability as for test-retest reliability.

Equivalence is evaluated in two major ways. The first of these predated the availability of high-speed computers and easily accessed statistical packages. This set of techniques deals with the comparison of scores on alternate or parallel forms of the instrument to which the subject responds at the same point in time. Parallelism means an item on one form has a comparable item on the second form, indexing the same aspect of the concept, and that the means and variances of these items are equal. These scores are compared through correlation or mean differences in a similar manner to stability. Consistency is assumed if the scores are equivalent. Assessment with alternative/parallel forms is not comparison with two different measures of the concept. It is comparison of two essentially identical tests that were developed at the same time through the same procedures. Therefore, a difficulty with this approach to equivalent reliability is obtaining a true parallel or alternative form of an instrument.

A more common way to look at equivalence is through internal consistency procedures. The assumption underlying internal consistency is that the response to a set of scale items should be equivalent. All internal consistency approaches are based in correlational procedures. An earlier form of internal consistency is split-half reliability, in which responses to half the items on a scale are randomly selected and compared to responses on the other half.

Currently Cronbach's (1951) alpha reliability coefficient is the most prevalent technique for assessing internal consistency. Developed in the 1950s, the formula basically computes the ratio of variability between individual responses to the total variability in responses, with total variability being a composite of the individual variability and the measurement error. As a ratio, the values obtained can range from 0 to 1, with 1 indicating perfect reliability and no measurement error. The ratio then reflects the proportion of the total variance in the response that is due to real differences between subjects. A general guideline for use of Cronbach's alpha to assess an instrument is that well-established instruments must demonstrate a coefficient value above .80, whereas newly developed instruments should reach values of .70 or greater. This should not be taken to indicate that the higher the coefficient, the better the instrument. Excessively high coefficients indicate redundancy and unnecessary items. A special case of alpha is the Kuder-Richardson 20, which is essentially alpha for dichotomous data.

As mentioned earlier, Cronbach's alpha is based on correlational analysis, which is highly influenced by the number of items and sample size. It is possible to increase the reliability coefficient of a scale by increasing the number of items. A small sample size can result in a reduced reliability coefficient that is a biased estimate. A limitation of alpha is that items are considered to be parallel, which means they have identical true scores. When this is not the case, alpha is a lower bound to reliability; and other coefficients for internal consistency, based within models of principal components and common factor analysis (e.g., Theta and Omega), are more appropriate (Ferketich, 1990). Obtaining an adequate alpha does not mean that examination of internal consistency is complete. Item analysis must be accomplished and focused on the fit of individual items with the other items and the total instrument. Guidelines outlined by Ferketich (1991) can be followed to accomplish this assessment.

Again, observational measures are a special case and require different formulas for the determination of equivalence. Interrater reliability refers to the need for ratings to be essentially equivalent across data collectors and not to differ due to individual rater variability. The most common assessment procedure, kappa, is based on percent agreement and controlling for chance (Cohen, 1960).

Any discussion of reliability as approached through classical test theory should note more recent proposals for test consistency. Of these proposals, generalizability theory (G theory) has received the most attention (Shavelson & Webb, 1991). Unlike classical test theory reliability, G theory can estimate several sources of random error in one analysis; in the process a generalizability coefficient is computed. Proponents of G theory believe that its concentration on dependability rather than reliability offers a more global and flexible approach to estimating measurement error.

PAULA M. MEEK
JOYCE A. VERRAN

See also
DATA COLLECTION METHODS
INSTRUMENTATION

MEASUREMENT AND SCALES
STATISTICAL TECHNIQUES
VALIDITY

REPLICATION STUDIES

Replication involves repeating or reproducing a research study to investigate whether similar findings will be obtained in different settings and with different samples. Replication is needed not only to establish the credibility of research findings but also to extend generalizability. Blomquist (1986) listed five reasons why replication studies should be encouraged in nursing: (a) scientific merit is established, (b) Type I and Type II errors are decreased, (c) construct validity is increased, (d) support for theory development is provided, and (e) acceptance of erroneous results is prevented. Replication studies are essential for developing a scientific knowledge base in nursing. Incorporating research findings into nursing practice has been seriously hampered by the limited number of replication studies. Clarification of replication terminology can assist in advancing replication research. Three of the most often cited classifications of replication research have been developed by Finifter (1975), LaSorte (1972), and Lykken (1968).

Lykken (1968) identified three methods of replication: literal, operational, and constructive. Literal replication is an exact duplication of the original researcher's sampling, procedure, experimental treatment, data collection techniques, and data analysis. Operational replication involves an exact duplication of only the sampling and experimental procedures in the original research to check whether the original design when used by another leads to the same results. In constructive replication duplicate methods are purposely avoided.

Finifter (1975) listed four replication strategies: identical, virtual, systematic, and pseudo. Identical replication involves a one-to-one duplication of the original study's procedures and conditions. In virtual replication the methods of the original study are re-created in varying degrees. In systematic replication neither the methods nor the substance of the original study are duplicated. Pseudoreplication is similar to identical and virtual replication;

however, data for pseudoreplication are collected at the same time as those for the original study. The simultaneous confirmation of the study is built into the original design.

LaSorte (1972) described retest, internal, independent, and theoretical replication. Retest replication involves repeating an original study with few, if any, significant changes in the research design. Internal replication is incorporated into the original study. Data for both the original study and its replicated study are collected simultaneously to provide a cross-check for the reliability of the original results. In independent replication, significant modifications in the design of the original study are made to verify the empirical generalization. In theoretical replication the inductive process is used to examine the feasibility of fitting the empirical findings into a general theoretical framework.

A comparison of these three replication classifications reveals that Finifter's (1975) identical replication is similar to Lykken's (1968) literal replication. The three classifications include strategies to approximate the original research design. Finifter calls this virtual replication, Lykken labels it operational, and LaSorte (1972) describes it as retest replication. The purpose of choosing this type of replication is to determine if the original findings can be confirmed when modest changes in the research conditions have been made. When original findings are replicated, confidence in the reliability of these results is enhanced.

All three classifications include an approach to increase empirical generalization by significantly modifying the original design. Finifter (1975) labels this systematic replication, Lykken (1968) describes it as constructive replication, and LaSorte (1972) calls it independent replication. This type of replication strategy is used when the researcher not only wants to validate earlier work but also wants to extend the results and determine the degree of generalizability.

Both Finifter (1975) and LaSorte (1972) specifically identify types of replication where data for both the original and replication studies are collected at the same time. According to Finifter, this is pseudoreplication, and to LaSorte it is internal replication. This type of replication provides additional data, which is used as a cross-check of the data's reliability. LaSorte's classification is the only one that includes a replication strategy to develop and verify theory.

Replication studies conducted in nursing have addressed topics such as nursing education, nurses' characteristics, perioperative nursing, body image during pregnancy, cardiac care, fetal monitoring, and time perception.

Campbell's research on family violence is an example of a program of nursing research that involved replication. A portion of this program focused on battering during pregnancy. In 1986 Campbell found that battering during pregnancy was associated with more frequent and severe abuse of the woman throughout the relationship. Campbell and colleagues' (Campbell, Poland, Walker, & Ager) 1992 study replicated this earlier research in terms of identifying the prevalence of prenatal partner assault. This replication study also extended the knowledge base by examining the relationship between battering during pregnancy and adequacy of prenatal care and investigating correlates of battering during pregnancy by category of abuse. Battering was divided into three categories: (a) partner assault during pregnancy, (b) partner assault prior to pregnancy only, and (c) assault by a person other than the partner either during or before the pregnancy. The replication process benefited nursing practice by first confirming the prevalence of battering during pregnancy (7%) found in earlier studies. Second, this replication revealed significant correlates of battering during pregnancy to be depression, anxiety, drug and alcohol abuse, inadequate prenatal care, and housing problems. It is essential that these correlates be recognized in the nursing assessment of pregnant women to help identify battering during pregnancy.

When publishing replicated studies nurse researchers should include the following information: (a) identification of the specific type of replication that is conducted, (b) provision of specific information on how a replicated study is the same as and different from the original study, and (c) explanation of what is replicated and how. This information will help readers to more clearly understand how the researchers methodically revised previous studies in a progressive manner. When publishing original studies, researchers also should explicitly detail the important points of their sampling and data collection techniques and their research design to aid replication of their work. Authors must be more diligent in identifying the minimum essential conditions and controls necessary for producing findings because replication is crucial for the further development of nursing knowledge.

CHERYL TATANO BECK

See also
STATISTICAL TECHNIQUES
THEORETICAL FRAMEWORK
VALIDITY

REPRESENTATION OF KNOWLEDGE FOR COMPUTATIONAL MODELING IN NURSING: THE *ARCS*© PROGRAM

There are a number of computational approaches to management and application of knowledge to clinical situations in medicine and, to a small degree, nursing. Computers can apply domain knowledge to data to diagnose and suggest treatment of diseases. Computers can also discover new knowledge. Much of this discovery research uses databases of observations of scientific phenomena and falls into two categories: empirical laws and formation of theories (Shrager & Langley, 1990). In contrast, *arcs*© uses the scientific findings reported in the research literature as data with which to propose theoretical models.

Historically, discovery of new knowledge in nursing has been more likely to start with theory than with clinical data. Many nursing observations (data) were discarded from the care record and thus not systematically available for inducing hypotheses. Thus, nurse researchers and theorists have traditionally used the scientific literature to develop theoretical models of a process or event, then empirically test the hypotheses suggested by these models.

Knowledge is found in experts, in the books and journals of a domain, and, one might say, in clinical databases if one knows how to acquire it. The process of searching the literature to find knowledge needed to build a testable theoretical model is an appalling task. Scientists want to know what variables were studied together with what result. For them to obtain this knowledge, they must sort through bibliographic databases and/or specific journals and/or work with their "invisible college." The "invisible college" is a term that refers generally to a self-selected group of researchers (or theorists) working in the same field who stay in touch to keep up with one another's work instead of waiting for publications to come out. Bibliographic searches are generally designed so that the searcher either finds too much that is not relevant or not enough that is. Upon finding the desired literature set, one must wade through pages that represent the knowledge in numeric relationship displays and text. An alternative would be to index research by variable names and findings. The scientist can then go directly to the literature that reports on the knowledge established between those variables.

Although *arcs* does not help the user directly with the literature search, *arcs* does demonstrate a methodology for indexing the research literature by variables studied so that all users could go directly to the studies that are of interest to them with 100% sensitivity and 100% specificity. Although *arcs* does not currently eliminate the work of wading through pages of prose to identify the knowledge contained within the research article, it does demonstrate an alternative methodology for reporting and storing research knowledge that immediately makes the knowledge and the salient characteristics obvious and a basis for computational modeling of nursing knowledge. These methods are now enjoying practical application at the Virginia Henderson International Nursing Library of Sigma Theta Tau International (STTI).

The *arcs* Program Development

The *arcs* program was developed initially as a knowledge engineering project. Knowledge engineering takes knowledge in one form (in this case the scientific literature) and processes it into a more easily used form (in this case textual and graphic

relational maps, also called causal/associational maps or concept maps). Knowledge must be represented in the computer so that the computer can process it predictably.

The first step of the *arcs* project was to identify and formalize a definition of knowledge by examining the way it is structured in the scientific literature. A further decision was made to delimit the project to knowledge expressed relationally and generated from empiricist designs, published in English-language journals, and involving only reports of research with humans. Numerous research articles from nursing, psychology, and sociology journals were used. For each article, the expression of the finding(s) was recorded. The overall structure of these knowledge expressions was virtually the same across disciplines. All contained names of variables, stated the relationship studied, and the results. On the basis of these investigations, a structure of scientific knowledge was defined grossly as *the result or finding about the (statistical) relationship between two or more variables, given the design, methods and conditions, and source* (Graves, 1990).

The second step of the project was to devise a knowledge-base structure that would store a unit of knowledge as defined above. In order to retain the original research language, variables are named as designated by the researcher at their operational (measured) level. To collect the potentially numerous variable names into manageable models, a higher level abstraction term may be assigned by the researcher or by the knowledge base builder. In addition to names, other attributes of variables (measurement, dependency [and thus directionality]) were added. Numerical relationships were largely statistical and were categorized as descriptive, associational, directional, difference, and structural. Together, these categories incorporated all types of statistical tests. A number of attributes were added to further describe the conditions of the study and the certainty associated with the finding, including direction and magnitude.

Next, this structure was implemented by using relational database software. Instead of calling the resulting product a database, it is called a knowledge base because it stores the entire unit of knowledge. Before it could be tested by anyone other than the author, however, a menu system had to be added to allow users to interact with the software without learning a database query language. The first program produced a text-based model of a focal variable with three levels of relationships. One had to draw one's own relational map, using the text model.

It was next necessary to test the generalizability of the knowledge structure. This was done by having selected doctoral students use the program in their dissertation literature reviews. It was found that they could use the program to store units of knowledge from very different domains, including research from multiple disciplines.

When it was established that there was sufficient generalizability between research domains, the software was then ported to a machine that could more easily be programmed to build graphical knowledge models. The name was changed from Arks© to *arcs* to denote the mathematical concept of *arc* as a relationship (directional or nondirectional) between two entities in the world—a natural model for representing relational knowledge.

Testing of this version consisted of entering subsets of knowledge in different domains to test the functionality of the program, the accuracy of the models, and the value of the graphics to a user. The program was modified to incorporate suggestions from users as appropriate. The *arcs* program was next converted to a Microsoft Windows™ environment and can be used on a Macintosh with Soft Windows™. It is in active use for building knowledge bases at Sigma Theta Tau.

How *arcs* Works

The *arcs* computer program uses the concept of a knowledge base that contains linked data about all essential elements of a unit of knowledge as defined above. Data must be entered into the program by the user, who must obtain the data from research studies published in a domain of knowledge. The *arcs* program builds the models of knowledge from the data entered by the user about *pairs of variables*, the *relationship* studied between then, *direction*, *sign*, and effect size of the finding. Each statistical relationship is represented by a different type of

line that includes the directionality of each relationship, if any. Indirect relationships can be modeled to two more levels. Discovery is supported only passively now; the user must examine models to identify gaps and conflicts in the modeled domain. However, the later version of *arcs* will use a mathematical approach to identifying gaps and conflicts. Work is also in progress to design and test an algorithm to provide an estimate of belief in models, depending on such things as research design and conflicting findings.

There are many more attributes of a unit of knowledge that can be stored in *arcs*. It is up to the user to decide how much detail will be of value in modeling. This, in turn, will depend on the characteristics of the domain being modeled. Virtually all of the attributes can be used to *condition* (restrict or specify) the model. For example, one can elect to model only studies that have certain validity scores or effect sizes or studies of a single sample type, such as children. By conditioning the model to address time of publication, *arcs* models will illustrate changes in what is being studied in a domain over time, changes in level of testing, and methodologies, even variable names. The amount of replication will be visible in the models. Because new findings can be added as they are published, the model stays up-to-date.

The *arcs Tracker* is a menu-guided interface for building queries. The results are reported as text and can be used to build text models as well as to summarize (count) various attributes in the knowledge base. The *arcs* program provides a guided validity review and produces a graph of validity distributions for the user who wishes to describe validities in a domain. Heuristic, internal, and external validities are graphed separately. In addition, *arcs* provides a metastructure map that graphs the frequency with which pairs of variables are studied, using the metastructure categories of person, environment (health or nursing) focus, intervention, and intervention outcome. The *arcs* program is laborintensive in the data input phase. Some research articles require up to an hour for extraction of all the relevant data about the knowledge, especially when the knowledge is embedded in text and not represented in numeric relationship displays. This limits usefulness.

The broader modeling concepts of *arcs*, however, are implemented in the STTI *Registry for Nursing Research*. In this case, the researchers themselves register their work and enter the details of their studies, so the data do not have to be extracted from published articles. This provides a new paradigm for publishing nursing knowledge and allows researchers access to unpublished as well as published nursing knowledge. Over time, the STTI *Registry for Nursing Research*, not a traditional library of documents, will be the knowledge base with which computational modeling of nursing knowledge will take place.

JUDITH R. GRAVES

See also
   BIBLIOGRAPHIC RETRIEVAL SYS-
      TEMS
   FORMAL LANGUAGES
   RESEARCH DISSEMINATION
   VIRGINIA HENDERSON INTERNA-
      TIONAL NURSING LIBRARY

RESEARCH CAREERS

Research as a Professional Obligation

Research expands the body of knowledge of a discipline and profession. To ensure that students have an opportunity to learn about the importance of nursing research to the profession, the National League for Nursing Accrediting Commission currently mandates that baccalaureate nursing programs teach nursing research methods and incorporate the utilization and evaluation of nursing research into their curricula. For baccalaureate nursing graduates, the expectations are to evaluate and utilize research in their practice. The expectation of master's program graduates is to participate in nursing research and to facilitate research utilization; the expectation of doctorally prepared graduates is that they conduct and disseminate their research. Every nurse has a professional obligation to use research findings to inform his or her practice. Some nurses choose a career in which the conduct

of research is one expectation, and others, nurse researchers, choose a career in which the primary expectation is the conduct of research, including the facilitation of research by others.

Development of a Research Career

As a result of their educational and practice experiences, nurses may decide to pursue research careers in a broad continuum of clinical and/or practice areas. Research careers in nursing, as in other disciplines, follow a developmental course, from novice to experienced to senior researcher, with each stage posing different demands and expectations and offering different satisfactions (Hinshaw & Ketefian, 1996).

The educational preparation for a nursing research career is an earned doctorate with specialized courses in statistics and research methodology. Generally, a nurse formally begins his or her research career with doctoral work. With the doctoral committee members, a research area of interest, a research problem, and senior research advisor are identified. In doctoral work the student has the opportunity to be actively involved in each step of the research process, to develop research skills, and to be formally socialized and mentored in the research environment.

Nurses at this beginning stage of a research career are intimately involved in building a sound foundation in research design, completing data collection and analysis, and starting to develop a scholarly identity through publication. The demands at this stage of a research career revolve around obtaining initial funding, prioritizing time for completing the research data collection and analysis, and working with peers to develop a network of research colleagues (Cole & Slocumb, 1990). The satisfaction of the novice researcher is in making a contribution to the body of knowledge in a specific area, acquiring a scholarly identity, and presenting and publishing the results of research studies that build the scientific base (LaMontagne, Pressler, & Salisbury, 1996).

Experienced nurses with evolving nursing research careers are challenged to maintain continued funding, serve as role models for students and other nurses, further develop their research trajectory, and extend their research network. Nurses at this level of their research careers find satisfaction in their growing reputation as researchers, the ability to extend their study to addressing new questions, and working with colleagues on multisite studies (Rankin, 1991).

The challenges facing the senior researchers are to continue and extend their own scholarly research, with interdisciplinary colleagues as appropriate, finding funding sources to support large studies and mentoring novice researchers and students. Senior researchers find career satisfaction in serving as consultants to other nurse researchers and interdisciplinary research teams, mentoring novice researchers, developing as nursing scholars, and making significant contributions to the body of nursing knowledge.

Centers for Nursing Research

For the nursing profession to remain viable in a changing world, the continuous development of nurse researchers is necessary. To promote this development, the National Institute of Nursing Research (NINR), the institute for nursing research within the National Institutes of Health, has funded core centers for research at universities across the nation. Examples of those funded are the University of Pittsburgh, University of California at San Francisco, University of North Carolina, University of Iowa, University of Pennsylvania, and University of Washington. The specific areas of research identified for each university center are chronic disorders, symptom management, chronic illness in vulnerable people, gerontological nursing interventions, advancing care in serious illness, and women's health, respectively.

These core centers support the creation of interdisciplinary collaborative nursing research programs in specific areas of basic and/or clinical nursing research and offer opportunities for nurses to consult with nursing experts in these areas, train with mentors, and develop professional networks with other interdisciplinary researchers (Hinshaw, 1996). Other schools of nursing have research centers (funded through other sources), and these also provide the infrastructure necessary to support the research careers of faculty.

NINR and Other Funding Resources

Financial support for individuals seeking a research career is also available from NINR. There are funding mechanisms to support nurses at various stages of research career development: (a) predoctoral fellowships for researchers beginning their research careers, (b) postdoctoral fellowships for nurses who want to expand the knowledge gained in their doctoral study, and (c) senior fellowships for investigators who have already been successful in a research arena and want to acquire new research capabilities or pursue new directions of research. For information about this funding source, contact National Institute for Nursing Research, 31 Center Drive, MSC 2178 Building 31, Bethesda MD 20892-2178. Professional nursing organizations are additional sources of research funding. Examples of these funding sources include Sigma Theta Tau International, Oncology Nursing Foundation, and American Association of Critical Care Nurses.

Settings Supporting Careers in Research

Research career development in nursing historically was confined to faculty in a university setting. With recent changes in the health care delivery systems, opportunities for research careers in industry, at clinical centers, and in outpatient care facilities are increasing. Hospitals and integrated systems of health care delivery are increasingly employing nurse researchers to study practice improvements, care quality, and health outcomes. Nurse researchers also assist in the development of the informatics systems used in these settings to support studies of comparison of practices, outcomes, and the benchmarking efforts required.

Summary

A research career offers nurses the opportunity to engage in a lifelong process of building a research program that attempts to find answers to the questions that are central to the discipline and professional practice. To pursue this career pathway requires a strong educational foundation, mentoring in the research environment, and available funding. Research centers established by the NINR and other sources serve as resources for beginning, experienced, and seasoned nurse researchers to extend their research trajectories. The future holds many opportunities for nursing research careers in integrated health systems, industry, and academe.

MARY J. MCNAMEE
ADA M. LINDSEY

See also
DOCTORAL EDUCATION
FUNDING
MENTORING IN NURSING RESEARCH
NATIONAL INSTITUTE OF NURSING
** RESEARCH**

RESEARCH DISSEMINATION

Research dissemination is the purposeful communication of research, particularly the findings and implications of those findings to members of society who can utilize them. Dissemination is initiated by those who "know" and extend to those who "do not know" but might apply the findings if they knew (Rogers, 1995). As a practice profession, nursing cannot be satisfied with just awareness but is always interested in the application prospects of the research.

Dissemination is sometimes differentiated from diffusion when the latter term is reserved for spontaneous spread and use of research. Most writers on dissemination and diffusion talk about a purposeful process aimed at spread and use of research. Utilization is another related term. Utilization is specifically focused on application and is more likely to be initiated at the user end, whereas dissemination is focused on knowledge acquisition and more likely is initiated at the researcher end. The two are obviously linked with overlapping phases in their processes.

Theory and Research

A principal writer/researcher whose work has directed research dissemination is Rogers, who writes on the "diffusion of innovations." Rogers (1995) noted that in 1962, at the time of his first book, 405 publications were found on innovation diffusion, whereas by 1995 the number approached 4,000. Recently, dissemination/diffusion is seen as a less linear process where the potential users of research have a responsibility to contribute to the dialogue so that the movement from innovation to application can occur (Rogers, 1995).

Rogers's (1995) innovation-decision process has five stages: knowledge, persuasion, decision, implementation, and confirmation. In the knowledge stage, whether the need for the innovation or the innovation occurs first is ambiguous. Three types of knowledge about innovations are essential: awareness, how-to, and principles. Each type represents a more thorough understanding of the innovation. In the persuasion stage a positive or negative impression of the innovation is formed. Here the potential user clearly engages in more active innovation information seeking, the outcome of this stage being formation of an attitude toward the innovation. Although knowledge and attitudes are important factors in the use of the innovation in practice, practice is clearly based on more. Major factors contributing to the knowledge-attitude-practice (KAP) gap include (a) whether the practice of the innovation is outside individual control; (b) whether the individual has interpersonal communication from a near-peer supporting the adoption; (c) individual characteristics toward being an early or late adopter, perhaps based on a sense of efficacy; and (d) whether the nature of the innovation is preventive. Adoption of prevention-focused innovations occurs more slowly.

The ultimate focus of this diffusion process is on the application of the innovation (Rogers, 1995) as evidenced by the last three stages. The adoption decision is made in the decision stage. At this stage the process begins to have more relevance for research utilization than for research dissemination. In the implementation stage the innovation is put to use. The final stage, confirmation, is where individuals seed reinforcement for their decision to adopt. In confirmation the innovation is evaluated, an outcome being continuation or discontinuation. The first two stages can guide dissemination; the latter stages, utilization.

The dissemination of research to nursing practice is weak. In a classic nursing study, Ketefian (1975) found nurses unfamiliar with well-published research findings related to temperature taking. Brett (1987) and Coyle and Sokop (1990) reported the rate of dissemination of specific nursing practices with solid research bases called innovations. Although these studies also looked at utilization, the initial survey questions asked about "knowing" about the innovation. They found "awareness" and "persuasion" to vary greatly, as did the gap between knowing and using. Michel and Sneed (1995) reported similar dissemination scores to the earlier writers even with a better educated sample. Graduate education and awareness of agency policy were associated with more dissemination. Nurses reported learning about innovations from reading, conferences, and colleagues.

Dissemination in Action

Explicit dissemination occurs as researchers present their findings, implications, and recommendations in articles, papers, and posters. Usually, these communications include details of the research process that facilitates a scholarly critique. The criticism is that too often these communications occur between researchers and that the nurse caregiver is not linked into the research communication networks. Fortunately, some practitioners do attend research conferences and some practice-focused conferences devote programming to research.

A model for dissemination reported by Funk, Tournquist, and Champagne (1989) included practice-oriented research conferences, edited (specifically for practice) monographs of presentations, and an information center. The evaluation of the conference found the general responses extremely positive, but still major communication problems existed in both oral and written reporting. These problems persisted even with a great deal of support to the research communicators. This communication deficit leaves a practitioner, who is unsure,

responsible for deciding about practice utility (persuasion). Because the "old way" is usually comfortable, the innovation may not move from knowledge awareness to the more advanced how-to or principles knowledge. Consequently, the nurse prepared at the graduate level has an important role in dissemination in a clinical agency. This nurse is usually the reader of research, can interpret the findings, and sees the application possibilities. Through means like continuing education and journal clubs, the nurse from a graduate program can assist in filtering the research literature to match closely the practicing nurses' concerns and interests.

Implicit dissemination also occurs. This dissemination occurs when educators (academe, staff development, and continuing education) incorporate relevant research into their offerings. Audiences frequently trust that presenters have carefully critiqued the research they cite. Although this assumption usually is well founded, the scholarly practitioner will seek references and do a personal review.

As more nurses are university educated, including nurse administrators, familiarity with the relevant research has become a standard of practice in some organizations. Although this practice is not yet the norm, practice policies, standards, and procedures should be written, with a literature review that includes applicable research from nursing and other relevant disciplines. With a policy or procedure focusing on the "need to know" for the practitioner, the review of relevant research can be productive in practical dissemination by providing a context for considering whether to move into the application/utilization phases of knowledge diffusion.

The Future

An additional means of dissemination is currently evolving, and that is via the Internet. Universities, professional organizations, and individuals have home pages that more and more are including research information. On-line journals also are available. Some of the home pages include only researcher names and topics; others include abstracts and findings. The book by Nicoll and Ouellette (1997), titled *Nurses' Guide to the Internet*, gives some of the more common nursing-related sites at the time of publication, but as the authors noted, the specifics are in a constant state of flux. The additional caveat needed is that few of the sites have any type of peer review for quality and should be read with that in mind. Sigma Theta Tau's *Online Journal of Knowledge Synthesis for Nursing* is an example of a site with peer-reviewed content.

With the pressure on health care providers to be effective and efficient, the responsibility to break the "knowledge creep and decision accretion" situation (Weiss, 1980) is incumbent upon providers. To speed the dissemination process and facilitate utilization, the outcomes of any research project must be communicated with clarity, especially for the practice implications and for future research. One approach is to "market" research findings. This is a persuasive approach and would require more than not speaking solely in "researcher terms" but also addressing the four factors in Rogers's KAP gap. Marketing also addresses who is the persuader; witness the number of nurses selling pharmaceuticals and medical supplies. Clinician partners, especially clinical nurse specialists, are appropriate disseminators of research. A larger proportion of research funds should be spent on dissemination, not just for the "telling" but also for the necessary dialogue for quality research (Backer & Koon, 1995). Although graduate education makes a substantial contribution to dissemination (Oddi, Griffith, Whitley, & Pool, 1994), students must know how to do more than tell. They should learn also to persuade and dialogue. Educators, administrators, and clinicians must all take responsibility with researchers for strengthening the dissemination process so that research can guide nursing practice.

PATRICIA A. MARTIN

See also

CLINICAL NURSE SPECIALIST
CONTINUING EDUCATION
INTERNET
THE ONLINE JOURNAL OF KNOWL-
  EDGE SYNTHESIS FOR NURSING
RESEARCH UTILIZATION

RESEARCH IN NURSING ETHICS

Recent developments in technology have created increased awareness on the part of society and health professionals about the ethical dimensions of high-tech care. It is now recognized that our ability to deal with human and ethical issues has not kept pace with the rapid advancements made possible through various technologies being applied in health care.

Nursing ethics has evolved from the use of etiquette or rules of conduct to the philosophical or empirical analysis of (1) the moral phenomena found in nursing practice, (2) the moral language and ethical foundations of nursing practice, and (3) the ethical judgments made by nurses (Fry, 1995).

It is a salutary development of the past two decades that nurse investigators in increasing numbers have engaged in ethical inquiry. Earlier studies on ethical inquiry were mainly philosophical and normative. In more recent years empirical and descriptive studies have predominated, utilizing both qualitative and quantitative methods. The aim of these studies, collectively, has been to understand nurses' ethical decision making and actions under a variety of conditions of ethical ambiguity and conflict, along with the factors that affect these actions and decisions (ethical practice, moral behavior). In addition, there has been interest in understanding how nurses reason about moral choice (moral reasoning) and what conditions promote high-quality reasoning.

Moral reasoning is defined as a cognitive and developmental process involving a sequential transformation in the way social arrangements and ethical problems are interpreted. Each successive stage (of six stages) is more complex, comprehensive, and differentiated than the preceding stage. It has been theorized that certain conditions stimulate moral development. These include cognitive development and the nature of the educational and social climates, such as when opportunities are provided for assumption of responsibility or when cognitive disequilibrium is created to show inadequacies in one's mode of thinking (Kohlberg, 1978).

This conception of morality is ostensibly based on notions of rights, obligations, and justice and is said to reflect a male-oriented perspective. Gilligan

(1982) challenged this perspective by proposing the ethic of care or care-based reasoning, reflecting the way women reason about moral choice. This mode of reasoning does not involve the application of abstract ethical principles; rather, moral conflict and possible choices of action are constructed and defined by the context of the situation and the relationship of self to others who are involved in the conflict. Research to date does not support the polarization of and gender identifications with care (as feminine) and justice (as masculine).

Further, Gilligan (1982) contended that moral problems can be viewed from both justice and care perspectives by the same person, and both perspectives contain important moral injunctions; they entail different (but not opposite) ways of approaching moral judgments. Several instruments have been developed to measure care orientation in women. In a few studies using the Ethic of Care Interview, significant relationships have emerged between age, ego identity, and use of care orientation among women.

In an integrative review published in 1989, Ketefian reported on empirical studies conducted in ethical practice and moral reasoning and updated this information by a literature search conducted in 1996. Nurse investigators have studied moral reasoning as a dependent variable, trying to predict its development from various educational, cognitive, environmental, and personal demographic variables. Recently, a number of studies have focused on qualitative descriptions of nurses' reasoning and whether they used the care or the justice conceptions of morality. No clear direction emerged.

Ethical practice refers to nursing decisions and actions that reflect high ethical standards, such as those set forth by the nursing profession. Various indices of ethical behavior have been proposed, which makes comparisons across studies difficult. The measures vary as well. The most frequently used tool is Judgments about Nursing Decisions (Ketefian, 1989), but many investigators have developed their own measures. Ethical practice, moral behavior, and ethical decision making are terms utilized interchangeably and have been studied as dependent variables. Educational variables, moral reasoning, and organizational and personal variables have been used as predictors of ethical practice with inconsistent and mixed results.

Caring Behaviors

Caring behaviors originate from a strong interest in something or someone that contributes to the good, worth, dignity, or comfort of others. A number of descriptive studies on nurses' caring behaviors have been conducted. In samples composed of patients or others, several aspects of nurses' caring behaviors have been identified—empathic communication, competence, providing continuity, meeting needs, and being respectful, nonjudgmental, and solicitous. These aspects of nurses' behaviors provide a starting point for further research on the effects of nurse behaviors on patient satisfaction and patient outcomes (Fry, Killen, & Robinson, 1996).

Description of Attitudes, Values, Roles, and Issues

A few studies have identified the attitudes and values of nurses concerning ethical issues, the extent to which nurses understand the concept of ethical dilemmas, physicians' and nurses' perceptions of ethical problems, how nurses address ethical concerns in their practice, nurses' perceptions of powerlessness in influencing ethical decisions, ethical conflicts related to pain management, and ethical issues in caring for patients receiving long-term tube feedings. Other studies have examined nurses' role in end-of-life treatment decisions, practices concerning assisted suicide and euthanasia, and differences among nurses and physicians in their ethical decision making.

In addition, studies have identified and compared the ethical decision making of nurses in various practice settings. Only a few studies have included variables such as the frequency with which nurses encounter specific ethical issues in their practice, how disturbed they are by them, the relationship of demographic and work-related variables to frequency and disturbance, the resources that nurses use to clarify ethical issues, and nurses' knowledge of patient care ethics committees.

A promising area of research relates to the way in which organizational variables impinge on the quality of nurses' reasoning, behavior, and judgments. There is a need for clearer definition and measurement. Typically, studies in nursing ethics tend to be isolated, individual projects; many are conducted as dissertations, and few are published. There is a need to move toward a programmatic and cumulative approach, along with a need for replications, so that a meaningful body of science can emerge, one in which we can have a degree of confidence.

SHAKÉ KETEFIAN
SARA T. FRY

See also

ATTITUDES

CARING

DECISION MAKING ABOUT END-OF-LIFE CHOICES

DECISION MAKING: ADVANCE DIRECTIVES

EMPATHY

RESEARCH INTERVIEWS (QUALITATIVE)

The interview is a major data collection strategy in qualitative research that aims to obtain textual, qualitative data reflecting the personal perspective of the interviewee. The interview creates an interactional situation in a face-to-face encounter between researchers and participants. In the study the interviewer acts as the instrument and through carefully designed questions, attempts to elicit the other person's opinions, attitudes, or knowledge about a given topic. Research interviews have historically provided the foundation for sociological and anthropological studies that attempted to understand other societies and cultures. As nurse scientists were trained in these methods in the late 1960s and the 1970s, they began using research interviews in nursing studies. Some researchers who seek quantitative data from questionnaires may refer to the structured, standardized survey that is administered face-to-face to large groups of people. The present definition, however, refers to the in-depth and generally less structured interview used in qualitative research.

The research method (e.g., grounded theory, phenomenology, ethnography) suggests the style and purpose of the interview questions. The research objectives are fundamental to the interview questions to maintain the integrity of the research. Grounded theory research intended to discover contexts, phases, and processes of a given phenomenon requires questions designed to acquire knowledge, such as, what is the context of death in a nursing home or at home or what are the phases of dying? Phenomenological research that aims to capture what is referred to as "the lived experience" may use only one general question: Please tell me all that you can about dying. Ethnographic research that is focused on culture may ask about which family members are involved in decisions concerning death and what their roles are.

Interviews are structured in phases—the introduction, the working phase, and termination. In the introduction the researcher gives a personal introduction, states the anticipated length of time of the interview, and makes some initial comments to relax the participant and to assist with the transition from social conversation to research interview. In the working phase the themes of the research are introduced, and the researcher and participant work toward generating a shared understanding. In the termination phase the interview draws to a close, and often brief social conversation occurs again.

The interview demands careful thought about the nature, wording, and sequence of questions. Generally, questions move from general to specific, becoming more focused as themes emerge and as data from other participants suggest additional leads. Questions should be unambiguous, meaningful, and successful in involving the interviewee in the process. The participants in the research are often helpful in critiquing the usefulness and appropriateness of the questions and suggesting others that may be more relevant or successful in obtaining the desired data.

Interviews are of two types: formal and informal. Formal interviews are scheduled as to time and place and generally occur over a period of 1 to 2 hours. Informal interviews are those used in participant observation, when the interviewer spends time in a specific environment and interviews participants as they appear on the scene or around a significant event. Although effective interviews, especially informal ones, may appear simple and comfortable, an expert interviewer is always both in and out of the interview. The interviewer listens carefully to the interviewee and anticipates how to direct the interview to accomplish the aims of the research.

Interviews are characterized as structured and focused when all questions are given in the same order to participants. Interviews in qualitative research studies are generally semifocused ones in which information about a certain subject is desired from all participants, but the phrasing and sequence of the questions may be varied to reflect the characteristics of the participants in the context. Time is permitted to encourage participants to introduce other subjects they believe are relevant and to elaborate, often with the help of interviewer's probes, on earlier comments. Participants' interpretations of meanings and definitions are valued. Such information is obtained only through open-ended questions and free-flowing conversation that follow the thinking of the interviewee. In a sense, the interviewee teaches the researcher about a particular experience or event.

Interviews are generally tape-recorded, and the researcher takes handwritten notes that jog his or her memory during the interview to return to a topic, to ask a hypothetical question, or to request new, related information. These taped interviews are transcribed as soon as possible by the researcher or a transcriptionist and cross-checked against the audiotape for accuracy.

Interviewing establishes the foundation for data analysis. The researcher's interview questions and responses to the interviewee must be analyzed in a reflexive manner to ascertain the quality of the interview. Is the interviewer cutting off the interviewee? Is the interviewer asking closed instead of open-ended questions? Is the interviewer asking relevant questions in a sensitive way? Is the interviewer giving the interviewee time to reflect and to complete his or her comments? Unfocused, insensitive interviewing yields poor data. Quality data result from the expression of affective responses and detailed personal information.

Qualitative research in nursing journals has been proliferating since the 1970s; currently, most of the major research journals have qualitative reviewers on their editorial boards. Some journals (*Research in Nursing and Health*) have a regular commentary from a qualitative expert. *Nursing Research*, in the "Methodology Corner," presents researchers' commentary about methodological issues confronted during the course of the research. Several articles have focused on the research interview (Hutchinson & Wilson, 1992). The subtleties and nuances and variations in form are discussed in nursing journal articles and in books that focus on qualitative research (Morse, 1992).

The complexity of interviewing becomes apparent in varied contexts. For example West, Bondy, and Hutchinson (1991) wrote about the difficulties they encountered when interviewing institutionalized elders. Cowles (1988) poignantly described interviewing individuals on sensitive topics such as being the adult survivor of a murder victim. Interviewing individuals from a culture different from that of the interviewer presents other issues; likewise interviewing the extremely poor or the extremely rich has it own sets of problems. Morse (personal communication, December 14, 1996) suggests that we "push the boundaries of our research practice," and it is with thoughtful attention to our methods that we do so. In the past, nurses have relied on sociological and anthropological researchers for guidance. Nurse methodologists agree that it is now time to identify and address issues in interviewing that are especially relevant to nursing topics and populations.

Good interviews provide access to the heart. Such personal information, essential to qualitative research that aims to access human meaning, is a gift. The researcher reciprocates by listening carefully and attempting to render or interpret the experience of the other as accurately as possible. An insensitive interviewer can harm the interviewee, leaving the person psychologically depleted or even wounded. Good interviewers leave interviewees feeling that they gained from the interview. Hutchinson, Wilson, and Wilson (1994) discovered that interviewees, when asked about the interview experience, described numerous unanticipated benefits, including catharsis, self-acknowledgment, sense of purpose, self-awareness, empowerment, healing, and the provision of a voice for the disenfranchised.

SALLY A. HUTCHINSON
HOLLY SKODOL WILSON

See also
ETHNOGRAPHY
GROUNDED THEORY
HERMENEUTICS
PHENOMENOLOGY
QUALITATIVE RESEARCH

RESEARCH ON INTERACTIVE VIDEO

Interactive video (IAV) is defined as a technology in which a video program is under the control of a computer, with user choices affecting program branching. The video source for IAV was videotape in early days of development, but current applications use the videodisk.

Development of IAV programs for nursing education began in the early 1980s, and commercially produced programs appeared in 1989. However, the body of research in this area is relatively small, and many studies were dissertations. Most of those mentioned here are described in more detail and referenced in Rizzolo (1994). Studies generally fall into six categories: cost-effectiveness, expert and usage surveys, effectiveness, learning in groups, learner attributes, and strategies to facilitate learning.

Cost-Effectiveness

Parker examined a large-scale IAV project initiated in 1981 to provide continuing education for nurses scattered across 30 different locations in Florida. She reported significant savings in time and money when IAV was compared with traditional workshops.

Expert and Usage Surveys

In 1987, Rizzolo solicited experts to participate in a three-round Delphi study. Twelve significant factors that were impeding the development of new programs in nursing were identified. Participants were able to identify clearly the content they wanted in IAV programs, especially applications for simulations. They agreed on the benefits of IAV for students but were less certain about how it might affect faculty roles. Conservative predictions were made about how technology might change nursing education in the future.

Two surveys examined the status of interactive video in nursing education. In 1989, Clark surveyed 504 BSN programs. Of the 369 respondents, 66 reported that they were using IAV. One year later Cambre and Castner conducted a study funded by FITNE, Inc. Of the 1,120 schools that responded, 207 were using IAV. Visits and phone interviews revealed positive attitudes about IAV but limited integration into the curriculum.

Effectiveness Studies

Several early studies compared IAV to another form of instruction, usually a linear videotape or lecture. Most found no significant differences in achievement. A few reported other positive findings attributable to IAV programs such as higher scores on retention, more positive attitudes toward content, or savings in time required to accomplish objectives.

Weiner et al. found that students who completed an IAV on labor and delivery, along with clinical experience, had significantly greater clinical confidence and learning than those who had only clinical experience. Wittstadt found no difference in confidence levels of nurses who used an interactive video program on infusion pumps as compared to those who learned the material in lecture. Froman et al. found that the sequence of lecture followed by IAV produced the largest gains in self-efficacy by students learning IV procedures.

Middlemiss evaluated IAV as a teaching strategy to help students develop ethical decision-making skills. Students wrote about and analyzed an ethical dilemma, then completed an IAV program and analyzed the event again. She found that students focused more on emotions in their first analysis and used a rational approach after completing the IAV program.

Learning in Groups

Conflicting results were reported in studies of students using IAV in groups. Rizzolo (1994) compared the pre- and posttest scores of students who worked though case study simulations in a large classroom situation to those who worked independently. Although both achieved significant increases in scores, the classroom group scored significantly higher on the posttest. Garcia's study used one case from the same IAV program and found no significant differences among students working individually, in groups of 2 or 3, and in groups of 10 to 12.

Battista-Calderone studied three groups who worked through an IAV tutorial. Some worked individually, some in groups of 2 or 3, the rest in groups of 7 to 10. Results revealed no significant differences in learning and attitude. Moyer (1996) audiotaped students in groups of two and four as they worked through six IAV programs and also had every student write journal entries. Content analysis revealed more problem-solving behaviors in the tetrad groups. Most felt the group experience was not as beneficial for those who learned more slowly nor for content like ethical decision making, particularly when a group member was very opinionated.

Learner Attributes

Several studies examined the interaction between learner attributes and achievement or attitudes. Glavin-Spiehs examined field dependence, and Hasset studied psychological type. Neither found significant differences.

Billings and Cobb evaluated the effects of learning style preferences, attitude, and GPA on learner achievement. The strongest predictor was attitude

toward computer-based instruction. In a later study, Billings assessed student learning style and attitude toward IAV instruction, then students worked through an IAV program either in a group or alone, as they wished. Students who studied in a group reported greater comfort, but there was no significant difference in learning outcomes.

Yoder's (1994) study measured preferred learning style, then randomly assigned students to IAV or linear videotape instruction. Students who preferred to learn through active experimenting learned better with IAV; those who preferred to learn by reflective observing scored higher after learning with linear videotape.

Strategies to Facilitate Learning

Two studies explored the use of organizers to facilitate learning while using IAV programs. Middlemiss found that graphic organizers facilitate retention for high-ability learners and facilitate immediate recall for both high- and lower-ability students. Renshaw (1996) found no significant difference when she examined the effect of content and structure organizers on student achievement and attitudes. Her qualitative focus groups revealed that students use a wide variety of approaches to work through programs. Every student said the IAV program was a valuable learning experience but very time-consuming to complete.

Future Research Directions

Most of the research on interactive video has implications for newer multimedia formats such as CD-ROM and interactive offerings on the World Wide Web. It seems clear that well-designed programs can teach content just as well if not better than traditional strategies. Some researchers are even using IAV programs as a tool for research. Predko tracked decisions made by cardiac care nurses as they worked through case study simulations to examine the effect of clinical experience and education on clinical decision-making skills.

Nurse researchers can look to instructional design and educational technology researchers for models and suggestions for future investigation. Their studies include approaches based on cognitive psychology, systems modeling, and instructional events and have suggested researchable propositions to test the validity of underlying assumptions about the technology to discover the conditions of effective use.

Although much additional research is needed on how people learn, nursing students are a diverse group, and qualitative studies might produce more useful data. Studies that identify ways to help students effectively choose and use technology-based applications to learn offer an important area of exploration.

Because studies found little integration of IAV into the curriculum and revealed that most faculty use IAV only for supplementary assignments, research on faculty use of technology is an important area of inquiry. Faculty can easily evaluate program content, but can they evaluate program design to determine if appropriate strategies and media are employed to match content and objectives? Can they decide if the degree of fidelity is appropriate for intended learners? These important questions must be answered so that faculty can select and use technology appropriately and design curricula that free the teacher to provide those experiences than only human interaction can accomplish.

MARY ANNE RIZZOLO

See also
CLINICAL DECISION MAKING
COMPUTER-AIDED INSTRUCTION
NURSING EDUCATION
VIRTUAL REALITY
WORLD WIDE WEB

RESEARCH UTILIZATION

Rodgers (1994) defined research utilization as a "process directed toward the transfer of research-based knowledge into nursing practice" (p. 907) with the ultimate goals of improving patient care and advancing the discipline of nursing. The importance of using research findings in clinical practice has been discussed for at least 45 years; however,

there are relatively few initiatives actually taking place in clinical or nursing education settings.

The first research utilization models were developed in the 1970s, beginning with the Western Interstate Commission for Higher Education in Nursing (WCHEN) Regional Program for Nursing Research Development (Krueger, 1978). Other models included the Conduct and Utilization of Research in Nursing (CURN) project (Horsley, Crane, Crabtree, & Wood, 1983), the Stetler/Marram model (Stetler, 1994), the Iowa model of research in practice (Titler et al., 1994), and the retrieval and application of research in nursing (RARIN) model (Bostrom & Wise, 1994). This list is not exhaustive; rather it is a representation of several well-known and referenced models found in the literature.

The WCHEN model was focused on cross-organizational planning and enhancing the value for research utilization. Nurses from a variety of clinical agencies were provided with 3 days of research training. Each clinician would identify a clinical problem, review the research in that area, and develop a plan for implementing and evaluating the outcomes of the practice change. The annual Communicating Nursing Research conferences also resulted from the initial WCHEN work group, with emphasis on dissemination of research results across academic and nursing service settings. There have been 30 conferences prior to 1997.

The CURN project was a federally funded initiative that focused on the use of a team approach for reviewing research results related to specific patient care problems, developing clinical protocols, and then testing the protocol in an acute care clinical setting. A key component of research utilization in this model was replication of previous studies. The focus of the Iowa model was similar to that of the CURN project, with particular attention to developing support for research utilization strategies at the organizational level. Both models were developed specifically to bridge the gap between research and practice. Both recommended that organizational resources such as personnel, equipment, time, and money be available to support the nursing staff. Policy, procedures, committee structures, and role expectations must exist in relation to staff involvement in research utilization activities. Both models also supported a fundamental belief that research can and must be applied to practice if patient care is to improve.

The Stetler/Marram model was developed primarily for use at the individual level and specifically outlined the role clinical specialists have in facilitating the application of research findings to clinical practice. The model includes specific steps related to the need for a sound foundation in the conduct of research, and what is more important, it demonstrates how to interpret and validate findings that can be used to change practice.

The RARIN model, funded by a National Library of Medicine grant, was developed at Stanford University Hospital in Palo Alto, California. Distinct from the other models, which focused on providing nurse education, skill building, and organization support strategies, the RARIN model focused on improving staff access to research findings through the use of computerized linkages to established research databases. Training a small set of nurses from each unit on the use of the computer network and the basics of the research critique was the other major component. The computer technology provided direct access to the MEDLINE citation system (including CINAHL) as well as databases of research abstracts that were written by experts. Hence, nurses could access almost any database, via use of the developed tools and technologies, while working in a patient care unit. The model assumption was based on a belief that if access to research findings was improved and the findings were represented in an easily understood yet clinically sound framework, then practicing nurses would be able to improve patient care.

Outcome results from these and other models have been limited. Numerous barriers to transferring research-based knowledge into nursing practice persist. Staff nurses reported the following as barriers to research utilization: (a) insufficient skills and knowledge about evaluating research, (b) lack of awareness or access to research, (c) minimal value of research for practice, (d) insufficient authority to actually change practice, (e) insufficient time to read research and to learn research skills and how to implement changes when necessary, (f) lack of cooperation and support from administration and other staff, (g) little personal benefit, (h) unclear and unhelpful statistical representation of results, (i) few replication studies to determine if sufficient evidence exists to change practice, and (j) lack of access to databases and research literature. Nurse administrators also reported barriers, such as (a) isolation from research colleagues, (b) lack of time because of heavy workloads, (c) difficulty in reading and interpreting research findings and statistics, (d) insufficient skills in research critique, (e) lack of replication studies to determine if practice requires change, and (f) lack of access to databases and research literature.

Facilitators for the research utilization process have also been identified. They include (a) creating practice environments that require research-based clinical standards, (b) providing expert consultation and activities such as research committees to increase adequacy of research skills, (c) improving access to computerized databases and research literature, (d) allotting time and money to support conference attendance and participation, (e) developing performance standards that include behavioral expectations to support research-based practice, and (f) obtaining grants to support research projects.

The literature related to research utilization is almost exclusively focused on nursing practice environments, with little attention to how research utilization is introduced into the nursing curricula at all levels. Research utilization is a critical professional accountability issue to resolve if the discipline of nursing is to advance. Therefore, it is essential for nursing educators to socialize students at all levels to the value of research utilization and to model the required skills. For example, most teaching about the research process at the baccalaureate level is isolated from discussions about actual caregiving and how that care might be improved by applying research findings. Graduate students are not adequately prepared for the integration of research into the care of specific patient populations and have little preparation in areas of quality improvement and outcomes-evaluation methodologies. Doctoral education continues to be focused on the conduct of research, with minimal emphasis on how to report results in ways that are understandable to practicing clinicians. Although learning a thesis format of writing is important, it is equally important to learn how to convert research jargon into useful, specific, and direct reports for clinicians. In addition, more value and attention should be given to replication research that would advance results that are more generalizable and easily applied to clinical practice.

The health care environment is changing rapidly, with increased attention to outcomes-based practice, evaluating patient outcomes, and demonstrating cost efficiency and effectiveness. Research utilization must become a matter of professional accountability for each nurse and every health care organization. Nurses must be better prepared to actively participate in and facilitate research utilization. More attention should be given to implementing strategies that remove the barriers identified in previous research. Technology is now available to provide much access to research and relevant databases; however, there is still need for timely and readable reports of completed research.

The critical challenge is how students, practitioners, educators, executives, and researchers can create learning environments in which research utilization will become an integral part of nursing practice. When nurse colleagues share a common vision related to improving the health of our communities, then research utilization becomes one method to ensure research-based care delivery models, with all nurses accountable for achieving optimal outcomes.

CAROL A. ASHTON

See also
CLINICAL INFORMATION SYSTEMS
CUMULATIVE INDEX TO NURSING
   AND ALLIED HEALTH LITERATURE
NURSING EDUCATION
REPLICATION STUDIES
RESEARCH DISSEMINATION

REVERSAL THEORY

Reversal theory, also known as the theory of psychological reversals, holds that personality is inherently inconsistent and that individuals reverse back and forth between the members of opposing pairs of states called metamotivational states. Developed by British psychologist Michael J. Apter (1982, 1989), reversal theory is a grand theory that describes motivation, emotion, and behavior. The theory states that psychological processes are bistable rather than homeostatic. Reversal theory has been used in nursing research to explain lapsing during smoking cessation. The theory also has been used in sports psychology, psychopathology, and psychophysiology.

According to Apter (1989), four pairs of metamotivational states describe experience: (1) telic versus paratelic, (2) negativistic versus conformist, (3) mastery versus sympathy, and (4) autic versus alloic. An individual is in one member of each of the pairs during all of waking life. Emotion and the experience of motivation differ, in fact are opposite to each other, in opposing states. An individual in the telic state is characterized by being serious-minded, oriented toward important goals, focused on the future, and usually preferring low felt arousal and high felt significance. High arousal is experienced as anxiety, and low arousal is experienced as a pleasant calmness. An individual in the paratelic state, on the other hand, is characterized by being playful, activity-oriented, focused on the present, and usually preferring high felt arousal and low felt significance. High arousal is experienced as pleasant excitement, and low arousal is experienced as unpleasant boredom in the paratelic state. In the negativistic state the individual desires to break rules; in the conformist state, adhering to rules is preferred. In the mastery state the individual is oriented to control and competition. In the sympathy state caring and cooperation are preferred. The autic state describes a self-centered orientation, whereas the alloic state describes an other-centered orientation. Reversal theory states have been assessed by self-report measures and by assessments made by trained raters of subjects' descriptions of specific episodes (reviewed in Cook, Gerkovich, Potocky, & O'Connell, 1993).

Reversals from each state to its opposite occur several times per day, and reversals are considered necessary for mental health. Reversals are caused by internal or external contingencies, frustration, and satiation. The tendency to remain in one state for longer periods than in its opposing state is termed state dominance.

Research applying reversal theory to smoking cessation (Cook, Gerkovich, O'Connell, & Potocky, 1995; O'Connell, Cook, Gerkovich, Potocky, & Swan, 1990; O'Connell, Gerkovich, & Cook, 1995) has demonstrated that individuals are more likely to lapse during highly tempting situations if they are in paratelic or sympathy states. Psychophysiological research suggests that smoking has different effects on the brain, as measured by EEG, in the telic state than in the paratelic state (Cook, Gerkovich, Hoffman, et al., 1995) and that telic-dominant subjects show EEG effects from smoking different from those of paratelic dominant subjects (Cook, Gerkovich, Hoffman, McClernon, & O'Connell, 1996).

More information about reversal theory can be found at the reversal theory website: www.swin.edu.au./ssb/rtconf/rthome.html.

KATHLEEN A. O'CONNELL

See also
**BEHAVIORAL RESEARCH
SMOKING/TOBACCO AS CARDIOVAS-
CULAR RISK FACTOR
THEORETICAL FRAMEWORK**

RIGHTS OF HUMAN SUBJECTS

Definition

Rights are just claims that are due to someone. Legal rights are valid claims recognized by a legal system. Moral rights are valid claims derived from customs, traditions, or ideals which may be upheld or protected by the law. Human rights are valid claims that are due to members of the human species and may be legal, moral, or both.

The rights of human subjects in research include the right to informed consent, the right to privacy, the right to refuse to participate in research, and the right to withdraw from a research study, without penalty, at any time (Fry, 1994). These four rights are all derived from a general right to liberty and are both moral and legal. They are supported by moral principles of the social community, profes-

sional codes of research ethics, and by legal protections. They become relevant in nursing research because all nurses have a responsibility to protect, and sometimes defend, the basic rights of patients within the health care system. When the nurse is also a researcher, the nurse has the added responsibility to make sure that these particular rights are not violated by the research process.

Informed Consent

Informed consent is a process that protects research subjects' autonomy, protects research subjects from harm, and assists the researcher to avoid fraud and coercion in the role of researcher. It is also a process that encourages researcher responsibility for how information is communicated in research, promotes rational decision making by human subjects, and involves the public in promoting self-determination as a social value. Informed consent has information elements and consent elements (Faden & Beauchamp, 1986).

Information Elements. For adequate disclosure of information, the research subject must be informed on the procedures to be used throughout the study. Information about available alternative treatment procedures, a discussion of risks and benefits of these procedures, and the opportunity for questions about or withdrawal from the project after treatment has begun, should all be provided to the research subject.

For adequate comprehension of information, the research subject must have time to consider the information and to ask questions. This means that when the ability to comprehend information is limited (such as when a subject's mental competence is limited), the researcher must allow the research subject additional opportunity to consider whether or not to participate in the study.

Consent Elements. Voluntary consent to participate in research means that the research subject has exercised choice, free of coercion and other forms of controlling influence by other persons. A research subject's consent is valid only if it is voluntarily given. Voluntariness protects the patient's right to choose goals and to choose among several goals when offered options. But consent cannot be given unless the research subject is "competent," or can make decisions based on rational reasons. Both competence and voluntariness are required for a subject's consent to be truly informed.

Nursing research on the informed consent of human subjects has focused on the comprehension of information by research subjects (Silva, 1985), subjects' competency for informed consent (i.e., adolescents, mentally retarded minors), and the factors that influence the informed consent of adolescents and adults. The study designs have been exploratory and quasi-experimental and have included relatively small sample sizes.

Basic Rights

Right to Privacy. The right to privacy includes the right to keep personal information about oneself private, undisclosed, and away from public scrutiny. It also includes the right to bodily integrity, or freedom from unwanted intrusions on body parts. One way that the research subject's right to privacy is protected is by following rules of confidentiality. For example, information about the research subject may not be disclosed without the subject's permission and then only under certain conditions. In a like manner, research data is not publicly connected to the research subject, thereby assuring subject privacy.

Another way that the research subject's right to privacy is protected is by obtaining an informed consent and signed permission for invasive procedures used during the research process. For example, informed consent must be obtained before passing a Levine tube to obtain gastric contents for analysis. Nursing research on the privacy of human subjects is not yet documented. Potential areas for nursing research are identifying how research studies protect or do not protect the privacy of human subjects, describing research subjects' perceptions of how their privacy was protected or not protected during a study, identifying researchers' attitudes toward rules of confidentiality under different research conditions, and identifying institutional review board (IRB) members' knowledge of and attitudes toward protection of human subject privacy in research studies.

Right to Refuse to Participate in Research. The right to refuse to participate in research protects the subject from being coerced to participate in research and assures that research subjects are truly voluntary. Nursing research on the right to refuse to participate in research is not yet documented. Potential areas for nursing research are identifying the conditions under which research subjects refuse to participate in a study and describing why subjects have refused to participate in particular types of research studies.

Right to Withdraw from a Research Study. Human subjects have the right to withdraw from a research study without any untoward treatment of them. Even though they had previously consented to participate in a research study, subjects have the right to change their minds and withdraw from the study at any time.

Nursing research on the right to withdraw from a research study is not yet documented. Potential areas for nursing research are identifying the conditions under which research subjects withdraw from a study and describing the course of treatment of subjects who do and do not withdraw from studies involving particular diseases.

Implications

The protection of human rights in research studies is important to the moral integrity of nursing research. International and professional codes of research ethics strongly support the morality of research, and the American Nurses Association's *Ethical Guidelines in the Conduct, Dissemination, and Implementation of Nursing Research* (Silva, 1995) supports the morality of nursing research. However, nursing research on the protection of human rights in research is at an early stage of development. As the 21st century approaches, nursing research should include studies of how human rights are protected in research and the factors that inhibit or promote their protection in various kinds of research designs.

SARA T. FRY

See also
CLINICAL TRIALS

ETHICS OF RESEARCH
HEALTH OF AFRICAN AMERICANS
INFORMED CONSENT

RISK FACTORS

Risk refers to the probability that a health problem will occur in a group of people who currently are free of that problem. Risk factors are characteristics or events that increase the probability that a health problem will develop. To determine risk factors, epidemiological researchers compare incidence and prevalence rates for a specified condition or health problem among various population groups. When higher levels of the characteristic are associated with higher incidence rates, the characteristic is considered a risk factor. For example, researchers have demonstrated that there is a higher incidence of low-birthweight babies born to women who smoke than women who do not smoke. Therefore, maternal smoking has been identified as a risk factor for low-birthweight babies.

Although risk factors are indicators of an increased risk of a health problem, they may or may not be directly related to the underlying causes of the health problem. For example, exposure to an infectious agent is known to be directly related to the cause of an infectious disease. In contrast, socioeconomic status may be a risk factor for some conditions, but it is not directly related to the cause of the problem. Use of this information, however, can be of assistance in planning preventive programs.

The presence of risk factors does not necessarily predict that the health problem will occur, nor does their absence provide a guarantee that the problem will not occur. However, knowledge of risk factors enables nurses to identify individuals and groups who have a high probability of developing a particular health problem. These individuals or groups are considered to be "at risk" in terms of that health problem.

Usually, a combination of biological characteristics, behavior, stressful life events, and environmental exposure can be identified that place people at high risk. For example, risk of coronary artery disease is associated with a sedentary lifestyle, smoking, obesity, and hypertension. These risk fac-

tors are potentially modifiable. Although advancing age is a risk factor, it is not modifiable. Following a health risk appraisal and nursing diagnosis, appropriate planning, implementation, and evaluation of primary preventive measures focused on modifiable risk factors can occur. Promotion of exercise, smoking-cessation clinics, and weight loss programs and an emphasis on the need to decrease stress and control blood pressure may result in the prevention of acute, premature heart attacks.

Based on prior risk factor research, recommendations for screening tests for early detection of disease, counseling for risk reduction, and immunizations to prevent infections have been detailed by the U.S. Preventive Services Task Force (1996a). A summary of the major risk factors found to be statistically associated with leading health problems is found in the accompanying Table 1.

TABLE 1   Major Risk Factors Associated With Selected Leading Health Problems in the United States

Coronary heart disease
  Nonmodifiable
    Advancing age
    Family history of heart disease
    Diabetes mellitus
  Potentially modifiable
    High blood lipids
    Hypertension
    Obesity
    Sedentary lifestyle
    Smoking
    Stressful lifestyle

Cerebral artery stenosis
  Nonmodifiable
    Advancing age
    Family history
    African descent
    Cardiac disease
    Diabetes mellitus
  Potentially modifiable
    Hypertension
    Atrial fibrillation
    High blood lipids
    Smoking
    Transient ischemic attacks

Hypertension
  Nonmodifiable

Advancing age
Males in young adulthood and early middle age
Females after 55
Family history
African descent
Diabetes mellitus
Potentially modifiable
Cigarette smoking
Elevated blood pressure
Elevated serum lipids
Excessive alcohol intake
High sodium intake
Lower socioeconomic status
Obesity, especially central abdominal obesity
Sedentary lifestyle
Stressful lifestyle

Non-insulin-dependent diabetes mellitus (Type II)
Nonmodifiable
Family history
Advancing age
Native American, Black, and Hispanic populations
Abnormality of glucose tolerance
Previous history of gestational diabetes
Potentially modifiable
Obesity

Breast cancer
Nonmodifiable
Age 55 years or older
Female gender
Menarche at 12 years or younger
Menopause at age 55 years or older
First full-term pregnancy after age 30
Nulliparity
Atypical breast changes
Family history
Potentially modifiable
Radiation exposure
Obesity
Alcohol consumption

Lung cancer
Nonmodifiable
Advancing age
Family history
Potentially modifiable
Cigarette smoking
Exposure to airborne environmental carcinogens
High socioeconomic class

Colon or rectum cancer
Nonmodifiable
Family history
Long-standing ulcerative colitis
Potentially modifiable

Large adenomatous colorectal polyps
Diet high in fat, low in fiber

Human immunodeficiency virus infection
Potentially modifiable
Injection drug users
Men who have sex with men
Heterosexual people with other sexually
transmitted diseases

Suicide
Nonmodifiable
More than one psychiatric hospital admission
Serious medical illness
Recent bereavement
Personal or family history of suicide attempt
Divorce
Potentially modifiable
Psychiatric illness
Substance abuse
Social adjustment problems
Living alone
Separation
Unemployment
Firearm in household
Alcohol intoxication

Risk factors are characteristics that have been identified through research to increase the probability that a specific state of health or illness will develop. The presence or absence of one or more risk factors does not necessarily predict the occurrence of the condition. Risk factors include a combination of biological characteristics, behavior, stressful life events, and environmental exposure that place people at high risk. Screening tests for early detection of disease, counseling for risk reduction, immunizations to prevent infections, and other primary and secondary prevention measures are based on this knowledge.

GAIL A. HARKNESS

See also
**CARDIOVASCULAR RISK FACTORS:
CHOLESTEROL
CHRONIC ILLNESS
CULTURAL/TRANSCULTURAL FOCUS
EPIDEMIOLOGY
OBESITY AS A CARDIOVASCULAR
RISK FACTOR**

ROGERS'S SCIENCE OF UNITARY HUMAN BEINGS

Rogers's science of unitary human beings is the most abstract of all the nursing models. Her science and its abstractness emerged from her synthesis of the scientific literature as well as through intuitive ways of knowing. Through her science, Rogers provides nurses a broad vision of people as unitary, not the narrow concrete view of people as fragmented objects that is prevalent in much of today's science.

It is the abstractness of Rogers's science that enriches creative and imaginative thinking for nurses to understand people and their environments. This abstractness also provides nurses an optimal structure and process for education, practice, and research, thus enhancing their power to create knowledge for the advancement of nursing science. The precision of her science is evident in the four postulates of energy fields, pattern, openness, and pandimensionality. These postulates are assumed to be true; their existence does not have to be proved.

Rogers saw the universe as energy and a whole, manifesting itself by energy fields. For Rogers, these energy fields are fundamental to everything in the universe, and they are dynamic and always in motion. According to Rogers, there are two energy fields of concern to nurses: human energy fields and environmental energy fields. She states that a person, as well as the environment, is an energy field and that the two are integral with each other. If a person has an energy field, one would be dealing with parts rather than wholeness. Moreover, because people and their environments are inseparable from the universe and infinite, Rogers gave nurses a new understanding of the word *unitary* in her science.

Unitary means undivided or whole, which Rogers refers to as indivisible and irreducible, thus specifying that each person is a unified phenomenon. Within the tenets of energy fields as delineated in Rogers's science, this means that people and the environment are different from a sum of their parts. In fact, when a thing is called unitary, parts do not exist. To obtain a Rogerian understanding of people, nurses cannot use ideas such as cell theory or the reductionist view of people from disciplines of biology, physiology, psychology, and sociology.

For example, nurses' knowledge of the parts of a person with AIDS gives no information about what that person as a whole is experiencing. In such situations, Rogers's science helps nurses to abandon outdated knowledge of parts and to understand the wholeness of people so that they can provide care that helps them to understand and appreciate the fullness of life.

Nurses have the responsibility to create concepts and theories that are meaningful in giving unitary nursing care to people. Such knowledge will help nurses to identify the distinctive attributes of each person, which are related to Rogers's postulate of pattern that distinguishes people and their environments. It is knowledge of pattern, the distinguishing characteristic of all energy fields, that is essential to nurses' care of people. Rogers states that each person, as well as his or her environment, has a unique pattern. Each person's pattern is different; therefore, nursing care cannot be the same for all people, even if they are experiencing a similar phenomenon such as AIDS or breast cancer.

Because Rogers's postulate of pattern is an abstraction that cannot be seen, people ask, "How does a nurse gain knowledge of it?" The answer is that a person's pattern is revealed through manifestations that come from the mutual person-environment process. Nurses are challenged when they realize that there are pattern manifestations invisible to the physical eye; these can be experienced by people in different ways. Once nurses know that there are other processes besides the five senses—sight, hearing, smell, taste, and touch—available to them, they will be open to such things as intuitive ways of knowing that help them to experience and understand invisible pattern manifestations.

Nurses may wonder how a person's pattern is manifested. Rogers's postulate of openness makes this possible. The person and the nurse are always open, as are their environmental fields. There are no degrees of openness to Rogers's energy fields; in fact, there are no closed energy fields in the universe. With this openness, people and their environments are integral. There is a mutual flow of energy through each other, not around each other. This mutual flow negates the traditional views of adaptation and causation; there can be only a continuous mutual patterning where everything changes simultaneously, where patterns are revealed through manifestations.

Rogers's postulate of pandimensionality offers nurses new ways to experience and understand a person's pattern and its manifestations, including the invisible ones. Because pandimensionality enables nurses to be aware of the infinite wholeness of energy fields, including their own, they are not confined to space and time. This signifies that nurses can experience the universe without boundaries or time constraints placed on their awareness of the actual and potential manifestations of people. In such instances, pandimensionality gives new meaning to experiences through such concepts as visualization, imagery, intuition, empathy, imagination, caring, and the paranormal. Pandimensionality helps nurses to create new forms of communicating with people and to enrich those that are important for unitary nursing care. This knowledge will give nurses an ability to experience manifestations that currently seem to be an impossibility; however, some nurses already know there is something other than the traditional space-time aspects of nursing that is nonphysical and that appears to be unmeasurable.

Rogers offers nurses ways to participate in the changes occurring in people and nursing today. Rogers's principles of hemodynamics give nurses an understanding of the nature and process of change. Rogers sees change as innovative: people become more diverse and have the capacity to participate knowingly in all of their actual and potential manifestations throughout the life process. People participate in their becoming by patterning an unending flow of energy in which change is unpredictable.

It is the responsibility of nurses to use Rogerian knowledge of change to conduct research that reveals the nature of pattern and its manifestations. Nurses can use this knowledge to create new ideas of nursing to replace outdated ones. As Rogers was a participator in enhancing the creativity of nursing, nurses can be creative in using her science for the advancement of nursing.

JOHN R. PHILLIPS

See also
CARING

EMPATHY
NONTRADITIONAL THERAPIES
NURSING THEORETICAL MODELS

ROLE OF GOVERNMENT

The first public health policy act was signed on July 16, 1798, by President John Adams. A public health service organization, later named the U.S. Public Health Service (USPHS), would operate hospitals and rest homes for sick merchant seamen. The act was expanded in 1877 as a result of a yellow fever epidemic in New Orleans that required the passage of the Quarantine Act of 1878.

In 1879 a National Board of Health was established to monitor public health regularly, especially in the area of sanitation. A weekly report that later became the *Public Health Reports* was published. The board had the authority to intervene in case of an epidemic. In the late 19th century, Robert Koch and Louis Pasteur made important discoveries about the nature of infectious diseases that explained the transmission of such diseases and aided in controlling their spread. In this control, government had a significant role.

Nursing Research

Nursing care research is defined as research directed to understanding the nursing care of individuals and groups and the biological, physiological, social, behavioral, and environmental mechanisms influencing health and disease that are relevant to nursing care. Nursing research develops knowledge about health and the promotion of health over the life span, care of persons with health problems and disabilities, and nursing actions that enhance the ability of individuals to respond effectively to actual or potential health problems.

Although the role of the federal government became significant in 1938 through grants-in-aid to universities under a research grants program, it is generally held that nursing research began after World War II, even though the work of Florence Nightingale (1820–1910) introduced the use of statistics in analyzing nursing data. Beginning in 1920, the Goldmark study was the first of the landmark studies of nursing. Research delved into nursing education, time studies, salaries, supply and demand, employment conditions, costs, status of nurses, job satisfaction, needs, and resources. In 1955 the Nursing Research Grants and Fellowship Program of the Division of Nursing, USPHS, was established; it awarded grants for nursing research projects, nursing research fellowships, and nurse-scientist graduate training. In 1978 the Division of Manpower Analysis to conduct research on manpower was established within the Division of Nursing in the Bureau of Health Manpower.

Thirty years after the idea was first proposed by the National Institutes of Health's National Advisory Council, the National Center for Nursing Research (NCNR) was established in 1986. Its mandate was "to advance science to strengthen nursing practice and health care that promotes health, prevents disease, and ameliorates the effects of illness and disability." The placement of the NCNR at the National Institutes of Health (NIH) moved nursing research into a broader based biomedical research environment and facilitated the collaboration between nursing and other research disciplines. On June 9, 1993, the NCNR was renamed and became the National Institute of Nursing Research, which placed nursing on an equal footing with other NIH institutes.

Role of Government in Current Nursing Research

The National Institute of Nursing Research is the key organ for funding nursing research grants and contracts and has approved priority areas for research as determined by its National Advisory Council for Nursing Research in 1986. The research priorities include (a) low birthweight (mothers and infants); (b) HIV infection, prevention and care; (c) long-term care for the elderly; (d) symptom management; (e) information systems; and (f) health promotion and technology dependency across the life span. Other issues identified for research are understanding the dysfunctioning bladder and bowel, nursing and biology interface, home health care supportive services for older adults,

interventions to manage Alzheimer's disease symptoms, community-based care for the chronically ill older person, biobehavioral symptom management, and minority youth health behavior. Additional focused areas of research have included community-based nursing models (1995); effectiveness of nursing interventions in HIV/AIDS (1996); cognitive impairment (1997); living with chronic illness (1998); and biobehavioral factors related to immunocompetence (1999).

The establishment of the Agency for Health Care Policy and Research (AHCPR) within USPHS in December 1988 has also contributed to the development of nursing research. This agency focuses on the development of clinical practice guidelines, outcome measures, and effectiveness research.

U.S. Public Health Service

The nursing programs of the USPHS stimulated the postwar expansion of nursing services through pilot studies, nursing research, and community health services. The Division of Nursing Resources, with a modest budget of $95,000 and a small staff, was able to undertake a number of landmark studies to find solutions to postwar nursing problems in hospitals and health agencies. During the years 1949 to 1955 a number of state surveys of nursing needs and resources were conducted in almost all states.

In 1954, among the many studies and tools developed by the USPHS Division of Nursing Resources (now the Division of Nursing) was a cooperative study carried out with the Commission on Nursing of Cleveland, Ohio, to discover the reasons for the understaffing of nursing departments. A byproduct of the study was that it produced the outcome measure patient satisfaction. Another study involved the use of disease classification for nursing planning. The diagnoses were then coded and classified into 58 groups representing discrete nursing problems. A similar methodological approach was followed in the development of the problem-oriented medical record more than a decade later and in the development of diagnostic related groups (DRGs). In 1955, Congress earmarked $625,000 for nursing research and fellowships that were awarded directly to universities, hospitals, health agencies, and professional associations.

History of Military Nursing

The Army Nurse Corps initiated nursing research in the military and has been a major contributor to the evolution of both military and civilian nursing research. The establishment of a Department of Nursing at Walter Reed Army Research Institute, with a Nursing Research Department in 1957, provided formal recognition and opportunities for growth of military nursing research. The army developed a program designed to concentrate on clinical nursing research in addition to fostering participation in the collaborative studies of other disciplines.

The history of nursing research in the navy (primarily unpublished master's theses) covers research topics that are broad and focus on various aspects of the organization and administration of nursing service. Further work to incorporate nursing research into the Navy Nurse Corps became prominent in 1987, when the navy conducted a review of billets and identified the need for doctorally prepared nurses.

The history of nursing research in the air force is found primarily through the review of unpublished mimeographed documents covering research at the School of Aerospace Medicine at Brooks Air Force Base, Texas. Among the research topics reported are the development of equipment for aeromedical evacuation (such as examination lamps, oxygen and humidity apparatus, hand disinfection devices, patient monitoring and blood pressure measurement, litter lift, and transportable airborne stations). Physiological and psychological changes experienced by air force nurses associated with flying duty on jet and propeller aircraft and ways to evaluate patient care in flight are other areas of research.

The TriService Nursing Research Program

In the fall of 1990, representatives from the army, navy and air force met to discuss collaborative research among the services. This group formed the Federal Nursing Research Interest Group, which later became the TriService Nursing Research Group (TSNR Group). The TSNR Group was made responsible for finding ways to promote military nursing research both collectively and individually, within and across the services. The initial appropriation for the TSNR program under S.R. 102-154 was $1 million for fiscal year (FY) 1992 and increased to $5 million in FY 1996, authorizing the TSNR program as part of the Department of Defense Health Care Program, administered by the TSNR Group and established at the Uniformed Services University of the Health Sciences.

FAYE G. ABDELLAH

See also
HISTORY OF NURSING RESEARCH
INFECTION CONTROL
NATIONAL INSTITUTE OF NURSING
   RESEARCH
NATIONAL INSTITUTES OF HEALTH

ROLE SUPPLEMENTATION: A NURSING THERAPEUTIC

Role supplementation is a nursing intervention designed to help individuals develop competence and mastery in new roles acquired because of health and illness experiences. Role supplementation is particularly indicated during transitions when used preventively or therapeutically to support healthy transitions and healthy outcomes for clients, their significant others, and their families. It is used when role insufficiency is anticipated, observed, or experienced. Role insufficiency is defined as any difficulty in carrying out the behaviors and the goals of new roles, such as caregiving, at risk, sick, well, or nonbattering, among other health- or illness-related roles. The difficulty may be experienced by the person undergoing the transition or observed by others who are able to articulate the responses of the person as well as their meanings.

Role supplementation is a deliberate and systematic nursing action designed to prevent role insufficiency or to therapeutically treat role insufficiency. Components of role supplementation are role clarification and role taking. To help clients and their families understand and develop the new roles needed because of changes in health or illness status, the nature of the role and the meaning of the sought identity require clarification. Role clarification, a component of role supplementation, is the process of uncovering the nature, meaning, processes, risks, and behaviors inherent in the new role, such as the caregiving role. Roles evolve through dialogues in conjunction with other roles, as they tend to be embedded in other roles. Therefore, acquisition of new roles could be considered only within the context of relationships with significant others. Another component of role supplementation is role taking. During the process of assuming each other's roles, that is, taking the role of the significant other, one can better understand how and why patients or partners respond in a certain way. As roles are clarified, roles that are mutually satisfying and complementary are created or modified in the process (Meleis, 1975).

Several strategies can be used to clarify and promote role-taking skills. Two such strategies are role modeling and role rehearsal. Clients undergoing transitions that require the acquisition of new roles (such as caregiving) or the development of new identities (such as mother) may benefit from hearing about the experiences of others or seeing others who have undergone the transition successfully (role modeling). They may also acquire the new role with more comfort if they have opportunities to practice some aspects of the new role (role rehearsal). Therefore, role modeling and role rehearsal may enhance role acquisition and facilitate the development of the desired identity. The components of role clarification and role taking and the strategies of rehearsal and modeling are connected with communication and interaction between nurses, clients, and significant others.

Role supplementation is the label given to the theory that describes each of these concepts and the interaction between them. Role supplementation was used and tested with couples assuming the new role of parenting (Meleis & Swendsen, 1978) and to help post–myocardial infarction patients develop an at-risk identity that led to compliance with a rehabilitation regimen (Dracup, Meleis, Baker, & Edlefsen, 1984). An explanatory framework using

role supplementation described how the elderly maintained their sexuality (Kass & Rousseau, 1983) and how parental caregiving roles were acquired (Brackley, 1992). Role supplementation was used in an intervention framework to ease the roles of caregivers for Alzheimer's disease patients (Kelly & Lakin, 1988). A theoretical framework was based on role supplementation to describe women who were not successful in becoming mothers and who manifested role insufficiency (Gaffney, 1992). Role supplementation has also been used in numerous master's and doctoral theses.

With patients being discharged earlier, nurses will play a major role in facilitating their transition to home care. Role supplementation provides an intervention framework for systematic care and evaluation. A future direction for further development of role supplementation is to critically analyze completed research results. Systematic testing of each component and strategy will help in refining this nursing therapeutic.

AFAF IBRAHIM MELEIS

See also
CAREGIVER
NURSE-PATIENT COMMUNICATION
NURSE-PATIENT INTERACTION
PREGNANCY
TRANSITIONAL CARE

ROY ADAPTATION MODEL

The Roy adaptation model for nursing defines *person* as a holistic adaptive system that is in constant interaction with the environment. As a holistic adaptive system the person can be described as a set of interrelated parts with inputs, control and feedback processes, and outputs functioning as a whole for some purpose. Inputs for the system are stimuli received externally from the environment (external stimuli) and internally from within the self (internal stimuli). These stimuli are classified as focal, contextual, or residual. The stimuli immediately confronting the person are called focal stimuli. All other stimuli in the situation that contribute to the effect of the focal stimuli are called contextual stimuli. Stimuli whose effects on the given situation are unclear are called residual stimuli.

The control processes of the system are two coping mechanisms, the regulator and cognator subsystems, to adapt or to cope with a changing environment. The process of perception links the regulator and cognator subsystems. Outputs of the system are responses, called behavior, that result from regulator and cognator activity. Behaviors are manifested in four adaptive modes: physiological, self-concept, role function, and interdependence. Behavior can be observed, measured, or subjectively reported and, in collaboration with the person, judged as adaptive or ineffective. Adaptive responses maintain or promote integrity or health, whereas ineffective responses disrupt integrity. Through feedback processes, behaviors (responses) provide further input for the person as a system.

The goal of nursing is to promote adaptation by enhancing the person-environment interaction through the use of the nursing process. Within the Roy adaptation model, nursing interventions are conceptualized as the management or manipulation of stimuli. Assumptions of the Roy adaptation model are both scientific and philosophical. The scientific assumption are derived from systems theory and adaptation-level theory, whereas the philosophical assumptions are related to humanism (Roy & Andrews, 1991).

The elements and assumptions of the Roy adaptation model provide a perspective for nursing research by suggesting what phenomena to study, identifying the research questions, and identifying appropriate methods of inquiry. The phenomena of study are persons as individuals or in groups. The distinctive nature of the research questions is related to basic life processes and patterns, coping with health and illness, and enhancing adaptive coping. Multiple methods are appropriate when conducting research based on the Roy adaptation model (Roy & Andrews, 1991).

A search of the literature revealed numerous studies that used the Roy adaptation model as the conceptual framework for the research, with considerable variability in the clarity and specificity of the links between the Roy adaptation model and the research. Some studies used the model in the development of data collection instruments within the four adaptive modes; other studies used the four adaptive modes as a framework for data analysis. Additional studies identified specific concepts from the model, such as interdependence mode or physical self, and used them as the basis for the research.

A number of studies identified specific links, conceptually and operationally, between the Roy adaptation model and the research variables. In these studies specific concepts were linked to the various aspects of the model, including focal, contextual, and residual stimuli; control processes; and adaptive modes. These concepts were then operationalized by identifying specific measurement tools. Several studies identified nursing interventions as the management or manipulation of stimuli, and some specifically tested propositions derived from the model.

Among the studies there were differences in methodologies, designs, data collection procedures, and data analysis techniques. A review of the research designs used in the studies revealed both cross-sectional and longitudinal designs, as well as prospective and ex post facto designs. Case study, single group, and comparison group designs were all represented in the studies reviewed. Additionally, designs ranged from exploratory, including descriptive-correlational and descriptive-comparative, to experimental and quasi-experimental.

Similarly, variety was found in the approaches used for data collection. Data were collected by record reviews, observation, interview, researcher-developed questionnaires, and standardized questionnaires such as the Norbeck Social Support Questionnaire and the State-Trait Anxiety Inventory. Methods of data analysis were both quantitative and qualitative. Several studies used qualitative data analysis procedures such as content analysis and the constant comparative method for grounded theory. The studies reviewed revealed that the Roy adaptation model was appropriate for guiding research in a variety of settings and populations.

Among those who have built a program of research using the Roy adaptation model are J. Fawcett, S. E. Pollock, and L. Tulman. Fawcett and Tulman (1990) conducted methodological (instrument development) and substantive research related to childbearing families. Retrospective and longitudinal studies examined factors associated with functional status during the postpartum period, and one study (Fawcett, 1990) tested an intervention derived from the Roy adaptation model.

The studies identified childbirth as the focal stimulus. Demographic variables, fear and anxiety, and father at delivery were among the contextual variables identified. The intervention, preparation for caesarean childbirth, was conceptualized as a contextual stimulus. The physiological mode was represented by health variables, pain, and distress; the self-concept mode was represented by individual psychosocial variables such as self-esteem. Family variables, feelings for baby, and marital relationship represented the interdependence mode, and functional status represented the role function mode.

Pollock (1993) and colleagues conducted a series of five longitudinal studies to examine human responses to chronic illness by identifying predictors of adaptation to chronic illness and determining whether adaptive responses differed by diagnostic group. Over a period of 7 years, 597 adults with various chronic health problems participated. The studies identified chronicity as the focal stimulus; and demographic characteristics, ability to tolerate stress, health promotion activities, participation in patient education programs, and health-related hardiness were considered contextual stimuli. Perceptions of illness impact represented the regulator and cognator mechanisms, and adaptation was represented by physiological and psychological integrity. Psychological integrity was examined in three modes: intrapsychic function (self-concept), role function, and social function.

These studies by Fawcett, Pollock, and Tulman demonstrate the usefulness of the Roy adaptation model as a guide for nursing research and support the credibility of the model. Using the Roy adaptation model to guide nursing research has contributed to both the basic and the clinical science of nursing. Increased understanding of the factors influencing adaptive and ineffective responses and the testing of nursing interventions designed to promote adaptive responses are examples. Studies have provided some confirmation for the model, demonstrated its ability to generate new information, and contributed to clinical practice.

Research that continues to test the model and the relationships among its components is needed.

One area that has been identified as a research concern is the overlap between the four adaptive modes. Further research may clarify this issue. Additional research should test nursing interventions to promote adaptive responses.

MARY E. TIEDEMAN

See also
BEHAVIORAL RESEARCH
COPING
NURSING PROCESS
NURSING THEORETICAL MODELS
ROLE SUPPLEMENTATION: A NURS-
ING THERAPEUTIC

RURAL HEALTH

Common usage of the word *rural* tends to imply a single dimension and universal image of rural life. Yet historic, cultural, economic, geographic, demographic, and occupational diversity is the hallmark of rural communities. Differences within rural areas and between rural areas are often as marked as differences between rural and urban settings. Understanding rural health needs has been hampered by the lack of a clear definition of rural to encompass the richness of the multiple dimensions of rural life, inadequate measurement of the degree of rurality, a fragmented and inadequate research base, and the absence of rural theory. This collection of factors inhibits the development of an adequate rural health profile, which can lead to a misdirection of resources and programs to address the health issues of rural communities. The challenge of grappling with the definition, description, and dimensions of the rural health faces not only rural nurses but those who plan community services, set policy, conduct research, or educate clinicians to work with rural dwellers.

Rural Diversity

Rurality can no longer be equated with agriculture as the typical rural occupations of farming, logging, fishing, and mining now account for less than 10 percent of non-metropolitan jobs. The economic base is highly diversified and includes manufacturing and service-related jobs associated with retirement communities, national parks, and recreational services. Computer modem and fax-linked workers now pursue urban careers from rural locations. The increasing variety in occupations and rapid advances in technology are blurring differences among urban and rural populations.

The enormous complexity and diversity of rural environments is possibly the most poorly understood fundamental factor in dealing with the health needs of rural communities. Because of the extent of the population and geographic diversity, a typical rural town is difficult to describe. As rural places are not all carbon copies of each other, neither are rural dwellers. For example, in Idaho there are few people with HIV infection, and those often have returned home for support in the final phases of the disease; whereas in Georgia, new cases of the HIV infection are discovered daily, especially among the rural poor (Berry, 1993).

Rural Definition

The diversity of rural settings contributes to the problem of developing an adequate definition of *rural*. The most frequently used classifications are rural/urban and metropolitan/non-metropolitan. These definitions imply clear-cut distinctions between opposing absolutes and gloss over the richness of the multiple dimensions of rural life. In using these two definitions, substantively different conclusions can be drawn. Hewitt (1992) noted that the elderly make up a larger proportion of the total population in non-metropolitan areas. However, if the urban/rural definition is applied, just the opposite is true: the proportion of elderly is greater in urban areas than in rural area.

A new interval-level research measure, the Montana State University Rurality Index, is designed to assign a degree of rurality to each participant in a study and is calculated using two pieces of easily obtained data: county population and distance to emergency care (Weinert & Boik, 1995). A degree of rurality is assigned to each family on a rural/urban continuum, avoiding artificial categorization, allowing for a finer urban/rural distinction, and permitting differentiation among residents in the same county.

Rural Health Profile

When considering rural health statistics, care must be taken not to generalize. For example, a global statistic such as "higher infant mortality rates in rural areas" is true. Yet for some rural areas the rates are actually lower than the national average.

In general, rural dwellers are more likely to suffer from chronic conditions such as arthritis, ulcers, thyroid, and renal disease and higher morbidity resulting from diabetes, hypertension, cardiac conditions, and pulmonary diseases. Childhood injury rates are higher, and farm machinery and tractor rollovers account for one half of the deaths of rural children. Machinery running in enclosed spaces may cause carbon monoxide poisoning, and harvesting equipment and power-take-off equipment can cause amputations, crushing, and suffocating injuries. There is a greater likelihood of hazardous occupations resulting in skin cancer from sun exposure, respiratory problems from exposure to pesticides, and hearing loss from the high noise levels of farm machinery. Factors unique to rural areas such as greater poverty, substandard living conditions, hazardous working conditions, health beliefs, and the scarcity of primary health care services intensify the magnitude of the health problems rural dwellers face (U.S. Department Health and Human Services, 1995).

Motor vehicle death rates are highest in sparsely populated counties and are attributed to variation in road conditions, not using seat belts, high speeds, types of vehicles, and limited emergency care. Accidents are complicated by the length of time before they are discovered, time needed for transfer to a health care facility, lack of availability of support equipment, and the level of expertise of health care personnel.

Other rural health concerns are domestic violence, use of smokeless tobacco, heavy drinking and smoking among adults, suicide, and unintentional firearms injuries. The death rate from unintentional shootings in rural areas is approximately

2.5 times the rates in central cities, and the rural suicide rate is 1.5 times higher.

Economic stressors such as the sagging farm economy take a heavy psychological toll and often force many rural dwellers to change from lifelong, multi generational careers in farming. A farmer's income for the year can be heavily dependent on rainfall, insects, and temperatures, and a hailstorm at harvest time can completely wipe out a year's income.

Rural residents are less likely to engage in preventive behaviors such as using seat belts, exercising, having Pap smears, or being immunized. Pregnant rural women are more likely to begin prenatal care later in their pregnancy and make fewer prenatal clinic visits. On some health indicators rural residents are clearly at risk, and on some there are no measurable urban/rural differences. Although the health of rural dwellers can be demonstrated to differ from that of urban residents, these differences are not universal across all health indicators or all rural population groups.

Rural Nursing Research

Rural America offers opportunities for focusing programs, targeting populations and locales, and testing well conceived ideas across a range of settings. Research-based rural practice should focus on (a) testing emerging rural nursing theory; (b) operationalizing and measuring rurality; (c) con-

ducting community-based interventions; (d) targeting research on specific topics with replication studies and multisite and collaborative studies; (e) designing studies to explore rural/urban differences; (f) developing measures that are valid, reliable, and sensitive to rural issues; (g) examining of the contextual factors that distinguish one rural area from another, as well as, those that are similar for all or most rural areas; and (h) exploring innovative methods to capture the picture of rural life and rural health needs (Weinert & Burman, 1994).

Rural is clearly a paradox. Evidence exists to support the classic bucolic, and healthy image of rural life. However, even after adjusting for compositional differences between rural and urban populations there remains a negative health effect associated with life in rural areas. The definition and measurement of rurality, an understanding of the vast diversity within and between rural settings, and an appreciation for the unique factors associated with the rural health profile are critical when conducting rural research, educating rural health care providers, and planning and providing services for rural communities.

CLARANN WEINERT

See also
ACCESS TO HEALTH CARE
CHRONIC ILLNESS
COMMUNITY HEALTH
TELEHEALTH
VULNERABLE POPULATIONS

S

SAMPLING

Sampling is a process or way in which one selects a representative part of the population of interest to make valid inferences and generalizations. A sample is not only more feasible, economical, and practical than using the whole population; it is often more accurate (Pedhazur & Schmelkin, 1991a). A

sample, in contrast to the greater number of cases in an entire population, decreases the likelihood of nonsampling errors such as measurement errors, nonresponse biases, and recording and coding errors. Most researchers think of sampling as important for accurately representing the population in descriptive terms, that is, external validity or generalization. Sampling, however, also is concerned with the relationships found. Therefore, sampling errors or biases may threaten internal validity as well. Also, strictly speaking, samples are not "representative," "unbiased," or "fair" (Stuart, 1968). Because the researcher never knows the true population values, one cannot determine if any given sample is truly representative of the population. It is the sampling *process* that is representative, unbiased, or fair.

There are several types of sampling. Simple random sampling is a procedure that may involve the use of a table of random numbers or the flip of a coin to determine who or what will be included in the sample. This approach, however, is often impractical and tedious and is infrequently used. Systematic random sampling involves the use of a random start and then the selection of every *k*th case or incidence. This approach is more convenient than simple random sampling, but it can have variance estimation problems (Kish, 1965).

A minimum of two systematic random samples with independent random starts is needed to estimate variance, unless one can assume a random distribution of the cases on the list used for sampling (Pedhazur & Schmelkin, 1991a). Also, when using systematic random sampling, one must be careful that the list does not have some systematic order or periodicity. If so, systematic random sampling may lead to a seriously misrepresented sample or pattern. For example, one might inadvertently select all head nurses if the sampling interval mimicked the sequencing of head nurses on the list. Or one might obtain blood samples only when certain hormones are at their peaks if the sampling time interval mimicked when the hormone peaked.

Stratified sampling is another method of random sampling. It involves identifying one or more classification variables for sampling purposes. With stratified sampling, one randomly samples within each nonoverlapping stratum of the classification variables (Pedhazur & Schmelkin, 1991a). For example, if sex is the classification variable, one randomly samples men and women separately. Stratified sampling is intended to decrease sampling variability by increasing the homogeneity of the strata. For research purposes, it is best to select classification variables on the basis of their assumed association with the dependent variable, choosing those that are uncorrelated with each other. Stratified sampling facilitates obtaining subgroup parameter estimates, may increase the statistical efficiency of estimates if proportional allocation is used, and may be more convenient if sampling lists are organized according to the selected strata. However, stratified sampling also may be more costly and complex and generally is applied to some, but not all, variables of interest (Pedhazur & Schmelkin, 1991a).

Cluster sampling is a fourth type of random sampling. Here the elements of interest for the study and the sampling units are not the same. The sampling unit or cluster is a convenient, practical, and economical grouping, such as practice sites, whereas the elements of interest for the study may be the individual patients obtained at the practice sites. Thus, one randomly samples the clusters and takes all elements (or a relevant, random subset) within each cluster. In contrast to stratified sampling, where one samples from all strata of the classification variable, one samples only some clusters in cluster sampling. In contrast to desiring homogeneous strata, clusters should be as heterogeneous as possible (Pedhazur & Schmelkin, 1991a). To the extent that the clusters are not heterogeneous, one loses some precision, and the cluster sample is less efficient than a simple random sample of the same size. At the extreme, if the cluster is completely homogeneous, one achieves no gain from more than one case per cluster.

Finally, convenience samples, or nonprobability samples, are frequently used in nursing research. However, it is not possible to estimate sampling errors with such samples (Pedhazur & Schmelkin, 1991a). Therefore, the validity of inferences drawn from nonprobability samples to the population remains unknown. Moreover, whenever nonrandom selection is used, the potential for serious sample selection biases exists. It is well known that sample selection bias may threaten internal as well as external validity. For this reason, sampling on one's dependent variable should never be done.

LAUREN S. AARONSON

See also
DATA ANALYSIS
PILOT STUDY
POPULATIONS AND AGGREGATES

REPLICATION STUDIES
VALIDITY

SCHIZOPHRENIA NURSING RESEARCH

The term *schizophrenia* evokes the most identifiable picture of a psychiatric illness. Of all the major mental disorders, schizophrenia probably exacts the most stigma, cost, family burden, and controversy. Over time, debate regarding the exact definition and presentation of schizophrenia has been a catalyst for research and innovation in treatment approaches. Various methods for diagnosis and treatment have been pursued over the years, changing to fit emerging technology and a better understanding of treatment effectiveness.

The contemporary focus for research in schizophrenia has become increasingly biological in nature, with a concomitant increase in inventive approaches that involve psychiatric rehabilitation and consumer-oriented programs. Nursing research in schizophrenia mirrors those changing paradigms. Historically, one of the early pioneers of psychiatric mental health nursing, Hildegard Peplau, wrote extensively on the nature of the one-to-one relationship and the helping model for psychiatric care, particularly inpatient care. Current nursing research on the understanding and treatment of schizophrenia reflects a variety of treatment settings, including acute inpatient care, partial hospitalization, outpatient groups, psychosocial rehabilitation, family and consumer education, and medication management. Increasingly, nursing research involves a better understanding of the broad place of health and illness for persons with a diagnosis of schizophrenia.

Review of major studies, researchers, and methodology in schizophrenia reveals a medley of foci. Nursing researchers have contributed to the understanding of symptoms and symptom self-monitoring by individuals with schizophrenia. In particular, nursing studies have validated or expanded findings in the area of prodromal symptoms (McClandless-Glimcher et al., 1986; O'Connor, 1991), delineation of the course of disorder (Harding, 1988), and the nature of family burden and expressed emotion (Loukissa, 1995). Nursing researchers have been forerunners in the area of understanding comorbidity issues such as the relationship between mental illness and physical health (Holmberg & Kane, 1995). In addition, because nursing interventions are directly related to knowledge of genetics and neurochemical disturbances, nursing research related to these areas has increased (Fox, 1990).

Additionally, nursing research has contributed to much of the program and policy literature in the post-deinstitutionalization era. The movement to community-based care has been advocated for, written about, and researched by nurses in federal, state, and local community agencies (Mann et al., 1993; Palmer-Erbs & Anthony, 1995).

Research appears to be important in the nursing practice arena. Review of a MEDLINE search on the topic of schizophrenia reveals 32,914 citations, only 278 with a nursing focus. Nursing specialty organizations such as the Society for Education and Research in Psychiatric Mental Health Nursing (SERPN) and the American Psychiatric Nurses Association (APNA) organize yearly conferences around research papers and innovative educational approaches. Other methods of dissemination include nursing journals specifically for or with specific features of nursing research findings. These include *Archives of Psychiatric Nursing* and *Journal of Psychiatric Nursing*. Additionally, nurse researchers are common contributors to interdisciplinary journals (i.e., *Psychiatric Services*, a journal with an interdisciplinary purpose and nurses as contributing editors and board members).

Future Directions

Scientific advances in schizophrenia, including genetic, neurobiological, cognitive, and psychosocial findings, have been increasingly integrated with nursing practice principles and interventions. Future research in treatment areas, including incorporation of ethnic and cultural differences, responses to a variety of treatments, and focus on outcome measures, seems likely. Given what we learn from the science of schizophrenia, nursing still consists of both the art and science of human responses. Therefore, gleaning from the biological sphere, nursing research must balance the need for new and improved information related to how to provide caring, supportive, and humane treatment with bi-opsychosocial information. How the disabilities from schizophrenia interact with physical health, family coping, and community adaptation continues to require research.

Economic concerns exist in many shapes. The decade of the 1990s has been labeled "the decade of the brain" to reflect the growing money and effort devoted to understanding the neurobiological nature of schizophrenia and other major mental illnesses. The personal and societal loss that accompanies such a persistent and disabling disorder has economic costs difficult to measure. Primary prevention research aimed at understanding earlier detection and treatment is needed.

Ethical issues in schizophrenia present a complicated picture. Informed consent issues take the forefront in both clinical and research arenas. Informed consent, the assumption that adults have the right to consent or refuse to consent to treatment, is complicated when one determines their judgment or competence to be altered by their illness. In the era of managed care, nursing research undoubtedly will explore the justice of the allocation of resources. Issues of access, quality, and cost are important variables for nursing research in the area of health care delivery systems.

SARAH P. FARRELL

See also
COMMUNITY MENTAL HEALTH
INFORMED CONSENT
MENTAL HEALTH IN PUBLIC SECTOR
  PRIMARY CARE
MENTAL HEALTH SERVICES RE-
  SEARCH
PEPLAU'S THEORETICAL MODEL

SCHLOTFELDT'S HEALTH-SEEKING NURSING MODEL

Rozella Schlotfeldt is truly a legend in her own time. She is cited by colleagues as an outstanding scholar, an original thinker, and an educator having innovative, progressive, and startling concepts for nursing (Safier, 1977). Schlotfeldt has published more than 120 scholarly works in books and journals. She has received numerous honors and awards, most notably election to the American Academy of Nursing and the Institute of Medicine, National Academy of Sciences. She was named a Living Legend by the American Academy of Nursing, received the Nell Watts Lifetime Achievement Award from Sigma Theta Tau International, and was awarded seven honorary doctorates.

What makes Schlotfeldt extraordinary is that she has made significant contributions to nursing research, nursing practice, nursing science, and nursing education. Three efforts that deserve recognition for their significance to the discipline of nursing but go beyond the scope of this article are (a) the development and implementation of the collaborative model between Frances Payne Bolton School of Nursing and University Hospitals of Cleveland in 1966, (b) the identification and use of factors that foster institutional support for nursing research, and (c) the development and implementation of the professional doctorate in nursing (ND). Major contributions to nursing research and nursing science include the development and refinement of the health-seeking nursing model, and the national and international leadership she provided in promoting critical analysis of nursing research, nursing science, and theory development via a sustained publication and presentation record.

Schlotfeldt's major influence on nursing research and nursing science arose from her writings in the 1960s and 1970s on the types of questions, designs, and methods appropriate for nursing research. Schlotfeldt addressed phenomena for the focus of nursing theories and the most promising approach to the development of theories significant for nursing.

In 1971, Schlotfeldt identified the central focus of practice as the care of people who need help in coping with problems along the continuum of health-illness. The origin of her health-seeking nursing model is defined by intervention modalities to enhance each individual's health-seeking behavior, to stimulate the avoidance of disease and disability, and to promote the productive use of inherent capacities for return to health and maximum capability in circumstances of disease, deprivation, genetic inadequacy, or trauma. She identified the focus of nursing inquiry as human behavior related to attaining, retaining, or regaining health and maximal function. The development of theories useful for nursing would focus on human behavior relative to the motivation to seek health, behavior in coping with crises encountered throughout life, and behavior to cope with diagnostic and therapeutic modalities (Schlotfeldt, 1971). Schlotfeldt reported in *Nursing Research* on a symposium held at Case Western Reserve in 1972. Whereas some of the nursing leaders contended there was no nursing science at the time, Schlotfeldt admonished them not to be defensive or self-conscious about using the term *nursing science*. She said, "We nurses also must put together, structure a body of verified knowledge, some from other disciplines and some that is verified, objective nursing knowledge per se; that is nursing science" (Schlotfeldt, 1972, p. 515).

Schlotfeldt's health-seeking nursing model was first described in its entirety in 1975. The model was developed to provide a conceptual framework for structuring nursing science and for directing nursing research. The major concepts of the model are person health-seeking behaviors, health-seeking mechanisms, intervening factors, health, nursing, and nursing strategies. A person is a biophysical, affective, cognitive, interpersonal, valuing human who possesses health assets (health-seeking behaviors and health-seeking mechanisms). Health-seeking behaviors are acquired and include physiological, psychological, social, cultural, institutional, philosophical, and spiritual activities that are essential to achievement of optimal health. Health-seeking mechanisms are inherent phenomena that are physiological, psychological, sociological, or genetically endowed.

Intervening factors are intrapersonal, interpersonal, and extrapersonal variables within the person's experience that may enhance or impede the attainment of optimal health. These factors include development and decline, environmental factors, educational and economic resources, belief, pathology-injury, illness, diagnosis, and medical treatment. Health is a dynamic state that may be inferred from one's level of physical and psychosocial functioning. Individuals seek optimal health throughout the life span. Optimal health is also sought by groups and the community.

Nursing care is provided when humans are unable to attain, maintain, or regain a level of optimal functioning. Nursing practice involves assisting people to maintain health, detecting deviations from health, helping to restore health, and supporting people during the life cycle. Nursing strategies are modalities used by nurses to stimulate or compensate for their client's health-seeking assets, such as assessing, compensating, sustaining-supporting, teaching-guiding, inspiring-stimulating, and motivating. Nursing strategies are also directed at intervening factors that may enhance or impede the person's attainment of health.

Schlotfeldt's health-seeking nursing model has been used for research purposes to explain results and to provide a nursing perspective, as a conceptual framework for specific research and as a predictive theoretical framework. Schlotfeldt's model primarily has been used to generate research questions and to explain research findings. Research based on Schlotfeldt's model encompassed family competence, nursing functions, coping processes of spouses of myocardial infarction patients, and prevention of confusion in hospitalized elderly persons. Other investigators explored health-seeking resources and adaptive functioning in depressed and nondepressed adults; factors associated with smoking cigarettes and health-seeking behaviors of mothers; guided imagery for enhancing health and health-seeking behaviors of employees in the work setting; nutrition knowledge and attitudes of weight maintainers, weight regainers, and normal weight women; and decision making by clients planning for continuing health care.

GREER GLAZER

See also
COMFORT
COPING
HEALTH CONCEPTUALIZATION
THEORETICAL FRAMEWORK

SCIENTIFIC DEVELOPMENT

Scientific development is a term defining the process of producing and making available new knowledge through systematically testing theories against empirical reality in order to solve problems. The term *scientific* is used as an attribute of the human knowledge interpreting natural, social, economical, historical, and psychological systems as parts of the empirical world. Scientific knowledge consists in systems of theories able to explain and solve scientific problems. Its essence is testability (Popper, 1969); it requires agreement among individuals about the nature of the problem and the validity of the explanation.

Controversies exist about what scientific knowledge is. For instance, the traditional empirical-ration-alism perspective holds the position that knowledge is scientific only when it has passed certain rigorous standards of method. Thus, only when reality has been defined in a measurable way and tested under sufficiently controlled conditions as an ''objective'' phenomenon (well protected from the investigators' subjective biases) can the generated knowledge be defined as scientific and therefore valid and reliable. Deductive reasoning facilitates objectivity by encouraging examination of a phenomenon in light of findings from previous . research, conceptualizations contributed by other scholars, and testing of more than one prediction. In this perspective, scientific knowledge progresses by a process of formulating bold conjectures and then subjecting them to equally bold criticism and test.

The main criticism against empirical rationalism comes from the phenomenological perspective originated by preeminent philosophers such as Husserl, Heidegger, and Merleau-Ponty. From the phenomenological point of view it does not make sense to objectify our knowledge because reality consists of the meanings one assigns throughout experiences. Therefore, to the phenomenologist there is no reality separated from the interaction of a person as a perceiving, meaning-giving being. Reality cannot be known independently of a person's experience with all its meanings: ''My knowledge of the world, even my scientific knowledge, is gained from my own particular point of view, or from some experience of the world without which the symbols of science would be meaningless'' (Merleau-Ponty, 1962, p. vii).

Theories of Rationality of the Scientific Development

The development of modern science can be defined from different theoretical perspectives; each one provides a rational framework (or a methodology) for understanding the historical development of human science. Each framework provides a set of rules for the validation of testable theories; those rules also can be used as criteria for demarcation between common and scientific knowledge. At least four different frameworks can be identified, each one characterized by a specific set of rules finalized to accept or reject theories or research programs.

Inductivism dictates that only those propositions describing hard facts or true generalizations of those facts (or very probable generalizations in the neoinductivist version) can be accepted as scientific. Inductivism's basic assumption is that primitive propositions can be directly derived from facts, and it has been widely criticized. An inductivist accepts a scientific proposition when proved true; otherwise it will be rejected. This approach has a very strict scientific rigor: a proposition has to be demonstrated by facts or inductively-deductively derived from propositions proved to be true. However, inductivism does not offer any explanation about directions of the scientific development, nor can it rationally explain the reasons for the main scientific progress of humankind.

Conventionalism defines science development as the building of systems organizing facts into a consistent whole. When inconsistencies arise, a conventionalist changes or modifies the system, assuming that it can be considered true or false by convention. According to this approach, science develops by accumulation on the level of facts and progresses through simplifications or better conventional explanations. For example, Einstein's theory was progressive because it provided a simpler explanation than former theories. For a conventionalist, false assumptions can lead to true conclusions; therefore, false theories may have great predictive power (this is a solid philosophical position, not to be confused with instrumentalism). Under conventionalism any idea can be acceptable and used for scientific inquiry; what cannot be used is not considered nonscientific, as in the inductivist approach.

Falsificationism admits that the basic assumptions about facts can be accepted by agreement, but it does not apply to the theories. According to this approach, a theory is scientific only if it can be tested against a basic assumption or if it can be experimentally falsified. Thus, a theory must be rejected if it conflicts with accepted assumptions. Popper (1969) stated that, in order to be considered scientific, a theory has to predict new facts (new because they are not considered by other rival theories), has to be empirically testable, and not be adjustable with ad hoc hypotheses. In the latter, more conventionalist version of this approach, some inductive principles are accepted. Falsificationists define the development of science as a process of falsifying the dominant theories: behind each important discovery there is a theory proved false. Scientific development is related to the importance of the falsified theories; the more important they are, the more progress that has been made.

Research programs have been proposed by Lakatos (1968) as methods of analysis for scientific development. Research programs are identified as testable results in terms of progressive and regressive "problemshifts." Scientific revolutions consist in substitution of a research program with a more advanced one. According to this approach a positive heuristic has to dictate the choice of problems for research instead of anomalies or incoherences, as in the falsificationism and inductivism methodologies. Therefore, the development of scientific theories is characterized by high degrees of freedom and is not influenced by the dominant paradigms. Thus, a research program progresses because its theoretical development anticipates the empirical one. It is regressing when it can provide only post hoc explanations because the empirical development is predominant over the theoretical one.

Each one of the four frameworks defines scientific development in a specific way. However, each perspective has to be integrated by external empirical theories able to explain the nonrational factors involved in scientific development, such as the social context and the historical period, because they are powerful forces driving or opposing any scientific development.

Scientific Development in Nursing Knowledge

A method of analysis that can define how knowledge evolves is essential for understanding scientific development in general as well as in a disciplinary field. Three approaches can be proposed to understand nursing's scientific development: (a) revolution, (b) evolution, and (c) integration.

Development by Revolution.   The concept of revolution was first used by Kant (1781/1991) to explain his idea that from an initial revolution a discipline will find a secure path for its scientific development. Kuhn (1970) introduced the idea that, under particular circumstances, the whole traditional paradigm (all theories, methods, applications, and instruments made available throughout a consistent tradition of research) is subject to change, not just a theory or a research program. Important progress in scientific development is possible through a series of transitions, from crisis or revolutions to normal science, when members of the field accept in a unified way a common, dominant paradigm (later defined as disciplinary matrix). Using a revolutionary perspective, nursing is in a preparadigmatic stage. Because there may not be periods of normal science (even if nursing knowledge is progressing), it is possible that the nursing scientific revolution may never come (Meleis, 1997).

Development by Evolution.   In this approach, knowledge progress is a gradual process of change and differentiation toward a higher level of complexity. It is a process of generating new ideas in continuity with the old ones and therefore systematically accumulating knowledge following a well-defined course. Propositions of one theory are used as premises for another; they are tested against the practice, and vice versa. As in the Darwinian process, environment continuously challenges the existent theories, and only the ones that interpret and meet its demands can temporarily survive. Using this approach to nursing, environmental demands for scientific development come from its practice and the scientific community. However, to date in nursing there are no recognizable trends of systematic development by accumulation.

Development by Integration. According to this approach, new ideas and theories are generated simultaneously without following any specific path. Thus, it is more than a process of testing, accepting, and rejecting theories; it is a process of developing agreement or disagreement about phenomena and methodologies that are most congruent with the subject matter of nursing. It follows, from this perspective, that nursing is much affected by external factors; nurses scientists gain insights mostly from the ongoing scientific developments in other fields. Therefore, nursing scientific development proceeds through a process of borrowing and repatterning ideas and theories across disciplines, as well as developing new ideas and differentiating them from the traditional ones; all are competing and coexisting.

From an evolutionist perspective, nursing has not accumulated enough knowledge to deserve the status of discipline; from an integrationist perspective, nursing is a discipline because it is able to provide new questions and answers, including repatterning, inventing, and testing knowledge through research and practice.

RENZO ZANOTTI

See also
  ACTION SCIENCE
  EPISTEMOLOGY
  MIDDLE-RANGE THEORY
  PHENOMENOLOGY
  THEORETICAL FRAMEWORK

SCIENTIFIC INTEGRITY

Scientific integrity is concerned with the principles of good science, which aim to promote the generation of knowledge that is both scientifically sound and ethically defensible. The principles are developed and operate within the frameworks of scientific community norms and ethical principles. Most authors conceive the domain of scientific integrity as concerned with the following: data management and access, publication practices, collaboration, mentorship, and conflict of interest. These areas collectively address scientists' duties and obligations toward science and society, fellow scientists, and their students.

Until recently, the rules governing the conduct of good science were implicit and understood among scientists. However, a number of highly publicized cases of scientific misconduct have heightened awareness of the public, legislative bodies, and professional groups. Given the scope of public funds devoted to science, demands for accountability have increased. As a result of these developments, policies and monitoring mechanisms have been created at every level to deal with ethical violations in research. A corollary development has occurred in educational institutions to systematically and formally teach good scientific practice during the training of future scientists. This has required the formalization and codification, by way of guidelines and policies, of canons of good science to guide the practice of science and the teaching of young scientists.

A survey of nursing found that instruction in scientific integrity varied greatly; the majority of schools limited coverage to the area of protection of human subjects, revealing a limited conception of scientific integrity. The norms regarding practices and data management varied greatly, with little consensus. The respondents saw varying roles for professional societies, institutions, and journals, but the need for common standards was frequently articulated (Ketefian & Lenz, 1995; Lenz & Ketefian, 1995).

Realizing the need for formal standards, the Midwest Nursing Research Society developed *Guidelines for Scientific Integrity* (MNRS, 1996). The guidelines are now being promulgated widely and are utilized by scientists in their research and teaching activities. The MNRS guidelines articulate general principles regarding relevant research practices that can be interpreted and applied to particular situations; it is recommended that institutions and research teams develop more specific guidelines for their unique situation. The main highlights of the MNRS guidelines are summarized below with permission of the society.

Data management and access. Research teams develop agreements among themselves regarding data access and use. The principal investigator has overall responsibility for the project. In the case of a grant, data belong to the institution; in the case of a contract, data belong to the funding agency. All team members have access to data and assume responsibility for safeguarding it. Following publication, relevant information is shared with qualified scientists within limits imposed by subject confidentiality. Steps are taken to assure that data are of high quality, making explicit any potential sources of bias. Procedures are developed for data collection, storage, and retrieval; data are reported accurately, avoiding intentional withholding or selective reporting; and data are kept for periods of 5–7 years or longer.

Authorship. Authors contribute substantively to published work and are able to defend it publicly, should the need arise. Substantive contribution may be operationalized in terms of assumption of responsibility for two or more of the following areas: conception and design, execution, analysis and interpretation of data, preparation and revision of manuscripts. Others who contribute in ways that are technical or financial are acknowledged. At the onset, teams should determine publication and authorship matters, such as how to report their results to avoid duplicative publications, ordering of authors, and the like. Status or rank of individuals should not be factors in authorship decisions.

Peer review. The best known current standards in the field are used in reviewing manuscripts or proposals. Peer reviewers maintain confidentiality, avoid conflicts of interest, and provide constructive and collegial comments. Any sources of bias that can jeopardize objectivity should be made known in advance.

Collaboration and mentorship. Teams determine, in advance, roles, responsibilities, and obligations of team members. Relationships are characterized by collegiality, respect, and openness. Senior team members provide mentorship and training opportunities for junior colleagues and students.

Mentors instruct trainees in the methods and values of the discipline through formal or informal means or by example. Mentors are advised to limit the number of trainees to the number for whom they can provide appropriate and meaningful supervision (National Institutes of Health, 1991a).

Conflict of interest. Individual professionals often engage in activities outside their employing institutions; such activities can enrich their teaching and other work, but they also increase the possibility of conflict of interest. Conflicts can occur when external relationships affect financial or other personal interests of the individual, who compromises professional judgment in carrying out work responsibilities. Such conflicts are to be avoided. Most institutions and governmental agencies now have policies in place that can help avoid these situations. Advice from appropriate officials also can provide guidance.

Institutional responsibilities. Institutions provide appropriate oversight to assure the generation of sound scientific knowledge. They take steps to assure that young scientists receive training in the ethical conduct of science, create a climate that prevents occurrence of dishonesty, and take prompt action to investigate allegations of misconduct.

Journal editor responsibilities. Journal editors serve a gatekeeping function in that they determine what manuscripts, letters, corrections, or retractions are published. Editorial policies provide for high-quality reviewers and assure prompt, fair, and collegial feedback to authors, with appropriate explanations for declining manuscripts.

The future. As a social enterprise, nursing science must be socially responsible and responsive to emergent social needs. Such social sensitivity may mean studying new health problems, new populations, or designing new approaches or methods to meet pressing demands. New social and scientific norms may evolve. Both scientists and professional societies must be sensitive to the need for flexibility and openness to enable the exploration of new frontiers. Thus, it is important that guidelines for scientific integrity be revised and updated periodically so that they reflect evolving thinking and practices.

SHAKÉ KETEFIAN

See also
ETHICS OF RESEARCH
MENTORING
RESEARCH DISSEMINATION
RIGHTS OF HUMAN SUBJECTS

SECONDARY DATA ANALYSIS

Definition

Secondary data analysis uses the analysis of data that the analyst was not responsible for collecting or data that was collected for a different problem from the one currently under analysis. The data that are already collected and archived in some fashion are referred to as secondary information (Stewart & Kamins, 1993). Statistical meta-analysis might be considered a special case of secondary analysis (see Meta-analysis).

Advantages

Secondary information is an inexpensive data source that facilitates the research process in several ways. It is also useful for generating hypotheses for further research. It is useful in comparing findings from different studies and examining trends. Stewart and Kamins (1993) point out that population data sets, such as Bureau of the Census data, may be used to compare sample to population characteristics in order to examine the representativeness of the study sample.

The analysis of secondary information is a useful strategy for learning the research process. The secondary data sets that have used optimum sampling techniques provide an optimum resource for students by virtue of the quality of sampling and the time and expense involved in data collection. Given that students are expected to understand, explain, and defend the data set in terms of purpose, sample selection, methods, and instruments, only the real-life collection and recording of data remain unexperienced by the student. A further virtue of using the analysis from secondary information while learning to do research is that it protects the pool of potential research participants and agencies for participation in studies conducted by qualified researchers.

Caveats

Every research study is conducted with a specific purpose in mind. Delimitations are specific to the original study and introduce specific types of sampling and other bias into the original study. Operational definitions may not be replicable in a second study. For learning purposes, differences in the original study and data set can be handled through careful critique processes by students. However, the biases and differences that exist may be too extreme to permit a valid secondary analysis outside the practice situation.

Archived data sets are rarely held in the form of raw data because the data are usually summarized. The summarization may or may not be appropriate for the research question under consideration for secondary analysis. To analyze such data further confounds results beyond acceptable limits.

The question of using clinical nursing data sets for secondary analysis comes with the advent of clinical nursing information systems. The use of clinical databases as research data sets must be examined carefully. One difficulty is that restricted data resources force clinicians to choose carefully which data to collect. These data are usually not identical with what the researcher needs. Zielstorff, Jette, and Barnett (1990) discuss how to design a database that will serve both clinicians and researchers.

Beyond data restrictions another major difficulty is that the sample biases of clinical databases and research data sets for randomized control studies are different. This difference in bias of the data from clinical databases and randomized controlled trial research data sets can be exploited as a strategy for doing cross-design synthesis (General Accounting Office, 1992). However, this special case aside, the issue is that of sample representativeness. The research sample is selected for a specific reason, with specific delimitations in mind, to be representative of the general population. In contrast, the clinical population from which the clinical data set is drawn is representative only of that type of patient or client on whom data are being collected in that location and rarely, if ever, typical of the general population or even all persons with that clinical problem. For example, patients with congestive heart failure in Alabama are not necessarily representative of patients with congestive heart failure in New England or California. The same is true of patients with congestive heart failure in a community hospital versus those in a teaching hospital in the same county.

These caveats necessitate close evaluation of data sets to be used for secondary analysis. The information needed for such evaluation must be archived along with the data set. Such information includes study purpose; data collection details, such as who collected the data, when, and where; sampling criteria and delimitations; known biases; operational definitions; and methods of data collection (see Stewart & Kamins, 1993).

Secondary Analysis in Nursing Research

Traditionally, nursing has not archived research data sets of its own for use in teaching or secondary analysis. Nursing students and nurse researchers do use large government databases, but none are collected specifically by nurse researchers to answer nursing research questions. This is a problem to the extent that learning takes place best when examples and experiences relate closely to daily (nursing) experience. Certainly, problems peculiar to but not exclusive to nursing research are more easily taught with examples from real life. This is a problem also to the extent that nursing research data sets can, in fact, generate new knowledge, whether by reanalysis or by stimulation of further investigation and hypothesis generation.

Sigma Theta Tau International has begun a program to archive selected research data sets of nurse researchers. The project is still in its infancy, with acquisition and dissemination policy still under study (see Data Stewardship). Descriptions of the research study will be required to fulfill criteria for data set evaluation mentioned above.

JUDITH RAE GRAVES

See also
DATA ANALYSIS
DATA STEWARDSHIP
RESEARCH DISSEMINATION
STATISTICAL TECHNIQUES

SELF-EFFICACY

Bandura's (1997) general self-efficacy construct provides a useful explanation for how people exercise influence over their own motivation and behavior. Perceived self-efficacy refers to beliefs in one's capabilities to organize and execute the courses of action required to produce given attainments. This influence may entail regulating one's motivation, thought processes, affective states, and actions; or it may involve changing environmental conditions, depending on what one seeks to manage. Self-efficacy judgments determine the behavior to be chosen and affect the amount of effort one devotes to a task, as well as the duration of one's persistence when difficulties are encountered. Bandura postulated four principal sources of self-efficacy information: (a) enactive mastery experiences that serve as indicators of capability; (b) vicarious experiences that alter efficacy beliefs through transmission of competencies and comparison with the attainments of others; (c) verbal persuasion (and allied types of social influences) that one possesses certain capabilities, and (d) physiological and affective states from which people partly judge their capability, strength, and vulnerability to dysfunction.

According to Bandura (1997), efficacy beliefs vary across activity domains, levels of demands within the domains, and different environmental circumstances of performance. Therefore, self-efficacy in psychosocial functioning is best determined by measures tailored to particular domains of functioning rather than by a global test. Self-efficacy scales must reflect these dimensions in their measurement and should include level, generality, and strength. Levels of task demands represent varying degrees of challenge or impediment to successful performance. These levels predict routine activities to be carried out regularly. Self-efficacy strength is a measure of an individual's ability to execute the requisite activity at different levels of task demands. The strength domains are presented as "can do" rather than "will do" because *can* is a measure of capability, whereas *will* is a statement of intention. Nursing knowledge of various developmental phenomena and life course events in health and illness has increased, using the construct of self-efficacy as an outcome or an intervention strategy incorporated into a nursing model.

Pender and Pender (1987) developed the health promotion model to explain the occurrence of behaviors directed toward increasing the level of wellness, rather than behaviors targeted specifically to decreasing the probability of illness. The health promotion model is a synthesis of findings from studies on factors related to health-promoting behaviors, and the model attempts to explain why individuals engage in health actions. Pender's model is appropriate for continued investigation because, being derived from social learning theory, it stresses the importance of cognitive mediating processes in behavior regulation.

Determinants of the health promotion model are cognitive-perceptual factors, modifying factors, and variables affecting the likelihood of action. The modifying factors indirectly influencing patterns of health behavior are demographic characteristics, biological characteristics, interpersonal influences, situational factors, and behavioral factors. The cognitive-perceptual factors are the primary motivational mechanisms for the acquisition and maintenance of health-promoting behaviors and include perceived self-efficacy. Nursing investigations of developmental phenomena and life course events have included self-efficacy as a predictor as well as an outcome of a tailored intervention.

Natural Disaster

Murphy (1987) investigated the influence of global self-efficacy and social support on the mental health of individuals who experienced a natural disaster, volcanic eruption. One to 3 years postdisaster, the victims continued to experience physical and mental distress. Self-efficacy was positively related to mental health; social support was not. The findings showed that the individuals relied more on themselves and believed in their own abilities to cope with their losses. Even though social support was not a predictor of mental distress, the findings suggested that if there was someone to turn to, the identified stressor was more manageable.

Cardiac Recovery

Self-efficacy was found to be a strong predictor of recovery from cardiac illness. It has been studied as a variable to predict exercise performance and as a theoretical framework for designing nursing interventions to increase exercise. Gortner (Gortner et al., 1988) was the first nurse researcher to design a self-efficacy-driven exercise intervention; it was tested in 67 patients recovering from cardiac surgery. The experimental intervention contained a counseling aspect focusing on emotional reactions. At 3 months postsurgery participants in the intervention group had higher self-efficacy than did participants in the control group. Gortner and Jenkins (1990) later tested education and telephone monitoring in 149 cardiac surgery patients during their recovery phase. Patients in the experimental group at 8 weeks had greater walking, lifting, and general activity. Self-efficacy expectations were a significant predictor for self-reported activity up to 24 weeks following surgery. These studies provide evidence of support for continued development of nursing interventions based on self-efficacy theory in patients recovering from cardiac surgery.

Family Roles

The parent role creates new stressors for individuals, and this phenomenon of parenting efficacy has long-term effects on both the parents and the child. The results of investigations by Gross and her colleagues (Gross, Fogg, & Tucker, 1995) showed that low perceived efficacy fosters depression in mothers of toddlers and may determine whether the mother goes on to develop chronic depression. The investigators created a program to build parenting confidence in ability to handle toddlers' behavioral problems using mastery modeling and self-efficacy theory. The mothers who participated in the program increased their sense of parenting efficacy and experienced lower familial stress and child behavior problems. The mothers who did not participate became more critical and had more negative interactions with their children.

Memory Aging

General or specific incidents of forgetting are often used by older adults to interpret the effectiveness of their memory ability and awareness. Self-efficacy in psychosocial functioning is best determined by measures tailored to particular domains of functioning, rather than by a global test. Memory self-efficacy is defined as beliefs about one's own capability to use memory effectively in various situations. Knowledge about memory is distinct from memory self-efficacy. Thus, it is possible that an older individual may have extensive and accurate knowledge about how memory functions but also may believe that his or her ability to remember in a given context is poor. More older adults than younger adults have poorer memory self-efficacy, and low memory self-efficacy has a number of adverse consequences. McDougall (1994) determined that healthy elders attending adult educational programs, without major chronic illness or depression, had decreased memory self-efficacy. This perception led them to believe that they had limited memory capacity, that they could do little to affect their memory, that anxiety and stress easily influenced their memory, and that it would inevitably decline with age.

If the individual perceives memory to be a decreasing function with age, then he or she is quick to interpret faulty performance as an indicator of declining memory capacity. Those who have low self-efficacy may give up trying because of doubts about achieving a desired level of performance. Conversely, the individual who views memory ability as a skill to be developed and practiced may achieve higher memory capacity. Nurses are able to assist older adults to view their cognitive abilities realistically and not promote negative views and stereotypes about cognitive aging. These studies offer examples in which nurse scientists investigated life-span phenomena incorporating self-efficacy theory as a component in the quest to develop nursing knowledge.

GRAHAM MCDOUGALL

See also
COGNITIVE INTERVENTIONS
DISASTER NURSING
PSYCHOSOCIAL INTERVENTIONS
REDUCING HIV RISK-ASSOCIATED
  SEXUAL BEHAVIOR AMONG ADO-
  LESCENTS

SEXUALITY RESEARCH

Attitudes of American nurses toward sexuality have gone through many phases (Bullough & Bullough, 1997). Before they could do major research in the area, nurses had to feel that the subject matter was worth researching and then gain the expertise to do the research. Through at least the first 50 years of modern nursing, they neither felt that the topic was worth researching nor had the knowledge to do more than repeat the standard prejudices and misconceptions of their time. In the first phase, which coincided with the emergence of the Nightingale schools, the topic was ignored; nurses wrote nothing on it.

The second phase could be called a hortatory one; the duty of nurses was to educate their patients to the dangers inherent in sexual activity (Robb, 1907), and this was believed to require little special knowledge. Representative of this phase are the writings of Lavinia Dock (1910), which emphasized the dangers of masturbation in children and the importance of the nurse in bringing this message to the mother. She taught that the "reproductive rituals" should "only be performed in the sincerity of aspiration to bring a new being in the world." In her attitudes, Dock simply mirrored the assumptions of the period.

A step forward was taken in the 1917 *Standard Curriculum Guide* of the National League of Nursing Education, which specified that sexual hygiene be included in the subjects covered by students. This seems like a real effort to gain some expertise, but unfortunately the sexual material was to be covered in a 1-hour lecture. It was extended to a whole unit in the curriculum guide of 1927. Still, nursing education was more influenced by the prohibitions and dangers of sex than by promotion of any real understanding (Smiley, Gould, & Melby, 1931).

The third phase was somewhat a reorientation of nursing education to coincide with some of the ongoing research into sexuality. The National League of Nursing Education set up a Committee on Social Hygiene in 1931 to draft a curriculum to better prepare nurses for the sexual problems they were likely to encounter. The result of this was a special curriculum guide in social hygiene for nurses (McCorkle 1934), and gradually elements of this report were integrated into nursing education. Although sex education in nursing remained mainly hortatory, there was more real information being given.

Nurses Margaret Sanger and Emma Goldman pushed for a different type of sex education; and although neither did much research themselves, Sanger was a key figure in promoting sex research, particularly on reproductive issues. She was instrumental in stimulating the research that led to oral contraceptives, bringing researchers and potential donors together (Bullough, 1994).

The fourth phase coincided with the formation in 1964 of the Sex Information and Education Council of the United States, which was a major factor in changing the nature of sex education. School nurses participated in this phase, which led to new demands for sex research by nurses. In part, the development and distribution of the pill gave women a new view of sexuality, and this coincided with the changing attitudes and receptiveness within the feminist movement on the importance of female sexuality.

Major evidence of change did not appear until the early 1970s. One sign of a new official nursing interest was a compilation of articles on sexuality by Browning and Lewis (1973). Articles were grouped under subsections of "mind-body continuum" (i.e., masturbation, homosexuality, transsexualism), sex education (emphasizing the role of the nurse in the education of the young person), fertility regulation (including family planning, contraceptives, sterilization), abortion (stressing attitudes as well as the procedures), and sexually transmitted diseases (including incidence, types, tests, and treatment). The fact that the compilation was published by the *American Journal of Nursing* gave encouragement to nurses to think about the topic and even begin to do tentative research. Shortly afterward, in 1974, *Nursing Clinics of North America* published a symposium with articles on various aspects of sexual behavior.

Nursing textbooks rapidly followed the new lead, and sophisticated textbooks on the subject of human sexuality appeared; they were specifically designed for nurses and authored by nurses who were doing research in human sexuality. Nancy Fugate Woods (1979), well known for her research into menstruation, published a sexuality text. Many nurses began to examine sexual markers in women's lives, from menarche to menopause; and in the process, they entered the mainstream of sex research. Among the major researchers in various aspects of sexuality were Bonnie Bullough, Beverly Whipple, and Vern Bullough. Whipple's (1982) work in sexual physiology, particularly her work with the G spot, made her one of the better known U.S. nurses. Although the G spot remains somewhat controversial, Whipple has gone beyond the controversy to do major research.

As with many other subjects of pertinence to nursing, nurses researching sexuality have moved from being disseminators of information and misinformation gathered by others to becoming researchers in their own right, although few have so far achieved recognition outside the nursing profession.

VERN L. BULLOUGH

See also
**FEMINIST RESEARCH METHOD-
   OLOGY
GENDER RESEARCH
MENSTRUAL CYCLE**

REDUCING HIV RISK-ASSOCIATED
SEXUAL BEHAVIOR AMONG ADO-
LESCENTS
WOMEN'S HEALTH RESEARCH

SHIVERING

Definitions

Shivering is defined as involuntary shaking of the body and is the adult human's primary defense against the cold. Characterized by a protracted generalized course of involuntary contractions of skeletal muscles that are usually under voluntary control, thermoregulatory shivering differs from transient tremors or "shivers" associated with fear, delight, or other forms of sympathetic arousal. Shivering occurs when heat loss stimulates specific heat-loss sensors in the skin, spinal cord, and brain. Sensory impulses are received and integrated at the preoptic area of the hypothalamus. Shivering is stimulated when integrated thermosensory information indicates body temperature is falling below optimal "set point" range (see Thermal Balance). The shivering center in the posterior hypothalamus is stimulated, sending impulses via anterior spinal routes of the gamma efferent system. Heat is generated by oscillation and friction of the fibrous muscle spindles of the fusimotor system. Shivering occurs in fever, despite rising temperatures, because the set point is raised to a higher level by circulating cytokines and other pyrogens.

Relevance to Nursing

Shivering is so ubiquitous that its consequences for seriously ill or vulnerable patients may be overlooked. The aerobic activity generated by vigorous shivering activity raises oxygen consumption three- to fivefold, approximately that of shoveling snow or riding a bicycle. Oxidative phosphorylation of glucose and fatty acids is required; this raises metabolic demands but is only about 11% efficient in raising body temperature. Although this energy expenditure is tolerated by healthy persons who shiver for short periods, specific patient groups are at risk for cardiorespiratory, metabolic, and thermal instability resulting from shivering. Uncontrollable shivering is distressful to patients, yet it occurs frequently in situations when ambient temperatures are cool, patients are exposed, or therapies induce fever. Shivering is often recalled by patients as a negative aspect of postoperative recovery, childbirth, antifungal drug administration, blood transfusions, and other hospital experiences. Nursing research has documented correlates and sequelae of shivering to determine adverse consequences in postoperative care, febrile illness, and induced hypothermia. Intervention studies have tested the efficacy of nursing measures to prevent shivering during surface cooling and febrile chills. Important to these studies was an effort to standardize the measurement of shivering by use of a shivering severity scale, originated by Abbey and co-workers (Abbey, Andrews, Avigliano, et al., 1973).

Historical Perspective

Although shivering had been studied extensively by physiologists in healthy humans and animals, little interest was evident in clinical settings until the 1970s. A group led by Abbey (1973) used wraps of ordinary terry cloth towels as insulation to protect thermosensitive regions of the skin during use of conductive cooling blankets. Shivering during surface cooling was a significant problem that was treated with chlorpromazine, a drug with severe side effects. The wrapping intervention was based on existing physiological research demonstrating dominance of the heat loss sensors on hands and feet in stimulating shivering. This landmark pilot study demonstrated that insulation of extremities diminishes shivering and improves comfort without drugs, even when surface cooling induces hypothermic temperatures.

Major Studies

Major studies by nurse investigators (Abbey et al., 1973; Holtzclaw, 1990) using more extensive temperature and electromyographic measurements further supported the usefulness of wrapping extremities. The theoretical perspective for much of the intervention research on shivering was based on Abbey's original work. Stated briefly, insulation blunts the neurosensory stimulus of heat loss from dominant sensors, whereas larger but less thermosensitive regions of the trunk allow heat exchange without inducing shivering.

In 1986, Holtzclaw demonstrated the hazardous increase in oxygen consumption, carbon dioxide production, and cardiovascular exertion during postoperative shivering following hypothermic cardiac surgery. Phillips (1996) found patients with left ventricular failure unable to compensate fully for this demand. A clinical predictor of shivering, the mandibular hum was detected by palpation of referred masseter vibrations over the ridge of the jaw (Holtzclaw, 1990; Holtzclaw & Geer, 1995). The changing ratio of gradients between pulmonary artery and bladder temperature was found to be associated with shivering in postoperative cardiac surgery patients (Earp & Finlayson, 1992).

In an effort to prevent postanesthesia shivering following general surgery, Heffline (1991) compared radiant heat alone with combinations of radiant heat and shivering-suppressant drugs. Radiant heat alone was as effective as combined therapy in rewarming patients. Extremity wraps were found to effectively reduce febrile shivering severity and duration in immunosuppressed cancer patients (Holtzclaw, 1990) and are under study as intervention for chills of AIDS-related fever.

Future Directions

As scientific evidence grows about the influence of neuroregulatory and immunological factors on shivering, new avenues of study emerge. Little is known about how shivering can be controlled in emergency situations such as rescue and evacuation. Few studies have examined outcomes of shivering among children. Surgery, trauma, circulatory bypass, and hypothermia have all been linked in preliminary studies to acute-phase reactions that stimulate febrile shivering. Although shivering is common during the last stage of labor, little attention has been paid to its origin and management.

Future directions in the study of shivering by nursing will likely address the biobehavioral interface of environmental stimuli, biochemical and neurotransmitter activity, energy expenditure, physics of heat exchange, and thermal comfort.

BARBARA J. HOLTZCLAW

See also
CARDIOVASCULAR NURSING
FEVER/FEBRILE RESPONSE
NURSE ANESTHETISTS AND RE-SEARCH
THERMAL BALANCE

SIGMA THETA TAU INTERNATIONAL *NURSING RESEARCH CLASSIFICATION SYSTEM*

The first nursing research classification system was developed during the project Survey and Assessment of Areas and Methods of Research in Nursing. It was conducted at Yale University under the direction of Leo W. Simmons, a sociologist. Two other sociologists and Virginia Henderson comprised the survey group (Cowan, 1956). This system formed the basis for the annotation of English language nursing studies in the *Nursing Studies Index* between the years 1900 and 1959 (Henderson & Yale University). The term *study* was broadly defined as "a structured effort to solve a problem" and included historical and biographical articles and monographs in addition to what Henderson called analytical (research) articles (Henderson & Yale University, 1959, p. vii). This classification system categorized the types of nursing research according to fields on which nurse researchers focused their work.

This research classification system was abandoned because there was a desire to index all the nursing literature, not just the research literature. To facilitate indexing and retrieval of this broad literature, it was decided to switch to a subject headings system. Subject headings permit articles to be located according to what the various articles are about. The headings describe important topics in a field and are usually organized into a tree structure to illustrate relationships between the various topics and subtopics. A subject heading system in and of itself does not enable comparison of studies according to aspects such as research design and methods and the myriad of other comparisons of interest in the body of nursing research.

The idea of a classification system for nursing research was not lost, however. Sigma Theta Tau, the International Honor Society of Nursing (STTI), began work on the *Nursing Research Classification System (NRCS)* in the early 1980s. In addition to categorizing the fields in which nurse researchers did studies and the research subjects and methods in which they had experience, an early purpose was to facilitate identification and location of the nurse researchers. Now in its third edition, the system includes description of studies, variables, and findings. The *NRCS* serves as the structure for the databases that were combined and came to be known as the (electronic) *Registry of Nursing Research* (Graves, 1994).

In this version it is a representation of the language and the structure of clinical nursing research knowledge as well as the language and structure of research knowledge in related domains in which nurses do research such as education, administration, management, and so forth (Graves, 1996, Summer; 2nd Quarter). In this usage, the term *language* refers to the names of research concepts and of variables studied together. The term *structure* refers to the descriptive details of the research describing any study: (a) the demographics (investigators, dissemination, funding, title, conceptual framework); (b) the sample, methodology and design, and analysis and results; and (c) the relationships (hierarchical arrangement) between these descriptors. Multiple knowledge (generation) theories are accommodated.

Definition

The STTI *Nursing Research Classification System* (NRCS) is a detailed description of the structured inquiry process used in individual nursing research studies. It identifies and logically relates salient characteristics of research studies in nursing. Sa-

lience is defined by whether a descriptive term (a) permits a comparison of studies according to the details of the research process, such as the design, the subjects, and the findings; (b) enables researchers and other users of research to make a preliminary judgment about the quality of a registered study, given the design; (c) enables direct indexing of the knowledge generated by each study (variable names and results); and (d) permits a comparison between studies that is of interest to the nursing profession, such as funding sources and amounts or domains of research that nurses investigate (education, administration, philosophy, culture, etc.).

In keeping with the original purpose of locating researchers, the category *Researcher* is the primary hierarchical element. The basic organization is described here:

- Each *researcher* may have many *research studies*. The single research study is the basic unit of analysis. A study may or may not be a part of a larger *research project*.
- Each *research study* is classified according to title, theoretical/conceptual framework, research domain, funding, keywords (subject headings), dissemination record, participants/sample, sampling plan, scope of sampling, data collection site, design type, extraneous variables.
- Each *study* may ask many *research questions*.
- Each *research question* may have many *analyses*.
- Each *analysis* is classified according to nature of the inquiry (knowledge theory), procedures, type of analysis, method of data analysis, research concept or names of variables studied together, relationship studied (if applicable), and findings.

The NRCS category *Domain of Research* is analogous to the first 9 of 10 categories of the Henderson nursing research classification system. Although not absolutely identical in detail, the categories are remarkably similar. Henderson's 10th category "Conducting Research," incorporates "Research methods and types including devices and techniques," whereas these characteristics form the primary corpus of the STTI NRCS, with domains being a secondary characteristic.

Relevance to Nursing

The NRCS provides a structure for a new archetype for storing and retrieving research knowledge in all disciplines. Of all the health science disciplines, only that of nursing has developed a research classification system. The classification system serves as the logical model for the database that organizes the Virginia Henderson Library's *Registry of Nursing Research*©. The Virginia Henderson International Nursing Library is the only known library to store research studies according to a research classification system and to index that research by the names of the variables or research concept studied.

The NRCS plays an active role in contributing the nursing subject headings maintained by the *Cumulative Index for Nursing and Allied Health Literature* (CINAHL). STTI has permission to use the subject headings from the CINAHL subject heading list in selected NRCS categories (i.e., funding sources, nursing theoretical framework, indexing terms, data collection sites). This prevents the development of still another subject heading system to describe the same topics, thus facilitating searching of both the CINAHL bibliographic database and the STTI *Registry of Nursing Research*. As the NRCS becomes more widely used, new terms in use by researchers will provide real data to influence updates of the CINAHL subject heading list. In turn, the CINAHL subject heading list will be used to maintain the descriptors in selected NRCS categories.

The NRCS identifies the data elements necessary for generating an index to the studies in the *Registry of Nursing Research*©, organized by variable name so that the index lists all studies in which a particular variable is studied.

JUDITH R. GRAVES

See also
BIBLIOGRAPHIC RETRIEVAL SYSTEMS

CUMULATIVE INDEX TO NURSING AND ALLIED HEALTH LITERATURE NURSING STUDIES INDEX VIRGINIA HENDERSON INTERNATIONAL NURSING LIBRARY

SMOKING/TOBACCO AS CARDIOVASCULAR RISK FACTOR

Smoking is an addictive behavior that causes both physiological and psychological dependence. Nicotine, the drug component leading to addiction, appears to have both stimulating and tranquilizing effects. Smokers tend to regulate the amount of nicotine delivered to the brain by varying the intensity, frequency, and depth of each puff. Smoking is also an "overlearned" habit. Success with quitting is dependent on identifying what triggers a person to smoke. Smoking is most often associated with many aspects of daily life, including habits such as driving in a car, eating a meal, talking on the telephone, or drinking coffee. Finally, smoking is used as a coping mechanism. Individuals smoke to deal with stress, boredom, anxiety, and many other emotions. Successful interventions must be directed to managing the complexity of the behavior, including nicotine addiction, the psychosocial influences, and the habit.

Prevalence in the United States

It is estimated that 49 million people, or at least one quarter of all Americans, are currently smoking. The prevalence of smoking in men is 28.2% and in women 23.1%. Smoking is highest in Black men (33.9%) and lowest in Hispanic and Asian women (15.2% and 7%, respectively). A strong relationship exists between smoking and level of education, the prevalence being several times higher among those with less than 12 years of education than among those with more than 16 years of education. Although smoking has declined by about 40% since 1965, recent data indicate that this downward trend may have leveled off. In fact, no decline has been seen in the number of cigarettes smoked since 1993 (American Heart Association, 1997).

According to the Centers for Disease Control and Prevention, 75% of all smokers begin smoking before the age of 18 and 90% before the age of 21 (American Heart Association, 1997). Approximately 3,000 teenagers begin smoking each day. The percentage of high school seniors now smoking is 22%, the highest since 1979. Teen smoking has not dropped since 1980, due heavily to the tobacco companies' targeting of minors through advertising. According to the U.S. Department of Health and Human Services, smokeless tobacco among youth also has increased, with about 1 million adolescents, including 20% of all high school boys, using this substance.

Economic Burden

Tobacco is an extremely important public health problem; smoking-related diseases cost the United States about $50 billion annually in medical care (American Heart Association, 1997). Smokers average $6,000 more in lifetime medical costs than do nonsmokers, are absent 6.5 more days per year from work, and make on average six more health care visits annually (MacKenzie, Bartecchi, & Schrier, 1994). The burden is compounded by the lack of work productivity associated with smoking. Approximately 50,000 additional fatalities from burns, pediatric diseases, and secondhand smoke are also attributed to smoking.

Health Effects

One in every five deaths in the United States is smoking-related. Almost every organ and tissue is damaged from smoking, the most common diseases being lung cancer, cardiovascular disease, and chronic obstructive pulmonary disease. On average, smokers will die 7 years earlier than nonsmokers, often suffering chronic debilitating conditions in the years prior to death. Although smokers are at risk for almost all diseases, the health benefits of smoking cessation are immediate and substantial

for all individuals regardless of age, gender, disease state, and smoking history. For example, smokers who quit smoking at the time of a myocardial infarction (MI) decrease their chances of a recurrent MI by 50% within the first year of quitting. Within 10 years this risk drops to only slightly above that of a nonsmoker.

Nonsmokers also are at risk from tobacco smoke. Cigarettes contain more than 4,000 chemicals and carcinogens, which are found in high concentrations in sidestream smoke. The risk of death from cardiovascular disease increases by about 30% in those who are exposed to environmental tobacco smoke (American Heart Association, 1997).

Smoking Interventions

Many interventions have been undertaken to help smokers quit: strong physician advice, hypnosis, acupuncture, use of medications such as nicotine replacement therapy, self-help materials, and smoking cessation behavioral counseling groups. Based on a meta-analysis of 39 studies conducted in clinical practice from the late 1970s to the early mid-1980s, Kottke, Battista, DeFriese, and Brekke (1988) found that, irrespective of the intervention or delivery system, smoking cessation is most often achieved by increasing reinforcement. That is, increasing the number of contacts made to the smoker who is trying to quit or remain abstinent after quitting, the type of contacts, and the number of people making contacts offers the greatest success.

Multiple components (i.e., strong physician advice, nicotine replacement therapy, counseling) and multiple methods of delivery (videotape, audiotapes, telephone follow-up) are more successful than a single intervention. This is reinforced in the recently released *Clinical Practice Guideline on Smoking Cessation* published by the Agency for Health Care Policy and Research (AHCPR) of the U.S. Department of Health and Human Services (1996b). All health care professionals can help people to stop smoking by (a) identifying them as smokers at every encounter; (b) asking if they are willing to make a quit attempt; (c) aiding them to quit by using such interventions as self-help materials, strong advice, nicotine replacement therapy;

and (d) arranging for follow-up, which should include at least two contacts in the month after quitting. Telephone contacts offer a convenient, effective, and inexpensive method of follow-up.

Pharmacological Therapy

The most effective pharmacological aid to help highly addicted smokers quit smoking is nicotine replacement therapy. Both nicotine chewing gum and the transdermal nicotine patch are now available over the counter and are highly beneficial in helping individuals to quit smoking. The patch is the preferred pharmacological aid; however, some people benefit from nicotine gum because of the oral stimulation the gum provides. Studies indicate that treatment with the patch for 8 weeks or less is as efficacious as longer treatment periods. The patch is very well tolerated, minor local skin reaction being the main side effect. Nicotine chewing gum requires appropriate instruction about administration and caution about the use of acidic beverages, which interfere with absorption. The gum is more effective if prescribed on a fixed-dose schedule. Little evidence exists about the value of nicotine replacement therapy in light smokers (< 15 cigarettes per day). For these individuals, starting at a lower dose may be appropriate (AHCPR, 1996b).

Nursing Practice and Research

As the largest group of health care professionals, nurses can play a major role in helping smokers to think about quitting. The hospital has become a unique setting to help smokers because bans on smoking prevent patients from continuing their habit. Smokers experience the worst of withdrawal effects during this time of enforced cessation. Interventions that focus on identification of patients, strong physician advice, and use of nurses to provide behavioral counseling at the bedside, with telephone follow-up, have proved highly efficacious in getting smokers to remain abstinent (Miller, Smith, DeBusk, Sobel, & Taylor, 1997; Taylor, Houston Miller, Killen, & DeBusk, 1990). Nursing research offers opportunities to improve interventions for smoking cessation. Nurses within community settings, schools, and clinics play a role in prevention, educating and counseling teenagers about not adopting the most addictive habit in the United States today.

NANCY HOUSTON MILLER

See also
ADOLESCENCE
CARDIOVASCULAR NURSING
DYSPNEA
RISK FACTORS

SNOMED INTERNATIONAL

SNOMED International is a compilation of nomenclatures organized into 11 modules or axes: (a) topography; (b) morphology; (c) living organisms; (d) chemicals, drugs, and biological products; (e) function; (f) occupation; (g) diagnosis; (h) procedure; (i) physical agents, forces, and attributes; (j) social context; and (k) general (Coté, Rothwell, Palotay, & Beckett, 1993). North American Nursing Diagnosis Association (NANDA) diagnoses are included in the functional axis of SNOMED, and a limited number of nursing procedures are included in the procedure module. In contrast to taxonomic vocabulary systems with the primary purpose of disjunctive classification (e.g., *International Classification of Diseases* or *Current Procedural Terminology Codes*), SNOMED terms can be combined for the purposes of concept representation for computer-based systems. For instance, the term "pain" from the function axis can be joined with a severity modifier from the general axis to represent the clinical expression "severe pain" or with an anatomic term from the topography axis to represent "back pain." This multiaxial approach is similar to the proposed architecture of the international classification of nursing practice (Nielsen & Mortensen, 1996).

Many investigations have demonstrated the usefulness of SNOMED for physician documentation, and a few have addressed the utility of SNOMED for nursing. Henry, Holzemer, Reilly, and Campbell (1994) demonstrated that nurses use both

NANDA diagnoses and other terms (i.e., symptoms, signs, medical diagnoses) to describe patient problems and that SNOMED terms other than those of NANDA diagnoses were exact matches for terms used by nurses in their clinical documentation. Lange (1996) found that SNOMED terms were useful for representing terms used by nurses in intershift reports. Campbell et al. (Campbell, Carpenter, Sneiderman, et al., 1997) compared SNOMED International with the Read Codes and the Unified Medical Language System (UMLS) on the attributes of completeness, clinical taxonomy, administrative mapping, term definitions, and clarity. Of the 1,929 records in the data set, 390 were nursing documents. Although no separate nursing analyses were reported, SNOMED was judged superior to Read and UMLS on the four categories of information (findings, diagnoses, interventions, and plans of care) that comprised greater than 97% of the nursing text sources and overall on the attributes of completeness, taxonomy, and compositional nature. It received lower ratings than Read and UMLS on administrative mappings. If the analyses related to nursing interventions and plans of care had been reported separately from other health care interventions and plans of care, the findings might have differed on the attribute of completeness because the UMLS includes nursing intervention schema from the *Omaha System*, the *Georgetown Home Health Care Classification*, and the *Nursing Interventions Classification*, although SNOMED does not.

Some utility has been demonstrated, but further work is needed to increase the usefulness of SNOMED for nursing. Two areas relate specifically to SNOMED itself, and the third is a more generic requirement for representing nursing concepts in computer-based systems. First, additional terms for nursing interventions must be added to SNOMED. Second, rules (grammars) for combining terms must be developed, using knowledge formalisms such as conceptual graphs. Third, data models that describe the attributes of nursing data must be developed. For instance, several authors have proposed attributes of nursing activities, including (a) target, (b) mode of action, (c) recipient, (d) time,

and (e) place (Henry & Mead, 1997; Nielsen & Mortensen, 1996).

SUZANNE BAKKEN HENRY

See also
HOME HEALTH CARE CLASSIFICATION SYSTEM
NANDA
NURSING INTERVENTIONS CLASSIFICATION
OMAHA SYSTEM
TAXONOMY

SOCIAL SUPPORT

Definition and Related Terms

Theorists and researchers began to describe the concept of social support in the mid 1970s. The term *social support* was identified as a separate term in the National Library of Medicine Medline data base in 1991 and has been indexed back to 1983. Prior to that time the primary indexing terms were *social environment* (1973–1982) and *social adjustment* (1969–1982).

The definition of the indexing term *social support* in Medline is "support systems that provide assistance and encouragement to individuals with physical or emotional disabilities in order that they may better cope. Informal social support is usually provided by friends, relatives, or peers, while formal assistance is provided by churches, groups, etc." This definition, with its explicit focus on individuals with physical or emotional disabilities, is not sufficiently broad to encompass social support as it is used in disciplines other than medicine. In the broader sense a basic level of social support is regarded as necessary for individuals to cope with the usual role demands of daily living. During times of crisis, stress, or illness, increased amounts of support or different kinds of support may be needed.

The term *social support* must be distinguished from the related but distinct term *social network*.

The members of a person's social support system are a subset of the wider social network that can include individuals who do not provide any social support.

Theoretical Underpinnings

Much social support research follows a simple model in which social support is held to have main effects on health outcomes as well as buffering effects modifying the effects of stress on health. Stewart (1989) outlined the more comprehensive theoretical approaches that some investigators have used for their research on social support, including attribution theory, coping theory, social exchange or equity theory, social comparison theory, and loneliness theory.

Issues in the Field

Early writings about social support posed the buffering theory: social support works only in the context of stress and that it buffers the negative effects of stress on health. Other models include main effects for social support and postulate that social support has beneficial effects regardless of the level of stress an individual is experiencing. Empirical findings from studies have not revealed a consistent pattern of results to clarify this issue.

A second issue is whether social support is best regarded as a perceived variable or whether researchers should try to capture what was actually provided. Theorists have tended to favor perceived support, perhaps because of the difficulty of determining whether an enacted supportive behavior is actually experienced as supportive by the recipient. Related to this question is the issue of hypothetical support versus either perceived or enacted support; the belief that support would be available when it is needed may in itself be protective.

A third issue is related to the paradox that not all socially supportive relationships are completely supportive; some relationships also provide a degree of conflict, negativity, or stress for the recipi-ent. Tilden and Galyen (1987) have contributed to this debate in discussing cost, conflict, and reciprocity issues of social support from the perspective of social exchange and equity theories.

Finally, as the weight of empirical evidence mounted, consistently showing a positive effect for social support in a variety of contexts and populations, researchers identified the need to study how social support might work or work most effectively. Issues such as the optimal timing of social support have been described, often in relation to known processes such as the phases of bereavement. Different types or qualities of support might be more beneficial at each phase of the grief process. Researchers have explored types and sources of support as differentially effective for people of different racial or ethnic groups, marital status, or gender.

Contributions of Nurse Scientists

The field of social support is highly interdisciplinary. Researchers from all of the social science disciplines, the health sciences, and other areas contribute to the field. There were over 10,000 citations of social support research in Medline from 1980 to 1996. During the period of 1992 to October 1996, of the 4,314 articles listed, 435 were from the International Nursing Index.

A nurse-epidemiologist can be credited with publishing one of the classic studies that opened the door to speculation about the protective effect of "psychosocial assets," which included social support resources (Nuckolls, Cassel, & Kaplan, 1972). An early review (Norbeck, 1988) showed that nurse investigators have made a contribution to the field through (a) studies of social support in clinical populations across the life span in the areas of life transitions, role performance, health behavior, and crisis or illness behavior; (b) instrument development; and (c) intervention studies.

The nurse investigators who have published the most extensively on social support from 1980 to the present are Jane S. Norbeck, Virginia P. Tilden, Miriam J. Stewart, and Clarann Weinert. Each of these authors has contributed empirical articles, and review, theoretical, or instrument development articles. Instruments developed by nurse investigators that have had extensive testing of reliability and validity are the Interpersonal Relationship Inventory by Tilden (Tilden, Nelson, & May, 1990); the Norbeck Social Support Questionnaire (Norbeck, Lindsey, & Carrieri, 1981); and the Personal Resource Questionnaire by Weinert (Weinert, 1987).

How Robust Is Social Support as a Variable?

Hundreds of studies have been published that demonstrate significant correlations between social support and positive health outcomes. On the other hand, intervention studies have had mixed results, many failing to find a significant effect for the support intervention. A recent meta-analysis (Smith, Fernengel, Holcroft, Gerald, & Marien, 1994) reported that the effect sizes on health outcomes for social support have been small, ranging from −.02 to .22. In addition to methodological issues, reasons for these modest effect sizes were postulated as the failure of most researchers to study support that matches the specific requirements of the situation of the study population. Studies adapting situation-specific support measures have shown higher effect sizes.

Methodological issues common to intervention studies contribute to uneven results, and it is premature to conclude that social support interventions are not effective until these flaws are corrected. For example, in studies that failed to show a significant effect for social support interventions to lower the rate of low birthweight, investigators (a) intervened with all pregnant women rather than identifying those women with inadequate social support for study, (b) failed to base the intervention on theoretical or empirical grounds, or (c) diluted the social support intervention with intervention elements that were incompatible with support. When these flaws were corrected in a study that used a culturally congruent, empirically based intervention, Norbeck, DeJoseph, and Smith (1996) found markedly reduced incidence of low birthweight for the intervention group (9.2% compared to 22.4% for the control group) among African American pregnant women who lacked adequate support.

Implications for Practice and Research

Many reports in the clinical literature describe the use of support groups, self-help groups, and the provision of support to individuals by nurses. Despite anecdotal reports of patient satisfaction, these interventions need empirical testing to validate their effectiveness.

The focus of research on social support should move beyond the plethora of correlational studies already completed. Research is required that is designed to explore the mechanisms of how social support works and then to test interventions based on these findings. Support specificity models hold the most promise for successful applications in the clinical arena.

JANE S. NORBECK

See also
ATTRIBUTION THEORY
CAREGIVER
COPING
ROLE SUPPLEMENTATION: A NURSING THERAPEUTIC
TRANSITIONS AND HEALTH

SOCIETY FOR RESEARCH IN CHILD DEVELOPMENT

Roots

The field of child development received formal recognition in 1922–1923 through the appointment of a Subcommittee on Child Development of the National Research Council. In 1925, under the direction of Robert S. Woodworth, an eminent experimental psychologist, this group became the Committee in Child Development, with offices and staff in the National Academy of Sciences. The purpose of the committee was to integrate research activities and to stimulate research in child development. The committee awarded fellowships, initiated conferences, and began publications. In 1927, 425 scientists were listed in the *Directory of Research in Child Development*, and that same year the first volume of *Child Development Abstracts and Bibliography* was published. In 1933 the Committee in Child Development disbanded and passed the torch to the newly organized Society for Research in Child Development (SRCD).

SRCD Today

The society is a multidisciplinary, not-for-profit, professional association with an international membership of approximately 5,000 researchers, practitioners, and human development professionals. The purposes of the society are to promote multidisciplinary research in the field of human development, to foster the exchange of information between scientists and other professionals of various disciplines, and to encourage applications of research findings. The goals are pursued through a variety of programs with the cooperation and service of our governing council, standing committees, and members.

Publications, Membership, and Activities.   In addition to its three journals, the society also publishes the *Social Policy Report*, a newsletter, and a membership directory. Membership is open to any individual actively engaged in research or teaching in human development of any of the related basic sciences or otherwise furthering the purposes of the society. Graduate and undergraduate students engaged in at least half-time study in child development or a related field may apply as student members with the sponsorship of a full member.

Almost 20% of SRCD's members are from nations outside the United States, representing nearly 50 countries throughout the world. Membership applications received prior to October 1 are considered eligible for membership effective in the current year. The society hosts an international biennial meeting with attendance of 5,000. The programs include individual research reports, symposia, invited lectures, and discussion sessions, among other timely and historical programs.

Ethical and Social Policies.   The Committee on Ethical Conduct in Child Development Research promulgates establishment and maintenance of eth-

ical standards for research with children. The society, through its Committee on International Relations, works to increase interaction and communication and fosters a commitment to research and training in diversity. The Committees on Ethnic and Racial Issues and the Committee on Interdisciplinary Affairs have made great progress in improving, increasing, and disseminating research to members. Under the guidance of the Committee on Child Development, Public Policy and Public Information, the society helps to bring the results of research to bear on the formulation of policy affecting children and families. One way in which this is done is through the Government Fellows Program in Child Development. Begun in 1978, this program is part of a larger fellowship program administered by the American Association for the Advancement of Science (AAAS). The goals of this program are to contribute to the effective use of scientific knowledge, to educate the scientific community about the development of public policy, and to establish a more effective liaison between scientists and federal offices. Fellows spend a year as aides or associates in various offices in federal agencies, working with staff in the translation of research to applied issues.

Future Directions

As research in human development expands, the need for coordination and integration among the disciplines grows. The society is constantly working to facilitate such coordination and integration and to assist in the dissemination of research findings. The society welcomes the increasing interest in child development research and seeks members who share this interest.

For information on nonmember journal subscriptions, contact the University of Chicago Press, Journals Division, P.O. Box 37005, Chicago, IL 60637. The SRCD offices can be reached by phone at (313) 998-6524; fax, (313) 998-6569; and E-mail, srcd@umich.edu.

GENE CRANSTON ANDERSON

See also
CHILD FAILURE TO THRIVE

CHILD LEAD EXPOSURE EFFECTS
NEUROBEHAVIORAL DEVELOPMENT
NUTRITION IN INFANCY AND CHILD-
HOOD
PRESCHOOL CHILDREN

SOCIETY OF BEHAVIORAL MEDICINE

The Society of Behavioral Medicine (SBM) is a multidisciplinary nonprofit organization. Founded in 1978, SBM has created a premier forum for cross-disciplinary research focused on health and human behavior across the life span and in diverse populations. From its inception the SBM has endeavored to integrate biomedical and behavioral research, with the ultimate goal of enhancing the health of the public. To this end, visionary leadership throughout the past two decades has recognized the unique and substantive contributions of numerous disciplines focused on the critical links between behavior and health. Composed of approximately 3,000 members, SBM disciplines include nursing, medicine, psychology, epidemiology, social work, health education, and nutrition. A common philosophy unites the disciplines and is best represented in the metaphor ''The whole is more and different from the sum of its parts.''

The society provides numerous benefits for its members and actively encourages cross-disciplinary collaboration in research, practice, and education. It maintains a research training-opportunities database, publishes a multidisciplinary training directory, provides peer consultation (on topics relevant to health and behavior) at each annual meeting, and maintains syllabi for relevant undergraduate and graduate courses. In addition, SBM advocates for behavioral medicine and represents relevant interests in Congress and the National Institutes of Health (NIH). SBM leaders were instrumental in advocating for the current Office of Behavioral and Social Sciences Research (OBSSR) at NIH; the president-elect of SBM, Dr. Norman Anderson, is the current director of OBSSR. SBM offices are at present located at 410 East Jefferson Street, Suite 205, Rockville, MD 20850-2617. E-mail address is info@socbehmed.org.

LAURA L. HAYMAN

See also
BEHAVIORAL RESEARCH
COLLABORATIVE RESEARCH
NATIONAL INSTITUTES OF HEALTH

STATISTICAL TECHNIQUES

Analysis of Covariance

Analysis of covariance (ANCOVA) is a statistical technique that combines analysis of variance (ANOVA) with regression to measure the differences among group means. The advantages of ANCOVA include the ability to reduce the error variance in the outcome measure and the ability to measure group differences after allowing for other differences between subjects. The error variance is reduced by controlling for variation in the dependent measure that comes from variables measured at the interval or ratio level (called covariates) that influence all the groups being compared. The covariate contributes to the variation and reduces the magnitude of the differences among groups. In ANCOVA the variation from this variable is measured and extracted from the within (or error) variation. The effect is the reduction of error variance and therefore an increase in the power of the analysis.

ANCOVA also has been used in both experimental and nonexperimental studies to ''equate'' the groups statistically. When the groups differ on some variable, ANCOVA is used to reduce the impact of that difference. Although ANCOVA has been widely used for such statistical ''equalization'' of groups, there is controversy about such efforts, and careful consideration should be given to the appropriateness of the manipulation.

As with ANOVA there are one or more categorical variables as independent variables; the dependent variable is continuous and meets the requirements of normal distribution and equality of variance across groups. The covariate is an interval- or ratio-level measure.

There are additional assumptions to be met in ANCOVA, and these are very important to the valid interpretation of results. There must be a linear relationship between the covariate and the dependent variable, and ANCOVA is most effective when the correlation is equal to or greater than .30. The direction and strength of the relationship between the covariate and dependent variable must be similar in each group. This assumption is called homogeneity of regression across groups.

ANCOVA is an extension of the ANOVA model that reduces the error term by removing additional sources of variation. It is a means of controlling extraneous variation. As with other types of analysis of variance, post hoc tests are used for pairwise comparison of group means.

Analysis of Variance

Analysis of variance (ANOVA) is a parametric statistical test that measures differences between two or more mutually exclusive groups by calculating the ratio of between- to within-group variance, called the F ratio. It is an extension of the t test, which compares two groups. The independent variable(s) are categorical (measured at the nominal level). The dependent variable must meet the assumptions of normal distribution and equal variance across the groups. A one-way ANOVA means that there is only one independent variable (often called factor), a two-way ANOVA indicates two independent variables, and an n-way ANOVA indicates that the number of independent variables is defined by n.

The null hypothesis in ANOVA is that all groups are equal and drawn from the same population. To test this assumption, three measures of variation are calculated. The total variation is a measure of the variability of all subjects around the grand mean and is composed of within-group variation and between-group variation. Within-group variation is a measure of how much the scores of subjects within a group vary around the group mean. Between-group variation is a measure of how much each group's mean varies from the grand mean or of how much difference exists between the groups. Quantifying total between- and within-group variation is accomplished by calculating a sum of squares (the sum of the squared deviations of each of the scores around the respective mean) for each component of the variation.

When the null hypothesis is true, the groups' scores overlap to a large extent, and the within-group variation is greater than the between-group variation. When the null hypothesis is false, the groups' scores show little overlapping, and the between-groups variation is greater.

When the ratio of between- to within-group variation (F ratio) is significant, the null hypothesis is rejected, indicating a difference among the groups. When more than two groups are being compared, however, it cannot be determined from the F test alone which groups differ from the others. In other words, a significant F test does not mean that every group in the analysis is different from every other group.

To determine where the significant differences lie, further analysis is required. Two types of comparisons can be made among group means. They include post hoc (after the fact) comparisons and a priori (planned) comparisons based on hypotheses stated prior to the analysis.

A variety of post hoc techniques exist. The purpose of all is to decrease the likelihood of making a Type I error when making multiple comparisons. The Scheffé test is reported frequently. The formula is based on the usual formula for the calculation of a t-test or F ratio, but the critical value for determining statistical significance is changed according to the number of comparisons to be made. A Bonferroni correction involves dividing the desired alpha (say .05) by the number of comparisons.

The least significant difference (LSD) test is equivalent to multiple t tests. The modification is that a pooled estimate of variance is used rather than variance common to groups being compared. Tukey's honestly significant difference (HSD) is the most conservative comparison test and as such is the least powerful. The critical values for Tukey remain the same for each comparison, regardless of the total number of means to be compared. Student

Newman-Keuls is similar to Tukey's HSD, but the critical values do not stay the same. They reflect the variables being compared. Tukey's wholly significant difference (WSD) uses critical values that are the average of those used in Tukey's HSD and Newman-Keuls. It is therefore intermediate in conservatism between those two measures.

Planned comparisons, or a priori contrasts, are based on hypotheses stated before data are collected. Prespecified contrasts that are orthogonal (statistically unrelated) to each other may be developed and tested. Such comparisons are more powerful than post hoc contrasts.

With two or more independent variables in an analysis, interactions between the independent variables can be tested. Testing for an interaction addresses the question of whether or not the results of a given treatment vary depending on the groups or conditions in which it is applied.

An ANOVA may include more than one dependent variable. Such an analysis usually is referred to as multivariate analysis of variance (MANOVA) and allows the researcher to look for relationships among dependent as well as independent variables. When conducting a MANOVA, the assumptions underlying the univariate model still apply, and in addition the dependent variable should have a "multivariate normal distribution with the same variance covariance matrix in each group" (Norusis, 1994, p. 58). The requirement that each group will have the same variance covariance matrix means that the homogeneity of variance assumption is met for each dependent variable and that the correlation between any two dependent variables must be the same in all groups (Bray & Maxwell, 1985). Box's M is a measure of the multivariate test for homogeneity of variance.

In the univariate model, the F value is tested for significance. In the multivariate model there are four outcome measures. They include Wilks's lambda, which represents the error variance; Pillai-Bartlett trace, which represents the sum of the explained variances; Roy's greatest characteristic root, which is based on the first discriminant variate; and Hotelling-Lawley trace, which is the sum of the between and within sums of squares for each of the discriminant variates. Wilks's lambda is the most widely used. Analysis of variance is commonly used to test for group differences. Multivariate analysis of variance includes more than one dependent variable.

Repeated Measures ANOVA

Repeated measures analysis of variance is an extension of analysis of variance (ANOVA) that reduces the error term by partitioning out individual differences that can be estimated from the repeated measurement of the same subjects. There are two main types of repeated measures designs (also called within-subjects designs). One involves taking repeated measures of the same variable(s) over time on a group or groups of subjects. The other involves exposing the same subjects to all levels of the treatment. This is often referred to as using subjects as their own controls.

Because the observations are not independent of each other, there is correlation among the outcome measures. This necessitates an assumption called compound symmetry. To meet this assumption, the correlations across the measurements (time points) must be the same, and the variances should be equal across measurements. This is important because the general robustness of the ANOVA model does not withstand much violation of this assumption.

Repeated measures ANOVA is a particularly interesting technique because health care providers tend to take repeated measures on clients, and it often makes sense to do so with research subjects as well. There are stringent requirements for this analysis, however. The most important is meeting the criteria for compound symmetry. This assumption is often violated, leading to improper interpretation of results. Most computer programs provide a test of this assumption. If the assumption is not met, several alternatives are available.

First, rather than the univariate approach, in which the repeated measures are treated as within-subjects factors, one might use a multivariate approach (MANOVA). In MANOVA, the repeated measures would be treated as multiple dependent variables. Another approach is to use an epsilon correction. The degrees of freedom are multiplied by the value of epsilon, and the new degrees of freedom, which are more conservative, are used to test the F value for significance.

Norusis (1994) summarizes the problems with repeated measures analyses as "the carry-over effect, the latent effect, and the order or learning effect" (pp. 107–108). When subjects are exposed to more than one treatment, previous treatments may still be having an effect, that is, may be carried over. An interaction with a previous treatment is referred to as a latency effect. This would occur if exposure to one treatment had an enhancing or depressing effect on a subsequent treatment. Randomization of the order of treatment is used to control the order of learning effect.

Repeated measures ANOVA is a very useful technique for research by health professionals. There are fairly stringent requirements for the analysis, however.

Correlational Techniques

Correlation is a procedure for quantifying the linear relationship between two or more variables. It measures the strength and indicates the direction of the relationship. The Pearson product-moment correlation coefficient (r) is the usual method by which the relation between two variables is quantified. There must be at least two variables measured on each subject; and although interval- or ratio-level data are most commonly used, it is also possible in many cases to obtain valid results with ordinal data. Categorical variables may be coded for use in calculating correlations and regression equations.

Although correlations can be calculated with data at all levels of measurement, certain assumptions must be made to generalize beyond the sample statistic. The sample must be representative of the population to which the inference will be made. The variables that are being correlated must each have a normal distribution. The relationship between the two variables must be linear. For every value of one variable, the distribution of the other variable must have approximately equal variability. This is called the assumption of homoscedasticity.

The correlation coefficient is a mathematical representation of the relationship that exists between two variables. The correlation coefficient may range from +1.00 through 0.00 to −1.00. A +1.00 indicates a perfect positive relationship, 0.00

indicates no relationship, and −1.00 indicates a perfect negative relationship. In a positive relationship, as one variable increases, the other increases. In a negative relationship, as one variable increases, the other decreases.

The strength of correlation coefficients has been described as follows:

.00–.25—little if any

.26–.49—low

.50–.69—moderate

.70–.89—high

.90–1.00—very high

(Munro, 1997, p. 235).

The coefficient of determination, r^2, often is used as a measure of the "meaningfulness" of r. This is a measure of the amount of variance the two variables share. It is obtained by squaring the correlation coefficient.

Correlational techniques may be used for control of extraneous variation. Partial correlation measures the relationship between two variables after statistically controlling for the influence of a confounding variable on both of the variables being correlated. It is usually expressed as $r_{12.3}$, which indicates the correlation between variables 1 and 2, with the effect of variable 3 removed from both 1 and 2. Semipartial correlation is the correlation of two variables with the effect of a third variable removed from only one of the variables being correlated. It is usually expressed as $r_{1(2.3)}$, which indicates the correlation between variables 1 and 2, with the effect of 3 removed only from variable 2.

Multiple correlation is a technique for measuring the relationship between a dependent variable and a weighted combination of independent variables. The multiple correlation is expressed as R. R^2 indicates the amount of variance explained in the dependent variable by the independent variables. Canonical correlation measures the relationship between two sets of variables and is expressed as R_c.

There are measures other than the Pearson r for measuring relationships. Before the advent of computers, "shortcut" methods of calculation were developed for certain circumstances. Three such measures are phi, point-biserial, and Spearman rho. These measures usually give the same result as r;

their only advantage is for doing hand calculations. Phi is used with two dichotomous variables and is often reported in conjunction with chi-square. Point-biserial can be used to calculate the relationship between one dichotomous and one continuous variable. Spearman rho can be used to measure the relationship between two rank-ordered variables.

There are also nonparametric measures of relationship. These are considered "distribution-free," that is, the assumption of normal distribution of the two variables does not have to be met. Kendall's tau is a nonparametric technique for measuring the relation between two ranked (ordinal) variables. The contingency coefficient can be used to measure the relationship between two nominal variables. It is based on the chi square statistic.

There are also formulas that can be used to estimate the correlation coefficient, r. Biserial can be used when one variable is dichotomized and the other is continuous. Dichotomized means that the variable has been made dichotomous—cut into two levels from a variable that would have been naturally continuous. Biserial estimates what r would be if you changed the dichotomized variable into a continuous variable. The tetrachoric coefficient is an estimate of r based on the relationship between two dichotomized variables.

Eta, sometimes called the correlation ratio, is referred to as the universal measure of the relationship between two variables. The values for eta range from 0 to 1. It can be used to measure nonlinear as well as linear relationships. When it is used with two continuous variables that have a linear relationship, it reduces to r.

Correlational techniques are used to explore and test relationships among variables. They serve as the basis for developing prediction equations through regression techniques.

Logistic Regression

Logistic regression is used to determine which variables affect the probability of the occurrence of an event. In logistic regression the independent variables may be at any level of measurement from nominal to ratio. The dependent variable is categorical, usually a dichotomous variable.

Although it is possible to code the dichotomous variable as 1/0 and run a multiple regression or use discriminant function analysis for categorical outcome measures (two or more categories), this is generally not recommended. Multiple regression and discriminant function are based on the method of least squares, whereas the maximum-likelihood method is used in logistic regression. Because the logistic model is nonlinear, the iterative approach provided by the maximum-likelihood method is more appropriate.

In addition to providing a better fit with the data, logistic regression results include odds ratios that lend interpretability to the data. The odds of an outcome being present as a measure of association has found wide use, especially in epidemiology, because the odds ratio approximates how much more likely (or unlikely) it is for the outcome to be present given certain conditions. An odds ratio is defined as the probability of occurrence over the probability of nonoccurrence.

The probability of the observed results, given the parameter estimates, is known as the likelihood. "Since the likelihood measure is a small number, less than 1, it is customary to use minus 2 times the log of the likelihood as a measure of how well the estimated model fits the data" (Norusis, 1994, p. 10). In logistic regression, comparison of observed to predicted values is based on the log likelihood (LL) function. A good model is one that results in a high likelihood of the observed results. A nonsignificant −2 LL indicates that the data fit the model.

The goodness of fit statistic compares the observed probabilities to those predicted by the model. Assessment of this is also provided in a classification table where percentages of correct predictions are provided. This statistic has a chi-square distribution. A nonsignificant statistic indicates that the data fit the model.

The model chi-square tests the null hypothesis that the coefficients for all the independent variables equal 0. It is equivalent to the F test in regression. A significant result indicates that the independent variables are contributing significantly. As in regression, one must assess the significance of each predictor. In multiple regression the b-weights are used in the calculation of the prediction equation.

In logistic regression the b-weights are used to determine the probability of the occurrence of an event.

As with all methods of regression it is of utmost importance to select variables for inclusion in the model on the basis of clear scientific rationale. Following the fit of the model, the importance of each variable included in the model should be verified (Norusis, 1994). This includes examination of the Wald statistic, which provides a measure of the significance (p) value for each variable. Additionally, one can test the model by systematically including and excluding the predictors. Variables that do not contribute to the model on the basis of these criteria should be eliminated and a new model fit. Once a model has been developed that contains the essential variables, the addition of interaction terms should be considered.

Logistic regression has been reported in the medical literature for some time, particularly in epidemiological studies. Recently, it has become more common in nursing research. This is the result of a new appreciation of the technique and the availability of software to manage the complex analysis. This multivariate technique for assessing the probability of the occurrence of an event requires fewer assumptions than does regression or discriminant function analysis and provides estimates in terms of odds ratios that add to the understanding of the results.

Nonparametric Techniques

Nonparametric statistics are techniques that are not based on assumptions about normality of data. When parametric tests of significance are used, at least one population parameter is being estimated from sample statistics. To arrive at such an estimation, certain assumptions must be made; the most important one is that the variable measured in the sample is normally distributed in the population to which a generalization will be made. With nonparametric tests there is no assumption about the distribution of the variable in the population. For that reason nonparametric tests often are called distribution-free.

At one time, level of measurement was considered a very important determinant in the decision to use parametric or nonparametric tests. Some authors said that parametric tests should be reserved for use with interval- and ratio-level data. More recent studies, however, have shown that the use of parametric techniques with ordinal data rarely distorts the results.

The calculations involved in nonparametric techniques are much easier than those associated with parametric techniques, but the use of computers makes that of little concern. Nonparametric techniques are valuable when using small samples and when there are distortions of the data that seriously violate the assumptions underlying the parametric technique.

Chi-square is the most frequently reported nonparametric technique. It is used to compare the actual number (or frequency) in each group with the "expected" number. The expected number can be based on theory, previous experience, or comparison groups. Chi-square tests whether or not the expected number differs significantly from the actual number. Chi-square is the appropriate technique when variables are measured at the nominal level. It may be used with two or more mutually exclusive groups.

When the groups are not mutually exclusive, as when the same subjects are measured twice, an adaptation of chi-square, the McNemar test, may be appropriate. The McNemar test can be used to measure change when there are two dichotomous measures on the subjects.

When comparing groups of subjects on ordinal data, two commonly used techniques are the Mann-Whitney U, which is used to compare two groups and is thus analogous to the t test, and Kruskal-Wallis H, which is used to compare two or more groups and is thus analogous to the parametric technique analysis of variance.

When one has repeated measures on two or more groups and the outcome measure is not appropriate for parametric techniques, two nonparametric techniques that may be appropriate are the Wilcoxon matched-pairs signed rank test and the Friedman matched samples. The Wilcoxon matched-pairs is analogous to the parametric paired t test, and the Friedman matched samples is analogous to a repeated-measures analysis of variance.

In addition to nonparametric techniques for making group comparisons, there are nonparametric techniques for measuring relationships. There is some confusion about these techniques. For example, point-biserial and Spearman rho are often considered nonparametric techniques but are actually shortcut formulas for the Pearson product-moment correlation (*r*). Biserial and tetrachoric coefficients are estimates of *r*, given certain conditions.

True nonparametric measures of relationship include Kendall's tau and the contingency coefficient. Kendall's tau was developed as an alternative procedure for Spearman rho. It may be used when measuring the relation between two ranked (ordinal) variables. The contingency coefficient can be used to measure the relationship between two nominal-level variables. The calculation of this coefficient is based on the chi-square statistic.

Nonparametric techniques should be considered if assumptions about the normal distribution of variables cannot be met. These techniques, although less powerful, provide a more accurate appraisal of group differences and relationships among variables when the assumptions underlying the parametric techniques have been violated.

Regression

Regression is a statistical method that makes use of the correlation between two variables and the notion of a straight line to develop an equation that can be used to predict the score of one of the variables, given the score of the other. In the case of a multiple correlation, regression is used to establish a prediction equation in which the independent variables are each assigned a weight based on their relationship to the dependent variable, while controlling for the other independent variables.

Regression is useful as a flexible technique that allows prediction and explanation of the interrelationships among variables and the use of categorical as well as continuous variables. Regression literally means a falling back toward the mean. With perfect correlations there is no falling back; using standardized scores, the predicted score is the same as the predictor. With less than perfect correlations there is some error in the measurement; the more error, the more regression toward the mean.

The regression equation consists of an intercept constant (a) and the b's associated with each independent variable. Given those elements and an individual's score on the independent variables, one can predict the individual's score on the dependent variable. The intercept constant (a) is the value of the dependent variable when the independent variable equals zero. It is the point at which the regression line intercepts the *Y* axis.

The letter *b* is called the regression coefficient or regression weight; it is the rate of change in the dependent variable with a unit change in the independent variable. It is a measure of the slope of the regression line, which is the "line of best fit" and passes through the exact center of the data in a scatter diagram. Beta is the standardized regression coefficient.

In multiple regression the multiple correlation (*R*) and each of the b-weights are tested for significance. In most reports the squared multiple correlation, R^2, is reported, as that is a measure of the amount of variance accounted for in the dependent variable. A significant R^2 indicates that a significant amount of the variance in the dependent variable has been accounted for. Testing the b-weight tells us whether the independent variable associated with it is contributing significantly to the variance accounted for in the dependent variable.

Although variables at all levels of measurement may be entered into the regression equation, nominal-level variables must be specially coded prior to entry. Three main types of coding are used: dummy, effect, and orthogonal. Regardless of the method of coding used, the overall *R* is the same, as is its significance. The differences lie in the meaning attached to testing the b-weights for significance. With dummy coding the b-weight represents the difference between the mean of the group represented by that b and the group assigned 0s throughout. In effect coding the b's represent the difference between the mean of the group associated with that b-weight and the grand mean. With orthogonal coding the b-weight measures the difference between two means specified in a hypothesized contrast. Interactions among variables also may be coded and entered into the regression equation.

When using regression, it is of utmost importance to select variables for inclusion in the model on the basis of clear scientific rationale. The method for entering variables into the equation is important, as it affects the interpretation of the results. Variables may be entered all at once, one at a time, or in subsets. Decisions about method of entry may be statistical, as in stepwise entry (where the variable with the highest correlation with the dependent variable is entered first), or theoretical. Stepwise methods have been criticized for capitalizing on chance related to imperfect measurement of the variables being correlated. It is generally recommended that decisions about the order of entry of variables into the regression equation should be made on the basis of the research questions being addressed.

Problems with multiple regression include a high degree of interrelatedness among the independent variables, referred to as multicollinearity. Selection of variables based on theoretical considerations, followed by careful screening of variables and testing of assumptions prior to analysis, can reduce potential problems. If multicollinearity is a problem, decisions must be made about which variables to eliminate. Residual analysis, conducted as part of the regression procedure, can contribute an additional check on whether or not the assumptions underlying the analysis have been met.

Multiple regression is the most commonly reported statistical technique in health care research. It can be used for both explanation and prediction but is more commonly reported as a method for explaining the variability in an outcome measure.

t Test

The *t* test involves an evaluation of means and distributions of two groups. The *t* test, or Student's *t* test, is named after its inventor, William Gosset, who published under the pseudonym Student. Gosset invented the *t* test as a more precise method of comparing groups. The *t* distributions are a set of means of randomly drawn samples from a normally distributed population. They are based on the sample size and vary according to the degrees of freedom.

The *t* test reflects the probability of getting a difference of a given magnitude in groups of a particular size with a certain variability if random samples drawn from the same population were compared. Three factors are included in the analysis: difference between the group means, size of each group, and variability of scores within the groups.

Given the same mean difference, an increase in group size increases the likelihood of a significant difference between two groups, and an increase in group variability decreases the likelihood of significant difference. Increased variability increases the error term and the likelihood of overlap between the scores of the two groups, thereby diminishing the difference between them.

There are three *t* tests. The first is used to compare two mutually exclusive groups when the dependent variable is normally distributed and the variances of the two groups are equal. The equal variance assumption is called homogeneity of variance and indicates that the groups are drawn from the same population. This version of the *t* test is referred to as the pooled or equal-variance *t* test because the denominator contains the variance for all the subjects.

If the assumption of homogeneity of variance is not met, a second formula, called the separate or unequal variance *t* test, can be used. In that case the variance is not pooled for all subjects; instead, the separate variances for each group are contained in the denominator.

When the two sets of scores are not independent, as when two measures are taken on the same subjects or matched pairs are used, a paired or correlated *t* test formula can be used. The formula incorporates the correlation between the two sets of scores.

The *t* tests are very useful when two groups or two correlated measures are being compared. Although analysis of variance can accomplish the same results, the *t* test continues to be used when appropriate as it is easy to present and to understand.

BARBARA MUNRO

See also
DATA ANALYSIS
DATA MANAGEMENT
MEASUREMENT AND SCALES
QUANTITATIVE RESEARCH METHOD-
  OLOGY
SECONDARY DATA ANALYSIS

STRESS

The term *stress* first appeared in the *Cumulative Index to Nursing and Allied Health Literature (CINAHL)* in 1956. Nursing's interest in stress as a focus of research has mushroomed since 1970. Although the word *stress* is familiar to many and has become part of our everyday vocabulary, the term conveys divergent meanings, and multiple theories have been proposed to explain it. Most of the theories attempting to describe and explain stress as a human phenomenon can be categorized under one of three very different orientations to the concept: response-based, stimulus-based, and transaction-based. The response-based orientation was developed by Hans Selye. Selye (1976) defined stress as a nonspecific response of the body to any demand. That is, regardless of the cause, situational context, or psychological interpretation of the demand, the stress response is characterized by the same chain of events or same pattern of physiological correlates.

Defined as a response, stress indicators become the dependent variables in research studies. Nurse researchers who have used the response-based orientation measure catecholoamines, cortisol, urinary Na/K ratio, vital signs, brain waves, electrodermal skin responses, and cardiovascular complaints as indicators of stress. The demand component of Selye's definition is treated as an independent variable, whereas hospitalization, surgery, or critical care unit transfer were commonly the assumed stressor in much of the nursing research using this orientation. The response-based model of stress is not consistent with the nursing philosophical presuppositions that each individual is unique and that individuals respond holistically and often differently to similar situations (Lyon & Werner, 1987).

The stimulus-based theoretical explanation treats stress as a stimulus that causes disrupted responses. As a stimulus, stress is viewed as an external force similar to the engineering use of the term to represent dynamics of strain in metals or an external force directed at a physical object. Defined in this way stress becomes the independent variable in research studies. The most frequently cited example of a stimulus-based theory is the life event theory proposed by Holmes and Rahe (1967). Stress is operationalized as a stable additive phenomenon that is measurable by researcher-selected life events or life changes that typically have preassigned normative weights. The tools most commonly used to measure stress from a stimulus-based orientation are the Social Readjustment Rating Scale (SRRS) and the Schedule of Recent Experiences (SRE). Nurse researchers who have used the stimulus-based orientation have used the SRRS or SRE or developed new tools such as the Hospital Stress Rating Scale (HSRS) (Volicer & Bohannon, 1975). The primary theoretical proposition of the stimulus-based orientation is that too many life events or changes increase vulnerability to illness. Results of studies using the life event perspective have failed to explain illness, accounting for only 2% to 4% of the incidence of illness.

The third way to conceptualize stress is a transaction between person and environment. In this context stress refers to uncomfortable tension-related emotions that arise when demanding situations tax available resources; and some kind of harm, loss, or negative consequence is anticipated. (Lazarus & Folkman, 1984). In the transactional orientation, stress represents a composite of experiences, including threatening appraisals, stress emotions (anxiety, fear, anger, guilt, depression), and coping responses. As such, the term *stress* has heuristic value but is a difficult construct to study. Use of a transactional theoretical orientation requires that the researcher clearly delineate which aspects of the person-environment transaction are to be studied. Commonly, the independent variables in experimental and quasi-experimental studies based on the transactional orientation are personal resources such as self-esteem, perceived control, uncertainty, social support, and hardiness. Appraisal of threat versus appraisal of challenge is commonly studied as a mediating factor between resource strength and coping responses. Dependent variables often include somatic outcomes such as pain, emotional disturbances such as anxiety and depression, and well-being. The transactional model was deemed by Lyon and Werner (1987) to be compatible with nursing's philosophical suppositions.

Lyon and Werner (1987) published a critical review of 82 studies conducted by nurses from 1974 to 1984. The studies reviewed fell evenly across the three different theoretical orientations, and approximately 25% of the studies were atheoretical in nature. In 1993, Barnfather and Lyon edited a monograph of the proceedings of a synthesis conference on stress and coping held in conjunction with the Midwest Nursing Research Society. This critical review of the research covered 296 studies published from 1980 to 1990. Both the 1987 and the 1993 critical reviews noted a disturbing absence of programs of research, making it difficult to identify what we have learned from the discipline's research efforts. Lyon (1993) noted in a preliminary synthesis of findings from the critical review that the transactional orientation has dominated nursing research studies since the late 1980s.

The significance of nursing research in the area of stress grows even more important in the era of managed care and capitated pay for health care services. It is widely recognized that as many as 65% of visits to physician offices are for illnesses that have no discernible medical cause, and many of those illness are thought to be stress-related. Furthermore, productivity in the workplace is thought to be greatly affected by the deleterious effects of stress. Future directions for nursing research in the area of stress will focus on (1) effects of psychological stress on the somatic sense of self, functional ability, the experience of illness, and aberrant behaviors such as abuse and use of alcohol and drugs; (2) the identification of patterns of variables that predict vulnerability or at-risk status for stress-related illness experiences and aberrant behaviors; (3) intervention studies designed to alter factors that make a person vulnerable to stress-related illnesses; and (4) intervention studies to evaluate the effects of various stress management strategies including cognitive restructuring on stress-related illnesses and aberrant behaviors.

BRENDA L. LYON

See also
COPING
JOB STRESS
NURSING OCCUPATIONAL INJURY
    AND STRESS
STRESS MANAGEMENT

STRESS MANAGEMENT

Stress management involves strategies to both decrease stress and prevent stress. Actions taken to decrease stress or alleviate it once experienced are commonly referred to as coping strategies or behaviors. Some of the coping strategies frequently used by nurses include taking action, drawing on past experiences, using problem-solving techniques, using humor, talking over problems with co-workers, accepting the situation, taking breaks (escaping from the situation), using diversions, using relaxation, and exercise (Lewis & Robinson, 1986; Petermann, Springer, & Farnsworth, 1995). Actions taken to prevent stress involve balancing demands and resources, focusing on the positive in difficult situations, maintaining perceived choice and sense of personal control, building social support, and viewing difficult situations as challenges that can bring gain or benefit through learning (Dionne-Proulz & Pepin, 1993; Lyon, 1996).

In addition to the research conducted on stress management strategies used by nurses, nurse researchers also have studied the effects of stress management interventions with various patient and client population groups. Snyder (1993) critically reviewed all 54 stress-related intervention studies appearing in the nursing literature from 1980 through 1990. The types of stress management interventions used included relaxation strategies (e.g., progressive muscle relaxation, imagery, meditation, breathing techniques, massage, music), educational strategies, and use of social support groups. A major flaw of most of the intervention studies was an inadequate description of the intervention used, and there was a lack of attempts to explain the theoretical link between the intervention and outcome measures. Manipulation checks as a way to assure that subjects mastered the intervention and to verify that subjects actually used the intervention also were lacking in the intervention studies. Studies using sensation information (e.g., Johnson, Rice, Fuller, & Endress, 1978) and studies using progressive relaxation techniques (e.g., Pender, 1985) have demonstrated positive effects on health-related outcomes such as less anxiety and an increased sense of well-being.

Future directions for nursing research should focus on the effectiveness of stress management interventions for both nurses and patients or clients. For meaningful results, however, it will be imperative that the researcher clearly define and delineate interventions and offer testable theoretical formulations that explain how the intervention affects outcome variables. It is also essential that the researcher incorporate manipulation checks into the methodology to verify that subjects have implemented a strategy correctly and that the intervention actually altered the target variable as proposed in the theoretical formulation.

BRENDA L. LYON

See also
  COPING
  MUSIC THERAPY
  RELAXATION TECHNIQUES
  SOCIAL SUPPORT
  STRESS

STRUCTURAL EQUATION MODELING

Structural equation modeling (SEM) is used to describe theoretical and analytic techniques for examining cause-and-effect relationships. It is used interchangeably with the terms causal modeling, covariance structure modeling, and LISREL modeling. The theoretical issues are discussed in "Causal Modeling." A description of the analytic issues when programs such as LISREL or EQS are used will ensue.

Types of Models

Structural equation modeling techniques are extremely flexible. Most models of cause can be estimated. In some models the causal flow is specified only between the latent variable and its empirical indicators, such as in a factor analysis model. This is known as confirmatory factor analysis. In other models, causal paths among the latent variables also are included.

Conducting a confirmatory factor analysis with SEM has many advantages. With SEM, the analyst

can specify exactly which indicators will load on which latent variables (the factors), and the amount of variance in the indicators not explained by the latent variable (due to error in either measurement or model specification) is estimated. Correlations between latent variables and among errors associated with the indicators can be estimated and examined. Statistics that describe the fit of the model with the data allow the analyst to evaluate the adequacy of the factor structure, make theoretically appropriate modifications to the structure based on empirical evidence, and test the change in fit caused by these modifications. Thus, confirmatory factor analysis provides a direct test of the hypothesized structure of an instrument's scales.

An advantage of using SEM to estimate models containing causal paths among the latent variables is that many of the regression assumptions can be relaxed or estimated. For example, with multiple regression, the analyst must assume perfect measurement (no measurement error); however, with SEM, measurement error can be specified and the amount estimated. In addition, constraints can be introduced based on theoretical expectations. For example, equality constraints, setting two or more paths to have equal values, are useful when the model contains cross-lagged paths from three or more time points. The path from latent variable A at Time 1 to latent variable B at Time 2 can be set to equal the path from latent variable A at Time 2 to latent variable B at Time 3. Equality constraints also are used to compare models for two or more different groups. For example, to compare the models of effects of maternal employment on preterm and full-term child outcomes, paths in the preterm model can be constrained to be equal to the corresponding paths in the full-term model.

Data requirements for SEM are similar to those for factor analysis and multiple regression in level of measurement but not sample size. Exogenous variables can have indicators that are measured as interval, near-interval, or categorical (dummy-, effect-, or orthogonally coded) levels, but endogenous variables must have indicators that are measured at the interval or near-interval level. The rule of thumb regarding the number of cases needed for SEM, 5 to 10 cases per parameter to be estimated, suggests considerably larger samples than usually needed for multiple regression; thus, samples of 100 for a very modest model to 500 or more for more complex models are often required. Despite the advantages of SEM, these larger samples can result in complex and costly studies.

Analysis Process

Structural equation modeling is generally a multistage procedure. First, the SEM implied by the theoretical model is tested and the fit of the model to the observed data is evaluated. A nonsignificant χ^2 indicates acceptable fit, but this is difficult to obtain because the χ^2 value is heavily influenced (increased) by larger sample sizes. Thus, most analytic programs provide other measures of fit (Bollen & Long, 1993). A well-fitting model is necessary before the parameter estimates can be evaluated and interpreted.

In most cases, the original theoretical model does not fit the data well, and modifications must be made to the model in order to obtain a well-fitting model. Although deletion of nonsignificant paths (based on t values) is possible, modifications generally focus on the inclusion of omitted paths (causal or correlational). Any path that is omitted specifies that there is no relationship, implying a parameter of zero; thus, analysis programs constrain these paths to be zero. After estimating the specified model, most programs provide a numerical estimate of the "strain" experienced by fixing parameters to zero or improvement in fit that would result from freeing the parameters (allowing them to vary). Suggested paths must be theoretically defensible before adding them to the respecified model.

Because model respecification is based on the data at hand in light of theoretical evidence and those data are repeatedly tested, the significance level of the χ^2 is actually higher than what the program indicates (Bollen, 1989). Thus, other criteria are necessary to evaluate the adequacy of the final model (Youngblut, 1994). First is the theoretical appropriateness of the final model. Comparison of the original model with the final model will indicate how much "trimming" has taken place. In addition, the values and signs of the parameters

are evaluated. The signs (positive or negative) of the parameters should be in the expected direction. Parameters on the paths between the latent variable and its indicators should be $\geq.50$ but ≤1.0 in a standardized solution. The lower the unexplained variance of the endogenous variables, the better the model performed in explaining those endogenous variables (similar to the $1-R^2$ value in multiple regression). Results that are consistent with a priori expectations and findings from previous research increase one's confidence in the model.

In summary, SEM is a powerful and flexible analysis technique for testing models of cause, investigating specific cause-and-effect relationships, and exploring the hypothesized process by which specific outcomes are produced. With SEM programs, the researcher has greater control over the analyses than with other factor analysis and multiple regression programs. Model respecification is usually necessary, but the role of theory in selecting appropriate modifications is crucial.

JoAnne M. Youngblut

See also
CAUSAL MODELING
DATA ANALYSIS
FACTOR ANALYSIS
MEASUREMENT AND SCALES
STATISTICAL TECHNIQUES

SUBSTRUCTION

Substruction is a heuristic technique, designed to be helpful in planning research and critiquing published research. It was first introduced to the nursing research literature by Hinshaw (1979). She outlined four steps in the process of substruction: (1) identify and isolate major concepts, (2) specify relationships among the concepts, (3) hierarchically order concepts by level of abstraction, and (4) pictorially present relationships among the variables. She provided guidelines for conducting theoretical substruction, and Dulock and Holzemer (1991) added a discussion of operational systems thus linking theory with methodology of research.

Substruction now comprises two components. The theoretical system explicates the relationship between constructs and concepts through articulating postulates or statements of relationships. For example, the construct of quality of life might postulate that it is composed of three dimensions or concepts, including physical, social, and spiritual. Thus, there is an implicit level of abstraction in substruction, moving vertically down from the most abstract (constructs) to less abstract notions (concepts). It is true that in the English language some authors will consider the words *constructs* and *concepts* to be interchangeable, and this must be recognized as a potential source of confusion when discussing substruction. The labels are less important than the idea of levels of abstraction.

In addition to examining vertical, conceptual relationships, the theoretical system examines across constructs through articulating axioms and propositions. Axioms are statements linking constructs; propositions are statements of relationships between or among concepts. For example, an investigator may hypothesize the relationship between the concepts of severity of illness and quality of life. The study might state as an axiom that there is an inverse, predictable relationship between severity of illness and quality of life. An author might hypothesize that as illness becomes more severe, quality of life diminishes.

The authors may conceptualize severity of illness to have related concepts, just as the construct quality of life had three concepts. Perhaps severity of illness is conceptualized to have two concepts, including physiological status and severity of symptoms. This example linking severity of illness and quality of life is summarized in the accompanying Figure 1. The theoretical system relates constructs and concepts and presents them pictorially in a fashion that demonstrates their relationships. The vertical axis represents level of abstraction. The horizontal axis is utilized to represent time, moving from left to right with the underlying assumption that the researchers are interested in causal relationships, and there may be an implicit understanding that the investigators are suggesting that change in severity of illness "causes" change in quality of life.

If one is reading or planning an intervention study, the construct may be the intervention itself, such as patient teaching. There also may be concepts related to the intervention, such as type of delivery technique (group vs. individual) or time spent on teaching activity as a measure of dose of the treatment. Each of these concepts may be operationalized in the operational system as strategies to assess the take of the treatment, even though the treatment may have as its empirical indicator Yes or No or "received treatment" or "did not receive treatment."

The operational system was added by Dulock and Holzemer (1991) in their article on the process of substruction. The operational system requires the investigator to link each concept identified in the theoretical substruction with an empirical indicator or measure. The process of identifying the measures for each concept (or subconcept) highlights for the reader how the investigator operationalized the constructs. Sometimes this process reveals that, although an investigator included a construct or concept, the variable was never actually measured in the study.

This process of identifying the empirical indicators or measures also helps the investigator to give attention to the validity and reliability of each measure selected to ensure confidence in the results of the measurement. Finally, a review of the empirical indicators assists with an analysis of the level of scaling of the measures so that the reader can have confidence that an appropriate statistical analysis was conducted. Labeling the obtained scores from empirical indicators or measures as continuous or discrete leads one directly to the discussion of parametric or nonparametric analyses and which approach might be appropriate.

Dulock and Holzemer (1991) outlined a series of questions that can be generated related to the process of substruction when either planning or critiquing research studies. These questions have been modified and include the following:

1. What is the evidence that supports the relationships between constructs and concepts in the study?
2. What is the evidence that supports the relationships between constructs and concepts?
3. How does the study propose to measure each of the identified concepts?
4. Is there evidence of the validity and reliability of the measures?

5. What level of measurement will result from these instruments?
6. Are the data analysis techniques appropriate for these measures?
7. Is there a logical consistency between the theoretical system and the operational system?

They wrote: "These questions are designed to guide the exploration of the relationships between the theoretical and operational aspects of a study. The analytical process of substructing helps one to focus upon the study as a Gestalt of interrelationships" (p. 86). Substruction has proved to be an extremely useful tool when developing a new research project as well as for analyzing published studies. As a heuristic technique, substruction helps the researcher to understand how to think about the relationships among the selected variables or to understand how the author conceptualized these relationships.

WILLIAM L. HOLZEMER

See also
MIDDLE-RANGE THEORY
THEORETICAL FRAMEWORK

SUICIDE

Suicide is defined as a death that is the result of an intentional self-destructive act. Nurses have demonstrated a great deal of clinical and theoretical interest in suicide, suicide attempts, attitudes toward suicide, and assisted suicide but have conducted very little research on these topics. A related topic that has been studied fairly extensively by nurses is suicide survivors, those family members and significant others who are bereaved by a suicide.

Suicide, Suicide Attempts, and Suicidal Thoughts

Few studies have addressed suicide specifically. Using a qualitative methodology, messages of psychiatric patients who attempted or committed suicide were compared by Valente (1994). She found that clear suicidal messages were sent by most psychiatric patients and that the messages of suicide completers and suicide attempters could be differentiated. Demi, Bakeman, Sowell, Moneyham, and Seals (1996) studied suicidality in HIV-infected women and found that suicidal thoughts were common among the women and that family cohesion moderated the effect of HIV-related symptoms on emotional distress. They also found that there were clear differences between women who neither thought about nor attempted suicide and those who thought about or attempted suicide, but there were no significant differences between those who thought about suicide and those who attempted it. Grabbe, Demi, Camann, and Potter (1997) used a national data base to assess suicidal risk factors among the elderly during their last year of life;

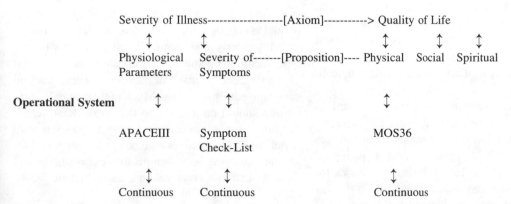

FIGURE 1   Sample substruction illustrating the theoretical and operation systems.

and using logistic regression, they confirmed the traditional risk factors of age, race, gender, alcohol use, and mental illness and provided preliminary evidence that cancer is also a risk factor among the elderly.

Two studies addressed adolescent suicide. Burge, Felts, Chenier, and Parrillo (1995), using a national data base, studied suicidal behaviors among U.S. high school students and found a significant positive relationship between cocaine use and severity of outcomes of suicide attempts. They also found a significant but less strong relationship between marijuana use, alcohol use, sexual activity, and suicide attempts. Conrad (1992) explored adolescents' beliefs about the causes of adolescent suicide and found that teens identified "too much pressure" as the major cause of teen suicide.

Attitudes toward Suicide

Several studies by nurses have investigated attitudes toward suicide in diverse groups, four studies addressed nurses' attitudes, and one studied elderly persons' attitudes. Oncology nurses' knowledge and misconceptions about suicide were explored through use of a vignette depicting a suicidal cancer patient (Valente, Saunders, & Grant, 1994). Although the nurses correctly identified a number of risk factors, few knew that race, age, and gender were risk factors. Further, few nurses assessed whether patients had a specific suicide plan, and less than one third identified appropriate interventions to prevent suicide in an at-risk patient. A second study compared nurses' attitudes toward suicide based on their clinical specialty, age, and highest degrees; they found no significant differences on any of the subscales based on clinical specialty, although age and degrees were significant on only the right to die subscale (Alston & Robinson, 1992).

When Irish casualty nurses' attitudes toward attempted suicide were assessed, older and more experienced nurses had better attitudes toward suicide attempters than did younger, less experienced nurses (McLaughlin, 1994). Positive attitudes toward suicide attempters were found among psychiatric nurses working in an acute psychiatric ward (Long & Reid, 1996). The only study of nonnurses explored attitudes toward suicide among low-income, elderly, inner city residents and compared attitudes toward suicide of men and women, African Americans and Whites, finding no significant differences. The researchers suggested that social class and place of residence may be better predictors of attitudes toward suicide in the elderly than race and gender (Parker, Cantrell, & Demi, 1997).

Suicide Survivors

Many studies have been conducted on suicide survivors, including parents, spouses, children, siblings, and therapists. Most of the studies of suicide survivors have been descriptive and have found that a death by suicide produces extreme distress in the survivors, with evidence of increased guilt, stigma, and resentment and a continuing questioning of "why" the suicide occurred. Several studies have compared those bereaved by suicide with those bereaved by other modes of death and have reported conflicting findings. Recently, an attempt was made to use a quasi-experimental design to study the effects of two group interventions on outcomes among spouse survivors of suicide (Constantino & Bricker, 1996). The researchers found that participants in both the social group intervention and the bereavement intervention experienced an overall reduction in distress; however, the bereavement intervention group experienced significantly lower levels of anger or hostility and guilt.

Future Directions

The suicide rates for the elderly are rising. At the same time, there is increased interest in euthanasia and assisted suicide. Nurses are intimately involved with elderly and terminally ill patients who are contemplating suicide and assisted suicide. At the same time, suicide rates among adolescents and young adults are rising. Much more research attention should be directed to this topic. Researchers should move beyond describing attitudes toward suicide and effects of suicide on survivors and toward studying interventions to prevent suicide and to assist those coping with a death by suicide.

ALICE S. DEMI

See also
ADOLESCENCE
ALCOHOLISM
CHRONIC MENTAL ILLNESS
DEPRESSION AMONG OLDER ADULTS
YOUNG WOMEN AND DEPRESSION

SURGERY: PREOPERATIVE PSYCHOLOGICAL PREPARATION

The preparation of patients for their experience with surgery is one of the largest bodies of clinical investigation relevant to the practice of nursing. The first report of an experimental study was published by a nurse, Rhetaugh Dumas (Dumas & Leonard, 1963), and the topic continued to attract researchers representing nursing, medicine, and psychology for over 20 years. The interest in psychological preparation for the surgical experience started with the discovery that when patients ambulated within hours after the operation, instead of being in bed for 7 to 10 days, morbidity and mortality decreased. This change in practice was anxiety-provoking for both patients and the people who cared for them. Preparing patients for the experience of getting out of bed soon after surgery was a way to deal with the anxiety. Much of the research stemmed from pragmatic concerns about how to help these anxious patients ambulate and perform behaviors believed to reduce postoperative complications. Psychological theories about *coping* with stressful events began to emerge in the late 1950s and 1960s, but most of the research on preparing patients for the stressful experience of undergoing surgery was atheoretical. Connections between the clinical research and theory, when attempted, were often vague.

Research on the effects of various approaches to preparing patients for surgery has been reviewed by a number of people, using meta-analysis (e.g., Devine & Cook, 1986; Hathaway, 1986) and narrative review (e.g., Johnson, 1984). It was difficult to conduct a tightly controlled study in the clinical settings, and there were methodological flaws in the studies. Nevertheless, there was consensus among the reviewers for the overall conclusion that preoperative interventions aimed at helping patients deal with their experiences postoperatively had a substantial positive effect on patients' welfare.

The interventions varied in content and focus. The most frequently tested intervention was instruction in the exercises and behaviors that patients were expected to engage in postoperatively to reduce complications. For abdominal and chest surgery patients, the intervention usually consisted of instruction in methods of deep breathing to effectively inflate the lungs, effective coughing techniques, leg exercises to increase circulation, and methods of getting out of bed to minimize incisional pain. The next most frequent intervention consisted of information that oriented patients to the routines of care. These descriptions were based on content in textbooks, manuals used by care providers, and providers' experiences. Patients were told, for example, that their skin would be prepared, that they would receive preoperative medication, and that they would go to the recovery room. The specifics of patients' experiences during those procedures were not included. This type of information has been referred to as procedural information.

In another type of informational intervention, the patient's perspective of the experience of undergoing surgery was emphasized. These descriptions focused on physical sensations associated with the events, when events would occur, and how long they would last. For example, the interventions included statements about how long patients could expect to be in the recovery room and about vital signs being checked frequently, descriptions of the sensations caused by preoperative medication (e.g., dry mouth and drowsiness), descriptions of sensations that abdominal surgery patients experienced when they coughed, and the expected progression of physical activities. This type of information was originally called sensory information and later called concrete objective information because that phrase more accurately described the content. Highly individualized nurse-patient interactions, hypnosis, relaxation, and positive thinking also have been used as interventions in a few studies of surgical patients. The impact of these studies on practice was decreased because of inconsistent findings and the special training required to deliver the intervention.

Clinical experience influenced the aspects of patient response, behaviors, and recovery selected as outcome measures in the research on preparing patients for surgery. Length of postoperative stay, pain medication use, complications, and ambulating behavior are representative of measures derived from clinical experience. Some researchers included patients' psychological responses, such as mood or emotions, pain reports, satisfaction with care, and well-being. Most researchers limited their measurement of outcomes to the time the patient was hospitalized. However, a few researchers were interested in the influence of the interventions on patients' long-term recovery and measured patients return to usual activities and psychological response after discharge from the hospital.

Although as many as 102 studies have been included in reviews, confident conclusions about relationships between content of interventions and specific outcomes cannot be drawn. The practice of combining content in interventions, instead of studying the effects of each type of content separately, contributes to the inability to sort out the content that was associated with specific outcomes. However, reviewers agree that combined interventions have the most consistent effects on outcomes. A frequently used combined content intervention consisted of instruction in postoperative exercises and behaviors and informing patients about routines of care (procedural information). This combined intervention appeared to have a positive effect on outcomes measured during hospitalization. A combination of descriptions of experiences from the patient's perspective (concrete objective information) and instruction in postoperative exercises and behavior also had a positive effect on outcomes measured during hospitalization. An additional benefit of the concrete objective information intervention was that it was associated with patients returning earlier to their usual activities after discharge.

The practice of preparing patients for surgery has been widely disseminated and is included in textbooks of nursing. It has become a part of care in most health care settings. The economic impact has been accepted as self-evident because of the reduction in complications and length of hospitalization and the early return to productive activities. In addition, the interventions had a positive effect on patients' subjective reports of well-being, such as mood and satisfaction with care. The combination of a practice activity having positive effects on cost and quality of care makes it an ideal practice to be widely adopted.

The recent practice of ambulatory surgery with discharge after patients awaken from anesthesia and that of admitting patients the day of surgery with brief hospital stays have changed the nature of patients' experiences when undergoing surgery. Patients and their families have to provide postoperative care. This includes assessing for complications, making decisions about the patient's status, progression of physical activities, and care of the incision. There has been little research on preparing patients for surgery since this change in practice.

Because the needs of surgical patients and their families have changed, new research on preparation for surgery is necessary. That research should draw on the prior research on preparing patients for surgery and advances in theory about coping with health care experiences. One such theory that has developed from a program of clinical research is self-regulation theory (Johnson, Fieler, Jones, Wlasowicz, & Mitchell, 1997; Leventhal & Johnson, 1983). Relying on informational processing explanations of behavior, self-regulation theory provides explanations for why specific types of information about an experience, combined with instruction in self-care and coping activities, can help patients and families to cope with the surgical experience.

In the current climate of containment of health care costs, insurance coverage decisions are informed primarily by data about cost of care. There is much less data about how coverage regulations affect patient welfare. Research on preparing surgical patients for their experience at this time has the potential of influencing policies about services covered by health insurance.

JEAN E. JOHNSON

See also
COPING
PATIENT EDUCATION
PSYCHOSOCIAL INTERVENTIONS
RELAXATION TECHNIQUES

T

TAXONOMY

Definition and Related Terms

The word *taxonomy* derives from the Greek *taxis-nomos*, meaning arrangement and rule; together, the two words lead to the idea of giving an order or classifying objects. The term *taxonomy* was first used in 1813 by de Condolle in his *Theorie Elementaire de la Botanique* as a system for classifying plants on the basis of natural relationships.

A distinction between taxonomy and classification was introduced by Sokol (1974), who defined classification as a process through which objects (or phenomena) are ordered into groups or sets based on their relationships. A process of classification produces a classification system. Taxonomy is a methodology that provides rules and principles on how to classify and identify objects, where identification means to assign additional objects to a correct class once a classification system has been established.

Taxonomy can also be defined as a field having as its object of inquiry theories, practical aspects, and rules for classifying organisms. Information for choosing name, description, and classification of a specific organism is derived from different disciplinary fields. For example, classic taxonomy is based on morphology and anatomy. Biochemical taxonomy studies analogies between structures of protein and nucleic acids.

Principles of Classification

Taxonomic theory provides two major principles of classification: (a) the principle of monothetic classification and (b) the principle of polythetic classification (Aydelotte & Peterson, 1991). The monothetic principle dictates that the established classes must differ by at least one property or characteristic that is common to the members of each class, for example, the classification of nursing students in the school of nursing. Undergraduate students are one class, and graduate students are another. Each class has a single property that all share in common (i.e., being a student) and that differentiates it from the other class. Other properties may be similar to those in the other class, such as age, marital status, income, and the like. The polythetic principle groups individuals (or objects) who share a large portion of their properties but do not necessarily agree on any one property (Sokal, 1974). This principle has been used in developing patients' classification systems based on activity. Patients in one class may share certain characteristics, but any one characteristic will not necessarily be observed in all members of the class. Therefore, following this principle, many properties may be necessary to classify objects.

Taxonomy requires, for classification purposes, the arrangement of the objects' properties by use of methods and techniques such as pairing, clustering, ordinating, or use of graphs and trees and other complex formulas to handle similarities and dissimilarities between objects.

Usefulness of a Taxonomy in Nursing

The World Heath Organization's *International Classification of Diseases*, diagnosis related groups, and other case mix groupings are being used to organize information about health care and make decisions for health care delivery and allocation of resources. All these systems are disease-oriented and may not include any nursing contribution.

The usefulness of defining a classification system in nursing depends on many factors, mainly the degree to which definitions systematize the knowledge in the field and lead to a standardized nomenclature and the degree to which simplicity characterizes the system. Aydelotte and Peterson (1991) define some requirements that must be met in order to use a taxonomy:

1. The purposes for the classifications must be clear and widely accepted in the discipline.
2. Procedures and rules for describing and naming properties (defined characteristics of phenomena) have been adopted and implemented.
3. Criteria for classes and subclasses have been identified, these have been defined and their definition and labels convey relationships that are logical and have meaning to the user; and the classes are exhaustive and mutually exclusive.
4. Format or structure of the system has been selected and shows a relationship between classes and subclasses.

Taxonomies in Nursing

In the past decades, nurses have produced several patients' classification systems in order to define nursing care requirements. The main difference between the early systems and the modern ones can be seen in the much higher measurability of the classification criteria and a better definition of the attributes used to define classes.

Hartley and McKibbin (1983) describe five types of classification systems traditionally used in nursing: (a) procedure-based; (b) acuity-based; (c) disease-based; (d) those that combine disease, procedures, and complications; and (e) intensity plus disease-based. For the most part, a nursing classification system will fall within the acuity-based grouping. The differences between the medical and the nursing classification systems relate to the variety of information contributing to the categories and the scope and depth of the information. The selection of categories and principles of division reflects the orientation toward, or perspective on,

the phenomena to be classified and the purpose of the classification. The underpinning classification system's conceptual framework must be consistent with the science of nursing in order to define the system as a nursing classification system. Bulechek and McCloskey's taxonomy of nursing practice, the Omaha classification scheme for interventions, the National Council of State Boards study's categories of nurse activities, and the North American Nursing Diagnosis Association's (NANDA) Taxonomy I for Nursing Diagnosis can be considered examples of nursing classification systems based on taxonomic rules.

Future Directions

NANDA's Taxonomy I for Nursing Diagnosis is probably the best known and most widely used taxonomy in nursing since 1973. It is a two-dimensional structure consisting of nine patterns of human responses on one dimension and two levels of abstractions to make them more concrete and clinically useful. NANDA's taxonomy II, currently under development, proposes the addition of multiple axes, which will change the structure from a two-dimensional orientation to a multidimensional structure based on four axes: unit of analysis, age group, wellness, and illness (Fitzpatrick, 1991a).

In 1996 an alpha version of *The International Classification for Nursing Practice* (ICNP) was released by the International Council of Nursing (ICN). The ICNP differs from the existing nursing classifications because it is built according to the rules of classification in which all of the concepts are placed within a framework of hierarchical relationships governed by one single principle of division and by a generic relationship between concepts (ICN, 1996).

Classification of phenomena helps to advance the knowledge base of the nursing field through the discovery of the principles governing what is known. Internationally standardized nursing taxonomies for diagnoses, activities, and outcomes are needed to create a common language in nursing, to develop compatible care systems, and to interface with other care provider information systems. More research is needed to evaluate and validate rules of classification and categories.

RENZO ZANOTTI

See also
INTERNATIONAL CLASSIFICATION
  FOR NURSING PRACTICE
NANDA
NURSING INTERVENTIONS CLASSIFI-
  CATIONS
NURSING OUTCOMES CLASSIFICA-
  TION
OMAHA SYSTEM

TELEHEALTH

Telehealth is a rapidly growing technology for health care delivery that holds the promise of improving access to health for people living in rural and underserved areas as well as improving the resources available to health care practitioners in those areas. Telehealth is an application of telecommunications technology. Historically, the use of telecommunications technology for aiding communications between health care practitioners has been occurring since the days of the telegraph. The 1990s has seen an exponential growth in the available technologies and the interest in their use for health care.

As yet there are no standard terms or definitions for the various aspects of this health care technology. Telecommunications refers to the transmission, emission, or reception of data or information, in the form of signs, signals, writings, images, and sounds or any other form, via wire, radio, visual, or other electromagnetic systems. Telehealth may be defined as the removal of time and distance barriers for the delivery of health care services or related health care activities. Some of the technologies used in telehealth include telephones, computers, interactive video transmissions, direct links to health care instruments, transmission of images (e.g., radiographic images), and teleconferencing by telephone or by video. The rapid development of new communications technologies and the discovery of new uses for existing technologies will continue to expand this list.

Telenursing is a subset of telehealth in which the focus is on nursing practice across the domains of nursing. Similarly, telemedicine is another telehealth subset and includes the domains of medical specialty practice, such as teleradiology, teledermatology, telepsychiatry, and so forth. As the use of telecommunications technologies became more popular and more prevalent during the early 1990s, *telemedicine* was the term most often used. All health care practitioners and activities were subsumed under the telemedicine label. In the health care literature during this time most descriptions of telemedicine projects addressed only physician-to-physician communications. Now *telehealth* is being adopted as it is more inclusive and more appropriate to a health care system focused on wellness, illness prevention, and health maintenance.

Many potential benefits are predicted from telehealth, including increased consumer access to primary care practitioners, health care specialists, and specialized or advanced care facilities; rapid access to client health records and related information; more accurate and faster diagnosis and care; decreased use of emergency rooms as consumers use direct video contact with a health care practitioner (e.g., the managed care "triage nurse"); and monitoring of health status between required in-person visits that will allow early identification of problems and initiation of appropriate interventions. The consistent belief among proponents of telehealth is better health outcomes for individuals and populations and a reduction in health care costs.

Unfortunately, empirical data to support the anticipated benefits of telehealth are lacking, as are methodologically sound evaluation studies. The federal government has recognized this lack and undertaken activities to resolve it. The Institute of Medicine (IOM) was requested to study the issue of evaluating telehealth projects. In its report, *Telemedicine: A guide to assessing telecommunications in health care* (Institute of Medicine, 1996), the IOM states that this technology must be subject to the same evaluation principles that apply to other technologies in health care.

Until recently, studies of telehealth were either pilot projects related to the feasibility of implementing a particular application or the implementation of large-scale projects. Reports on these studies were focused on technological issues and factors affecting success or failure. This is beginning to change. In late 1996 the National Library of Medicine (NLM) funded 19 telehealth projects affecting rural, inner-city, and suburban areas, with a total budget of $42 million. The projects were focused on evaluating the impact of telehealth on cost, quality, and access to health care; assessing approaches to ensuring the confidentiality of health data transmitted via electronic networks; and testing health data standards.

In addition to the NLM-funded projects, the Office of Rural Health Policy directs a telehealth grant program designed to study rural telehealth by gathering the data needed for a systematic evaluation of its applications. As of 1997, 11 projects in 10 states have received $5.1 million to provide services to rural residents and to facilitate the development of rural health networks. This office also funds an additional seven telehealth projects under an outreach grant program. Along with increased federal interest in telehealth research, state governments and private funding sources are interested in evaluating this technology. This widespread interest in the evaluation of telehealth provides enhanced opportunities for nurse scientists interested in studying telehealth in its broadest sense or telenursing as a specific arena.

Telenursing applications may be examined within four domains: education, administration, research, and clinical practice. Nursing educators have made use of telecommunications technology for many years in the provision of distance learning to remote areas where the travel distance to the nearest college or university makes it difficult for registered nurses to continue their education. In nursing administration, telehealth offers the opportunity for peer conferences and consultations among administrators situated in diverse facilities of an integrated health care system. Nurse researchers may provide research consultation services to health care settings, set up discussions with groups of nurse researcher colleagues, experience enhanced opportunities for collaborative research across distances, have access to expanded populations for recruitment, and collect data from remote sites.

As with other health care professions, it is clinical nursing practice for which telenursing interest is greatest and most likely to be funded. Nursing staff can consult with remote peers and specific clinical expert nurses. Registered nurses may conduct multimedia assessments of clients at remote sites or at the client's home (e.g., telephone triage, home care monitoring). Nurses from a client's community health care facility may participate in clinical care conferences. Nurses have improved access to on-line health care databases and scientific knowledge, sometimes at the point of care. The home health nurse can consult directly with a client's primary care practitioner, a pharmacist, or others as necessary. Telenursing enables the professional nurse to monitor and assess a client's health status and responses to health care interventions between personal visits. Nurses may provide support to lay caregivers as well.

Future directions for research in telehealth involve the legal and regulatory implications of practicing health care (nursing, medicine, psychology) across state boundaries and payment for health care services provided from a distance. Other research interests would include impact on the therapeutic practitioner–client relationship; ethical obligations of the practitioner; privacy and confidentiality; informed consent related to participation in telehealth; and development, implementation, and evaluation of practice guidelines for telehealth. The effectiveness of telehealth on short-term and long-term health outcomes, including the client's health status, well-being, functional status, reintegration into the community, and adaptation to a changed health state, will provide a challenge to researchers in all disciplines. Thus, telehealth and telenursing offer rich opportunities from many perspectives for nurse researchers.

D. KATHY MILHOLLAND

See also
ACCESS TO HEALTH CARE
HEALTH SYSTEMS DELIVERY
RURAL HEALTH
TELENURSING/TELEPRACTICE
TELEPRESENCE

TELENURSING/TELEPRACTICE

Telenursing is the use of telemedicine technology to deliver nursing care and conduct nursing practice.

Telemedicine is defined as the practice of health care delivery, diagnosis, consultation, treatment, transfer of medical data and education using interactive audio, visual, and data communications. The origin of the term *telemedicine* is the Latin *tele*, meaning "distance," and *mederi*, meaning "healing." The power of telemedicine technology for nursing practice and nursing science lies within the context of distance healing. Telenursing combines telecommunications and computer technologies to project nursing expertise to patients, other nurses, multidisciplinary health team members, health care organizations, and policymakers. Geography and location of the nurse are irrelevant; the focus is on the practice of nursing via "distance healing."

Telenursing and telepractice occur by the application of emerging telemedicine technologies to the field of nursing. Descriptions of telenursing in the literature are few. Muller and colleagues (Muller et al., 1977) tested the cost-effectiveness of a pediatric nurse practitioner primary care program, linking autonomous nurse practitioners to consulting pediatricians by television. Muller concluded that the nurse practitioner could be a "physician substitute" if there was TV backup. This article was the earliest documented evidence of nursing's participation in telemedicine, and it had a strong medical influence and evaluative aspect.

Telenursing is emerging as a new nursing role of the 1990s (Nelson & Schlachta, 1995). The roots of telenursing lie in the history of telemedicine. In the early 1960s and 1970s the efficacy of long-distance diagnosis, consultation, education, and patient care in the fields of telepsychiatry, teledermatology, and telecardiology were explored (Dwyer, 1973; Gravenstein, Berzina-Moettus, Regan, & Pao, 1974; Murphy, Block, Bird, & Yurchak, 1973). Thirty years ago, however, the fiscal incentive for widespread use of telemedicine was not present. Affordable computer technology with capabilities for satellite, fiberoptic, and telephone communications, combined with the fiscal impetus to reorganize the way health care is provided, results in telemedicine.

Within the capabilities of telemedicine are a wide range of applications based on clinical need that encompasses nursing as well as medical care. Telecommunications technology ranges from POTS (plain old telephone service) to satellites.

In between there is a myriad of opportunities for conveying clinical information. In the planning of a telemedicine clinical application, it is important to identify the clinical requirement of the practitioner and select the appropriate telemedicine medium to meet the clinical need (Swartz, 1994). Experience shows that the most successful telemedicine projects are those that use the lowest form of technology for the clinical application required. A satellite or fiberoptic system is not necessary or appropriate for every clinical application.

Current Telenursing Applications

Providing interactive video and audio patient care in the patient's home is a new concept currently being explored. The "electronic house call" initiative of Dr. Jay Sanders at Medical College of Georgia provides telenursing care to patients with multiple medical and nursing problems (Sanders, 1995). Through the Electronic Housecall Project, 25 chronically ill patients' homes are being accessed by computers running over the traditional cable TV lines. With the addition of a "black box" the usual one-way TV cable coming into the home is used for two-way communication, allowing the patient to electronically visit a telenurse. Various peripheral assessment devices, such as a stethoscope, blood pressure cuff, oxygen saturation monitor, temperature probe, three-lead ECG, and scale, enable telenurses to conduct remote physical assessment, provide medical consultation, and conduct patient teaching, virtually in the patient's home. Telenurses are located at central computer stations at Eisenhower Army Medical Center and the Medical College of Georgia.

Elsewhere in the United States, telenurses conduct electronic home visits in Minnesota and California as part of pilot programs in large managed care organizations. Telenursing is at times a substitute for an in-person home visit and allows more frequent yet less resource-intensive nursing intervention.

In 1994 the International Telenurses Association was formed. It is a listserv (discussion group on the Internet), a truly virtual nursing organization. In 1994 approximately 10 nurses in the United States were involved in telemedicine; today the listserv membership has grown to over 250, and multitudes of telenursing applications, such as tele-critical care, telepediatric multidisciplinary team evaluation of medically involved children, and nurse managers of growing telehealth programs, are occurring. Members are international civilian and military nurses, nursing students, and nurse practitioners interested and involved in telenursing and telepractice.

Nurses at Sheppard Center, a spinal cord specialty center in Atlanta, conduct wound assessments in patients' homes by using telemedicine technology over regular phone lines. A nursing student at the University of Michigan linked a young boy in isolation after a bone marrow transplant with his schoolmates, using video over the Internet and a laptop computer in the boy's hospital room.

Telenursing applications are limited only by the reluctance of nurses to embrace technology and the paradigm of our current practice and current health care system. Opportunities for support groups, education of patients, postpartum electronic visits and teaching, ostomy care, medication monitoring, and psychiatric nursing care of the mentally ill in group homes scattered across communities are some examples of future telenursing applications. Interstate licensure, practice standards and guidelines, reimbursement, malpractice, and changing roles of health care providers are all issues yet to be defined as telenursing emerges. The evolution of these issues will have an impact on the practice of nursing.

Telemedicine, telenursing, and telepractice are not simply a mixing of computers and telecommunications with health care. Rather, they encompass a system for delivery of health care that requires a paradigm shift in order to see new and more productive interrelationships among health care professionals, patients, policymakers, and communities (Preston, 1993).

The opinions expressed are those of the author(s) and do not reflect the official position of the author's organizations and/or the Department of Defense.

LORETTA M. SCHLACHTA
SUSAN M. SPARKS

See also
ACCESS TO HEALTH CARE

HEALTH SYSTEMS DELIVERY
INTERNET
TELEHEALTH
TELEPRESENCE

TELEPRESENCE

Telepresence is the ability of a health care provider to touch, palpate, or manipulate a patient without being physically present with that patient. Telepresence is most commonly depicted in the image of telerobotic surgery, when a surgeon wearing virtual-reality glasses operates via robotics on a patient in a remote geographic location (Gagner, Begin, Hurteau, & Pomp, 1994; Perednia & Allen, 1995; Simon, 1993). Although the image may seem futuristic, the ability of telepresence is today a reality, albeit in a very primitive form. At the Joint Warrior Interoperability Demonstration, an annual U.S. military telecommunications and technology testing exercise, telepresence surgery was conducted by surgeons in one tent on a goat in another tent located approximately 60 feet away.

As technology becomes more reliable and advanced, the current limitations experienced by telenursing will be solved by telepresence. Currently, only nursing practice that does not involve touch can occur via telemedicine technology. With telepresence, the ability to touch patients, change dressings, do wound care, offer back rubs, soothe, and conduct therapeutic touch will be available to nurses. Emerging technologies include a palpation device, which would allow remote palpation of patients by a provider in another location (Burrows, M. J., personal communication, 1995).

It is thought that one of the severe technical limitations of telenursing currently is the inability to touch. Intuitively, nursing involves touch as a key element of the caring profession. However, data do not document the amount of touch that occurs in a given health care setting by nurses. In one study of Department of Defense beneficiaries, community health nurses at Wilford Hall Air Force Medical Center in San Antonio, Texas, identified patients with three or more hospital admissions in the prior year and began doing periodic home visits on discharge. The results of this 9-month study involving 37 patients who received a total of 138 home visits showed a decrease in hospital admission rate from 17% to 4% (Williams, Blue, & Langlois, 1993). Most important, this study characterized the nursing interventions that occurred during the home visits, including patient education, referral to clinic, medication refill, and patient and family support. It is interesting to note that not one documented patient intervention required touch by the nurse. This does not imply that nurses did not use touch during home visits; rather it was not required to accomplish interventions, according to the reported results.

The Wilford Hall Air Force Medical Center study suggests that frequent monitoring and support of chronically ill patients can affect their health care utilization. It also suggests that these outcomes may occur without the use of touch by nurses. The role of touch and the value of telepresence to an electronic home visit or to telenursing and telepractice is yet to be determined through research as telepresence technology continues to evolve.

The opinions expressed are those of the author(s) and do not reflect the official positions of the author's organizations and/or the Department of Defense.

LORETTA M. SCHLACHTA
SUSAN M. SPARKS

See also
TELEHEALTH
TELENURSING/TELEPRACTICE
VIRTUAL REALITY

TERMINAL ILLNESS

A terminal illness is defined as one in which a patient's remaining life is judged to be limited. The last phase of such an illness is the phase that eventuates in death. Usually, conventional therapies have been unsuccessful in effecting a cure, and care is directed toward the palliation of symptoms. Terminal illness implies that there has been an onset and a termination with various phases in between. It also suggests a history of chronicity. Thus, a death resulting from an acute insult to the body's functioning in which death ensues within hours or days thereafter would not be construed as having been the outcome of a terminal illness.

Florence Wald engaged in pioneering work in this area. Wald was dean of the School of Nursing in 1963 when Dame Cicely Saunders first came to Yale's School of Medicine to explore care of the dying in the United States. A series of visits by Dr. Saunders, the founder of St. Christopher's Hospice in London, culminated in a study of the care of the dying in New Haven by Wald and her colleagues, which resulted in the development of what is now the Connecticut Hospice (Wald, 1994).

The research undertaken by Wald investigated the adequacy and efficacy of the care of the dying. Other investigators have continued to explore this topic by contrasting settings for care as well as the comparative effectiveness of different approaches to symptom control. Although there continues to be a major concern with pain control, other troublesome symptoms such as anorexia, pressure ulcers, delirium, and dyspnea also have been studied. Much of this research has taken place in the setting of cancer care.

The experience of dying and the fact of death as a field of scholarly inquiry was stimulated by the work of Herman Feifel with the publication of his book *The Meaning of Death* in 1959. Feifel's endeavors and those of Robert Fulton in sociology, Elizabeth Kubler Ross in psychiatry, Robert Kastenbaum in psychology, Jean Quint Benoliel in nursing, and a small coterie of colleagues resulted in a renewed interest in the field and subsequently an increase in research. A number of the initial studies in the field of terminal illness concerned the attitudes of providers toward caring for the dying. This is not entirely surprising given the fact that nurses' attitudes in general were a subject for investigation at the time.

In one of the first studies conducted by a nurse researcher in terminal illness, Jan Folta (1965) found that staff nurses showed higher levels of anxiety about caring for dying patients than did nurses in other positions. This continues to be a subject of interest to researchers and clinicians, but the emphasis has shifted to questions of the prevention of burnout and more recently spirituality. There also has been a recent surge of studies about the knowledge and attitudes of health care providers toward the care of those infected with the human immunodeficiency virus (HIV).

The study of terminal illness in the hospital has been an important part of the life work of Anselm Strauss. His emphasis was on the staff and the manner in which they handled dying patients. Strauss, with his colleague Barney Glaser, found that health care providers have to answer questions regarding certainty and the time of death for every terminally ill person (Glaser & Strauss, 1965, 1968). Another important contribution has been the work on trajectory, which schematically depicts the path and shape of a chronic illness with its disease-specific perturbations, culminating in a terminal phase (Corbin & Strauss, 1991). By way of contrast, Benita Martocchio (1980) introduced a categorical approach to defining the health-illness course of patients, with such distinctions as well, acutely ill, chronically ill, high risk of dying, dying, and dead.

Another early researcher in the field of terminal illness, Jeanne Quint Benoliel (1994) joined Glaser and Strauss as an associate after her prior studies on women who had mastectomies. She contributed to their work (cited above), which she described as being concerned with

> the influence of cultural values and social context characteristics on (1) what patients were or were not told about their situation, (2) different patterns of dying associated with different diseases, and (3) the education of student nurses for work involving death and dying patients. (Benoliel, 1994, p. 6; see also Quint, 1967)

Benoliel and her students continued their interest in death education for student nurses and also developed a transition service that would allow terminally ill persons to die at home. The transition service provided the clinical base for further research.

Ida Martinson also was concerned with allowing individuals to die at home, but the subjects for her investigation were children. The impact of children dying at home on the children themselves, their parents, and in more recent studies, on their siblings has opened the door for the home care of dying children (Martinson et al., 1978).

The focus of research on the adult terminally ill has broadened to include studies of their family caregivers and the support required by these individuals. A number of studies have explored the congruence of expectations and perceptions between the terminally ill and either the professional or the family caregiver, as well as the needs of the terminally ill and their satisfaction with care and quality of life.

Research on the terminally ill person with acquired immunodeficiency syndrome (AIDS) has examined the needs of those dying from this disease, their partners, and family members. Although there have been papers on multiple loss, the literature on living and dying as a result of AIDS has not sufficiently exposed the experience of terminal illness in the context of an epidemic, as contrasted with dying of a disease without the public attention given to HIV/AIDS. Further research also is needed on the dying family, that is, the family where two or more generations are infected or where all of the siblings are infected.

Other areas requiring investigation include the impact of managed care on the care of the terminally ill; the manner in which care of the terminally ill will be affected by the presence or absence of health care provider–assisted suicide; and the nature of terminal illness care in an aging society. If the research on symptom control leads to the desired improvements in care, then future researchers will find that the terminally ill are able to live and die well.

INGE B. CORLESS

See also
CAREGIVER
CHRONIC ILLNESS
DECISION MAKING ABOUT END-OF-LIFE CHOICES
HIV/AIDS: CARE AND TREATMENT
HOSPICE

THEORETICAL FRAMEWORK

A theoretical framework is a group of statements composed of concepts related in some way to form an overall view of a phenomenon. As constructions of our mind, theoretical frameworks provide explanations about our experiences of phenomena in the world. The explanations provided by theoretical frameworks are of two types: descriptive (understanding the interaction among a set of variables) or prescriptive (anticipating a particular set of outcomes) (Dubin, 1978). The term *theoretical framework* often is used interchangeably with the terms *theory*, *theoretical model*, and *theoretical system*. Conceptual frameworks and conceptual models are related to but different from theoretical frameworks in that conceptual frameworks and models are more abstract and more comprehensive than theoretical frameworks and usually are not able to be tested empirically (Fawcett, 1995).

Theoretical frameworks consist of the following components: (a) concepts that are identified and defined, (b) assumptions that clarify the basic underlying truths from which and within which theoretical reasoning proceeds, (c) the context within which the theory is placed, and (d) relationships between and among the concepts that are identified (Chinn & Kramer, 1995). Theoretical frameworks serve as guides for practitioners and researchers in that they organize existing knowledge and aid in making new discoveries to advance nursing practice.

It is important to distinguish an empirical system from a theoretical one. An empirical system is what we apprehend, through senses, in the environment. A theoretical system is what we construct in our mind's eye to model the empirical system (Dubin, 1978). The scientist focuses on making the empirical world and the theoretical world (represented by theoretical frameworks) as congruent as possible. Linkages between the theoretical world and the empirical world to which it applies are made through the formulation and testing of hypotheses. As long as the abstraction of the theoretical framework can be represented with empirical indicators, hypotheses can be generated and empirically tested (Chinn & Kramer, 1995). Theoretical frameworks are developed and tested through theory-linked research (Chinn & Kramer, 1995). Theory-generating research is designed to discover and describe concepts and relationships for the construction of theory. Once theory is constructed, theory-testing research is used to validate how accurately the theory depicts empirical phenomena and their relationships.

Generation of theoretical frameworks in nursing has followed an evolutionary process. Initially, nursing grappled with defining theory for a developing discipline. In the 1960s and 1970s early nurse theorists attempted to answer questions such as:

1. Around what phenomena do nurses develop theory?
2. What are the things nurses think about and take action on?
3. What are the boundaries of the discipline?

In response to these questions, a proliferation of conceptual models and philosophies of practice of nursing were developed. These nursing conceptual models are considered at the grand theory level, examples of which are the theories of Johnson, Roy, Neuman, Rogers, and Watson.

The discipline also addressed the question of how to develop theory for nursing and proposed definitions emphasizing the structure, purpose, and use of theory. Nurse scientists and theorists debated methods of developing theory, including reformulation of borrowed theories and development of unique nursing theories based on quantitative and qualitative research. These discussions have led to the acceptance of multiple approaches to theory development in nursing (Walker & Avant, 1995), including both inductive and deductive methods. Recent attention has focused on the need to develop knowledge about the substance of nursing. In response to this call, theoretical frameworks that address specific nursing phenomena and that focus on the clinical processes in nursing are being developed. This knowledge is referred to as middle- and micro-range theory.

The notion of different levels of theory has been a useful to way to develop knowledge in nursing. Each level of theory has characteristics and purposes that are specific to that level. The scope or breadth of the concepts and goals of a theoretical framework determine its usefulness for research and practice. As the goal of a theory narrows in scope, it moves from grand to middle range to micro range. Grand theories provide global perspectives of the discipline and offer ways of looking at nursing phenomena based on these perspectives. However, because of the broad scope and abstract concepts of grand theories, they are not testable and therefore are limited in their usefulness to researchers.

Unlike grand theories, the scope of middle-range theories is not as broad as the full range of phenomena of concern to the discipline but involves more concepts than micro-range theories. Middle-range theories are sufficiently abstract to generalize yet specific enough to be empirically tested. In contrast to grand theories, middle-range theories contain concepts close to observed data, from which hypotheses may be logically derived and empirical tested. Examples of middle-range theoretical frameworks are Mishel's theory of uncertainty in illness, Pender's theory of health promotion, and Lenz and colleagues' theory of unpleasant symptoms.

Micro-range theory (also called practice theory) is more specific than middle-range theory and refers to precise goals and actions to achieve goals in a particular nursing practice situation. Examples of micro-range theories are those addressing catheter care and care of decubitus ulcers (Fitzpatrick & Whall, 1996). Although micro-range theory offers specific guidelines for practitioners, it is often situation-specific and thus limited in generalizability. It is generally agreed that the development of theoretical frameworks at all three levels—grand, middle range, and micro range—are needed and will enhance the knowledge base of nursing.

The process of developing theoretical frameworks that inform nursing practice and drive nursing research is ongoing. Several challenges prevail in the development of nursing theoretical frameworks. One challenge is how to integrate related theoretical frameworks that have arisen from the multiple ways of developing knowledge in nursing. For example, how does the theory about stages of behavior change, developed from grounded theory methods, relate to theories of self-efficacy for health behaviors that were developed using empirical methods? Additionally, what mechanisms are needed to enhance communication between practitioners and researchers about the knowledge produced by both using divergent methods? Also, how do different levels of theory relate to each other? How can one level of theory be used to develop related theories at another level? Another challenge

is the need to build programs of research that are substantially large enough to accrue sufficient knowledge around a particular set of phenomena. Such programs of research will require greater use of collaborative approaches to knowledge development than those previously used within the discipline. The efficient development of nursing theoretical frameworks will require extensive collaboration among institutions, disciplines, researchers, and practitioners.

SHIRLEY M. MOORE

See also
EPISTEMOLOGY
MIDDLE-RANGE THEORY
NURSING THEORETICAL MODELS
SCIENTIFIC DEVELOPMENT

THERMAL BALANCE

Definitions

Thermal balance is defined as a thermal steady state in which the loss of body heat is equal to the heat gain. In health this balance produces a thermoneutral state, optimal for cellular function. In humans this state averages about $37°C \pm 0.05$ for internal temperatures and $33.5°C \pm 0.05$ for skin. Hypothalamic thermoregulatory controls keep internal temperatures fairly stable despite environmental changes and the propensity of heat to escape to cooler regions. Metabolic and physical activity continually generate heat while it is constantly lost to the cooler environment. Current theory is that elaborate thermoregulatory control systems maintain temperatures within the optimal "set point" range. Compensatory cooling or warming mechanisms respond to deviations above or below this range. Temperatures rising above this range evoke vasodilation and sweating, whereas falling temperatures cause vasoconstriction, shivering, and increased metabolic activity.

Each physiological response augments or inhibits the transfer of heat by affecting the thermodynamics of conduction, convection, radiation, and evaporation. Vasodilation warms the skin, where heat is more easily lost to air, contact surfaces, or liquids. Vasoconstriction creates a poorly perfused insulative layer of tissue that conserves heat. In infants cold exposure causes metabolic breakdown of brown fat to generate heat. In older children and adults, the primary means of heat generation is shivering.

Relevance to Nursing

Nursing has recognized the importance of assessing thermal balance as a vital health indicator for as long as the profession has existed. Body temperature provides an important vital sign of metabolic, neurological, and infectious activity. Circadian rhythms, monthly cycles, and daily body temperature ranges are assurances of healthy variations. The pregnant mother provides heat exchange both for herself and the fetus; therefore, high maternal body temperatures from fever, hyperthermia, or prolonged ''hot tub'' use puts the unborn infant at risk for neurological damage.

Temperature elevations in the acutely ill and injured may indicate either fever or hyperthermia. Each has its own dynamics and treatment. Thermoregulatory control remains intact during fever, and cell mediators usually limit excessively high temperature elevations. Thermoregulatory control is lost during hyperthermia and requires aggressive cooling treatment. If temperatures rise above 42°C, irreversible neural cellular damage is likely. Conductive cooling blankets, ice packs, and cooling fans are used to lower core temperatures. In immunosuppression associated with cancer treatment, fevers may indicate fulminating systemic infection. However, the immunosuppressed HIV-infected patient may become febrile from high cytokine levels, without obvious secondary infection. In both groups, constant assessment of other indicators is necessary to rule out infection.

Situations that promote heat loss or interfere with heat generation place certain patients at risk for hypothermia. The neonatal nurse must be extremely sensitive to the low-birthweight infant's need for external heat source. Unable to shiver, the neonate expends oxygen to metabolize brown fat and can easily become hypoxic from cold exposure. Declining metabolic and vasomotor activity makes elders particularly susceptible to heat loss during surgery, trauma, or outdoor exposure. Hypothermic states can destabilize thermoregulatory function further, leading eventually to death.

Historical Perspective

Fever patterns have been used to detect the onset and progress of infections since early times (see Fever/Febrile Response). It was recognized that high temperatures could lead to brain damage, so nurses routinely cooled patients with fever or heat stroke with ice packs, cooling sponge baths, or circulating fans. In the 1970s, nurses used conductive cooling blankets with refrigerated circulating coolant to treat refractory hyperthermia. Sharp gradients between skin and core temperatures stimulated vigorous and distressful shivering. Interventions to prevent shivering were among the earliest to be tested by nurses (see Shivering).

Interest in and awareness of temperature variations became more acute among nurse researchers when advanced technology in thermometry was introduced to clinical settings. In the 1970s thermistor probes in hemodynamic monitoring systems made pulmonary artery temperatures possible in some critical care settings. As probes became available for bladder, tympanic membrane, and skin temperatures, studies of gradients between body regions and measurement sites were common. Variation in quality and precision of instruments made studies of reliability and accuracy important. Recognition of malignant hyperthermia, a rare but lethal, genetically linked disorder occurring when susceptible persons receive anesthetic agents, led to closer surveillance of perioperative body temperature. The precaution not only reduced mortality from hyperthermia in this uncommon condition, it brought to awareness the high incidence of low body temperatures in most surgical patients. Increased survival of preterm infants in the 1970s created increased concern for thermal balance of vulnerable infants. Studies of environmental influences, warming devices, and skin-to-skin contact were made possible by sophisticated continuous skin temperature monitors.

Major Studies

Measurement issues dominate nursing research related to thermal balance. Research in body temperature measurement by Erickson (1980; Erickson & Yount, 1991) compared oral, rectal, and tympanic membrane measurement sites in children and adults. Findings reassured nurses that oral measurement provided reliable intermittent thermal assessment in afebrile patients. Placement site and method of insertion yield statistically significant differences, but they are of less importance clinically. Erickson's work differs from many contemporary studies in its appropriate statistical treatment beyond simple correlations and its meaningful interpretation of device reliability, accuracy, and linearity. In the past decade nurse researchers began drawing inferences from observed relationships between thermal changes and other variables. Earp and Finlayson (1991) observed gradients between bladder and pulmonary artery temperatures to establish baseline differences. These investigators later predicted shivering by observing bladder and pulmonary artery temperature ratios (see Shivering). Caruso et al. (Caruso, Hadley, Shukla, Frame, & Khoury, 1992) recognized the importance of thermal gradients in stimulating warming responses and distress in a comparison of cooling blanket temperatures.

Nursing research also has tested methods to alleviate adverse effects of warming and cooling in patients of all ages. Particularly vulnerable are the preterm infant, the elderly, and patients recovering from surgery, cardiopulmonary bypass, or traumatic injury. Anderson (1991a) and colleagues drew from perinatal practices of Western Europe to test skin-to-skin care for preterm infants. Thermal balance was maintained when infants were held "kangaroo" style under the mother or father's clothing. Self-demand breast feeding and lactation was promoted by close constant maternal contact. Henker's dissertation work compared two patterns of cooling on human responses in young adults; in a more recent study he compared methods of warming intravenous fluids (Henker, Bernardo, O'Connor, & Sereika, 1995). Numerous small studies in nursing have tested various products that prevent or restore heat loss in perioperative patients, but they are often empirical in nature. By contrast, the investigations mentioned above are theoretically based on principles of thermodynamics and physiological responses. They seek to explain mechanisms, predict consequences, and alleviate hazards of altered thermal balance.

Future Directions

New avenues for nursing research in thermal balance emerge with new situations of vulnerability and advances in measurement techniques. At particular risk is the rapidly growing population of the frail elderly. Declining metabolic rate, lower vasomotor sensitivity, and diminishing insulation from body fat make this group vulnerable to extremes of heat or cold. The existence and treatment of thermoregulatory failure in homebound patients is an area that nursing has not studied systematically. Improved survival of individuals with neurological, vasomotor, and endocrine impairments or extensive burns creates new situations where thermal balance is altered. Study and intervention are needed to address thermal balance, thermal perception, and thermal comfort during a variety of life events and health alterations.

BARBARA J. HOLTZCLAW

See also
FEVER/FEBRILE RESPONSE
HIV/AIDS: CARE AND TREATMENT
INFECTION CONTROL
NICU PRETERM INFANT CARE
SHIVERING

TIME SERIES ANALYSIS

Time series analysis and statistical time series models are basic to describing and studying change in human responses and behavior. They are appropriate to cyclical patterns as well as periodic or systematic variance across time. Many of the phenomena of interest to nursing are intimately related to time. Thus, time series statistical models are an appropriate and powerful methodology for longitudinal nursing studies of intraindividual differences in rate and patterns of change.

In contrast to inferential statistical models, where aggregate data are generalized to describe changes in human behavior, time series analysis uses individual patterns of change to predict future behavior. Thus, the subject is a unitary entity or system whose behavioral state can be isolated within a given point and measured through a specified window of time. For the purpose of time series analysis, the singular system can be defined at many different levels of complexity and inclusiveness. Examples of individual systems that are legitimate subjects for time series nursing research include cardiovascular response to a cardiac stressor, individuals, families, communities, health care systems, even political institutions.

The characteristic feature of time series analysis is that the phenomenon to be studied has a distinctive temporal component—the behavioral state will vary predictably with the passage of time. Obviously, the passage of time can not be manipulated, thus, differences in patterns of change are not a direct function of time. Time is not the independent variable; it is, instead, a necessary temporal frame or marker in any time series analysis study.

Time series studies can be either univariate or multivariate. However, a time series variable always consists, by definition, of a series of observations that occur in temporal order. Thus, multivariate time series analysis is accomplished by identifying the relationship between or among two or more pairs of univariate time series.

Unlike inferential statistical models, time series data points are not intended to be independent of one another. Each value is highly correlated with every successive value. Thus, any observation in a time series has significantly less individual predictive significance than its inferential counterpart. In time series analysis, predictive power is not a direct function of sample size. Instead, predictive power depends on an accurate hypothesis of the internal temporal structure of the phenomenon, selection of a sampling time window of sufficient length to capture multiple expressions of the change being studied, and identification of a sampling frequency that will adequately capture all critical phases of the evolving pattern.

Although change in behavior is an essential characteristic of many of the phenomena of interest to nursing science (Metzger & Schultz, 1982), the use of statistical time series models is not always appropriate or feasible. However, although time series analyses are complex and costly, they permit nurse scientists to more completely examine and evaluate trends, cycles, and patterns of change that are framed within predictable spaces of time.

BONNIE L. METZGER

See also
DATA ANALYSIS
EPIDEMIOLOGY
STATISTICAL TECHNIQUES

TRANSITIONAL CARE

Definition

Transitional care refers to care and services required in the safe and timely transfer of patients from one level of care to another or from one type of health care setting to another (Brooten, 1993). Transitional environments include the hospital, home, nursing home, rehabilitation center, and hospice. Some authors differentiate subacute care from transitional care; others use the terms interchangeably. Those who make the distinction view subacute care as a unit or component of inpatient care in an acute care facility, skilled nursing facility, or free-standing medical or rehabilitation center. Transitional care ideally ends with normal functioning and recovery, functional independence, or stabilization of the patient's condition (Brooten, 1993). In the case of many frail children or adults, transitional services end in long-term care.

Key features of transitional care include comprehensive discharge planning from one site of care to another, coordination of postdischarge services, provision of in-home services on a short-term basis, and continued health care follow-up. The most important components of transitional care services are continuity of care across sites of care, communication of the plan of care among the differing providers, and matching patient needs and knowledge with skills of the care providers (Brooten, 1993).

Trends and Issues

Transitional care services have increased significantly over the past 10 to 15 years in response to changes in health care delivery, especially earlier hospital discharge of patients. Home care agencies, for example, have increased from approximately 1,100 in 1963 to 17,561 in 1995 (National Association for Home Care, 1995).

Research issues in transitional care include determining the nature and needed length of the service, risk profiles of patients who need the service, type and level of providers needed, and cost-effectiveness of the service compared to alternative services. The length of transitional services should vary with the specific needs of the patients or group of patients rather than being dictated by the reimbursement plan. However, data are not available demonstrating the most effective and cost-efficient endpoint for services to achieve optimal patient outcomes in specific patient groups or subgroups.

It is generally agreed that vulnerable groups such as the elderly, the technologically dependent, the disabled, and some high-risk infants and children should receive transitional services. Decisions regarding which patients should receive these services are currently based on the patient's functional ability, available caretakers at home, ethnicity, age, previous hospitalization, and technology dependence.

Currently, there is wide variation in the type and level of transitional care provider, and there is disagreement about who should provide the care (Kornowski et al., 1995). The work of Brooten (Brooten, Kumar, Brown, et al., 1986; Brooten, Naylor, York et al., 1995; Brooten, Roncoli, Finkler et al., 1994), Naylor (Naylor, Brooten, Jones et al., 1994) and others using master's degreed–prepared advanced practice nurses (APNs) to provide transitional care for high-risk groups have consistently demonstrated improved patient outcomes with reduced health care costs for the patient groups followed. Use of a master's degree–prepared nurse assumes that the nurse has advanced knowledge and skill in the care of the specific patient groups

followed, an assumption that cannot be made of a nurse generalist. APNs with advanced knowledge and skills can function under general protocols, they require less direct supervision, and in nonadministrative roles they have annual salaries approximately $5,500 higher than that of a registered nurse (American Nurses Association, 1994b). Whether APNs are needed for transitional services to all patient groups has not yet been tested. Home care provided by professional nurses (RNs) has been reported to decrease the negative psychosocial impact on parents caring for medically fragile children at home. Improved patient outcomes using home care provided by RNs also has been reported with ventilator-dependent children, with oncology patients, and with elders.

Data also are needed on the cost-effectiveness of transitional care compared to alternative approaches to care. Although the direct costs for transitional care have been calculated in some studies, costs such as prevention of rehospitalization, acute care visits, decreased employment, and burden on family caregivers are less well documented. These data are important in examining the overall cost benefit or cost-effectiveness of transitional services.

Models of Transitional Care Services

Transitional care services are provided through public agencies; private, not-for-profit agencies; free-standing and privately operated proprietary agencies; free-standing and operated for profit, hospital-based agencies; and dedicated units or departments operated by a hospital. Transitional services are provided by community nursing services, hospital home care services, health maintenance organization (HMO) follow-up services, and subacute care units established within hospitals or skilled nursing facilities or as free-standing subacute care hospitals.

Community or public health nurses have historically provided home follow-up to high-risk patients with complex health needs. Their services are well known and accepted by the general public and health care providers. Unfortunately, over the past 10 to 15 years, budget reductions for community nursing services have virtually eliminated home follow-up services to many patient groups. Current challenges for community nursing services include updating the specialty knowledge and skills of agency nurses with a generalist preparation, maintaining continuity of patient care from the hospital to the home, providing sufficient services to maintain continuity of patient care from the hospital to the home, and providing sufficient services to maintain good patient outcomes as insurers reimburse for fewer services.

As reimbursed length of stay for even high-risk patients decreases, the hospitals' need for improved discharge planning and postdischarge home care services for these groups increases. Documented discharge planning is mandatory for hospitals, and many have hired discharge planners to facilitate earlier discharge. Some hospitals contract with community nursing services or independent home care agencies to provide home care services for their high-risk patients. An increasing number of hospitals are establishing their own home care services.

HMOs have a clear financial incentive for discharging patients early and for preventing costly rehospitalizations. They have used case managers and nurses with specialty knowledge and skills to review patients' discharge and home care needs. Because realizing a profit is essential in the for-profit HMOs, their approach has been one of minimal hospital length of stay and postdischarge services. Home follow-up services vary in number of visits provided, type of nurse provider (nurse generalist or specialist), and length of follow-up. More than the routine allowable for home visits may be reimbursable for a patient, but this must be negotiated between provider and insurer.

Gaps and Recommendations

Research is needed to determine: the nature, intensity, and length of transitional services required to optimize patient and family outcomes; the profile of patients who would benefit most from these services; the type and level of providers needed to deliver these services; and the costs of such services. Continued study of existing and emerging models of transitional care also is necessary to determine which of these models achieves the highest quality and most cost-effective outcomes.

Study findings suggest that, for selected patient groups or subgroups, discharge planning and home care protocols designed to meet their unique needs are more effective than the general protocols designed for all patients that is currently used by many hospitals and home care agencies. Targeted protocols should be derived from empirical data regarding the unique needs of specific patient groups and their caregivers after hospital discharge. Transitional care protocols should be based on an empirical understanding of the nature of the patients' and caregivers' needs (e.g., lack of knowledge, complexity of therapeutic regimen), strengths (e.g., supportive family) or barriers (e.g., language) to meeting needs, timing of needs (e.g., 24 hours after discharge), most cost-effective strategy to meet needs (e.g., telephone contact vs. home visit), and length of follow-up needed. Unfortunately, for many patient groups, this research base is limited. For these patient groups, research efforts should be targeted first at identifying patients' and caregivers' needs and subsequently at the design and testing of interventions to meet their unique needs.

There is a need for studies that compare and contrast existing and emerging models of transitional care, focusing on differences in both processes and outcomes of care. Knowledge generated from studies of these models would contribute to the ongoing discussion and debate about which providers are most effective and efficient in coordinating transitional care services and providing continuity of care for patients and their caregivers. Study findings also would advance our understanding about effective ways to engage a multidisciplinary team of providers in transitional services. Finally, the knowledge generated from this research would determine the processes of care that available data suggest are important to positive patient outcomes: assessing, communicating, clinical decision making, teaching, collaborating, referring, monitoring, and evaluating.

DOROTHY BROOTEN
MARY DUFFIN NAYLOR

See also
**HEALTH MAINTENANCE ORGANIZA-
TIONS
HEALTH SYSTEMS DELIVERY**

HOME HEALTH SYSTEMS
MANAGED CARE
VULNERABLE POPULATIONS

TRANSITIONS AND HEALTH

Nurses provide care to patients and families who are experiencing many kinds of transitions. Developmental transitions (pregnancy, birth, parenthood), situational transitions (immigration, widowhood, relocation), and health/illness transitions (diagnosis of a chronic disease, recovery from surgery, rehabilitation) are examples of the many types of transitions encountered in clinical practice. Transitions also occur in the work setting of nurses and can be classified as organizational transitions. Examples include changes in leadership, new staffing patterns, implementation of new models for nursing care, and structural reorganization. A focus on transitions is so central to nursing practice that it has been argued that the mission of nursing is to facilitate transitions (Meleis & Trangenstein, 1994).

Transition is defined as a passage between two relatively stable periods of time. In this passage the individual moves from one life phase, situation, or status to another (Chick & Meleis, 1986; Schumacher, Jones, & Meleis, in press). Transitions often are conceptualized in terms of stages in order to capture their movement and direction as they evolve over time. A classic description of transition stages is found in Bridge's (1991) work. He identified three stages: (a) a period of ending or disconnectedness from what had been before, (b) a neutral period characterized by a sense of disruption and disorientation as well as discovery, and (c) a period of new beginnings in which the individual finds new meanings and a sense of control and challenge. Transitions also can be conceptualized in terms of critical points. Critical points are turning points that can lead to either healthy or unhealthy outcomes. The identification of stages, critical points, and strategies for coping during the transition experience provides the basis for nursing therapeutics to support healthy transitions processes and outcomes and to prevent unhealthy transitions.

When using a transition framework in clinical practice or research, several universal properties of transitions must be taken into account. First, transitions are precipitated by significant marker events or turning points that require new patterns of response. These markers prompt the recognition that new strategies are needed to handle familiar daily life experiences. Second, transitions are processes that occur over time. Transition processes encompass the period of time from the first anticipation of a transition until a new identity is formed at the completion of the transition. During this process the context, history, and future of the person are important. A sense of disconnectedness from one's familiar world is another universal property of transition. There is often a sense of loss or alienation from what had been familiar and valued. Another property is that transitions involve fundamental changes in one's view of oneself and the world. During transitions, changes in identity, roles, and patterns of behavior occur. New skills, new relationships, and new coping strategies must be developed (Schumacher, Jones, & Meleis, in press).

Persons in transition experience a wide range of responses. They may experience losses or gains, suffer from physical debilitation, have lower or higher immune responses, feel an emergence or loss of spirituality, discover new meanings, or experience traumatic stress symptoms. Indicators of a healthy transition include a sense of well-being, the development of a new identity, mastery of new roles, well-being in relationships, harmony with the environment, renewed energy, and positive quality of life. Indicators of unhealthy transitions may be protracted transitional periods or the continuation of responses, such as role insufficiency or isolation, during the transition period. Previous life patterns may be maintained that are incongruent with the demand for new identities and life patterns (Chick & Meleis, 1986; Schumacher & Meleis, 1994).

Goals for knowledge development about transitions include increased understanding of the following: (a) the processes and experiences of human beings who are in transition; (b) the nature of life patterns and new identities that emerge during transitions; (c) the processes or conditions that promote healthy transition outcomes; (d) environments that constrain, support, or promote healthy transitions; and (e) the structure and components of nursing therapeutics that deal with transitions (Meleis, 1993). Numerous theories of family, ecology, problem solving, and self-care can be used to facilitate such knowledge development.

Research has begun to contribute to development of knowledge about transitions. Transition frameworks have been used in research to uncover the experiences of persons living with chronic illness, new mothers, patients recovering from surgery, and persons taking on the caregiving role. Nursing therapeutics tested in research include debriefing, transition services, and role supplementation. Further research is needed to identify the types and dimensions of transitions and the consequences of transition for individuals, families, and communities. Because transitions are processes, appropriate research methods include qualitative and longitudinal approaches.

As a discipline, nursing is concerned with the process and the experiences of human beings undergoing transitions where health and perceived well-being are the outcomes (Meleis & Trangenstein, 1994). The concept of transition was developed as a framework particularly appropriate for viewing nursing phenomena from the perspective of a human science and a practice-oriented discipline. A transition framework provides a way of understanding human responses to events that affect growth and development, health, and person/environment interaction. A transition framework also provides a focus for understanding the content and timing of nursing interventions. From a transition perspective, both the timing and the duration of nursing interventions are of utmost importance. Further, a transition perspective is focused on clients and nurses as dynamic, changing beings evolving within the context of an environment that may be healthy or unhealthy. During the process of transition, clients experience losses and gains. They need new skills to develop new lifestyles or modify lifestyles, prevent illness or live with illness, and enhance or maintain well-being. Nurses and nurses' actions are instrumental in the process of developing these skills.

In summary, the use of transition as a framework facilitates the development of knowledge related to changes in persons, health, and environment. Within this framework, scholarship should focus on uncovering and explaining patterns of responses and critical points in transitions that require nursing interventions.

AFAF IBRAHIM MELEIS
KAREN L. SCHUMACHER

See also
CHRONIC ILLNESS
COPING
IMMIGRANT WOMEN
**ROLE SUPPLEMENTATION: A NURS-
 ING THERAPEUTIC**
TRANSITIONAL CARE

TRIANGULATION

Triangulation, as it is most commonly used in nursing research, refers to the combination of qualitative and quantitative research methods within a single study. There are a number of approaches to triangulation, and it can serve a number of purposes. According to Duffy (1987), triangulation is "the use of multiple methods, theories, data and/or investigators in the study of a common phenomenon" (p. 130). The term *triangulation* has its roots in surveying and navigation and describes the idea of using known points and angles in a triangular fashion to locate an unknown point. Campbell and Fiske (1959) are credited as the first to apply this approach in their use of the multitrait-multimethod matrix to establish convergent validity.

Types of Triangulation

Denzin (1989) identified four different approaches to triangulation: methodological, data, theoretical, and investigator. Methodological triangulation, currently the most commonly used triangulation approach in nursing research, involves the use of two or more different methods within a single study. Denzin points out that this approach can involve within-method or between-method triangulation. Mitchell (1986) emphasized the need for complementarity in the methods used with this approach. Within-method triangulation refers to the use of several different instruments to measure a construct, for example, the use of the Peabody Picture Vocabulary Test—Revised (PPVT-R) as well as the Kaufman Assessment Battery for Children (KABC) to measure different dimensions of child development. Between-method (also known as across-method) triangulation refers to the use of more than one research method to study a phenomenon, for example, the use of a qualitative approach such as phenomenology in concert with a quantitative approach such as a descriptive survey. Between-method triangulation can be accomplished simultaneously or sequentially.

A second type of triangulation, theoretical triangulation, involves analysis of data using several related yet perhaps contradictory theories or hypotheses. The hypothesis supported by the data can be strongly supported because other theories and hypotheses have been discounted (Mitchell, 1986). This type of triangulation can be utilized within a quantitative or a qualitative methodology; it seeks to avoid a narrow, specialized interpretation of the data (Denzin, 1989). Denzin described this approach, explaining that theoretical triangulation encourages an awareness of the multiple ways data can be interpreted.

A third type, data triangulation, involves data collected from different sources, for example, different time points, different types or groups of people, or different locations. In Mitchell's (1986) study of food cravings, data were collected from women at many time points throughout the day, throughout a woman's menstrual cycle, and throughout the seasons of the year. The study was designed to uncover more about the dimensions of food cravings. A fourth type of triangulation is investigator triangulation. Denzin (1989) suggested that the use of more than one data collector helps to ensure the reliability of the data and the uses of multiple analysts to interpret the data guards against the risk of bias associated with only one point of view. Mitchell (1986) added a fifth variety of triangulation, multiple triangulation, or the combining of two or more types of triangulation, for example, the use of methodological, data, and investigator triangulation within a single study.

Goals of Triangulation

Originally, triangulation was carried out mainly for purposes of confirmation. Confirmation is analogous to convergent validity and refers to the idea that through the use of multiple methods, data sources, or investigators, a single, obvious conclusion or representation of reality can be researched. Recently, triangulation has been conducted to achieve completeness. Breitmayer, Ayres, and Knafl (1993) posited that this approach can illuminate many of the individual facets of a multidimensional construct. These researchers used qualitative and quantitative methods as they sought both confirmation and completeness in their study of families with a critically ill child. However, not all scholars agree with the notion of triangulation for completeness. Sandelowski (1995) acknowledged the use of triangulation for purposes of convergent validity or confirmation but stressed that completeness is unreachable because "no vision of a phenomenon is ever complete" (p. 573).

Limitations of Triangulation

Mitchell (1986) identified a number of concerns with multiple triangulation that also apply to other triangulation approaches. First, Mitchell noted that a common unit of analysis is essential in any form of triangulation. Second, some forms of triangulation, especially data and investigator triangulation, can be especially costly in terms of time and money. In addition, triangulation places special demands on the investigator because combining methods requires, as Mitchell noted, "a broad knowledge base in research methodology including both qualitative and quantitative methods" (p. 24). Perhaps the greatest challenge of triangulation, however, is found in the area of analysis. Mitchell noted that analysis in a triangulated study presents special challenges, such as the difficulties of combining numerical and textual data. Problems can also arise in interpreting divergent results from these types of data and in weighing data collected from different sources and from different methods.

In spite of these challenges, triangulation of method, data, theories, or investigators can be an important tool in developing nursing science. The concepts of interest to nursing are generally complex, multidimensional human constructs and are difficult to examine by means of a singular research approach. Triangulation is a means to a deeper understanding of these constructs.

THERESA STANDING

See also
DATA ANALYSIS
DATA COLLECTION METHODS
QUALITATIVE RESEARCH
QUANTITATIVE RESEARCH

U

UNIFIED LANGUAGE SYSTEMS

A unified language system is a network of linked terms that allows integration of existing sets of machine-readable terms, such as thesauri, classification systems, and nomenclatures for the purposes of information retrieval. Whereas a *uniform* language system would necessitate that a common set of terms is utilized for multiple purposes, a *unified* language system builds on the strengths of existing systems that have been designed from a variety of perspectives and for a broad range of purposes (McCormick et al., 1994). The primary unified language systems of relevance to nursing are the Unified Medical Language System (UMLS) (Lindberg, Humphreys, & McCray, 1993) and the Unified Nursing Language System (UNLS) (McCormick et al., 1994).

In 1986 the National Library of Medicine began a long-term research and development project to build the UMLS, utilizing the strategy of successive approximations of the capabilities ultimately desired. The UMLS currently comprises four knowledge sources: the *Metathesaurus*, the *Semantic Network*, the *SPECIALIST Lexicon*, and the *Information Sources Map*. All sources are available via the Internet through the Knowledge Source Server (McCray, Razi, Bangalore, Browne, & Stavri, 1996).

The *Metathesaurus* is a database of information on concepts that appear in at least one of a set of controlled source vocabularies. Thirty source vocabularies provide the 252,892 concepts and 542,723 concept names in the 1996 *Metathesaurus* (http://wwwlst.nlm.nih.gov:8000/Docs). These include Medical Subject Headings (MeSH), *International Classification of Diseases: Clinical Modification*, and SNOMED International. Four systems specifically designed for use by nurses are source vocabularies in the Metathesaurus: the North American Nursing Diagnosis Association (NANDA) *Taxonomy 1*, the *Omaha System*, the *Georgetown Home Health Care Classification*, and the *Nursing Interventions Classification* (NIC). The *Metathesaurus* is organized by concept, with entries connecting alternative names for the same concept (e.g., synonyms, lexical variants, translations) from different vocabularies. Thus, shortness of breath, breathlessness, and dyspnea share a common concept identifier but different lexical identifiers in the *Metathesaurus*.

The UMLS *Semantic Network* provides a consistent categorization of concepts represented in the *Metathesaurus* and a set of relationships between the concepts. The 1996 version includes 135 semantic types (http://wwwlst.nlm.nih.gov:8000/Docs). Concepts are broadly categorized into the semantic types of entity or event. Examples of semantic types of relevance to nursing are "Finding," "Individual Behavior," "Therapeutic or Preventive Procedure," and "Disease or Syndrome." The primary relationship among concepts is "IS__A," for example, "Pain Management IS__A Therapeutic or Preventive Procedure." Other relationships include temporal—for example, "Diabetes Mellitus PRECEDES Diabetic Retinopathy"—and causal, for example, "CMV Retinitis is CAUSED__BY cytomegalovirus."

The *SPECIALIST Lexicon* comprises a set of commonly used English and biomedical terms. Entries include the base form of the term and its lexical variants, for example, *assess*, *assesses*, and *assessed*. The *Information Sources Map* describes the publicly available databases of the National Library of Medicine and selected expert systems and databases from outside the National Library of Medicine.

TABLE 1 Elements of NMDS in Systems Comprising the Current UNLS

System	Diagnosis	Intervention	Outcome
NANDA	x		
Omaha	x	x	x
Georgetown	x	x	x
NIC		x	

Several studies have examined the ability of the *Metathesaurus* terms to capture nursing concepts. Zielstorff, Cimino, Barnett, Hassan, and Blewett (1993) demonstrated the lack of nursing terminology in Version 1.0 of the *Metathesaurus* and supported the inclusion of the four nursing vocabularies that are now part of the *Metathesaurus*. Lange (1996) examined the ability of the *Metathesaurus* to represent the everyday language of nurses used in intershift report. She found exact matches for 56% of the terms in the dataset. The matches comprised 59 semantic types and 24 source vocabularies. Through the sponsorship of the National Library of Medicine and the Agency for Health Care Policy and Research, a large-scale vocabulary test that utilized UMLS technology to determine the

extent to which existing controlled vocabularies covered the terminology required for health care and public health was undertaken in 1996 (Humphreys, Hole, McCray, & Fitzmaurice, 1996).

The American Nurses Association Steering Committee on Databases to Support Nursing Practice has endorsed the concept of a unified nursing language system within the structure of the UMLS (McCormick et al., 1994; McCormick & Zielstorff, 1995). The nursing care elements of the nursing minimum data set (NMDS) define the data elements of a UNLS: nursing diagnosis, nursing intervention, nursing outcome, and nursing care intensity (see Table 1). The current UNLS comprises the four nursing systems in the UMLS: NANDA *Taxonomy 1*, the *Omaha System*, the *Georgetown Home Health Care Classification*, and NIC. Extensive research is underway to enhance and refine the existing UNLS, for example, the *Nursing Intervention Lexicon and Taxonomy*, the *Patient Care Data Set*, the *Nursing Outcomes Classification*, and the *International Classification of Nursing Practice*.

Suzanne Bakken Henry

See also
HOME HEALTH CARE CLASSIFICATION
NANDA
NURSING MINIMUM DATA SET
OMAHA SYSTEM
SNOMED INTERNATIONAL

UNINTENTIONAL INJURY OF INFANTS

Definitions

Injuries are defined in two ways: (a) the physical damage to the body caused by the transfer of mechanical, chemical, or thermal energy (e.g., a broken bone, salicylate-related poisoning, or frostbite to a toe); and (b) as the event that caused the damage (e.g., motor vehicle crash, aspirin ingestion, or prolonged exposure to cold). When talking about unintentional injuries, it is still common to use the word *accident* as if unexpectedness or lack of intent were the primary feature of the injurious process. However, although the moment of occurrence of an injury may not be precisely known, its likelihood of occurring is usually predictable. If events are predictable, they are not called accidents; rather, the term *injury* is used.

It is crucial that those who study injury and collect injury data recognize that the term *injury* can refer both to the physical damage caused to the body and to the predictable causative event. In fact, the *International Classification of Disease* (ICD-9- or -10-CM) uses two separate systems to classify injuries. One is a set of physical damage codes (N-codes, e.g., humerus fracture); the other is a set of event codes (E-codes, or External Cause of Injury Codes, e.g., fall on stairs). Together these two systems of classification provide a fuller picture of an injury episode than does either alone (knowing that an infant fell on stairs is important; knowing that the fall resulted in head trauma provides a more complete description) (see Baker, O'Neill, Ginsburg, & Li, 1992, for a complete review).

Injury Data

Unintentional injuries are the principal cause of death in the United States for individuals from the newborn period, 29 days, to age 44 years. For infants in particular they represent the predominant cause of nonbirth-related death. Fatal injuries are usually recorded according to the events that cause them, such as the number of deaths from motor vehicle crashes or house fires; whereas nonfatal injuries usually have been reported by physical damage groups. This is because fatality data are derived from death certificates, which classify cause of death by circumstances and facilitate E-coding. Morbidity data generally are gathered from medical records and often are derived from N-coding.

National mortality data are routinely available from death certificate reviews. These vital statistics mortality data from 1994 show the principal causes of infant (under age 1 year) injury death as homicide, 7.92 deaths/100,000; suffocation and choking, 7.82 deaths/100,000; motor vehicle, 4.40 deaths/100,000; other, 5.63 deaths/100,000 (Centers for Disease Control, 1997).

National data are not routinely available regarding the incidence of and associated risk factors for nonfatal injuries in infants, which means that most morbidity data by type of injury event are generated only by special studies. Siegel and colleagues (Siegel et al., 1996), investigating the association between maternal age and other risk factors for infant deaths in the state of Colorado from 1986 to 1992, found that rates peaked at a maternal age of 22 years for unintentional infant injury deaths. Among the unintentional injury deaths, more mothers had inadequate education, higher proportion of low-birthweight infants, more siblings in the family, and a higher proportion of interpartum intervals of less than 2 years.

Data from studies by Jordan, Dugan, and Hardy (1993) and O'Sullivan and Schwarz (1997) documented the nonfatal injury rate specifically for infants (< 15 months) of adolescent mothers as 15.7 and 16.3 per 100 children, respectively. Falls and burns were the leading two causes of injury in both studies. Additional studies on injury rates for infants through age 18 months of life also documented falls, burns, and ingestions as the leading causes of nonfatal injuries, as shown by the work of O'Sullivan and Schwarz (1997) with infants of teenage mothers and Schwarz and co-workers (Schwarz, Grisso, Holmes, et al., 1994) in an urban African American population.

Injury researchers bemoan the flaws in external causes in fatal injuries and the fact that existing mortality data do not give a good picture of how injuries occur. To target intervention efforts, nurses must know how injuries are occurring. These data do not exist because fatal injuries are relatively infrequent events. The few studies on injury risk factors usually use data on nonfatal and minor injuries (which are relatively more frequent) to identify risk factors for injury. Unfortunately, we do not know whether nonfatal and fatal injuries involved the same causative factors and sequence of injury (see Peterson & Brown, 1994, for review).

Injury Prevention Research

In addition to these data-specific barriers to effective injury prevention, there are others. Many injuries occur because of an interaction between environmental and behavioral risks, for example, burns from hot water could not occur if water heaters were all set at a safe temperature (below 125°F). Environmental change strategies that avoid change in behavior have been favored by injury prevention professionals (e.g., air bags in cars, sprinkler systems in buildings). For many infant injuries, the behavioral piece in injury prevention must be addressed with parents, but there is sparse information about changing parental behavior with regard to injury or most other infant health-promoting activities. Unfortunately, injury often has no meaning to families until after an injury has already affected a child. Moreover, parents can often repeatedly behave in a relatively risky fashion without injury occurring. This leads to complacency and denial of risk. In fact, as parents obtain more experience with the environment around the infant, there is evidence that their expectations of severity of injury decreases. They become more willing to take risks. This adds to the difficulty of undertaking successful behavior change with parents to improve infant safety.

To provide a framework for injury prevention strategies, Haddon and Baker (1980) described the occurrence of injuries through the interaction of three factors: an agent that can do harm, a vector or vehicle that conveys the agents, and a host. Knowledge exists on how to change the agents, vehicles, and hosts to prevent death and disability. The value of these options for nurses is that they specify the various stages in the injury process in which intervention could be considered, and they address both behavioral and environmental approaches.

At present, other than for motor vehicle injuries, where passenger restraints, drunk-driving laws, and road and automotive safety standards have been shown to reduce infant injury and death, there are few proven injury-prevention interventions. Much more work is needed by nurses and other researchers to define and evaluate injury control strategies. In the meantime, research to understand injury etiology and better data collection systems are urgently needed.

ANN L. O'SULLIVAN
DONALD F. SCHWARZ

See also
CHILD LEAD EXPOSURE EFFECTS
EMERGENCY NURSING RESEARCH
FAMILY HEALTH
MOTHER-INFANT/TODDLER RELATIONSHIPS
PARENTING RESEARCH IN NURSING

URBAN HEALTH RESEARCH: NURSING RESEARCH IN URBAN NEIGHBORHOODS

Urban communities are home to heterogeneous ethnic, age, and socioeconomic groups, populations that make up a large share of the underserved in this country. These underserved populations face daunting hurdles that challenge their ability to maintain healthy lifestyles. Moreover, urban environments may provide limited or inaccessible support for individuals seeking health-promotion and disease-prevention information and services. Many urban environments are marred by poverty, strained school systems, crowded housing, unemployment, a pervasive drug culture, periodic street violence, and high levels of stress (Scally, 1996). Some health issues resulting from the urban environment include high rates of HIV infections and AIDS, increased morbidity and mortality due to violence, increased morbidity and mortality secondary to substance abuse, the resurgence of infectious diseases (tuberculosis and hepatitis B), chronic illness, and maternal/child health problems.

Many of the health problems experienced by residents in urban neighborhoods are preventable, at least in part, through lifestyle changes. Steps also can be taken to reduce health disparities through early identification and treatment. Unfortunately, statistics demonstrate that urban populations do not routinely receive early screening and preventive health care.

Urban Defined

When thinking about what *urban* means, we are confronted with a number of images, ranging from shining tall buildings, greater opportunities for employment, upscale housing, and community parks to dilapidated buildings, vacant lots sewn with rubble, high rates of unemployment, congested expressways, youth gangs, drug dealers and drug addicts, and, most of all, people. Perhaps the images include the stark difference between cultures—African, Asian, Caribbean, European, Hispanic, Middle Eastern—expressing the diversity and cosmopolitan atmosphere of everyday life in big cities. In some cases the images are those of opportunity; in others, of despair. Historically, urban images in the United States have tended to oscillate between the positive (cities as innovative, progressive, and modern) and the negative (cities as alienated, pathological, and decadent). Today, popularly depicted urban images include culture, arts, and music; recreation and leisure; and the hustle and bustle of commerce, as well as violent crime, rampant drug abuse, crumbling infrastructure, transportation gridlock, and pollution. These images not only depict sharp contrasts between rich and poor but suggest that the worst states of health are found among urban dwellers exposed to substandard housing, poverty, unemployment, and drug abuse (Andranovich & Irposa, 1993; Scally, 1996).

The process of attaching meaning to these images is multifaceted. However, there is no consensus on a common definition of *urban*. Most definitions include an interrelationship between people (demography) and space: political and administrative boundaries, social and cultural arrangements, economic and technological restructuring. The process of urbanization in the United States has resulted in political, social, economic, environmental, and health changes; at the same time, political, social, economic, environmental, and health changes have influenced the process of urbanization. Urbanization is a dynamic process, and its effects on health are seen and felt in different ways within particular cities and across the nation.

Health Issues of Urban Neighborhoods

Striking disparities in health outcomes among urban populations provide compelling evidence of the significant health risk these groups experience. The health outcomes described below are observed in nonurban populations but are disproportionally seen in urban populations (Gemson, Ashford, Dickey, et al., 1997; Prewitt, 1997; U.S. Department of Health and Human Services, 1990).

Chronic Illnesses

Hypertension and heart disease: Thirty-eight percent of Blacks suffer from hypertension; of those, only 25% are managing their disease.

Obesity: Forty-four percent of Black and Latino women ages 20 and older are obese, compared to 27% for all women and 37% for low-income women.

Diabetes: The disease is 33% more common among Blacks than among the general population. Latino and Native American populations report elevated morbidity rates from diabetes, often exacerbated by poor nutrition and exercise habits.

Cancer: Major disparity in cancer rates exist among Blacks, Latinos, Native Americans, the elderly, and poor Americans. Failure to screen is often due to fatalism, lack of knowledge, or limited access.

General health habits: Poor nutrition, smoking, alcohol and drug abuse, minimal exercise and stress management, along with other risk factors, appear to be more common among persons with low incomes, who tend to be urban residents.

Violence

Men, young adults, and teenagers within minority populations, particularly Blacks and Latinos, are most likely to be murder victims.

Domestic violence accounts for one of six homicides, particularly among young adults and Blacks.

Child abuse cases make up a significant portion of urban violence, affecting mostly poor families.

Maternal and Child Health

Black, Native American, and Latino infants have the highest morbidity and mortality rates in the

United States. Low-birthweight Black babies account for most of these deaths, but even normal-weight Black babies have a greater risk of death.

Asthma risk is increased for poor, minority urban residents, both initial attacks and exacerbations. Environmental factors such as air pollution and cockroach allergens have been correlated with emergency room visits for asthma.

Teen pregnancy has risen for all girls, particularly among poor and ethnic minority groups, with significant social, economic, and health consequences.

HIV and AIDS

The rate of AIDS among Blacks and Latinos are more than triple that of the general population.

Women and their children are one of the largest groups infected.

Sexually active teens are a fast-growing population at risk for HIV infection.

Urban Health Research

Urban Health Research focuses on the following processes, which form a circular link:

Identifying methodologies and models for developing culturally sensitive research approaches, data collection instruments, and program evaluation instruments.

Building partnerships with community members, nurses, and other health professionals who have community-based practices and with transdisciplinary researchers to identify and prioritize urban health issues that need investigating.

Determining the most effective, culturally sensitive health-promotion and disease-prevention intervention strategies and best-practice models for the targeted urban setting.

Implementing the most effective health-promotion and disease-prevention intervention strategies and best-practice models within the targeted urban community while simultaneously collect-

ing evaluation data that will be used to modify the implementation process as needed.

An example of urban health research was recently documented by Steigman (1996). Although Romieu and others (Romieu et al., 1995) found that emergency room visits for asthma correlated with levels of air pollution, Gottlieb, Beiser, and O'Conner (1995) showed that severity varied within the urban area of Boston; for instance, there were much higher rates of asthma-related hospital admissions in poor, minority areas than in other areas of the city. Upon examining the practice-based data, they also noted a much higher rate of beta-agonist use than anti-inflammatory use in the poor areas versus the other parts of the city.

The following questions that the researchers raised should be addressed by a collective partnership of community members (potential or actual victims), practice-based health care professionals who work within the geographical setting, and transdisciplinary researchers. Could the increased incidence in asthma be due to an environmental stimulus such as cockroach allergy that is not present in other parts of the city? Could limited or lack of access to medical care be responsible? Could health promotion models assist in preventing this problem? How can nurses use research data and political advocacy to foster environmental modification efforts within such communities to help eliminate this health problem?

As nurses we must be concerned about how the issues of urbanization affect the health of urban communities. Residents of such communities are the most reliable sources for this information. However, they are not likely to volunteer this information either because of distrust of researchers or the perception that their opinions or facts are not valued by nurses or researchers. Hence, one of the early steps in the urban health research process is to empower and recruit urban community members, especially minorities, to become active research partners, not just participants, in research programs.

Nursing Research in Urban Health

The overall goal of urban-related nursing research is to integrate scientific knowledge, professional skill, community input and support, and political advocacy of health promotion and disease prevention in an effort to create and maintain healthy urban communities. To achieve this goal, nurse researchers in urban settings, with community input, must seek to develop, test, and disseminate health care interventions, tailored to address the major urban health care issues, that are found to be scientifically sound, culturally relevant, and effective. Once identified, the urban-related nursing research process continues with the implementation of effective interventions and best practices within the community while maintaining overall health care costs. When logistically feasible, it is advisable to take the programs or practices to the target populations because this approach tends to foster participant.

Nurses' Role in Urban Health Research

Nurses can meet the challenges of addressing the needs of urban community residents by using a multidimensional approach that focuses on their social, psychological, biological, and environmental needs. Historically, nurses have viewed the recipients of their care in a holistic manner, taking into account all domains that have an impact on their lives. This approach is particularly useful with urban minority populations, who tend to experience many different stressors and who also tend to value the interpersonal process.

Through innovative research projects, innovative educational programs, and new strategies for providing services, we can meet their needs. For today, urban health is a priority. With the recent economic trend that is moving health care from hospitals to the community, current nursing students are being prepared to shift their work setting to the community and to interact with clients in their "home environment." This educational preparation should result in better health care as well as stronger client advocacy, another important aspect in the process. Nurses in the future will increasingly work in community-based settings such as homeless shelters, community clinics, small independent practices, schools, and church clinics.

Conclusion

To summarize, for programs of nursing research to be effective in urban communities the researcher must do the following:

Design programs that are based on a comprehensive needs assessment, including an identification of the target population.

Make programs accessible and affordable to the target population.

Ensure that the programs are culturally competent and relevant to the target population (i.e., consistent with norms, attitudes, beliefs, and attitudes). Members of the target populations should be included in program design, implications, and evaluation.

Ensure that the programs are consistent with the social and community norms of the target population so that program participants will receive consistent messages and reinforcement for the prescribed health behavior plan.

Address the linguistic needs of the target population (i.e., with translators and health and education reading materials in the community's native language and at the appropriate reading levels).

When applicable, ensure that programs meet the needs of the deaf and hearing-impaired members of the target population, as well as those with developmental disabilities.

Residents of urban communities have numerous health care challenges. Fortunately, nurses with the proper education and training emerge to provide excellent compassionate and innovative care and to design culturally competent and theory-driven intervention that will produce positive healthy outcomes. One advantage of meeting this need is the fact that most schools of nursing are located in urban communities, which enhances the interaction between and among nurses, community members, and researchers. Nurse researchers are not the only ones who benefit from such interaction; students and the people in the community also benefit. Nursing research projects designed and implemented by building bridges with the community can provide the most effacious and cost-effective community-based health care.

LORETTA SWEET JEMMOTT
EMMA J. BROWN

See also
CULTURAL/TRANSCULTURAL FOCUS
REDUCING HIV RISK-ASSOCIATED
  SEXUAL BEHAVIOR AMONG ADO-
  LESCENTS
RISK FACTORS
VIOLENCE AS A NURSING AREA OF IN-
  QUIRY
VULNERABLE POPULATIONS

URINARY INCONTINENCE

Definition

Urinary incontinence was defined by the International Continence Society Committee on Standardisation of Terminology in 1973 as "involuntary loss of urine which is objectively demonstrable and a social or hygienic problem" (ICS, 1990). The committee defined four specific types of incontinence: (a) genuine stress, (b) urge as described by the patient, (c) reflex, and (d) overflow incontinence, as evidenced by urodynamic demonstration of urine loss.

In 1992 an Agency for Health Care Policy and Research (AHCPR) expert panel defined incontinence as "involuntary loss of urine which is sufficient to be a problem" (Diokno, McCormick, Colling, et al., 1992, p. 1). The expert panel deleted the words "objectively demonstrable and a social or hygienic problem." It was the judgment of the panel that the literature would not support science-based evidence that changes in outcomes of urinary incontinence were "objectively demonstrable." For several days the AHCPR panel deliberated what outcomes could be measured in incontinence. If involuntary loss of urine is the problem, then it was determined the outcome was dryness or no voluntary loss of urine. Dryness was measured in

episodes or accidents per day, per week, or per month. To measure dryness, a toileting diary was recommended as the tool to collect measurable outcomes of dryness.

Four Types of Incontinence

The four types of incontinence result from four different pathophysiological mechanisms. Therefore, the correct nursing diagnosis is important because the treatment must be specific to the diagnosis to achieve an appropriate outcome.

The symptom of urge incontinence is the involuntary loss of urine associated with a strong desire to void (urgency). Urge incontinence is usually, but not always, associated with urodynamic findings of involuntary detrusor contractions, referred to as detrusor instability (DI). When this symptom is associated with a neurological lesion, it is called detrusor hyperreflexia (DH), which is seen in patients with stroke. In patients with multiple sclerosis and suprasacral spinal cord lesions, DH is accompanied by detrusor sphincter dyssynergia (DSD), inappropriate contraction of the external sphincter with detrusor contraction. In older adults this symptom is associated with detrusor hyperactivity with impaired bladder contractility (DHIC).

The symptom of stress incontinence is seen in patients who involuntarily lose urine during coughing, sneezing, laughing, or other physical activities that increase intraabdominal pressure. Stress urinary incontinence is defined as urine loss that occurs with an increase in intraabdominal pressure, in the absence of a detrusor contraction or an overdistended bladder. The most common cause of stress incontinence in women is a floppy uterus or urethral hypermobility. It is also common in men after prostatectomy.

Reflex incontinence occurs without any warning or sensory awareness, often in patients with paraplegia. It is also called unconscious incontinence.

Overflow incontinence is involuntary loss of urine associated with overdistention of the bladder. This type of incontinence causes constant dribbling. Overflow may be caused by an underactive or acontractile detrusor. The bladder may be underactive or acontractile secondary to use of drugs, to neurological conditions such as diabetic neuropathy or low spinal cord injury, or to radical pelvic surgery that interrupts the motor innervation of the detrusor muscle.

Nursing research has contributed to the definition of functional incontinence, which is urine loss caused by factors outside the lower urinary tract, such as a physical or cognitive impairment. A patient who is immobile and cannot toilet in time is functionally incontinent.

Prevalence and Costs

Urinary incontinence affects approximately 13 million Americans, with the highest prevalence in the elderly in both community and institutional settings (National Kidney and Urologic Diseases Advisory Board, 1994). Urinary incontinence is estimated to cost $11.2 billion annually in community-dwelling persons and $5.2 billion in nursing homes (based on 1994 dollars) (Fantl et al., 1996).

Risk Factors

Nursing research has provided identification of important risk factors in adult urinary incontinence. The risk factors validated by nurses are low fluid intake, environmental barriers, estrogen depletion, and pelvic muscle weakness (Fantl et al., 1996). These are in addition to other risk factors, including immobility, impaired cognition, medications, morbid obesity, diuretics, smoking, fecal impaction, delirium, high-impact physical activities, diabetes, stroke, childhood nocturnal enuresis, race, and pregnancy, vaginal delivery, or episiotomy.

Nursing Assessment and Diagnosis

The diagnosis of incontinence is based on a structured history, physical exam, urinalysis, and postvoid residual volume measurement. Recommended questions for the history include frequency of episodes, duration of the problem, volume of accidents, precipitating factors and questions related to risk factors. The physical exam should include tests for neurological abnormalities, abdominal examination, rectal examination, genital and pelvic examinations, and direct observation of urine loss using a cough stress test.

Treatment

There are three basic treatments of incontinence: medications and behavioral and surgical interventions. The most significant contributions of nursing science have been in the behavioral interventions. Nurse researchers have conducted research on toileting assistance, bladder retraining, and pelvic muscle rehabilitation.

Toileting assistance includes scheduled toileting, habit training, and prompted voiding. Studies have been conducted in outpatient populations and in nursing home residents. Nursing staff have achieved significant reductions in urinary incontinence during a 4–9-week intervention—about 80% improvement. Four clinical trials in nursing homes, three controlled and one uncontrolled, demonstrated that prompted voiding reduced incontinence by 0.8–1.8 episodes per patient per day (Fantl et al., 1996).

Bladder training is a procedure that includes education, scheduled voiding with systematic delay, and positive reinforcement. A controlled, randomized clinical trial of 131 women with sphincteric incompetence and unstable detrusor function showed that of the 60 women in the treatment group, 12% became dry, and 75% had a 50% reduction in incontinent episodes (Fantl et al., 1996).

Pelvic muscle rehabilitation (Kegel exercises) may be done alone or augmented with bladder biofeedback therapy or vaginal weight training. This type of intervention is most beneficial in patients with stress urinary incontinence. In a study of 65 women aged 35 to 75, a 62% reduction in incontinence episodes was documented. In another uncontrolled study, 20 women aged 35 to 65 were reported to have a 95% reduction in urinary incontinence episodes. In a nurse-directed project, when pelvic muscle exercise was compared with phenylpropanolamine hydrochloride treatment, patients experienced a 77% reduction with exercise and 84% with drugs (Fantl et al., 1996).

When pelvic muscle exercise is augmented by bladder inhibition with biofeedback therapy, a range of 54%–87% improvement has been demonstrated. Biofeedback that uses feedback from pelvic muscle contraction and abdominal and detrusor activity shows the greatest improvement, with a 75.9%–82% improvement rate across six studies involving 166 subjects. Overall, the literature indicates that pelvic muscle exercise and other behavioral strategies, with or without biofeedback, can cure or reduce incontinent episodes.

Pelvic muscle exercise also can be augmented with vaginal weight training. Women insert cone-shape weights (20–100 g) into the vagina. They try to retain the cone by contracting the pelvic muscle for up to 15 minutes. Research from 103 premenopausal women indicated a subjective cure or improved status of 68%–80% after 4–6 weeks of treatment.

Pelvic floor electrical stimulation is another intervention used by nurses and supported by nursing research. Pelvic muscle electrical stimulation produces a contraction of the levator ani and external urethral and anal sphincters, accompanied by a reflex inhibition of the detrusor. Two randomized controlled trials have been conducted. Using electrical stimulation, 86% of patients improved or were cured, compared to 33% in the control group. Behavioral therapies are very effective and carry no risks.

Pharmacological and Surgical Treatments, and Other Management Options

Several medications have been tested in clinical trials for specific types of urinary incontinence. As with most drugs, there is a risk of side effects, and persons taking more than one drug should be observed for adverse drug interactions. Various procedures have been described in AHCPR clinical practice guidelines (Fantl et al., 1996) to treat incontinence surgically. The objectives of surgical treatments depend on the underlying anatomical and physiological etiology; the purpose is to circumvent the underlying pathophysiology that is causing urine loss. As with any surgery, there are possible complications and risks.

Other measures and supportive devices can be used to manage rather than treat or cure incontinence. Nursing has contributed to the development and evaluation of several measures, including intermittent catheterization, indwelling urethral catheterization, suprapubic catheters, external collection systems, penile compression devices, pelvic organ support devices, and absorbent pads or garments.

Psychological Impact of Incontinence

Nursing research has identified the quality-of-life and psychological impact of incontinence on the adult and the nursing staff or other caregiver (Palmer, 1996). Incontinent adults often remove themselves from social situations where the risk of an accident would be embarrassing. Family members caring for the incontinent patient often find the care burdensome or tiring, and they become resentful. Health care providers are consumed by the labor-intensive care required by the incontinent patient. They may avoid the person, complain about the burden of care, or even blame the patient for accidents. Standardized questionnaires have been developed by nurse researchers to determine the psychological impact of incontinence.

KATHLEEN A. McCORMICK

See also
ACTIVITIES OF DAILY LIVING
FAMILY CAREGIVING TO FRAIL ELDERS
GERONTOLOGIC CARE
PREGNANCY
WOMEN'S HEALTH RESEARCH

V

VALIDITY

Validity refers to the accuracy of responses on self-report, norm-referenced measures of attitudes and behavior. Validity arises from classical measurement theory, which holds that any score obtained from an instrument will be a composite of the individual's true pattern and error variability. The error is made up of random and systematic components. Maximizing the instrument's reliability helps to reduce the random error associated with the scores (see "Reliability"), although the validity of the instrument helps to minimize systematic error. Reliability is necessary but not a sufficient requirement for validity.

Validity and theoretical specification are inseparable, and the conceptual clarification (see "Instrumentation") performed in instrument development is the foundation for accurate measurement of the concept. Broadly stated, validity estimates how well the instrument measures what it purports to measure. Underlying all assessment of validity is the relationship of the data to the concept of interest. This affects the instrument's ability to differentiate between groups, predict intervention effects, and describe characteristics of the target group.

Literature usually describes three forms of validity: content, criterion, and construct. These forms vary in their value to nursing measurement, and unlike reliability, singular procedures are not established that lead to one coefficient that gives evidence of instrument validity. Instead, validity assessment is a creative process of building evidence to support the accuracy of measurement.

Content validity determines whether the items sampled for inclusion adequately represent the domain of content addressed by the instrument. The assessment of content validity spans the development and testing phases of instrumentation and supersedes formal reliability testing. Examination of the content focuses on linking the item to the purposes or objective of the instrument, assessing the relevance of each item, and determining if the item pool adequately represents the content. This process is typically done by a panel of experts, which may include professional experts or members of the target population. Lynn (1986) has provided an excellent overview of the judgment-quantification process of having judges assert that each item and the scale itself is content-valid. The results of the process produce a content validity index (CVI), which is the most widely used single measure for supporting content validity. Content validity should not be confused with the term *face validity*, which is an unscientific way of saying the instrument looks as if it measures what it says it measures. Although content validity is often considered a minor component for instrument validation, researchers have repeatedly found that precise attention to this early step has dramatic implications for further testing.

Criterion validity is the extent to which an instrument may be used to measure an individual's present or future standing on a concept through comparison of responses to an established standard. Examination of the individual's current standing is usually expressed as concurrent criterion validity, although predictive criterion validity refers to the individual's future standing. It is important to note that rarely can another instrument be used as a criterion. A true criterion is usually a widely accepted standard of the concept of interest. Few of these exist within the areas of interest to nursing.

Construct validity has become the central type of validity assessment. It is now thought that construct validity really subsumes all other forms. In essence, construct validation is a creative process that rarely achieves completion. Instead, each piece of evidence adds to or detracts from the support of construct validity, which builds with time and use.

Nunnally (1978) proposes three major aspects of construct validity: (a) specification of the domain of observables; (b) extent to which the observables tend to measure the same concept, which provides a bridge between internal consistency, reliability, and validity; and (c) evidence of theoretically proposed relationships between the measure and predicted patterns. The first aspect is similar to content validity and is essentially handled through formalized concept clarification in instrument development. The inclusion of this specification of the domain under construct validity supports the contention that construct validity is the primary form, with other types forming subsets within its boundaries.

The other two aspects of construct validity are examined formally through a series of steps, as described by Goodwin and Goodwin (1991). These steps form a hypothesis-testing procedure in which the hypotheses are based on the theoretical underpinnings of the instrument. Hypotheses can relate to the internal structure of the items on the instrument. Hypotheses can also refer to the instrument's anticipated relationship with other concepts, based on a theoretical formulation. The first set of hypotheses fall into the second aspect of construct validity testing; the latter relate to the third aspect.

Although there are no formalized ways to examine the hypothesis proposed for construct validity testing, some typical approaches have been identified in nursing research. Primarily, the internal structure of an instrument is tested through factor analysis and related factor analytic procedures, such as latent variable modeling. Factor analysis has become one of the major ways in which nursing researchers examine the construct validity of an instrument. It is important to note that this approach addresses only the second aspect of construct validity testing and in itself is insufficient to support the validity of an instrument. Factor analysis simply provides evidence that the underlying factor structure of the instrument is in line with the theoretically determined structure of the construct.

The third aspect of construct validation provides an opportunity for more creative approaches to testing. Hypotheses proposed have to do with the relationship of the concept being measured with other concepts that have established methods of measurement. These hypotheses deal with convergent and discriminate construct validity, subtypes that examine the relationship of the concept under study with similar and dissimilar concepts. If data evidence a strong relationship with similar concepts and no relationship with dissimilar concepts, evidence is built for the construct validity of the instrument. Should data not support similarities and differences, several options are possible: (a) the instrument under construction may not be accurately measuring the concept, (b) the instruments for the other concepts may be faulty, or (c) the theory on which the testing was based may be inaccurate. The multitrait-multimethod (MTMM) matrix has been proposed as a way to formally test convergent and discriminate construct validity. This approach has been discussed by Ferketich, Figueredo, and Knapp (1991), and the same authors provide an extension of the method through confirmatory factor analysis (Figueredo, Ferketich, & Knapp, 1991).

Another approach to examining the relationship among concepts involves a known group technique. In this method, the researcher hypothesizes that the instrument will provide a certain level of data from groups with known levels on the concept the instrument has been designed to measure.

The above approaches to testing construct validity are only samples of techniques that can be used. As mentioned, construct validity testing is creative. Researchers can design unique ways to support the validity of their instruments. The important point is that whatever is designed must be based in theory and must be intuitively and logically supported by the investigator.

JOYCE A. VERRAN
PAULA MEEK

See also
FACTOR ANALYSIS
INSTRUMENTATION
MEASUREMENT AND SCALES
RELIABILITY
THEORETICAL FRAMEWORK

VIOLENCE AS A NURSING AREA OF INQUIRY

Violence is well recognized as an important health problem in the United States, and nursing research, practice, policy, and advocacy have all been instrumental in addressing the problem. The United States is one of the most violent countries in the industrialized world. Each year homicide and suicide claim more than 50,000 lives, and 2.2 million people are injured by violent assaults. If the trend continues, death rates from firearms will surpass motor vehicle crashes by the year 2003 (U.S. Public Health Service, 1995). Since the 1985 Surgeon General's Conference on Violence, a public health approach has been recognized as an important framework for research and interventions to reduce violence and ameliorate its effects.

The term *violence* originates from the Latin *violare*, to violate. The victims of violence are violated, physically, emotionally, spiritually, and socially. Nurses encounter victims and perpetrators of violence in every health care setting, with a variety of injuries and other health problems. The holistic approach of nursing addresses all aspects of human responses to violence. Nursing scholarship has also recognized the complex interaction of community factors (structural inequalities and erosion, residential mobility, poverty, lack of career opportunities, housing, cultural norms and biases, and population density) and individual and family risk factors for violence that require preventive measures.

Violence against Women

The largest body of nursing research is focused on violence against women. Ann Burgess's groundbreaking studies of rape in the early 1970s initiated a program of nursing research to address the cognitive processing of trauma and later focused on the concerns of rape victims about HIV infection (Campbell, Anderson, Fulmer, et al., 1993). Nurse researchers have studied children who have been sexually abused and have done work on identifying response patterns in children and adolescents exploited in sex rings and pornography as well as the development of a model of children's responses to sexual abuse that explains their acute and chronic symptoms.

Other nurse researchers have focused on incest survivors, exploring both the long-term difficulties they experience and the positive aspects of adaptation, healing, and empowerment. Work with rape victims has included examination of self-esteem and primary prevention techniques.

Battered Women. Nursing studies related to domestic violence have resulted in a diverse but impressive body of nursing knowledge. A recently published review (Campbell & Parker, in press) of 20 years of nursing research on domestic violence documented a significant prevalence of abused women in a variety of health care settings with significant physical (chronic pain, headaches, and backaches; risk of sexually transmitted disease; and sleep disturbances) and mental health problems (depression, low self-esteem, substance abuse, and anxiety). Battered women's perceptions of less than adequate care given by health professionals has been supported by studies of the attitudes of physicians and nurses that identified the paternalistic and blaming attitudes of many of these professionals. Related to these issues, an experimental nursing intervention study tested a training program for emergency room nurses that resulted in a significant increase in appropriate identification and documentation of battered women in the nurses who received the training.

Judy McFarlane and Barbara Parker (Campbell & Parker, in press) have documented a higher prevalence of abuse during pregnancy (16% to 17%) than was shown in other research studies. This higher prevalence may be related to the use of nurse-conducted personal interviews. Findings of various studies have suggested that universal screening of all women (including adolescents) for intimate partner abuse at *each* health system encounter should become routine nursing practice. Nursing research has also supported the link between abuse during pregnancy and low-birthweight infants, substance abuse, smoking, and depression.

There was also substantiation in nursing research of the significant strengths of battered women, indication of normal processes of grieving and recovering, and the fact that leaving battering relationships is a process that occurs over time, the majority of women leaving or making the violence end. Landenburger (Campbell & Humphreys, 1993) used grounded theory to develop a theory of entrapment and recovery from an abusive relationship that was later used as a basis for clinical nursing intervention.

Understanding dating violence among adolescents is recognized as significant not only because of the injuries and suffering experienced at the time but also because of its relationship to adult domestic violence. The prevalence of dating violence varied between 9% and 61% in various studies. These differences may be related to differences in definition. One nursing study of adolescent dating violence in North Carolina revealed that many adolescents denied abusive relationships but reported numerous abusive events. Twenty-four percent of these adolescents reported extreme violence, including episodes of rape or use of weapons. In one midwestern city a nursing study found the prevalence of dating violence among nursing students to be similar to the prevalence among American women overall, thus the need for nursing faculty to be alert for signs of abuse.

The contribution of nursing research to the field of domestic violence is noteworthy because of its activist and feminist (i.e., woman-centered) assumptions and stance. Nursing scholars have developed close collaboration with shelters for abused women, paid particular attention to the safety and empowerment of women and their children, and documented strengths as well as problems. Nursing research has proceeded from the assumption that the locus of responsibility for battering lies not only with individual perpetrators but also with our societal structures and attitudes that facilitate or fail to prevent the battering of female partners. There has also been a beginning sensitivity and inquiry about ethnic and cultural differences in women's responses to battering from nursing investigators such as Doris Campbell, Sara Torres, Rachel Rodriguez, and Diane Bohn (Campbell & Parker, in press).

Children of Battered Women. In the United States at least 3.3 million children ages 3 to 17 witness domestic violence each year. There is a strong correlation (40% to 77% concordance) between domestic violence and violence against children. Nurse researchers have studied some of the effects on children witnessing or experiencing family violence. These effects include more physical health problems, higher levels of internalizing behaviors (depression, social withdrawal), low self-esteem and self-efficacy, lower social competence, higher levels of externalizing behaviors (aggression, hyperactivity, conduct problems), anxiety re-

actions, posttraumatic stress symptoms, and school problems. Children who were abused also showed a high incidence of subsequent violent behavior and arrests. The qualitative studies of Humphreys and Henderson (Campbell & Parker, in press) have provided new insights into the experience of children living with domestic violence and into their concerns, for example, worries about their mother's actual (battering) or potential (smoking, pregnancy) health problems.

Child Abuse

According to 1990 data, over 2.7 million children in the United States were victims of child maltreatment in that year, and this number has remained high (U.S. Public Health Service, 1995). Nurses have contributed to the view that child abuse is the result of a complex interaction of individual, family, environmental, and societal factors (Campbell & Humphreys, 1993) and to the recognition that disability and twinship place children at risk for abuse. Factors that influenced clinicians' identification and management of child abuse and family violence were found to be education and attitudes towards the abuser. Nurse researchers in the United States and the United Kingdom have demonstrated the effectiveness of home visits in screening, intervening, and preventing child abuse.

Adolescent Violence

Youths are increasingly involved as perpetrators and victims of violence. Homicide is a leading cause of death among 15–19-year-olds nationally. Risk behavior surveys indicated that a large percentage of students in grades 9 through 12 reported carrying a weapon in the 30 days preceding the surveys. These indicators, along with the increase in juvenile arrests, raise concerns about our youth and their access to firearms. In recognition of these trends, the midcourse review of Healthy People 2000 includes a new objective addressing physical fighting by adolescents (U.S. Public Health Service, 1995).

More research on youth violence by nurses and social scientists is needed. The research in this area by nurses has been rather limited. Cull (Campbell, Harris, & Lee, 1995) examined the influence of being a victim of violence on self-care practices of adolescents, and Lee used epidemiological methods to examine the effects of gun violence on youths and adults. More studies are needed to examine the etiology and prevention of youth violent behavior and the effects on our children of witnessing violence. Nurses play a significant role in schools and in the community and have the opportunity to evaluate interventions in these settings.

Elder Abuse

Elder maltreatment is an important topic that has received very little attention. It is estimated that 700,000 to 1 million older Americans experience mistreatment each year. Nursing research on this topic has focused on an understanding of predictive factors, instrument development, and clinical decision making. This research, led by Fulmer and Phillips (Campbell, Anderson, Fulmer, et al., 1993), has influenced policy on such issues and leads the way to an important avenue of nursing research.

Summary, Critique, and Future Directions

Nursing research has made substantial contributions to the health problem of violence. There have been methodological shortcomings in terms of relatively small sample sizes and unsophisticated designs. There is also a scattering of studies in many different directions, impeding accumulation of nursing knowledge in specific areas. However, many study findings have been corroborated by findings from other disciplines.

Attention to culture and ethnicity, use of qualitative and quantitative data, a holistic perspective, strong clinical grounding, and the advocacy positions of prior nursing research should be continued to advance the body of nursing knowledge about the causes and interventions related to violence. More longitudinal, comparison group, and large sample studies are needed, especially those that develop and test midrange nursing theory. Further documentation and investigation of health conse-

quences and costs of violence must build on existing nursing research. The effects of violence should be incorporated in other programs of nursing research in maternal-child health, substance abuse, HIV/AIDS, gerontology, international health, and community health. Studies that test nursing interventions with victims of violence, their families, and groups at risk are needed to demonstrate the value of nursing care in making the health care system a primary, secondary, and tertiary prevention site.

JACQUELYN C. CAMPBELL
JOAN KUB
LINDA LEWANDOWSKI

See also
   ELDER ABUSE
   EMERGENCY NURSING RESEARCH
   REDUCING HIV RISK-ASSOCIATED
      SEXUAL BEHAVIOR AMONG ADO-
      LESCENTS
   VULNERABLE POPULATIONS
   YOUNG WOMEN AND DEPRESSION

VIRGINIA HENDERSON INTERNATIONAL NURSING LIBRARY

The Virginia Henderson International Nursing Library is an electronic library whose resources are digital, not physical. It is supported by Sigma Theta Tau International (STTI), the international honor society of nursing, and is housed at the Center for Nursing Scholarship, international headquarters of STTI in Indianapolis, Indiana. The holdings are distributed worldwide via the Internet and the World Wide Web (WWW).

The goal for the Virginia Henderson Library is encompassed in the mission statement of STTI: "to improve the health of people worldwide by improving nursing scholarship." Three of four objectives for achieving this mission speak directly to nursing knowledge: knowledge development, knowledge dissemination, and knowledge utilization. Of all the nursing organizations in the United States, only the International Nursing Library and

Sigma Theta Tau together have the unique mission of nursing scholarship.

The Virginia Henderson Library began early in the 1980s under the sponsorship of STTI in response to continuing dissatisfaction with the limitations of extant bibliographic services to locate nursing literature, particularly nursing research and theory. Bibliographic services distribute information about where knowledge might be found, not the knowledge itself (see Bibliographic Retrieval Systems). Addressing this identified need, the library was envisioned as a repository of nursing research, and collection of biographical data and summary information about nurse researchers began almost immediately, forming the core resource of the library. The first *Directory of Nurse Researchers* was printed in 1983.

In 1989 the library was named for one of the most respected nurse leaders, Virginia Henderson, who developed the first nursing research classification system. In that same year, the library became a computer-based electronic resource. Over the next decade, the *Directory of Nurse Researchers* evolved into the *Registry of Nursing Research*, changing in intent from the networking and location of other nurse researchers to the intent of registering all nurse researchers and nursing research, including findings.

The Virginia Henderson Library now has many resources, including data, information, and knowledge, which are designed to serve the scholarship and knowledge mission of STTI. Data services include archived nursing research data sets contributed by various researchers. Although these research data sets may be used for teaching research, their primary purpose is for generating knowledge via secondary analysis by qualified students and researchers. Information services include the STTI *International Book Service*, which provides peer reviews of newly published nursing books in partnership with Doody Publishing, Inc., a leading independent reviewer of health science books. Knowledge services include the Registry of Nursing Research© and the Online Journal of Knowledge Synthesis for Nursing© (OJKSN).

The Registry of Nursing Research© is the premier resource of the Virginia Henderson Library to such an extent that library and Registry are sometimes used synonymously, though incorrectly. Both published and fugitive research are sought for the Registry. Rather than the narrative reporting of knowledge as in published scientific journals, the Registry presents research knowledge as data describing researchers, their studies, and the findings generated by the studies. The data base of the Registry is organized by the STTI *Nursing Research Classification System*, third edition. The knowledge (findings) is indexed directly by variable name. Data for the Registry is submitted by researchers with a special registration form on the WWW or on disks for Macintosh and Windows. Minimum information required is biographical data about the researcher and a structured abstract of each study. More data about the study and findings are required of registrants whose work is funded by STTI. In addition, detailed data are requested of researchers who work in a domain that has been identified as a primary focus area by the STTI research and library committees.

The Online Journal of Knowledge Synthesis for Nursing provides critical reviews (i.e., narrative meta-analysis, integrative review, qualitative knowledge synthesis) of research pertinent to clinical nursing practice problems. Author teams composed of a clinical specialist and a clinical researcher provide the reviews in an area of expertise and are expected to update the review when required by new knowledge in the area. A traditional peer review process is used. A major difference in the electronic publication format is that distribution takes place within hours of acceptance, rather than the months required to bring a print version of a publication to subscribers. Articles can be printed at the user's local printer or ordered from a document delivery service. In addition to being able to browse the articles, a user can search for a keyword of interest. Such a search produces all articles that contain the keyword. It is anticipated that the Online Journal of Knowledge Synthesis for Nursing is only the first of many electronic publications that will be offered by the Virginia Henderson Library.

Communication services offer an electronic conferencing/bulletin board service for networking, group publishing, group bibliographic citation management, and conducting multisite research. These services are all in the support of knowledge development, dissemination, and utilization goals of STTI.

The Henderson International Library is not the only major nursing library in the world; however, it is the only major nursing library that is completely electronic. It is the only library to register details of nursing research and findings. The Registry can be searched by researcher name, keywords, and research variable or concept names. It is the only known library in the world to index research knowledge by variables studied together.

JUDITH R. GRAVES

See also
> BIBLIOGRAPHIC RETRIEVAL SYSTEMS
> THE ONLINE JOURNAL OF KNOWLEDGE SYNTHESIS FOR NURSING
> REPRESENTATION OF KNOWLEDGE FOR COMPUTATIONAL MODELING IN NURSING: THE *ARCS©* PROGRAM
> SIGMA THETA TAU INTERNATIONAL NURSING RESEARCH CLASSIFICATION SYSTEM
> WORLD WIDE WEB

VIRTUAL REALITY

Definition

Virtual reality is a computer-simulated technique that allows an individual to hear and feel stimuli that correspond with a visual image. The term *virtual reality* was first used by Jaron Lanier in 1989 to refer to a collection of technological equipment capable of creating an alternative environment (Steuer, 1992). A typical equipment-driven definition of virtual reality is ''virtual reality is electronic simulations of environments experienced via head-mounted eye goggles and wired clothing enabling the end user to interact in realistic three dimensional situations'' (Coates, 1992, cited in Steuer, 1992).

An alternative to an equipment- or technology-driven definition is an experience-driven definition. Steuer (1992) advocated use of an experience-driven definition based on the concepts of presence, which is viewed as being in an environment, and telepresence, which is the ''experience of presence in an environment by means of a communication medium'' (p. 76). Combining these experience-related concepts, Steuer defined virtual reality as ''a real or simulated environment in which a perceiver experiences telepresence'' (pp. 76–77). In this situation virtual reality is viewed as a psychological variable that is not limited by specific technological hardware. Steuer concluded that virtual reality is composed of two interdependent components, human experience and a technologically mediated environment.

Research Using Virtual Reality

Virtual reality technology is so new that studies on its effects are small in scale and lack scientific rigor. Mon-Williams, Wann, and Rushton (1993) conducted a study to determine the short-term effects on binocular stability. Some subjects in the small sample ($N = 20$) showed signs of induced binocular stress. More research is needed to determine if visual effects of virtual reality are harmful or any different from those produced by television or video games.

Another experiment compared the value of virtual reality training, real-world training, and no training (Kozak, Hancock, Arthur, & Chrysler, 1993). In this study, 21 subjects performed a pick-and-place sequence task. There was no significant difference between the group that received no training and the virtual reality training group. The real-world training group performed significantly better than the other two groups. This study challenges the notion that virtual reality task training can be transferred to a real-world situation.

These two experiments question whether our current expectations for the potentials of virtual reality are valid. Scientists must consider the possible detriments, such as visual changes or altered perceptions that may occur as a result of the use of virtual reality equipment.

Examples of Virtual Reality Applications

A variety of medical applications for virtual reality are currently being tested. One of the most common applications is to enhance surgical techniques. Virtual reality surgical simulators can help surgeons learn to control hand tremors or obtain more practice on rarely performed techniques. Another possible application is remote surgery. A surgeon could perform surgery without being physically present in the operating room. The surgeon operates in a virtual reality workstation, and the movements are transmitted to the actual surgical site.

Virtual reality systems are also being used for motion analysis and physical therapy applications. In Palo Alto, California, physical therapists are using a virtual reality body suit to understand body movements. The suit could be programmed to slow movements to help reteach individuals how to walk or eat. Suzanne Weghorst at the University of Washington in Seattle, uses virtual reality glasses to enhance gait control in individuals with Parkinson's disease (LeFevre, 1994). Virtual reality systems also can help with rehabilitation and improving quality of life for quadriplegic patients. Using only their eyes, quadriplegic patients have been able to use virtual instruments to move objects and to communicate (Dutton, 1992).

In educational applications, virtual reality simulations can help students learn about client care prior to real-life experiences in the clinical setting. Virtual reality can be used to help students understand how people react in crisis situations or the physiological changes that occur in septic shock. Research is needed regarding how virtual reality systems can help to improve classroom learning.

Virtual Reality as Tool for Nurses

One can hypothesize many ways in which nurses will be able to use virtual reality. Professional and patient teaching could be improved by using virtual reality models to practice dressing changes and hygiene care or to administer medication. Virtual reality environments could be created that would allow nurses to practice decision making. For example, a nurse could practice how to set priorities when caring for seven patients, all of whom require differing levels of nursing intervention.

Nurses could use virtual reality as a distraction intervention during painful procedures or to prevent boredom during long periods of hospitalization.

The distraction literature indicates that various techniques such as music, humor, and relaxation have been tested, but all of these require that the person consciously and continuously focus on the distraction strategy. Virtual reality may be effective as a distraction intervention because it blocks competing environmental stimuli and does not require practice. Currently, the author is conducting a nursing study that examines the effects of a virtual reality distraction intervention on symptom distress in children receiving cancer chemotherapy.

For those patients who would benefit from confronting reality rather than escaping it, virtual reality could be therapeutic. Individuals could use virtual reality to replace disruptive thoughts or to practice effective problem solving. Virtual reality could help decrease anxiety related to unknown procedures. Young women could use virtual reality to "experience" a Pap smear prior to the actual clinical exam.

Barrett (1993) explains how virtual reality is congruent with Martha Rogers's science of unitary human beings. Rogers's theory states that "nurses pattern the environment to promote comfort, well-being, health, and healing" (Barrett, 1993, p. 14). Virtual reality can be used to pattern the environment for health. The Rogerian view is that the person as an energy field is infinite and is not bound by the physical body. Virtual reality "allows a person to experience their energy field in a place where the physical body is not present" (Barrett, 1993, p. 15). Virtual reality experiences may increase nursing's understanding of human perceptions, transcendence, and the human-environmental mutual process.

In the next decade virtual reality will influence the way individuals learn, work, and receive health care. Phillips (1993) writes that "when virtual reality becomes an actuality in health care, nurse researchers will have to evaluate its usefulness for and application to nursing" (p. 5).

SUSAN M. SCHNEIDER

See also
RESEARCH ON INTERACTIVE VIDEO
ROGERS'S SCIENCE OF UNITARY HUMAN BEINGS

TELEHEALTH
TELENURSING/TELEPRACTICE
TELEPRESENCE

VULNERABLE POPULATIONS

Definition

Vulnerable populations are those social groups who are at increased relative risk for adverse health-related outcomes. Groups commonly considered vulnerable to increased risk of poor health include women and children, the elderly, ethnic people of color, immigrants and refugees, gay men and lesbians, homeless persons, disabled persons, and chemically dependent persons. These groups are socially and politically marginalized, disenfranchised, and subject to social and racial inequality, intolerance, injustice, and stigma.

Factors that contribute to the relative risk of poor health for vulnerable populations are personal and community health needs and resource availability. These factors may be categorized as socioeconomic and demographic conditions, physiological processes and genetic traits, psychosocial and behavioral characteristics, and environmental and health system constraints. Socioeconomic and demographic conditions include poverty, substandard housing, unemployment, and lower educational level. Physiological processes and genetic traits are defined by developmental stage, age, gender, biology, resistance, immunity, family history of disease, and genetic inheritance. Psychosocial and behavioral characteristics are represented by cultural ideology and practices, social networks, family structure, lifestyle practices, and psychological traits. Environmental and health system constraints are reflected in access to health care, availability and proximity of health care, quality of care, availability of insurance, and environmental stressors such as crowding, mobility, migration, occupational hazards, and area of residence. In most instances, several of the factors contributing to vulnerability are operating together and interactively.

Adverse health-related outcomes are evidenced in increased comparative morbidity and mortality rates and decreased life expectancy. Nursing research has contributed additional indicators of poor health, such as decreased quality of life, decreased functional and mental status, decreased ability to work, and limitation of activity.

Community Perspective

For nursing research and practice purposes, vulnerable populations are viewed from a community health perspective. Community-based care models and intervention strategies include direct community participation, cultural and linguistic competence, comprehensive and coordinated services, and multiorganizational collaboration. A community framework for research and practice interventions with vulnerable populations encompasses primary, secondary, and tertiary levels of prevention. These levels of prevention consist of health promotion and disease prevention; early diagnosis and prompt treatment of disease and human responses to illness; rehabilitation, restoration, and resocialization to limit disease progression; and palliation. Outcomes of community-based models of care and intervention strategies are analyzed on the basis of changes in the incidence or prevalence of health problems among the vulnerable populations studied.

A community perspective acknowledges the essential social and political origins of vulnerability and requires that research planning, design, and outcomes be related to societal conditions, public policy, ethical decision making, and economic costs. The economic and social value of supportive public policies to facilitate the provision of community resources and services must be emphasized. The staggering social and economic costs of continued risk to vulnerable groups is critical for public policy formulation. The ethical issues of societal racism, discrimination, and bias must be faced, and the ethical foundations of equal care must be delineated.

Scientific Development

Distinguished scholars from a number of disciplinary perspectives have contributed to the recent focus on vulnerable populations. Social scientists from the Nelson A. Rockefeller Center for the Social Sciences at Dartmouth College produced a series of lectures on populations at risk in America at the end of the 20th century (Demko & Jackson, 1995). LuAnn Aday (1993), at the University of Texas School of Public Health, developed a framework for studying vulnerable populations, including who the vulnerable groups are; predictors of populations at risk; programs, cost, quality of care, and barriers to care; and needed community programs and policies. The U.S. Public Health Service Bureau of Primary Care (1995) funded and published a compendium of innovative primary health care programs for underserved and vulnerable populations. A community-based practice model (Sebastian, 1996) designates when and how nurses intervene with vulnerable populations.

The National Institute of Nursing Research funds an institutional pre- and postdoctoral research training grant at the UCLA School of Nursing to study the health-related problems of vulnerable populations, health policy issues, and ethical decision making associated with vulnerable populations (Flaskerud & Chang, 1994). In fall 1996 the National Institute for Nursing Research requested proposals for research into the clinical application of intervention strategies designed to reduce risks at the community level, especially targeted to rural residents and underserved minorities (*Health Risk Reduction: Community-Based Strategies*, 1996).

Research Issues

Several conceptual and methodological problems in research on vulnerable populations remain to be solved. Conceptual issues—identifying who is vulnerable and why, health status, relative risk, and resource availability—must be clarified. Methodological issues involve selecting correlates and indicators of vulnerability and identifying vulnerable group subjects. It is necessary to measure changes in health status and to use both biological and be-

havioral markers of change. Equally important is measuring a comprehensive variety of health outcomes. The strength and dose of the intervention strategy and sustaining change overtime are other critical aspects of study. The use of standard instruments and replication and generalization of shared intervention strategies will facilitate progress in research.

Future directions for research on vulnerable populations should focus on community-based interventions and health outcomes. To date, the research in this area has been descriptive and correlational. In the future, studies must develop and test interventions based on the results of the multitude of correlational studies that have been done. Evaluating links between vulnerability factors and health outcomes requires complex multivariate models that ultimately are tested prospectively. Minimally, such models will demand objective measures of the range of vulnerability factors and a repertoire of health outcomes that includes categorical clinical disease, preclinical disease markers, health care utilization data, and self-reported health. The most challenging aspect of these models is identifying the large number of intervening variables that may moderate health outcomes. In developing and testing such models, the observed morbidity and mortality effects must exceed some minimal absolute standard for classifying disease or longevity. Documenting changes in the incidence and prevalence of disease and changes in mortality and longevity in vulnerable populations will demonstrate the effectiveness of community-based prevention strategies.

JACQUELYN H. FLASKERUD

See also
COMMUNITY EMPOWERMENT
CULTURAL/TRANSCULTURAL FOCUS
HOMELESS HEALTH
IMMIGRANT WOMEN
WOMEN'S HEALTH RESEARCH

W

WATSON'S HUMAN CARE MODEL

The human care model (Watson, 1979, 1985a, 1989, 1997) focuses on the spiritual nature of human beings, specifically the patient and nurse as spiritual beings. Watson (1990) explained that "the ideas and ideals associated with my philosophy and theory of human caring are concerned with spirit rather than matter, flux rather than form, inner knowledge and power, rather than circumstance" (p. 219). Humanistic caring is the ethic on which the human care model is based. The author of the model was influenced by the writings of Hegel, Marcel, Whitehead, and Kierkegaard; works in nursing by Peplau and Gadow; personal experiences with other cultures; and Eastern philosophy. The significance of the human care model for nursing is that Watson has described a philosophy and ethic of nursing that recognizes and affirms the spiritual essence of human beings.

A person is viewed as a magnificent spiritual being (Watson, 1989) whose power for healing and transcendence dwells in the soul, or inner self (Watson, 1985a). The meaning of living in the world is experienced through self-awareness. The knowledge of meaning results in evolutionary movement to higher levels of consciousness and becoming. Health is equated with unity and harmony of "mind-bodyspirit" (Watson, 1985a, 1989). The experience of health is associated with congruence between "self as perceived and self as experienced" (Watson, 1989, p. 226). Illness is a manifestation of disharmony and the subjective experience of inner turmoil and suffering (Watson, 1985a). Illness is not disease but can lead to disease if a lack of congruence with self and the world and the soul of the person remains distressed.

Watson has delineated eleven values of the human care perspective that include

deep respect for the wonders and mysteries of life; the power of humans to grow and change; acknowledgment of a spiritual dimension to life; acknowledgment of the internal power of the human care process; high regard and reverence for the spiritual-subjective center of the person; high value on how the person (patient and nurse) is perceiving and experiencing health-illness conditions; nonpaternalistic values that recognize human autonomy and freedom of choice; emphasis placed upon helping a person gain more self-knowledge, self-control, and readiness for self-healing regardless of the present health-illness condition; high value is placed on the relationship between the nurse and the person; the nurse is a co-participant in the human care process. (Watson, 1985a, pp. 34–35)

The definitive value of the model is that "caring is presented as the moral ideal of nursing with a concern for preservation of humanity, dignity and fullness of self" (Watson, 1985a, p. 73).

Eleven assumptions direct the human care model and are briefly paraphrased here. (For a more complete presentation, see Watson, 1979, pp. 32–33.) The assumptions include the following:

1. Care and love are universal forces.
2. If our humanness is to survive, there is a need to become more caring and loving to nourish our humanity.
3. Nursing is a caring profession whose practice can influence human development.
4. One must focus on one's own behavior and respect self before one can care for others with respect and dignity.
5. Historically, nursing has valued caring in addressing people's health.
6. Caring is the essence of nursing and practice.
7. The focus on human care has decreased in the health care delivery system.

8. The caring values of nursing have been submerged in modern technological society.
9. Human care is a significant epistemic and practice concern for nursing.
10. Human care can be practiced only in an interpersonal, intersubjective human encounter.
11. Nursing's contributions to humankind and society is its commitment to human care ideals.

In addition, Watson (1985a) described seven premises of the human care model:

1. The mind and emotion are windows to the human soul.
2. The mind and body are not limited by the physical universe and transcend time and space.
3. The nurse can access a person's mind, emotions, and inner self indirectly through mind, body, or soul, which are inseparable spheres of the human being.
4. The inner self, or soul, of a person exists in and for itself.
5. People need the love and care of each other to survive.
6. To find solutions to overt and covert illnesses it is necessary to identify meanings in the context of the human predicament.
7. The wholeness of human experience at any moment comprises a phenomenal field.

Human care and transpersonal caring relationships are key components of the model. Self, phenomenal field, event, and actual caring occasion are concepts specific to the transpersonal caring relationship. Human care is a way of knowing self (nurse) and the other (patient) as a result of an intersubjective, intentional human to human contact. A transpersonal caring relationship is a specific professional, human-to-human contact with the goal of promoting a patient's experience of health, or inner harmony. Self is a process that synthesizes experiences and transforms experience into what is known of being in the world. This knowing includes awareness of the ideal self and one's relationship with the other (Watson, 1985a). A phenomenal field

is the subjective experience of the person (Morris, 1996). Another's phenomenal field is known indirectly through empathetic understanding. When human beings choose to engage in an transpersonal caring relationship, a new and unique phenomenal field is created. An actual caring occasion is the result of a transpersonal caring relationship and is exclusive to the newly co-created phenomenal field (Watson, 1985a). The patient and nurse both become more human, and transcendent healing is obtained and continues beyond the actual caring occasion.

Nursing activities focus on the use of the carative factors described by Watson, originally in 1979, as a modalities for achieving nursing's goals in a transpersonal caring relationship. The carative factors include

> formation of a humanistic-altruistic system of values; faith-hope; sensitivity to self and others; helping-trusting, human care relationship; expressing positive and negative feelings; creative problem-solving caring process; transpersonal teaching-learning; supportive, protective, or corrective mental, physical, societal, and spiritual environment; human needs assistance; and existential-henomenological-spiritual forces. (Watson, 1985b, p. 75)

In 1986 the Center for Human Caring was established at the University of Colorado Health Science Center, School of Nursing, in Denver, Colorado. One of the goals of the center is to develop knowledge of human caring and healing. Research activities at the center include collaborative research on caring needs and behaviors, development of practice modalities, and guidance of master's theses and dissertations. In addition, a summer visiting fellows program for academics who want to be mentored in caring-healing theory and research methods has been developed.

The human care model is being used as a practice model in the United Sates and Canada in acute, community, and long-term care settings (J. Watson, personal communication, December, 1994). Implementation of the model in practice is supported through consultation activities provided by Watson and through videotapes. Clinicians also can study at the Center for Human Caring and obtain a certificate in caring skills.

In addition, the human care model is the basis for the nursing doctor (ND) program curriculum at the University of Colorado and for at least four nursing education programs in the United States and Canada (J. Watson, personal communication). An advanced postgraduate program of study is available through the Center for Human Caring; it includes mentored study of caring-healing for educators.

DIANA LYNN MORRIS

See also
CARING
NURSING THEORETICAL MODELS

WEIGHT MANAGEMENT

Weight management, defined as deliberate actions to reduce body weight to normal ranges, can be classified as formal and informal. Formal weight management consists of paying for organized services to assist individuals with weight reduction. Informal weight management includes personal weight loss methods without professional assistance or attending groups for the purpose of losing weight. Weight management in American society most often is targeted at reducing weight, rather than increasing weight, because of the high incidence of overweight, obesity, and associated diseases.

Body mass index (BMI = kg/m^2) is the current means of describing overweight and obesity by most health professionals. Overweight is defined as a BMI of 24 to 29, obesity is a BMI of 30 to 39, and morbid obesity is a BMI of 40 or more. Traditionally, overweight has been defined as greater than 10% above ideal weight and obesity as greater than 20% above ideal weight from insurance height and weight tables. Women, particularly those in advanced years, gained more weight than men did (Kuczmarski, Flegal, Campbell, & Johnson, 1994). Among Mexican American and African American women, 48% were overweight, whereas 32% of European American women were overweight. Recently, body composition has been considered a more specific and accurate means of describing excessive adipose tissue versus lean body mass, including measures of hydrostatic weighing, skinfold calipers, bioelectrical impedance, and radioisotope. A percentage of body fat greater than 17–21 for men and 22–31 for women is considered excessive, depending on age.

Background and Prevalence

In the United States losing weight has become a $40 billion-plus industry. Nevertheless, 5 of the 10 leading causes of death are linked to fat intake and obesity. In 1985 a National Institutes of Health (NIH) panel on obesity concluded that the need for future research in obesity assumes great significance and demands attention because of its prevalence and associated major health problems. The panel recommended more obesity research to explore effective prevention and treatment programs. The panel noted the increased risk of morbidity and mortality for overweight compared to normal-weight individuals.

The 1990 U.S. Department of Health and Human Services *Healthy People 2000* report noted major declines in death rates for two leading obesity-related causes of death, heart disease and stroke. In spite of these improved mortality rates, overweight people remain at greater risk for heart disease and stroke compared to normal-weight individuals. Obesity has been associated with hypertension, hypercholesterolemia, noninsulin-dependent diabetes mellitus, gallbladder disease, pulmonary function impairment, endocrine abnormalities, obstetric and surgical complications, osteoarthritis and trauma to weight-bearing joints, gout, cutaneous disease, hernias, proteinuria, and menstrual disturbances.

In the 16-year Nurse's Health Study (Mason et al., 1995), obese women were found to have four times the risk of death caused by cardiovascular disease compared to the leanest women. Weight gain greater than 22 pounds after 18 years of age increased risk of death from heart disease, cancer, and all causes. Despite these surprising statistics, women appear to have been less studied than men in terms of reduction of weight and cardiovascular risk.

Weight Cycling

Individuals who gain and lose body weight frequently over a prolonged period present a pattern called yo-yo dieting, or weight cycling. In 1993 about 45% of men and 75% of women were trying actively to lose weight (Wing, 1993). Most diets and approaches for reducing can lead to weight loss; however, body weight often is regained after overeating in response to restricted intake while dieting. Formal weight management failure rates have been estimated to be higher than 90%.

In 1992 the NIH convened a panel to examine existing methods for voluntary weight loss, weight control, and health effects of weight cycling. Researchers believed that weight cycling caused rapid excessive weight regain, higher percentage of fat in regained pounds, and lower metabolic rate. The panel encouraged further study to confirm the longer-term negative effects of weight cycling on psychological and physical health.

Then, in 1994 the NIH called together the National Task Force on the Prevention and Treatment of Obesity to address concerns about weight cycling and direct researchers and practitioners in weight management. The task force summarized work published from 1988 to 1994 and found no convincing evidence of harmful effects of human weight cycling on body composition, energy expenditure, cardiovascular risk, or future efforts at weight loss. New studies should be designed to correct deficits in sample size and methodological limitations (Brownell & Rodin, 1994; National Task Force on the Prevention and Treatment of Obesity, 1994). Sensitive and long-term measures to study weight management as a multidimensional problem may shed light on the physical and psychological reasons for regaining weight.

Unidimensional versus Multidimensional Interventions

Nurses and health care professionals are confused about appropriate interventions for weight management. Most weight loss treatments have been unidimensional and aimed at reducing caloric intake or metabolizing stored fat. The treatments may include fasts, food restrictions, supplements, and regular exercise. Medical treatments include surgical reduction of the gastrointestinal tract, stomach expansion devices to simulate feeling full, and drugs to suppress the appetite.

According to Brownell and Wadden (1992), traditional weight management based on unidimensional approaches is not viable for promoting long-term weight loss. The 1992 NIH panel suggested seven essential program dimensions for healthy and successful weight loss and control: (1) a mix of diet, exercise, and behavior modifications; (2) individual and closed group counseling; (3) multidisciplinary expertise availability; (4) training for relapse prevention to deal with high-risk emotional and social situations; (5) a maintenance phase; (6) flexibility of food choices; and (7) weight goal setting cooperatively with program director. Panelists believed that long-term clinical trials on weight control would provide evidence about the long-term health effects of weight loss. They emphasized the paucity of well-designed long-term clinical trials evaluating various methods for voluntary weight loss, particularly in minority populations and persons who are mildly to moderately overweight.

Nurses and health promoters are responsible for designing multidimensional programs to correct what researchers know causes people to drop out of weight programs, namely feelings of restrictions and deprivations, no time for exercise, and life stressors that habitually send them to seek temporary relief from food (Brownell & Wadden, 1992). Although formal programs designed to help people stop overeating and increase exercise can promote weight loss, the psychological components often are not considered and may be the reasons that diet and exercise programs fail. Although Bartlett, Wadden, and Vogt (1996) found no statistical relationships among depression, psychopathology, and weight cycling, their subjects reported numerous negative psychological factors related to their weight cycling.

Because lifestyle changes occur over years, long-term intervention studies must be designed to track strategies that assist overweight and obese individuals to make permanent weight changes. Both qualitative and quantitative measurement of physical and psychological progress should be employed to accurately measure the multivariate weight problem of modern American society.

SUE POPKESS-VAWTER

See also
HYPERALIMENTATION
OBESITY AS A CARDIOVASCULAR
    RISK FACTOR
NUTRITION
NUTRITION IN INFANCY AND CHILD-
    HOOD

WELLNESS

Definition

Wellness is an integrated method of functioning directed toward maximizing the potential of which an individual is capable within the environment where functioning occurs. Wellness is both a process and a goal that can be chosen by anyone of any age, in any setting, and with any condition of illness or disability. As a process, wellness is a movement toward greater awareness and satisfaction derived from engaging in activities that move the whole person toward fitness, positive nutrition, positive relationships, stress management, clear life purpose, consistent belief systems, commitment to self-care, and environmental comfort. The goal of wellness is the actualization of the person that results from learning how to remain healthy and the personal assumption of health-promoting behaviors.

Relevance to Nursing

Nursing is concerned with the phenomena of human responses to illness and health. Although it has been difficult to move nursing language systems such as that of the North American Nursing Diagnosis Association (NANDA) to descriptors of wellness and its maintenance and promotion, progress has been made. The wellness model focuses on what is "right" with the person; quality of life is more important that just being alive. The integration of body, mind, and spirit is the orientation of wellness. Nurses in all arenas of practice are in strategic positions to assist patients in making positive lifestyle changes directed toward wellness.

Nursing pioneers in the wellness movement adopted a holistic approach and promoted wellness through self-care and self-responsibility. Dimensions of a health-promoting lifestyle, encompassing behaviors that serve to maintain or enhance the wellness and fulfillment of the individual, were identified and scientifically validated. Those dimensions include health responsibility, nutrition, exercise, stress management, interpersonal support, and self-actualization. Later, wellness practitioners developed this theme into wellness practices. Promotion of health is an appropriate term for the wellness model because it emphasizes improving one's general state of health.

Historical Perspective

Dunn (1961) was the first to use the term *wellness* nearly two decades before the concept of high-level wellness and holistic health were popularized by Ardell, Travis, and others in the late 1970s and early 1980s. Dunn's writings reflect and acknowledge the ideas of thinkers such as Eric Fromm, Carl Rogers, Abraham Maslow, and Hans Selye, who were also concerned about how individuals might achieve their full potential within their world. Dunn equated health with the integration of person-mind-body-spirit and maintained that what people feel, believe, and think affects their physical capabilities, and vice versa.

The wellness and holistic health movement of the 1970s evolved outside the traditional health professions. Major threads throughout the movement today continue to reflect the integration of body, mind, and spirit; the ethic of self-responsibility and choice; and the interdependence of individual, social, and environmental wellness originally conceptualized. These terms have become popularized and used by lay persons and health professionals alike, often without clear conceptual understanding of what the concepts really mean. The dichotomy between the characteristics of the medical model and the wellness model creates dissonance and makes the use of wellness language inaccurate and confusing in the context of a medically driven system of illness care.

Major Studies

Smith (1983) described distinctive models of health, which include a clinical orientation, a role-performance or functional definition of health, a eudaemonistic definition of health as exuberant well-being or high-level wellness, and an adaptive definition of health. The Laffrey Health Conception Scale (Laffrey, 1986), based on Smith's work, was developed to measure the perception of health held by individuals. The Health Promoting Lifestyle Profile, the work of Walker, Sechrist, and Pender (1987), contributed further to the development of the science of wellness and its defining variables.

Relationship to Nursing Practice

Well persons who want to learn to maintain and improve their health will not find answers to their questions in the medical system, which is characterized by diagnosis and cure of disease. Well persons are often unrecognizable in medical systems. They are, however, increasingly recognized in nursing systems of care, where health promotion and wellness diagnoses are commonly made and where interventions designed to assist clients to greater levels of wellness are based on rapidly accumulating evidence.

MARION M. HEMSTROM

See also
FUNCTIONAL HEALTH
HEALTH CONCEPTUALIZATION
QUALITY OF LIFE
SELF-EFFICACY
STRESS MANAGEMENT

WOMEN'S HEALTH RESEARCH

Definition

''Women's health'' is a phrase that has come to signal movement away from a focus on gynecology—synonymous with traditional reproductive matters—to gyn-ecology, meaning a focus on the fit between the woman and her environment (Matthews et al., 1997). Women's health research is sensitive to the relationships between and among genetic, physiological, psychosocial, economic, political, cultural, generational, developmental, and lifestyle factors.

History

Women's health research, as a subset of women's studies, began as a critique of patriarchal practices and their effects on women's well-being (McBride, 1993). Women frequently were not included as subjects in health research. For example, studies of alcoholism or cardiovascular disease traditionally did not include women as subjects. Moreover, women have historically been excluded from the first two stages of drug testing, and female animals have typically not been used in animal model research because of ''their hormonal fluctuations.''

The sociocultural factors shaping health problems in girls and women have been too often ignored—for example, the relationships between learned helplessness and some kinds of depression; between anorexia and the popular admonition that you can never be too rich nor too thin; and between cigarette advertising that links smoking to chic slimness and the resulting increase in lung cancer as more women took up the habit, seeking to be as sophisticated as magazine images. There has been sex bias in treatment choices based on skewed assessments and the extent to which women were perceived to deserve a voice in shaping their treatment. For example, women's symptoms have been too often dismissed as primarily psychological, and until recent times, the biopsy diagnosis of breast cancer was typically combined with surgical treatment of breast cancer, with the physician deciding alone how radically to proceed.

Health has been construed so that male behavior has been regarded as normative. Research on males has typically been generalized to all human beings. From Freud to Kohlberg, theoretical models have been constructed so that women are regarded as less morally developed when they do not act in fashion similar to men. Social/health systems also have been prejudicial in important respects. Women have not been in research and policy making positions proportionate to their numbers, responsibilities, and educational preparation. The burden of family caregiving that women bear has been invisible, notably in estimates of the Gross National Product (GNP). Moreover, men have not been studied much in some situations, thus reinforcing the notion that some health issues are of concern only to women, for example, parenting, contraception, cyclic change, role stress and strain.

A Call to New Research

Women's health, however, has been concerned with more than a critique of the extent to which women's experience has been constituted by others; it has signaled a call to research informed by how women constitute themselves (McBride & McBride, 1993). Women's special health concerns have begun to be studied seriously. Some of the conditions and diseases that solely or disproportionately affect women are now receiving attention: urinary incontinence, menstrual cycle changes, violence, poverty, sexually transmitted diseases, osteoporosis, breast cancer, autoimmune diseases, aging, comorbidity, and lesbian health. The notion of the constituting self has led to feminist innovations in therapy—consciousness raising, self-in-relation perspective on development, feminist psychoanalysis—and to new concepts, for example, sexual harassment, date rape, coerced caring, and role rewards. A feminist ethic has been much discussed that is neither concerned with "doing good" nor "doing unto others what one would wish for oneself" but with providing care that builds on the patient's perceptions of what is good for her.

Awareness of health as a social construction has meant rethinking shibboleths about body image and the so-called eating disorders—for example, that diets are the principal means to lose weight and that weight-reduction efforts cannot be regarded as successful unless one achieves "normal" weight. Critical reconstitution of the meaning of women's experience as mothers has resulted in an emphasis on the growth and development of mothers along with their children and has demonstrated the importance of fathers to child development.

The substantially different health trajectories of women and men over a lifetime—women report more illness and health care use than men at every stage but consistently live longer—has led to new research on this gender paradox and to focusing on morbidity as a feminist issue. The lifestyle issues undergirding the expression of symptoms have begun to call into question drugs and surgery, with their frequent iatrogenic consequences, as the treatments of choice and to increase interest in self-care and noninvasive alternative therapies. Health is increasingly not conceptualized as the absence of disease, nor is the presence of disease automatically assumed to preclude well-being.

Accomplishments

Often led by nurses, women's health research has become relatively mainstream in the past three decades. Many new professional organizations, annuals, and journals dedicated to women's health research have come into existence; the latter include *Annual Review of Women's Health, Health Care for Women International, Journal of Women's Health, Menopause: The Journal of the North American Menopause Society, Psychology of Women Quarterly, Sex Roles, Update on Women's Health Issues, Women and Health, Women's Health: Research on Gender, Behavior and Policy,* and *Women and Therapy.* Graduate programs in women's health have developed (McElmurry, 1993), and a center for women's health research, sponsored by the National Institute of Nursing Research, has been established at the University of Washington under the leadership of Nancy Fugate Woods.

Considerable effort has gone into the development of a women's health research agenda (USPHS Office on Women's Health, 1991). Woods (1994b) eloquently described principal efforts, summarized recommendations, and provided an overview of additional criteria for designating priorities. At this time, researchers in women's health are advantaged by a considerable infrastructure, including some agreement about national research priorities. Topics of traditional interest to women are being analyzed from a fresh perspective, and subjects traditionally considered to be the province of men only or women only are being studied for insights into how they affect all human beings in similar fashion or differentially.

Future Directions

There are many challenges remaining, not the least of which is the tendency to treat women as a monolithic group without proper regard for the extent to which women vary by race, culture, age, employment status, education, caregiving obligations, sexual orientation, available resources, and so forth. In an attempt to reject "biology as destiny," women's health research may also have inadvertently minimized the physiological pathways involved in responses to stressful psychosocial conditions. Larger health delivery issues, such as the closing of Planned Parenthood clinics and the impact of managed care on women's health, also have been either unstudied or understudied. These challenges collectively call for the development of research programs that move away from an emphasis only on status variables to one that deciphers underlying interactive processes.

ANGELA BARRON MCBRIDE

See also
FEMINIST RESEARCH METHOD-
  OLOGY
GENDER RESEARCH
IMMIGRANT WOMEN

VIOLENCE AS A NURSING AREA OF IN-
  QUIRY
VULNERABLE POPULATIONS

WORKFORCE

Webster's unabridged dictionary defines *workforce* as "the total number of workers in a specific undertaking" or "the total number of persons employed or employable" (Webster's, 1989). The latter concept is the one used when referring to the study of the nurse workforce. The Interagency Conference on Nursing Statistics referred to the workforce as the "registered nurse population," encompassing all those with current licenses to practice as registered nurses (Interagency Conference on Nursing Statistics, 1993).

Research on the nurse workforce has a twofold purpose. First, it is crucial to the understanding of the effects of various policy decisions on the workforce itself and on the availability of resources to provide for the health care needs of the population. Second, this type of research is vital to the development of such policies. The research carried out on the workforce has many aspects. It encompasses an examination of the so-called pipeline, that is, the characteristics of the nursing student body and the educational resources, the characteristics of those practicing and available for practice, the milieu in which they practice, and future resources and requirements for such resources.

The collection of data on the educational resources has been ongoing for many years. Annual data are available on the number and characteristics of the schools providing nursing education and on the number of students and graduates. Less developed are data on the characteristics of the students, with the exception of information on racial and ethnic background and gender. More comprehensive information has been available on new licensees. These data reflect the successful candidates, however, and little is known about the characteristics of those who do not achieve that success.

Initial efforts to obtain data on the registered nurse population involved working through the licensing agencies and state nurses associations to identify all those who were considered registered nurses. These efforts often were joint efforts of the federal government and the American Nurses' Association. Because there is no one list of all available nurses with licenses to practice as registered nurses, the actual collection of data was decentralized so that each state would survey its own licensees. The data would then be merged into a single data base after accounting for duplication of licenses from state to state. Of necessity, the scope of the data that could be collected through this mechanism was limited.

The issues underlying the need for data on registered nurses called for far more comprehensive information than was possible from the limited data set available. This prompted the Division of Nursing, the federal entity responsible for the Nurse Training Act (Title VIII), to begin looking for alternative approaches. The importance of this search was reinforced by a legislative mandate from Congress, Public Law 94-63, which contained the Nurse Training Act of 1975 (Title VIII). Title IX, Section 951, of the law required the examination of the current and future supply and distribution of nurses within states and in the country as a whole. The legislative requirements were broad and encompassed data on all nurses with licenses to practice, including requirements for such data as the numbers of nurses with advanced training or graduate degrees by specialty and average rates of compensation by type of employment.

The Division of Nursing developed a survey plan to satisfy the congressional requirements. Baseline data to satisfy models for estimates and projections of the nurse supply in the country and in each state would provide data on nurse characteristics needed for program planning, administration, monitoring, and evaluating by Congress, state legislators, and federal and state agencies and associations. The study design included the selection of a carefully developed sample and was completed in June 1976. The first National Sample Survey of Registered Nurses was conducted in 1977. Five subsequent studies were carried out, the latest in March 1996.

Over the years, data collection geared to provide information on registered nurses has evolved from attempts to reach every nurse and collect basic and minimal information to a sophisticated sampling approach with a comprehensive, detailed survey instrument. This last approach to the study of the numbers and characteristics of registered nurses has been effective in obtaining a large measure of the information required. Valid and statistically reliable estimates are prepared on a variety of measures of nursing resources. However, limitations do exist. From a geographical perspective, only broad-based information can be derived from most states except those that have a sufficient number of nurses to provide statistically sound estimates. The study cannot provide data on individual counties within states, although it can be used to examine aggregates of counties with similar characteristics. The ability to provide detailed information of selected groups of nurses with specific characteristics is limited unless the group is of substantial size or the sample is augmented to assure a sufficient sample for that particular group.

The National Sample Survey of Registered Nurses has also provided the base for the development of a model used to make annual estimates of the supply during interim years between sample surveys and projections for the future supply. In keeping with the data requirements spelled out in the congressional mandate, estimates are made on a state-by-state basis and according to highest educational level.

The examination of the supply is one aspect of the workforce picture. The other aspect to be examined is the determination of whether the workforce is adequate to achieve what is required of it. Requirements may be from a judgment view, that is, how many would be required if a given level of quality and service were to be achieved; or from a market viewpoint, how many would be required at a given level of available financial resources and actual utilization patterns. Both types of methodologies have been used to generate what the future requirements for nurses might be. A major modeling effort was made in the mid-1970s that identified several alternative approaches (U.S. Department of Health, Education and Welfare, 1979). Again in response to the congressional mandate, these efforts projected requirements on a state-by-state basis and, in some instances, according to nurse educational level. The results of models that looked at requirements from both the judgment and the market perspectives can be found in the nursing portions of the biennial reports to Congress on the status of health personnel in the United States. In the more recent analyses of the number of nurses required, the Division of Nursing followed an economic or market-demand modeling perspective.

The examination of nursing requirements, regardless of the viewpoint taken, was based on the settings in which nurses were employed, the development of projections for the services provided within each setting, and utilization of nurses. Therefore, the most appropriate data base for these models involves setting-by-setting studies as well as overall studies on health services to the public and the distribution of nurses throughout the health care delivery system. In recent years the lack of trend data for most health care delivery settings has required some modifications in the approach taken to requirements modeling.

The blending of studies of the educational system and registered nurse population and the models projecting the future supply of and demand for nurses provide a base for the analysis of issues and appropriate policy decisions on the nurse workforce. Comparative analyses of the results of modeling future supply and future requirements indicates that the supply would be in balance with requirements until about 2010, and then requirements would outstrip the anticipated supply. Data on nurse workforce and the concentration of the educational system suggest that, given the direction of the future health care delivery system, the educational base of the registered nurse workforce will not match the knowledge and skills necessary for managing and providing nursing services to individuals, families, groups, and populations. The data on the nurse workforce also suggest that meeting the requirements for nurses in the future is significantly challenged by the "aging" of the nurse workforce.

MARLA E. SALMON
EVELYN B. MOSES
DENISE H. GEOLOT

See also
AMERICAN NURSES ASSOCIATION
NATIONAL LEAGUE FOR NURSING
NURSE STAFFING
NURSING EDUCATION

WORLD HEALTH ORGANIZATION

The World Health Organization (WHO) is an international organization devoted to enhancing the health of people globally. The WHO promotes and coordinates research and programs that advance the cause of disease prevention and primary health care. The organization provides technical assistance to improve national health education, nutrition, water, sanitation, and maternal and child health; conducts immunization campaigns, and is currently coordinating a global program to control and conquer AIDS. The WHO is composed of 190 Member States. Although the WHO is part of the United Nations (UN) family, it maintains autonomy as an intergovernmental agency functioning with its own staff under its own charter and budget. Formally, the WHO falls under the Economic and Social Council (ECOSOC) branch of the UN.

The idea for such an organization was first spawned by UN delegates from China and Brazil at the UN conference in San Francisco in May 1945. The proposal by the delegates prompted the UN to arrange an international conference to establish an international organization devoted entirely to health. This conference was held in New York City during the summer of 1946. It yielded the development and signing of the constitution that was to govern the newly formed WHO. The constitution came into effect on April 7, 1948, the day now commemorated annually as World Health Day.

The WHO constitution states: "The enjoyment of the highest attainable standard of health is one of the fundamental rights of every human being without distinction of race, religion, political belief, economic or social condition" (WHO, 1948). The ultimate objective of the organization and its member countries is the "attainment by all peoples of the highest possible level of health" (WHO, 1994). The constitution places emphasis on the importance of governmental responsibility to provide adequate social, environmental, and health measures for their constituents. It also recognizes the importance of the informed opinion and active cooperation of the public in improving the health of a population.

According to the WHO constitution, the organization has two main functions: (1) to act as the directing and co-coordinating authority on national and international health work and (2) to foster technical cooperation in the area of health in member states (WHO Press Office, 1996). The functions are complementary and include advocating measures to improve health, stimulating and mobilizing specific health action, disseminating information, developing norms and standards, developing plans and policies, providing training, promoting research, mobilizing resources, and technical consultation (WHO, 1994).

Structure

The central authority in the WHO is the World Health Assembly, which meets once a year and is composed of national delegations from all member states. The World Health Assembly determines the organization's policies. The executive board is composed of 30 public health experts designated by their countries for 3-year terms. The executive board advises the World Health Assembly and gives effect to its policies. The secretariat of the WHO is the director general, the chief technical and administrative officer, who is elected by the World Health Assembly.

The WHO functions in six regions of the globe: (1) the AMRO region (all countries of the Americas), (2) the AFRO region (sub-Sahara Africa), (3) the EMRO region (the countries of the eastern Mediterranean), (4) the EURO region (Europe and the countries of the newly independent states of the former Soviet Union), (5) the WPRO region (the countries of the Pacific Rim), and (6) the SEARO region (the countries of Southeast Asia). Representatives of the member states of each region meet yearly as a regional committee to formulate policies for the region and to monitor regional activities.

The WHO is financed by the direct contribution of member states based on a scale of assessments similar to that of the UN. Other funds include voluntary contributions by countries or philanthropic organizations, non-governmental organizations, and individuals.

Health for All by the Year 2000

The WHO defines health as "a state of complete physical, mental, social well-being and not merely the absence of disease and infirmity" (WHO, 1994). "Health for All by the Year 2000" (HFA) is a global strategy that was developed in 1977 by the World Health Assembly. HFA seeks a commitment by all governments to a level of health for all people that permits them to lead socially and economically productive lives. HFA provides the policy framework for worldwide health action until the turn of the century and is thereby the basis for WHO's work during this period.

In 1978 the International Conference on Primary Health Care in Alma-Ata identified primary health care as the means by which HFA could be achieved. Primary health care is defined as, "essential health care that is practical, scientifically sound and socially acceptable and that is accessible and affordable to the country and community" (WHO, 1994). Primary health care will continue to be WHO's strategy of choice beyond the year 2000, as reaffirmed at a 1988 conference in Riga, Latvia.

The WHO's HFA global health policy is expressed in three general programs of work. Programs of work are plans developed by the WHO that outline in greater detail the tasks before the WHO and the world community for certain periods of time. Since the adoption of HFA, the programs of work (7th, 8th, and 9th) have been devoted to setting forth tasks that would bring the goals of HFA to realization. The Seventh General Program of Work (1984–1989) emphasized the systematic building of the infrastructure of health systems; the Eighth General Program of Work (1990–1995) stressed action at country level; the Ninth (1996–2001) focuses on supporting countries and the international community in concerted, sustained, and complementary action to bring about greater equity in health (WHO, 1994).

Since its inception the WHO has made many significant contributions to world health. It has been instrumental in the eradication of small pox as well as the radical declension of the incidence of polio and many other age old diseases. The WHO has provided and coordinated emergency services for outbreaks of communicable diseases for many countries and facilitated global research programs throughout the world. The WHO has access to the services of approximately 1,900 scientists in 90 developing countries and about 1,600 scientists in

27 developing countries. The organization's commitment is not to establish itself as a research institution but rather that "research in the field of health is best advanced by assisting, coordinating and making use of the activities of existing institutions" (WHO, 1987, p. 4). The organization issues a variety of publications, including *World Health*, *WHO Chronicle*, and the *Bulletin of the World Health Organization*.

The WHO can be reached on the World Wide Web at http://www.who.or.jp.documents.hq/.

DORIS MODLY

See also
EPIDEMIOLOGY
HEALTH CONCEPTUALIZATION
VULNERABLE POPULATIONS
WELLNESS
WORLD HEALTH ORGANIZATION COLLABORATING CENTERS

WORLD HEALTH ORGANIZATION COLLABORATING CENTERS

A World Health Organization (WHO) Collaborating Center is an already existing institution that has been designated by the director general of the WHO to form part of an international collaborative network. The purpose of collaborating centers is to carry out activities in support of the WHO and its programs—locally, nationally, and internationally. Additionally, collaborating centers must participate in the strengthening of country resources in information, services, and research and training to support national health development. There are over 700 WHO collaborating centers located in many areas of the world and representing many, if not all, of the major health disciplines, including nursing.

The idea of using national institutions for international purposes, or as collaborating centers, began with the League of Nations reference centers established for the standardization of biological products. After the inception of the WHO, more reference centers were appointed; the World Influenza Center, established in London in 1947, was the first. This policy of designating already existing institutions as collaborating centers is secondary to the organization's commitment to *not* consider "the establishment, under its own auspices, of international research institutions" and that "research in the field of health is best advanced by assisting, coordinating and making use of the activities of existing institutions" (WHO, 1987).

Collaborating centers operate under the following seven prescribed functions:

1. Standardization of terminology and nomenclature of diagnostic, therapeutic and preventive substances and technologies, and procedures and methods beneficial for the attainment of the organization's goals
2. Synthesis and dissemination of the scientific and technical information needed to (a) conduct the activities of the Collaborating Center and (b) promote the country's national health development to the WHO in the implementation of its program
3. Provision of services to the Organization in support of the worldwide program (i.e., epidemiological surveillance, identification of causal agents, and development of preventive services) and the development of technical cooperation for national health development
4. Development of research objectives, programs and collaborative efforts
5. Training and strengthening of researchers and research programs in developing countries
6. Coordination, promotion, and support of collaborative schemes developed by other centers; this function is limited to select Centers
7. Contribution of technical aid in cooperation with other countries through the provision of information, services, and advice and by stimulating and supporting research and training

(World Health Organization, 1987)

Designation as a WHO collaborating center must be attained through two processes. First, the candidate institution or organization must enter into direct negotiation with the staff of the respective regional WHO office or the WHO headquarters in Geneva. Second, the candidate must gain regional approval, approval from the government office invested with international affairs of the country where the institution is located, and the approval of the director general of the WHO. To be designated as a WHO collaborating center an institution must demonstrate scientific and technical standing (national and international); a high level of scientific and technical leadership; stability in terms of personnel, activity, and funding; and ability, capacity, and readiness to contribute to WHO program activities.

WHO Collaborating Centers for Nursing

It has been only recently that nursing institutions have received recognition as WHO collaborating centers. In the early 1980s the European Regional Office of WHO-EURO designated seven nursing institutions or agencies in Europe to facilitate nursing research and practice in that Region. There are now 32 WHO collaborating centers for nursing worldwide, assuming an important role in furthering the goals of the WHO.

The Global Network of Collaborating Centers

The Global Network of the World Health Organization Collaborating Centers for Nursing and Midwifery Development is an independent organization founded by a network of collaborating centers. Its purpose is to support the efforts of participating members to improve nursing development toward "Health for All by the Year 2000" (HFA), thereby improving the quality of nursing services to meet health care needs of all people. The network has the primary goal of strengthening membership institutions in their efforts to improve nursing development in education, practice, research, and leadership—to achieve the goal of HFA through primary health care.

The formation of a global network of nursing institutions and organizations to support the goal of HFA was first discussed in March 1987 at an interregional workshop organized by WHO. The workshop was attended by 23 nursing leaders representing 20 different institutions, agencies, and organizations, a number of which are now represented in the network. At that time only five nursing institutions had been designated as WHO collaborating centers; four in Europe and one in the United States.

The 3-day meeting culminated in a "unanimous agreement to establish a global network of WHO Collaborating Centers for Nursing Development as an integral part of national and international strategies for achieving 'Health for All by the Year 2000 through Primary Health Care' " (*Report of the Secretariat*, 1992). The first general meeting of the network was held in April of 1988.

A brief description of the Global Network of WHO Collaborating Centers and their functions is outlined in notes distributed by Dr. M. J. Kim (personal communication, April 1990), then current head of the WHO. The notes also provide information about the process of attaining center designation. The functions of the network are as follows:

1. Coordination and technical cooperation
2. Dissemination and exchange of information
3. Research
4. Promotion and support of efforts of the network members in nursing development
5. Identification and securing of resources for network activities
6. Monitoring trends in health services development and assessment of these trends in terms of their implication for nursing development.

DORIS MODLY

See also
INTERNATIONAL CENTER FOR NURSING SCHOLARSHIP
INTERNATIONAL NURSING RESEARCH
RESEARCH CAREERS
WORLD HEALTH ORGANIZATION

WORLD WIDE WEB

The World Wide Web (WWW or Web) is one of several electronic networking protocols supported by the Internet. The Web was originally developed to allow information sharing about physics within internationally dispersed teams as well as the dissemination of information by support groups. The technologies of the Web have spread to other areas and attracted much interest in user support, resource discovery, and collaborative work areas. It has changed the way people view, create, and interact with information, data, and each other.

The Web is mostly used on the Internet, but they do not mean the same thing. The Web refers to a global body of information, an abstract space of knowledge; whereas the Internet refers to the physical side of the global network of information, a giant mass of cables and computers. Internet access is necessary in order to make full use of and participate in the Web.

The Web provides users of disparate computers, via client-server technology, with a consistent means to access a variety of media in a very simple manner. Using a graphic software interface, a browser on the user-client computer connects with host computers, the server. Both the client (browser) and server perform functions that enable hypertext file transfers and display on the client computer. The Web protocol enables the transfer of text, graphics, audio, and still images. The Web uses the Internet to transmit hypermedia documents between local or international computer users. Currently, there is much effort directed at solving the problems of transferring moving images and other media features.

Nursing and the Web

Because Web software was not developed until 1993, there is limited research addressing nursing use of the Web, specifically its unique incorporation of multimedia. The Web holds tremendous potential for nursing. Areas such as home care will come to include real-time, voice-activated, portable systems for patient access to nursing services. Hospital-based nurses will carry portable devices for real-time linkage with their patients. Nursing knowledge will be dispersed by consulting with virtual nurse experts. Nursing research of the Web and its potential as a new nursing care modality is necessary to maintain focus on the ultimate goal, patient care.

W. Scott Erdley
Susan M. Sparks

See also
COMPUTER SIMULATION
INTERNET
INTRANET
TELEPRESENCE
VIRTUAL REALITY

Y

YOUNG WOMEN AND DEPRESSION

Major depressive disorder (MDD) is common among premenopausal women. The National Co-Morbidity Study showed a 12-month MDD prevalence in women of 12.9% and a lifetime prevalence of 21.3% (Kessler, McGonagle, Zhao, et al., 1994). Depressive disorder begins early in adolescence for many women, and its incidence peaks before menopause. Women most commonly experience the chronic recurrent form of the disorder and often have comorbid seasonal affective disorder, premenstrual syndrome (PMS), and anxiety disorder. Recurrent MDD is characterized by its spontaneous

onset, severity, and longevity and is accompanied by significant impairment of familial, social, and occupational functioning. For women managing demanding familial and occupational careers, MDD is a powerful barrier to personal success and well-being.

Despite its impact, MDD often is not detected or appropriately treated in women. One reason is women's tendency to seek health care in primary care settings, where physicians do not often recognize or treat MDD. This is lamentable because effective treatment modalities have been developed and evaluated through empiricism, and guidelines exist for practice in primary care settings. Neither these treatment modalities nor the derived guidelines, however, are gender-specific. Depression treatment for women often does not address their specific relational needs and is not culturally sensitive, nor does it consider specific barriers like poverty, child care needs, or transportation (Hauenstein, 1996). Because of this, women frequently stop treatment before securing symptom remission.

Descriptive studies of women with MDD have linked the disorder to biological phenomena and interpersonal distress (Weissman & Olfson, 1995). Researchers using data from female twins have identified at least four interacting risk factor domains: early traumatic experiences, genetic factors, temperament, and interpersonal relationships (Kendler, Kessler, Neale, Heath, & Eaves, 1993). Recently, Hauenstein (1996a) has developed a theory-based, biopsychosocial causal model of depression for rural disadvantaged women to guide nursing intervention.

The Nursing Practice Paradigm for Depressed Women depicts two major pathways leading to depression. One portrays depression as occurring relatively spontaneously in vulnerable women. Excessive stress reactivity, early trauma, and the cyclical mood disturbance attendant on PMS are widely regarded as altering specific neurotransmitter and hormonal physiological systems. These alterations lead to MDD without an apparent external precipitating event.

Uncompensated environmental or personal stress triggers these same physiological mechanisms in the second pathway. Emphasized here is the role of physical, cognitive, emotional, and social resources in reducing the deleterious effects of external and internal stressors. This perspective permits nursing intervention to be directed to both reducing stressor effects and augmenting personal resources. Empiricism supporting the model is described elsewhere (Hauenstein, 1996a, 1997).

The model depicts four goals of nursing intervention: depression prevention, reduction in stress responsiveness, prevention of stress dysregulation, and promotion of recovery from MDD. Outcomes from several major research clinical trials of MDD treatment demonstrate that both somatic and psychosocial intervention are key to enacting these goals of treatment.

Nonpharmacological, somatic interventions for depressed women are supported by the nursing practice paradigm and are an important area for nursing research. Predominant among these are stress-reduction modalities, sleep-restoration techniques, dietary manipulation, and exercise. Stress-reduction techniques, including deep-breathing exercises, meditation, and progressive muscle relaxation, have shown promising effects in reducing excessive stress responses that initiate central neurotransmitter and peripheral cortisol changes antecedent to MDD.

Regular aerobic exercise improves neurotransmitter and hormonal responses to stress, thereby creating a more dynamic and effective stress response system. Diet regulation also is necessary, to manage cyclical weight gain associated with carbohydrate craving that is seen in 75% of women with affective disturbance. Sleep-restoration techniques and diet address circadian and appetite disturbances prominent in depression. One nursing researcher is pioneering research in sleep deprivation and phase variation interventions that promote circadian rhythm restoration in women (McEnany, 1990). Still, significant nursing research demonstrating improvement in physiological and psychological functioning with the use of nonpharmacological somatic therapies is sorely needed.

Psychosocial therapies are requisite to achieving the goals of the nursing practice paradigm and are critical in effectively treating women's depression. There is vigorous debate about what strategies are most effective in reducing depressive symptoms and improving functioning. Research has shown that cognitive-behavioral therapy is most effective in those with prominent cognitive dysfunction, and interpersonal therapy works best for those with predominately social dysfunction. Because women's relationships are critically important to them and pessimism and poor self-esteem are common, it often is impossible to determine where the greater source of dysfunction lies. Nursing has much to contribute in identifying factors that lead to an effective match between treatment modalities and specific characteristics of young women.

The nursing practice paradigm does not provide guidance about the needed intensity of treatment for depressed women. Most clinical trials have shown that brief treatment of 3–6 months is adequate to secure symptom remission. There are several issues germane to women's depression, however, that are not addressed in these studies. Women with comorbid personality disorder often require sustained intervention beyond that supported by outcomes of these trials. Needed treatment intensity also may vary among groups of women. Women with a history of current or past trauma may require frequent, sustained psychosocial treatment during different phases of treatment while the biological, psychological, and social concomitants of trauma are addressed. Women with recurrent MDD may require much different intensity and duration of treatment than do women who are early in their trajectory for recurrent illness or experiencing a first episode.

Somatic and psychosocial treatment for premenopausal rural women with MDD based on the nursing practice paradigm is currently under investigation (Hauenstein, 1997). Each aspect of the model is tested, with the basic premise of reducing risks for depression while augmenting client resources. Somatic therapies implemented include stress reduction modalities, sleep restoration, dietary regulation, exercise, and augmentation of social support. Antidepressant medication is provided according to specific criteria. Psychosocial treatment is provided as well, aimed at increasing personal resiliency, problem solving, and use of social support. Cognitive-behavioral therapy and psychoeducation predominate among treatment strategies used.

Treatment is implemented according to a structured protocol in 12 sessions delivered in 3 months, with a protracted period of maintenance and follow-up for 12 months. Treatment is administered by clinical nurse specialists in collaboration with each woman's primary care provider and is offered in the client's home to overcome specific barriers to treatment.

Early outcomes indicate that women show symptomatic improvement with the described nursing intervention. Functional role limitations also are reduced with intervention. Treatment gains appear to be maintained for at least 6 months. Preliminary data indicate, however, that rural, low-income women may not tolerate the intensity of treatment involved in the 12-week sequence. About half of women entering treatment fail to complete the 12 sessions.

Early findings from this study illustrate the numerous challenging problems for nurses in providing depression treatment for women. Novel nursing approaches that illuminate unique etiological factors in specific populations of women are needed as well as innovative programs that match therapies to discrete populations. Intervention intensity and longevity also are fruitful areas for nursing research. Because nurses are often positioned to care for depressed women, nursing research and practice can contribute to reducing this health care need.

EMILY J. HAUENSTEIN

See also
BEHAVIORAL RESEARCH
CHRONIC MENTAL ILLNESS
NUTRITION
RELAXATION TECHNIQUES
WOMEN'S HEALTH RESEARCH

REFERENCES

Aaronson, L. S., Teel, C., Cassmeyer, V., Neuberger, G. B., Pallikkathayil, L., Pierce, J., Press, A. N., Williams, P. D., & Wingate, A. (in press). Defining and measuring fatigue. *Image: The Journal of Nursing Scholarship.*

Abbey, J. C., Andrews, C., Avigliano, K., Blossom, R., Bunke, B., Clark, E., Engberg, N., Healy, P., Halliburton, P., & Peterson, J. (1973). A pilot study: The control of shivering during hypothermia by a clinical nursing measure. *Journal of Neurosurgical Nursing, 5,* 78–88.

Abdellah, F. (1959). Improving the teaching of nursing through research in patient care. In L. E. Heidgerken (Ed.), *Improvement of nursing through research.* Washington, DC: Catholic University of America Press.

Abdellah, F., & Levine, E. (1965). *Better patient care through nursing research.* New York: Macmillan.

Abdellah, F. G., & Levine, E. (1979). *Better patient care through nursing research* (2nd ed.). New York: Macmillan.

Abdellah, F. G., & Levine, E. (1986). *Better patient care through nursing research* (3rd ed.). New York: Macmillan.

Abdellah, F. G., & Levine, E. (1994). *Preparing nursing research for the 21st century.* New York: Springer Publishing.

Abraham, I. L., Chalifoux, Z., & Evers, G. C. M. (1992). Conditions, interventions, and outcomes: A quantitative analysis of nursing research (1981–1990). In P. Moritz (Ed.), *Patient outcomes research: Examining the effectiveness of nursing practice* (NIH Publication No. 93-3411, pp. 70–87). Bethesda, MD: National Institutes of Health.

Abraham, I. L., Currie, L. J., Neese, J. B., Yi, E. S., & Thompson-Heisterman, A. A. (1994). Risk profiles for nursing home placement of rural elderly: A cluster analysis of psychogeriatric indicators. *Archives of Psychiatric Nursing, 8,* 262–271.

Abraham, I. L., Neundorfer, M. M., & Currie, L. J. (1992). Effects of group interventions on cognition and depression in nursing home residents. *Nursing Research, 41,* 196–202.

Achenbaum, W. A. (1995). *Crossing frontiers: Gerontology emerges as a science.* Cambridge: Cambridge University Press.

Acute Pain Management Panel. (1992). *Acute pain management: Operative or medical procedures and trauma: Clinical practice guideline* (DHHS Publication No. [AHCPR]91-0046). Rockville, MD: U.S. Department of Health and Human Services, Agency for Health Care Policy and Research.

Adams, M. (1986). Aging: Gerontological nursing research. In H. H. Werley, J. J. Fitzpatrick, & R. L. Taunton (Eds.), *Annual review of nursing research* (pp. 77–103). New York: Springer.

Aday, L. A. (1993). *At risk in America: The health and health care needs of vulnerable populations in the United States.* San Francisco: Jossey-Bass.

Aday, L. (1994). Health status of vulnerable populations. *Annual Review of Public Health, 15,* 487–509.

Affonso, D. D. (1992). Postpartum depression: A nursing perspective on women's health and behaviors. *Image: Journal of Nursing Scholarship, 24,* 215–221.

Affonso, D. D. (1996). Passion for improving the health, health care system and health professional training of APIAs. *Asian American and Pacific Islander Journal of Health, 4,* 199–205.

Affonso, D. D., DeLeon, P. H., Raymond, J. S., & Mayberry, L. J. (1994). Promoting community partnerships: Public policy initiatives related to prenatal care. *Clinical Psychology: Science and Practice, 1,* 13–24.

Affonso, D. D., Mayberry, L. J., Graham, K., Shibuya, J., & Kunimoto, J. (1993). Prenatal and postpartum care in Hawaii: A community-based approach. *Journal of Obstetric, Gynecologic, and Neonatal Nursing, 22,* 320–325.

Affonso, D. D., Mayberry, L. J., Graham, K., Shibuya, J., Kunimoto, J., & Kunimoto, M. (1992). Adaptation themes for prenatal care delivered by public health nurses. *Public Health Nursing, 9,* 172–176.

Affonso, D. D., Mayberry, L. J., Lovett, S., Paul, S., Johnson, B., Nussbaum, R., & Newman, L. (1993). Pregnancy and postpartum symptoms. *Journal of Women's Health, 2,* 157–163.

Agency for Health Care Policy and Research (AHCPR). (1995). *Cardiac rehabilitation clinical practice guidelines* (AHCPR Publication No. 96-0672). Washington, DC: U.S. Department of Heath and Human Services.

Agency for Health Care Policy and Research. (1996a). Making vaccines free to providers may not improve childhood immunization rates. *Research Activities, 195,* 10.

Agency for Health Care Policy and Research. (1996b). *Smoking cessation* (Publication No. 96-0692). Rockville, MD: Author.

Ahern, D. K., Gorkin, L., Anderson, J. L., Tierney, C., Hallstrom, A., Ewart, C., Capone, R. J., Schron, E., Kornfeld, D., Herd, J. A., Richardson, D. W., & Follick, M. J., for the CAPS investigators. (1990). Biobehavioral variables and mortality or cardiac arrest in the Cardiac Arrthymia Pilot Study (CAPS). *American Journal of Cardiology, 66*(1), 59–62.

Ahrens, T., Pennick, J. C., & Tucker, M. K. (1995). Frequency requirements for zeroing transducers in hemodynamic monitoring. *American Journal of Critical Care, 4,* 466–471.

Aish, A. E., & Isenberg, M. (1996). Effects of Orem-based nursing intervention on nutritional self-care of myocardial infarction patients. *International Journal of Nursing Studies, 33,* 259–270.

Ajzen, I. (1985). From intentions to actions: A theory of planned behavior. In J. Kuhl & J. Beckman (Eds.), *Action-control: From cognition to behavior* (pp. 11–39). Heidelberg: Springer Verlag.

Ajzen, I. (1988). *Attitudes, personality and behavior.* Chicago: Dorsey Press.

Akers, P. A. S. (1991). An algorithmic approach to clinical decision making. *Oncology Nursing Forum, 18,* 1159–1163.

Alford-Smith, D. L. (1997). *Health attitudes and practices of low income Blacks and Whites in Cleveland, OH.* Unpublished manuscript, Frances Payne Bolton School of Nursing, Case Western Reserve University at Cleveland, OH.

Algase, D. L., Beck, C., Kolanowski, A., Whall, A., Berent, S., Richards, K., & Beattie, E. (1996). Need-driven dementia-compromised behavior: An alternative view of disruptive behavior. *American Journal of Alzheimer's Disease, 11*(6), 10–19.

Allan, J. D. (1988). Knowing what to weigh: Women's self-care activities related to weight. *Advances in Nursing Science, 11*(1), 47–60.

Allan, J. D. (1989). Women who successfully manage their weight. *Western Journal of Nursing Research, 11,* 657–675.

The Alma-Ata conference on primary health care. (1978). *WHO Chronicle, 32,* 409–430.

Als, H. (1991). Neurobehavioral organization of the newborn: Opportunity for assessment and intervention. *NIDA Research Monographs, 114,* 106–116.

Alston, M. H., & Robinson, B. H. (1992). Nurses' attitudes toward suicide. *Omega: Journal of Death and Dying, 25,* 205–215.

American Academy of Nursing. (1976). *Primary care by nurses: Sphere of responsibility and accountability.* Kansas City, MO: American Nurses Association.

American Academy of Nursing. (1995). *Promoting cultural competence in and through nursing education.* Washington, DC: Author.

American Academy of Nursing. (1996). *Official bylaws of the American Academy of Nursing.* Unpublished document.

American Academy of Pediatrics, Committee on Nutrition. (1993). *Pediatric nutrition handbook.* Elk Grove, IL: American Academy of Pediatrics.

American Academy of Pediatrics, Committee on Practice and Ambulatory Medicine. (1997). Pediatrician's responsibility for infant nutrition. *Pediatrics, 99,* 749–751.

American Association of Colleges of Nursing. (1986). *Essentials of colleges and university education for nursing.* Washington, DC: American Association of Colleges of Nursing.

American Association of Critical Care Nurses. (1993). Evaluation of the effects of heparinized and nonheparinized flush solutions on the patency of arterial pressure monitoring lines: The AACN Thunder Project. *American Journal of Critical Care, 2,* 3–15.

American College of Nurse-Midwives. (1978). *Definition of a certified nurse-midwife and nurse-midwifery practice.* Washington, DC: Author.

American College of Nurse-Midwives. (1992). *Standards for the practice of nurse-midwifery.* Washington, DC: Author.

American Colleges of Nurse-Midwives. (1993). *Core competencies for basic nurse-midwifery practice.* Washington, DC: Author.

American Colleges of Nurse-Midwives. (1996). *Education programs accredited by the ACNM division of accreditation.* Washington, DC: Author.

American College of Obstetricians and Gynecologists. (1989). Intrapartum fetal heart rate monitoring. *ACOG Technical Bulletin.* Washington, DC: Author.

American Heart Association. (1993). Human blood pressure determination by sphygmomanometry. *Circulation, 88,* 2462–2465.

American Heart Association. (1997). *Heart and stroke statistical update.* Dallas, TX: Author.

American Journal of Nursing, in conjunction with the National Library of Medicine. (1966). *International nursing index.* New York: Author.

American Medical Informatics Association, Board of Directors. (1994). Standards for medical identifiers, codes, and messages needed to create an efficient computer-stored medical record. *Journal of the American Medical Informatics Association, 1,* 1–7.

American Nurses Association. (1975). *Human rights guidelines for nurses in clinical and other research.* Kansas City, MO: Author.

American Nurses Association. (1976). *One strong voice: The story of the American Nurses Association.* Kansas City, MO: Lowell Press.

American Nurses Association. (1980). *Nursing's social policy statement*. Kansas City, MO: Author.

American Nurses Association. (1982). *A challenge for change: The role of gerontological nursing*. Kansas City, MO: Author.

American Nurses Association. (1985a). *Code for nurses*. Washington, DC: Author.

American Nurses Association. (1985b). *Code for nurses with interpretive statements*. Kansas City, MO: Author.

American Nurses Association. (1985c). *Human rights guidelines for nurses in clinical and other research*. Kansas City, MO: Author.

American Nurses Association. (1989). *Education for participation in nursing research*. Kansas City, MO: Author.

American Nurses Association. (1990). *American Nurses Association continuing education program*. Washington, DC: Author.

American Nurses Association. (1991a). *Nursing's agenda for health care reform*. Washington, DC: Author.

American Nurses Association. (1991b). *Standards of clinical nursing practice*. Washington, DC: Author.

American Nurses Association. (1992a). *Compendium of position statements on the nurse's role in end-of-life decisions*. Washington, DC: Author.

American Nurses Association. (1992b). *Nursing and the American Nurses Association*. Washington, DC: Author.

American Nurses Association. (1992c). *Nursing's agenda for health care reform*. Washington, DC: Author.

American Nurses Association. (1993). *Nursing facts ANA*. Washington, DC: Author.

American Nurses Association. (1994a). *The scope of practice for nursing informatics*. Washington, DC: Author.

American Nurses Association. (1994b). *Today's registered nurse: Numbers and demographics*. Washington, DC: Author.

American Nurses Association. (1995a). In N. Lang (Ed.), *An emerging framework: Data system advances for clinical nursing practice*. Washington, DC: American Nurses Publishing.

American Nurses Association. (1995b). *Nursing: A social policy statement*. Washington, DC: American Nurses.

American Nurses Association. (1995c). *Position statement on restructuring, work redesign, and the job and career security of registered nurses*. Washington, DC: Author.

American Nurses Association. (1995d). *Summary of the Lewin-VHI, Inc. report: Nursing report card for acute care settings*. Washington, DC: Author.

American Nurses Association. (1997). *End of life care: Ethical dimensions*. A Continuing Education Monograph for Nurses. Research Triangle Park, NC: Glaxco Wellcome Health Care Education.

American Nurses Association Cabinet on Nursing Research. (1985). *Directions for nursing research: Toward the twenty-first century*. Kansas City, MO: American Nurses Association.

American Nurses Association Center for Nursing Research. (1980). Generating a scientific basis for nursing practice: Research priorities for the 1980's. *Nursing Research, 29*, 219.

American Pain Society, Quality of Care Committee. (1995). Quality improvement guidelines for the treatment of acute pain and cancer pain. *Journal of the American Medical Association, 274*, 1874–1880.

American Psychiatric Association. (1994). *Diagnostic and statistical manual of mental disorders* (DSM-IV) (4th ed. rev.). Washington, DC: Fiest, M. B. (ed.).

Anderson, G. C. (1977). The mother and her newborn: Mutual caregivers. *Journal of Obstetric, Gynecologic, and Neonatal Nursing (JOGNN), 6*(5), 50–57.

Anderson, G. C. (1989). Risk in mother-infant separation postbirth. *Image: Journal of Nursing Scholarship, 21*, 196–199.

Anderson, G. C. (1991a). Current knowledge about skin-to-skin (kangaroo) care for preterm infants. *Journal of Perinatology, 11*, 216–226.

Anderson, G. C. (1995). Touch and the kangaroo method. In T. Field (Ed.), *Touch and infancy* (pp. 35–51). Hillsdale, NJ: Erlbaum.

Anderson, G. C. (in press). Kangaroo care of the premature infant. In E. Goldson (Ed.), *Nurturing the premature infant: Developmental interventions in the neonatal intensive care nursery*. New York: Oxford University Press.

Anderson, I. (1997). The Malmo mammography screening trial: Update on results and a harm-benefit analyses. In *NIH Consensus Development Conference: Breast cancer screening for women ages 40–49: Program and abstracts* (pp. 51–53). Bethesda, MD: National Institutes of Health.

Anderson, J. (1991b). Immigrant women speak of chronic illness: The social construction of the devalued self. *Journal of Advanced Nursing, 16*, 710–717.

Anderson-Loften, W., Wood, D., & Whitefield, L. A. (1995). Case study of nursing case management in a rural hospital. *Nursing Administration Quarterly, 19*(3), 33–40.

Andranovich, G., & Irposa, G. (1993). *Doing urban research: Vol. 33. Applied social research methods*. Newbury Park, CA: Sage.

Andrews, C., & Andrews, E. (1983). Nursing, maternal postures and fetal position. *Nursing Research, 32*, 336–340.

Ansell, D., Lacey, L., Whitman, S., Chen, E., & Phillips, C. (1994). A nurse-delivered intervention to reduce barriers to breast and cervical cancer screening in Chicago inner cities. *Public Health Reports, 1,* 104–111.

Apter, M. J. (1982). *The experience of motivation: The theory of psychological reversals.* London: Academic Press.

Apter, M. J. (1989). *Reversal theory: Motivation, emotion, and personality.* London: Routledge.

Aravanis, S. C., Adelman, R. D., Breckman, R., Fulmer, T., Holder, E., Lachs, M., O'Brien, J. G., & Sanders, A. B. (1992). *Diagnostic and treatment guidelines on elder abuse and neglect.* Chicago: American Medical Association.

Archbold, P. G., & Stewart, B. J. (1996). The nature of the family caregiving role and nursing interventions for caregiving families. In E. A. Swanson & T. Tripp-Reimer (Eds.), *Advances in gerontological nursing* (Vol. 1, pp. 133–157). New York: Springer Publishing.

Archer, S. B., Burnett, R. J., & Fischer, J. E. (1996). Current uses and abuses of total parenteral nutrition. *Advances in Surgery, 29,* 165–189.

Argyris, C. (1987). Seeking truth and actionable knowledge: How the scientific method inhibits both. *Philosophica, 40,* 5–21.

Argyris, C., Putnam, R., & Smith, D. M. (1985). *Action science.* San Francisco: Jossey-Bass.

Argyris, C., & Schön, D. (1974). *Theories in practice: Increasing professional effectiveness.* San Francisco: Jossey-Bass.

Arras, J. D. (1994). The technologic tether: An introduction to ethical and social issues in high-tech home care. *Hastings Center Report, 24* (Special suppl.), 51–52.

Arthur, C. (1992). Did reality move for you? *New Scientist, 134,* 22–27.

Artinian, N. T. (1993). Resources: Factors that mediate the stress-outcome relationship. In J. Barnfather & B. Lyon (Eds.), *Stress and coping: State of the science and implications for nursing theory, research and practice.* Indianapolis: Center Nursing Press of Sigma Theta Tau International.

Atterbury, J. L., Groome, L. J., & Baker, S. I. (1996). Elevated midtrimester mean arterial blood pressure in women with severe pre-eclampsia. *Applied Nursing Research, 9,* 161–166.

Augustyn, M., & Maiman, L. A. (1994). Psychological and social barriers to prenatal care. *Women's Health Issues, 5,* 1049–1067.

Austin, J. K. (1991). Family adaptation to a child's chronic illness. *Annual Review of Nursing Research, 9,* 103–120.

Austin, J. (1996a). A model of family adaptation to new-onset childhood epilepsy. *Journal of Neuroscience Nursing, 28*(2), 82–92.

Austin, J. K. (1996b). Behavior problems in children with epilepsy. In A. B. McBride & J. K. Austin (Eds.), *Psychiatric–mental health nursing: Integrating the behavioral and biological sciences* (pp. 107–132). Philadelphia: W. B. Saunders.

Austin, J. K., Risinger, M. W., & Beckett, L. A. (1992). Correlates of behavior problems in children with epilepsy. *Epilepsia, 33,* 1115–1122.

Austin, J. L. (1975). *How to do things with words* (2nd ed.). Oxford: Oxford University Press.

Auvil-Novak, S. E. (1997). A middle range theory of chronotherapeutic intervention for post-surgical pain. *Nursing Research, 46,* 66–71.

Auvil-Novak, S. E., Novak, R. D., & El Sanadi, N. (1996). Twenty-four-hour pattern in emergency room presentation for sickle cell vaso-occlusive pain crisis. *Chronobiology International, 13,* 449–456.

Aydelotte, M. (1973). *Nurse staffing methodology: A review and critique of selected literature* (DHEW Publication No. 73-433). Washington, DC: National Institutes of Health.

Aydelotte, M. K., & Peterson K. H. (1991). Nursing taxonomies: State of the art. In R. M. Carroll-Johnson (Ed.), *Classification of nursing diagnoses: Proceedings of the Ninth Conference.* Philadelphia: Lippincott.

Baar, A., Moores, B., & Rhys-Hearn, C. (1973). A review of the various methods of measuring the dependency of patients on nursing staff. *International Journal of Nursing Studies, 10,* 195–203.

Backer, T., & Koon, S. (1995). Sharing the wealth of ideas: Demonstrate, evaluate, disseminate, repeat. *Foundation News and Commentary, 36*(2), 28–34.

Bailey, K. D. (1994). *Typologies and taxonomies: An introduction to classification techniques.* Thousand Oaks, CA: Sage.

Bain, R. J. I., Fox, J. P., Jagger, J., Davies, M. K., Littler, W. A., & Murray, R. G. (1992). Serum cortisol levels predict infarct size and patient mortality. *International Journal of Cardiology, 37,* 145–150.

Baker, C. (1995). The development of the self-care ability to detect early signs of relapse among individuals who have schizophrenia. *Archives of Psychiatric Nursing, 9,* 261–268.

Baker, S. P., O'Neill, B., Ginsburg, M. J., & Li, G. (1992). *The injury fact book* (2nd ed.). New York: Oxford University Press.

Baltes, P. B., & Danish, S. J. (1980). Intervention in life-span development and aging. In R. R. Turner & H. W. Reese (Eds.), *Life-span developmental psychology* (pp. 49–78). New York: Academic Press.

Bandura, A. (1986). *Social foundations of thought and action: A social cognitive theory.* Englewood Cliffs, NJ: Prentice-Hall.

Bandura, A. (1997). *Self-efficacy: The exercise of control.* New York: W. H. Freeman.

Bankert, K., Daughtridge, S., Meehan, M., & Colburn, L. (1996). The application of collaborative benchmarking to the prevention and treatment of pressure ulcers. *Advances in Wound Care: The Journal for Prevention and Healing, 9*(2), 21–29.

Bankert, M. (1989). *Watchful care: A history of America's nurse anesthetists.* New York: Continuum.

Barkauskas, V. (1990). Home health care. In J. J. Fitzpatrick, R. L. Taunton, & J. Q. Benoliel (Eds.), *Annual Review of Nursing Research* (Vol. 8, pp. 103–132). New York: Springer Publishing.

Barnard, K. E. (1983). Nursing research related to infants and young children. In H. Werley & J. J. Fitzpatrick (Eds.), *Annual Review of Nursing Research* (Vol. 1, pp. 3–25). New York: Springer Publishing.

Barnard, K. E., & Bee, H. (1983). The impact of temporally-patterned stimulation on the development of preterm infants. *Child Development, 54,* 1156–1167.

Barnard, K. E., & Eyres, S. J. (1979). *Child health assessment: Part 2. The first year of life.* Hyattsville, MD: U.S. Department of Health, Education, and Welfare, Public Health Service.

Barnard, K. E., Hammond, M. A., Booth, C. L., Bee, H. L., Mitchell, S. K., & Spieker, S. (1989). Measurement and meaning of parent child interaction. In F. Morrison, C. Lord, & D. Keating (Eds.), *Applied developmental psychology* (Vol. 3, pp. 287–296). New York: Academic Press.

Barnard, R. M., & Reame, N. E. (1996). Perimenopause. In J. A. Lewis & J. Bernstein (Eds.), *Women's health: A relational perspective across the life cycle* (pp. 144–191). Boston: Jones and Bartlett.

Barnes, C. M. (1975). Levels of consciousness indicated by responses of children to phenomena in the intensive care unit. *Maternal-Child Nursing Journal, 4,* 215–285.

Barnes, D., Eribes, C., Juarbe, T., Nelson, M., Proctor, D., Sawyer, L., Shaul, M., & Meleis, A. I. (1995). Primary health care and primary care: A confusion of philosophies. *Nursing Outlook, 43,* 7–16.

Barnfather, J. S., & Lyon, B. L. (1993). *Stress and coping: State of the science and implications for nursing theory, research and practice.* Indianapolis, IN: Sigma Theta Tau International.

Barnsteiner, J. H. (1993). The online journal of knowledge synthesis for nursing. *Reflections, 19*(1), 8, Spring.

Baron, R. A., & Byrne, D. (1994). *Social psychology: Understanding human interaction* (7th ed.). Boston: Allyn and Bacon.

Barrett, E. A. M. (1993). Virtual reality: A health patterning modality for nursing in space. *Visions, 1*(1), 10–21.

Barthes, R. (1974). *Introduction to the structural analysis of the narratives* (R. Miller, Trans.). New York: Hill & Wang.

Bartlett, E. E. (1985). At last, a definition. *Patient Education and Counseling, 7,* 323.

Bartlett, S. J., Wadden, T. A., & Vogt, R. A. (1996). Psychosocial consequences of weight cycling. *Journal of Consulting and Clinical Psychology, 64,* 587–592.

Barton, J. A. (1991). Parental adaptation to adolescent drug abuse: An ethnographic study of role formulation in response to courtesy stigma. *Public Health Nursing, 8,* 39–45.

Bassett, K. (1996). Anthropology, clinical pathology and the electronic fetal monitor: Lessons from the heart. *Social Science and Medicine, 42,* 281–292.

Basson, P. (1967). The gerontological nursing literature. *Nursing Research, 16*(3), 267–272.

Bates-Jensen, B. (1990). New pressure ulcer status tool. *Decubitus, 3*(3), 14–15.

Baumann, L. J., Zimmerman, R. S., & Leventhal, H. (1989). An experiment in common sense: Education at blood pressure screening. *Patient Education and Counseling, 14,* 53–67.

Bearn, J., & Wessely, S. (1994). Neurobiological aspects of the chronic fatigue syndrome. *European Journal of Clinical Investigation, 24,* 79–90.

Beck, A. T. (1978). *Cognitive therapy and emotional disorders.* New York: International Universities Press.

Beck, C., Heacock, P., Rapp, C. G., & Mercer, S. O. (1993, November/December). Assisting cognitively impaired elders with activities of daily living. *American Journal of Alzheimer's Care and Related Disorders and Research,* pp. 11–20.

Beck, C. K., Cronin-Stubbs, D., Buckwalter, K. C., & Rapp, C. G. (in press). Managing cognitive impairment and depression in the elderly. In A. S. Hinshaw, S. Feetham, & J. Shaver (Eds.), *Handbook of clinical nursing research.*

Beck, C. T. (1992a). Caring between nursing students and physically/mentally handicapped children: A phenomenological study. *Journal of Nursing Education, 31,* 1–6.

Beck, C. T. (1992b). The lived experience of postpartum depression: A phenomenological study. *Nursing Research, 41,* 166–170.

Beck, C. T. (1993). Teetering on the edge: A substantive theory of postpartum depression. *Nursing Research, 42,* 42–48.

Beck, C. T. (1996a). A meta-analysis of predictors of postpartum depression. *Nursing Research, 45,* 297–303.

Beck, C. T. (1996b). The effects of postpartum depression on maternal-infant interaction: A meta-analysis. *Nursing Research, 44,* 298–304.

Beck, C. T. (1996c). Postpartum depressed mothers' experiences interacting with their children. *Nursing Research, 45,* 98–104.

Becker, D. M., Hill, D. R., Jackson, J. S., Levine, D. M., Stillman, F. A., & Weiss, S. M. (1992). *Health behavior research in minority populations: Access, design, and implementation* (NIH Publication No. 92-2965). Washington, DC: U.S. Government Printing Office.

Becker, L. B., Han, B. H., Meyer, P. M., Wright, F. A., Rhodes, K. V., Smith, D. W., & Barrett, J. (1993). Racial differences in the incidence of cardiac arrest and subsequent survival: The CPR Chicago Project. *New England Journal of Medicine, 329,* 600–606.

Becker, P. T., Grunwald, P. C., Moorman, J., & Stuhr, S. (1993). Effects of developmental care on behavioral organization in very-low-birth-weight infants. *Nursing Research, 42,* 214–220.

Beezhold, D. M., Koystal, D. A., & Wiseman, J. (1994). The transfer of protein allergies from latex gloves. *AORN Journal, 59,* 605–613.

Beisser, A. R., & Rose, G. (1972). *Mental health consultations and education.* Los Angeles: Institute Press.

Bell, K. E., & Mills, J. I. (1989). Certified nurse-midwife effectiveness in the health maintenance organization obstetric team. *Obstetrics and Gynecology, 74,* 112–116.

Bell, R. P., & McGrath, J. (1996). Implementing a research based kangaroo care program in the NICU. In L. Brown (Ed.), *Nursing clinics of North America: Maternal/fetal nursing* (Vol. 31, pp. 387–403). Philadelphia: Saunders.

Bellack, J., & Fleming, J. (1996). The use of projective techniques in pediatric nursing research from 1984–1993. *Journal of Pediatric Nursing, 11,* 10–28.

Bem, S. L. (1974). The measurement of psychological androgyny. *Journal of Consulting and Clinical Psychology, 42,* 155–162.

Benarroch, E. E. (1993). The central autonomic network: Functional organization, dysfunction and perspective. *Mayo Clinic Proceedings, 68,* 908–1001.

Benenson, A. S. (1995). *Control of communicable diseases in man* (16th ed.). Washington, DC: American Public Health Association.

Benner, P. (1984). *From novice to expert: Power and excellence in nursing practice.* Palo Alto, CA: Addison-Wesley.

Benner, P. (1985). Quality of life: A phenomenological perspective on explanation, prediction, and understanding in nursing science. *Advances in Nursing Science, 8*(1), 1–14.

Benner, P. (Ed.). (1994). *Interpretive phenomenology: Embodiment, caring and ethics in health and illness.* Thousand Oaks, CA: Sage.

Benner, P., Panner, C. A., & Chesla, C. (1996). *Expertise in nursing practice: Caring, clinical judgment, and ethics.* New York: Springer.

Bennett, J. A. (1995). "Methodological notes on empathy": Further considerations. *Advances in Nursing Science, 18,* 35–50.

Bennett, L. (1991). Adolescent girls' experience of witnessing marital violence: A phenomenological study. *Journal of Advanced Nursing, 16,* 431–438.

Benoliel, J. Q. (1983). Nursing research on death dying and terminal illness: Development, present state, and prospects. In H. Werley & J. Fitzpatrick (Eds.), *Annual Review of Nursing Research* (Vol. 1, pp. 105–123). New York: Springer Publishing.

Benoliel, J. Q. (1994). Death and dying as a field of inquiry. In I. B. Corless, B. B. Germino, & M. Pittman (Eds.), *Dying, death and bereavement: Theoretical perspectives and other ways of knowing* (pp. 3–14). Boston: Jones & Bartlett.

Berenson, R. A. (1984). *Intensive care units: Clinical outcomes, costs, and decision making* (OTA-HCS-28). Washington, DC: U.S. Government Printing Office.

Berg, L. (1994). Alzheimer's disease. In J. C. Morris (Ed.), *Handbook of dementing illnesses* (pp. 229–242). New York: Marcel Dekker.

Bergstrom, N., Bennett, M. A., & Carlson, C. E. (1994). *Treating pressure ulcers.* Clinical practice guideline No. 15 (AHCPR Publication No. 94-0047). Rockville, MD: U.S. Department of Health and Human Services, Agency for Health Care Policy and Research.

Bergstrom, N., Braden, B., Laguzza, A., & Holman, V. (1987). The Braden Scale for Predicting Pressure Sore Risk. *Nursing Research, 36,* 205–210.

Bernard-Bonnin, A. C., Stachenko, S., Bonin, D., Charette, C., & Rousseau, E. (1995). Self-management teaching programs and morbidity of pediatric asthma: A meta-analysis. *Journal of Allergy and Clinical Immunology, 1,* 34–41.

Berrio, M., & Levesque, M. (1996). Advance directives: Most patients don't have one—do yours? *American Journal of Nursing, 96*(8), 25–29.

Berry, D. (1993). The emerging epidemiology of rural AIDS. *Journal of Rural Health, 2,* 293–302.

Berry, D. L., & Catanzaro, M. (1992). Persons with cancer and their return to the workplace. *Cancer Nursing, 13,* 40–46.

Biegel, D. E., Sales, E., & Schulz, R. (1991). *Family caregiving in chronic illness: Alzheimer's disease, cancer, heart disease, mental illness, and stroke.* Newbury Park, CA: Sage.

Bierman, E. (1992). Atherogenesis in diabetes. *Arteriosclerosis and Thrombosis, 12,* 647–656.

Bigos, S., Bowyer, O., Braen, G., Brown, K., Deyo, R., Haldeman, S., Hart, J. L., Johnson, E. W., Keller, R., Kido, D., Liang, M. H., Nelson, R. M., Nordin, M., Owens, B. D., Schwartz, R., Stewart, D. H., Jr., Susman, J., Triano, J. J., Tripp, L. C., Turk, D. C., Watts,

C., & Weinstein, J. N. (1994). *Acute low back problems in adults* (Clinical Practice Guideline No. 14). Rockville, MD: U.S. Department of Health and Human Services, Agency for Health Care Policy and Research, Public Health Service.

Binstock, M. A., & Wolde-Tsadik, G. (1995). Alternative prenatal care: Impact of reduced visit frequency, focused visits, and continuity of care. *Journal of Reproductive Medicine, 40,* 507–512.

Bishop, S., & Ingersoll, G. (1989). Effects of marital conflict and family structure on the self-concepts of pre- and early adolescents. *Journal of Youth and Adolescence, 18*(1), 25–38.

Bishop, W., & Goldie, S. (1962). *A bio-bibliography of Florence Nightingale.* London: Dawson's, for the International Council of Nurses.

Bissell, R. A., Becker, B. M., & Burkle, F. M. (1996). Health care personnel in disaster response: Reversible roles or territorial imperatives? *Emergency Medicine Clinics of North America, 14,* 267–288.

Bjurstam, N., Bjorneld, L., & Duffy W. S. (1997). The Gothenburg breast screening trial: Results from 11 years follow up. In *NIH Consensus Development Conference: Breast cancer screening for women ages 40–49: Program and abstracts* (pp. 63–64). Bethesda, MD: National Institutes of Health.

Blackburn, S. T., & Barnard, K. E. (1985). Analysis of caregiving events relating to preterm infants in the special care unit. In A. W. Gottfried & J. L. Gaiter (Eds.), *Infant stress under intensive care* (pp. 113–129). Baltimore: University Park Press.

Blackmon, P. W., Marino, C. A., Aukward, R. K., Bresnahan, R. E., Carlisle, R. G., Goldenberg, K. L., Hiller, J. M., Lowke, G. A., & Patterson, J. T. (ANSER Analytic Services). (1982). *Evaluation of the medical information system at the NIH Clinical Center* (Vols. 1–6). Springfield, VA: National Technical Information Service.

Blake, J., Carter, M., O'Brien-Pallas, L., & McGillis-Hall, L. (1995). A surgical process management tool. In *Proceedings of MedInfo '95* (pp. 527–531).

Blalock, H. M. (1960). *Social statistics.* New York: McGraw-Hill.

Blau, P. (1964). *Exchange and power in social life.* New York: Wiley.

Blegen, M. A. (1993). Nurses' job satisfaction: A meta-analysis of related variables. *Nursing Research, 42,* 36–41.

Blegen, M. A., & Tripp-Reimer, T. (1997). Implications of nursing taxonomies for middle-range theory development. *Advances in Nursing Science, 19*(3), 37–49.

Blesch, K., Paice, J., Wickham, R., Harte, N., Schnoor, D., Purl, S., Rehwalt, M., Kopp, P., Manson, S., Coveny, S., McHale, M., & Cahill, M. (1991). Correlates of fatigue in people with breast or lung cancer. *Oncology Nursing Forum, 18,* 81–87.

Bleyer, A. (1990). The impact of childhood cancer on the United States and the world. *Ca: A Cancer Journal for Clinicians, 40,* 355–367.

Bliss-Holtz, J. (1995). Methods of newborn infant temperature monitoring: A research review. *Issues in Comprehensive Pediatric Nursing, 18,* 287–298.

Blomquist, K. (1986). Replication of research. *Research in Nursing and Health, 9,* 193–194.

Bloom, B. L. (1984). *Community mental health: A general introduction* (2nd ed.). Belmont, CA: Brooks/Cole.

Blos, P. (1979). The second individuation process. In P. Blos (Ed.), *The adolescent passage: Developmental issues of adolescence* (pp. 141–170). New York: International University Press.

Bodkin, N. L., Hannah, J. S., Ortmeyer, H. K., & Hansen, B. C. (1993). Central obesity in rhesus monkeys: Association with hyperinsulinemia, insulin resistance and hypertriglyceridemia? *International Journal of Obesity and Related Metabolic Disorders, 17,* 53–61.

Boehm, S. (1992). Patient contracting. In G. M. Bulechek & J. C. McCloskey (Eds.), *Nursing interventions: Essential nursing treatments* (2nd ed., pp. 425–433). Philadelphia: W. B. Saunders.

Boehm, S., Schlenk, E. A., Raleigh, E., & Ronis, D. (1993). Behavioral analysis and behavioral strategies to improve self-management of type II diabetes. *Clinical Nursing Research, 2,* 327–344.

Bollen, K. A. (1989). *Structural equations with latent variables.* New York: Wiley.

Bollen, K. A., & Long, J. S. (Eds.). (1993). *Testing structural equation models.* Newbury Park, CA: Sage.

Bonica, J. J. (1990). *The management of pain* (2nd ed.). Philadelphia: Delea and Febiger.

Bookbinder, M., Coyle, N., & Thaler, H. (in press). Implementing national standards for cancer pain management. *Journal of Pain and Symptom Management.*

Borgman, C. L. (1990). Editor's introduction. In C. L. Borgman (Ed.), *Scholarly communication and bibliometrics* (pp. 10–27). Newbury Park, CA: Sage Publications.

Bornstein, M. H. (1995). Parenting infants. In M. H. Bornstein (Ed.), *Handbook of parenting: Children and parenting* (Vol. 1, pp. 3–39). Mahwah, NJ: Lawrence Erlbaum.

Bostrom, J., & Wise, L. (1994). Closing the gap between research and practice. *Journal of Nursing Administration, 24*(5), 22–27.

Bottorff, J. L. (1993). The use and meaning of touch in caring for patients with cancer. *Oncology Nursing Forum, 20,* 1531–1538.

Bottorff, J. L., & Morse, J. M. (1994). Identifying types of attending: Patterns of nurses' work. *Image: Journal of Nursing Scholarship, 26,* 53–60.

Boumans, N. P., & Landeweerd, J. A. (1994). Working in intensive care or nonintensive care unit: Does it make any difference? *Heart and Lung, 23,* 71–79.

Brackley, M. H. (1992). A role supplementation group pilot study: A nursing therapy for potential parental care givers. *Clinical Nurse Specialist, 6*(1), 14–19.

Bradlyn, A. S., Ritchey, A. K., Harris, C. V., Moore, I. M., O'Brien, R. T., Parsons, S. K., Patterson, K., & Pollock, B. H. (1996). Quality of life research in pediatric oncology: Research methods and barriers. *Cancer, 78,* 1333–1339.

Brady, P. F. (1987). Labeling confusion in the elderly. *Journal of Gerontological Nursing, 13*(6), 29–32.

Braithwaite, R. L., & Taylor, S. E. (Eds.). (1992). *Health issues in the Black community.* San Francisco: Jossey-Bass.

Braithwaite, V. (1992). Caregiving burden: Making the concept scientifically useful and policy relevant. *Research on Aging, 14,* 3–27.

Brandstater, B., & Muallem, M. (1969). Atelectasis following tracheal suction in infants. *Anesthesiology, 31,* 468–472.

Bray, J. H., & Maxwell, S. E. (1985). *Multivariate analysis of variance.* Quantitative Applications in the Social Sciences, No. 54. Newbury Park, CA: Sage.

Brayfield, A., & Rothe, H. (1951). An index of job satisfaction. *Journal of Applied Psychology, 35,* 307–311.

Breitmayer, B., Ayres, L., & Knafl, K. (1993). Triangulation in qualitative research: Evaluation in completeness and confirmation purposes. *Image: Journal of Nursing Scholarship, 25,* 237–244.

Brennan, P. F., Moore, S. M., & Smyth, K. A. (1991). ComputerLink: Electronic support for the home caregiver. *Advances in Nursing Science, 13*(4), 14–27.

Brennan, P. F., Moore, S. M., & Smyth, K. A. (1995). The effects of a special computer network on caregivers of persons with Alzheimer's disease. *Nursing Research, 44,* 166–172.

Brett, J. (1987). Using nursing practice research findings. *Nursing Research, 36,* 344–349.

Bridges, W. (1991). *Managing transitions: Making the most of change.* Menlo Park, CA: Addison Wesley.

Brimmer, P. F. (1979). Past, present and future in gerontological nursing research. *Journal of Gerontological Nursing, 5*(6), 27–34.

Brink, P. J. (1976). *Transcultural nursing: A book of readings.* New York: Haworth Press.

Brink, P., & Wood, M. (1989). *Advanced design in nursing research.* Newbury Park: Sage.

Brink, P. J., & Wood, M. J. (1993). Toward a definition of a successful dieter. *Clinical Nursing Research, 2,* 345–359.

Broering, L. (1993). The adolescent, health, and society: Commentary from the perspective of nursing. In S. G. Millstein, A. C. Peterson, & E. O. Nightingale (Eds.), *Promoting the health of adolescents: New directions for the twenty-first century* (pp. 151–157). New York: Oxford University Press.

Bromley, D. (1986). *The case-study method in psychology and related disciplines.* Chichester, England: Wiley.

Bronner, Y. L. (1996). Nutritional status outcomes for children: Ethnic, cultural and environmental contexts. *Journal of the American Dietetic Association, 96,* 891–900.

Brooten, D. (1993). Assisting with transitions from hospital to home. In S. Funk, E. Tornquist, M. Champagne, & R. Wiese (Eds.), *Key aspects of caring for the chronically ill: Hospital and home.* New York: Springer Publishing.

Brooten, D. (1995). Perinatal care across the continuum: Early discharge and nursing home follow-up. *Journal of Perinatal and Neonatal Nursing, 9*(1), 38–44.

Brooten, D., Brown, L. P., Hazard-Munro, B., York, R., Cohen, S. M., Roncoli, M., & Hollingsworth, A. (1988). Early discharge and specialist transitional care. *Image: The Journal of Nursing Scholarship, 20,* 64–68.

Brooten, D., Brown, L., Munro, B., York, R., Cohen, S., Ronocoli, M., & Hollingsworth, A. (1988). Early discharge and nurse specialist transitional care. *Image: Journal of Nursing Scholarship, 20,* 64–68.

Brooten, D., Gennaro, S., Brown, L. P., Butts, P., Gibbons, A. L., Bakewell-Sachs, S., & Kumar, S. P. (1988). Anxiety, depression, and hostility in mothers of preterm infants. *Nursing Research, 37,* 213–216.

Brooten, D., Kumar, S., Brown, L. P., Butts, P., Finkler, S. A., Bakewell-Sachs, S., Gibbons, A., & Deliveria-Papadopoulos, M. (1986). A randomized clinical trial of early hospital discharge and home follow-up of very low-birthweight infants. *New England Journal of Medicine, 315,* 934–939.

Brooten, D., & Naylor, M. D. (1995). Nurses' effect on changing patient outcomes. *Image: Journal of Nursing Scholarship, 27,* 95–99.

Brooten, D., Naylor, M., York, R., Brown, R., Roncoli, M., Hollingsworth, A., Cohen, S., Arnold, L., Finkler, S., Munro, B., & Jacobsen, B. (1995). Effects of nurse specialist transitional care on patient outcomes and cost: Results of five randomized trials. *American Journal of Managed Care, 1,* 45–51.

Brooten, D., Roncoli, M., Finkler, S., Arnold, L., Cohen, A., & Mennuti, M. (1994). A randomized trial of early hospital discharge and home follow-up of women having cesarean birth. *Obstetrics and Gynecology, 84,* 832–838.

Brown, E. L. (1948). *Nursing for the future.* New York: Russell Sage Foundation.

Brown, L. (Ed.). (1993a). *The New Shorter Oxford English Dictionary.* Oxford, England: Clarendon Press.

Brown, S. A. (1990). Studies of educational interventions and outcomes in diabetic adult: A meta-analysis revisited. *Patient Education and Counseling, 16,* 189–215.

Brown, S. A., & Grimes, D. E. (1995). A meta-analysis of nurse practitioners and nurse-midwives in primary care. *Nursing Research, 44,* 332–339.

Brown, S. A., & Hedges, L. V. (1994). Predicting metabolic control in diabetes: A pilot study using meta-analysis to estimate a linear model. *Nursing Research, 43,* 362–368.

Brown, S. C. (1993b). Revitalizing "handicap" for disability research. *Journal of Disability Policy Studies, 4*(2), 57–75.

Brownell, K. D., & Rodin, J. (1994). The dieting maelstrom: Is it possible and advisable to lose weight? *American Psychologist, 49,* 781–791.

Brownell, K. D., & Wadden, T. A. (1992). Etiology and treatment of obesity: Understanding a serious, prevalent, and refractory disorder. *Journal of Consulting and Clinical Psychology, 60,* 505–517.

Browning, M., & Lewis, E. (1973). *Human sexuality: Nursing implications.* New York: American Journal of Nursing.

Buchanan, G. M., & Seligman, M. E. P. (Eds.). (1995). *Explanatory style.* Hillsdale, NJ: Lawrence Erlbaum.

Buckwalter, K. C. (1989). Caring and Alzheimer's disease: The nursing perspective. In G. Gilmore, P. Whitehouse, & M. Wykle (Eds.), *Memory, aging and dementia.* New York: Springer Publishing.

Buckwalter, K. C., Hartsock, J., & Gaffney, J. (1985). Music therapy. In G. M. Bulecheck & J. C. McCloskey (Eds.), *Nursing interventions: Treatments for nursing diagnoses* (pp. 58–74). Philadelphia: W. B. Saunders.

Bullock, L., & McFarlane, J. (1989). The birth-weight/battering connection. *American Journal of Nursing, 89,* 1153–1155.

Bullough, V. L. (1994). *Science in the bedroom: A history of sex research.* New York: Basic Books.

Bullough, V. L., & Bullough, B. (1993). *Cross dressing, sex, and gender.* Philadelphia: University of Pennsylvania Press.

Bullough, V. L., & Bullough, B. (1997). Sex education in American nursing: A historical review. *Nursing History Review, 6,* 199–217.

Bureau of Primary Health Care, US DHHS, Public Health. (1995). *Models that work: The 1995 compendium of innovative primary health care programs for underserved and vulnerable populations.* Bethesda, MD: U.S. Health Resources and Services Administration.

Burge, V., Felts, M., Chenier, T., & Parrillo, A. V. (1995). Drug use, sexual activity, and suicidal behavior in U.S. high school students. *Journal of School Health, 65,* 222–227.

Burgener, S., Jirovec, M., Murrell, L., & Barton, D. (1992). Caregiver and environmental variables related to difficult behaviors in institutionalized, demented elderly persons. *Journal of Gerontology: Psychological Sciences, 47*(4), 242–249.

Burgess, E. (1926). The family as a unity of interacting personalities. *Family, 7,* 3–9.

Burke, L. E., Dunbar-Jacob, J., & Hill, M. N. (1997). Compliance with cardiovascular disease prevention strategies: A review of the research. *Annals of Behavioral Medicine, 19*(3).

Burns, D., Burns, D., & Shively, M. (1996). Critical care nurses' knowledge of pulmonary artery catheters. *American Journal of Critical Care, 5,* 49–54.

Burns, J. P., Reardon, F. E., & Truog, R. D. (1994). Using newly deceased patients to teach resuscitation procedures. *New England Journal of Medicine, 331,* 1652–1655.

Burns, K., Cunningham, N., White-Traut, R., Silvestri, J., & Nelson, M. N. (1994). Infant stimulation: Modification of an intervention based on physiologic and behavioral cues. *Journal of Obstetric, Gynecologic, and Neonatal Nursing, 23,* 581–589.

Burns, N., & Grove, S. (1993). *The practice of nursing research: Conduct, critique, and utilization* (2nd ed.). Philadelphia: W. B. Saunders.

Burns, N., & Grove, S. K. (1997). *The practice of nursing research: Conduct, critique and utilization* (3rd ed.). Philadelphia: W. B. Saunders.

Burns, Y., Roger, Y., Neil, M., Brazier, K., Croker, A., Behnke, L., & Tudehope, D. (1987). Development of oral function in preterm infants. *Physiotherapy Practice, 3,* 168–178.

Burnside, I. M. (1988). *Nursing and the aged: A self-care approach.* New York: McGraw-Hill.

Burt, B. L., Whelton, P. K., Rocella, E. J., Brown, C., Cutler, J. A., Higgins, M., Horan, M., & Labarthe, D. (1995). Prevalence of hypertension in the U.S. adult population: Results from the third national health and nutrition survey, 1988–1991. *Hypertension, 25,* 305–309.

Byerly, E. L. (1990). The nurse-researcher as participant-observer in a nursing setting. In P. J. Brink (Ed.), *Transcultural nursing* (pp. 143–162). Prospect Heights, IL: Waveland Press. (Original work published in 1969)

Cadman, E. C. (1994). The academic physician-investigator: A crisis not to be ignored. *Annals of Internal Medicine, 120,* 401–410.

Cairns, R. B., Elder, G. H., & Costello, E. J. (1996). *Developmental science.* Cambridge: Cambridge University.

Callister, L. C. (1995). Cultural meanings of childbirth. *Journal of Obstetric, Gynecologic and Neonatal Nursing, 24,* 327–331.

Campbell, D., & Fiske, D. (1959). Convergent and discriminant validation by the multitrait-multimethod matrix. *Psychological Bulletin, 56,* 81–105.

Campbell, D. T., & Stanley, J. C. (1963). Experimental and quasi-experimental designs for research on teaching. In N. L. Gage (Ed.), *Handbook of research on teaching* (pp. 171–246). Chicago: Rand-McNally.

Campbell, J. C. (1986). Nursing assessment for risk of homicide with battered women. *Advances in Nursing Science, 8,* 36–51.

Campbell, J. C., Anderson, E., Fulmer, T. L., Girourd, S., McElmurry, B., & Raff, B. (1993). Violence as a nursing priority: Policy implications. *Nursing Outlook, 41,* 89–92.

Campbell, J., Carpenter, P., Sneiderman, C., Cohn, S., Chute, C., & Warren, J. (1997). Phase II evaluation of clinical coding schemes: Completeness, taxonomy, mapping, definitions, and clarity. *Journal of the American Medical Informatics Association, 4,* 238–251.

Campbell, J. C., Harris, M. J., & Lee, R. K. (1995). Violence research: An overview. *Scholarly Inquiry for Nursing Practice: An International Journal, 9,* 104–125.

Campbell, J., & Humphreys, J. (1993). *Nursing care of survivors of family violence.* St. Louis: C. V. Mosby.

Campbell, J., & Parker, B. (in press). Clinical nursing research on battered women and their children: A review. In A. S. Hinshaw, S. Feetham, & J. Shaver (Eds.), *Handbook of clinical nursing research.* Newbury Park, CA: Sage.

Campbell, J. C., Poland, M., Walker, J., & Ager, J. (1992). Correlates of battering during pregnancy. *Research in Nursing and Health, 15,* 219–226.

Campbell, T. L., & Patterson, J. M. (1995). The effectiveness of family interventions in the treatment of physical illness. *Journal of Marital and Family Therapy, 21,* 545–583.

Caplan, G., Mason, E. A., & Kaplan, D. M. (1965). Four studies of crisis in parents of prematures. *Community Mental Health Journal, 1,* 149–161.

Capossela, C., & Warnock, S. (1995). *Share the care: How to organize a group to care for someone who is seriously ill.* New York: Fireside.

Care of the aged [Editorial]. (1925). *American Journal of Nursing, 25,* 394.

Caring for our future: The content of prenatal care. A report of the public health service expert panel on the content of prenatal care (1989). Washington, DC: U.S. Department of Health and Human Services.

Carman, J. M., Shortell, S. M., Foster, R. W., Hughes, E. F., Boerstler, H., O'Brien, J. L., & O'Connor, E. J. (1996). Keys for successful implementation of total quality management in hospitals. *Health Care Management Review, 21*(1), 48–60.

Carnegie Council on Adolescent Development. (1995). *Turning points preparing American youth for the 21st century: Recommendations for transforming middle grade school* (abridged version). Washington, DC: Author.

Carney, R. M., Freedland, K. E., Rich, M. W., & Jaffe, A. S. (1995). Depression as a risk factor for cardiac events in established coronary heart disease: A review of possible mechanisms. *Annals of Behavioral Medicine, 17,* 142–149.

Carper, B. A. (1978). Fundamental patterns of knowing in nursing. *Advances in Nursing Science, 1*(1), 13–23.

Carr, D. B., Jacox, A. K., Chapman, C. R., Ferrell, B., Fields, H. L., Heidrich III, G., Hester, N. K., Hill, C. S., Jr., Lipman, A. G., McGarvey, C. L., Miaskowski, C., Mulder, D. S., Payne, R., Schecter, N., Shapiro, B. S., Smith, R. S., Tsou, C. V., & Vecchiarelli, L. (1992). *Acute pain management: Operative or medical procedures and trauma* (Clinical Practice Guidelines). Rockville, MD: U.S. Public Health Service, Agency for Health Care Policy and Research.

Carrier, V. K., Janson-Bjerklie, S., & Jacobs, S. (1984). The sensation of dyspnea: A review. *Heart and Lung, 13,* 436–447.

Carroll-Johnson, R. M., & Paquette, M. (Eds.). (1994). *Classification of nursing diagnoses: Proceedings of the Tenth Conference, North American Nursing Diagnosis Association.* Philadelphia: J. B. Lippincott.

Carter, J. H., Moorhead, S. A., McCloskey, J. C., & Bulechek, G. M. (1995). Using the Nursing Interventions Classification to implement Agency for Health Care Policy and Research guidelines. *Journal of Nursing Care Quality, 9*(2), 76–86.

Caruso, C. C., Hadley, B. J., Shukla, R., Frame, P., & Khoury, J. (1992). Cooling effects and comfort of four cooling blanket temperatures in humans with fever. *Nursing Research, 41,* 68–72.

Cassem, N. H., & Hackett, T. P. (1971). Psychiatric consultation in a coronary care unit. *Annals of Internal Medicine, 75,* 9–14.

Cataldi-Betcher, E. L., Seltzer, M. H., Slocum, B. A., & Jones, K. W. (1983). Complications occurring during enteral nutrition support: A prospective study. *JPEN: Journal of Parenteral and Enteral Nutrition, 7,* 546–552.

Catolico, O., Navas, C. M., Sommer, C. K., & Collins, M. A. (1996). Quality of decision making by registered nurses. *Journal of Staff Development, 12,* 149–154.

Cattell, R. B. (1966). The scree test for the number of factors. *Multivariate Behavioral Research, 1,* 245–276.

The Center for Human Caring. (1997). *Colorado Caring Praxis Project.* Denver: University of Colorado Health Sciences Center.

Centers for Disease Control. (1991). *HIV/AIDS surveillance report.* Atlanta, GA: Author.

Centers for Disease Control. (1992). *Preventing lead poisoning in young children: A statement from the Centers for Disease Control.* Atlanta, GA: Author.

Centers for Disease Control. (1996a). *AIDS information: Reported cases of AIDS and HIV infection in health care workers.* Atlanta: CDC Fax Information Service.

Centers for Disease Control. (1996b). *Disease burden from viral hepatitis A, B, and C in the United States.* Atlanta: CDC Fax Information Service.

Centers for Disease Control. (1996c). *HIV/AIDS surveillance report: U.S. HIV and AIDS cases reported through June 1996.* Atlanta: Centers for Disease Control, Center for Infectious Disease.

Centers for Disease Control. (1997). Mortality/population data request. [On-line]. Available Internet: http://wonder.cdc.gov/rchtml/Convert/data/AdHoc.html.

Centers for Disease Control and Prevention. (1992). Public health focus: Surveillance, prevention, and control of nosocomial infections. *Morbidity and Mortality Weekly Report, 41,* 783.

Centers for Disease Control and Prevention. (1994). *Standard precautions, No. 55552 (Federal Register,* 59, 214). Washington, DC: U.S. Government Printing Office.

Centers for Disease Control and Prevention. (1996). *Evaluation handbook.* Atlanta: Author.

Champion, V. (1991). The relationship of selected variables to breast cancer detection behaviors in women 35 and older. *Oncology Nursing Forum, 18,* 733–739.

Champion, V. L. (1995). Results of a nurse-delivered intervention on proficiency and nodule detection with breast self-examination. *Oncology Nursing Forum, 22,* 819–824.

Chang, B. L., & Hirsch, M. (1991). Knowledge acquisition and knowledge representation in a rule-based expert system. *Computers in Nursing, 9,* 174–178.

Chapman, R. H., Reiley, P., McKinney, J., Welch, K., Toomey, B., & McCausland, M. (1994). Implementing a local area network for nursing in a large teaching hospital. *Computers in Nursing, 12,* 82–88.

Charlton, B. G. (1995). Mega-trials: Methodological issues and clinical implications [Review]. *Journal of the Royal College of Physicians of London, 29*(2), 96–100.

Chase, S. K. (1988). Knowledge representation in expert systems: Nursing diagnosis applications. *Computers in Nursing, 6,* 58–64.

Chavetz, L. (1996). The experience of severe mental illness: A life history approach. *Archives of Psychiatric Nursing, 10,* 24–31.

Chen, H. T. (1990). *Theory-driven evaluations.* Newbury Park, CA: Sage.

Chenitz, W. C., Sater, B., Davies, H., & Friesen, L. (1990). Developing collaborative research between clinical agencies: A consortium approach. *Applied Nursing Research, 3,* 90–97.

Chick, N., & Meleis, A. I. (1986). Transitions: A nursing concern. In P. L. Chinn (Ed.), *Nursing research methodology: Issues and implementation* (pp. 237–257). Rockville, MD: Aspen.

Chinn, P. L., & Kramer, M. K. (1995). *Theory and nursing: A systematic approach.* St. Louis: C. V. Mosby.

Chlan, L. L. (1998). Music therapy. In M. Snyder & R. Lindquist (Eds.), *Alternative/complementary therapies in nursing.* New York: Springer Publishing.

Chodorow, N. (1978). *The reproduction of mothering: Psychoanalysis and the sociology of gender.* Berkeley: University of California Press.

Choi, E. C. (1986). Unique aspects of Korean-American mothers. *Journal of Obstetric Gynecology Nursing, 15,* 394–400.

Chute, C. G., Cohn, S. P., Campbell, K. E., Oliver, D. E., & Campbell, J. R. (1996). The content coverage of clinical classifications. *Journal of the American Medical Informatics Association, 3,* 224–233.

Chyba, M. M., & Washington, L. R. (1990). Questionnaires from the National Health Interview Survey, National Center for Health Statistics. *Vital Health Statistics, 1,* 24.

Cimprich, B. (1992). Attentional fatigue following breast cancer surgery. *Research in Nursing and Health, 15,* 199–207.

Clare, M., Sargent, D., Moxley, R., & Forthman, T. (1995). Reducing health care delivery costs using clinical paths: A case study on improving hospital profitability. *Journal of Health Care Finance, 21*(3), 48–58.

Claridge, A. (1996). My turn: Harnessing intranet technology. *Healthcare Informatics, 13*(6), 144.

Clark, J., & Lang, N. (1992). Nursing's next advance: An international classification for nursing practice. *International Nursing Review, 3,* 109–112.

Clark, P. N., Williams, C. A., Percy, M. A., & Kim, Y. S. (1995). Health and life problems of homeless men and women in the Southeast. *Journal of Community Health Nursing, 12,* 101–110.

Clarke, A. (1994). What is chronic disease? The effects of the re-definition of HIV and AIDS. *Social Science and Medicine, 39,* 591–597.

Clifford, J., & Horvath, K. (1990). *Advancing professional nursing practice at Boston's Beth Israel Hospital.* New York: Springer Publishing.

Clinton, J., & McCormick, K. (1987). *Research in nursing: Toward a science of nursing.* Kansas City, MO: American Nurses Association.

Cockerill, R., Pallas, L. O., Bolley, H., & Pink, G. (1993). Measuring nursing workload for case costing. *Nursing Economics, 11,* 342–349.

Coenen, A., & Wake, M. (1996). Developing a database for an international classification for nursing practice (ICNP). *International Nursing Review, 43,* 183–187.

Cohen, E. L., & Cesta, T. G. (Eds.). (1997). *Nursing case management: From concept to evaluation.* St. Louis: Mosby Year Book.

Cohen, I. B. (1984). Florence Nightingale. *Scientific American, 250,* 128–137.

Cohen, J. (1960). A coefficient of agreement for nominal scales. *Educational and Psychological Measurement, 20,* 37–46.

Cohen, J. (1988). *Statistical power analysis for the behavioral sciences* (2nd ed.). Hillsdale, NJ: Erlbaum.

Cohen, J. (1994). The earth is round ($p < .05$). *American Psychologist, 49,* 997–1003.

Colaizzi, P. (1978). Psychological research as the phenomenologist views it. In R. Valle & M. King (Eds.), *Existential phenomenological alternative for psychology* (pp. 48–71). New York: Oxford University Press.

Cole, F. L., & Slocumb, E. N. (1990). Collaborative nursing research between novices: Productivity through partnership. *Nursing Forum, 25*(4), 13–18.

Collins, C. E., Givens, B. A., & Givens, C. W. (1994). Interventions with family caregivers of persons with Alzheimer's disease. *Nursing Clinics of North America, 29,* 195–207.

A comprehensive program for nationwide action. (1945). *American Journal of Nursing, 45,* 707–713.

Conn, V. S., Taylor, S. G., & Wiman, P. (1991). Anxiety, depression, quality of life, and self-care among survivors of myocardial infarction. *Issues in Mental Health Nursing, 12*(4), 321–331.

Connelly, C. E. (1987). Self care and the chronically ill patient. *Nursing Clinics of North America, 22,* 621–629.

Connor, R. J. (1960). A hospital inpatient classification system. *Dissertation Abstracts International, 21,* 565. (University Microfilms No. 60-3319)

Connor, R. J., Flagle, C. D., Hsieh, R. K. C., Preston, R., & Singer, S. (1961). Effective use of nursing resources: A research report. *Hospitals, 35*(9), 30–39.

Conrad, N. (1992). Stress and knowledge of suicidal others as factors in suicidal behavior of high school adolescents. *Issues in Mental Health Nursing, 13,* 95–104.

Constantino, R. E., & Bricker, P. L. (1996). Nursing post intervention for spousal survivors of suicide. *Issues in Mental Health Nursing, 17,* 151–152.

Constantinople, A. (1973). Masculinity-femininity: An exception to a famous dictum? *Psychological Bulletin, 80,* 389–407.

Conti, R. M. (1993). Role behaviors of nurse case managers. George Mason University. Dissertation Abstracts International, Vol. 54, no. 2 (DA9316549).

Cook, J. D. (1981).The therapeutic use of music: A literature review. *Nursing Forum, 20,* 252–266.

Cook, M. R., Gerkovich, M. M., Hoffman, S. J., McClernon, F. J., Cohen, H. D., Oakleaf, K. L., & O'Connell, K. A. (1995). Smoking and EEG power spectra: Effects of differences in arousal seeking. *International Journal of Psychophysiology, 19,* 247–256.

Cook, M. R., Gerkovich, M. M., Hoffman, S. J., McClernon, F. J., & O'Connell, K. A. (1996). Effects of smoking and telic/paratelic dominance on the contingent negative variation (CNV). *International Journal of Psychophysiology, 23,* 101–110.

Cook, M. R., Gerkovich, M. M., O'Connell, K. A., & Potocky, M. (1995). Reversal theory constructs and cigarette availability predict lapse early in smoking cessation. *Research in Nursing and Health, 18,* 217–224.

Cook, M. R., Gerkovich, M. M., Potocky, M., & O'Connell, K. A. (1993). Instruments for assessment of reversal theory states. *Patient Education and Counseling, 22,* 99–106.

Cook, T., & Campbell, D. (1979). *Quasi-experimentation: Design and analysis issues for field studies.* Chicago: Rand McNally.

Cooke, R., & Rousseau, D. (1987). Behavioral norms and expectations: A quantitative approach to the assessment of organizational culture. *Group and Organizational Studies, 13,* 245–273.

Coons, D. H. (1983). The therapeutic milieu. In W. Reichel (Ed.), *Clinical aspects of aging* (pp. 137–159). Baltimore: Williams & Wilkins.

Cooper, D. M. (1990). Optimizing wound healing. A practice within nursing's domain. *Nursing Clinics of North America, 25,* 165–180.

Corbin, J. M., & Strauss, A. (1991). A nursing model for chronic illness management based upon the trajectory framework. *Scholarly Inquiry for Nursing Practice: An International Journal, 5,* 155–174.

Corless, I. B. (1994). Dying well: Symptom control within hospice care. In J. Fitzpatrick & J. Stevenson (Eds.), *Annual Review of Nursing Research* (Vol. 12, pp. 125–146). New York: Springer Publishing.

Corless, I. B. (1995). A new decade for hospice. In I. B. Corless, B. B. Germino, & M. A. Pittman (Eds.), *A challenge for living: Dying, death, and bereavement* (pp. 77–94). Boston: Jones & Bartlett.

Costa, P. T. Jr., Williams, T. F., Somerfield, M., et al. (1996). *Early identification of Alzheimer's disease and related dementias: Clinical practice guideline, quick reference guide for clinicians,* No. 19 (AHCPR Publication No. 97-0704). Rockville, MD: U.S. Department of Health and Human Services, Public Health Service, Agency for Health Care Policy and Research.

Cotanch, P., & Strum, S. (1987). Progressive muscle relaxation as antiemetic therapy for cancer patients. *Oncology Nursing Forum, 14*(1), 33–37.

Coté, J. J., Morse, J. M., & James, S. G. (1991). The pain response of the postoperative newborn. *Journal of Advanced Nursing, 16,* 378–387.

Coté, R. A., Rothwell, D. J., Palotay, J. L., & Beckett, R. S. (1993). *SNOMED international*. Northfield, IL: College of American Pathologists.

Cowan, M. (1990). Cardiovascular nursing research. In J. J. Fitzpatrick, R. L. Taunton, & J. Q. Benoliel (Eds.), *Annual review of nursing research* (Vol. 8, pp. 3–33). New York: Springer Publishing.

Cowan, M. C. (Ed.). (1956). *The yearbook of modern nursing*. New York: G. P. Putnam's Sons.

Cowan, M. J., Heinrich, J., Lucas, L., Sigmon, H., & Hinshaw, A. S. (1993). Integration of biological and nursing sciences: A 10-year plan to enhance research and training. *Research in Nursing and Health, 16,* 3–9.

Cowan, M. J., Kogan, H., Burr, R., Hendershot, S., & Buchanan, L. (1991). Power spectral analysis of heart rate variability after biofeedback training. *Journal of Electrocardiology, 23*(Suppl.), 85–94.

Cowles, K. (1988). Issues in qualitative research on sensitive topics. *Western Journal of Nursing Research, 10,* 163–179.

Coyle, L., & Sokop, A. (1990). Innovation adoption behavior among nurses. *Nursing Research, 39,* 176–180.

Cronbach, L. J. (1951). Coefficient alpha and the internal structure of tests. *Psychometrika, 16,* 297–334.

Cronin-Stubbs, D. (1996). Delirium intervention research in acute care settings. In J. J. Fitzpatrick & J. Norbeck (Eds.), *Annual review of nursing research* (Vol. 14, pp. 57–73). New York: Springer Publishing.

Cronin-Stubbs, D., & Rooks, C. A. (1985). The stress, social support, and burnout of critical care nurses: The results of research. *Heart and Lung, 14,* 31–39.

Crosby, L. J., & Parsons, L. C. (1992). Cerebrovascular response of closed head-injured patients to a standardized endotracheal tube suctioning and manual hyperventilation procedure. *Journal of Neuroscience Nursing, 24,* 40–49.

Cuddigan, J. E., Logan, S., Evans, D., & Hoesing, H. (1988). Evaluation of an artificial intelligence–based nursing decision support system in a clinical setting. In N. Daly & K. J. Hannah (Eds.), *Nursing and computers: Proceedings of the Third International Symposium on Nursing Use of Computers and Information Science* (pp. 629–636). St. Louis: C.V. Mosby.

Cugliari, A. M., Miller, T., & Sobol, J. (1995). Factors promoting completion of advance directives in the hospital. *Archives of Internal Medicine, 155,* 1893–1898.

Curtin, L. L. (1994). Restructuring: What works—and what does not! *Nursing Management, 25*(10), 7–8.

Czarnecki, M. T. (1996). Benchmarking: A data-oriented look at improving health care performance. *Journal of Nursing Care Quality, 10*(3), 1–6.

Czarnik, R. E., Stone, K. S., Everhart, C. C., & Preusser, B. A. (1991). Differential effects of continuous versus intermittent suction on tracheal tissue. *Heart and Lung, 20,* 144–151.

Daley, J., Mitchell, G. J., & Jonas-Simpson, C. M. (1996). Quality of life and human becoming theory: Exploring discipline-specific contributions. *Nursing Science Quarterly, 9,* 170–174.

Daltroy, L. H., & Laing, M. H. (1993). Arthritis education: Opportunities and state of the art. *Health Education Quarterly, 20,* 3–16.

Dan, A. (1994). *Reframing women's health: Multidisciplinary research and practice*. Thousand Oaks, CA: Sage.

Danford, S. (1982). Therapeutic design for aging. In A. M. Horton (Ed.), *Mental health interventions for aging* (pp. 163–169). South Hadley, MA: J. F. Bergin.

Dartmouth Medical School. (1996). *The Dartmouth atlas of health care*. Chicago: American Hospital.

D'Auria, J. P. (1994). A bibliometric analysis of published maternal and child health nursing research from 1976 to 1990. In S. J. Grobe & E. S. P. Pluyter-Wenting (Eds.), *Nursing informatics: An international overview for nursing in a technological era* (pp. 471–475). Amsterdam: Elsevier.

D'Avanzo, C. E. (1992). Barriers to health care for Vietnamese refugees. *Journal of Professional Nursing, 8,* 245–253.

Davis, B. J., & Voegtle, K. H. (1994). *Culturally competent health care for adolescents*. Chicago: American Medical Association.

Davis, J. A. (1996). Sadness, tragedy and mass disaster in Oklahoma City: Providing critical incident stress debriefings to a community in crisis. *Accident and Emergency Nursing, 4,* 59–64.

Davis, K. A. (1995). AIDS nursing care and standardized language: An application of the Nursing Interventions Classification. *Journal of the American Nurses in AIDS Care, 6*(6), 37–44.

Dawber, T. R. (1980). *The Framingham study: The epidemiology of atherosclerotic disease*. Cambridge, MA: Harvard University Press.

Day, J. C. (1996). Population projections of the United States by age, sex, race, and hispanic origin: 1995 to 2050. In U.S. Bureau of the Census, *Current Population Reports* (P26-1130). Washington, DC: U.S. Government Printing Office.

DeBusk, R. F., Houston-Miller, N., Superko, R., Dennis, C. A., Thomas, R. J., Lew, H. T., Berger, W. E., Heller, R. S., Rompf, J., Gee, D., Kraemer, H. C., Bandura, A., Ghandour, G., Clark, M., Shah, R. V., Fisher, L., & Taylor, C. B. (1994). A case-management system for coronary risk modification after acute myocardial infarction. *Annals of Internal Medicine, 120,* 721–729.

De Geest, S., Borgermans, L., Gemoets, H., Abraham, I., Vlaminck, H., Evers, G., & Vanrenterghem, Y.

(1995). Incidence, determinants, and consequences of non-compliance with immunosuppressive therapy in renal transplant patients. *Transplantation, 59,* 340–347.

De Geest, S., Kesteloot, K., Degryse, I., & Vanhaecke, J. (1995). Hospital costs of protective isolation procedures in heart transplant recipients. *Journal of Heart and Lung Transplantation, 14,* 544–552.

De Geest, S., Kesteloot, K., Adriaenssen, G., Lenaerts, K., Thelissen, M. J., Mekers, G., Sergeant, P., & Daenen, W. (1996). Clinical and cost comparison of three preoperative skin preparation protocols in CABG-patients. *Progress in Cardiovascular Nursing, 11,* 4–16.

Deiriggi, P. M., & Miles, K. E. (1995). The effects of waterbeds on heart rate in preterm infants. *Scholarly Practice for Nursing Practice: An International Journal, 9,* 245–262.

Delbecq, A., Van de Ven, A., & Gustafsen, D. (1975). Group techniques for program planning: A guide to nominal group and Delphi processes. Glenview, IL: Scott Foresman.

Delgado, J., & Estrada, L. (1993). Improving data collection strategies. *Public Health Reports, 108,* 540–545.

Dellefield, K. S., & McDougall, G. J. (1996). Increasing metamemory in community elderly. *Nursing Research, 45,* 284–290.

Demi, A., Bakeman, R., Sowell, R., Moneyham, L., & Seals, B. (1996, October). Suicidality among HIV-infected women. Paper presented at Ninth Annual Association of Nurses in AIDS Care, Chicago, IL.

Demi, A. S., Meredith, C. E., & Gray, M. (1996). Research priorities for urological nursing: A Delphi study. *Urological Nursing, 16,* 3–8.

Demi, A. S., & Miles, M. S. (1986). Bereavement. In H. H. Werley, J. J. Fitzpatrick, & R. L. Taunton (Eds.), *Annual Review of Nursing Research* (Vol. 4, pp. 105–123). New York: Springer.

Demi, A. S., & Miles, M. S. (1987). Parameters of normal grief: A Delphi study. *Death Study, 11,* 397–412.

Demitrack, M. A., Dale, J. K., Straus, S. E., Laue, L., Listwak, S. J., Kruesi, M. J., Chrousos, G. P., & Gold, P. W. (1991). Evidence for impaired activation of the hypothalamic-pituitary-adrenal axis in patients with chronic fatigue syndrome. *Journal of Clinical Endocrinology and Metabolism, 73,* 1224–1234.

Demko, G. J., & Jackson, M. C. (1995). *Populations at risk in America: Vulnerable groups at the end of the twentieth century.* Boulder, CO: Westview Press.

Denmark, F., Russo, N. F., Frieze, I. H., & Sechzer, J. A. (1988). Guidelines for avoiding sexism in psychological research: A report of the ad hoc committee on nonsexist research. *American Psychologist, 43,* 582–585.

Dennis, K. E., & Goldberg, A. P. (1993). Differential effects of body fatness and body fat distribution on risk factors for cardiovascular disease in women: Impact of weight loss. *Arteriosclerosis and Thrombosis, 13,* 1487–1494.

Dennis, K. E., & Goldberg, A. P. (1996). Weight control self- efficacy types and positive transitions affect weight loss in obese women. *Addictive Behaviors, 21,* 103–116.

Denzin, N. (1989). *The research act: A theoretical introduction to sociological methods.* Englewood Cliffs, NJ: Prentice-Hall.

Denzin, N. K., & Lincoln, Y. S. (1994). *Handbook of qualitative research.* Newbury Park, CA: Sage Publications.

D'Eramo-Melkus, G., Wylie-Rosett, J., & Hagan, J. (1992). Metabolic impact of education in NIDDM. *Diabetes Care, 15,* 864–869.

DeSisto, M. J., Harding, C. M., McCormick, R. V., Ashikaga, T., & Brooks, G. W. (1987). The Maine-Vermont three decade studies of serious mental illness: Longitudinal course comparisons. *British Journal of Psychiatry, 167,* 338–342.

de Villers, A. S., Russell, V. A., Carstens, M. E., Aalbers, C., Gagiano, C. A., Chalton, D. O., & Taljaard, J. J. F. (1987). Noradrenergic function and hypothamamic-pituitary-adrenal axis activity in primary unipolar major depressive disorder. *Psychiatry Research, 22,* 127–140.

Devine, E. C. (1992). Effects of psychoeducational care for adult surgical patients: A meta-analysis of 191 studies. *Patient Education and Counseling, 19,* 129–142.

Devine, E. C. (1996). Meta-analysis of the effects of psychoeducational care in adults with asthma. *Research in Nursing and Health, 19,* 367–376.

Devine, E., & Cook, T. (1983). A meta-analytic analysis of effects of psychoeducational interventions on length of postsurgical hospital stay. *Nursing Research, 32,* 267–274.

Devine, E. C., & Cook, T. D. (1986). Clinical and cost-saving effects of psychoeducational interventions with surgical patients: A meta-analysis. *Research in Nursing and Health, 9,* 89–105.

Devine, E. C., & Pearcy, J. (1996). Meta-analysis of the effects of psychoeducational care in adults with chronic obstructive pulmonary disease. *Patient Education and Counseling, 26,* 167–178.

Devine, E. C., & Reifschneider, E. (1995). A meta-analysis of the effects of psychoeducational care in adults with hypertension. *Nursing Research, 44,* 237–245.

Devine, E. C., & Westlake, S. K. (1995). The effects of psychoeducational care provided to adults with cancer: Meta-analysis of 116 studies. *Oncology Nursing Forum, 22,* 1369–1381.

Diabetes Control and Complications Trial (DCCT) Research Group. (1993). The effect of intensive treatment of diabetes on the development and progression of long-term complications in insulin-dependent diabetes mellitus. *New England Journal of Medicine, 329,* 977–986.

Diamond, M. (1965). A critical evaluation of the ontogeny of human sexual behavior. *Quarterly Review of Biology, 40,* 147–175.

Dickoff, J., James, P., & Wiedenbach, E. (1968). Theory in a practice discipline: Part 1. Practice oriented theory. *Nursing Research, 17,* 415–435.

Diers, D., & Schmidt, R. L. (1977). Interaction analysis in nursing research. In P. J. Verhonick (Ed.), *Nursing research II* (pp. 77–132). Boston: Little, Brown.

Diers, D., Schmidt, R. L., McBride, M. A., & Davis, B. L. (1972). The effect of nursing interaction on patients in pain. *Nursing Research, 21,* 419–428.

DiIorio, C. (1990). An analysis of trends in neuroscience nursing research. *Journal of Neuroscience Nursing, 22,* 139–146.

Dillman, A. (1978). *Mail and telephone surveys: The total design method.* New York: Wiley.

Diokno, A., McCormick, K. A., Colling, J., Fantl, J. A., Loughery, R., Newman, D. K., Ouslander, J., Pearson, B., Raz, S., Resnick, N. M., Rohner, R. J., Schnelle, J., Tries, J., Urich, V., & Vernon, M. (1992). *Urinary incontinence in adults: AHCPR Clinical Practice Guideline* (Publication No. 92-0038). Rockville, MD: U.S. Department of Health and Human Services, Public Health Service, Agency for Health Care Policy and Research.

Dionne-Proulz, J., & Pepin, R. (1993). Stress management in the nursing profession. *Journal of Nursing Management, 1,* 75–81.

Dock, L. (1910). *Hygiene and morality: A manual for nurses and others.* New York: Putnam.

Dock, L. L. (1912). *A history of nursing* (Vol. 3). New York: G. P. Putnam's Sons.

Dodd, M. J. (1984). Patterns of self-care in cancer patients receiving radiation therapy. *Oncology Nursing Forum, 11,* 23–27.

Dodd, M. J., & Ahmed, N. (1987). Preference for type of information in cancer patients receiving radiation therapy. *Cancer Nursing, 10,* 244–251.

Dodge, B. (1997). *Schools, skills and scaffolding on the Web* [On-line]. Available: http://edweb.sdsu.edu/people/bdodge/scaffolding.html

Doll, R., & Hill, A. G. (1950). Smoking and carcinoma of the lung: Preliminary report. *British Medical Journal, 2,* 739.

Donabedian, A. (1969). Part 2: Some issues in evaluating the quality of nursing care. *American Journal of Public Health, 59,* 1833–1836.

Donabedian, A. (1980). Explorations in quality assessment and monitoring (Vols. 1–3). Ann Arbor, MI: Health Administration Press.

Donald, R. A., Crozier, I. G., Foy, S. G., Richards, A. M., Livesey, J. H., Ellis, M. J., Mattioli, L., & Ikram, H. (1994). Plasma corticotropin releasing hormone, vasopressin, ACTH and cortisol responses to acute myocardial infarction. *Clinical Endocrinology, 40*(4), 499–504.

Donaldson, M. S., Yordy, K. D., Lohr, K. N., & Vanselow, N. A. (Eds.). (1996). *Primary care: America's health in a new era.* New York: National Academy Press.

Donaldson, S. K., & Crowley, D. M. (1978). The discipline of nursing. *Nursing Outlook, 26,* 113–120.

Dougherty, M. C., & Tripp-Reimer, T. (1990). Nursing and anthropology. In T. M. Johnson & C. F. Sargent (Eds.), *Medical anthropology: A handbook of theory and method* (pp. 174–186). New York: Greenwood.

Douglas, S., Daly, B., Rudy, E., Song, R., Dyer, M. A., & Montenegro, H. (1995). The cost-effectiveness of a special care unit to care for the chronically critically ill. *Journal of Nursing Administration, 25*(11), 47–53.

Doyle, J. B. (1986). How experts scan journals: Implications for expert systems in text retrieval. In R. Salamon, B. Blum, & M. Jorgensen (Eds.), *MEDINFO 86* (pp. 540–544). North-Holland, The Netherlands: Elsevier.

Dracup, K., Meleis, A. I., Baker, K., & Edlefsen, P. (1984). Family-focused cardiac rehabilitation: A role supplementation program for cardiac patients and spouses. *Nursing Clinics of North America, 19*(1), 113–124.

Dreifuss, F. E. (1996). Classification of the epilepsies: Influence on management. In N. Santilli (Ed.), *Managing seizure disorders: A handbook for health care professionals* (pp. 19–28). Philadelphia: Lippincott-Raven.

Dretske, F. (1988). *Explaining behavior: Reasons in a world of causes.* Cambridge, MA: MIT Press.

Drossman, D. A., Funch-Jensen, P., Janssens, J., Talley, N. J., Thompson, W. G., & Whitehead, W. E. (1990). Identification of subgroups of functional disorders. *Gastroenterology International, 3,* 159–172.

Drossman, D. A., Li, Z., Andruzzi, E., Temple, R. D., Talley, N. J., Thompson, W. G., Whitehead, W. E., Janssens, J., Funch-Jensen, P., Corazziari, E., Richter, J. E., & Kock, G. G. (1993). U.S. householder survey of functional gastrointestinal disorders: Prevalence, sociodemography, and health impact. *Digestive Diseases and Sciences, 38,* 1569–1580.

Drossman, D. A., & Thompson, W. G. (1992). The irritable bowel syndrome. *Annals of Internal Medicine, 116,* 1009–1016.

Dubignon, J., Campbell, D., Curtis, M., & Partington, M. (1969). The relation between laboratory measures of sucking, food intake, and perinatal factors during the newborn period. *Child Development, 40,* 1107–1120.

Dubin, R. (1978). *Theory building* (rev. ed.). New York: Macmillan.

DuBois, K., & Rizzolo, M. A. (1994). Cruising the "information superhighway." *American Journal of Nursing, 94*(12), 58–60.

Dubos, R. (1965). *Man adapting*. New Haven, CT: Yale University Press.

Duffy, M. (1987). Methodological triangulation: A vehicle for merging quantitative and qualitative research methods. *Image: Journal of Nursing Scholarship, 19*, 130–133.

Dulock, H. L., & Holzemer, W. L. (1991). Substruction: Improving the linkage from theory to method. *Nursing Science Quarterly, 4*, 83–87.

Dumas, R. G., & Leonard, R. C. (1963). The effect of nursing on the incidence of post-operative vomiting: A clinical experiment. *Nursing Research, 12*, 12–15.

Dunbar, S. B., & Farr, L. (1996). Temporal patterns of heart rate and blood pressure in elders. *Nursing Research, 45*, 43–49.

Dunbar-Jacob, J., & Schlenk, E. (1996). Treatment adherence and clinical outcome: Can we make a difference? In *Health psychology over the life span* (pp. 323–343). Washington, DC: American Psychological Association.

Duncan, L. (1987). *The medical department of the United States Army in the Civil War*. Gaithersburg, MD: Olde Soldiers Books. (Original work published 1905)

Dungee-Anderson, D., & Beckett, J. O. (1992). Alzheimer's disease in African-American and White families: A clinical analysis. *Smith College Studies in Social Work, 62*(2), 155–168.

Dunn, H. L. (1961). *High level wellness*. Emmaus, PA: Rodale.

Dunn, M. E. (1980). *High-level wellness*. Thorofare, NJ: Charles B. Slack.

Dupont, H., Chappell, C., Sterling, C., Okhuysen, P., Rose, J., & Jakubowski, W. (1995). The infectivity of *Cryptosporidium parvum* in healthy volunteers. *New England Journal of Medicine, 332*, 855–889.

Dutton, G. (1992). Medicine gets closer to virtual reality. *IEE Software, 9*, 108.

Dwyer, T. F. (1973). Telepsychiatry: Psychiatric consultation by interactive television. *American Journal of Psychiatry, 130*, 865–869.

Eagly, A. H. (1992). Uneven progress: Social psychology and the study of attitudes. *Journal of Personality and Social Psychology, 63*, 693–710.

Early Alzheimer's Disease Guideline Panel. (1996). *Recognition and initial assessment of Alzheimer's disease and related dementias* (AHCPR Publication No. 97-0702). Washington, DC: U.S. Government Printing Office.

Early Treatment Diabetic Retinopathy Study Research Group. (1991). Early photocoagulation for diabetic retinopathy. *Ophthalmology, 98*, 766–785.

Earp, J. K., & Finlayson, D. C. (1991). Relationship between urinary bladder and pulmonary artery temperatures: A preliminary study. *Heart and Lung, 20*, 265–270.

Earp, J. K., & Finlayson, D. C. (1992). Urinary bladder/pulmonary artery temperature ratio of less than 1 and shivering in cardiac surgical patients. *American Journal of Critical Care, 1*, 43–52.

Eckhart, J. G. (1993). Costing out nursing services: Examining the research. *Nursing Economics, 11*, 91–98.

Edenfield, S., Thomas, S., Thompson, W., & Marcotte, J. (1995). Validity of the Creasy risk appraisal instrument for prediction of preterm labor. *Nursing Research, 44*, 76–81.

Edwardson, S., & Giovannetti, P. (1994). Nursing workload measurement systems. *Annual Review of Nursing Research, 12*, 95–123.

Eisenberg, D. M., Kessler, R. C., Foster, C., Norlock, F. E., Calkins, D. R., & Delbanco, T. L. (1993). Unconventional medicine in the United States: Prevalence, costs, and patterns of use. *New England Journal of Medicine, 32*, 246–252.

Eland, J. M., & Anderson, J. E. (1977). The experience of pain in children. In A. K. Jacox (Ed.), *Pain: A source book for nurses and other health professionals* (pp. 453–476). Boston: Little Brown.

Elfrink, V. L., & Martin, K. S. (1996). Educating for community nursing practice: Point of care technology. *Healthcare Information Management, 10*(2), 81–89.

Elkind, D. (1984). *All grown up and no place to go*. Menlo Park, CA: Addison-Wesley.

Ellison, S. L., Vidyasagar, D., & Anderson, G. C. (1979). Sucking in the newborn infant during the first hour of life. *Journal of Nurse Midwifery, 24*, 18–25.

Ellwood, P. M., & Enthoven, A. C. (1995). Responsible choice: The Jackson Hole group plan for health reform. *Health Affairs, 14*, 24–39.

Elster, A. B., & Kuznets, N. J. (Eds.). (1994). *AMA guidelines for adolescent preventive services (GAPS)*. Chicago: American Medical Association.

Emergency medical services for children: There's still a long way to go. (1993). *Institute of Medicine News, 1*(4), 1.

Employee Benefit Research Institute. (1994). *The effectiveness of health care cost management strategies: A review of the evidence* (Issue Brief No. 154). Washington, DC: Author.

Engebretson, J., & Wardell, D. W. (1997). The essence of partnership in research. *Journal of Professional Nursing, 13*, 38–47.

Engle, V. F. (1996). Newman's theory of health. In J. J. Fitzpatrick & A. L. Whall (Eds.), *Conceptual models of nursing: Analysis and application* (pp. 275–288). Stamford, CT: Appleton and Lange.

Erickson, J. I. (1997). Collaborative governance is here. *Caring Headlines, 3*(12), 2.

Erickson, R. S. (1980). Oral temperature differences in relation to thermometer and technique. *Nursing Research, 29,* 157–164.

Erickson, R. S., & Yount, S. T. (1991). Comparison of tympanic and oral temperatures in surgical patients. *Nursing Research, 40,* 40–90.

Erikson, E. H. (1959). Identity and the life cycle. *Psychological Issues, 1,* 18–164.

Ersek, M., Ferrell, B. R., Hassey Dow, K., & Melancon, C. H. (1997). Quality of life in women with ovarian cancer. *Western Journal of Nursing Research, 19,* 334–350.

Estabrooks, C. A. (1989). Touch: A nursing strategy in the intensive care. *Heart and Lung, 18,* 392–401.

Estes, C. L., Binney, E. A., & Culbertson, R. A. (1992). The gerontological imagination: Social influences on the development of gerontology, 1945–present. *International Journal of Aging and Human Development, 35,* 49–65.

Estok, P. H., Rudy, E. B., Kerr, M. E., & Menzel, L. (1993). Menstrual response to running: Nursing implications. *Nursing Research, 42,* 158–165.

Ethridge, P., & Lamb, G. (1989). Professional nursing case management improves quality, access, and costs. *Nursing Management, 20*(3), 30–35.

Evans, D. A., Cimino, J. J., Hersh, W. R., Huff, S. M., & Bell, D. S. (1994). Toward a medical-concept representation language. *Journal of the American Medical Informatics Association, 1,* 207–217.

Evans, L. K. (1987). Sundown syndrome in institutionalized elderly. *Journal of the American Geriatrics Society, 35,* 101–108.

Evans, L. K. (1996). Knowing the patient: The route to individualized care. *Journal of Gerontological Nursing, 22*(3), 15–19.

Evans, L., & Strumpf, N. (1989). Tying down the elderly: A review of the literature on physical restraint. *Journal of the American Geriatrics Society, 37,* 65–74.

Evans, L., & Strumpf, N. (1990). Myths about elder restraint. *Image: Journal of Nursing Scholarship, 22,* 124–128.

Evans, L., Strumpf, N., Allen-Taylor, S., Capezuti, E., Maislin, G., & Jacobson, B. (1997). A clinical trial to reduce restraints in nursing homes. *Journal of the American Geriatrics Society, 45,* 675–681.

Evans, L., Strumpf, N., Williams, C., Williams, T., Middleton, W., Jacobsen, B., Allen-Taylor, S., & Capezuti, E. (1993). A comparison of physical restraints in American and European nursing homes. *Gerontologist, 34*(Special issue 1), 271.

Expert Panel on Electronic Networks, Community-based Health Services, and Public Health. (1996). *Nursing services for the public's health in an electronic world* (final report to the American Academy of Nursing). Washington, DC: American Academy of Nursing.

Faden, R. R., & Beauchamp, T. L. (1986). *A history and theory of informed consent.* New York: Oxford University Press.

Falck, K., Grohn, P., Sorsa, M., Vanio, H., Heinonen, E., & Holsti, L. R. (1979). Mutagenicity in urine of nurses handling cytostatic drugs. *Lancet, 1,* 1250–1251.

Fantl, J. A., Newman, D. K., Colling, J., DeLancey, J. O. L., Keeys, C., Loughery, R., McDowell, B. J., Norton, P., Ouslander, J., Schnelle, J., Staskin, D., Tries, J., Urich, V., Vitousek, S. H., Weiss, B. D., & Whitmore, K. (1996). *Urinary incontinence in adults: Acute and chronic management: AHCPR Clinical Practice Guideline* (Publication No. 96-0682). Rockville, MD: U.S. Department of Health and Human Services, Public Health Service, Agency for Health Care Policy and Research.

Farr, L., Keene, A., Samson, D., & Michael, A. (1984). Alterations in circadian excretion of urinary variables and physiological indicators of stress following surgery. *Nursing Research, 33,* 140–146.

Fawcett, J. (1990). Preparation for caesarean childbirth: Derivation of a nursing intervention from the Roy adaptation model. *Journal of Advanced Nursing, 15,* 1418–1425.

Fawcett, J. (1993). *Analysis and evaluation of nursing theories.* Philadelphia: F. A. Davis.

Fawcett, J. (1995). *Analysis and evaluation of conceptual models of nursing* (3rd ed.). Philadelphia: F. A. Davis.

Fawcett, J., & Buhle, E. L. Jr. (1995). Using the Internet for data collection. An innovative electronic strategy. *Computers in Nursing, 13,* 273–279.

Fawcett, J., Pollio, N., & Tully, A. (1992). Women's perceptions of cesarean and vaginal delivery: Another look. *Research in Nursing and Health, 15,* 439–446.

Fawcett, J., & Tulman, L. (1990). Building a programme of research from the Roy adaptation model. *Journal of Advanced Nursing, 15,* 720–725.

Fazio, R. H., & Williams, C. J. (1986). Attitude accessibility as a moderator of the attitude-perception and attitude-behavior relations: An investigation of the 1984 presidential election. *Journal of Personality and Social Psychology, 51,* 505–514.

The Federal Register, 61(192), 51497–51532. (1996).

Feetham, S. (1993). Family outcomes: Conceptual and methodological issues. In P. Moritz (Ed.), *Patient outcomes research: Examining the effectiveness of nursing practice.* Bethesda, MD: National Center for Nursing Research.

Feetham, S. (1997). Families and health in the urban environment: Implications for programs, research, and policy. In H. J. Walberg, O. Reyes, & R. P. Weissberg (Eds.), *Children and youth: Interdisciplinary perspective* (Vol. 7, pp. 321–362). Issues in Children's and Families' Lives. Thousand Oaks, CA: Sage.

Fehring, R. J. (1986). Validating diagnostic labels: Standardized methodology. In M. E. Hurley (Ed.), *Classification of nursing diagnoses: Proceedings of the Sixth Conference.* St. Louis: C. V. Mosby.

Feifel, H. (Ed.). (1959). *The meaning of death.* New York: McGraw-Hill.

Feldman, M. J., Ventura, M. R., & Crosby, F. (1987). Studies of nurse practitioner effectiveness. *Nursing Research, 36,* 303–308.

Feldstein, M. A., & Gemma, P. B. (1995). Oncology nurses and chronic compounded grief. *Cancer Nursing, 18,* 228–236.

Feldstein, P. J. (1994). *Health policy and issues: An economic perspective on health reform.* Ann Arbor, MI: AUPHA Press/Health Administration Press.

Ferketich, S. (1990). Internal consistency estimates of reliability. *Research in Nursing and Health, 13,* 437–440.

Ferketich, S. (1991). Aspects of item analysis. *Research in Nursing and Health, 14,* 165–168.

Ferketich, S. L., Figueredo, A. J., & Knapp, T. R. (1991). The multitrait-multimethod approach to construct validity. *Research in Nursing and Health, 14,* 315–320.

Ferketich, S., & Muller, M. (1990). Factor analysis revisited. *Nursing Research, 39,* 59–62.

Ferrans, C. E., & Powers, M. J. (1992). Psychometric assessment of the quality of life index. *Research in Nursing and Health, 15,* 29–38.

Ferrell, B. R., & Hassey Dow, K. (1997). Quality of life in long-term cancer survivors. *Oncology, 11,* 565–571.

Ferrell, B. R., Hassey Dow, K., & Grant, M. (1995). Measurement of the quality of life of cancer survivors. *Quality of Life Research, 4,* 523–531.

Ferrell, B. R., Hassey Dow, K., Leigh, S., Ly, J., & Gulasekaram, P. (1995). Quality of life among long-term cancer survivors. *Oncology Nursing Forum, 22,* 915–922.

Fetter, B. J., & Lowery, B. J. (1992). Psychiatric rehospitalization of the severely mentally ill: Patient and staff perspectives. *Nursing Research, 41,* 301–305.

Fickeissen, J. L. (1995). Nursing resources on the Internet. *New Jersey Nurse, 25*(8), 5.

Field, P. A., & Morse, J. M. (1985). *Nursing research: The application of qualitative approaches.* Rockville, MD: Aspen.

Fielding, J., & Weaver, S. M. (1994). A comparison of hospital- and community-based mental health nurses: Perceptions of their work environment and psychological health. *Journal of Advanced Nursing, 19,* 1196–1204.

Figueredo, A. J., Ferketich, S. L., & Knapp, T. R. (1991). More on MTMM: The role of confirmatory factor analysis. *Research in Nursing and Health, 14,* 387–391.

Fillmore, A., Sheahan, M. W., & Miller, J. O. M. (1953). The NLN is everybody's business. *Nursing Outlook, 1,* 22–27.

Finifter, B. (1975). Replication and extension of social research through secondary analysis. *Social Science Information, 14,* 119–153.

Fiser, D. H. (1992). Assessing the outcome of pediatric intensive care. *Journal of Pediatrics, 121,* 68–74.

Fishbein, M., & Ajzen, I. (1975). *Belief, attitude, intention, and behavior: An introduction to theory and research.* Reading, MA: Addison-Wesley.

Fisher, R. A. (1935). *The design of experiments.* London: Oliver & Boyd.

Fitzpatrick, J. J. (1989). A life perspective rhythm model. In J. J. Fitzpatrick & A. L. Whall (Eds.), *Conceptual models of nursing: Analysis and application* (2nd ed., pp. 401–407). Princeton, NJ: Appleton-Century-Crofts.

Fitzpatrick, J. J. (1990). Conceptual basis for the organization and advancement of nursing knowledge: Nursing diagnosis/taxonomy. *Nursing Diagnosis, 1,* 102–106.

Fitzpatrick, J. J. (1991a). Taxonomy II: Definitions and development. In R. M. Carroll-Johnson (Ed.), *Classification of nursing diagnoses: Proceedings of the Ninth Conference.* Philadelphia: Lippincott.

Fitzpatrick, J. J. (1991b). The translation of the NANDA taxonomy into ICD code. In R. M. Carroll-Johnson (Ed.), *Classification of nursing diagnoses: Proceedings of the Ninth Conference* (pp. 19–22). Philadelphia: Lippincott.

Fitzpatrick, J. J., & Abraham, I. (1987). Toward the socialization of scholars and scientists. *Nurse Educator, 12,* 23–25.

Fitzpatrick, J. J., & Donovan, M. J. (1978). Temporal experience and motor behavior among the aging. *Research in Nursing and Health, 1,* 60–68.

Fitzpatrick, J. J., & Whall, A. L. (Eds.). (1989). *Conceptual models of nursing: Analysis and application.* Norwalk, CT: Appleton & Lange.

Fitzpatrick, J. J., & Whall, A. L. (1996). *Conceptual models of nursing: Analysis and application* (3rd ed.). Stanford, CT: Appleton & Lange.

Fitzpatrick, J. J., Wykle, M. L., & Morris, D. L. (1990). Collaboration in care and research. *Archives of Psychiatric Nursing, 4,* 53–61.

Flaskerud, J. H., & Chang, B. (1994). *Health-related problems of socially vulnerable populations.* Unpublished manuscript.

Fleming, C. M., & Scanlon, C. (1994). The role of the nurse in the Patient Self Determination Act. *Journal of the New York State Nurses Association, 25,* 19–23.

Fleming, J. (1986). Preschool children. In H. H. Werley, J. J. Fitzpatrick, & R. L. Taunton (Eds.), *Annual review of nursing research,* (Vol 4, pp. 21–54). New York: Springer Publishing.

Fleming, M. F., & Barry, K. L. (1992). *Addictive disorders.* St. Louis: Mosby.

Fleury, J., Kimbrell, L. C., & Kruszewski, M. A. (1995). Life after a cardiac event: Women's experiences in healing. *Heart and Lung: Journal of Critical Care, 24,* 474–482.

Flick, L. H., Reese, S. G., Rogers, G., Fletcher, P., & Sonn, J. (1994). Building community for health: Lessons from a seven-year-old neighborhood/university partnership. *Health Education Quarterly, 2,* 369–380.

Floyd, J. A. (1982). Rhythm theory: Relationship to nursing conceptual models. In J. J. Fitzpatrick, A. L. Whall, R. L. Johnston, & J. A. Floyd (Eds.), *Nursing models and their psychiatric mental health applications* (pp. 95–116). Bowie, MD: R. J. Brady.

Flynn, B. C., Ray, D. W., & Rider, M. S. (1994). Empowering communities: Action research through healthy cities. *Health Education Quarterly, 21,* 395–405.

Folta, J. R. (1965). The perception of death. *Nursing Research, 14,* 232–235.

Forchuk, C. (1994). The orientation phase of the nurse-client relationship: Testing Peplau's theory. *Journal of Advanced Nursing, 20,* 532–537.

Foreman, M. D. (1989). Confusion in the hospitalized elderly: Incidence, onset, and associated factors. *Research in Nursing & Health, 12,* 21–29.

Foreman, M. D. (1993). Acute confusion in the elderly. In J. J. Fitzpatrick & J. S. Stevenson (Eds.), *Annual review of nursing research* (Vol. 11, pp. 3–30). New York: Springer Publishing.

Foster, F. B., & Jones, D. A. (1997). The development and preliminary testing of the functional health pattern assessment screening tool. In M. Rantz & P. LeMone (Eds.), *Classification of the 12th Nursing Diagnoses Proceedings.* Glendale, CA: CINAHL Information Systems.

Foster, S. B., Kloner, J. A., & Stengrevics, S. S. (1984). Cardiovascular nursing research: Past, present and future. *Heart and Lung, 13,* 111–116.

Foucault, M. (1972). *The archeology of knowledge.* London: Tavistock.

Foundation for Health Services Research. (1992). *Health outcomes research: A primer.* Washington, DC: Author.

Fowler, B. A., & Padgett, J. J. (1994). Ideological shifts needed in primary care delivery: Removing barriers through reform. *American Black Nurses Foundation Journal, 5,* 126–129.

Fox, J. (1990, November). *Etiologic factors and information processing deficits associated with schizophrenia: A review of findings.* Paper presented at National Institute of Mental Health, Washington, DC.

Fox, J., Merwin, E., & Blank, M. (1995). De facto mental health services in the rural south. *Journal of Health Care for the Poor and Underserved, 6,* 434–468.

Francis, P., Merwin, E., & Fox, J. (1995). Relationship of clinical case management to hospitalization and service delivery for seriously mentally ill clients. *Issues in Mental Health Nursing, 16,* 57–274.

Frank-Stromberg, M., & Olsen, S. (1997). *Instruments for clinical health-care research* (2nd ed.). Sudbury, MA: Jones and Bartlett.

Frasure-Smith, N. (1991). In-hospital symptoms of psychological stress as predictors of long-term outcome after acute myocardial infarction in men. *American Journal of Cardiology, 67*(2), 121–127.

Frasure-Smith, N., Lesperance, F., & Talajic, M. (1993). Depression following myocardial infarction: Impact on 6-month survival. *Journal of the American Medical Association, 270,* 1819–1825.

Frasure-Smith, N., & Prince, R. (1989). Long-term follow-up of the ischemic heart disease life stress monitoring program. *Psychosomatic Medicine, 51,* 485–513.

Fraulo, E., Munster, M., & Pathman, D. (1991). Preterm labor in critical care nurses. *Heart and Lung: Journal of Critical Care, 20,* 299–302.

Freda, M., Damus, K., & Merkatz, J. (1991). What do pregnant women know about preventing preterm birth? *Journal of Obstetric, Gynecologic and Neonatal Nursing, 20,* 140–143.

Freedland, K. E., Carney, R. M. Lustman, P. J., Rich, M. W., & Jaffe, A. S. (1992). Major depression in coronary artery disease patients with or without a prior history of depression. *Psychosomatic Medicine, 54,* 416–421.

Freire, P. (1970). *Pedagogy of the oppressed.* New York: Seabury Press.

French, J. R. P., Jr., Rodgers, W., & Cobb, S. (1974). Adjustment as person-environment fit. In G. V. Coelho, D. A., Hamburg, & J. E. Admans (Eds.), *Coping and adaptation* (pp. 316–333). New York: Basic Books.

Frenn, M., Lundeen, S. P., Martin, K. S., Riesch, S. K., & Wilson, S. A. (1996). Symposium on nursing centers: Past, present, and future. *Journal of Nursing Education, 35*(2), 54–62.

Freud, S. (1957). *Mourning and melancholia: Standard edition of the complete psychological works of Sigmund Freud* (Vol. 14). London: Hogarth Press.

Frey, M. (1995). Toward a theory of families, children and chronic illness. In M. A. Frey & C. Gieloff (Eds.), *Advancing King's system framework and theory of nursing* (pp. 109–125). Newbury Park, CA: Sage.

Frey, M. A., & Sieloff, C. L. (Eds.). (1995). *Advancing King's systems framework and theory of nursing.* Thousand Oaks, CA: Sage.

Friedman, E. (1996). Capitation, integration, and managed care: Lessons from early experiments. *Journal of the American Medical Association, 275,* 957–962.

Friedman, M., Thoresen, C. E., Gill, J. J., Ulmer, D., Powell, L. H., Price, V. A., Brown, B., Thompson, L., Rabin, D. D., Breal, W. S., Bourg, E., Levy, R., & Dixon, T. (1986). Alteration of Type A behavior and its effect on cardiac recurrences in post myocardial infarction patients: Summary results of the recurrent coronary prevention project. *American Heart Journal, 112,* 663–665.

Fry, S. T. (1994). *Ethics in nursing practice: A guide to ethical decision making.* Geneva: International Council of Nurses.

Fry, S. T. (1995). Nursing ethics. In W. Reich (Ed.), *Encyclopedia of bioethics* (2nd ed., pp. 1822–1827). New York: Macmillan.

Fry, S. T., Killen, A. R., & Robinson, E. M. (1996). Care-based reasoning, caring, and the ethic of care: A need for clarity. *Journal of Clinical Ethics, 7,* 41–47.

Fukuda, K., Straus, S. E., Hickie, I., Sharpe, M. C., Dobbins, J. G., Komaroff, A., & the International Chronic Fatigue Syndrome Study Group. (1994). The chronic fatigue syndrome: A comprehensive approach to its definition and study. *Annals of Internal Medicine, 121,* 953–959.

Fullerton, C. S., & Ursano, R. J. (1997). The other side of chaos: Understanding the patterns of posttraumatic responses. In C. S. Fullerton & R. J. Ursano (Eds.), *Posttraumatic stress disorder* (pp. 3–18). Washington, DC: American Psychiatric Press.

Fullerton, J. T., & Wingard, D. (1990). Methodological problems in the assessment of nurse-midwifery practice. *Applied Nursing Research, 3,* 153–160.

Fulmer, T., & Gurland, B. J. (1996). Restriction as elder mistreatment: Differences between caregiver and elder perceptions. *Journal of Mental Health and Aging, 2,* 89–100.

Funk, S., Tournquist, E., & Champagne, M. (1989). Application and evaluation of the dissemination model. *Western Journal of Nursing Research, 11,* 486–491.

Funk, S., Tornquist, E., Champagne, M., & Wiese, R. (Eds.). (1993). *Key aspects of caring for the chronically ill.* New York: Springer Publishing.

Fuster, V., & Pearson, T. A. (1996). 27th Bethesda Conference: Matching the intensity of risk factor management with the hazard for coronary disease events. *Journal of the American College of Cardiology, 27,* 957–1047.

Gabriel, H. P., & Danilowicz, D. (1978). Postoperative response in "prepared" child after cardiac surgery. *British Heart Journal, 40,* 1046–1051.

Gadamer, H. (1989). *Truth and method* (rev. ed.) (J. Weinsheimer & D. G. Marshall, Trans.). New York: Continuum. (Original work published 1960)

Gaffney, K. F. (1992). Nursing practice model for maternal role sufficiency. *Advances in Nursing Science, 15*(2), 76–84.

Gagan, J. J. (1983). Methodological notes on empathy. *Advances in Nursing Science, 5,* 65–72.

Gagner, M., Begin, E., Hurteau, R., & Pomp, A. (1994). Robotic interactive laparoscopic cholecystectomy. *Lancet, 343,* 596–597.

Gallagher, D., Lovett, S., & Zeiss, A. (1989). Interventions with caregivers of frail elders: Current research status and future research directions. In M. Ory & K. Bond (Eds.), *Aging and health care: Social science and policy perspectives* (pp. 167–190). New York: Routledge.

Gallo, A. M., Breitmayer, B. J., & Knafl, K. A. (1992). Well siblings of children with chronic illnesses: Parents' reports of their psychological adjustment. *Pediatric Nursing, 18,* 23–27.

Gardner, K. (1991). A summary of findings of a five-year comparison study of primary and team nursing. *Nursing Research, 40,* 113–117.

Garfield, E. (1985). Citation patterns in nursing journals, and their most-cited articles. In E. Garfield, *Essays of an information scientist: 1984* (Vol. 7, pp. 336–345). Philadelphia: ISI Press.

Garg, A., Owen, B. D., & Carlson, N. (1992). An ergonomic evaluation of nursing assistants' job in a nursing home. *Ergonomics, 35,* 979–995.

Garlinghouse, J., & Sharp, L. J. (1968). The hemophiliac child's self-concept and family stress in relation to bleeding episodes. *Nursing Research, 17,* 32–37.

Garris, R., & Jewell, D. (1995). Comparison of outcomes between acute care general hospital transfers and direct admissions to a detoxification unit. *Addictions Nursing, 7,* 117–120.

Garvin, B. J., & Ryan-Wenger, N. (1997, April). *Coping with health-illness concerns: Knowledge synthesis and implications.* Paper presented at the Midwest Nursing Research Society Stress and Coping Synthesis Conference, Minneapolis.

Gassert, C. A. (1991). Defining nursing information systems requirements: A linked model. In L. C. Kingsland III (Ed.), *Proceedings of the Thirteenth Annual Symposium on Computer Applications in Medical Care* (pp. 779–782). Washington, DC: IEEE Computer Society Press.

Gaston, E. T. (1951). Dynamic music factors in mood change. *Music Educators Journal, 3,* 42–44.

Gastrin, G., Miller, A. B., To, T., Aronson, K. J., Wall, C., Hakama, M., Louhivuori, K., & Pukkala, E. (1994). Incidence and mortality from breast cancer in the Mama program for breast screening in Finland, 1973–1986. *Cancer, 73,* 2168–2174.

Gates, S. J., & Brooks, M. (1991). Imaging of the orthopaedic patient: Implications for primary care. *Nurse Practitioner Forum, 2,* 225–230.

Gatsonis, C. A., & Needleman, H. L. (1992). Recent epidemiologic studies of low-level lead exposure and the IQ of children: A meta-analytic review. In H. L. Needleman (Ed.), *Human lead exposure* (pp. 243–255). Boca Raton, FL: CRC Press.

Gebbie, K. M. (1976). *Summary of the Second National Conference Classification of Nursing Diagnosis.* St. Louis, MO: National Group for Classification of Nursing Diagnosis.

Gebbie, K. M., & Lavin, M. A. (1975). *Classification of nursing diagnoses: Proceedings of the First National Conference.* St. Louis: C. V. Mosby.

Gee, J. P. (1991). A linguistic approach to narrative. *Journal of Narrative and Life History, 1,* 15–39.

Gegor, C. L., & Paine, L. L. (1992). Antepartum fetal assessment techniques: An update for today's perinatal nurse. *Journal of Perinatal and Neonatal Nursing, 5*(4), 1–15.

Gelinas, L. S., & Boston, C. (1995). *The impact of organizational redesign on nurse executive leadership.* Irving, TX: VHA Inc.

Gemsom, D., Ashford, A., Dickey, L., Raymore, S., Roberts, J., Ehrlich, M., Foster, B., Ganz, M., Moun-Howard, J., Field, L., Bennett, B., Elinson, J., & Francis, C. (1997). Putting prevention into practice: Impact of a multifaceted physician education program on preventive services in the inner city. *Archives of Internal Medicine, 155,* 2210–2216.

General Accounting Office. (1992). *Cross design synthesis: A new strategy for medical effectiveness research* (B-244808). Washington, DC: Author.

Genette, G. (1988). *Narrative discourse revisited.* Ithaca, NY: Cornell University Press.

George, L. K., & Gwyther, L. P. (1986). Caregiver well-being: A multidimensional examination of family caregivers of demented adults. *Gerontologist, 26,* 253–259.

Germain, C. B., & Dodd, M. J. (Eds.). (1993). *Developing taxonomies for nursing research.* Washington, DC: American Nurses Publishing.

Geronimus, A. T., Bound, J., Waidmann, T. A., Hillemeier, M. M., & Burns, P. B. (1996). Excess mortality among Blacks and Whites in the United States. *New England Journal of Medicine, 335,* 1552–1558.

Gibson, J. L., Love, W., Hardie, D., Bancroft, P., & Turner, A. J. (1892). Notes on lead poisoning as observed among children in Brisbane. In L. Huxtable (Ed.), *Transactions from the Third Intercolonial Medical Congress of Australasia* (pp. 76–77). Sydney, Australia: Charles Potter.

Gift, A., Moore, T., & Soeken, K. (1992). Relaxation to reduce dyspnea and anxiety in COPD patients. *Nursing Research, 41,* 242–246.

Gift, A. G., & Soeken, K. L. (1988). Assessment of physiologic instruments. *Heart and Lung, 17,* 128–133.

Gilligan, C. (1982). *In a different voice: Psychological theory and women's development.* Cambridge: Harvard University Press.

Gilliss, C., & Knafl, K. (1997). Nursing care of families in non-normative transitions: The state of science and practice. In A. S. Hinshaw, S. L. Feetham, & J. Shaver (Eds.), *Handbook of clinical nursing research.* Thousand Oaks, CA: Sage.

Giorgi, A. (1985). *Phenomenology and psychological research.* Pittsburgh, PA: Duquesne University Press.

Giovannetti, P. (1978). Patient classification systems in nursing: A description and analysis (DHEW Publication No. HRA 78/22). Washington, DC: U.S. Government Printing Office.

Giovannetti, P. (1980). A comparison of team and primary nursing care delivery systems. *Nursing Dimensions, 7*(4), 96–100.

Giovannetti, P. (1984). Staffing methods: Implications for quality. In L. Willis & P. Lindwood (Eds.), *Measuring the quality of nursing care* (pp. 123–150). London: Churchill Livingstone.

Giovannetti, P. (1986). Evaluation of primary nursing. In H. H. Werley, J. J. Fitzpatrick, & R. L. Taunton (Eds.), *Annual Review of Nursing Research* (Vol. 4, pp. 127–151). New York: Springer Publishing.

Giovannetti, P. (1994). Measurement of nursing workload. In J. M. Hibberd & M. E. Kyle (Eds.), *Nursing management in Canada* (pp. 331–349). Toronto: W. B. Saunders.

Givens, B. A., & Givens, C. W. (1991). Family caregiving for the elderly. In J. J. Fitzpatrick & J. S. Stevenson (Eds.), *Annual review of nursing research* (Vol. 9, pp. 77–92). New York: Springer Publishing.

Glaser, B. (1978). *Theoretical sensitivity.* Mill Valley, CA: Sociology Press.

Glaser, B. G., & Strauss, A. L. (1965). *Awareness of dying.* Chicago: Aldine.

Glaser, B., & Strauss, A. (1967). *The discovery of grounded theory.* Chicago: Aldine.

Glaser, B. G., & Strauss, A. L. (1968). *Time for dying.* Chicago: Aldine.

Glass, G. (1976). Primary, secondary, and meta-analysis of research. *Educational Researcher, 5,* 3–8.

Glass, P. (1990). Light and the developing retina. *Documenta Ophthalmologica, 74,* 195–203.

Glick, O. J., & Tripp-Reimer, T. (1996). The Iowa conceptual model of gerontological nursing. In E. A. Swanson & T. Tripp-Reimer (Eds.), *Advances in gerontological nursing* (Vol. 1, pp. 11–55). New York: Springer Publishing.

Glick, W. H., Huber, G. P., Miller, C. C., Doty, D. H., & Sutcliffe, K. M. (1990). Studying changes in organizational design and effectiveness: Retrospective event histories and periodic assessments. *Organization Science, 1,* 293–312.

Glick, W. H., Huber, G. P., Miller, C. C., Doty, D. H., & Sutcliffe, K. M. (1993). Studying changes in organizational design and effectiveness: Retrospective event histories and periodic assessments. In G. P. Huber & W. H. Glick (Eds.), *Organizational change and redesign. Ideas and insights for improving performance* (pp. 411–433). New York: Oxford University Press.

Goddaer, J., & Abraham, I. L. (1994). Effects of relaxing music on agitation during meals among nursing home residents with severe cognitive impairment. *Archives of Psychiatric Nursing, 8,* 150–158.

Gold, D. R., Rogacz, S., Bock, N., Tosteson, T. D., Baum, T. M., Speizer, F. E., & Czeisler, C. A. (1992). Rotating shift work, sleep and accidents related to sleepiness in hospital nurses. *American Journal of Public Health, 82,* 1011–1014.

Goldie, S., & Bishop, W. J. (1983). *A calendar of the letters of Florence Nightingale.* Oxford: Wellcome Institute for the History of Medicine, Oxford Microform.

Goldmark, J. (1923). *Nursing and nursing education in the United States.* New York: Macmillan.

Good, M., & Moore, S. M. (1996). Clinical practice guidelines as a new source of middle-range theory: Focus on acute pain. *Nursing Outlook, 44,* 74–79.

Goodwin, J. O., & Edwards, B. S. (1975). Developing a computer program to assist the nursing process: Phase I—from systems analysis to an expandable program. *Nursing Research, 24,* 299–305.

Goodwin, L. D., & Goodwin, W. L. (1991). Estimating construct validity. *Research in Nursing and Health, 14,* 235–243.

Gordon, M. (1982). *Nursing diagnosis: Process and application.* New York: McGraw-Hill.

Gorham, W. (1962). Staff nursing behaviors contributing to patient care and improvement. *Nursing Research, 11,* 68–79.

Gorsuch, R. L. (1983). *Factor analysis* (2nd ed.). Hillsdale, NJ: Lawrence Erlbaum Associates.

Gortner, S. R., Gillis, C. L., Shinn, T. A., Sparacino, P. A., Rankin, S., Leavitt, M., Price, M., & Hudes, M. (1988). Improving recovery following cardiac surgery: A randomized clinical trial. *Journal of Advanced Nursing, 13,* 649–661.

Gortner, S. R., & Jenkins, L. S. (1990). Self-efficacy and activity level following cardiac surgery. *Journal of Advanced Nursing, 15,* 1132–1138.

Gosnell, D. (1973). An assessment tool to identify pressure sores. *Nursing Research, 22,* 5–59.

Gothler, A. W. (1988). *Nurse faculty socioeconomic trends.* New York: National League for Nursing.

Gottlieb, D., Beiser, A., & O'Conner, G. (1995). Poverty, race, and medication use are correlates of asthma hospitalization rates. *Chest, 108,* 28–35.

Grabbe, L., Demi, A., Camann, M., & Potter, L. (1997). The health status of elderly persons in the last year of life: A comparison of deaths by suicide, injury, and natural causes. *American Journal of Public Health, 87,* 434–437.

Grady, P. A., Harden, J. T., Moritz, P., & Amende, L. (1997). Incorporating environmental sciences and nursing research: An NINR initiative. *Nursing Outlook, 45,* 73–75.

Grahl, C. (1994). Improving compliance: Solving a $100 billion problem. *Managed Health Care,* S11–S13.

Grandbois, M. (1964). The nursing literature index: Its history, present needs, and future plans. *Bulletin of the Medical Library Association, 52,* 676–683.

Grant, J. A., & Kennedy-Caldwell, C. (Eds.). (1987). *Nutrition and nursing.* Orlando, FL: Grune and Stratton.

Grant, J. P., Curtas, M. S., & Kelvin, F. M. (1983). Fluoroscopic placement of nasojejunal feeding tubes with immediate feeding using a nonelemental diet. *JPEN: Journal of Parenteral and Enteral Nutrition, 7,* 299–303.

Gravenstein, J. S., Berzina-Moettus, L. A., Regan, Y. H., & Pao, Y. H. (1974). Laser mediated telemedicine in anesthesia. *Anesthesia and Analgesia, 53,* 605–608.

Graves, J. (1990). A research-knowledge systems (ARKS) for storing, managing, and modeling knowledge from the scientific literature. *Advances in Nursing Science, 13*(2), 34–45.

Graves, J. R. (1993). Data versus information versus knowledge. *Reflections, 19*(1), 4–5, Spring.

Graves, J. R. (1994). STTI Library: A registry of nursing research. *Reflections, 20*(2), 9.

Graves, J. R. (1996, Summer). Announcing the third edition of the Sigma Theta Tau International Research Classification System. *Sigma Theta Tau International Reflections,* pp. 4–5.

Graves, J. R. (1996, 2nd quarter). New classification system announced. *Reflections,* pp. 24–28.

Graves, J. R. (1997). The Virginia Henderson International Nursing Library: Resource for nurse administrators. *Nursing Administration Quarterly, 21*(3), 76–83.

Graves, J. R., & Corcoran, S. (1989). The study of nursing informatics systems. *Image: Journal of Nursing Scholarship, 21,* 227–231.

Gray, D. P. (1995). A journey into feminist pedagogy. *Journal of Nursing Education, 34,* 77–81.

Gray-Toft, P. A., & Anderson, J. G. (1981). Stress among hospital nursing staff: Its causes and effects. *Social Science and Medicine, 15,* 639–647.

Graydon, J. (1994). Women with breast cancer: Their quality of life following a course of radiation therapy. *Journal of Advanced Nursing, 19,* 617–622.

Green, M., & Solnit, A. J. (1964). Reactions to the threatened loss of a child: A vulnerable child syndrome. *Pediatrics, 34,* 58–66.

Green, N. (1994). *Bright futures: Guidelines for health supervision of infants, children and adolescents.* Arlington, VA: National Center for Education in Maternal and Child Health.

Greenwood, J. (1996). *Nursing theory in Australia: Development and application.* New South Wales, Australia: Harper.

Greiner, A. (1995). *Cost and quality matters: Workplace innovations in the health care industry.* Washington, DC: Economic Policy Institute.

Grey, M., Cameron, M. E., Lipman, T. H., & Thurber, F. W. (1995). Psychosocial status of children with diabetes over the first two years. *Diabetes Care, 18,* 1330–1336.

Griffith, H. M., & Robinson, K. R. (1992). Survey of the degree to which critical care nurses are performing Current Procedural Terminology-coded services. *American Journal of Critical Care, 1,* 91–98.

Griffith, H. M., & Robinson, K. R. (1993). Current Procedural Terminology (CPT) coded services provided by nurse specialists. *Image: Journal of Nursing Scholarship, 25,* 178–186.

Griffith, H. M., Thomas, N., & Griffith, L. (1991). MDs bill for these routine nursing tasks. *American Journal of Nursing, 91*(1), 22–25, 27.

Grobe, S. J. (1996). The Nursing Intervention Lexicon and Taxonomy: Implications for representing nursing care data in automated records. *Holistic Nursing Practice, 11*(1), 48–63.

Grondin, J. (1995). *Sources of hermeneutics.* Albany: State University of New York Press.

Gross, D., & Conrad, B. (1995). Temperament in toddlerhood. *Journal of Pediatric Nursing, 10,* 146–151.

Gross, D., Conrad, B., Fogg, L., Willis, L., & Garvey, C. (1995). A longitudinal study of maternal depression and preschool children's mental health. *Nursing Research, 44,* 96–101.

Gross, D., Fogg, L., & Tucker, S. (1995). The efficacy of parent training for promoting positive parent-toddler relationships. *Research in Nursing and Health, 18,* 489–499.

Grossman, J. A., Clark, D. C., Gross, D., Halstead, L., & Pennington, J. (1995). Child bereavement after paternal suicide. *Journal of Child and Adolescent Psychiatric Nursing, 8*(2), 5–17.

Grossman, P. (1991). Respiratory mediation of cardiac function within a psychophysiological perspective. In J. G. Carlson & A. R. Seifert (Eds.), *International perspectives on self-regulation and health* (pp. 17–39). New York: Plenum Press.

Grossman, S., Campbell, C., & Riley, B. (1996). Assessment of clinical decision-making ability of critical care nurses. *Dimensions of Critical Care Nursing, 15,* 272–279.

Grossman, S. A., Piantadosi, S., & Couchey, C. (1994). Are informed consent forms that describe clinical oncology research protocols readable by most patients and their families? *Journal of Clinical Oncology, 12,* 2211–2215.

Gunn, I. P. (1974). Preparing today's nurse anesthetist to meet contemporary needs: A philosophic and pragmatic approach. *AANA Journal, 42,* 25–38.

Gunn, I. P., Jenecik, J. A., Lewis, B. J., & Meyer, J. A. (1965). Expiratory resistance of oxygen catheters in patients with tracheostomies. *Journal of the American Medical Association, 193,* 737–739.

Gunn, I. P., Sullivan, E. F., & Glor, B. A. K. (1966). Blood pressure measurement as a quantitative research criterion. *Nursing Research, 15,* 4–11.

Gunter, L., & Estes, C. (1979). *Education for gerontic nursing.* New York: Springer Publishing.

Gunther, L. M., & Miller, J. C. (1977). Toward a nursing gerontology. *Nursing Research, 26,* 208–221.

Gurney, J. G., Davis, S., Severson, R. K., Fang, J., Ross, J. A., & Robison, L. L. (1996). Trends in cancer incidence among children in the U.S. *Cancer, 78,* 532–541.

Gustafson, Y., Brannstrom, B., Berggren, D., Ragnarsson, J. I., Sigaard, J., Bucht, G., Reiz, S., Norberg, A., & Winblad, B. (1991). A geriatric anesthesiologic program to reduce acute confusional states in elderly patients treated for femoral neck fractures. *Journal of the American Geriatrics Society, 89,* 655–662.

Guttman, L. (1954). Some necessary conditions for factor analysis. *Psychometrika, 19,* 149–161.

Guzzetta, C. E. (1988). Music therapy: Hearing the melody of the soul. In B. M. Dossey, L. Keegan, C. E. Guzzetta, & L. G. Kolkmeier (Eds.), *Holistic nursing: A handbook for practice* (pp. 263–288). Rockville, MD: Aspen.

Haber, L., & Austin, J. (1992). How married couples make decisions. *Western Journal of Nursing Research, 14,* 322–342.

Hack, M., Estabrook, M., & Robertson, S. (1985). Development of sucking rhythm in preterm infants. *Early Human Development, 11,* 133–140.

Hackett, T. P. (1985). Depression following myocardial infarction. *Psychosomatics, 26,* 23–28.

Haddon, W., Jr., & Baker, S. P. (1980). Injury control. In D. Clark & B. MacMahon (Eds.), *Preventive medicine.* Boston: Little, Brown.

Hagey, R. (1984). The phenomenon, the explanations, and the responses: Metaphors surrounding diabetes in urban Canadian Indians. *Social Science and Medicine, 18,* 265–272.

Hall, G. R., & Buckwalter, K. C. (1987). Progressively lowered stress threshold: A conceptual model for care of adults with Alzheimer's disease. *Archives of Psychiatric Nursing, 1,* 399–406.

Hall, G. R., Gerdner, L., Zwycart-Stauffacher, M., & Buckwalter, K. C. (1995). Principles of nonpharmacological management: Caring for people with Alzheimer's disease using a conceptual model. *Psychiatric Annals, 25,* 432–440.

Hall, L., Gurley, D., Sachs, B., & Kryscio, R. (1991). Psychosocial predictors of maternal depressive symptoms, parenting attitudes, and child behavior in single-parent families. *Nursing Research, 40,* 214–220.

Hall, L., Kotch, J., Browne, D., & Rayens, M. K. (1996). Self-esteem as a mediator of the effects of stressors and social resources on depressive symptoms in postpartum mothers. *Nursing Research, 45,* 231–237.

Halloran, E. (Ed.). (1995). *A Virginia Henderson reader: Excellence in nursing.* New York: Springer Publishing.

Halloran, E. J., & Hadley-Vermeersch, P. (1987). Variability in nurse setting research. *Journal of Nursing Administration, 17,* 26–32.

Halstead, J., Hayes, R., Reising, D., & Billings, D. M. (1995). Nursing student information network: Fostering collegial communications using a computer conference. *Computers in Nursing, 13,* 55–59.

Hamera, E. K., Peterson, K. A., Handley, S. M., Plumlee, A. A., & Frank-Ragan, E. (1991). Patient self-regulation and functioning in schizophrenia. *Hospital and Community Psychiatry, 42,* 630–631.

Hamera, E. K., Peterson, K. A., Young, L. M., & Schaumloffel, M. M. (1992). Symptoms monitoring in schizophrenia: Potential for enhancing self-care. *Archives of Psychiatric Nursing, 6,* 324–330.

Hamilton, J. A., & Harberger, P. N. (1992). *Postpartum psychiatric illness: A picture puzzle.* Philadelphia: University of Pennsylvania Press.

Hammond, K. R. (1964). Part 2. Clinical inference in nursing—a methodological approach. *Nursing Research, 13,* 315–319.

Hamric, A. B., & Spross, J. (1989). *The clinical nurse specialist in theory and practice* (2nd ed.). New York: Grune & Stratton.

Hamric, A. B., Spross, J. A., & Hanson, C. M. (1996). *Advanced practice nursing: An integrated approach.* Philadelphia: W. B. Saunders.

Hansen, B. C., Ortmeyer, H. K., & Bodkin, N. L. (1995). Prevention of obesity in middle-aged monkeys: Food intake during body weight clamp. *Obesity Research, 3*(Suppl. 2), 199s–204s.

Happ, M. B., Williams, C. C., Strumpf, N. E., & Burger, S. G. (1996). Individualized care for frail elders: Theory and practice. *Journal of Gerontological Nursing, 22*(3), 7–14.

Harding, C. M. (1988). Course types in schizophrenia: An analysis of European and American studies. *Schizophrenia Bulletin, 14,* 633–643.

Harding, C. M., Brooks, G. W., Ashikaga, T., Strauss, J. S., & Breier, A. (1987). The Vermont Longitudinal Study of persons with severe mental illness: 1. Methodology, study sample, and overall status 32 years later. *American Journal of Psychiatry, 144,* 718–726.

Harkness, G. A. (1995). *Epidemiology in nursing practice.* St. Louis: Mosby Yearbook.

Harmer, B., & Henderson, V. (1939). *Textbook of the principles and practice of nursing* (4th ed.). New York: Macmillan.

Harmer, B., & Henderson, V. (1955). *Textbook of the principles and practice of nursing* (5th ed.). New York: Macmillan.

Harrell, J. S., McMurray, R. G., Bangdiwala, S. I., Frauman, A. C., Gansky, S. A., & Bradley, C. B. (1996). The effects of a school-based intervention to reduce cardiovascular disease risk factors in elementary school children: The Cardiovascular Health in Children (CHIC) Study. *Journal of Pediatrics, 128,* 797–805.

Harris, Z. S. (1952). Discourse analysis. *Lg, 28,* 1–30.

Harrison-Woermke, D., & Graydon, J. (1993). Perceived informational needs of breast cancer patients receiving radiation therapy after excisonal biopsy and axillary node dissection. *Cancer Nursing, 16,* 44–45.

Hartley, L. A. (1988). Congruence between teaching and learning self-care: A pilot study. *Nursing Science Quarterly, 1,* 161–167.

Hartley, S. S., & McKibbin, R. C. (1983). *Hospital payment mechanisms, patient classification systems and nursing: Relationships and implications.* Kansas City, MO: American Nurses Association.

Hartweg, D. L. (1991). *Dorothea Orem: Self-care deficit theory.* Newbury Park, CA: Sage.

Haskell, W. L., Alderman, E. L., Fair, J. M., Maron, D. J., Mackey, S. F., Superko, H. R., Williams, P. T., Johnstone, I. M., Champagne, M. E., Krauss, R. M., & Farquhar, J. (1994). Effects of intensive multiple risk factor reduction on coronary atherosclerosis and clinical cardiac events in men and women with coronary artery disease. *Stanford Coronary Risk Intervention Project (SCRIP), 84,* 975–990.

Hasselmeyer, E. G. (1961). *Behavior patterns of premature infants* (USPHS Publication No. 840). Washington, DC: U.S. Government Printing Office.

Hassey, D., Ferrell, B. R., Leigh, S., & Melancon, C. (in press). The cancer survivor as co-investigator: The benefits of collaborative research with advocacy groups. *Cancer Practice.*

Hassey Dow, K. (1994). Having children after breast cancer. *Cancer Practice, 2,* 407–413.

Hassey Dow, K. (1997). Nursing research in radiation oncology. In K. Hassey Dow, J. Dunn Bucholtz, R. Iwamoto, V. Fieler, & L. Hilderley (Eds.), *Nursing care in radiation oncology* (2nd ed., chap. 25). Philadelphia: W. B. Saunders.

Hathaway, D. (1986). Effect of preoperative instruction on postoperative outcomes: A meta-analysis. *Nursing Research, 35*, 269–275.

Hathaway, D., Abell, T., Cardoso, S., Hartwig, M., Elmer, D., Horton, J., Lawrence, D., Gaber, L., & Gaber, A. O. (1993). Improvement in autonomic function following pancreas-kidney versus kidney-alone transplantation. *Transplantation Proceedings, 25*(1 Pt. 2), 1306–1308.

Hauenstein, E. (1992). Shifting the paradigm: Toward integrating research on mothers and children. *Journal of Child and Adolescent Psychiatric Nursing, 5*(4), 18–29.

Hauenstein, E. (1996a). A nursing practice paradigm for depressed rural women: Theoretical basis. *Archives of Psychiatric Nursing, 10*, 283–292.

Hauenstein, E. (1996b). Testing innovative nursing care: Home intervention with depressed rural women. *Issues in Mental Health Nursing, 17*, 33–50.

Hauenstein, E. (1997). A nursing practice paradigm for depressed rural women: The women's affective illness treatment program. *Archives of Psychiatric Nursing, 11*, 1–9.

Hauser, W. A., & Hesdorffer, D. C. (1990). *Epilepsy: Frequency, causes, and consequences.* New York: Demos Publications.

Hawley, D. J. (1995). Psycho-educational interventions in the treatment of arthritis. *Bailliere's Clinical Rheumatology, 9*, 803–823.

Hayman, L. L., Cleves, M. A., & Meininger, J. C. (1997, November). *Diet-lipid profile associations in school-age twins.* Paper presented at the American Heart Association 70th Scientific Sessions, Orlando, FL.

Hayman, L. L., Mcininger, J. C., Coates, P. M., & Gallagher, P. R. (1995). Nongenetic influences of obesity on risk factors for cardiovascular disease during two phases of development. *Nursing Research, 44*, 277–283.

Hayman, L. L., Meininger, J. C., Stashinko, E. E., Gallagher, P. R., & Coates, P. M. (1988). Type A behavior and physiological cardiovascular risk factors in school-age twin children. *Nursing Research, 37*, 290–296.

Haynes, R. B., Taylor, D. W., & Sackett, D. L. (Eds.). (1979). *Compliance in health care.* Baltimore: Johns Hopkins University Press.

Hays, B., Norris, J., Martin, K., & Androwich, I. (1994). Informatics issues for nursing's future. *Advances in Nursing Science, 16*(4), 71–81.

Head, B., Maas, M., & Johnson, M. (1997). Outcomes for home and community nursing in integrated delivery systems. *Caring, 16*(1), 50–56.

Health Care Financing Administration. (1980). *Medicare: Provider reimbursement manual: Part 2. Provider cost reporting forms and instructions* (1728, DHHS). Baltimore: HCFA.

Health Care Financing Administration and Bureau of Data Management and Strategy. (1990). *HCFA, BDMS, BMAD system procedure file.* Washington, DC: U.S. Department of Health and Human Services.

Health Risk Reduction: Community Based Strategies (Fall, 1996). (RFA PA 96037). National Institute of Nursing Research.

Heffline, M. S. (1991). A comparative study of pharmacological versus nursing interventions in the treatment of postanesthesia shivering. *Journal of Post Anesthesia Nursing, 6,* 311–320.

Heidegger, M. (1962). *Being and time* (J. Macquarrie & F. Robinson, Trans.). New York: Harper & Row. (Original work published 1927)

Heidegger, M. (1993). In D. Krell (Ed.), *Basic writings* (rev. ed.). San Francisco: Harper. (Original work published 1977)

Heidegger, M. (1996). *Being and time: A translation of Sein und Zeit* (J. Stambaugh, Trans.). New York: Harper and Row. (Original work published 1927)

Heitkemper, M. M., Jarrett, M., Cain, K., Shaver, J. F., Bond, E. F., Woods, N. F., & Walker, E. (1996). Increased urine catecholamines and cortisol in women with irritable bowel syndrome. *American Journal of Gastroenterology, 91,* 906–913.

Heitkemper, M. M., Levy, R., Jarrett, M., & Bond, E. F. (1995). Interventions for irritable bowel syndrome: A nursing model. *Gastroenterology Nursing, 18,* 224–230.

Henderson, M. G., & Wallack, S. S. (1987). Evaluating case management for catastrophic illness. *Business and Health, 4*(3), 7–11.

Henderson, V. (1966). *The nature of nursing.* New York: Macmillan.

Henderson, V. (1978). The concept of nursing. *Journal of Advanced Nursing, 3,* 113–130.

Henderson, V. (1991). *The nature of nursing: Reflection after 25 years.* New York: National League of Nursing. (Original work published 1966)

Henderson, V. (1997). *Basic principles of nursing care.* Geneva: International Council of Nurses. (Original work published 1960)

Henderson, V., & Nite, G. (1997). *Principles and practice of nursing* (6th ed.). New York: Macmillan. (Original work published 1978)

Henderson, V., & the Yale University School of Nursing Index Staff. (1963–1972, 1984). *Nursing studies index* (Vols. 1–4). Philadelphia: J. B. Lippincott.

Hendrickson, M. H., & Paganelli, B. (1994). Facing the challenges of nurse expert systems in the future. In S. J. Grobe & E. S. P. Pluyter Wenting (Eds.), *Nursing informatics: Enhancing patient care* (NIH Publication No. 93-2419). Bethesda, MD: U.S. Department of Health and Human Services.

Henker, R., Bernardo, L. M., O'Connor, K., & Sereika, S. (1995). Evaluation of four methods of warming intravenous fluids. *Journal of Emergency Nursing, 21,* 385–390.

Henley, W. (1888). In hospital 1872–1875, in *A Book of Verses.* London: David Nutt.

Henry, B., Moody, L. E., Pendergast, J. F., O'Donnell, J., Moody, L. E., & Hutchinson, S. A. (1987). Delineations of nursing administration research priorities. *Nursing Research, 36,* 309–314.

Henry, J. P. (1992). Biological basis of the stress response. *Integrative Physiological and Behavioral Science, 27,* 66–83.

Henry, S. B. (1989). Evaluation in staff development. In W. L. Holzemer (Ed.), *Review of research in nursing education* (Vol. 11, pp. 129–153). New York: National League for Nursing.

Henry, S. B., Holzemer, W. L., Randell, C., Hsieh, S.-F., & Miller, T. J. (1997). Comparison of Nursing Interventions Classification and Current Procedural Terminology codes for categorizing nursing activities. *Image: Journal of Nursing Scholarship, 29,* 133–138.

Henry, S. B., Holzemer, W. L., Reilly, C. A., & Campbell, K. E. (1994). Terms used by nurses to describe patient problems: Can SNOMED III represent nursing concepts in the patient record? *Journal of the American Medical Informatics Association, 1,* 61–74.

Henry, S. B., & Mead, C. N. (1997). Nursing classification systems: Necessary but not sufficient for representing "what nurses do" for inclusion in computer-based patient record systems. *Journal of the American Medical Informatics Association, 4*(3), 222–232.

Herron, M., Katz, M., & Creasy, R. (1982). Evaluation of a preterm birth prevention program: A preliminary report. *Obstetrics and Gynecology, 59,* 452–454.

Herth, K. (1990). Relationship of hope, coping styles, concurrent losses, and setting to grief resolution in the elderly widow(er). *Research in Nursing and Health, 13,* 109–117.

Hester, N. O. (1979). The preoperational child's reaction to immunizations. *Nursing Research, 28,* 250–255.

Hewitt, M. (1992). Defining "rural" areas: Impact on health care policy and research. In W. Gesler & T. Ricketts (Eds.), *Health in rural North America,* (pp. 25–54). New Brunswick, NJ: Rutgers University Press.

Higgins, J. M., Ponet, P. R., James, J. R., Fay, M., & Madden, M. J. (1994). Restructuring the CNS role for a managed care environment. *Clinical Nurse Specialist, 8,* 163–166.

Highfield, M. F., & Cason, C. (1983). Spiritual needs of patients: Are they recognized? *Cancer Nursing, 6,* 187–192.

Hill, J. P. (1987). Research on adolescent and their families: Past and prospect. In C. E. Irwin, Jr. (Ed.), *Adolescent social behavior and health: New directions in child development* (Vol. 37, pp. 13–31). San Francisco: Jossey-Bass.

Hill, M. N., & Becker, D. M. (1995). Role of nurses and health care workers in cardiovascular health promotion. *American Journal of the Medical Sciences, 310,* S123–S126.

Hill, R. (1958). Social stresses on the family. *Social Casework, 39,* 139–150.

Hinds, P. S. (1988). Adolescent hopefulness in illness and health. *Advances in Nursing Science, 10*(3), 79–88.

Hinshaw, A. S. (1979). Theoretical substruction: An assessment process. *Western Journal of Nursing Research, 1,* 319–324.

Hinshaw, A. S. (1996). Research traditions: A decade of progress. *Journal of Professional Nursing, 12*(2), 68.

Hinshaw, A., & Atwood, J. (1982). A patient satisfaction instrument: Precision by replication. *Nursing Research, 31,* 170–175.

Hinshaw, A. S., & Atwood, J. R. (1983–1985). *Anticipating turnover among nursing staff study: Final report.* Rockville, MD: U.S. Department of Health and Human Services, Division of Nursing.

Hinshaw, A. S., & Ketefian, S. (1996). A missing research tradition. *Journal of Professional Nursing, 12*(4), 196.

Hobson, J. A. (1989). *Sleep.* New York: Scientific American Library.

Hockenberry-Eaton, M., Kemp, V., & DiIorio, C. (1994). Cancer stressors and protective factors: Predictors of stress experienced during treatment for childhood cancer. *Research in Nursing and Health, 17,* 351–361.

Hogue, C. C. (1984). Falls and mobility in late life: An ecological model. *Journal of the American Geriatrics Society, 32,* 858–861.

Holaday, B. (1987). Patterns of interaction between mothers and their chronically ill infants. *Maternal Child Nursing Journal, 16,* 29–46.

Holditch-Davis, D. (in press). Neonatal sleep-wake states. In C. Kenner, J. Loh, & A. Bruggemeyer (Eds.), *Comprehensive neonatal nursing care: A physiologic perspective* (2nd ed.). Philadelphia: W. B. Saunders.

Holditch-Davis, D., & Miles, M. S. (1997). Parenting the prematurely-born child. In J. J. Fitzpatrick & J. Norbeck (Eds.), *Annual Review of Nursing Research* (Vol. 15, pp. 3–34). New York: Springer Publishing.

Holloran, S. (1989). Mentoring: The experience of nursing service executives (Doctoral Dissertation, Boston University, 1989). *Dissertation Abstracts International, 25,* 199.

Holmberg, S. K., & Kane, C. F. (1995). Severe psychiatric disorder and physical health risks. *Clinical Nurse Specialist, 9,* 287–292.

Holmes, G. L. (1987). *Diagnosis and management of seizures in children.* Philadelphia: W. B. Saunders.

Holmes, O. W. (1860). *Currents and counter-currents in medical science.* Boston: Massachusetts Medical Society.

Holmes, T. H., & Rahe, R. (1967). The social readjustment rating scale. *Journal of Psychosomatic Research, 12,* 213–218.

Holt, L. E. (1897). *Diseases of infancy and childhood.* New York: D. Appleton.

Holtzclaw, B. J. (1990). Effects of extremity wraps to control drug induced shivering: A pilot study. *Nursing Research, 39,* 280–283.

Holtzclaw, B. J. (1996). AIDS-related fever: Hydration and cardiorespiratory effects. In *Proceedings: Sigma Theta Tau International, Eighth International Nursing Research Congress at Ocho Rios, Jamaica.* Indianapolis, IN: Sigma Theta Tau International (p. 72).

Holtzclaw, B. J., & Geer, R. T. (1995). Clinical predictors and metabolic consequences of postoperative shivering after cardiac surgery. In S. G. Funk, E. M. Tornquist, M. T. Champagne, & R. A. Wiese (Eds.), *Key aspects of caring for the acutely ill* (pp. 226–233). New York: Springer Publishing.

Holzemer, B., Henry, S., Stewart, A., & Janson-Bjerklie, S. (1993). The HIV quality audit marker (HIV-QAM): An outcome measure for hospitalized AIDS patients. *Quality of Life Research, 2,* 99–107.

Holzemer, W. L., Henry, S. B., Dawson, C., Sousa, K., Bain, C., & Hsieh, S. F. (1997, September). *An evaluation of the utility of the Home Health Care Classification for categorizing patient problems and nursing interventions from the hospital setting.* Paper presented at the NI97, Stockholm.

Holzemer, W. L., & Reilly, C. A. (1994). Variables, variability, and variations research: Implications for medical informatics. In *Informatics: The infrastructure for quality assessment and improvement in nursing. Proceedings of the Fifth International Nursing Informatics Symposium Post-Conference* (pp. 47–51). San Francisco: University of California Nursing Press.

Homans, G. (1961). *Social behavior: Its elementary forms.* New York: Harcourt, Brace, and World.

Hoover, H. C., Jr., Ryan, J. A., Anderson, E. J., & Fischer, J. E. (1980). Nutritional benefits of immediate postoperative jejunal feeding of an elemental diet. *American Journal of Surgery, 139,* 153–159.

Horn, S., Ashton, C., & Tracy, D. (1994). Prevention and treatment of pressure ulcers by protocol. In S. Horn & D. Hopkins (Eds.), *Clinical practice improvement: A new technology for developing cost-effective quality health care.* New York: Faulkner & Gray.

Horowitz, A. (1985). Family caregiving to the frail elderly. In C. Eisdorfer (Ed.), *Annual review of gerontology* (Vol. 5, pp. 194–246). New York: Springer Publishing.

Horowitz, R. S., & Fuller, S. S. (1982). Concurrence in content descriptions: Author vs. medical subject headings (MeSH). *Proceedings of the American Society for Information Science Annual Meeting, 19,* 139–140.

Horsley, J. A., Crane, J., Crabtree, M. K., & Wood, D. J. (1983). *Using research to improve nursing practice: A guide.* New York: Grune & Stratton.

Hudson, M. F. (1989). Analysis of the concepts of elder mistreatment: Abuse and neglect. *Journal of Elder Abuse and Neglect, 1*(1), 5–25.

Hudson, M. F. (1991). Elder mistreatment: A taxonomy with definitions by Delphi. *Journal of Elder Abuse and Neglect, 3*(2), 1–20.

Hudson, M. F. (1994). Elder abuse: Its meaning to middle-aged and older adults: Part 2. Pilot results. *Journal of Elder Abuse and Neglect, 6*(1), 55–83.

Hudson, M. F., & Carlson, J. (1994). Elder abuse: Its meaning to middle-aged and older adults: Part 1. Instrument development. *Journal of Elder Abuse and Neglect, 6*(1), 29–55.

Hueston, W. J., Knox, M. A., Eilers, G., Pauwels, J., & Lonsdorf, D. (1995). The effectiveness of preterm-birth prevention educational programs for high-risk women: A meta-analysis. *Obstetrics and Gynecology, 86,* 705–712.

Hugo, M. (1992). Left or right, up or down: A case for positioning of unconscious head-injured patients. *Curationis: South African Journal of Nursing, 15*(1), 1–7.

Humenick, S., & Marchbanks, P. (1981). Validation of a scale to measure relaxation in childbirth education classes. *Birth and Family Journal, 8,* 3–6.

Humphreys, B. L., Hole, W. T., McCray, A. T., & Fitzmaurice, M. J. (1996). Planned NLM/AHCPR large-scale vocabulary test: Using UMLS technology to determine the extent to which controlled vocabularies cover terminology needed for health care and public health. *Journal of the American Medical Informatics Association, 3,* 281–287.

Hurley, A., Volicer, B., Hanrahan, P., Houde, S., & Volicer, L. (1992). Assessment of discomfort in advanced Alzheimer patients. *Research in Nursing and Health, 15,* 367–377.

Husserl, E. (1962). *Ideas: General introduction to pure phenomenology.* New York: Macmillan.

Hutchinson, S. (1993). Grounded theory: The method. In P. Munhall & C. Oiler Boyd (Eds.), *Nursing research: A qualitative perspective* (pp. 180–212). New York: NLN Publications.

Hutchinson, S., & Wilson, H. (1992). Validity threats in scheduled semistructured research interviews. *Nursing Research, 41,* 117–119.

Hutchinson, S., Wilson, M., & Wilson, H. (1994). Benefits from participating in research interviews. *Image: Journal of Nursing Scholarship, 26,* 161–164.

Huttlinger, K. W. (1985). Keeping adolescents health: Face-care. Unpublished manuscript, University of Arizona, Tucson.

Hyman, R. B., Feldman, H. R., Harris, R. B., Levin, R. F., & Malloy, G. B. (1989). The effects of relaxation training on clinical symptoms: A meta-analysis. *Nursing Research, 38,* 216–220.

Hymes, D. (1964). Introduction toward ethnographies of communication. *American Anthropologist, 66,* 6–56.

Iberti, T. J., Daily, E. K., Leibowitz, A. B., Schecter, C. B., Fischer, E. P., & Silverstein, J. H. (1994). Assessment of critical care nurses' knowledge of the pulmonary artery catheter. *Critical Care Medicine, 22,* 1674–1678.

Ibrahim, M. A., Feldman, J. G., Sultz, H. A., Staiman, M. G., Young, L. I., & Dean, D. D. (1974). Management after myocardial infarction: A controlled trial of the effect of group psychotherapy. *International Journal of Psychiatric Medicine, 5,* 253–268.

ICN—International Council of Nurses. (1996). *The international classification for nursing practice: A unifying framework.* Geneva: ICN Press.

Iglehart, J. K. (1992). The American health care system. Managed care. *New England Journal of Medicine, 327,* 742–747.

Inglehart, J. K., Hiebert-White, J., & Zuercher, A. (Eds.). (1995). Mental health in the age of managed care. *Health Affairs, 14*(3), 7–286.

Immunizing America's children: Strategies and partnerships to remove barriers to immunization. (1995, September). *Children's Action Network, 1.*

Ingersoll, G. L. (1996a). Evaluation research. *Nursing Administration Quarterly, 20*(4), 28–39.

Ingersoll, G. L. (1996b). Organizational redesign: Effect on institutional and consumer outcomes. In. J. J. Fitzpatrick & J. Norbeck (Eds.), *Annual review of nursing research* (Vol. 14, pp. 121–143). New York: Springer Publishing.

Institute of Medicine. (1985). *Preventing low birth weight.* Washington, DC: National Academy Press.

Institute of Medicine. (1988). *Homelessness, health, and human needs.* Washington, DC: National Academy Press.

Institute of Medicine. (1994). Report of the Task Force on Clinical Research in Nursing and Clinical Psychology. In W. Kelley & M. Randolph (Eds.), *Careers in clinical research: Obstacles and opportunities* (pp. 251–278). Washington, DC: National Academy Press.

Institute of Medicine. (1996). *Telemedicine: A guide to assessing telecommunications in health care.* Washington, DC: National Academy Press.

Institute of Medicine. (1997a). *The computer-based patient record: An essential technology for health care* (rev. ed.). Washington, DC: National Academy Press.

Institute of Medicine. (1997b). *For the record: Protecting electronic health information.* Washington, DC: National Academy Press.

Institute of Medicine Staff. (1989). *Quality of life and technology assessment.* Washington, DC: National Academy Press.

Interagency Conference on Nursing Statistics. (1993, June). *Research on Nursing Resources, Definitions and Calculations.*

International Association for the Study of Pain, Subcommittee on Taxonomy. (1979). Pain terms: A list with definitions and usage. *Pain, 3,* S216–221.

International Association for the Study of Pain. (1986). Pain terms: The current list with definitions and notes on usage. *Pain, 3,* S216–S221.

International Continence Society Committee for the Standardisation of Terminology of the Lower Urinary Tract Function. (1990). *British Journal of Obstetrics and Gynaecology,* (Suppl. 6), 1–16.

International Council of Nurses. (1992). *Nursing's next advance: An international classification for nursing practice (ICNP).* Unpublished manuscript. Geneva: Author.

International Council of Nurses. (1996). *The international classification for nursing practice: A unifying framework* (alpha version). Geneva: Author.

Intrieri, R., Cerdas, M., & Morse, J. M. (1994, June). *Indices of distress in the trauma patient.* Paper presented at the 2nd Qualitative Health Research Conference, Hershey, PA.

Iowa Intervention Project. (1996). *Nursing interventions classification (NIC)* (2nd ed.). (J. C. McCloskey & G. M. Bulechek, Eds.). St. Louis: Mosby Year Book.

Iowa Outcomes Project. (1997). *Nursing outcomes classification NOC,* ed. M. Johnson & M. Maas. St. Louis: C. V. Mosby.

Irvine, D., & Evans, M. (1992). *Job satisfaction and turnover among nurses: A review and meta-analysis.* University of Toronto (Canada) Faculty of Nursing Monograph Series, Quality of Nursing Worklife Research Unit Monograph 1.

Irvine, D. M., Vincent, L., Bubela, N., Thompson, L., & Graydon, J. (1991). A critical appraisal of the research literature investigating fatigue in the individual with cancer. *Cancer Nursing, 14,* 188–199.

Israel, B. A., Checkoway, B., Schulz, A., & Zimmerman, M. (1994). Health education and community empowerment: Conceptualizing and measuring perceptions of individual, organizational, and community control. *Health Education Quarterly, 21,* 149–170.

Israel, M. J., & Mood, D. W. (1982). Three media presentations for patients receiving radiation therapy. *Cancer Nursing, 5,* 57–63.

Jacobs, J. (1995, Fall). Statement of purpose for the Alternative and Complementary Health Section of the American Public Health Association. *SPIG Newsletter, APHA,* pp. 2–3.

Jacobs, S. R. (1996). The grief experience of older women whose husbands had hospice care. *Journal of Advanced Nursing, 24,* 280–286.

Jacobsen, B. S., Lowery, B. J., & McCauley, K. (1992). Why me? Causal thinking, affect, and expectations in myocardial infarction patients. *Journal of Cardiovascular Nursing, 6*(2), 57–65.

Jacobson, S. F. (1994). Native American health. In J. J. Fitzpatrick & J. S. Stevenson (Eds.), *Annual review of nursing research* (Vol. 12, pp. 193–213). New York: Springer Publishing.

Jacobson, S. P., & McGraw, H. M. (1983). *Nurses under stress.* New York: John Wiley.

Jacox, A. (1970). Issues in construction of nursing theory. In *Proceedings, Kansas Theory Conference.*

Jacox, A. K., Carr, D. B, Payne, R., Berde, C. B., Brietbart, W., Cain, J. M., Chapman, C. R., Cleeland, C. L., McGavery, C. L., Miaskowski, C. A., Mulder, D. S., Paice, J. A., Shapiro, B. S., Silberstein, E. B., Smith, R. S., Stover, J., Tsou, C. V., Vecchiarelli, L., & Weissman, D. E. (1994). *Management of cancer pain* (Clinical Practice Guideline No. 9). Rockville, MD: Agency for Health Care Policy and Research.

Jaffe, C. C., & Lynch, P. J. (1995). Computer-aided instruction in radiology: Opportunities for more effective learning. *American Journal of Radiology, 164,* 463–467.

Jagger, J. (1994). A new opportunity to make the health care workplace safer. *Advances in Exposure Prevention, 1*(1), 1–2.

Jalowiec, A. (1992). Multidimensional assessment of QOL in clinical studies. *Progress in Cardiovascular Nursing, 7*(2), 7–12.

Jalowiec, A. (1993). Coping with illness: Synthesis and critique of the nursing literature from 1980–1990. In J. Barnfather & B. Lyon (Eds.), *Stress and coping: State of the science and implications for nursing theory, research and practice.* Indianapolis: Center Nursing Press of Sigma Theta Tau International.

Jambunathan, J., & Stewart, S. (1995). Hmong women in Wisconsin: What are their concerns in pregnancy and childbirth? *Birth, 22,* 204–210.

Janz, N. K., & Becker, M. H. (1984). The health belief model: A decade later. *Health Education Quarterly, 11,* 1–47.

Jarrett, M., Heitkemper, M. M., Cain, K., Tuftin, M., Walker, E., Bond, E., & Levy, R. (in press). The relationship between psychological distress and gastrointestinal symptoms in women.

Jarrett, N., & Payne, S. (1995). A selective review of the literature on nurse-patient communication: Has the patient's contribution been neglected? *Journal of Advanced Nursing, 22,* 72–78.

Jelovsek, F. R., & Adebonojo, L. (1993). Learning principles as applied to computer-assisted instruction. *MD Computing, 10,* 165–172.

Jemmott, J. B., & Jemmott, L. S. (1996). Strategies to reduce the risk of HIV infection, sexually transmitted diseases, and pregnancy among African American adolescents. In R. Resnick & R. Rozensky (Eds.), *Health psychology through the life span* (pp. 395–422). Washington, DC: American Psychological Association.

Jemmott, J. B., Jemmott, L. S., & Fong, G. (1992). Reductions in HIV risk-associated sexual behaviors among Black male adolescents: Effects of an AIDS prevention intervention. *American Journal of Public Health, 82,* 372–377.

Jemmott, J. B., Jemmott, L. S., Fong, G., & McCaffree, K. (1997). Reducing the risk of HIV in young Black adolescents: Evidence for the generality of intervention effects. *Journal of Community Psychology.*

Jemmott, J. B., Jemmott, L. S., & Hacker, C. I. (1992). Predicting intentions to use condoms among African-American adolescents: The theory of planned behavior as a model of HIV risk-associated behavior. *Ethnicity and Disease, 2,* 371–380.

Jemmott, J. B., Jemmott, L. S., Spears, H., Hewitt, N., & Cruz-Collins, M. (1992). Self-efficacy, hedonistic expectancies, and condom-use intentions among inner-city, Black adolescent women: A social cognitive approach to AIDS risk behavior. *Journal of Adolescent Health, 13,* 512–519.

Jemmott, L. S., & Jemmott, J. B. (1991). Applying the theory of reasoned action to AIDS risk behavior: Condom use among Black women. *Nursing Research, 40,* 228–234.

Jemmott, L. S., & Jemmott, J. B. (1992). Increasing condom-use intentions among sexually active Black adolescent women. *Nursing Research, 41,* 273–279.

Jemmott, L. S., Jemmott, J. B., & McCaffree, K. (1995). *Be proud! Be responsible! Strategies to empower youth to reduce their risk for AIDS* (2nd ed.). New York: Select Media Publications.

Jenkins, J. (1996). Oncology nursing practice. In M. B. Burke, G. Wilkes, & K. Ingwersen (Eds.), *Cancer chemotherapy: A nursing process approach* (2nd ed., pp. 3–19). Boston: Jones and Bartlett.

Jensen, D. M. (1955). *History and trends of professional nursing* (3rd ed.). St. Louis: C. V. Mosby.

Jette, A. M. (1994). How measurement techniques influence estimates of disability in older populations. *Social Science and Medicine, 38*(7), 937–942.

Jezewski, M. (1993). Culture brokering as a model for advocacy. *Nursing and Health Care, 14,* 78–85.

John, R. (1990). The uninvited researcher in Indian country: Problems of process and product conducting research among Native Americans. *Mid-American Review of Sociology, 13*(1 & 2), 113–133.

Johnson, B., & Gross, J. (1982). Handling methotrexate—a safety problem? *American Journal of Nursing, 82,* 1531.

Johnson, C. L., Rifkind, B. M., Sempos, C. T., Carroll, M. D., Bachorik, P. S., Briefel, R. R., Gordon, D. J., Burt, V. L., Brown, C. D., Lippel, K., & Cleeman, J. (1993). Declining serum cholesterol levels among U.S. adults: The National Health and Nutrition Examination Surveys. *Journal of the American Medical Association, 269,* 3002–3008.

Johnson, D. (1959). A philosophy of nursing. *Nursing Outlook, 7,* 198–200.

Johnson, D. E. (1980). The behavioral system model for nursing. In J. P. Riehl & C. Roy (Eds.), *Conceptual models for nursing practice* (2nd ed., pp. 207–216). New York: Appleton-Century-Crofts.

Johnson, D. E. (1990a). The behavioral system model for nursing. In M. E. Parker (Ed.), *Nursing theories in practice* (pp. 23–32). New York: National League for Nursing.

Johnson, J. E. (1984). Coping with elective surgery. In H. H. Werley & J. J. Fitzpatrick (Eds.), *Annual review of nursing research* (Vol. 2, pp. 107–132). New York: Springer Publishing.

Johnson, J. E., Fieler, V. K., Jones, L. S., Wlasowicz, G. S., & Mitchell, M. L. (1997). *Self-regulation theory: Applying theory to practice.* Pittsburgh: Oncology Nursing Press.

Johnson, J. E., Rice, V. H., & Endress, M. P. (1978). Sensory information, instruction in a coping strategy, and recovery from surgery. *Research in Nursing and Health, 1,* 4–17.

Johnson, J. E., Rice, V. H., Fuller, S. S., & Endress, M. P. (1978). Sensory information, instruction in coping strategy and recovery from surgery. *Research in Nursing and Health, 1,* 4–17.

Johnson, M. B. (1990b). The holistic paradigm in nursing: The diffusion of an innovation. *Research in Nursing and Health, 13,* 129–139.

Johnson, M. K., & Schumann, L. (1995). Comparison of three methods of measurement of pulmonary artery catheter readings in critically ill patients. *American Journal of Critical Care, 4,* 300–307.

Johnson, M. R., & Maas, M. (Eds.). (1997). *Nursing outcomes classification (NOC).* St. Louis: Mosby.

Johnson, R. J., & Wolinsky, F. D. (1993). The structure of health status among older adults: Disease, disability, functional limitation and perceived health. *Journal of Health and Social Behavior, 34,* 105–121.

Johnson, W. L. (1976). Educational preparation for nursing—1975. *Nursing Outlook, 24,* 568–573.

Joint Commission on Accreditation of Health Care Organizations. (1994). *Lexicon dictionary of health care terms, organizations, and acronyms for the era of reform.* Chicago: Author.

Joint Commission on the Accreditation of Healthcare Organizations. (1997). *Oryx outcomes: The next evolution in accreditation.* Oakbrook Terrace, IL: Author.

Joint National Committee. (1993). The fifth report of the Joint National Committee on the Detection, Evaluation and Treatment of High Blood Pressure (JNC V). *Archives of Internal Medicine, 153,* 154–183.

Jones, S. M., Fiser, D. H., & Livingston, R. L. (1992). Behavioral changes in pediatric intensive care units. *American Journal of Diseases in Children, 146,* 375–379.

Jordan, E. A., Dugan, A. K., & Hardy, J. B. (1993). Injuries in children of adolescent mothers: Home safety education associated with decreased injury risk. *Pediatrics, 91,* 481–487.

Jowers, L. T., & Herr, K. (1990). A review of literature on mentor-protégé relationships. In G. M. Clayton & P. A. Baj (Eds.), *Review of research in nursing education* (Vol. 3, pp. 49–77). New York: National League for Nursing.

Kahn, D., & Steeves, R. (1993). Spiritual well-being: A review of the research literature. In M. Whedon (Ed.), *Quality of life: A nursing challenge* (pp. 60–64). Philadelphia: Meniscus Ltd.

Kandolin, I. (1993). Burnout of female and male nurses in shiftwork. *Ergonomics, 36,* 141–147.

Kant, I. (1991). *Critique of pure reason.* London: Dent. (Original work published 1781)

Kaplan, N. M. (1994). *Clinical hypertension.* Baltimore: Williams and Wilkins.

Kaplun, A. (Ed.). (1992). *Health promotion and chronic illness: Discovering a new quality of life.* Copenhagen: World Health Organization.

Karasek, T., & Theorell, T. (1990). *Healthy work.* New York: Basic Books.

Karvetti, R. L., & Hamalainen, H. (1993). Long-term effect of nutrition education on myocardial infarction patients: A 10-year follow-up study. *Nutrition Metabolic Cardiac Disease, 3,* 185–192.

Kasper, C. E., Maxwell, L. C., & White, T. P. (1996). Alterations in skeletal muscle related to short-term impaired physical mobility. *Research in Nursing and Health, 19,* 133–142.

Kass, M. J., & Rousseau, G. K. (1983). Geriatric sexual conformity: Assessment and intervention. *Clinical Gerontologist, 2*(1), 31–44.

Katon, W., & Gonzales, J. (1994). A review of randomized trials of psychiatric consultation-liaison studies in primary care [Review]. *Psychosomatics, 35,* 268–278.

Kayser-Jones, J. S. (1981). Gerontological nursing research revisited. *Journal of Gerontological Nursing, 7,* 217–223.

Kayser-Jones, J. (1990). The use of nasogastric feeding tubes in nursing homes: Patient, family and health care provider perspectives. *Gerontologist, 30,* 469–479.

Keddy, B., Sims, S. L., & Stern, P. N. (1996). Grounded theory as feminist research methodology. *Journal of Advanced Nursing, 23,* 448–453.

Keefe, M., Kotzer, A. M., Froese-Fretz, A., & Curtin, M. (1996). A longitudinal comparison of irritable and nonirritable infants. *Nursing Research, 45,* 4–11.

Kelleghan, S. I., Salemi, C., Padilla, S., McCord, M., Mermilliod, G., Canola, T., & Becker, L. (1993). An effective continuous quality improvement approach to the prevention of ventilator-associated pneumonia. *American Journal of Infection Control, 21,* 322–330.

Kelly, L. S., & Lakin, J. A. (1988). Role supplementation as a nursing intervention for Alzheimer's disease: A case study. *Public Health Nursing, 5,* 146–152.

Kelly, M. J. (1964). An approach to the study of clinical inference in nursing. *Nursing Research, 13,* 314–315.

Kendall, M. G., & Buckland, W. R. (1960). *A dictionary of statistical terms.* New York: Hofner.

Kendler, K. S., Kessler, R. C., Neale, M. C., Heath, A. C., & Eaves, L. J. (1993). The prediction of major depression in women: Toward an integrated etiologic model. *American Journal of Psychiatry, 150,* 1139–1148.

Kennedy, C. (in press). Childhood nutrition. *Annual Review of Nursing Research, 16.*

Kerlinger, F. N. (1986). *Foundations of behavioral research* (3rd ed.). New York: Holt, Rinehart & Winston.

Kerr, M. E., Rudy, E. B., Brucia, J., & Stone, K. S. (1993). Head-injured adults: Recommendations for endotracheal suctioning. *Journal of Neuroscience Nursing, 25,* 86–91.

Kerr, R. B. (1994). Meanings adult daughters attach to a parent's death. *Western Journal of Nursing Research, 16,* 347–365.

Kessler, R. C., McGonagle, K. A., Zhao, S., Nelson, C. B., Hughes, M., Eshleman, S., Wittchen, H., & Kendler, K. S. (1994). Lifetime and 12 month prevalence of DSM-III-R psychiatric disorders in the United States: Results from the national comorbidity survey. *Archives of General Psychiatry, 51,* 8–19.

Ketefian, S. (1975). Application of selected nursing research findings into nursing practice: A pilot study. *Nursing Research, 24,* 89–92.

Ketefian, S. (1989). Moral reasoning and ethical practice in nursing. In J. J. Fitzpatrick & R. L. Taunton (Eds.), *Annual review of nursing research* (Vol. 7, pp. 173–195). New York: Springer Publishing.

Ketefian, S., & Lenz, E. (1995). Promoting scientific integrity in nursing research: Part 2. Strategies. *Journal of Professional Nursing, 11,* 263–269.

Killeen, M. (1993). Parent influences on children's self-esteem in economically disadvantaged families. *Issues in Mental Health Nursing, 14,* 323–336.

Killien, M. G. (1993). Returning to work after childbirth: Considerations for health policy. *Nursing Outlook, 41,* 73–78.

Kim, H. S. (1994). Action science as an approach to develop knowledge for nursing practice. *Nursing Science Quarterly, 7,* 134–138.

Kim, M. J. (1989). Nursing diagnosis. In J. J. Fitzpatrick & R. L. Taunton (Eds.), *Annual review of nursing research* (Vol. 7, pp. 117–142). NY: Springer Publishing.

Kim, M. J., McFarland, G. K., & McLane, A. M. (1995). *Pocket guide to nursing diagnoses* (2nd ed.). St. Louis, MO: Mosby.

King, I. M. (1981). *A theory for nursing: Systems, concepts, process.* New York: Wiley.

King, I. M. (1986). *Curriculum and instruction in nursing.* Norwalk, CT: Appleton-Century-Crofts.

King, I. M. (1992). King's theory of goal attainment. *Nursing Science Quarterly, 5,* 19–26.

King, K. B., Nail, L. M., Kraemer, K., Strohl, R., & Johnson, J. (1985). Patients' descriptions of the experience of receiving radiation therapy. *Oncology Nursing Forum, 12,* 55–61.

Kinney, M. R. (1985). Trends in cardiovascular nursing research. *Cardiovascular Nursing, 21*(5), 25–30.

Kirchhoff, K. T. (1993). The role of nurse researchers employed in clinical settings. *Annual Review of Nursing Research, 11,* 169–181.

Kirchhoff, K. T., & Mateo, M. A. (1996). Roles and responsibilities of clinical nurse researchers. *Journal of Professional Nursing, 12,* 86–90.

Kish, L. (1965). *Survey sampling.* New York: Wiley.

Kleiber, C. (1986). Clinical implications of deep and shallow suctioning in neonatal patients. *Focus on Critical Care, 13*(4), 36–39.

Kleiger, R. E., Miller, J. P., Bigger, I. T. Jr., Moss, A. L. J., & the Multicenter Postinfarction Research Group. (1987). Decreased heart rate variability and its association with increased mortality after acute myocardial infarction. *American Journal of Cardiology, 59,* 256–262.

Klein, D., & White, J. (1996). *Family theories: An introduction.* Thousand Oaks, CA: Sage.

Kleinbaum, D. G., Kupper, L. L., & Morgenstern, H. (1982). *Epidemiologic research: Principles and quantitative methods.* Belmont, CA: Wadsworth.

Knafl, K. A., Bevis, M. E., & Kirchhoff, K. T. (1987). Research activities of clinical nurse researchers. *Nursing Research, 36,* 249–252.

Knafl, K. A., & Deatrick, J. A. (1990). Family management style: Concept analysis and development. *Journal of Pediatric Nursing, 5,* 4–14.

Knapp, T. R. (1995). Ten measurement commandments that often should be broken. *Research in Nursing and Health, 18,* 465–469.

Knapp, T. R., & Brown, J. K. (1995). Ten measurement commandments that often should be broken. *Research in Nursing and Health, 18,* 465–469.

Knebel, A. R., Janson-Bjerklie, S. L., Malley, J. D., Wilson, A. G., & Marini, J. J. (1994). Comparison of breathing comfort during weaning with two ventilatory modes. *American Journal of Respiratory and Critical Care Medicine, 149,* 14–18.

Knight, B. G., Lutzky, S. M., & Macofsky-Urban, F. (1993). A meta-analytic review of interventions for caregiver distress: Recommendations for future research. *Gerontologist, 33,* 240–248.

Knobf, T., & Durivage, H. (1993). Chemotherapy: Principles of therapy. In S. Groenwald, M. Frogge, M. Goodman, & C. Yarbro (Eds.), *Cancer nursing: Principles and practice* (3rd ed., pp. 270–292). Boston: Jones and Bartlett.

Koehn, M. (1992). Effectiveness of prepared childbirth and childbirth satisfaction. *Journal of Perinatal Education, 1*(2), 35–43.

Koestenbaum, P. (1968). *Philosophy: A general introduction.* New York: Van Nostrand Reinhold.

Kohlberg, L. (1978). The cognitive-developmental approach to moral education. In P. Scharf (Ed.), *Readings in moral education* (pp. 36–51). Minneapolis: Winston Press.

Kolanowski, A. M., & Whall, A. L. (1996). Life-span perspective of personality in dementia. *Image: Journal of Nursing Scholarship, 28,* 315–320.

Kolcaba, K. (1991). A taxonomic structure for the concept of comfort. *Image: Journal of Nursing Scholarship, 23,* 237–240.

Kolcaba, K. (1994). A theory of holistic comfort for nursing. *Journal of Advanced Nursing, 19,* 1178–1184.

Kolcaba, K. (1995). The art of comfort care. *Image: Journal of Nursing Scholarship, 27,* 287–289.

Kolcaba, K., & Fisher, E. (1996). A holistic perspective on comfort care as an advance directive. *Critical Care Nursing Quarterly, 18*(4), 66–76.

Kolcaba, K., & Kolcaba, R. (1991). An analysis of the concept of comfort. *Journal of Advanced Nursing, 16,* 1301–1310.

Kongsvedt, P. R. (1995). *Essentials of managed health care.* Rockville, MD: Aspen.

Koopman, C., Classen, C., & Spiegel, D. (1997). Multiple stressors following a disaster and dissociative symptoms. In C. S. Fullerton & R. J. Ursano (Eds.), *Posttraumatic stress disorder* (pp. 21–35). Washington, DC: American Psychiatric Press.

Kornowski, R., Zeeli, D., Averbuch, M., Finkelstein, A., Schwartz, D., Moshkovitz, M., Weinreb, B., Hershkovitz, R., Eyal, D., Miller, M., Levo, Y., & Pines, A. (1995). Intensive home-care surveillance prevents hospitalization and improves morbidity rates among elderly patients with severe congestive heart failure. *American Heart Journal, 129,* 762–766.

Kottke, T. E., Battista, R. N., DeFriese, G. H., & Brekke, M. L. (1988). Attributes of successful smoking cessation interventions in medical practice. A meta-analysis of 39 controlled trials. *Journal of the American Medical Association, 259,* 2883–2889.

Kovar, M. G. (1989). Data systems of the National Center for Health Statistics. *Vital Health Statistics, 1,* 23.

Kovarsky, R. S. (1989). Loneliness and disturbed grief: A comparison of parents who lost a child to suicide or accidental death. *Archives of Psychiatric Nursing, 3,* 86–96.

Kozak, J. J., Hancock, P. A., Arthur, F. J., & Chrysler, S. T. (1993). Transfer of training from virtual reality. *Ergonomics, 36,* 777–784.

Kramer, J., Yellin, E., & Epstein, W. (1983). Social and economic impacts of four musculoskeletal conditions: A study using national community based data. *Journal of Rheumatology, 26,* 901–907.

Kramer, M., & Haffner, L. P. (1989). Shared values: Impact on staff nurse job satisfaction and perceived productivity. *Nursing Research, 38,* 172–177.

Kramer, R. F. (1987). Living with childhood cancer: Impact on the healthy siblings. In T. Krulik, B. Holaday, & I. M. Martinson (Eds.), *The child and family facing life-threatening illness* (pp. 258–272). Philadelphia: J. B. Lippincott.

Kraus, W. A., Dryer, E. A., Wagner, D. P., & Zimmerman, J. E. (1986). An evaluation of outcome from intensive care in major medical centers. *Annals of Internal Medicine, 104,* 410–418.

Krawczak, J., & Bersky, A. (1995). The development of automated client responses for computerized clinical simulation testing. *Computers in Nursing, 13,* 295–300.

Krieger, D. (1975). Therapeutic touch: The imprimator of nursing. *American Journal of Nursing, 75,* 784–787.

Krieger, N. (1994). Epidemiology and the web of causation. *Social Science and Medicine, 39,* 887–903.

Kristjanson, L. J., & Ashcroft, T. (1994). The family's cancer journey: A literature review. *Cancer Nursing, 17,* 1–17.

Krueger, J. C. (1978). Utilization of nursing research: The planning process. *Journal of Nursing Administration, 8*(1), 6–9.

Kuczmarski, R. J., Flegal, K. M., Campbell, S. M., & Johnson, C. L. (1994). Increasing prevalence of overweight among U.S. adults: The national health and nutrition examination surveys, 1960–1991. *Journal of the American Medical Association, 272,* 205–211.

Kuhn, T. S. (1970). *The structure of scientific revolution* (2nd ed.). Chicago: University of Chicago Press.

Labov, W. (1972). *Language in the inner city: Studies in the Black English vernacular.* Philadelphia: University of Pennsylvania Press.

Labovitz, S. (1970). The nonutility of significance tests: The significance of tests of significance reconsidered. *Pacific Sociological Review, 13,* 141–148.

Laffrey, S. C. (1986). Development of a health conception scale. *Research in Nursing and Health, 9,* 107–113.

Lakatos, I. (1968). *The problem of inductive logic.* Amsterdam: North-Holland.

Lamberty, G., Papai J., & Kessell, J. W. (Eds.). (1996). *Proceedings of the Fourth National Title V Maternal and Child Health Priorities Conference* (pp. 35–37). Arlington, VA: National Center for Education in Maternal and Child Health.

Lamerato, L. E., Ye, E., & Tilley, B. C. (1996). Using administrative data and a diagnosis clustering program to assess healthcare needs of African Americans: Healthcare utilization. *American Journal of Managed Care, 2,* 495–501.

La Monica, E., Oberst, M., Madea, A. R., & Wolf, R. M. (1986). Development of a patient satisfaction scale. *Research in Nursing and Health, 31,* 43–50.

LaMontagne, L. L., Pressler, J. L., & Salisbury, M. H. (1996). Scholarly mission: Fostering scholarship in research, theory, and practice. *Nursing and Health Care, 17,* 299–302.

Lancaster, J. (1980). *Community mental health nursing: An ecological perspective.* St. Louis: C. V. Mosby.

Landefeld, C., Palmer, R., Kresevic, D., Fortinsky, R., & Kowal, J. (1995). A randomized trial of care in a hospital medical unit especially designed to improve the functional outcomes of acutely ill older patients. *New England Journal of Medicine, 332,* 1338–1344.

Landgridge, D. W. (1992). *Classification: Its kinds, elements, systems and applications.* New York: Bowker-Saur.

Lang, N. M. (Ed.). (1995). *Nursing data systems: The emerging framework.* Washington, DC: American Nurses Association.

Lang, N. (Ed.). (1996). *Nursing data systems: The emerging framework.* Washington, DC: American Nurses Association.

Lang, N. M., & Marek, K. D. (1990). The classification of patient outcomes. *Journal of Professional Nursing, 6,* 158–163.

Lange, L. (1996). Representation of everyday clinical nursing language in UMLS and SNOMED. In J. J. Cimino (Ed.), *Proceedings of the American Medical Informatics Association, Fall Symposium* (pp. 140–144). Philadelphia: Hanley & Belfus.

Larese, F., & Fiorito, A. (1994). Musculoskeletal disorders in hospital nurses: A comparison between two hospitals. *Ergonomics, 37,* 1205–1211.

Larsen, J. F. (1996). Why has conventional intrapartum cardiotocography not given the expected results? *Journal of Perinatal Medicine, 24,* 15–23.

Larson, E. (1988). Nursing research and AIDS. *Nursing Research, 37,* 60–62.

Larson, E., & Ropka, M. (1990). Nursing research and HIV infection: Nursing and the HIV epidemic—a national action agenda. Washington, DC: U.S. Department of Health and Human Services, Division of Nursing and the National Center for Nursing Research.

Larson, E., & Ropka, M. (1991). An update on nursing research and HIV infection. *Image: Journal of Nursing Scholarship, 23,* 4–12.

Larson, O. J., & Ferketich, S. L. (1993). Patient satisfaction with nurses' caring during hospitalization. *Western Journal of Nursing Research, 15,* 690–707.

Larsson, B., Svardsudd, K., Welin, L., Wilhelmsen, L., Bjorntorp, P., & Tibblin, G. (1984). Abdominal adipose tissue distribution, obesity and risk of cardiovascular disease and death: 13 year follow-up of participants in the study of men born in 1913. *British Medical Journal, 288,* 1401–1404.

LaSorte, M. (1972). Replication as a verification technique in survey research: A paradigm. *Sociological Quarterly, 13,* 218–227.

Lauterbach, S. (1993). In another world: A phenomenological perspective and discovery of meaning in mothers' experience with death of a wished-for baby: Doing phenomenology. In P. L. Munhall & C. O. Boyd (Eds.), *Nursing research: A qualitative perspective* (pp. 133–179). New York: NLN Press.

Lauver, D. (1992). Psychosocial variables, race, and intentions to seek care for breast cancer symptoms. *Nursing Research, 41,* 236–241.

Lauver, L. S. (1996). Benchmarking: Improving outcomes for the congestive heart patient population. *Journal of Nursing Care Quality, 10*(3), 7–11.

Lawhon, G. (1986). Management of stress in premature infants. In D. Angelini, C. Whelan Knapp, & R. Gibbs, *Perinatal/neonatal nursing: A clinical handbook* (pp. 319–328). Boston: Blackwell.

Lawrence, R. H., & Jette, A. M. (1996). Disentangling the disablement process. *Journals of Gerontology: Social Sciences, 51,* S173–S182.

Lawson, S., & Adamson, H. (1995, September–December). Informed consent readability: Subject understanding of 15 common consent form phrases. *IRB,* pp. 16–19.

Lawton, M. (1975). Competence, environmental press and the adaptation of older people. In P. Windley, T. Byerts, & F. Ernst (Eds.), *Theory development in environments and aging* (pp. 13–83). Washington, DC: Gerontological Society.

Lawton, M. P. (1991). A multidimensional view of quality of life in frail elders. In J. E. Birren, J. C. Rowe, & D. E. Deutchman (Eds.), *The concept and measurement of quality of life in the frail and elderly* (pp. 4–27). San Diego, CA: Academic Press.

Lazarus, R. S., & Folkman, S. (1984). *Stress, appraisal, and coping.* New York: Springer Publishing.

League, D. (1995). Interactive, image-guided, stereotactic neurosurgery systems. *AORN Journal, 61,* 360–370.

Lee, K. A. (1992). Self-reported sleep disturbances in employed women. *Sleep, 15,* 493–498.

Lee, K. A., & DeJoseph, J. F. (1992). Sleep disturbances, vitality, and fatigue among a select group of employed childbearing women. *Birth, 19*(4), 208–213.

Lee, K. A., Shaver, J. F., Giblin, E. C., & Woods, N. F. (1990). Sleep patterns related to menstrual cycle phase and premenstrual affective symptoms. *Sleep, 13,* 403–409.

LeFevre, C. (1994, Spring/Summer). Altered states. *Four Seasons Hotels and Resorts Magazine,* pp. 64–67.

LeFort, S. M. (1993). The statistical versus clinical significance debate. *Image: Journal of Nursing Scholarship, 25,* 57–62.

Leidy, N. (1994). Functional status and the forward progress of merry-go-rounds: Toward a coherent analytical framework. *Nursing Research, 43,* 196–202.

Leininger, M. M. (1985). *Qualitative research methods in nursing.* New York: Grune and Stratton.

Leininger, M. (1991). *Culture care diversity and universality: A theory of nursing.* New York: National League for Nursing.

Leininger, M. (1995). Rebuttal excerpts on the American Academy of Nursing panel report on culturally competent health care. *Journal of Transcultural Nursing, 4*(2), 45.

Lenfant, C., & Ernst, N. (1994). Daily dietary fat and total food-energy intakes: Third Health and Nutrition Examination Survey, phase 1, 1988–1991. *Morbidity and Mortality Weekly Reports, 43,* 116.

Lentz, M., & Woods, N. F. (1989). Women's health research: Implications for design, measurement and analysis. In I. L. Abraham, D. M. Nadzam, & J. J. Fitzpatrick (Eds.), *Statistics and quantitative methods in nursing: Issues and strategies for research and education* (pp. 84–93). Philadelphia: W. B. Saunders.

Lenz, E., & Ketefian, S. (1995). Promoting scientific integrity in nursing research: Part 1. Current approaches in doctoral programs. *Journal of Professional Nursing, 11,* 213-219.

Leventhal, H., & Johnson, J. E. (1983). Laboratory and field experimentation: Development of a theory of self-regulation. In P. J. Wooldridge, M. H. Schmitt, J. K. Skipper, Jr., & R. C. Leonard (Eds.), *Behavioral science and nursing theory* (pp. 189–262). St. Louis: C. V. Mosby.

Levine, M. E. (1967). The four conservation principles. *Nursing Forum, 1,* 45–49.

Levine, M. E. (1988). Antecedents from adjunctive disciplines: Creation of nursing theory. *Nursing Science Quarterly, 1,* 26–21.

Levine, M. E. (1989). The four conservation principles: Twenty years later. In J. Riehl-Sisca (Ed.), *Conceptual models for nursing practice* (3rd ed., pp. 325–337). Norwalk, CA: Appleton-Lange.

Levine, M. E. (1991). The conservation principles: A model for health. In K. M. Schaefer & J. B. Pond (Eds.), *Levine's conservation model: A framework for nursing practice* (pp. 1–11). Philadelphia: F. A. Davis.

Levkoff, S. E., Besdine, R. W., & Wetle, T. (1986). Acute confusional states (delirium) in the hospitalized elderly. In C. Eisdorfer (Ed.), *Annual review of geriatrics and gerontology* (pp. 1–26). New York: Springer Publishing.

Levy, R., Jarrett, M. J., Cain, K., & Heitkemper, M. M. (1997). The relationship between daily life stress and gastrointestinal symptoms in women. *Journal of Behavioral Medicine, 20,* 177–193.

Lewandowski, L., & Kositsky, A. (1983). Research priorities for critical care nursing: A study by the American Association of Critical Care Nurses. *Heart and Lung: Journal of Critical Care, 12,* 35–44.

Lewis, B. J., & Gunn, I. P. (1964). Tracheostomy, oxygen administration, and expiratory airflow resistance: Evaluation of a nursing procedure in a laboratory model. *Nursing Research, 13,* 301–308.

Lewis, D. J., & Robinson, J. A. (1986). Assessment of coping strategies of ICU nurses in response to stress. *Critical Care Nurse, 6*(6), 38–43.

Lewis, E. N. (1989). *Manual of patient classification: Systems and techniques for practical application.* Rockville, MD: Aspen.

Lewis, J. E. (1995). How big should an integrated health care delivery system be at an academic medical center? *Academic Medicine, 70,* 569–577.

Liaschenko, J. (1997). Ethics and the geography of the nurse-patient relationship: Spatial vulnerabilities and gendered space. *Scholarly Inquiry for Nursing Practice: An International Journal, 11,* 47–59.

Libbus, M., & Sable, M. (1991). Prenatal education in a high-risk population: The effect on birth outcomes. *Birth: Issues in Perinatal Care and Education, 18,* 78–82.

Lierman, L., Kaspryzyk, D., & Benoliel, J. (1991). Understanding adherence to breast self-examination in older women. *Western Journal of Nursing Research, 13,* 46–61.

Light, E., Niederehe, G., & Lebowitz, B. D. (Eds.). (1994). *Stress effects on family caregivers of Alzheimer's patients: Research and interventions.* New York: Springer Publishing.

Lincoln, Y., & Guba, E. (1985). *Naturalistic inquiry.* Beverly Hills, CA: Sage.

Lindberg, D. A. B., Humphreys, B. L., & McCray, A. T. (1993). The Unified Medical Language System. *Methods of Information in Medicine, 32,* 281–291.

Lindeman, C. (1981). *Priorities within the health care system: A Delphi survey*. Kansas City, MO: American Academy of Nursing.

Linden, M., Habib, T., & Radojevic, V. (1996). A controlled study of the effects of EEG biofeedback on cognition and behavior of children with attention deficit disorder and learning disabilities. *Biofeedback and Self-Regulation, 21,* 35–49.

Linden, W., Stossel, C., & Maurice, J. (1996). Psychosocial interventions for patients with coronary artery disease: A meta-analysis. *Archives of Internal Medicine, 156,* 745–752.

Lindenberg, C. S., Gendrop, S. C., Nencioli, M., & Adames, Z. (1994). Substance abuse among inner-city Hispanic women: Exploring resiliency. *Journal of Gynecologic and Neonatal Nursing, 23,* 609–616.

Lindquist, R., Banasik, J., Barnsteiner, J., Beccroft, P. C., Prevost, S., Reigel, B., Sechrist, K., Strzelecki, C., & Titler, M. (1993). Determining AACN's research priorities for the 90s. *American Journal of Critical Care, 2,* 110–117.

Lindsey, A. M. (1984). Research for clinical practice: Physiological phenomena. *Heart and Lung, 13,* 496–507.

Lindsey, A. (1995). Physical health of homeless adults. In J. J. Fitzpatrick & J. Norbeck (Eds), Publishing, *Annual review of nursing research,* (Vol 13, pp 31–61). New York: Springer.

Linneman, C. C., Cannon, C., DeRonde, M., & Lanphear, B. (1991). Effect of educational programs, rigid sharps containers, and universal precautions on reported needlestick injuries in health care workers. *Infection Control and Hospital Epidemiology, 12,* 214–219.

Lipman, T. H., & Deatrick, J. A. (1997). Preparing advanced practice nurses for clinical decision making in specialty practice. *Nurse Educator, 22,* 47–50.

Lipson, J. (1993). Afghan refugees in California: Mental health issues. *Issues in Mental Health Nursing, 14,* 411–423.

Lipson, J. G., & Meleis, A. I. (in press). Immigrants and refugees. In A. S. Hinshaw, S. Feetham, & J. Shaver (Eds.), *Handbook of clinical nursing research.* Newbury Park, CA: Sage.

Llewellyn-Thomas, H., Thiel, E., Sem, F., & Woermke, D. (1995). Presenting clinical trial information: A comparison of methods. *Patient Education and Counseling, 25,* 97–107.

Lobo, M. L., Barnard, K. E., & Coombs, J. B. (1992). Failure to thrive: A parent-infant interaction perspective. *Journal of Pediatric Nursing, 7,* 251–261.

Loftus, G. R. (1993). A picture is worth a thousand *p* values: On the irrelevance of hypothesis testing in the microcomputer age. *Behavior Research Methods, Instruments, and Computers, 25,* 250–256.

Long, A., & Reid, W. (1996). An exploration of nurses attitudes to the nursing care of the suicidal patient in an acute psychiatric ward. *Journal of Psychiatric and Mental Health Nursing, 3,* 29–37.

Longman, A. J., Saint-Germain, M. A., & Modiano, M. (1992). Use of breast cancer screening by older Hispanic women. *Public Health Nursing, 9,* 118–124.

Longstreth, G. F., & Wolde-Tsadik, G. (1993). Irritable bowel–type symptoms in HMO examinees: Prevalence, demographics, and clinical correlates. *Digestive Diseases and Sciences, 38,* 1581–1589.

Loos, F. D., Shortridge, H. A., Adaskin, E. J., & Rock, B. L. (1994). When industry courts your clinical research skills, should you collaborate? *Clinical Nurse Specialist, 8,* 85–89.

Lorig, K. (1996). *Patient education: A practical approach.* Thousand Oaks, CA: Sage.

Lorig, K., Chastain, R. L., Ung, E., Shoor, S., & Holman, H. R. (1989). Development and evaluation of a scale to measure perceived self-efficacy in people with arthritis. *Arthritis and Rheumatism, 32,* 37–44.

Lorig, K., Stewart, A., Ritter, P., Gonzalez, V., Laurent, D., & Lynch, J. (1996). *Outcome measures for health education and other health care interventions.* Thousand Oaks, CA: Sage.

Loukissa, D. A. (1995). Family burden in chronic mental illness: A review of research studies. *Journal of Advanced Nursing, 21,* 248–255.

Lowenberg, J. S. (1994). The nurse-patient relationship reconsidered: An expanded research agenda. *Scholarly Inquiry for Nursing Practice: An International Journal, 8,* 167–184.

Lowery, B. (1991). Resources to maintain the academic culture. *Journal of Professional Nursing, 7,* 177–183.

Lubar, J. (1991). Discourse on development of EEG diagnostics and biofeedback for attention deficit/hyperactivity disorders. *Biofeedback and Self-Regulation, 16,* 201–224.

Lubkin, I. M. (1995). *Chronic illness impact and interventions.* Boston: Jones and Bartlett.

Ludington-Hoe, S., Thompson, C., Swinth, J., Hadeed, A., & Anderson, G. C. (1994a). Kangaroo care: Research results, and practice implications and guidelines. *Neonatal Network, 11*(1), 2–9.

Ludington-Hoe, S. M., Thompson, C., Swinth, J., Hadeed, A. J., & Anderson, G. C. (1994b). Kangaroo care: Research results and practice implications and guidelines. *Neonatal Network, 13,* 19–27.

Lueckenotte, A. G. (1996). *Gerontologic nursing.* St. Louis: C. V. Mosby.

Lukens, J. N. (1994). Progress resulting from clinical trials. *Cancer, 74*(Suppl.), 2710–2718.

Lusk, S. L., Ronis, D. L., & Hogan, M. M. (1997). Test of the health promotion model as a causal model of construction workers use of hearing protection. *Research in Nursing and Health, 20,* 183–194.

Lykken, D. (1968). Statistical significance in psychological research. *Psychological Bulletin, 70,* 151–159.

Lynbaugh, J. E., & Fairman, J. (1992). New nurses, new spaces: A preview of the AACN history study. *American Journal of Critical Care, 1,* 19–24.

Lynn, M. R. (1986). Determination and quantification of content validity. *Nursing Research, 35,* 382–385.

Lyon, B. (1993). Summary and preliminary synthesis. In J. S. Barnfather & B. L. Lyon (Eds.), *Stress and coping: State of the science and implications for nursing theory, research and practice.* Indianapolis: Sigma Theta Tau.

Lyon, B. L. (1996). *Conquering stress in changing times.* Research Triangle Park, NC: Glaxo Wellcome Inc.

Lyon, B. L., & Werner, J. S. (1987). Stress. In J. J. Fitzpatrick & R. L. Taunton (Eds.), *Annual Review of Nursing Research* (Vol. 5, pp. 3–22). New York: Springer Publishing.

Lyotard, J. (1984). *The postmodern condition: A report on knowledge.* Manchester, England: Manchester University Press.

Maas, M., & Buckwalter, K. (1990). *Nursing evaluation research: Alzheimer's care unit. Final report.* Rockville, MD: National Institutes of Health, National Center for Nursing Research.

Maas, M. L., & Buckwalter, K. C. (1991). Alzheimer's disease. In J. J. Fitzpatrick & J. S. Stevenson (Eds.), *Annual review of nursing research* (Vol. 9, pp. 19–55). New York: Springer Publishing.

Maas, M., Swanson, E., Reed, D., & Specht, J. (1996, November). *Nursing staff perceptions of family involvement in care in SCUs.* Paper presented at the 49th Annual Meeting of the Gerontological Society of America, Washington, DC.

MacKenzie, T. D., Bartecchi, C. E., & Schrier, R. W. (1994). The human costs of tobacco use. *New England Journal of Medicine, 330,* 975–980.

Mackey, M., & Coster-Schultz, M. (1993). Women's views of the preterm labor experience. *Clinical Nursing Research, 1,* 366–384.

MacPherson, K. I. (1981). Menopause as disease: The social construction of a metaphor. *Advances in Nursing Science, 3,* 95–113.

MacPherson, K. I. (1983). Feminist methods: A new paradigm for nursing research. *Advances in Nursing Science, 5*(2), 17–25.

MacVicar, M., Winningham, M., & Nickel, J. (1989). Effects of aerobic interval training on cancer patients' functional capacity. *Nursing Research, 38,* 348–351.

Magaw, A. (1899). Observations in anaesthesia. *Northwestern Lancet, 19,* 207–210.

Magaw, A. (1906). A review of over fourteen thousand surgical anesthesias. *Surgery, Gynecology and Obstetrics, 3,* 795–799.

Mahon, S. (1991). Managing the psychosocial consequences of cancer recurrence: Implications for nurses. *Oncology Nursing Forum, 18,* 577–583.

Management of Cancer Pain Panel. (1994). *Management of Cancer Pain: Adults.* (Quick Reference Guide for Clinicians, No. 9 [AHCPR Publication No. 94-0593]). Rockville, MD: U.S. Department of Health and Human Services, Agency for Health Care Policy and Research.

Mann, N. A., Tandon, R. J., Butler, J., Boyd, M., Eisner, W. H., & Lewis, M. (1993). Psychosocial rehabilitation in schizophrenia: Beginnings in acute hospitalization. *Archives of Psychiatric Nursing, 7,* 154–162.

Manson, J. E., Colditz, G. A., Stampfer, M. J., Willett, W. C., Rosner, B., Monson, R. R., Speizer, F. E., & Hennekens, C. H. (1990). A prospective study of obesity and risk of coronary heart disease in women. *New England Journal of Medicine, 322,* 882–889.

Manthey, C., Ciske, K., Robertson, P., & Harris, I. (1970). Primary nursing: A return to the concept of "my nurse" and "my patient." *Nursing Forum, 9,* 64–83.

Margolin, S., Breneman, J., Denman, D., LaChapelle, P., & Weckbach, L. (1990). Management of radiation-induced moist skin desquamation using hydrocolloid dressing. *Cancer Nursing, 13,* 71–80.

Marion, L. N. (1996). *Nursing's vision for primary health care in the 21st century.* Washington, DC: American Nurses Publishing.

Marks, R. M., & Sachar, E. G. (1973). Undertreatment of medical in patients with narcotic analgesics. *Annals of Internal Medicine, 78,* 173–181.

Markson, L. J., Kern, D. C., Annas, G. J., & Glantz, L. H. (1994). Physician assessment of patient competence. *Journal of the American Geriatrics Society, 42,* 1074–1080.

Marston, M. (1970). Compliance with medical regimen: A review of the literature. *Nursing Research, 19,* 312–323.

Martin, K. S., & Martin, D. L. (1997). How can the quality of nursing practice be measured? In J. C. McCloskey & H. K. Grace (Eds.), *Current issues in nursing* (5th ed., pp. 315–321). St. Louis: C. V. Mosby.

Martin, K. S., & Norris, J. (1996). The Omaha System: A model for describing practice. *Holistic Nursing Practice, 11*(1), 75–83.

Martin, K. S., & Scheet, N. J. (1992). *The Omaha System: Applications for community health nursing.* Philadelphia: W. B. Saunders.

Martin, K. S., Scheet, N. J., & Stegman, M. R. (1993). Home health clients: Characteristics, outcomes of care, and nursing interventions. *American Journal of Public Health, 83*(12), 1730–1734.

Martin, P. (1988). Organizational influence on research by hospital nurses (Doctoral dissertation, Case Western Reserve University, 1988). *Dissertation Abstracts International, 49*(08), 3106B.

Martin, P. (1993). Clinical settings need organizational support for research. *Applied Nursing Research, 6,* 103–104.

Martinson, I. M. (1995). Pediatric hospice nursing. In J. Fitzpatrick & J. Stevenson (Eds.), *Annual review of nursing research* (Vol. 13, pp. 195–214). New York: Springer Publishing.

Martinson, I. M., Armstrong, G. D., Geis, D. P., Anglim, M. A., Gronseth, E. C., MacInnis, H., Kersey, J. H., & Nesbitt, M. E. (1978). Home care for children dying of cancer. *Pediatrics, 62,* 106–113.

Martocchio, B. C. (1980). *Living while dying.* Bowie, MD: Robert J. Brady.

Mason, J. E., Willett, W. C., Stampfer, M. J., Colditz, G. A., Hunter, D. J., Hankinson, S. E., Hennekens, C. H., & Speizer, F. E. (1995). Body weight and mortality among women. *New England Journal of Medicine, 333,* 677–685.

Masten, Y., & Conover, K. P. (1990). Automated continuing education and patient education—KARENET—linking rural Texas. *Computers in Nursing, 8,* 144–150.

Matthews, K. A., Shumaker, S. A., Bowen, D. J., Langer, R. D., Hunt, J. R., Kaplan, R. M., Klesges, R. C., & Ritenbaugh, C. (1997). Women's health initiative. Why now? What is it? What's new? *American Psychologist, 52,* 101–116.

Maurer, J. D., Rosenberg, H. M., & Keemer, J. B. (1990). Deaths of Hispanic origin: 15 reporting states, 1979–1981. *Vital Health Statistics, 20*(18) (DHHS Publication No. 91-1855). Washington, DC: U.S. Government Printing Office.

Mausner, J. S., & Kramer, S. (1985). *Epidemiology: An introductory text.* Philadelphia: W. B. Saunders.

May, C. (1990). Research on nurse-patient relationships: Problems of theory, problems of practice. *Journal of Advanced Nursing, 15,* 307–315.

May, C. (1991). Affect neutrality and involvement in nurse-patient relationships: Perceptions of appropriate behavior among nurses in acute medical and surgical wards. *Journal of Advanced Nursing, 16,* 552–558.

May, C. R., & Purkis, A. A. (1995). The configuration of nurse-patient relationships: A critical view. *Scholarly Inquiry for Nursing Practice: An International Journal, 9,* 283–295.

May, K. (1994). Impact of maternal activity restriction for preterm labor on the expectant father. *Journal of Obstetric, Gynecologic and Neonatal Nursing, 23,* 246–251.

Mays, D., Devitt, K., Gottlieb, T., Kemble, S., Merrill, R., Torres, G., Asderian, E., & Becnel, B. (1992). Nursing research in the VA system: A consortium approach. *Journal of Nursing Administration, 22*(10), 54–59.

McBride, A. B. (1985). Differences in women's and men's thinking about parent-child interactions. *Research in Nursing and Health, 8,* 389–396.

McBride, A. B. (1993). From gynecology to gyn-ecology: Developing a practice-research agenda for women's health. *Health Care for Women International, 14,* 316–325.

McBride, A. B., & McBride, W. L. (1981). Theoretical underpinnings for women's health. *Women and Health, 6*(1/2), 37–55.

McBride, A. B., & McBride, W. L. (1993). Women's health scholarship: From critique to assertion. *Journal of Women's Health, 2,* 43–47.

McCarthy, R. T. (1985). *History of the American Academy of Nursing.* Kansas City, MO: American Academy of Nursing.

McClandless-Glimcher, L., McKnight, S., Hamera, E., Smith, B. I., Peterson, K. A., & Plumlee, A. A. (1986). Use of symptoms by schizophrenics to monitor and regulate their illness. *Hospital and Community Psychiatry, 37,* 929–933.

McCloskey, J. C., & Bulechek, G. M. (1992). *Nursing interventions classifications (NIC).* St. Louis: Mosby Year Book.

McCloskey, J. C., & Bulechek, G. M. (1996). *Nursing interventions classifications (NIC)* (2nd ed.). St. Louis: C. V. Mosby.

McClure, M., Poulin, M. L., Sovie, M. D., & Wandelt, M. A. (1983). *Magnet hospitals: Attraction and retention of professional nurses.* Kansas City, MO: American Academy of Nursing.

McCorkle, M. D. (1934). *A curriculum study in social hygiene for nurses.* New York: American Social Hygiene Association and NLNE.

McCormick, K. A., Lang, N., Zielstorff, R., Milholland, D. K., Saba, V., & Jacox, A. (1994). Toward standard classification schemes for nursing language: Recommendations of the American Nurses Association Steering Committee on Databases to Support Nursing Practice. *Journal of the American Medical Informatics Association, 1,* 421–427.

McCormick, K. A., & Zielstorff, R. (1995). Building a unified nursing language system. In N. Lang (Ed.), *Nursing data systems: The emerging framework* (pp. 19–30). Washington, DC: American Nurses Publishing.

McCowan, D. E., & Davies, B. (1995). Patterns of grief in young children following the death of a sibling. *Death Studies, 19,* 41–53.

McCray, A. T., Razi, A. M., Bangalore, A. K., Browne, A. C., & Stavri, P. Z. (1996). The UMLS knowledge source server: A versatile Internet-based research tool. In J. J. Cimino (Ed.), *AMIA Fall Symposium* (pp. 164–168). Philadelphia: Hanley & Belfus.

McCubbin, H., & Patterson, J. (1983). The family stress process: The Double ABCX model of adjustment and adaptation. In H. McCubbin, M. Sussman, & J. Patterson (Eds.), *Social stress and the family: Advances and developments in family stress theory and research* (pp. 7–37). New York: Haworth Press.

McDaniel, C. (1995). Organizational culture and ethics work satisfaction. *Journal of Nursing Administration, 25*(11), 15–21.

McDaniel, C., & Nash, J. (1990). Compendium of instruments measuring patient satisfaction with nursing care. *Quality Review Bulletin, 16*(5), 182–188.

McDaniel, C., & Stumpf, L. (1993). Organizational culture: Implications for nursing service. *Journal of Nursing Administration, 17*(3), 54–60.

McDougall, G. J. (1990). A review of screening instruments for assessing cognition and mental status in older adults. *Nurse Practitioner, 15*, 18–28.

McDougall, G. J. (1994). Predictors of metamemory in older adults. *Nursing Research, 43*, 212–218.

McDougall, G. (1995). A critical review of research on cognitive function/impairment in older adults. *Archives of Psychiatric Nursing, 9*, 22–33.

McDowell, I., & Newell, C. (1996). *Measuring health* (2nd ed.). New York: Oxford University.

McElmurry, B. J. (1993). Introduction. In B. J. McElmurry & R. S. Parker (Eds.), *Annual review of women's health* (pp. 1–7). New York: National League for Nursing Press.

McEnany, G. W. (1990). Psychobiological indices of bipolar mood disorder: Future trends in nursing care. *Archives of Psychiatric Nursing, 4*, 29–38.

McFadden, E. A., & Miller, M. A. (1994). Clinical nurse specialist practice: Facilitators and barriers. *Clinical Nurse Specialist, 8*, 27–33.

McFarlane, J., & Fehir, J. (1994). De Madres a Madres: A community, primary health care program based on empowerment. *Health Education Quarterly, 21*, 381–394.

McGee, H. M., O'Boyle, C. A., Hickey, A., O'Malley, K., & Joyce, C. R. B. (1991). Individual quality of life in patients undergoing hip replacement. *Lancet, 339*, 1088–1091.

McGinnis, B. G., & Axford, R. (1997). Exploring nursing knowledge by using digital photography. In M. Talberg & U. Gerden (Eds.), *Proceedings, NI97: The impact of nursing knowledge on health care informatics.* International Medical Informatics Association.

McHugh, M. (1988). Comparison of four nurse staffing patterns using computer simulation. In *Nursing and computers: Third International Symposium on Nursing Use of Computers and Information Science* (pp. 787–795). St. Louis: C. V. Mosby.

McHugh, M. (1989). Computer simulation as a method for selecting nurse staffing levels in hospitals. In E. MacNair, K. Musselman, & P. Heidelberger (Eds.), *Proceedings of the 1989 Simulation Conference* (pp.

1121–1129). New York: Association for Computing Machinery.

McHugh, M. (1994). *Conceptual definition and measurement of the concept, "intensity of nursing care."* Manuscript submitted for publication.

McKay, S., & Roberts, J. (1990). Obstetrics by ear: Maternal and caregiver perceptions of the meaning of maternal sounds during second stage labor. *Journal of Nurse-Midwifery, 35*, 266–273.

Mckenna, H. P. (1994). *Nursing theories and quality of care.* Brookfield: Avebury.

McKhann, G., Drachman, D., Folstein, M., Katzman, R., Price, D., & Stadian, E. (1984). Clinical diagnosis of Alzheimer's disease: Report of the NINCDS-ADRDA work group. *Neurology, 34*, 939–944.

McKinney-Edmonds, M. (1993). Physical health. In J. S. Jackson, L. M. Chatters, & R. J. Taylor (Eds.), *Aging in Black America* (pp. 151–166). Newbury Park, CA: Sage.

McLaughlin, C. (1994). Casualty nurses' attitudes toward attempted suicide. *Journal of Advanced Nursing, 20*, 1111–1118.

McPhillips, R. (1988). Essential elements for the nursing minimum data set as seen by federal officials. In H. H. Werley & N. M. Lang (Eds.), *Identification of the nursing minimum data set* (pp. 233–238). New York: Springer Publishing.

McQueen, J. (1995). Evolution of patient-focused care within the contextual framework of an integrated delivery system (IDS). *Journal of Society for Health Systems, 5*, 5–9.

Medical Outcomes Trust. (1993). *How to score the SF-36 health survey.* Boston: Author.

Medoff-Cooper, B. (1991). Changes in nutritive sucking patterns with increasing gestational age. *Nursing Research, 40*, 245–247.

Medoff-Cooper, B. (1995). Infant temperament: Implications for parenting from birth through 1 year. *Journal of Pediatric Nursing, 10*, 141–145.

Medoff-Cooper, B., & Gennaro, S. (1996). The correlation of sucking behaviors and Bayley Scales of Infant Development at six months of age in VLBW infants. *Nursing Research, 45*, 291–296.

Medoff-Cooper, B., Verklan, T., Meyer, N., & Kaplan, J. (1996). *State and sucking behaviors in 1 and 2 day old infants.* Manuscript submitted for publication.

Medoff-Cooper, B., Weininger, S., & Zukowsky, K. (1989). Neonatal sucking as a clinical assessment tool: Preliminary findings. *Nursing Research, 39*, 162–165.

Meehan, M. (1994). National pressure ulcer prevalence survey. *Advanced Wound Care, 7*(3), 27–30, 34, 36–38.

Meek, P. A., & Lareau, S. C. (1997). Comparison of actual and recalled rating of dyspnea and fatigue.

American Journal of Respiratory and Critical Care Medicine, 155, A200.

Meininger, J. C. (1989). Epidemiologic designs. In P. F. Brink & M. J. Wood (Eds.), *Advanced design in nursing research* (pp. 201–222). Newbury Park, CA: Sage.

Meininger, J. C., Hayman, L. L., Coates, P. M., & Gallagher, P. R. (in press). Genetic and environmental influences on cardiovascular risk factors in adolescents. *Nursing Research.*

Meleis, A. I. (1975). Role insufficiency and role supplementation: A conceptual framework. *Nursing Research, 24,* 264–271.

Meleis, A. I. (1987). International nursing research. In J. J. Fitzpatrick & Taunton, R. L. (Eds), *Annual review of nursing research* (Vol. 5, pp 205–223). New York: Springer Publishing.

Meleis, A. I. (1993, June). *A passion for substance revisited: Global transitions and international commitments.* Paper presented at the 1993 National Doctoral Forum, St. Paul, MN.

Meleis, A. I. (1994). Transcending national boundaries: Empowerment through international collaboration. In O. Strickland & D. Sishman (Eds.), *Nursing issues in the 1990s* (pp. 544–555). Albany, NY: Delmar.

Meleis, A. I. (1995). Immigrant women in borderless societies: Marginalized and empowered. *Asian Journal of Nursing Studies, 2*(4), 39–47.

Meleis, A. I. (1996). Culturally competent scholarship: Substance and rigor. *Advances in Nursing Science, 19*(1), 1–16.

Meleis, A. I. (1997). *Theoretical nursing: Development and progress* (3rd ed.). Philadelphia: J. B. Lippincott.

Meleis, A. I., Lipson, J., Muecke, M., & Smith, G. (in press). Immigrant women and their health. Indianapolis, IN: Center Nursing Press of Sigma Theta Tau International.

Meleis, A. I., Omidian. P., & Lipson, J. (1993). Women's health status in the United States: An immigrant women's project. In B. McElmurry, K. F. Norr, & R. S. Parker (Eds.), *Women's health and development: A global challenge* (pp. 163–181). Boston: Jones and Bartlett.

Meleis, A. I., & Swendsen, L. (1978). Role supplementation: An empirical test of a nursing intervention. *Nursing Research, 27,* 11–18.

Meleis, A. I., & Trangenstein, P. A. (1994). Facilitating transitions: Redefinition of a nursing mission. *Nursing Outlook, 42,* 255–259.

Meltzer, H. Y. (1990). The role of serotonin in depression. In P. M. Whitaker-Asmitia & S. J. Peroutka (Eds.). The neuropharmacology of serotonin. *Annals of New York Academy of Science, 600,* 486–500.

Melzack, R., Ofiesh, J. G., & Mount, B. M. (1976). The Brompton mixture: Effects on pain in cancer patients.

Canadian Medical Association Journal, 115, 125–128.

Melzack, R., & Wahl, P. D. (1965). Pain mechanisms: A new theory. *Science, 150,* 971–979.

Mendez-Bauer, C., & Wadell, D. (1983). The effects of maternal position on uterine contractility and efficiency. *Birth, 10,* 243–246.

Mendoza, F. S., Ventura, S. J., Valdez, R. B., Castillo, R. O., Salvidar, L. E., Baisden, K., & Martorell, R. (1991). Selected measures of health status for Mexican-American, mainland Puerto Rican, and Cuban-American children. *Journal of the American Medical Association, 265,* 227–232.

Mercer, R. (1995). *Becoming a mother.* New York: Springer Publishing.

Mercer, R., Ferketich, S., DeJoseph, J., May, K., & Sollid, D. (1988). Effect of stress on family functioning during pregnancy. *Nursing Research, 37,* 268–275.

Merleau-Ponty, M. (1962). *Phenomenology of perception.* London: Routledge & Kegan Paul.

Merleau-Ponty, M. (1964). *The primacy of perception* (J. Edie, Trans.). Evanston, IL: Northwestern University Press.

Merrill, J. C. (1985). Designing case management. *Business and Health, 3*(5-9), 5–9.

Merton, R. K. (1957). *On sociological theories of the middle range: Social theory and social structure.* New York: Free Press.

Merwin, E. (1995). Building interdisciplinary mental health services research teams: A case example. *Issues in Mental Health Nursing, 16,* 547–554.

Merwin, E., Goldsmith, H., & Manderscheid, R. (1995). Human resource issues in rural mental health services. *Community Mental Health Services, 31,* 525–537.

Merwin, E., & Mauck, A. (1995). Psychiatric nursing outcome research: The state of the science. *Archives of Psychiatric Nursing, 9,* 311–331.

Messler, E. C. (1974). Transforming information into nursing knowledge: A study of maternity nursing practice (Doctoral dissertation: Columbia University, 1974). *Dissertation Abstracts International, 35,* 4B.

Metheny, N. A., Eisenberg, P., & Spies, M. (1986). Aspiration pneumonia in patients fed through nasoenteral tubes. *Heart and Lung, 15,* 256–261.

Metzger, B. L., & Schultz, S., II. (1982). Time series analysis: An alternative for nursing. *Nursing Research, 31,* 375–378.

Meyer, A. D., Goes, J. B., & Brooks, G. R. (1993). Organizations reacting to hyperturbulence. In G. P. Huber & W. H. Glick (Eds.), *Organizational change and redesign: Ideas and insights for improving performance* (pp. 66–111). New York: Oxford University Press.

Meyer, L. (1956). *Emotion and meaning in music.* Chicago: University of Chicago Press.

Mezey, M., Mitty, E., Rappaport, M., & Ramsey, G. (1997). Implementation of the Patient Self Determination Act in nursing homes in New York City. *Journal of the American Geriatric Society, 45,* 43–49.

Mezey, M., Ramsey, G., Mitty, E., & Leitman, R. (1995, October–November). *The Patient Self Determination Act: Cultural and socio-economic differences among recently discharged hospital patients.* Paper presented at the American Public Health Association, 123rd annual meeting, San Diego, CA.

Mezey, M. D., Stokes, S., & Rauckhurst, L. (1995). *Health assessment in the older adult.* New York: Springer Publishing.

Mezey, M. D., Teresi, J., Mitty, E., Ramsey, G., & Goldstein, T. (1997). *Determination of decision-making capacity sufficient to execute a health care proxy.* Manuscript submitted for publication.

Miaskowski, C., Nichols, R., Brody, R., & Synold, T. (1994). Assessment of patient satisfaction utilizing the American Pain Society's quality assurance standards on acute and cancer-related pain. *Journal of Pain and Symptom Management, 9,* 5–11.

Michel, Y., & Sneed, N. (1995). Dissemination and use of research findings in nursing practice. *Journal of Professional Nursing, 11,* 306–311.

Midwest Nursing Research Society. (1996). *Guidelines for scientific integrity.* Glenview, IL: Author.

Miles, M. S., D'Auria, J., & Avant, K. (1997). A conceptual framework of parental responsibilities. Manuscript under review.

Miles, M. S., Funk, S. G., & Carlson, J. (1993). Parental Stressor Scale: Neonatal Intensive Care Unit. *Nursing Research, 42,* 148–152.

Miles, M. S., Funk, S., & Kasper, M. A. (1992). The stress response of mothers and fathers of preterm infants. *Research in Nursing and Health, 15,* 261–269.

Miles, M. S., & Holditch-Davis, D. (1997). Parenting the prematurely-born child: Pathways of influence. *Seminars in Perinatology, 213,* 254–266.

Milio, N. (in press). Promoting community-based prevention policy. *Journal of Public Health Management and Practice.*

Miller, N. H., Smith, P. M., DeBusk, R. F., Sobel, D. S., & Taylor, C. B. (1997). Smoking cessation and hospitalized patients: Results of a randomized trial. *Archives of Internal Medicine.*

Milligan, R. A., & Pugh, L. C. (1994). Fatigue during the childbearing period. In J. J. Fitzpatrick & J. S. Stevenson (Eds.), *Annual review of nursing research* (Vol. 12, pp. 33–49). New York: Springer Publishing.

Millstein, S. G., Petersen, A. C., & Nightingale, E. O. (1993). *Promoting the health of adolescents.* New York: Oxford University Press.

Minarik, P. A. (1992). Second license for advanced nursing practice? *Clinical Nurse Specialist, 6,* 221–222.

Ministère de la Santé Publique et de l'Environnement Administration des Etablissements de Soins. (1988). *National statistics 1988: Medical acuities in the general hospitals.* Leuven, Belgium: Katholieke Universiteit Leuven.

Mishel, M. H. (1988). Uncertainty in illness. *Image: The Journal of Nursing Scholarship, 20,* 225–232.

Mishler, E. G. (1995). Models of narrative analysis: A typology. *Journal of Narrative and Life History, 5,* 87–123.

Mitchell, E. S. (1986). Multiple triangulation: A methodology for nursing science. *Advances in Nursing Science, 8*(3), 18–26.

Mitchell, E. S., Woods, N. F., & Lentz, M. J. (1994). Differentiation of women with three perimenstrual symptom patterns. *Nursing Research, 43,* 25–30.

Mitchell, P. H., Kirkness, C., Burr, R., March, K., & Newell, D. W. (in press). Waveform predictors of adverse responses to nursing care. *Acta Neurochirurgica.*

Mock, V., Dow, K. H., & Meares, C. (1986). Exercise effects on fatigue, physical functioning, and emotional distress during radiotherapy treatment for breast cancer. In *Proceedings: 8th International Research Congress,* Sigma Theta Tau International.

Mock, V., Hassey Dow, K., Meares, C., Grimm, P., Dieneman, J., Haisfield-Wolfe, M., Quitasol, W., Mitchell, S., Chakravarthy, A., & Gage, I. (1997). Effects of exercise on fatigue, physical functioning, and emotional distress during radiation therapy for breast cancer. *Oncology Nursing Forum, 24.*

Money, J. (1955). Linguistic resources and psychodynamic theory. *British Journal of Medical Psychology, 28,* 264–266.

Money, J., & Ehrhardt, A. A. (1972). *Man and woman, boy and girl.* Baltimore: Johns Hopkins University Press.

Montag, M. (1959). *Community college education for nursing.* New York: McGraw-Hill.

Montgomery, C. L. (1993). *Healing through communication: The practice of caring.* Newbury Park, CA: Sage.

Mon-Williams, M., Wann, J. P., & Rushton, S. (1993). Binocular vision in a virtual world: Visual deficits following the wearing of a head mounted display. *Ophthalmic and Physiologic Optic, 13,* 387–391.

Moody, L. E., Wilson, M. E., Smyth, K., Schwartz, R., Tittle, M., & VanCott, M. L. (1988). Analysis of a decade of nursing practice research: 1977–1986. *Nursing Research, 37,* 374–379.

Moore, I. J., Kramer, J., & Ablin, A. (1986). Late effects of central nervous system prophylactic leukemia therapy on cognitive functions. *Oncology Nursing Forum, 18,* 1381–1390.

Moore, I. M. (1995). Central nervous system toxicity of cancer therapy in children. *Journal of Pediatric Oncology Nursing, 12,* 203–210.

Moore, P., Fenlon, N., & Hepworth, J. T. (1996). Indicators of differences in immunization rates of Mexican American and White non-Hispanic infants in a Medicaid managed care system. *Public Health Nursing, 13,* 21–30.

Moore, R. D., Stanton, D., Gopalan, R., & Chaisson, R. E. (1994). Racial differences in the use of drug therapy for HIV disease in an urban community. *New England Journal of Medicine, 330,* 763–768.

Moore, S., Kuhrik, M., Kuhrik, N., & Katz, B. (1996). Coping with downsizing: Stress, self-esteem and social intimacy. *Nursing Management, 27*(3), 28–30.

Morgan, S. P (1990). A comparison of three methods of managing fever in the neurologic patient. *Journal of Neuroscience Nursing, 22,* 19–24.

Morin, K. H. (1995). Obese and nonobese postpartum women: Complications, body image, and perceptions of the intrapartal experience. *Applied Nursing Research, 8,* 81–87.

Morris, D. L. (1996). Watson's theory of caring. In J. J. Fitzpatrick & A. L. Whall (Eds.), *Conceptual models of nursing: Analysis and application* (3rd ed., pp. 289–303). Stamford, CT: Appleton & Lange.

Morris, J. N. (1964). *Uses of epidemiology.* Baltimore: Williams and Wilkins.

Morse, J. M. (1991). Negotiating commitment and involvement in the nurse-patient relationship. *Journal of Advanced Nursing, 16,* 455–468.

Morse, J. (1992). *Qualitative health research.* Newbury Park, CA: Sage.

Morse, J. M. (1995). Exploring the theoretical basis of nursing using advanced techniques of concept analysis. *Advances in Nursing Science, 17*(3), 31–46.

Morse, J. M., Anderson, G., Bottorff, J. L., Yonge, O., O'Brien, B., Solberg, S. M., & McIlveen, K. H. (1992). Exploring empathy: A conceptual fit for nursing practice. *Image: Journal of Nursing Scholarship, 24,* 173–280.

Morse, J. M., & Bottorff, J. L. (1990). The use of ethology in clinical nursing research. *Advances in Nursing Science, 12,* 53–64.

Morse, J. M., Bottorff, J. L., Anderson, G., O'Brien, B., & Solberg, S. (1992). Beyond empathy: Expanding expressions of caring. *Journal of Advanced Nursing, 17,* 809–821.

Morse, J. M., & Field, P. A. (1995). *Qualitative research methods for health professionals.* Newbury Park, CA: Sage.

Morse, J. M., Miles, M. W., Clark, D. A., & Doberneck, B. M. (1994). "Sensing" patient needs: Exploring concepts of nursing insight and receptivity used during nursing assessment. *Scholarly Inquiry for Nursing Practice: An International Journal, 8,* 233–254.

Mortensen, R. A., & Nielsen, G. H. (1996). *International classification of nursing practice (version 0.2).* Geneva: International Council of Nursing.

Moses, E. (1992). *The registered nurse populations: Findings from the National Sample Survey of Registered Nurses, March 1992.* Bethesda, MD: U.S. Department of Health and Human Services, Division of Nursing.

Motzer, S., Moseley, J., & Lewis, F. (1997). Recruitment and retention of families in clinical trials with longitudinal designs. *Western Journal of Nursing Research, 19,* 314–333.

Moyer, B. (1996) *The effects of interactive video on the problem-solving abilities of senior level nursing students in group settings.* Unpublished doctoral dissertation, Lehigh University.

Mudd, S. A., Boyd, C. J., Brower, K. J., Young, J. P., & Blow, F. C. (1994). Alcohol withdrawal and related nursing care in older adults. *Journal of Gerontological Nursing, 20*(10), 17–26.

Mueller, C. W., & McCloskey, J. C. (1990). Nurses' job satisfaction: A proposed measure. *Nursing Research, 39,* 113–117.

Muller, C., Marshall, C. L., Krasner, M., Cunningham, N., Wallerstein, E., & Thomstad, B. (1977). Cost factors in urban telemedicine. *Medical Care, 15,* 251–259.

Munoz, K. A., Krebs-Smith, S. M., Ballard-Babash, & Cleveland, L. E. (1997). Food intakes of U.S. children and adolescents compared with recommendations. *Pediatrics, 100,* 323–329.

Munro, B. H. (1997). *Statistical methods for health care research* (3rd ed.). Philadelphia: J. B. Lippincott.

Munro, B., Jacobsen, D., & Brooten, D. (1994). Reexamination of the psychometric characteristics of the La Monica–Oberst Patient Satisfaction Scale. *Research in Nursing and Health, 17,* 119–125.

Murnaghan, J. H. (1978). Uniform basic data sets for health statistical systems. *International Journal of Epidemiology, 7,* 263–269.

Murphy, E., & Fenton, M. S. (1991). An analysis of theory-research linkages in published gerontologic nursing studies, 1983–1989. *Advances in Nursing Science, 13*(4), 1–13.

Murphy, L. (1978). *Methods for studying nurse staffing on a patient unit* (DHEW Publication No. HRA 78-3). Washington, DC: U.S. Department Health and Human Services.

Murphy, L. N., Gass-Sternas, K., & Knight, K. (1995). Health of the chronically mentally ill who rejoin the community: A community assessment. *Issues in Mental Health Nursing, 16,* 239–256.

Murphy, R. L., Block, P., Bird, K. T., & Yurchak, P. (1973). Accuracy of cardiac auscultation by microwave. *Chest, 63,* 578–581.

Murphy, S. A. (1987). Self-efficacy and social support mediators of stress on mental health following a natural disaster. *Western Journal of Nursing Research, 9,* 58–86.

Murray, P. J. (1995). Connecting points. Internet. Using the Internet for gathering data and conducting research: Faster than the mail, cheaper than the phone. *Computers in Nursing, 13,* 206, 208–209.

Naegle, M. A. (1995). Education, research, and theory development. In E. J. Sullivan (Ed.), *Nursing care of clients with substance abuse.* St. Louis: Mosby.

Nagi, S. Z. (1991). Disability concepts revisited. In A. M. Pope & A. R. Tarlov (Eds.), *Disability in America: Toward a national agenda for prevention* (pp. 309–327). Washington, DC: National Academy Press.

Napholz, L., & McCanse, R. (1994). Interactive video instruction increases efficiency in cognitive learning in a baccalaureate nursing education program. *Computers in Nursing, 12,* 149–153.

National Association for Home Care. (1995). *Basic statistics about home care 1995.* Washington, DC: Author

National Center for Human Genome Research. (1996). *The Human Genome Project: From maps to medicine* (DHHS Publication No. NIH 96-3897). Bethesda, MD: National Institutes of Health.

National Center for Nursing Research. (1992). *Patient outcomes research: Examining the effectiveness of nursing practice* (NIH Publication No. 93-3411). Washington, DC: U.S. Government Printing Office.

National Center for Nursing Research. (1993). *Nursing informatics: Enhancing patient care* (NIH Publication No. 93-2419). Bethesda, MD: National Institutes of Health.

National Cholesterol Education Program. (1988). Report of the National Cholesterol Education Program Expert Panel on Detection, Evaluation and Treatment of High Blood Cholesterol in Adults. *Archives of Internal Medicine, 148,* 36–69.

National Cholesterol Education Program. (1991). *Report of the Expert Panel on Blood Cholesterol Levels in Children and Adolescents* (NIH Publication No. 91-2732). Bethesda, MD: U.S. Department of Health and Human Services, National Heart, Lung, and Blood Institute.

National Cholesterol Education Program. (1993). *Second report of the Expert Panel on Detection, Evaluation, and Treatment of High Blood Cholesterol in Adults* (NIH Publication No. 93-3095). Bethesda, MD: U.S. Department of Health and Human Services, National Heart, Lung, and Blood Institute.

National Commission for the Protection of Human Subjects of Biomedical and Behavioral Research. (1979). *The Belmont report* (GPO No. 887-809). Washington, DC: U.S. Government Printing Office.

National Health Service. (1982). *Steering group on health services information.* London: Author.

National Institute of Mental Health. (1991). *Caring for people with severe mental disorders: A national plan of research to improve services* (DHHS Publication No. ADM 91-1762). Washington, DC: U.S. Government Printing Office.

National Institute of Nursing Research. (1993). *Health promotion of older children and adolescents.* Bethesda, MD: Author.

National Institute of Nursing Research Priority Expert Panel. (1995). *Community-based health care: Nursing strategies* (NIH Publication No.95-3917). Bethesda, MD: U.S. Department of Health and Human Services.

National Institute of Nursing Research Priority Expert Panel on Health Promotion. (1993). *Health promotion for older children and adolescents.* Bethesda, MD: U.S. Department of Health and Human Services, Public Health Service.

National Institute on Alcohol Abuse and Alcoholism (NIAAA). (1993). *Eighth special report to US Congress: Alcohol and health* (DHHS Publication No. ADM 281-88-003). Alexandria, VA: Editorial Experts.

National Institutes of Health. (1991a). *Guidelines for the conduct of research in the intramural research program at the NIH.* Bethesda, MD: Author.

National Institutes of Health. (1991b). *Helpful hints on preparing a research grant application to the National Institutes of Health.* Bethesda, MD: NIH Office of Grants Inquiries, Division of Research Grants.

National Institutes of Health, Office of the Director. (1996). *NIH almanac 1995–1996* (NIH Publication No. 96-50). Washington, DC: Author.

National Kidney and Urologic Diseases Advisory Board. (1994). *Barriers to rehabilitation of persons with end-stage renal disease or chronic urinary incontinence* (Workshop summary report). Bethesda, MD: Author.

National League for Nursing. (1953). Student enrollment in 1953. *Nursing Outlook, 1,* 635–639.

National League for Nursing. (1954). Factors in the success of students in schools of practical nursing. *Nursing Outlook, 2,* 423–427.

National League for Nursing. (1991). *Nursing data review 1991.* New York: National League for Nursing, Division of Research.

National League of Nursing Education, Department of Studies. (1947). Student enrollment. *American Journal of Nursing, 47,* 489–490.

National Library of Medicine. (1960). *Medical subject headings.* Washington, DC: Author.

National Research Council. (1989). *Recommended dietary allowances.* Washington, DC: National Academy Press.

National Safety Council. (1996). *Accident prevention manual* (10th ed.). Chicago: Author.

National sample survey of registered nurses. (1997). Washington, DC: Division of Nursing, Bureau of

Health Professions, Health Resources and Services Administration.

National Task Force on the Prevention and Treatment of Obesity. (1994). Weight cycling. *Journal of the American Medical Association, 272,* 1196–1202.

Naylor, M., Brooten, D., Jones, R., Lavizzo-Mourey, R., Mezey, M., & Pauly, M. (1994). Comprehensive discharge planning for hospitalized elderly: A randomized clinical trial. *Annals of Internal Medicine, 120,* 999–1006.

Needleman, H. L., Gunnoe, C., Leviton, A., Peresie, H., Maher, C., & Barrett, P. (1979). Deficits in psychological and classroom performance of children with elevated dentine lead levels. *New England Journal of Medicine, 300,* 689–695.

Neelon, V. J., & Champagne, M. T. (1992). Managing cognitive impairment: The current bases for practice. In S. G. Funk, E. M. Tornquist, M. T. Champagne, & R. A. Wiese (Eds.), *Key aspects of elder care: Managing falls, incontinence, and cognitive impairment* (pp. 239–250). New York: Springer Publishing.

Neighbors, H. W., & Jackson, C. S. (1996). Mental health in Black America: Psychosocial problems and help-seeking behavior. In H. W. Neighbors & J. S. Jackson (Eds.), *Mental health in Black America* (pp. 1–13). Thousand Oaks, CA: Sage.

Nelson, R., & Schlachta, L. (1995). Nursing and telemedicine: Merging the expertise into telenursing. *Journal of the Healthcare Information and Management System Society, 9*(3), 17–23.

Nemcek, M. (1989). Factors influencing Black women's breast self-examination practice. *Cancer Nursing, 12,* 339–343.

Neufeldt, V. (Ed.). (1990). *Webster's new world dictionary.* Cleveland, OH: Simon & Schuster.

Neugarten, B. (1968). *Middle age and aging.* Chicago: University of Chicago Press.

Newacheck, P. W., & Taylor, W. R. (1992). Childhood chronic illness: Prevalence, severity, and impact. *American Journal of Public Health, 82,* 364–371.

Newell, A., & Simon, H. A. (1972). *Human problem solving.* Englewood Cliffs, NJ: Prentice-Hall.

Newman, M. (1997). Evolution of the theory of health as expanding consciousness. *Nursing Science Quarterly, 10*(1), 22–25.

Newman, M. A. (1979). *Theory development in nursing.* Philadelphia: F. A. Davis.

Newman, M. A. (1986). *Health as expanding consciousness.* St. Louis: C. V. Mosby.

Newman, M. A. (1990). Newman's theory of health as praxis. *Nursing Science Quarterly, 3,* 37–41.

Newman, M. A. (1994). *Health as expanding consciousness* (2nd ed.). New York: National League for Nursing Press.

Newman, M. A., Sime, A. M., & Corcoran-Perry, S. A. (1991). The focus of the discipline of nursing. *Advances in Nursing Science, 14*(1), 1–6.

Nicoll, L., & Ouellette, T. (1997). *Nurses' guide to the Internet.* New York: J. B. Lippincott.

Nielsen, G. H., & Mortensen, R. A. (1996). The architecture for an international classification of nursing practice (ICNP). *International Nursing Review, 43,* 175–182.

Nightingale, F. (1858). *Notes on matters affecting the health, efficiency, and hospital administration of the British army, founded chiefly on the experience of the late war.* London: Harrison and Sons.

Nightingale, F. (1860). *Notes on nursing.* New York: Appleton. (Original work published 1859)

Nightingale, F. (1862). *Army Sanitary Administration and its reform under the late Lord Herbert.* London: McCorquodale & Co.

Nightingale, F. (1863). *Notes on hospitals* (3rd ed.). London: Longman, Green, Longman, Roberts and Green.

Nightingale, F. (1969). *Notes on nursing: What it is and what it is not.* New York: Dover. (Original work published 1860)

Nightingale, F. (1992). *Notes on nursing: What it is and what it is not.* Philadelphia: J. B. Lippincott. (Original work published 1859)

NINR Priority Expert Panel on Nursing Informatics. (1993). *Nursing informatics: Enhancing patient care.* United States Department of Health and Human Services. Publication #93-2419.

Nite, G., & Willis, F. (1964). *The coronary patient: Hospital care and rehabilitation.* New York: Macmillan.

Noble, M. A. (Ed.). (1982). *The ICU environment: Directions for nursing.* Reston, VA: Reston Publishing.

Nokes, K., Wheeler, K., & Kendrew, J. (1994). Development of an HIV assessment tool. *Image: Journal of Nursing Scholarship, 26,* 133–138.

Norbeck, J. S. (1988). Social support. In J. J. Fitzpatarick, R. L. Taunton, & J. Q. Benoliel (Eds.), *Annual review of nursing research* (Vol. 6, pp. 85–109). New York: Springer Publishing.

Norbeck, J. S., DeJoseph, J. F., & Smith, R. T. (1996). A randomized trial of an empirically-derived social support intervention to prevent low birthweight among African American women. *Social Science and Medicine, 43,* 947–954.

Norbeck, J. S., Lindsey, A. M., & Carrieri, V. L. (1981). The development of an instrument to measure social support. *Nursing Research, 30,* 264–269.

North American Nursing Diagnosis Association. (1992). *NANDA nursing diagnoses: Definitions and classification, 1992–1993.* St. Louis: Author.

North American Nursing Diagnosis Association. (1994). *Taxonomy I revised—1990, with official nursing diagnoses.* St. Louis: Author.

North American Nursing Diagnosis Association. (1996). *Nursing diagnoses: Definitions and classification.* Philadelphia: Author.

Northouse, L. (1981). Mastectomy patients and the fear of cancer recurrence. *Cancer Nursing, 4,* 213–220.

Northouse, L. (1995). The impact of cancer in women on the family. *Cancer Practice, 3,* 134–142.

Northridge, M. E., Nevitt, M. C., Kelsey, J. L., & Link, B. (1995). Home hazards and falls in the elderly: The role of health and functional status. *American Journal of Public Health, 85,* 509–515.

Norton, D., McLaren, R., & Exton-Smith, A. N. (1975). *An investigation of geriatric nursing problems in hospital.* London: Churchill Livingstone. (Original work published in 1962)

Norusis, M. J. (1994). *SPSS for Windows 6.1 advanced statistics.* Chicago: SPSS.

Noureddine, S. N. (1995). Research review: Use of activated clotting time to monitor heparin therapy in coronary patients. *American Journal of Critical Care, 4,* 272–277.

Novak, R. D., & Auvil-Novak, S. E. (1996). Focus group evaluation of night nurse shiftwork difficulties and coping strategies. *Chronobiology International, 13,* 457–463.

Nuckolls, K. B., Cassel, J., & Kaplan, B. H. (1972). Psychosocial assets, life crisis, and the prognosis of pregnancy. *American Journal of Epidemiology, 95,* 431–441.

Nunnally, J. C. (1978). *Psychometric theory* (2nd ed.). New York: McGraw-Hill.

Nunnally, J. C., & Bernstein, I. H. (1994). *Psychometric theory* (3rd ed.). New York: McGraw-Hill.

Nurses Association of the American College of Obstetrics and Gynecology. (1991). *Antepartum fetal surveillance and intrapartum fetal heart monitoring* (2nd ed.). Washington, DC: Author.

Nyamathi, A. M. (1991). Relationship of resources to emotional distress, somatic complaints, and high-risk behaviors in drug recovery and homeless minority women. *Research in Nursing and Health, 14,* 269–277.

Oakley, D., Murray, M. E., Murtland, T., Hayashi, R., Andersen, H. F., Mayes, F., & Rooks, J. (1996). Comparisons of outcomes of maternity care by obstetricians and certified nurse-midwives. *Obstetrics and Gynecology, 88,* 823–829.

O'Brien-Pallas, L. L., Cockerill, R., & Leatt, P. (1991). A comparison of the workload estimated by five patient classification systems in nursing (Final report No. 6606-3706-57). Ottawa, Ontario: Health and Welfare Canada.

O'Connell, K. A., Cook, M. R., Gerkovich, M. M., Potocky, M., & Swan, G. E. (1990). Reversal theory and smoking: A state-based approach to ex-smokers' highly tempting situations. *Journal of Consulting and Clinical Psychology, 58,* 489–494.

O'Connell, K. A., Gerkovich, M. M., & Cook, M. R. (1995). Reversal theory's mastery and sympathy states in smoking cessation. *Image: Journal of Nursing Scholarship, 27,* 311–316.

O'Connor, F. W. (1991). Symptom monitoring for relapse prevention in schizophrenia. *Archives of Psychiatric Nursing, 5,* 193–201.

O'Connor, G. T., Plume, S. K., Olmstead, E. M., Morton, J. R., Maloney, C. T., Nugent, W. C., Hernandez, F. Jr., Clough, R., Leavitt, B. J., Coffin, L. H., Marrin, C. A., Wennberg, D., Birkmeyer, J. D., Charlesworth, D. C., Malenka, D. J., Quinton, H. B., & Kasper, J. F. (1996). A regional intervention to improve the hospital mortality associated with coronary artery bypass graft surgery. *Journal of the American Medical Association, 275,* 841–846.

Oddi, L., Griffith Whitley, G., & Pool, B. (1994). Contribution of graduate students to the creation and dissemination of nursing knowledge. *Image: Journal of Nursing Scholarship, 26,* 7–11.

Office of Alternative Medicine. (1992). *Alternative medicine: Expanding medical horizons. A report to the National Institutes of Health on alternative medical systems and practices in the United States* (NIH Publication No.94-066). Washington, DC: U.S. Government Printing Office.

Office of Communications, Office of the Director. (1996). *National Institutes of Health.* Washington, DC: National Institutes of Health.

Office of Technology Assessment, U.S. Congress. (1986). *Nurse practitioners, physician assistants, and certified nurse-midwives: A policy analysis* (Health Technology case study No. 37). Washington, DC: U.S. Congress.

Office of Technology Assessment. (1987). *Losing a million minds: Confronting the tragedy of Alzheimer's disease and other dementias.* Washington, DC: U.S. Government Printing Office.

O'Flynn, A. (1982). Meta-analysis. *Nursing Research, 31,* 314–316.

Ohlsson, A. (1994). Systematic reviews: Theory and practice. *Scandinavian Journal of Clinical and Laboratory Investigation, 219,* 25–32.

Olds, D., Eckenrode, J., Henderson, C., Kitzman, H., Powers, J., Cole, R., Sidora, K., Morris, P., Pettitt, L., & Luckey, D. (1997). Long term effects of home visitation on maternal life course and child abuse and neglect. *Journal of the American Medical Association, 278,* 637–643.

Olds, D., & Kitzman, H. (1990). Can home visitation improve the health of women and children at environmental risk? *Pediatrics, 86,* 108–116.

Olds, D. L., & Kitzman, H. (1993). Review of research on home visiting for pregnant women and parents of young children. In R. E. Behrman (Ed.), *Home visiting: The future of our children* (pp. 53–92). Los Angeles: Center for the Future of Our Children, The David and Lucille Packer Foundation.

Olson, D. H. L. (1995). *Marriage and family: Diversity and strength.* Mountain View, CA: Mayfield Publishers.

Olson, R. K., & Vance, C. (1993). *Mentorship in nursing: A collection of research abstracts with selected bibliographies, 1977–1992.* Houston: University of Texas Printing Services.

Olson, R. K., & Vance, C. (in press). Mentorship in nursing education. In K. A. Stevens (Ed.), *Review of research in nursing education* (Vol. 8). New York: National League for Nursing.

Omar, M. A., & Schiffman, R. F. (1995). Pregnant women's perceptions of prenatal care. *Maternal-Child Nursing Journal, 23,* 132–142.

Omery, A., Kasper, C., & Page, G. (1995). *In search of nursing science.* Thousand Oaks, CA: Sage Publications.

Omnibus Budget Reconciliation Act of 1990. (1991). *Patient Self Determination Act* (Pub.L. No. 101-508 [4206, 4751, codified in scattered sections of 42 U.S.C., esp. 1395cc, 1396a], West Supp.).

Opie, N. (1992). Childhood and adolescent bereavement. In J. J. Fitzpatrick & J. S. Stevenson (Eds.), *Annual review of nursing research* (Vol. 10, pp. 127–141). New York: Springer Publishing.

Orem, D. (1980). *Nursing: Concepts of practice.* New York: McGraw-Hill.

Orem, D. E. (1991). *Nursing: Concepts of practice* (4th ed.). St. Louis: Mosby Year Book.

Orem, D. E. (1995). *Nursing: Concepts of practice.* St. Louis: C. V. Mosby.

Orlando, I. J. (1961). *The dynamic nurse-patient relationship.* New York: Putnam.

O'Sullivan, A. L., & Schwarz, D. F. (1997, March). *Infant injuries and teenage mothers.* Workshop presentation at meeting of the Society for Adolescent Medicine, San Francisco.

O'Toole, A., & Welt, S. (Eds.). (1989). *Interpersonal theory in nursing practice: Selected works of Hildegard E. Peplau.* New York: Springer Publishing.

Ozbolt, J. F., Fruchtnight, J. N., & Hayden, J. R. (1994). Toward data standards for clinical nursing information. *Journal of the American Medical Informatics Association, 1,* 175–185.

Ozbolt, J. G. (1996). From minimum data to maximum impact: Using clinical data to strengthen patient care. *Advanced Practice Nursing Quarterly, 1*(4), 62–69.

Ozer, E. M., Brindis, C. D., Millstein, S. G., Knopf, D. K., & Irwin, C. E., Jr. (1997). *American adolescents: Are they healthy?* San Francisco: University of California, National Adolescent Health Information Center.

Pabst, M. K., Scherubel J. C, & Minnick, A. F. (1996). The impact of computerized documentation on nurses' use of time. *Computers in Nursing, 14,* 25–30.

Padilla, G. V., & Grant, M. M. (1987). Quality of life as a cancer nursing outcome variable. *Nln Publications, 21*(2194), 169–185.

Padilla, G. V., Presant, C., Grant, M. M., Metter, G., Lipsett, J., & Heide, F. (1983). Quality of life index for patients with cancer. *Research in Nursing and Health, 6,* 117–126.

Palmateer, L. M., & McCartney, J. R. (1985). Do nurses know when patients have cognitive deficits? *Journal of Gerontological Nursing, 11*(2), 6–16.

Palmer, M. H. (1996). *Urinary continence: Assessment and promotion.* Gaithersburg, MD: Aspen Publications.

Palmer, R. (1969). *Hermeneutics: Interpretation theory in Schleiermacher, Dilthey, Heidegger, and Gadamer.* Evanston, IL: Northwestern University Press.

Palmer-Erbs, V. K., & Anthony, W. A. (1995). Incorporating psychiatric rehabilitation principles into mental health nursing. *Journal of Psychosocial Nursing and Mental Health Services, 33*(3), 36–44.

Panel for the Prediction and Prevention of Pressure Ulcers in Adults. (1992). *Pressure ulcers in adults: Prediction and prevention.* Clinical practice guideline No. 3 (AHCPR Publication No. 92-0047). Rockville, MD: U.S. Department of Health and Human Services, Agency for Health Care Policy and Research.

Paolella, L. P., Dorfman, G. S., Cronan, J. J., & Hasan, F. M. (1988). Topographic location of the left atrium by computed tomography: Reducing pulmonary artery calibration error. *Critical Care Medicine, 16,* 1154–1156.

Pappas, G., Queen, S., Hadden, W., & Fisher, G. (July 8, 1993). The increasing disparity in mortality between socioeconomic groups in the United States, 1960 and 1986. *New England Journal of Medicine, 329,* 1139.

Parker, L. D., Cantrell, C., & Demi, A. S. (1997). Older adults' attitudes toward suicide: Are there race and gender differences? *Death Studies, 21,* 289–298.

Parker, S., Tong, T., Bolden S., & Wingo, S. (1997). Cancer statistics 1996. *CA: A Cancer Journal for Clinicians, 47*(1), 5–27.

Parlocha, P. K. (1995). *Examination of a critical path for psychiatric home care patients with a diagnosis of major depressive disorder.* Unpublished doctoral dissertation, University of California, San Francisco.

Parse, R. R. (1981). *Man-living-health: A theory of nursing.* New York: Wiley.

Parse, R. R. (1987). *Nursing science: Major paradigms, theories, and critiques.* Philadelphia: W. B. Saunders.

Parse, R. R. (1992). Human becoming: Parse's theory of nursing. *Nursing Science Quarterly, 5,* 35–42.

Parse, R. R. (1995). The human becoming practice methodology. In R. R. Parse (Ed.). *Illuminations: The hu-*

man becoming theory in practice and research (pp. 81–85). New York: National League for Nursing Press.

Parse, R. R. (1996). The human becoming theory: Challenges in practice and research. *Nursing Science Quarterly, 9,* 55–60.

Parse, R. R. (1997). The human becoming theory: The was, is, and will be. *Nursing Science Quarterly, 10,* 32–38.

Parsons, L. C., & Wilson, M. M. (1984). Cerebrovascular status of severe closed head injured patients following passive position changes. *Nursing Research, 33,* 68–75.

Paterson, J., & Zderad, L. (1976). *Humanistic nursing.* New York: John Wiley and Sons.

Paterson, J. G., & Zderad, L. T. (1988). *Humanistic nursing.* New York: National League for Nursing Press. (Original work published 1976; New York: John Wiley & Sons)

Patterson, E., Douglas, A., Patterson, P., & Bradle, J. (1992). Symptoms of preterm labor and self-diagnostic confusion. *Nursing Research, 41,* 367–372.

Patton, M. Q. (1990). *Qualitative evaluation and research methods.* Newbury Park, CA: Sage Publications.

Peden, A. R., Rose, H., & Smith, M. (1992). Transfer of continuing education to practice: A test of an evaluation model. *Journal of Continuing Education in Nursing, 23,* 152–155.

Pedhazur, E. J. (1982). *Multiple regression in behavioral research* (2nd ed.). New York: Holt, Rinehart, and Winston.

Pedhazur, E. J., & Schmelkin, L. P. (1991a). Introduction to sampling. In *Measurement, design, and analysis: An integrated approach* (pp. 318–341). Hillsdale, NJ: Lawrence Erlbaum Associates.

Pedhazur, E. J., & Schmelkin, L. P. (1991b). *Measurement, design and analysis.* Hillsdale, NJ: Lawrence Erlbaum Associates.

Pender, N. (1985). Effects of progressive muscle relaxation training on anxiety and health locus of control among hypertensive adults. *Research in Nursing and Health, 8,* 67–72.

Pender, N. J. (1990). Expressing health through lifestyle patterns. *Nursing Science Quarterly, 3,* 115–122.

Pender, N. J. (1996). *Health promotion in nursing practice* (3rd ed.). Norwalk, CT: Appleton & Lange.

Pender, N. J., & Pender, A. J. (1987). *Health promotion in nursing practice.* Norwalk, CT: Appleton & Lange.

Pennebaker, J. W., Burnam, M. A., Schaeffer, M. A., & Harper, D. C. (1977). Lack of control as a determinant of perceived physical symptoms. *Journal of Personality and Social Psychology, 35,* 167–174.

Peplau, H. (1952). *Interpersonal relations in nursing.* New York: G. P. Putnam & Sons.

Peplau, H. (1988). The art and science of nursing: Similarities, differences, and relations. *Nursing Science Quarterly, 1,* 8–15.

Peplau, H. (1992). Interpersonal relations: A theoretical framework for application in nursing practice. *Nursing Science Quarterly, 5,* 13–18.

Perednia, D., & Allen, A. (1995). Telemedicine technology and clinical applications. *Journal of the American Medical Association, 273,* 483–488.

Perese, E. F. (1997). Unmet needs of persons with chronic mental illnesses: Relationship to their adaptation to community living. *Issues in Mental Health Nursing, 18,* 19–34.

Perrin, E. C., Newacheck, P., Pless, I. B., Drotar, D., Gortmaker, S. L., Leventhal, J., Perrin, J. M., Stein, R. E. K., Walker, D. K., & Weitzman, M. (1993). Issues involved in the definition and classification of chronic health conditions. *Pediatrics, 91,* 787–793.

Perry, C. L., Kelder, S. H., Murray, D. M., & Klepp, K. I. (1992). Communitywide smoking prevention: Long-term outcomes of the Minnesota Heart Health Program and the class of 1989 study. *American Journal of Public Health, 82,* 1210–1216.

Peterman, B. A., Springer, P., & Farnsworth, J. (1995). Analyzing job demands and coping techniques. *Nursing Management, 26*(2), 51–53.

Peterman, T., Drotman, D. P., & Curran, J. W. (1985). Epidemiology of the acquired immunodeficiency syndrome (AIDS). *Epidemiology Review, 7,* 1.

Peters, K. L. (1996). Dinosaurs in the bath. *Neonatal Network, 15,* 71–73.

Peterson, C., Maier, S. F., & Seligman, M. E. P. (1993). *Learned helplessness.* New York: Oxford University Press.

Peterson, L., & Brown, D. (1994). Integrating child injury and abuse-neglect research: Common histories, etiologies and solutions. *Psychological Bulletin, 116,* 293–315.

Petrucci, K., Petrucci, P., Canfield, K., McCormick, K. A., Kjerulff, K., & Parks, P. (1992). Evaluation of UNIS: Urological nursing information systems. In P. D. Clayton (Ed.), *Proceedings of the Fifteenth Annual Symposium on Computer Applications in Medical Care* (pp. 43–47). New York: McGraw-Hill.

Philipson, S., Doyle, M. A., Gabram, S. G. A., Nightingale, C., & Philipson, E. H. (1995). Informed consent for research: A study to evaluate readability and processability to effect change. *Journal of Investigative Medicine, 43,* 459–467.

Phillips, C. Y., Castorr, A., Prescott, P. A., & Soeken, K. (1992). Nursing intensity: Going beyond patient classification. *Journal of Nursing Administration, 22*(4), 46–52.

Phillips, J. R. (1993). Virtual reality: A new vista for nurse researchers? *Nursing Science Quarterly, 6*(1), 5–7.

Phillips, R. A. (1996). Shivering effects on left ventricular performance and mixed venous oxygen saturation. *Southern Nursing Research Society: Southern Connections, 9*(1), 5–6. Miami Beach, FL.

Picot, S. J. (1995). Rewards, costs, and coping of African American caregivers. *Nursing Research, 44*(3), 147–152.

Pike, A. W. (1990). On the nature and place of empathy in clinical nursing practice. *Journal of Professional Nursing, 6,* 235–241.

Pillemer, K. A., & Finkelhor, D. A. (1988). The prevalence of elder abuse: A random sample survey. *Gerontologist, 28,* 51–57.

Piper, B. F. (1989). Fatigue: Current bases for practice. In S. G. Funk, E. M. Tornquist, M. T. Champagne, L. A. Copp, & R. Wiese (Eds.), *Key aspects of comfort* (pp. 187–240). New York: Springer Publishing.

Ploeg, J., Dobbins, M., Hayward, S., Ciliska, D., Thomas, H., & Underwood, J. (1995). *A systematic overview of the effectiveness of public health nursing interventions.* Working paper 95-12. Hamilton, Ontario: McMaster University & University of Toronto, Quality of Nursing Worklife Research Unit.

Polit, D., & Hungler, B. (1983). *Nursing research.* Philadelphia: Lippincott.

Polit, D., & Hungler, B. (1995). *Nursing research: Principles and methods* (5th ed.). Philadelphia: J. B. Lippincott.

Pollack, M. M., Cuerdon, T. C., & Getson, P. R. (1993). Pediatric intensive care units: Results of a national survey. *Critical Care Medicine, 21,* 607–614.

Pollock, S. E. (1993). Adaptation to chronic illness: A program of research testing nursing theory. *Nursing Science Quarterly, 6,* 86–92.

Poole, K., & Jones, A. (1996). A re-examination of the experimental design for nursing research. *Journal of Advanced Nursing, 24,* 108–114.

Popper, K. (1969). *Conjectures and refutations.* London: Routledge & Kegan Paul.

Potempa, K. M. (1993). Chronic fatigue. In J. J. Fitzpatrick & J. S. Stevenson (Eds.), *Annual review of nursing research* (Vol. 11, pp. 57–76). New York: Springer Publishing.

Pravikoff, D. S. (1993). Commentary. *Nursing Forum, 28*(4), 33–35.

Prescott, P. (1991). Nursing intensity: Needed today for more than staffing. *Nursing Economics, 9,* 409–414.

Prescott, P., Ryan, J., Soeken, K., Castorr, A., Thompson, K., & Phillips, C. (1991). The Patient Intensity for Nursing Index (PINI). *Research in Nursing and Health, 14,* 213–221.

Pressler, J. L., Wells, N., & Hepworth, J. T. (1993). *Methodological issues in preterm infant outcomes.* Unpublished manuscript. Vanderbilt University, Nashville, TN.

Preston, J. (1993). *The telemedicine handbook: Improving health care with interactive video.* Austin, TX: Telemedical Interactive Consultative Services.

Prewitt, E. (1997). Inner-city health care. *Annals of Internal Medicine, 126,* 485–490.

Priority Expert Panel. (1994). *National nursing research agenda: Vol. 4. Symptom management—pain* (NIH Publication No. 93-2420). Bethesda, MD: National Institutes of Health, National Institute of Nursing Research.

Priority Panel on Nursing Informatics. (1993). *Nursing informatics: Enhancing patient care.* Bethesda, MD: U.S. Department of Health and Human Services, U.S. Public Health Service, National Institutes of Health.

Pritchard, A. (1969). Statistical bibliography or bibliometrics? *Journal of Documentation, 25,* 348–349.

Prochaska, J. O., Velicer, W. F., Rossi, J. S., Goldstein, M. G., Marcus, B. H., Rakowski, W., Fiore, C., Harlow, L. L., Redding, C. A., Rosenblook, D., & Rossi, S. R. (1994). Stages of change and decisional balance for 12 problem behaviors. *Health Psychology, 13,* 39–46.

Proctor, A., Morse, J. M., & Khonsari, E. S. (1996). Sounds of comfort in the trauma center: How nurses talk to patients in pain. *Social Science and Medicine, 42,* 1669–1680.

Propp, V. (1968). *Morphology of the Russian folktale.* Austin: University of Texas Press.

Protection of human subjects; informed consent and waiver of informed consent requirements in certain emergency research: Final rules. (1966). *Federal Register, 61*(192), 51497–51532.

Protopapas, Z., Siegel, E. L., Reiner, B. I., Pomerantz, S. M., Pickar, E. R., Wilson, M., & Hooper, F. J. (1996). Picture archiving and communication system training for physicians: Lessons learned at the Baltimore VA Medical Center. *Journal of Digital Imaging, 9,* 131–136.

Province, M. A., Hadley, E. C., Hornbrook, M. C., Lipsitz, L. A., Miller, J. P., Mulrow, C. D., Ory, M. G., Sattin, R. W., Tinetti, M. E., & Wolf, S. L. (1995). The effects of exercise on falls in elderly patients. A preplanned meta-analysis of the FICSIT trials. *Journal of the American Medical Association, 273,* 1381–1383.

Purfield, P., & Morin, K. (1995). Excessive weight gain in primigravidas with low-risk pregnancy: Selected obstetric consequences. *Journal of Obstetric, Gynecologic and Neonatal Nursing, 24,* 434–439.

Putnam, R. (1992, October). *Theory of action from the action science perspective.* A paper presented at the Third Knowledge Development Symposium, University of Rhode Island College of Nursing, Newport.

Putnam, R. (1996). The reflective mode: Interpersonal reflections regarding espoused theories and theories in use. In *Building a cumulative knowledge base for nursing: From fragmentation to congruence of philosophy, theory, methods of inquiry and practice* (Invited papers of the 4th and 5th symmposia of the Knowledge Development Series) (pp. 45–52). Kingston, RI: University of Rhode Island, College of Nursing.

Quinn, J. (1984). Therapeutic touch as energy exchange: Testing the theory. *Advances in Nursing Science, 6*(2), 42–49.

Quint, J. C. (1967). *The nurse and the dying patient.* New York: Macmillian.

Radloff, L. (1977). The CES-D Scale: A self-report depression scale for research in the general population. *Applied Psychological Measurement, 1,* 385–401.

Ragucci, A. T. (1990). The ethnographic approach and nursing research. In P. J. Brink (Ed.), *Transcultural nursing* (pp. 163–174). Prospect Heights, IL: Waveland Press. (Original work published in 1972)

Rahe, R. H., Ward, H. W., & Hayes, V. (1979). Brief group therapy in myocardial infarction rehabilitation: Three-to-four-year follow-up study. *Psychosomatic Medicine, 41,* 229–242.

Rains, J. W., & Ray, D. W. (1995). Participatory action research for community health promotion. *Public Health Nursing, 12,* 256–261.

Raisig, M. (1964). The index to current nursing periodical literature in the United States. *Nursing Forum, 3,* 97–109.

Rakowski, W., Dube, C., Marcus, B. H., Prochaska, J. O., Velicer, W., & Abrams, D. (1992). Assessing elements of women's decisions about mammography. *Health Psychology, 11,* 111–118.

Rankin, E. A. (1991). Mentor, mentee, mentoring: Building career development relationships. *Nursing Connections, 4*(4), 50–57.

Rantz, M. J. (1995). *Nursing quality measurement: A review of studies.* Washington, DC: American Nurses Publishing.

Rantz, M. J., & LeMone, P. (Eds.). (1997). *Classification of nursing diagnoses: Proceedings of the Twelfth Conference, North American Diagnosis Association.* Glendale, CA: Cumulative Index of Nursing and Allied Health.

Raval, D., Yeh, R. F., Mora, A., & Pildes, R. S. (1980). Changes in transcutaneous PO_2 during tracheobronchial hygiene in neonates. *Perinatology Neonatology, 4,* 41–44.

Ray, C. (1991). Chronic fatigue syndrome and depression: Conceptual and methodological ambiguities. *Psychological Medicine, 21,* 1–9.

Raymond, S. J. (1995). Normal saline instillation before suctioning: Helpful or harmful? A review of the literature. *American Journal of Critical Care, 4,* 267–271.

Reame, N. E., Kelch, R. P., Beitins, I. Z., Yu, M. Y., Zawacki, C., & Padmanabha, V. (1996). Age effects on FSH and pulsatile LH secretion across the menstrual cycle of premenopausal women. *Journal of Clinical Endocrinology and Metabolism, 81,* 1512–1518.

Redman, B. K. (1993). Patient education at 25: Where we have been and where we are going. *Journal of Advanced Nursing, 18,* 725–730.

Redman, R., & Ketefian, S. (1995). Defining and measuring work redesign: A field study. In K. Kelly (Ed.), *Health care work redesign: Series on nursing administration* (Vol. 7, pp. 2–20). Thousand Oaks, CA: Sage.

Reed, P. (1996a). Peplau's interpersonal relations model. In J. Fitzpatrick & A. Whall (Eds.), *Conceptual models of nursing* (3rd ed., pp. 55–76). Norwalk, CT: Appleton & Lange.

Reed, P. (1996b). Transforming practice knowledge into nursing knowledge: A revisionist analysis of Peplau. *Image: Journal of Nursing Scholarship, 29,* 29–33.

Rehm, L. P. (1977). A self-control model of depression. *Behavior Therapy, 8,* 787–804.

Reif-Lehrer, L. (1995). *Grant application writer's handbook.* Boston: Jones and Bartlett.

Reiley, P., Iezzoni, L. I., Phillips, R., Davis, R. B., Tuchin, L. I., & Calkins, D. (1996). Discharge planning: Comparison of patients' and nurses' perceptions of patients following hospital discharge. *Image: Journal of Nursing Scholarship, 28,* 143–147.

Reiner, B. I., Siegel, E. L., Hooper, F., Pomerantz, S. M., Protopapas, Z., Pickar, E., & Killewich, L. (1996). Picture archiving and communication systems and vascular surgery: Clinical impressions and suggestions for improvement. *Journal of Digital Imaging, 9,* 167–171.

Reisberg, B. (1984). Alzheimer's disease: Stages of cognitive decline. *American Journal of Nursing, 84,* 225–228.

Reitz, J. (1988). The relationship of intensity and severity factors to the nursing minimum data set. In H. Werley & N. Lang (Eds.), *Identification of the nursing minimum data set* (pp. 313–324). New York: Springer Publishing.

Reizian, A., & Meleis, A. I. (1987). Symptoms reported by Arab American patients on the Cornell Medical Index. *Western Journal of Nursing Research, 9,* 368–384.

Rempusheski, V. F. (1991). Historical and futuristic perspectives on aging and the gerontological nurse. In E. M. Baines (Ed.), *Perspectives on gerontological nursing* (pp. 3–28). Newbury Park, CA: Sage.

Renshaw, S. (1996). *The effect of content vs. structure graphic organizers on nursing student achievement and attitudes when using computer interactive videodisc simulations.* Unpublished doctoral dissertation, Temple University.

Report of the Secretariat to the 1992 general meeting of the Global Network of WHO Collaborating Centers for Nursing Development in PHC. (1992). Unpublished manuscript, College of Nursing, University of Illinois at Chicago.

Reynolds, N. R., Timmerman, G., Anderson, J., & Stevenson, J. S. (1992). Meta-analysis for descriptive research. Research in Nursing and Health, 15, 467–475.

Richards, S. M. (1995). Meta-analyses and overviews of randomized trials [Review]. Blood Reviews, 9, 85–91.

Richie, M. F. (1996). Meeting the challenge of disruptive behaviors in the nursing home. Journal of Gerontological Nursing, 22(11), 3.

Ricoeur, P. (1984). Time and narrative. Chicago: University of Chicago Press.

Riehl-Sisca, J. (1989). Conceptual models for nursing practice (3rd ed.). Norwalk, CT: Appleton & Lange.

Ries, J. B., & Leukefeld, C. G. (1995). Applying for research funding: Getting started and getting funded. Thousand Oaks, CA: Sage.

Riesch, S. K. (1992). Nursing centers. In J. J. Fitzpatrick, R. L. Taunton, & A. K. Jacox (Eds.), Annual review of nursing research (Vol. 10, pp. 143–162). New York: Springer Publishing.

Riesch, S. K., Tosi, C. A., Thurston, C. A., Forsyth, D. M., Kuenning, T. S., & Kestly, J. A. (1993). Effects of communication training on parents and young adolescents. Nursing Research, 42, 10–16.

Riessman, C. K. (1993). Qualitative research methods series. Vol. 30. Narrative analysis. Newbury Park, CA: Sage Publications.

Ripich, S., Moore, S. M., & Brennan, P. F. (1992). A new nursing medium: Computer networks for group intervention. Journal of Psychosocial Nursing and Mental Health Services, 30(7), 15–20.

Rizzolo, M. A. (Ed.). (1994). Interactive video: Expanding horizons in nursing. New York: American Journal of Nursing Co.

Rizzuto, C., & Mitchell, M. (1988a). Research in service settings: Part 1. Consortium project outcomes. Journal of Nursing Administration, 18(2), 32–37.

Rizzuto, C., & Mitchell, M. (1988b). Research in service settings: Part 2. Consortium project. Journal of Nursing Administration, 18(3), 19–24.

Rizzuto, C., & Mitchell, M. (1990). Outcomes of research consortium project. Journal of Nursing Administration, 20(4), 13–17.

Robb, I. H. (1907). Nursing: Its principles and practice for hospital and private use. Toronto: J. A. Carveth.

Roberson, M. H. B. (1992). The meaning of compliance: Patient perspectives. Qualitative Health Research, 2(1), 7–26.

Roberts, B. L., Anthony, M. K., Matejczyk, M., & Moore, D. (1994). The relationship of social support to functional limitations, pain and well-being among men and women. Journal of Women and Aging, 6, 3–19.

Roberts, B. L., & Fitzpatrick, J. J. (1983). Improving balance: Therapy of movement. Journal of Gerontological Nursing, 9, 151–156.

Roberts, J., While, A., & Fitzpatrick, J. (1996). Clinical problem-solving using video simulation: An investigation. Medical Education, 29, 347–354.

Robin, A. L., & Koepke, T. (1990). Behavioral assessment and treatment of parent-adolescent conflict. In M. Hersen, R. M. Eisler, & P. M. Miller (Eds.), Progress in behavior modification (Vol. 25, pp. 178–215). Newbury Park, CA: Sage.

Robins, R. W., Mendelsohn, G. A., & Spranca, M. D. (1996). The actor-observer effect revisited: Effects of individual differences and repeated social interactions on actor and observer attributions. Journal of Personality and Social Psychology, 71, 375–389.

Robinson, J. C. (1996). Decline in hospital utilization and cost inflation under managed care in California. Journal of the American Medical Association, 276, 1060–1064.

Robinson, J. H. (1995). Grief responses, coping processes, and social support of widows: Research with Roy's model. Nursing Science Quarterly, 8, 158–164.

Robinson, L. D. (1981). Gerontological nursing research. In I. M. Burnside (Ed.), Nursing and the aged (2nd ed., pp. 654–666). New York: McGraw-Hill.

Rodgers, B. L., & Knafl, K. A. (1993). Concept development: Foundations, techniques, and applications. Philadelphia: W. B. Saunders.

Rodgers, S. (1994). An exploratory study of research utilization by nurses in general medical and surgical wards. Journal of Advanced Nursing, 20, 904–911.

Roffwarg, H. P., Muzio, J. N., & Dement, W. C. (1995). Annals of research: What do infants dream about? Neonatal Intensive Care, 8, 54–56.

Rogers, A. E., & Aldrich, M. S. (1993). The effect of regularly scheduled naps on sleep attacks and excessive daytime sleepiness associated with narcolepsy. Nursing Research, 42, 111–117.

Rogers, A. E., Aldrich, M. S., & Caruso, C. C. (1994). Patterns of sleep and wakefulness in treated narcoleptic subjects. Sleep, 17, 590–597.

Rogers, B. (1994). Occupational health nursing: Concepts and practice. Philadelphia: W. B. Saunders.

Rogers, B., & Emmett, E. A. (1987). Handling antineoplastic agents: Urine mutagenicity in nursing personnel. Image: Journal of Nursing Scholarship, 19, 108–113.

Rogers, B., & Travers, P. (1991). Occupational hazards of critical care nursing: Overview of work-related hazards in nursing: Health and safety issues. Heart and Lung, 20, 486–499.

Rogers, E. (1995). Diffusion of innovations (4th ed.). New York: Free Press.

Rogers, M. (1970). *An introduction to the theoretical basis of nursing.* Philadelphia: F. A. Davis.

Rogers, M. E. (1983). *Science of unitary human beings: A paradigm for nursing.* Unpublished manuscript, New York University.

Rogers, M. E. (1990). Nursing: Science of unitary, irreducible human beings: Update. In E. A. M. Barrett (Ed.), *Visions of Rogers' science-based nursing* (pp. 5–11). New York: National League for Nursing.

Romieu, I., Meneses, F., Sienra-Monge, J., Huerta, J., Ruiz Velasco, S., White, M., Etzel, R., & Hernandez-Avila, M. (1995). Effects of urban air pollutants on emergency visits for childhood asthma in Mexico City. *American Journal of Epidemiology, 141,* 546–553.

Rooks, J. P., Weatherby, N. L., Ernst, E. K., Stapleton, S., Rosen, D., & Rosenfield, A. (1989). Outcomes of care in birth centers: The national birth center study. *New England Journal of Medicine, 321,* 1804–1811.

Rosenstock, I. M. (1966). Why people use health services. *Milbank Memorial Fund Quarterly, 44,* 94–121.

Rosenthal, G., Halloran, E., Kiley, M., & Landefeld, S. (1995). Validation of the nursing severity index in the assessment of hospital outcomes in patients with musculoskeletal disease. *Journal of Clinical Epidemiology, 48,* 179–188.

Rosenthal, G., Halloran, E., Kiley, M. L., Pinkley, C., & Landefeld, S. (1992). Development and validation of the nursing severity index: A new method for measuring severity of illness using nursing diagnosis. *Medical Care, 30,* 1127–1141.

Rosenthal, R. (1979). The file drawer problem and tolerance for null results. *Psychological Bulletin, 86,* 638–641.

Ross, D. (1995). "letter." *Skeptical Inquirer, 19*(4), 58–60.

Rossi, M., & Lindell, S. (1986). Maternal position and pushing techniques in a nonprescriptive environment. *Journal of Obstetric, Gynecologic and Neonatal Nursing, 15,* 203–208.

Rossi, P. H., & Freeman, H. E. (1985). *Evaluation: A systematic approach* (3rd ed.). Beverly Hills, CA: Sage.

Rosswurm, M. A. (1991). Attention-focusing program for persons with dementia. *Clinical Gerontologist, 10*(2), 3–16.

Rotheram-Borus, M. J., Koopman, C., Haignere, C., & Davies, M. (1991). Reducing HIV sexual risk behaviors among runaway adolescents. *Journal of the American Medical Association, 26,* 1237–1241.

Rothert, M., Rover, D., Holmen, M., Schmitt, N., Talarczyk, G., Knoll, J., & Gogato, J. (1990). Women's use of information regarding hormone replacement therapy. *Research in Nursing and Health, 13,* 355–366.

Rovner, B. W., Lucas-Blaustein, J., Folstein, M., & Smith, S. W. (1990). Stability over one year in patients admitted to a nursing home dementia unit. *International Journal of Geriatric Psychiatry, 5,* 77–82.

Rowles, G. D., & Dallas, M. (1996). Individualizing care: Family roles in nursing home decision making. *Journal of Gerontological Nursing, 22*(3), 20–25.

Roy, C. (1980). *Introduction to nursing: An adaptation model.* Englewood Cliffs, NJ: Prentice-Hall.

Roy, C., & Andrews, H. A. (1991). *The Roy adaptation model: The definitive statement.* Norwalk, CT: Appleton & Lange.

Rozeboom, W. W. (1960). The fallacy of the null hypothesis significance test. *Psychological Bulletin, 57,* 416–428.

Ruccione, K. S., Waskerwitz, M., Buckley, J., Perin, G., & Hammond, G. D. (1994). What caused my child's cancer? Parents' responses to an epidemiology study of childhood cancer. *Journal of Pediatric Oncology Nursing, 11,* 71–84.

Rudy, E. B., & Grenvik, A. (1992). Future of critical care. *American Journal of Critical Care, 1,* 33–37.

Rush, A. J., Gullion, C. M., & Prien, R. F. (1996). A curbside consult to applicants for National Institute of Mental Health grant support. *Psychopharmacology Bulletin, 32,* 311–320.

Russo, J. M., & Landcaster, D. R. (1995). Evaluating unlicensed assistive personnel models: Asking the right questions, collecting the right data. *Journal of Nursing Administration, 25*(9), 51–57.

Rutala, W. A., & Hamory, B. H. (1989). Expanding role of hospital epidemiology: Employee health—chemical exposure in the health care setting. *Infection Control and Hospital Epidemiology, 10*(6), 261–266.

Rybash, J. M., Hoyer, W. J., & Roodin, P. A. (1986). *Adult cognition and aging: Developmental changes in processing, knowing, and thinking.* New York: Pergamon Press.

Ryden, M., Bossenmaier, M., & McLachlan, C. (1991). Aggressive behavior in cognitively impaired nursing home residents. *Research in Nursing and Health, 14*(2), 87–95.

Saba, V. K. (1991). *Home health care classification project* (NTIS Publication No. PB92-177013/AS). Washington, DC: Georgetown University.

Saba, V. K. (1992a). The classification of home health care nursing: Diagnoses and interventions. *Caring, 11*(3), 50–57.

Saba, V. K. (1992b). Home health care classification: Part 2. *Caring, 11*(5), 58–60.

Saba, V. K. (1994). *Home health care classification (HHCC) of nursing diagnoses and interventions* (rev. ed.). Washington, DC: Author.

Saba, V., O'Hare, P. A., Zuckerman, A. E., Boondas, J., Levine, E., & Oatway, D. M. (1991). A nursing intervention taxonomy for home health care. *Nursing and Health Care, 12,* 296–299.

Saba, V. K., & McCormick, K. A. (1996). *Essentials of computers for nurses* (2nd ed.). New York: McGraw-Hill.

Saba, V. K., & Zuckerman, A. E. (1992). A new home health reclassification method. *Caring, 11*(10), 27–34.

Sackett, D. L., & Cook, D. J. (1993). Can we learn anything from small trials? [Review]. *Annals of the New York Academy of Sciences, 703,* 25–32.

Sacks, H. (1967). *The search for help: No one to turn to.* In E. S. Schneidman (Ed.), *Essays in self destruction* (pp. 203–223). New York: Science House.

Sacks, H. S., Reitman, D., Pagano, D., & Kupelnick, B. (1996). Meta-analysis: An update [Review]. *Mount Sinai Journal of Medicine, 63*(3–4), 216–224.

Safier, G. (1977). *Contemporary American leaders in nursing: An oral history.* New York: McGraw-Hill.

Samarel, N., & Fawcett, J. (1992). Enhancing adaptation to breast cancer: The addition of coaching to support groups. *Oncology Nursing Forum, 19,* 591–596.

Samples, J. F., Van Cott, M. L., Long, C., King. I., & Kersenbrock, A. (1985). Circadian rhythms: Basis for screening for fever. *Nursing Research, 34,* 377–379.

Sandelowski, M. (1995). Triangles and crystals: On the geometry of qualitative research. *Research in Nursing and Health, 18,* 569–574.

Sanders, J. H. (1995). *A dual-use telecommunications system for delivering medical care.* Proposal to U.S. Army Medical Research and Research Command, Medical College of Georgia Research Institute, Inc., 1–44.

Sarna, L. (1989). *Impact of chemotherapy on the quality of life and functional states of older adults with non-small-cell lung cancer.* Unpublished doctoral dissertation, University of California, San Francisco.

Savedra, M. (1976). Coping with pain: Strategies of severely burned children. *Maternal-Child Nursing Journal, 5,* 197–203.

Sawyer, L., Regev, H., Proctor, S., Nelson, M., Messias, D., Barnes, D., & Meleis, A. I. (1995). Matching versus cultural competence in research: Methodological considerations. *Research in Nursing and Health, 18,* 557–567.

Scally, G. (1996). Citizen health. *Lancet, 134,* 3–4.

Scanlon, C., & Fibison, W. (1995). *Managing genetic information: Implications for nursing practice.* Washington, DC: American Nurses Association.

Schaefer, K. M., & Potylycki, M. J. (1993). Fatigue associated with congestive heart failure: Use of Levine's conservation model. *Journal of Advanced Nursing, 18,* 260–268.

Schaefer, K. M., Swavely, D., Rothenberger, C., Hess, S., & Williston, D. (1996). Sleep disturbances post coronary artery bypass surgery. *Progress in Cardiovascular Nursing, 11*(1), 5–14.

Schaie, K. W., Campbell, R. D., Meredith, W., & Rawlings, S. W. (Eds.). (1989). *Methodological issues in aging research.* New York: Springer Publishing.

Schlotfeldt, R. (1971). The significance of empirical research for nursing. *Nursing Research, 20,* 140–142.

Schlotfeldt, R. (1972). Approaches to the study of nursing questions and the development of nursing science discussion. *Nursing Research, 21,* 513–517.

Schlotfeldt, R. (1975). The need for a conceptual framework. In P. Verhonic (Ed.), *Nursing research* (pp. 3–25). Boston: Little, Brown

Schnelle, J. F., McNees, P., Crooks, V., & Ouslander, J. G. (1995). The use of a computer-based model to implement an incontinence management program. *Gerontologist, 35,* 656–665.

Schön, D. (1983). *The reflective practitioner: How professionals think in action.* New York: Basic Books.

Schriber, T. (1991). *An introduction to simulation using GPSS/H.* New York: John Wiley & Sons.

Schultz, A. (1973). *Collected Papers I: The problem of social reality.* The Hague: Martinus Nijhoff.

Schutz, A. (1973). Collected Papers I: The Problem of Social Reality. The Hague, Netherlands: Martinus Nijhoff.

Schumacher, H., Kippel, J., & Koopman, W. (Eds.). (1993). *Primer on the rheumatic diseases* (10th ed.). Atlanta: Arthritis Foundation.

Schumacher, K. L., Jones, P. S., & Meleis, A. I. (in press). The elderly in transition: Needs and issues of care. In T. Tripp-Reimer & E. Swanson (Eds.), *Advances in gerontological nursing: Vol. 4. Chronic illness and the older adult.* New York: Springer Publishing.

Schumacher, K. L., & Meleis, A. I. (1994). Transitions: A central concept in nursing. *Image: Journal of Nursing Scholarship, 26,* 119–127.

Schutzenofer, K. K., & Potter, P. (1989). Collaboration by consortium. *Nursing Connections, 2*(2), 39–47.

Schwartz, C. E., & Fox, B. H. (1995). *Social Science and Medicine, 40,* 359–370.

Schwartz, C. L., Hobbie, W. L., Constine, L. S., & Ruccione, K. S. (Eds.). (1994). *Survivors of childhood cancer: Assessment and management.* St. Louis: Mosby-Year Book.

Schwarz, D. F., Grisso, J. A., Holmes, J. H., Miles, C. G., Wishner, A. R., & Sutton, R. L. (1994). Injuries in an urban African American population. *Journal of the American Medical Association, 271,* 755–760.

Scott, J. D. (1996). *Hypothesis generating research: The role of medical treatment effectiveness research in hypothesis generation.* Rockville, MD: U.S. Public Health Services, Center for Medical Effectiveness Research, Agency for Health Care Policy and Research.

Scupholme, A., Paine, L. L., Lang, J. M., Kumar, S., & DeJoseph, J. F. (1994). Time associated with components of clinical services rendered by nurse-midwives: Sample data from phase II of Nurse-Midwifery Care to Vulnerable Populations in the United States. *Journal of Nurse-Midwifery, 39*(1), 5–12.

Searle, J. R., Kiefer, F., & Bierwisch, M. (Eds.). (1980). *Speech act theory and pragmatics.* Dordrecht, Netherlands: Reidel.

Sebastian, J. (1996). Vulnerability and vulnerable populations: An introduction. In M. Stanhope & J. Lancaster (Eds.), *Community health nursing: Promoting health of aggregates, families, and communities* (4th ed., pp. 623–646). St. Louis: C. V. Mosby.

Segeren, C. (1994). Transatlantic cooperation. *COHE-HRE Newsletter, 2,* 4–5.

Seligman, M. (1975). *Helplessness: On depression, development, and death.* San Francisco: W. H. Freeman.

Selye, H. (1976). *The stress of life* (2nd ed.). New York: McGraw-Hill.

Sempos, C., Fulwood, R., Haines, C., Carroll, M., Anda, R., Williamson, D. F., Remington, P., & Cleeman, J. (1989). The prevalence of high blood cholesterol levels among adults in the United States. *Journal of the American Medical Association, 262,* 45–52.

Sempos, C. T., Cleeman, J. I., Carroll, M. D., Johnson, C. L., Bachorik, P. S., Gordon, D. J., Burt, V. L., Briefl, R. R., Brown, C. D., Lippel, K., & Rifkind, B. M. (1993). Prevalence of high blood cholesterol among U.S. adults: An update based on guidelines from the second report of the National Cholesterol Education Program adult treatment panel. *Journal of the American Medical Association, 269,* 3009–3014.

Seventh Day Adventist Hospital Association. (1961–1967). *Cumulative index to nursing literature.* Glendale, CA: Author.

Shamian, J. (1991). Effect of teaching decision analysis on student nurses' clinical intervention decision making. *Research in Nursing and Health, 14,* 59–66.

Shanas, E. (1979). Social myth as hypothesis: The case of the family relations of old people. *Gerontologist, 19,* 3–9.

Shaughnessy, P., Crisler, K., Schlenker, R. E., Arnold, A. G., Kramer, A., Powell, M. C., & Hittle, D. F. (1994). Measuring and assuring the quality of home health care. *Health Care Financing Review, 16*(1), 35–68.

Shavelson, R. J., & Webb, N. M. (1991). *Generalizability theory: A primer.* Newbury Park, CA: Sage.

Shaver, J. L. F., Giblin, E., Lentz, M., & Lee, K. (1988). Sleep patterns and stability in perimenopausal women. *Sleep, 11,* 556–561.

Shaver, J., Giblin, E., & Paulsen, V. (1991). Sleep quality subtypes in midlife women. *Sleep, 14,* 18–23.

Shaver, J., & Woods, N. F. (1986). Consistency of perimenstrual symptoms across two cycles. *Research in Nursing and Health, 8,* 313–319.

Shepard, J., & Faust, S. (1994). Refugee health care and the problem of suffering. *Bioethics Forum, 9,* 3–7.

Sherwood, G. (1996). Nurse administrators' perceptions of the impact of continuing nursing education in underserved areas. *Journal of Continuing Education in Nursing, 27,* 124–130.

Sherwood, G. D. (1997). Meta-synthesis of qualitative analyses of caring: Defining a therapeutic model of nursing. *Advanced Practice Nursing Quarterly, 3*(1), 32–42.

Shortell, S. M., O'Brien, J. L., Carman, J. M., Foster, R. W., Hughes, E. F., Boerstler, H., & O'Connor, E. J. (1995). Assessing the impact of continuous quality improvement/total quality management: Concept versus implementation. *Health Services Research, 30,* 377–401.

Shortell, S., Zimmerman, J., Rousseau, D., Gillies, R., Wagner, D., Draper, E., Knaus, W., & Duffy, J. (1994). The performance of intensive care units: Does good management make a difference? *Medical Care, 32,* 508–525.

Shrager, J., & Langley, P. (1990). *Computational models of scientific discovery and theory formation.* San Mateo, CA: Morgan Kaufmann.

Siegel, C. D., Graves, P., Maloney, K., Norris, J. M., Colonge, B. N., & Lezotte, D. (1996). Mortality from intentional and unintentional injury among infants of young mothers in Colorado, 1986 to 1992. *Archives of Pediatric and Adolescent Medicine, 150,* 1077–1083.

Silva, M. C. (1985). Comprehension of information for informed consent by spouses of surgical patients. *Research in Nursing and Health, 8,* 117–124.

Silva, M. C. (1986). Research testing nursing theory: State of the art. *Advances in Nursing Science, 9*(1), 1–11.

Silva, M. C. (1995). *Ethical guidelines in the conduct, dissemination, and implementation of nursing research.* Washington, DC: American Nurses Publishing of the American Nurses Association.

Silva, M. C. (1997). Philosophy, theory, and research in nursing: A linguistic journey to nursing practice. In I. M. King & J. Fawcett (Eds.), *The language of nursing theory and metatheory* (pp. 52–53). Indianapolis, IN: Sigma Theta Tau's International Center Nursing Press.

Simmons, L., & Henderson, V. (1964). *Nursing research: A review and assessment.* New York: Macmillan.

Simon, I. (1993). Surgery 2001: Concepts of telepresence surgery. *Surgical Endoscopy, 7,* 462–463.

Simon, P. M., Schwartzstein, R. M., Weiss, J. W., Fencl, V., Teghtsoonian, M., & Weinberger, S. E. (1990). Distinguishable types of dyspnea in patients with shortness of breath. *American Review of Respiratory Disease, 142,* 1009–1014.

Sittig, D. F., Jiang, Z., Manfre, S., Sinkfeld, K., Ginn, R., Smith, L., Olsen, A., & Borden, R. (1995). Evaluating a computer-based experiential learning simulation: A case study using criterion-referenced testing. *Computers in Nursing, 13,* 17–24.

Skiba, D. (1993). Collaborative tools. *Reflections, 19*(1), 10–12.

Slavinsky, A. T., & Krauss, J. B. (1982). Two approaches to the management of long-term psychiatric outpatients in the community. *Nursing Research, 33,* 284–289.

Slavitt, D. B., Stamps, P. L., Piedmont, E. B., & Haase, A. M. (1978). Nurses' satisfaction with their work situation. *Nursing Research, 27,* 114–120.

Smart, C. R., Hendrick, R. L., Rutledge, J. H., III, & Smith, R. A. (1995). Benefit of mammography screening in women ages 40–49 years. Current evidence from randomized controlled trials. *Cancer, 75,* 1619–1626.

Smeltzer, C. H., Leighty, S., & Williams-Brinkley, R. (1997). In J. C. McCloskey & H. K. Grace (Eds.), *Current issues in nursing* (5th ed., pp. 93–98). St. Louis: C. V. Mosby.

Smets, E. M. A., Garssen, B., Schuster-Uitterhoeve, A. L. J., & de Haes, J. C. J. M. (1993). Fatigue in cancer patients. *British Journal of Cancer, 68,* 220–224.

Smiley, D. F., Gould, A. G., & Melby, E. (1931). *The principles and practice of hygiene.* New York: Macmillan.

Smith, C. E. (1993). Quality of life in long-term total parenteral nutrition patients and their family caregiver. *Journal of Parenteral and Enteral Nutrition, 17,* 501–506.

Smith, C. E. (1994a). A model of caregiving effectiveness for technologically dependent adults residing at home. *Advances in Nursing Science, 17,* 27–40.

Smith, C. E. (1994b). *Technological home care: Costs and quality of life.* Unpublished manuscript.

Smith, C. E. (1995). Technology and home care. In J. J. Fitzpatrick & J. S. Stevenson (Eds.), *Annual review of nursing research* (Vol. 13, pp. 137–167). New York: Springer Publishing.

Smith, C. E. (1996). Quality of life and caregiving in technological home care. In J. J. Fitzpatrick & J. Norbeck (Eds.), *Annual review of nursing research* (Vol. 14, pp. 95–118). New York: Springer Publishing.

Smith, C. E., Fernengel, K., Holcroft, C., Gerald, K., & Marien, L. (1994). Meta-analysis of the associations between social support and health outcomes. *Annals of Behavioral Medicine, 16,* 352–362.

Smith, C. E., & Kleinbeck, S. V. M. (1996). Nutrition and quality of life measurement. In B. Spilker (Ed.), *Quality of life and pharmacoeconomics in clinical trials* (2nd ed., pp. 1063–1075). Philadelphia: Raven Press.

Smith, E. (1979). Nonclinical practice: CE meeting the needs of the demanding nursing profession. *CE Focus, 2,* 8–10.

Smith, J. A. (1981). The idea of health. *Advances in Nursing Science, 3*(3), 43–50.

Smith, J. A. (1983). *The idea of health implications for the nursing professional.* New York: Columbia University.

Smith, M. A., Ruffin, M. T., & Green, L. A. (1993). The rational management of labor. *American Family Physician, 47,* 1471–1481.

Smith, P. C., Kendall, L. M., & Hulin, C. L. (1969). *The measurement of satisfaction in work and retirement.* Chicago: Rand McNally.

Snow, J. (1855). *On the mode of communication of cholera* (2nd ed.). London: Churchill.

Snyder, M. (1993). The influence of interventions on the stress-health outcome linkage. In J. S. Barnfather & B. L. Lyon (Eds.), *Stress and coping: State of the science and implications for nursing theory, research and practice* (pp. 159–170). Indianapolis, IN: Sigma Theta Tau International.

Snyder, M. (1997, April). *The influence of interventions on the stress-health outcomes linkage.* Paper presented at Midwest Nursing Research Society preconference. Minneapolis, MN.

Sokal, R. R. (1974). Classification: Purposes, principles, progress, prospects. *Science, 185,* 1115–1123.

Solberger, A. (1965). *Biological rhythm research.* New York: Elsevier.

Solon, J. A., Kilpatrick, N. S., & Hill, M. F. (1988). Aging-related education: A national survey. *Journal of Gerontological Nursing, 14*(9), 21–26, 38–39.

Sparks, S. M. (1993). Electronic networking for nurses. *Image: Journal of Nursing Scholarship, 25,* 245–248.

Sparks, S. M., & Lien-Gieschen, T. (1994). Modification of the diagnostic content validity model. *Nursing Diagnosis, 5,* 31–35.

Spence, J. T., & Helmreich, R. L. (1978). *Masculinity and femininity.* Austin: University of Texas Press.

Spilker, B., Simpson, R. L. Jr., & Tilson, H. H. (1991). Quality of life bibliography and indexes: 1991 update. *Journal of Clinical Research in Pharmacoepidemiology, 6,* 205–266.

Spitz, R. (1945). Hospitalism: An inquiry into the genesis of psychiatric conditions in early childhood. *Psychoanalytic Study of the Child, 1,* 52–74.

Spitzer, V., Ackerman, M. J., Scherzinger, A. L., & Whitlock, D. (1996). The visible human male: A technical report. *Journal of the American Medical Informatics Association, 3,* 118–130.

Spradley, J. (1980). *Participant observation.* New York: Holt, Rinehart and Winston.

St. Lawrence, J. S., Brasfield, T. L., Jefferson, K. W., Alleyne, E., O'Bannon, R. E., & Shirley, A. (1995). Cognitive-behavioral intervention to reduce African American adolescents' risk for HIV infection. *Journal of Consulting and Clinical Psychology, 63,* 221–237.

Stake, R. (1994). Case studies. In N. Denzin & Y. Lincoln (Eds.), *Handbook of qualitative research.* Thousand Oaks, CA: Sage.

Stanhope, M. (1990). An innovative approach to health care for the homeless/very poor: A nurse managed clinic. Washington, DC: U.S. Department of Commerce, National Technical Information Service.

Stanhope, M., & Lancaster, J. (1988). *Community health nursing: Process and practice for promoting health* (2nd ed.). St Louis: Mosby.

Starfield, B. (1992). *Primary care: Concept, evaluation, and policy.* New York: Oxford University Press.

Starr, P. (1982). *The social transformation of American medicine.* New York: Basic Books.

Steckel, S. B. (1974). The use of positive reinforcement in order to increase patient compliance. *American Association of Nephrology Nurses and Technicians Journal, 1,* 39–41.

Steckel, S. B. (1982). *Patient contracting.* Norwalk, CT: Appleton-Century-Crofts.

Steckel, S. B., & Funnell, M. M. (1981). *Increasing adherence of outpatients to therapeutic regimens* (Final report on Veterans Administration Health Service Research and Development Project No. 343). Ann Arbor, MI: VA Hospital.

Steefel, L. (1993). The World Trade Center disaster: Healing the unseen wounds. *Journal of Psychosocial Nursing and Mental Health Services, 3*(6), 5–7.

Steeman, E., Abraham, I., & Godderis, J. (in press). Risk profiles for institutionalization in a cohort of elderly people with dementia or depression. *Archives of Psychiatric Nursing.*

Steigman, D. (1996). Is it "urban" or is it "asthma"? *Lancet, 348,* 143–144.

Stein, R. E. K. (1996). To be or not to be . . . noncategorical. *Developmental and Behavioral Pediatrics, 17,* 36–37.

Steinberg, L., & Silverberg, S. B. (1986). The vicissitudes of autonomy in early adolescence. *Child Development, 57,* 841–851.

Steptoe, A. (1991). The links between stress and illness. *Journal of Psychosomatic Research, 35,* 633–644.

Stetler, C. B. (1994). Refinement of the Stetler/Marram model for application of research findings to practice. *Nursing Outlook, 42,* 15–25.

Steuer, J. (1992). Defining virtual reality: Dimensions determining telepresence. *Journal of Communication, 42*(4), 73–93.

Stevens, R., & Heide, F. (1977). Analgesic characteristics of prepared childbirth techniques: Attention focusing and systematic relaxation. *Journal of Psychosomatic Research, 21,* 429–438.

Stevenson, J. S. (1988). Nursing knowledge development. *Journal of Professional Nursing, 4,* 152–162.

Stevenson, J. S. (1990). Quantitative care research: Review of content, process, and product. In J. S. Stevenson & T. Tripp-Reimer (Eds.), *Knowledge about care and caring: State of the art and future developments* (pp. 97–118). Kansas City, MO: American Academy of Nursing.

Stevenson, J. S. (1993). Adult development is NOT (JUST) a demographic variable: A call for contextual content in doctoral programs. In M. Snyder & M. Newman (Eds.), *Annual Forum on Doctoral Nursing Education: 1993 Proceedings* (pp. 23–31). Minneapolis: University of Minnesota.

Stewart, B., & Krueger, L. (1996). An evolutionary concept analysis of mentoring in nursing. *Journal of Professional Nursing, 12,* 311–321.

Stewart, D. W., & Kamins, M. A. (1993). *Secondary research: Information sources and methods.* Newbury Park, CA: Sage.

Stewart, J. (1995). Balancing learner control and realism with specific instructional goals: Case studies in fluid balance for nursing students. In *Proceedings of MedInfo '95* (p. 1715).

Stewart, M. J. (1989). Social support: Diverse theoretical perspectives. *Social Science and Medicine, 28,* 1275–1282.

Stillman, M. J. (1977). Women's health beliefs about breast cancer and breast self-examination. *Nursing Research, 26,* 121–127.

Stone, K. S. (1990). Ventilator versus manual resuscitation bag as the method for delivering hyperoxygenation before endotracheal suctioning. *AACN's Clinical Issues in Critical Care Nursing, 1,* 289–299.

Stone, K. S., Bell, S. D., & Preusser, B. A. (1991). The effect of repeated endotracheal suctioning on arterial blood pressure. *Applied Nursing Research, 4,* 150–158.

Stone, K., & Turner, B. S. (1989). Endotracheal suctioning in the adult and newborn. In J. J. Fitzpatrick & R. L. Taunton (Eds.), *Annual review of nursing research* (Vol. 7, pp. 27–49). New York: Springer Publishing.

Strickland, O. L. (1993a). Measuring well to study well [Editorial]. *Journal of Nursing Measurement, 1,* 3–4.

Strickland, O. L. (1993b). Qualitative or quantitative: So what is your religion? [Editorial]. *Journal of Nursing Measurement, 1,* 103–105.

Strickland, O. L. (1995). Assessment of perinatal indicators for the measurement of programmatic effectiveness. *Journal of Perinatal and Neonatal Nursing, 9*(1), 52–67.

Strickland, O., & Waltz, C. (1986). Measurement of research variables in nursing. In P. Chinn (Ed.)., *Nurs-*

ing research methodology: Issues and implementation (pp. 79–90). Rockville, MD: Aspen Publishers.

Stroebe, W., & Stroebe, M. S. (1995). *Social psychology and health*. Buckingham, England: Open University Press.

Strube, M., & Hartman, D. (1983). Meta-analysis: Techniques, applications, and functions. *Journal of Consulting and Clinical Psychology, 51,* 14–27.

Strumpf, N., & Tomes, N. (1993). Restraining the troublesome patient: An historical perspective on a contemporary debate. *Nursing History Review, 1*(1), 3–24.

Stuart, A. (1968). Sample surveys: Non-probability sampling. In D. L. Sills (Ed.), *International Encyclopedia of the Social Sciences* (Vol. 13, pp. 612–616). New York: Macmillan.

Stuhlmiller, C. M. (1994). Occupational meanings and coping practices of rescue workers in an earthquake disaster. *Western Journal of Nursing Research, 16,* 268–287.

Suarez, L., Nichols, D. C., Pully, L., Brady, L., & McAlister, C. A. (1993). Theory based models. *Public Health Reports, 108,* 477–482.

Sullivan, E. J. (1995). *Nursing care of clients with substance abuse*. St. Louis: Mosby.

Sullivan-Marx, E. M., & Mullinix, C. (1998). Payment for advanced practice nurses: Economic structures and systems. In M. D. Mezey & D. O. McGivern (Eds.), *Nurses, nurse practitioners*. New York: Springer Publishing.

Sullivan-Marx, E., & Strumpf, N. (1996). Restraint-free care for acutely ill hospitalized patients. *AACN: Advanced Practice in Acute and Critical Care, 7,* 572–578.

Suppe, F. (1996). *Middle-range theories: Historical and contemporary perspectives*. Paper presented at Summer Nursing Theory Conference, Wayne State University, Detroit.

Suppe, F. (1997). *Middle-range theories and knowledge development*. Manuscript submitted for publication.

Surgeon General's National Workshop on Hispanic/Latino Health. (1992). *Blueprint for improving Hispanic/Latino health: Implementation strategies* [Workshop proceedings]. Washington, DC: Office of the Surgeon General.

Survey of Income and Program Participation. (1995). Disabilities among children aged ≤17 years—United States, 1991–1992. *Journal of the American Medical Association, 274,* 1112–1113.

Suserud, B., & Haljamae, H. (1997). Acting at a disaster site: Experiences expressed by Swedish nurses. *Journal of Advanced Nursing, 25,* 155–162.

Susman, E., Dorn, L., & Fletcher, J. (1992). Participation in biomedical research: The consent process as viewed by children, adolescents, young adults, and physicians. *Journal of Pediatrics, 121,* 547–552.

Sutherland, J. A. (1993). The nature and evolution of phenomenological empathy in nursing: An historical treatment. *Archives of Psychiatric Nursing, 7,* 369–376.

Sveinsdottir, H., & Reame, N. E. (1991). Symptom patterns in women with premenstrual syndrome complaints: A prospective assessment using a marker for ovulation and screening criteria for adequate ovarian function. *Journal of Advanced Nursing, 16,* 689–700.

Swain, M. A., & Steckel, S. B. (1981). Influencing adherence among hypertensives. *Research in Nursing and Health, 4,* 213–233.

Swan, J. H. C., Ganz, W., Forrester, J., Marcus, H., Diamond, G., & Chonette, D. (1970). Catheterization of heart in man with use of flow-directed balloon tipped catheter. *New England Journal of Medicine, 283,* 447–451.

Swanson, K. M. (in press). What's known about caring in nursing science: A literary meta-analysis. In A. S. Hinshaw, S. Feetham, & J. Shaver (Eds.), *Handbook of clinical nursing research*.

Swartz, D. (1994). Tech talk. *Telemedicine Today, 2*(2), 6–8.

Swartz, K., & Tiffany, C. R. (1994). Evaluating Bhola's configuration theory of planned change. *Nursing Management, 25*(6), 56–61.

Taft, L. B. (1995, March/April). Interventions in dementia care: Responding to the call for alternatives to restraints. *American Journal of Alzheimer's Disease,* pp. 30–38.

Taft, L. B., & Cronin-Stubbs, D. (1995). Behavioral symptoms in dementia: An update. *Research in Nursing and Health, 18,* 143–163.

Taliaferro, D. H., & Richmond, C. R. (1996). Monitoring fever patterns and hydration in hospitalized PLWA. In *Proceedings: Ninth Annual Conference, Association of Nurses in AIDS Care, Chicago*. Reston, VA: ANAC (p. 100).

Talley, N. J., Phillips, S. F., Melton, J., Wiltgen, C., & Zinsmeister, A. R. (1989). A patient questionnaire to identify bowel disease. *Annals of Internal Medicine, 111,* 671–674.

Tappen, R., & Barry, C. (1995). Assessment of affect in advanced Alzheimer's disease: The Dementia Mood Picture Test. *Journal of Gerontological Nursing, 21*(3), 44–46.

Tatara, T. (1993). Understanding the nature and scope of domestic elder abuse with the use of state aggregate data: Summaries of the key findings of a national survey of state APS and aging agencies. *Journal of Elder Abuse and Neglect, 5*(4), 35–57.

Taylor, C. B., Houston Miller, N., Killen, J. D., & DeBusk, R. F. (1990). Smoking cessation after acute myocardial infarction: Effects of a nurse-managed intervention. *Annals of Internal Medicine, 113,* 118–123.

Taylor, D. (1990). Time-series analysis: Use of autocorrelation as an analytic strategy for describing pattern and change. *Western Journal of Nursing Research, 12,* 254–261.

Taylor, D. L. (1994). Evaluating therapeutic change in symptom severity at the level of the individual woman experiencing severe PMS. *Image: Journal of Nursing Scholarship, 26,* 25–33.

Taylor, D., & Woods, N. (Eds.). (1991). *Menstruation, health and illness.* New York: Hemisphere.

Taylor, F. W. (1911). *The principles of scientific management.* New York: Harper.

Tetrick, L. E., & LaRocco, J. M. (1987). Understanding, prediction and control as moderators of the relationships between perceived stress, satisfaction and psychological well being. *Journal of Applied Psychology, 72,* 538–543.

Thatcher, V. S. (1953). *History of anesthesia with emphasis on the nurse specialist.* Philadelphia: J. B. Lippincott.

Thibaut, J., & Kelley, H. (1959). *The social psychology of groups.* New York: Wiley.

Thiele, J. R. (1989). Guidelines for collaborative research. *Applied Nursing Research, 2,* 150–153.

Thoman, E. B. (1982). A biological perspective and a behavioral model for assessment of premature infants. In L. A. Bond & J. M. Joffee (Eds.), *Primary prevention of psychopathology: Facilitating infant and early childhood development* (Vol. 6, pp. 159–179). Hanover, NH: University Press of New England.

Thomas, C. L. (Ed.). (1997). *Taber's cyclopedic medical dictionary* (18th ed., p. 363). Philadelphia: F. A. Davis.

Thomas, D., Gao, D., Self, S., Allison, C., Toa, Y., Mahloch, J., Ray, R., Qin, Q., Presley, R., & Porter, P. (1997). Randomized trial of breast self examination in Shanghai: Methodology and preliminary results. *Journal of the National Cancer Institute, 89,* 355–365.

Thomas, K. A. (1990). Design issues in the NICU: Thermal effects of windows. *Neonatal Network, 9,* 23–26.

Thomas, S. A., & DeKeyser, F. (1996). Blood pressure. In J. J. Fitzpatrick & J. Norbeck (Eds.), *Annual review of nursing research* (Vol. 14, pp. 3–22). New York: Springer Publishing.

Thompson, C. L. (1990). Examination of walking distance by patients with chronic obstructive pulmonary disease. *American Review of Respiratory Disease, 141,* A326.

Thompson, C. L. (1997). Dyspnea, airway resistance, positive end expiratory pressure, heart rate, blood pressure, and mucus weight with tracheal suction in ICU patients. *Critical Care Medicine, 25*(Suppl.), A77.

Thompson, J. E. (1986). Nurse-midwifery care: 1925–1984. In H. H. Werley, J. J. Fitzpatrick, & R. L. Taunton (Eds.), *Annual review of nursing research* (Vol. 4, pp. 153–173). New York: Springer Publishing.

Thompson, J. (1991). Exploring gender and culture with Khmer refugee women: Reflections on participatory feminist research. *Advances in Nursing Science, 13*(3), 30–48.

Thompson, J. E., Walsh, L. V., & Merkatz, I. R. (1990). History of prenatal care: Cultural, social and medical contexts. In I. R. Merkatz & J. E. Thompson (Eds.), *New perspectives on prenatal care* (pp. 9–30). New York: Elsevier Science.

Thompson, R. J., & Gustafson, K. E. (1996). *Adaptation to chronic childhood illness.* Washington, DC: American Psychological Association.

Thornton, N. (1996). Congruence between parent satisfaction with nursing care of their children and nurses' perceptions of parent satisfaction. *Axon, 18*(2), 27–37.

Thurber, F., Berry, B., & Cameron, E. (1991). The role of school nursing in the United States. *Journal of Pediatric Health Care, 5,* 135–140.

Tichy, A. M., Braam, C. M., Meyer, T. A., & Rattan, N. S. (1988). Stressors in pediatric intensive care unit. *Pediatric Nursing, 14,* 40–42.

Tilden, V. P., & Galyen, R. D. (1987). Cost and conflict: The darker side of social support. *Western Journal of Nursing Research, 9*(1), 9–18.

Tilden, V. P., Nelson, C. A., & May, B. A. (1990). The Interpersonal Relationship Inventory: Development and psychometric characteristics. *Nursing Research, 39,* 337–343.

Tinetti, M. E., Baker, D. I., McAvay, G., Claus, E. B., Garrett, P., Gottschalk, M., Koch, M. L., Trainor, K., & Horwitz, R. I. (1994). A multifactorial intervention to reduce the risk of falling among elderly people living in the community. *New England Journal of Medicine, 331,* 821–827.

Titler, M. G., Kleiber, C., Steelman, V., Goode, C., Rakel, B., Barry-Walker, J., Small, S., & Buckwalter, K. (1994). Infusing research into practice to promote quality care. *Nursing Research, 43,* 307–313.

Todd, C., Robinson, G., & Reid, N. (1993). 12-hour shifts: Job satisfaction of nurses. *Journal of Nursing Management, 1,* 215–220.

Topf, M. (1992). Effects of personal control over hospital noise on sleep. *Research in Nursing and Health, 15,* 19–28.

Torgerson, D. J., Ryan, M., & Ratcliffe, J. (1995). Economics of sample size determination for clinical trials. *Quarterly Journal of Medicine, 88,* 517–521.

Torrance, G. W. (1987). Utility approach to measuring health-related quality of life. *Journal of Chronic Diseases, 40,* 593–603.

Traska, M. R. (1995). *Managed care strategies 1996.* New York: Faulkner & Gray.

Tripp-Reimer, T. (1994). *Gerontologic Nursing Interventions Research Center overview* (P30-NR03979). Iowa City: University of Iowa College of Nursing.

Tryon, P. (1966). Use of comfort measures as support during labor. *Nursing Research, 15,* 109–113.

Tucker, K. (1996). The use of epidemiologic approaches and meta-analysis to determine mineral element requirements. *Journal of Nutrition, 126*(Suppl. 9), 2365S–2372S.

Tulman, L., & Fawcett, J. (1990). Maternal employment following childbirth. *Research in Nursing and Health, 13,* 181–188.

Turner, P. (1991). Benefits and costs of continuing nursing education: An analytical survey. *Journal of Continuing Education in Nursing, 22,* 104–108.

UCSF Symptom Management Faculty Group. (1992). *Symptom management proceedings: Symposium I and II.* San Francisco: UCSF School of Nursing.

Umlauf, M. G. (1990). How to produce around-the-clock CPR certification without losing any sleep. *Journal of Continuing Education in Nursing, 21,* 248–251.

Underwood, P. W., & Ruiz-Bueno, J. (1997, April). *Resources as moderators/mediators of the stress-health outcome linkage.* Paper presented at the Midwest Nursing Research Society Stress and Coping Synthesis Conference, Minneapolis.

United States Health Care Financing Administration. (1997a). [On-line]. Available: http://www.hcfa.gov/facts/F960100.htm

United States Health Care Financing Administration. (1997b). [On-line]. Available: http://www.hcfa.gov/medicaid/mover.htm

United States Health Care Financing Administration. (1997c). [On-line]. Available: http://www.hcfa.gov/medicaid/mservice.htm

United States Health Care Financing Administration. (1997d). [On-line]. Available: http://www.hcfa.gov/scripts/gotourl.exe#whatis

Ursano, R. J., & Fullerton, C. S. (1997). Trauma, time, and recovery. In C. S. Fullerton & R. J. Ursano (Eds.), *Posttraumatic stress disorder* (pp. 269–274). Washington, DC: American Psychiatric Press.

U.S. Bureau of the Census. (1992). *1990 census of population: Vol. 1. Characteristics of the population.* Washington, DC: U.S. Government Printing Office.

U.S. Bureau of the Census. (1993a). Hispanic Americans today. *Current population reports* (P23-183). Washington, DC: U.S. Government Printing Office.

U.S. Bureau of the Census. (1993b). Poverty in the United States: 1992. *Current population reports* (P60-185). Washington, DC: U.S. Government Printing Office.

U.S. Bureau of the Census. (1996). *Statistical abstract of the United States* (116th ed.). Washington, DC: U.S. Government Printing Office.

U.S. Department of Health and Human Services. (1983). Protection of human subjects. *Code of Federal Regulation,* title 45, part 46.

U.S. Department of Health and Human Services. (1990). *Healthy people 2000: Full report with commentary.* Boston: Jones & Bartlett.

U.S. Department of Health and Human Services. (1995). *Community-based health care: Nursing strategies* (NINR Publication No. 95-3917). Bethesda, MD: Author.

U.S. Department of Health and Human Services. (1996). Protection of human subjects: Informed consent and waiver of informed consent requirement in certain emergency research: Final rules. *Code of Federal Regulation,* title 21, part 50.

U.S. Department of Health and Human Services. (1997). *Fiscal year 1998, justification of estimates for appropriations committees (Vol. 1. National Institutes of Health).* Washington, DC: National Institutes of Health.

U.S. Department of Health and Human Services, National Center for Health Statistics. (1996). *Healthy people 2000 review, 1995–1996.* Hyattsville, MD: Public Health Service.

U.S. Department of Health and Human Services, Public Health Service. (1990). *Healthy people 2000: National health promotion and disease prevention objectives.* Washington, DC: Author.

U.S. Department of Health and Human Services, Public Health Service. (1991). *Healthy people 2000: National health promotion and disease prevention objectives* ([PHS]91-50212). Washington, DC: Author.

U.S. Department of Health, Education and Welfare, Division of Nursing. (1979). *Second report to the Congress, March 15, 1979 (revised), Nurse Training Act of 1975* (DHEW Publication No. HRA 79-45). Washington, DC: Author.

U.S. Department of Labor. (1991). *Occupational exposure to bloodborne pathogens (Federal Register,* 58). Washington, DC: U.S. Government Printing Office.

U.S. Preventive Services Task Force. (1996a). *Guide to clinical preventive services* (2nd ed.). Washington, DC: U.S. Department of Health and Human Services, Office of Disease Prevention and Health Promotion.

U.S. Preventive Services Task Force. (1996b). *Guide to clinical preventive services: Counseling to prevent unintended pregnancy* (pp. 739–753). Baltimore: Williams and Wilkins.

U.S. Public Health Service. (1995). *Healthy people 2000: Midcourse review and 1995 revisions.* Washington, DC: U.S. Department of Health and Human Services.

USPHS Office on Women's Health. (1991). *Action plan for women's health* (PHS-91-50214). Washington, DC: U.S. Department of Health and Human Services.

Utz, S. W., & Ramos, M. C. (1994). Mitral valve prolapse and its effects: A program of inquiry within Orem's self-care deficit theory of nursing. In J. P. Smith (Ed.), *Models, theories and concepts* (pp. 115–130). London: Blackwell.

Vachon, M. L. S. (1987). *Occupational stress in the care of the critically ill, the dying and the bereaved.* Washington, DC: Hemisphere.

Vachon, M. L. S., Lyall, W. A. L., & Freeman, S. J. J. (1978). Measurement and management of stress in health professionals working with advanced cancer patients. *Death Education, 1,* 365–375.

Valanis, B., & Shortridge, L. (1987). Self-protective practices of nurses handling antineoplastic drugs. *Oncology Nursing Forum, 14*(3), 23–27.

Valente, S. M. (1994). Messages of psychiatric patients who attempted or committed suicide. *Clinical Nursing Research, 3,* 316–333.

Valente, S. M., Saunders, J. M., & Grant, M. (1994). Oncology nurses knowledge and misconceptions about suicide. *Journal of Cancer Care, 2,* 209–216.

Vance, C. (1977). A group profile of contemporary influentials in American nursing (Doctoral dissertation, Teachers College, Columbia University, 1977). *Dissertation Abstracts International, 38,* 4734B.

Vance, C. (1982). The mentor connection. *Journal of Nursing Administration, 12*(4), 7–13.

Vance, C. (1986). The role of mentorship in the leadership development of nurse influentials. In W. A. Gray & M. M. Gray (Eds.), *Mentoring: Aid to excellence in career development, business, and the professions* (Vol. 2, pp. 177–184). Vancouver, BC: International Association for Mentoring.

Vance, C., & Olson, R. K. (1991). Mentorship. In J. J. Fitzpatrick, R. L. Taunton, & A. K. Jacox (Eds.), *Annual review of nursing research* (Vol. 9, pp. 175–200). New York: Springer Publishing.

Vance, C., & Olson, R. K. (1998). *The mentor connection in nursing.* New York: Springer Publishing.

VanCott, M. L., Tittle, M. B., Moody, L. E., & Wilson, M. E. (1991). Analysis of a decade of critical care nursing practice research: 1979 to 1988. *Heart and Lung, 20,* 394–397.

van Dijk, T. A. (Ed.). (1985). *Handbook of discourse analysis: Vol. 1. Disciplines of discourse.* London: Academic Press.

van Dixhoorn, J., Duivenvorden, J., Stall, J. A., Pool, J., & Verhage, F. (1987). Cardiac events after myocardial infarction: Possible effect of relaxation therapy. *European Heart Journal, 8,* 1210–1214.

Van Dover, L. (1986). Influence of nurse-client contracting on family planning knowledge and behaviors in a university student population. *Dissertation Abstracts International, 46,* 3787B.

Van Kaam, A. (1966). *Existential foundations of psychology.* Pittsburgh, PA: Duquesne University Press.

Van Manen, M. (1990). *Researching lived experience.* New York: State University of New York Press.

Vargas, J. H., Ament, M. E., & Berquist, W. E. (1987). Long-term home parenteral nutrition in pediatrics: Ten years of experience in 102 patients. *Journal of Pediatric Gastroenterology and Nutrition, 6,* 24–32.

Veith, R. C., Barnes, R. F., Villacres, E. C., Murburg, M. M., Raskind, M. A., Borson, S., Backus, F., & Halter, J. B. (1988). Plasma catecholamines and norepinephrine kinetics in depression and panic disorder. In R. Belmaker (Ed.), *Catecholamines: Clinical aspects* (pp. 197–202). New York: Alan R. Liss.

Veith, R. C., Lewis, M., Linares, O. A., Barnes, R. F., Taskind, M. A., Villacres, E. C., Murburg, M., Ashleigh, E. A., Castillo, S., Peskind, E. R., Pascualy, M., & Halter, J. B. (1994). Sympathetic nervous system activity in major depression: Basal and desipramine-induced alterations in plasma norepinephrine kinetics. *Archives of General Psychiatry, 51,* 411–422.

Verbrugge, L. M., & Jette, A. M. (1994). The disablement process. *Social Science Medicine, 38,* 1–14.

Verhaegen, P., Marcoen, A., & Goosens, L. (1992). Improving memory performance in the aged through mnemonic training: A meta-analytic study. *Psychology and Aging, 7,* 242–251.

Viscoli, C., Bruzzi, P., & Glauser, M. (1995). An approach to the design and implementation of clinical trials of empirical antibiotic therapy in febrile and neutropenic cancer patients [Review]. *European Journal of Cancer, 31A,* 2013–2022.

Voda, A. M. (1997). *Menopause me and you: The sound of women pausing.* New York: Haworth Press.

Voda, A. M., & George, T. (1986). Menopause. *Annual Review of Nursing Research, 4,* 55–75.

Voda, A. M., & Mansfield, P. K. (1993). Changes in the pattern of menstrual bleeding. In D. Golgert (Ed.), *Proceedings of the 9th Conference, Society for Menstrual Cycle Research.* Seattle, WA: Hamilton and Cross.

Volicer, B. J., & Bohannon, M. W. (1975). A hospital stress rating scale. *Nursing Research, 24,* 352–359.

Vredevoe, D., Brecht, M., Shuler, P., & Woo, M. (1992). Risk factors for disease in a homeless population. *Public Health Nursing, 9,* 263–269.

Wadd, L. (1983). Vietnamese postpartum practices: Implications for nursing in the hospital setting. *Journal of Gynecology Nursing, 12,* 252–258.

Waddell, D. (1991). The effects of continuing education on nursing practice: A meta-analysis. *Journal of Continuing Education in Nursing, 22,* 113–118.

Waechter, E. H. (1987). Children's awareness of fatal illness. In T. Krulik, B. Holaday, & I. M. Martinson (Eds.), *The child and family facing life-threatening illness* (pp. 101–107). Philadelphia: J. B. Lippincott.

Wake, M. M., Murphy, M., Affara, F. A., Lang, N. M., Clark, J., & Mortensen, R. (1993). Toward an international classification for nursing practice: A literature review and survey. *International Nursing Review, 40,* 77–80.

Walcott-McQuigg, J. A. (1995). The relationship between stress and weight-control behavior in African-American women. *Journal of the National Medical Association, 87,* 427–432.

Wald, F. (1994). Finding a way to give hospice care. A nurse's diary. In I. B. Corless, B. B. Germino, & M. Pittman (Eds.), *Dying, death and bereavement: Theoretical perspectives and other ways of knowing* (pp. 31–47). Boston: Jones & Bartlett.

Walker, A. J., Pratt, C. C., & Eddy, L. (1995). Informal caregiving to aging family members: A critical review. *Family Relations, 44,* 402–411.

Walker, A. M. (1986). Reporting the results of epidemiologic studies. *American Journal of Public Health, 76,* 556–558.

Walker, L. O. (1992). *Parent-infant nursing science: Paradigms, phenomena, methods.* Philadelphia: F. A. Davis.

Walker, L. O., & Avant, K. C. (1988). *Strategies for theory construction in nursing.* Norwalk, CT: Appleton & Lange.

Walker, L. O., & Avant, K. C. (1995). *Strategies for theory construction in nursing* (3rd ed.). Norwalk, CT: Appleton & Lange.

Walker, P. H. (1994). Dollars and sense in health reform, interdisciplinary practice and community centers. *Nursing Administration Quarterly, 19*(1), 1–11.

Walker, S. N., Sechrist, K. R., & Pender, N. (1987). The Health Promoting Lifestyle Profile: Development and psychometric characteristics. *Nursing Research, 36,* 76–81.

Wallerstein, N., & Bernstein, E. (1994). Introduction to community empowerment, participatory education, and health. *Health Education Quarterly, 21,* 141–148.

Walter, H. J., Vaughan, R. D., Ragin, D. F., Cohall, A. T., Kasen, S., & Fullilove, R. E. (1993). Prevalence and correlates of AIDS-risk behaviors among urban minority high school students. *Preventive Medicine, 22,* 813–824.

Waltz, C. F., & Strickland, O. L. (1988). *Measurement of nursing outcomes: Vol.1. Measuring client outcomes.* New York: Springer.

Waltz, C. F., Strickland, O. L., & Lenz, E. R. (1991). *Measurement in nursing research* (2nd ed.). Philadelphia: F. A. Davis.

Wandelt, M. (1970). *Guide for the beginning researcher.* New York: Appleton-Century Crofts.

Ward, S. E., & Gordon, D. (1994). Application of the American Pain Society quality assurance standards. *Pain, 56,* 299–306.

Ware, J. E., Bayliss, M. S., Rogers, W. H., Kosinski, M., & Tarlov, A. R. (1996). Differences in 4-year health outcomes for elderly and poor, chronically ill patients treated in HMO and fee-for-service systems. *Journal of the American Medical Association, 276,* 1039–1047.

Wasserbauer, L. I., & Abraham, I. L. (1995a). Quantitative designs. In L. A. Talbot (Ed.), *Principles and practice of nursing research* (pp. 217–239). St. Louis: Mosby Yearbook.

Wasserbauer, L. I., & Abraham, I. L. (1995b). Research design: Purpose, major concepts, and selection. In L. A. Talbot (Ed.), *Principles and practice of nursing research* (pp. 197–216). St. Louis: Mosby Yearbook.

Watson, J. (1979). *Nursing: The philosophy and science of caring.* Boston: Little, Brown.

Watson, J. (1985a). *Nursing: Human science and human care: A theory of nursing.* Norwalk, CT: Appleton-Century-Crofts.

Watson, J. (1985b). *Nursing: The philosophy and science of caring.* Boulder, CO: Colorado Associated University Press.

Watson, J. (1988). *Nursing: Human science and human care: A theory of nursing.* New York: National League for Nursing.

Watson, J. (1989). Watson's philosophy and theory of human caring in nursing. In J. Riehl-Sisca (Ed.), *Conceptual models for nursing practice* (pp. 219–236). Norwalk, CT: Appleton & Lange.

Watson, J. (1990). The moral failure of the patriarchy. *Nursing Outlook, 38*(2), 62–66.

Watson, J. (1995). Nursing's caring-healing paradigm as exemplar for alternative medicine? *Alternative Therapies in Health and Medicine, 1*(3), 64–69.

Watson, J. (1997). The theory of human caring: Retrospective and prospective. *Nursing Science Quarterly, 10,* 49–52.

Watson, J. (in press). Caring as a basis of healing. In W. Jonas & J. Levin (Eds.), *Textbook of complementary and alternative medicine.* Baltimore: Williams and Wilkins.

Webb, D. J., Fayad, P. B., Wilbur, C., Thomas, A., & Brass, L. M. (1995). Effects of a specialized team on stroke care: The first two years of the Yale Stroke Program. *Stroke, 26,* 1353–1357.

Webster's American dictionary (college ed.). (1997). New York: Random House.

Webster's Encyclopedic Unabridged Dictionary of the English Language. (1989). NJ: Gramercy Books.

Weil, M., & Karls, J. (1985). Historical origins and recent developments. In M. Weil & J. Karls (Ed.), *Case management in human service practice* (pp. 1–28). San Francisco: Jossey-Bass.

Weinberg, B. H. (1987). Why indexing fails the researcher. *Proceedings of the 50th Annual Meeting of the American Society for Information Science, 24,* 241–244.

Weinberg, N. (1995). Does apologizing help? The role of self-blame and making amends in recovery from bereavement. *Health and Social Work, 20,* 292–299.

Weiner, B. (1986). *An attributional theory of motivation and emotion.* New York: Springer.

Weiner, J. M., Stowe, S. M., Shirley, S., & Gilman, N. J. (1981). Information processing using document data management techniques. *Proceedings of the 44th Annual Meeting of the American Society for Information Science, 18,* 291–294.

Weinert, C. (1987). A social support measure: PRQ85. *Nursing Research, 36,* 273–277.

Weinert, C. & Boik, R. (1995). MSU Rurality Index: Development and evaluation. *Research in Nursing and Health, 18,* 453–464.

Weinert, C., & Burman, M. (1994). Rural health and health seeking behaviors. In J. J. Fitzpatrick & J. S. Stevenson (Eds.), *Annual review of nursing research* (Vol. 12, pp. 65–92). New York: Springer Publishing.

Weinert, C., & Burman, M. (1996). Nurturing longitudinal samples. *Western Journal of Nursing Research, 18,* 360–364.

Weinert, C., & Catanzaro, M. (1994). [Family health study]. Unpublished raw data.

Weisensee, M. G., Kjervik, D. K., & Anderson, J. B. (1994). Impairment of short-term memory as a criterion for determination of incompetency. *Geriatric Nursing: American Journal of Care for the Aging, 15*(1), 35–40.

Weiss, C. (1980). Knowledge creep and decision accretion. *Image: Journal of Nursing Scholarship, 1,* 381–404.

Weissman, M., & Olfson, M. (1995). Depression in women: Implications for health care research. *Science, 269,* 279–801.

Wells, Y., & Jorm, A. (1987). Evaluation of a special nursing home unit for dementia sufferers: A randomized controlled comparison with community care. *Australian and New Zealand Journal of Psychiatry, 21,* 524–531.

Werley, H. H. (1988). Introduction to the nursing minimum data set and its development. In H. H Werley & N. M. Lang (Eds.), *Identification of the nursing minimum data set* (pp. 1–15). New York: Springer Publishing.

Werley, H. H., Devine, E. C., & Zorn, C. R. (1988). *Nursing minimum data set data collection manual.* Milwaukee: University of Wisconsin, School of Nursing.

Werley, H. H., Devine, E. C., Zorn, C. R., Ryan, P., & Westra, B. L. (1991). The nursing minimum data set: Abstraction tool for standardized, comparable, essential data. *American Journal of Public Health, 81,* 421–426.

Werley, H. H., & Lang, N. M. (Eds.). (1988). *Identification of the nursing minimum data set.* New York: Springer Publishing.

Werner, J. S. (1993). Stressors and health outcomes: Synthesis of nursing research, 1980–1990. In J. Barnfather & B. Lyon (Eds.), *Stress and coping: State of the science and implications for nursing theory, research and practice.* Indianapolis: Center Nursing Press of Sigma Theta Tau International.

West, M., Bondy, E., & Hutchinson, S. (1991). Interviewing institutionalized elders: Threats to validity. *Image: Journal of Nursing Scholarship, 23,* 154–159.

Wetle, T., Walker, L., & Blechner, B. (1994). Developing model policies for implementing the Patient Self Determination Act in nursing homes [Special issue]. *Gerontologist, 14*(Suppl.), 251.

Whipple, B. (1982). *The G spot and other recent discoveries about human sexuality.* New York: Holt, Rinehart and Winston.

White, J. (1988). The perceived role of mentoring in the career development and success of academic nurse administrators. *Journal of Professional Nursing, 4,* 178–185.

White, J. E., Nativio, D. G., Kobert, S. N., & Engberg, S. J. (1992). Content and process in clinical decision making by nurse practitioners. *Image: Journal of Nursing Scholarship, 24,* 153–158.

White, M. A., Williams, P. D., Alexander, D. J., Powell-Cope, G. M., & Conlon, M. (1990). Sleep onset latency and distress in hospitalized children. *Nursing Research, 39,* 134–139.

Whittle, J., Conigliaro, J., Good, C. B., & Lofgren, R. P. (1993). Racial differences in the use of invasive cardiovascular procedures in the Department of Veterans Affairs medical system. *New England Journal of Medicine, 329,* 621–627.

Wilbur, J., Holm, K., & Dan, A. (1992). The relationship of energy expenditure to physical and psychologic symptoms in women at midlife. *Nursing Outlook, 40,* 269–276.

Wilcock, A., Kobayashi, K., & Murray, I. (1997). Twenty-five years of obstetric patient satisfaction in North America: A review of the literature. *Journal of Perinatal and Neonatal Nursing, 10*(4), 36–47.

Wilford, S. L. (1989). Knowledge development in nursing: Emergence of a paradigm (Doctoral dissertation: University of Minnesota, 1989). *Dissertation Abstracts International, 50,* 8B.

Williams, C. A. (1977). Community health nursing—what is it? *Nursing Outlook, 25,* 250–254.

Williams, C. A. (1996). Community-based population—focused practice: The foundation of specialization in public health nursing. In M. K. Stanhope & J. Lancaster (Eds.), *Community health nursing* (pp. 21–33). St. Louis: C. V. Mosby.

Williams, H., Blue, B., & Langlois, P. (1993). Do follow-up home visits by military nurses of chronically ill medical patients reduce readmissions? *Military Medicine, 159,* 141–144.

Williams, J. S., & Engle, V. F. (1995). Staff evaluation of nursing home residents' competence. *Applied Nursing Research, 8,* 18–22.

Williams, P. D., Williams, P. D., & Griggs, C. (1990). Children at home on mechanical assistive devices and their families: A retrospective study. *Maternal-Child Nursing Journal, 19,* 297–311.

Williams, T. F. (1988). Research and care: Essential partners in aging. *Gerontologist, 28,* 579–585.

Wilson, H. (1993). *Introducing nursing research.* Redwood City, CA: Addison-Wesley.

Wilson, H., & Hutchinson, S. (1996). *The consumer's guide to nursing research: Exercises, learning activities, tools and resources.* Albany, NY: Delmar.

Wilson, H., Hutchinson, S., & Holzemer, W. (1997). Salvaging quality of life in ethnically diverse patients with advanced HIV/AIDS. *Qualitative Health Research, 7,* 75–97.

Wing, D. M., & Thompson, T. (1995). Causes of alcoholism: A qualitative study of traditional Muscogee (Creek) Indians. *Public Health Nursing, 12,* 417–423.

Wing, R. R. (1993). Obesity and related eating and exercise behaviors in women. *Annals of Behavioral Medicine, 15,* 124–134.

Wing, R., & Jeffery, R. (1995). Effect of modes of weight loss on changes in cardiovascular risk factors: Are there differences between men and women or between weight loss and maintenance? *International Journal of Obesity, 19,* 67–73.

Wing, R. R., Matthews, K. A., Kuller, L. H., Meilahn, E. N., & Plantinga, P. (1991). Waist to hip ratio in middle-aged women: Associations with behavioral and psychosocial factors and with changes in cardiovascular risk factors. *Arteriosclerosis and Thrombosis, 11,* 1250–1257.

Winningham, M., MacVicar, M., Bondoc, M., Anderson, J., & Minton, J. (1989). Effect of aerobic exercise on body weight and composition in patients with breast cancer on adjuvant chemotherapy. *Oncology Nursing Forum, 16,* 683–689.

Winningham, M. L., Nail, L. M., Burke, M. B., Brophy, L., Cimprich, B., Jones, L. S., Pickard-Holley, S., Rhodes, V., St. Pierre, B., Beck, S., Glass, E. C., Mock, V. L., Mooney, K. H., & Piper, B. (1994). Fatigue and the cancer experience: The state of the knowledge. *Oncology Nursing Forum, 21,* 23–36.

Winslow, E. H., Lane, L. D., & Gaffney, F. A. (1985). Oxygen uptake and cardiovascular responses in control adults and acute myocardial infarction patients during bathing. *Nursing Research, 34,* 164–169.

Wisner, K. L., Perel, J. M., & Findling, R. L. (1996). Antidepressant treatment during breast-feeding. *American Journal of Psychiatry, 153,* 1132–1137.

Wolanin, M. O. (1983). Clinical geriatric nursing research. In H. H. Werley & J. J. Fitzpatrick (Eds.), *Annual review of nursing research* (Vol. 1, pp. 77–99). New York: Springer.

Wolf, S. (1981). Introduction: The role of the brain in bodily disease. In H. Weiner, M. A. Hofer, & A. J. Stunkard (Eds.), *Brain, behavior and bodily disease* (pp. 1–9). New York: Raven Press.

Wolff, P. (1968). The serial organization of sucking in young infants. *Pediatrics, 42,* 945–956.

Wood, J., & Estes, C. (1990). Impact of DRGs on community-based service providers: Implications for the elderly. *American Journal of Public Health, 80,* 840–843.

Woodham-Smith, C. (1951). *Florence Nightingale.* New York: McGraw-Hill.

Woods, N. F. (1979). *Human sexuality in health and illness.* St. Louis: Mosby.

Woods, N. F. (1993). Midlife women's health: There's more to it than menopause. In B. J. McElmurry & R. S. Parker (Eds.), *Annual review of women's health* (pp. 164–196). New York: National League for Nursing Press.

Woods, N. F. (1994a). Menopause: Challenges for future research. *Experimental Gerontology, 29,* 237–242.

Woods, N. F. (1994b). The United States women's health research agenda analysis and critique. *Western Journal of Nursing Research, 16,* 467–479.

Woods, N., & Catanzaro, M. (1988). *Nursing research: Theory and practice.* St. Louis: C. V. Mosby.

Woods, N. F., Lentz, M. J., Mitchell, E. S., & Kogan, H. (1994). Arousal and stress response across the menstrual cycle in women with three perimenstrual symptom patterns. *Research in Nursing and Health, 17,* 99–110.

Woods, N. F., & Mitchell, E. S. (1996). Patterns of depressed mood in midlife women: Observations from the Seattle Midlife Women's Health Study. *Research in Nursing and Health, 19,* 111–123.

Woods, N. F., Most, A., & Dery, G. K. (1982). Prevalence of perimenstrual symptoms. *American Journal of Public Health, 72,* 1257–1264.

Woods, N., Most, A., & Longenecker, G. D. (1985). Major life events, daily stressors and perimenstrual symptoms. *Nursing Research, 34,* 263–267.

Woods, N. M., Haberman, M. R., & Packard, N. J. (1993). Demands of illness and individual, dyadic, and family adaptation in chronic illness. *Western Journal of Nursing Research, 15*(1), 10–30.

Woods, S. L., Felver, L., & Hoeksel, R. (1996). Temporal patterns of heart rate and selected arrhythmias for 48 hours after cardiac surgery. *American Journal of Critical Care Nursing, 2,* 359–370.

Woolery, L., Grzymala-Busse, J., Summers, S., & Budihardjo, A. (1991). The use of machine learning program LERS LB 2.5 in knowledge acquisition for expert system development in nursing. *Computers in Nursing, 9,* 227–234.

Work Group on Research and Evaluation of SCUs (WRESCU). (1996, November). *Alzheimer's disease special care units: Findings from the National Institute on Aging SCU WRESCU Investigators.* Paper presented at the 49th Annual Meeting of the Gerontological Society of America, Washington, DC.

World Health Organization. (1948). *WHO constitution.* Geneva: Author.

World Health Organization. (1976). *Statistical indices of family health* (Report No. 589). Geneva: Author.

World Health Organization. (1977). *Development of designs in, and the documentation of the nursing process* (Report on a Technical Advisory Group, Regional Office for Europe, Copenhagen). Geneva: Author.

World Health Organization. (1978). Primary health care: Report of the International Conference on Primary Health Care, Alma Ata, USSR (Serican No. 1). Geneva: Author.

World Health Organization. (1980). *International classification of impairment, disabilities and handicaps.* Geneva: Author.

World Health Organization. (1985). *Evolution of primary health care* (HFA Leadership/IM.1). Geneva: Author.

World Health Organization. (1986). *Regulatory mechanisms for nursing training and practice: Meeting primary health care needs* (Technical Report Series #738). Geneva: Author.

World Health Organization. (1987). *WHO collaborating centers: General information.* Geneva: World Health Organization Office of Research and Development.

World Health Organization. (1992). *International statistical classification of diseases and related health problems* (10th rev. ed.). Geneva: Author.

World Health Organization. (1994). *Forty-seventh World Health Assembly: Executive summary.* Geneva: Author.

World Health Organization Press Office. (1996, July 22). *WHO press.* Geneva: WHO.

Wright, T. F., Blache, C. F., Ralph, J., & Luterman, A. (1993). Hardiness, stress, and burnout among intensive care nurses. *Journal of Burn Care and Rehabilitation, 14,* 376–381.

Wunderlich, G. S., Sloan, G. A., & Davis, C. K. (Eds.). (1996). *Nursing staff in hospitals and nursing homes: Is it adequate?* Washington, DC: National Academy Press.

Wyatt, R. J., Portnoy, B., Kupfer, D. J., Snyder, F., & Engelman, K. (1971). Resting plasma catecholamine concentrations in patients with depression and anxiety. *Archives of General Psychiatry, 24,* 65–70.

Wykle, M., & Kaskel, B. (1991). Increasing the longevity of minority older adults through improved health status. *Minority elders: Longevity, economics, and health: Building a public policy base* (pp. 24–31). Washington, DC: Gerontological Society of America.

Wykle, M. L., & Morris, D. L. (1994, May). Nursing care in Alzheimer's Disease. *Clinics in Geriatric Medicine,* Vol. 10, Number 2, pp. 351–365.

Yeates, D. A., & Roberts, J. E. (1984). A comparison of two bearing-down techniques during the second stage of labor. *Journal of Nurse-Midwifery, 29,* 3–11.

Yelin, E. H., Criswell, L. A., & Feigenbaum, P. G. (1996). Health care utilization and outcomes among persons with rheumatoid arthritis in fee-for-service and prepaid group practice settings. *Journal of the American Medical Association, 276,* 1048–1053.

Yensen, J. (1996). Connecting points. Project CyberNurse: Part 2. Implementation. *Computers in Nursing, 14,* 17–18.

Yensen, J., & Woolery, L. (1995). A demonstration of the virtual nursing college. In *Proceedings of MedInfo '95* (p. 1716).

Yin, R. (1989). *Case study research: Design and methods* (rev. ed.). Newbury Park, CA: Sage.

Yoder, M. E. (1994). Preferred learning style and educational technology: Linear vs. interactive video. *Nursing and Health Care, 15*(3), 128–132.

Young, J., Giovanetti, P., Lewison, D., & Thoms, M. (1981). *Factors affecting nurse staffing in acute care hospitals: A review and critique of the literature* (DHEW Publication No. HRA 81-10). Washington, DC: U.S. Department of Health and Human Services.

Youngblut, J. M. (1994a). A consumer's guide to causal modeling: Part 1. *Journal of Pediatric Nursing, 9,* 268–271.

Youngblut, J. M. (1994). A consumer's guide to causal modeling: Part 2. *Journal of Pediatric Nursing, 9,* 409–413.

Youngblut, J. M. (1995). Consistency between maternal employment attitudes and employment status. *Research in Nursing and Health, 18,* 501–513.

Youngblut, J. M., & Jay, S. S. (1991). Emergent admission to the pediatric intensive care unit: Parental concerns. *AACN Clinical Issues in Critical Care Nursing, 2,* 329–337.

Youngblut, J. M., & Shiao, S-Y. P. (1993). Child and family reactions during and after pediatric ICU hospitalization. *Heart and Lung, 22,* 46–54.

Zabin, L. S., Hirsch, M. D., Smith, E. A., Streett, R., & Hardy, J. B. (1986). Evaluation of a pregnancy prevention program for urban teenagers. *Family Planning Perspectives, 18,* 119–126.

Zalar, M. K., Welches, L. J., & Walker, D. D. (1985). Nursing consortium approach to increase research in service settings. *Journal of Nursing Administration, 15*(7–8), 36–41.

Zander, K. (1988). Nursing case management: Strategic management of cost and quality outcomes. *Journal of Nursing Administration, 18*(5), 23–30.

Zauszniewski, J. A. (1995). Severity of depression, cognitions, and functioning among depressed inpatients with and without coexisting substance abuse. *Journal of the American Psychiatric Nurses Association, 1,* 55–60.

Zelickson, B. D., & Homan, L. (1997). Teledermatology in the nursing home. *Archives of Dermatology, 133,* 171–174.

Zielstorff, R. D., Cimino, C., Barnett, G. O, Hassan, L., & Blewett, D. R. (1993). Representation of nursing terminology in the UMLS Metathesaurus: A pilot study. In M. Frisse (Ed.), *16th Annual Symposium on Computer Applications in Medical Care* (pp. 392–396). New York: McGraw-Hill.

Zielstorff, R. D., Hudgings, C. I., & Grobe, S. J. (1993). *Next-generation nursing information systems: Essential characteristics for professional practice.* Washington, DC: American Nurses Publishing.

Zielstorff, R. D., Jette, A. M., & Barnett, G. O. (1990). Issues in designing an automated record system for clinical care and research. *Advances in Nursing Science, 13*(2), 75–88.

SUBJECT INDEX

CONTRIBUTOR INDEX